Interventional Pain Management

A Practical Approach

Interventional Pain Management

A Practical Approach

Third Edition

Editors

Dwarkadas K Baheti MD
Consultant Pain Physician
Lilavati, Shushrusha, Raheja and Holy Family Hospitals
Mumbai, Maharashtra, India

Sanjay Bakshi MD MBA
Director-at-Large
American Society of Interventional Pain Physicians
New York, USA

Sanjeeva Gupta MBBS MD Dip NB FRCA FIPP FFPMRCA
Consultant
Bradford Teaching Hospitals NHS Foundation Trust
Bradford, England, UK

Raghbir Singh P Gehdoo MD DA
Ex-Professor
Department of Anesthesia
Tata Memorial Hospital
Mumbai, Maharashtra, India

Foreword

Subhash Jain

JAYPEE

JAYPEE BROTHERS MEDICAL PUBLISHERS
The Health Sciences Publisher
New Delhi | London

JAYPEE **Jaypee Brothers Medical Publishers (P) Ltd.**

Headquarters
EMCA House
23/23-B, Ansari Road, Daryaganj
New Delhi 110 002, India
Landline: +91-11-23272143, +91-11-23272703
+91-11-23282021, +91-11-23245672
E-mail: jaypee@jaypeebrothers.com

Corporate Office
Jaypee Brothers Medical Publishers (P) Ltd.
4838/24, Ansari Road, Daryaganj
New Delhi 110 002, India
Phone: +91-11-43574357
Fax: +91-11-43574314
E-mail: jaypee@jaypeebrothers.com

Overseas Office
JP Medical Ltd.
83, Victoria Street, London
SW1H 0HW (UK)
Phone: +44-20 3170 8910
E-mail: info@jpmedpub.com

EU GPSR Authorised Representative
Logos Europe, 9 rue Nicolas Poussin
17000, La Rochelle, France
Phone: +33 (0) 6 67 93 73 78
E-mail: Contact@logoseurope.eu

Website: www.jaypeebrothers.com
Website: www.jaypeedigital.com

Inquiries for bulk sales may be solicited at: jaypee@jaypeebrothers.com

Interventional Pain Management: A Practical Approach

First Edition: 2009

Second Edition: 2016

Third Edition: 2025

Reprint: ***2026***

ISBN: 978-93-5696-943-8

Printed in India

Dedicated to

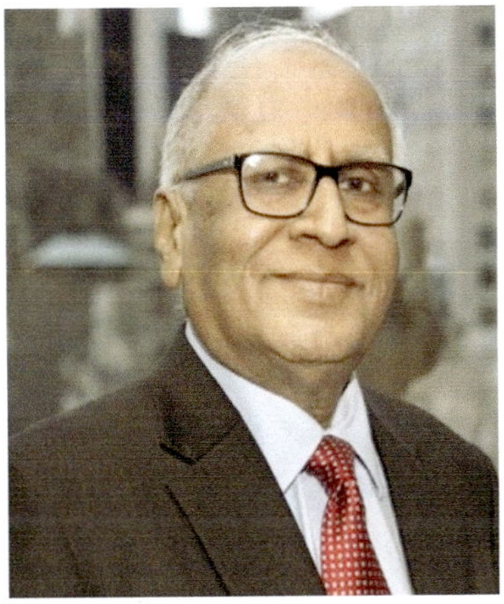

Dr. Subhash Jain MD

A Mentor, Friend, Philosopher and Guide
to
Many Pain Physicians from India and Globally

ब्रह्मानंदं परमसुखम केवलं ज्ञानमूर्ति
द्वन्दातीतं गगनसद्दृशं तत्वमस्यादिलकश्यम्।
एकं नित्यं विमलचलं सर्वधीसाक्षिमूतं
भावातीतं त्रिगुणरहित सदगुरं तं नमामी।

Contributors

Gerard W Abrahamsen PA-C
Physician Assistant
Manhattan Spine and Pain
New York, USA

Gaurav Agarwal
MBBS DNB FIPM CCEPC PGDHA
Senior Consultant
Department of Anesthesia and Pain Management
Care Hospitals
Bhubaneshwar, Odisha, India

Arthur Atchabahian MD
Professor
Department of Anesthesiology
New York University School of Medicine
New York, USA

Steve M Aydin DO
Clinical Assistant Professor
Hofstra North Shore-LIJ School of Medicine
New York, USA

Dwarkadas K Baheti MD
Consultant Pain Physician
Lilavati, Shushrusha, Raheja and Holy Family Hospitals
Mumbai, Maharashtra, India

Sanjay Bakshi MD MBA
Director-at-Large
American Society of Interventional Pain Physicians
New York, USA

Vijay B Bandikatla
MBBS DA FRCA MBA FFPMRCA
Senior Consultant and Director
Pain Medicine
Indo British Advanced Pain Clinic
Hyderabad, Telangana, India

Kevin K Bernard MD
Department of Physical Medicine and Rehabilitation
Rusk Rehabilitation, New York University Langone Medical Center
New York City, New York, USA

Sarath Bethapudi MBBS MRCP FRCR
Consultant
Department of Radiology
University Hospital of North Durham
Durham, England, UK

Surbhi Bhagat MBBS MD FIAPM PG
Diploma in MSK Ultrasound
Director
Department of Anesthesia and Pain Management
Prabhi Speciality Centre
Visiting Consultant HCG Cancer Care and Wockhardt Hospital
Mumbai, Maharashtra, India

Amit Bharath
MA BMBCh PG Cert FRCR
Specialist Registrar
Leeds Teaching Hospitals
Leeds General Infirmary
England, UK

Dhruv Bibra MBBS DA DNB
Senior Consultant
Delhi Pain Management Centre
New Delhi, India

Christopher V Boudakian DO
Department of Physical Medicine and Rehabilitation
Rusk Rehabilitation, New York University Langone Medical Center
New York City, New York USA

George C Chang Chien DO
Medical Director
Department of Pain Management
Ventura County Medical Center
California, USA

Jianguo Cheng MD PhD
Professor and Director
Department of Pain Management
Cleveland Clinic
Cleveland, Ohio, USA

Nayeema Chowdhury DO
Resident Physician
Department of Physical Medicine and Rehabilitation
New York University School of Medicine
New York, USA

Gautam Das MD
Director of Pain Clinic
Daradia, The Pain Clinic
Kolkata, West Bengal, India

Girish Datar MBBS D Ortho MS Ortho
Consultant
Endoscopic Spine Surgery and Interventional Spine and Pain Management
Sushruta Hospital for Orthopedics and Traumatology
Miraj, Maharashtra, India

Samyadev Datta MD FRCA
Director
Center for Pain Management
Hackensack, New Jersey, USA

Gerard DeGregoris III MD
Clinical Assistant Professor
Department of Anesthesiology
Hofstra North Shore-LIJ School of Medicine
New York, USA

Richard Derby MD FIPP
Medical Director
Department of Anesthesiology
Spinal Diagnostics and Treatment Center
California, USA

Prakash Deshmukh
FIAPM FIPP FPCI DA MBBS
Director, Pain Clinic of India Pvt Ltd
Visiting Pain Consultant
LTMGH and LTMMC
Mumbai, Maharashtra, India

Sudhir Diwan MD
Director, Division of Pain Medicine
Director, Pain Medicine Fellowship Program
New York Presbyterian Hospital
Weill Medical College of Cornell University
New York, USA

Lisa V Doan MD
Assistant Professor
Department of Anesthesiology
New York University School of Medicine
New York, USA

Kritika M Doshi MD DA FIPP ISSP-Pain Fellowship
Consultant in Charge Pain Clinic
Jupiter Hospital and Bethany Hospital
Thane, Maharashtra, India

Preeti P Doshi MD FRCA FIPP
Consultant and In-Charge of Pain Clinic
Jaslok Hospital & Research Centre
Wockhardt Hospital, and Bhatia Hospital
Mumbai, Maharashtra, India

GP Dureja MBBS MD
Director
Delhi Pain Management Centre
New Delhi, India

Jason D Freeman DO
Resident Physician
Department of Physical Medicine and Rehabilitation
New York University School of Medicine
New York, USA

Pratik J Gandhi DO
Resident
Department of Physical Medicine and Rehabilitation
Rusk Rehabilitation, New York
University Langone Medical Center
New York City, New York, USA

Kingsuk Ganguly MD
Fellow
Department of Anesthesiology and Pain Medicine
Weill Cornell School of Medicine
New York City, USA

Raghbir Singh P Gehdoo MD DA
Ex-Professor
Department of Anesthesia
Tata Memorial Hospital
Mumbai, Maharashtra, India

Evan C Grant MD
Resident
Department of Physical Medicine and Rehabilitation
Rusk Rehabilitation, New York
University Langone Medical Center
New York City, New York, USA

Harun Gupta MBBS MD DNB MRCP FRCR
Consultant
Leeds Teaching Hospitals
Leeds General Infirmary
Leeds, England, UK

Risha Gupta
Medical Student
University College
London, UK

Sanjeeva Gupta
MBBS MD Dip NB FRCA FIPP FFPMRCA
Consultant
Bradford Teaching Hospitals NHS Foundation Trust
Bradford, England, UK

Madouna G Hanna DO
Resident
Department of Physical Medicine and Rehabilitation
Hofstra North Shore-LIJ School of Medicine
New York, USA

Corey Hunter MD
CEO
Ainsworth Institute of Pain Management
New York City, New York, USA

Shoji Ishigami MD PhD
Resident
Department of Physical Medicine and Rehabilitation
Hofstra North Shore-LIJ School of Medicine
New York, USA

Madhavi Joshi MD DNB (Anesthesiology) FCPM FIAPM
Fellowship in Chronic Pain Medicine and Indian Academy of Pain Medicine
Consultant Pain Physician
LTMMC and Sion Hospital, IIT Bombay Hospital, Nirali Hospital, and Sushrusha Hospital
Mumbai, Maharashtra, India

Ramkumar Kalaiyarasan
MBBS MD DNB FRCA FFPMRCA
Anesthetics and Pain Medicine,
Neuromodulation and Pain Medicine
The Walton Centre NHS Foundation Trust
Liverpool, UK

Jan Willem Kallewaard MD FIPP
Consultant
Department of Anesthesiology and Pain Medicine
Rijnstate Hospital
Arnhem, The Netherlands

Neemish N Kamat MD DMRD
Radiologist, HOD and Consultant Radiologist of CT and Pet-CT
Nanavati Max Super Speciality Hospital
Mumbai, Maharashtra, India

Shruti G Kapoor MD MPH
Assistant Professor
Department of Anesthesiology
Stony Brook University
New York, USA

Rishi Khanna MBChB FRCA FFPMRCA
Consultant
Department of Anesthesia and Pain Medicine
Bradford Teaching Hospitals NHS Foundation Trust
Bradford, England, UK

Kailash Kothari MD
Interventional Pain Consultant
Director, Pain Clinic of India Pvt Ltd
Honorary Pain Consultant KEM Hospital, Fortis, Global, and Apollo Spectra Hospitals
Mumbai, Maharashtra, India

Kyriacos Kyriakides
BSc MBChB FRCA FPMRCA
Consultant in Pain Management and Anesthesia
Department of Pain Management and
Bradford Royal Infirmary
Bradford, England, UK

Eric Lee MD MA
Director of Musculoskeletal Care
Chief Operations Officer, Ainsworth Institute of Pain Management
Lenox Hill Hospital, North Shore LIJ
New York, USA

Jeong-Eun Lee PT
Research Analyst
Department of Anesthesiology
Spinal Diagnostics and Treatment Center
California, USA

Thomas P Lione DO
Resident Physician
Department of Physical Medicine and Rehabilitation
Hofstra North Shore-LIJ School of Medicine
New York, USA

Laxmaiah Manchikanti MD
Clinical Director
Department of Anesthesiology and Perioperative Medicine
University of Louisville
Medical Director, Pain Management Center of Paducah
Kentucky, USA

Amod Manocha FRCA FFPMRCA EDRA
PG Diploma in Musculoskeletal Ultrasound, PG Diploma (Rheumatology)
Head
Department of Pain Management
Max Hospital and International Pain Centre
New Delhi, India

Khushnuma Mansukhani MBBS
Head
Department of Clinical Neurophysiology
Bombay Hospital and Research Centre
Mumbai, Maharashtra, India

Neel Mehta MD
Medical Director, Division of Pain Medicine
Fellowship Director, Pain Medicine Fellowship
Weill Cornell Medical College
New York, USA

Irina Melnik MD
Staff Physician
Department of Anesthesiology Physical Medicine and Rehabilitation
Spinal Diagnostics and Treatment Center
California, USA

Mona Mirchandani DO
Resident Physician
Department of Physical Medicine and Rehabilitation
Rusk Rehabilitation, New York
University Langone Medical Center
New York City, New York, USA

Alex Moroz MD
Resident Physician
Department of Physical Medicine and Rehabilitation
Rusk Rehabilitation, New York
University Langone Medical Center
New York City, New York, USA

Yashwant L Nankar MD
Director
Department of Pain Management
Niramaya Hospital Pvt Ltd
Pune, Maharashtra, India

Kristina Natan MD
Department of Anesthesiology
New York University Medical Center
New York, USA

Annu H Navani MD
Medical Director
Comprehensive Spine and Sports Center
Adjunct Clinical Associate Professor
Stanford University School of Medicine
California, USA

Beatriz Nistal-Nuño MD
Anesthesiologist
Department of Cardiac and Thoracic Anesthesiology
The John Radcliffe Hospital, Oxford
University Hospitals NHS Trust
Oxford, Oxfordshire, UK

Omobonike O Olowosuko DO
Resident Physician, Hofstra North Shore-LIJ School of Medicine
New York, USA

Shefali Panjwani MBBS MD
Pain Fellow
Department of Pain Management
Max Hospital and International Pain Centre
New Delhi, India

Edward Papa DO
Resident
Department of Physical Medicine and Rehabilitation
Hofstra North Shore-LIJ School of Medicine
New York, USA

Jacob R Peacock MD
Resident
Department of Physical Medicine and Rehabilitation
Rusk Rehabilitation, New York
University Langone Medical Center
New York City, New York, USA

Nikhitha Peechera MD (Anesthesiology)
Pain Medicine, Fellow in Pain Medicine
Indo British Advanced Pain Clinic|
Hyderabad, Telangana, India

Sushama R Phanse MD
Consultant
Sushama Phanse's Pain Clinic
HJ Doshi Hindu Sabha Hospital, Asian Institute of Oncology
Mumbai, Maharashtra, India

Mohammed Piracha MD
Department of Anesthesiology and Pain Medicine
New York, USA

Gabor B Racz MD
Professor and Chairman Emeritus
Texas Tech University Health Sciences Center
Texas, USA

Manjiri N Ranade MBBS DA FIAPM FISSP
Director and Pain Physician
Palash Pain and Palliative Care
Consultant at Jupiter Hospital
Thane, Maharashtra, India

Emilia Ravski DO
Sports Medicine Fellow
University of Pittsburgh Medical Center
Pittsburgh, Pennsylvania, United States

Jonathan Richardson
MD FRCA FRCP FIPP
Consultant
Bradford Teaching Hospitals
NHS Foundation Trust
Bradford, England, United Kingdom

Ritesh Roy MBBS MD FRA
Clinical Director and Head
Department of Anesthesia and Pain Management
Care Hospitals
Bhubaneshwar, Odisha, India

Mahendra Sanapati MD
Co-Director of the Pain Management Centres of America and
Medical Director of Pain Management Centres of America
Evansville, Indiana, USA

Rajiv Shah MD
Fellow
Department of Anesthesiology and Pain Medicine
Weill Cornell School of Medicine
New York City, New York, USA

Samir N Shah MD
Resident
Department of Anesthesiology
Stony Brook Medicine
New York, USA

Anil K Sharma MD DABPM
President, Spine and Pain Centers
Director of Pain Management
Monmouth Medical Center
New Jersey, USA

Beamy S Sharma MD MBA
Resident Physician
Department of Anesthesiology
NYU Langone Medical Center
New York City, New York, USA

Manohar L Sharma
MBBS MD FRCA FFPMRCA MSc
Clinical Director
Department of Pain Medicine
The Walton Centre NHS Foundation Trust
Liverpool, UK

Puneet Sharma MBBS MD CCEPC
Head
Department of Anesthesia and Pain Management
Max Hospital
New Delhi, India

Vince Z Si MD
Resident Physician
Department of Physical Medicine and Rehabilitation
New York University School of Medicine
New York, USA

Sadiah Siddiqui MD
Fellow
Department of Anesthesiology and Pain Medicine
Weill Cornell School of Medicine
New York City, New York, USA

Harpreet Singh MBBS MD
Fellow
Department of Pain Management
Cleveland Clinic Foundation
Cleveland, Ohio, United States

Prit Anand Singh
MBBS FRCA FFPMRCA MSc (Pain Management)
Senior Consultant
Department of Anesthesia
Changi General Hospital, Singapore
Clin Assistant Professor
Sing Health
Duke—NUS Medical School, Singapore

James Taylor
BSc MBChB MRCS FRCA FFPMRCA
Consultant
Department of Anesthesia and Pain Management
Bradford Teaching Hospitals NHS Foundation Trust
Bradford, England, UK

Kevin H Trinh MD
Chief Resident
Department of Physical Medicine and Rehabilitation
Hofstra North Shore - LIJ School of Medicine
New York, USA

Dellene E Troy DO
Department of Physical Medicine and Rehabilitation
Rusk Rehabilitation, New York
University Langone Medical Center
New York City, New York, USA

Sanjay Varma MBBS FRCA FFPMRCA
Consultant
Department of Anesthesia
Sunderland Royal Hospital
Sunderland, UK

Chaitanya Veera
MD (Anesthesiology) IDCCM, Pain Medicine
Fellow in Pain Medicine
Indo British Advanced Pain Clinic
Hyderabad, Telangana, India

Bruce M Vrooman MD FIPP
Staff Physician
Department of Pain Management
Cleveland Clinic
Ohio, USA

Julia M Webb MD
Resident
Department of Physical Medicine and Rehabilitation
Rusk Rehabilitation, New York
University Langone Medical Center
New York City, New York, USA

Annie Wong MBBS MMed (Anesthesiology)
Associate Consultant
Department of Anesthesia
Changi General Hospital
Singapore

Foreword

The subject of intervention for various painful conditions has been given sufficient attention in the last two decades. A large percentage of specialties of medicine have professed various treatment modalities in which they are familiar with.

A surgeon will offer some surgical intervention for intractable pain, while a psychologist might recommend psychological intervention, or pharmacotherapy might be the main support for a neurologist or internist. Even on the bias of physicians or leaders of various pain organizations that do not recommend the interventional therapy, early interventional therapy was reported with multiple complications for achieving long-term benefits from these therapies. Even the World Health Organization (WHO) presented and recommended biased steps for treatment of pain.

The pain management field has made great stride in assessment of pain, diagnosis, and specific therapy for various kinds of pain syndromes or conditions. During the last 35 years, I have had the pleasure and the opportunity of teaching exclusively in this field and witnessing the development in the field of pain management. During these years, the development of various techniques, modalities, and support from radiological equipment such as X-rays, sonographic imaging, and CT-guided imaging has improved the various techniques both in accuracy in the placement of needles and the outcome of procedures.

The development of various techniques such as spinal cord stimulation, implantable devices, and nerve ablation has improved the overall quality of life of our patients. In both the developed and underdeveloped countries, these techniques have provided an immense improvement in the quality of treatment for patients. These techniques have been immensely helpful in underdeveloped nations where various pharmacological therapies are unavailable.

This book edited by Dr Baheti, Dr Bakshi, Dr Gupta, and Dr Gehdoo, is an extensive well-balanced text which fulfills an important need in this rapidly changing field. The various authors who have contributed their chapters are well-known players in the field of pain management. These book chapters represent various tools to help various conditions of pain with the most recent developments. The book will be very insightful for readers, and it will enhance their knowledge in providing safe treatment options to their patients.

Subhash Jain MD
Medical Director, Institute of Pain and Palliative Care, New York City, New York, USA
Attending Physician and Consultant, Memorial Sloan Kettering Cancer Center, New York City, New York, USA
Former Chief of Pain Service, Memorial Sloan Kettering Cancer Center, New York City, New York, USA
Former Clinical Associated Professor, Cornell University Medical Center, New York City, New York, USA
Former Chairman of the Department of Pain of Palliative Care at Hackensack University Hospital, Hackensack New Jersey, USA

Preface to the Third Edition

The editorial team feels privileged to come out with the second edition of their first ever book on "Interventional Pain Management: A Practical Approach." We express our heartfelt gratitude to our readers for the stupendous response to that book which gave us much needed courage and responsibility to bring out the second edition.

Interventional pain treatment procedures have become an integral part of a multimodal approach to provide relief of chronic pain. Interventional pain treatment procedures must be performed correctly to have maximum pain relief with minimum morbidity and mortality. Recent advances in the understanding of imaging such as fluoroscopy, ultrasound and CT scan, has become a great asset in performing interventional pain treatment procedures more accurately.

Many pain physicians are enthusiastic to learn the art of interventional techniques for managing pain, but do not have access to appropriate reference books. The availability and cost of the books add to further constraints.

We, the practicing pain physicians, have recognized the problem and realize the need for a book on Interventional Pain Management techniques, which can be both comprehensive and affordable. Our first book filled this void partly.

This book fulfills all the needs of present day pain physicians as it has a stepwise description of most of the interventional pain treatment procedures. The images of the book are self-explanatory which will hopefully make performing these procedures relatively easy. The highlight is the DVDs provided with this book. The editors are confident that the second edition will fill the void at all levels from postgraduate to university libraries all over.

It is our sincere attempt to come out with this second edition by adding many procedures and DVDs of the procedures.

We express our heartfelt gratitude to all the contributors, without whose support this Herculean task would have been impossible.

We have taken utmost care to bring out this book of international standards, at an affordable price. We sincerely hope that our efforts to come out with this book will benefit the pain physicians as well as the chronic pain patients.

Dwarkadas K Baheti
Sanjay Bakshi
Sanjeeva Gupta
Raghbir Singh P Gehdoo

Preface to the First Edition

Interventional pain management is one of the most important components of managing chronic intractable pain. It is mandatory that interventional procedures need to be performed correctly right from the time of diagnosis to the relief of pain, so as to provide the best possible results.

Many universities in India as well as abroad do not have appropriate pain training program in their curriculum not only at the undergraduate but, also at postgraduate levels. There are very few pain certification programs or pain specialists or pain training facilities across the world.

Even in the countries where such programs exist, there are significant inadequacies and lacunae in teaching of the techniques. Although there are courses run by various organizations, they only incorporate a few common techniques and hence can never be comprehensive.

Many pain physicians are enthusiastic to learn the art of interventional techniques for managing pain, but do not have an access to appropriate reference books. The availability and cost of the books add to further constraints.

We, the practicing pain physicians, have recognized the problem and realized the need for a book on Interventional Pain Management techniques, which can be both comprehensive and affordable.

It is our sincere attempt to come out with a book on interventional pain procedures due to existing vacuum in this field.

We express our heartfelt gratitude to all the contributors, without whose support this Herculean task would have been impossible.

We have taken utmost care to bring out this book with an international quality at an affordable price.

We sincerely hope that our efforts to come out with this book will benefit the pain physicians as well as the chronic pain patients.

Dwarkadas K Baheti
Sanjay Bakshi
Sanjeeva Gupta
Raghbir Singh P Gehdoo

Contents

SECTION 9: Alternate Therapies

SECTION 10: Miscellaneous

Video Contents

Chapter 13: Trigeminal Nerve Block

Ramkumar Kalaiyarasan, Manohar L Sharma

Video 1: Trigeminal Ganglion Block RF

Chapter 15: Mandibular Nerve Block

Yashwant L Nankar

Video 2: Mandibular Nerve Block

Part 1

Part 2

Chapter 18: Stellate Ganglion Block

Preeti P Doshi

Video 3: Stellate Ganglion

Chapter 22: Intrapleural Block

Dwarkadas K Baheti

Video 4: Intra pleural Block

Chapter 23: T2/T3 Sympathetic Block

Prakash Deshmukh

Video 5: T2-3 Sympathetic Block

Chapter 24: Celiac Plexus Block

Dwarkadas K Baheti

Video 6: CT Guided Neurolytic Coeliac Plexus Block

Chapter 34: Lumbar and Caudal Epidural Blocks

Sanjay Bakshi, Gerard W Abrahamsen

Video 7: Trans Foraminal Lumbar Epidural

Video 8: Lumbar Epidural-inter Laminar

Video 9: Caudal Epidural

Chapter 35: Lumbar Facet Joint, Medial Branch, and Radiofrequency Procedures

Annu H Navani, Irina Melnik, Richard Derby, Jeong-Eun Lee

Video 10: Median Branch Block (Lumbar)

Chapter 39: Coccygeal Nerve Block

Yashwant L Nankar

Video 11: Coccygeal Nerve Block

Chapter 41: Piriformis Muscle Injection

Yashwant L Nankar

Video 12: Piriformis Muscle Injection

Chapter 42: Popliteal Nerve Block of Sciatic Nerve

Yashwant L Nankar

Video 13: Popliteal Nerve Block of Sciatic Nerve

Chapter 56: Subarachnoid or Intrathecal Neurolysis

Kritika M Doshi

Video 14: Intra Thecal Neurolysis

Chapter 68: Dry Needling and Ultrasound-guided Dry Needling

Sushama R Phanse, Madhavi Joshi

Video 15: US Guided Dry Needling Twitch

Chapter 69: Myofascial Pain Syndrome and Trigger Point Injections

Vince Z Si, Mona Mirchandani, Kevin K Bernard, Emilia Ravski, Dellene E Troy, Christopher V Boudakian, Nayeema Chowdhury, Jason D Freeman

Video 16: Trigger point injection

1 SECTION

Basics of Interventional Pain Management

1

CHAPTER

Understanding Magnetic Resonance Imaging for Spinal and Pelvic Pain

Neemish N Kamat

INTRODUCTION

Back pain is the most common pain in clinical practice. It can be evaluated by magnetic resonance imaging (MRI). The role of MRI has increased in imaging of spinal, abdominal, musculoskeletal, and neurological causes of pain.

CAUSES OF BACK PAIN

- *Mechanical causes:*
  - Muscle strain/spasm
  - Degenerative disk disease
    - Disk herniation
    - Intervertebral osteochondrosis (Modic type 1 changes)
  - Sacroiliac joint disease, e.g., sacroiliitis, osteoarthritis, instability
    - ~10% of patients will have sacroiliitis findings on computed tomography (CT)
  - Facet joint osteoarthritis
  - Vertebral fractures
- *Nonmechanical causes:*
  - Spinal tumors and bone metastases
  - Spinal infections
- *Extravertebral causes of back pain:*
  - Abdominal and visceral processes (cholecystitis, pancreatitis)
  - Pelvic causes [prostatitis, endometriosis, pelvic inflammatory disease (PID)].

Degenerative Spinal disease[1,2]

Disk Herniations (Figs. 1 and 2)

The normal intervertebral disk has peripheral annulus fibrosus and central nucleus pulposus. The nucleus pulposus consists of collagen and hydrophilic proteoglycans. The normal hydrated disk has high-signal

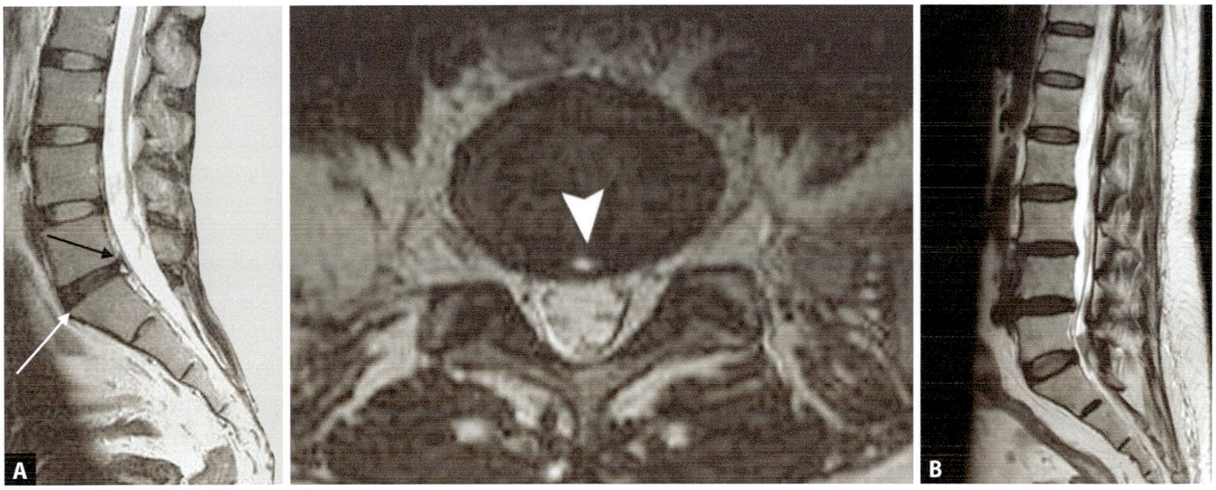

Figs. 1A and B: (A) T2W sagittal image shows hyperintense tear (black arrow) and desiccated L5-S1 disk (white arrow), T2W axial image at L5-S1 with annular tear (white arrowhead); (B) Desiccated disks at various levels.

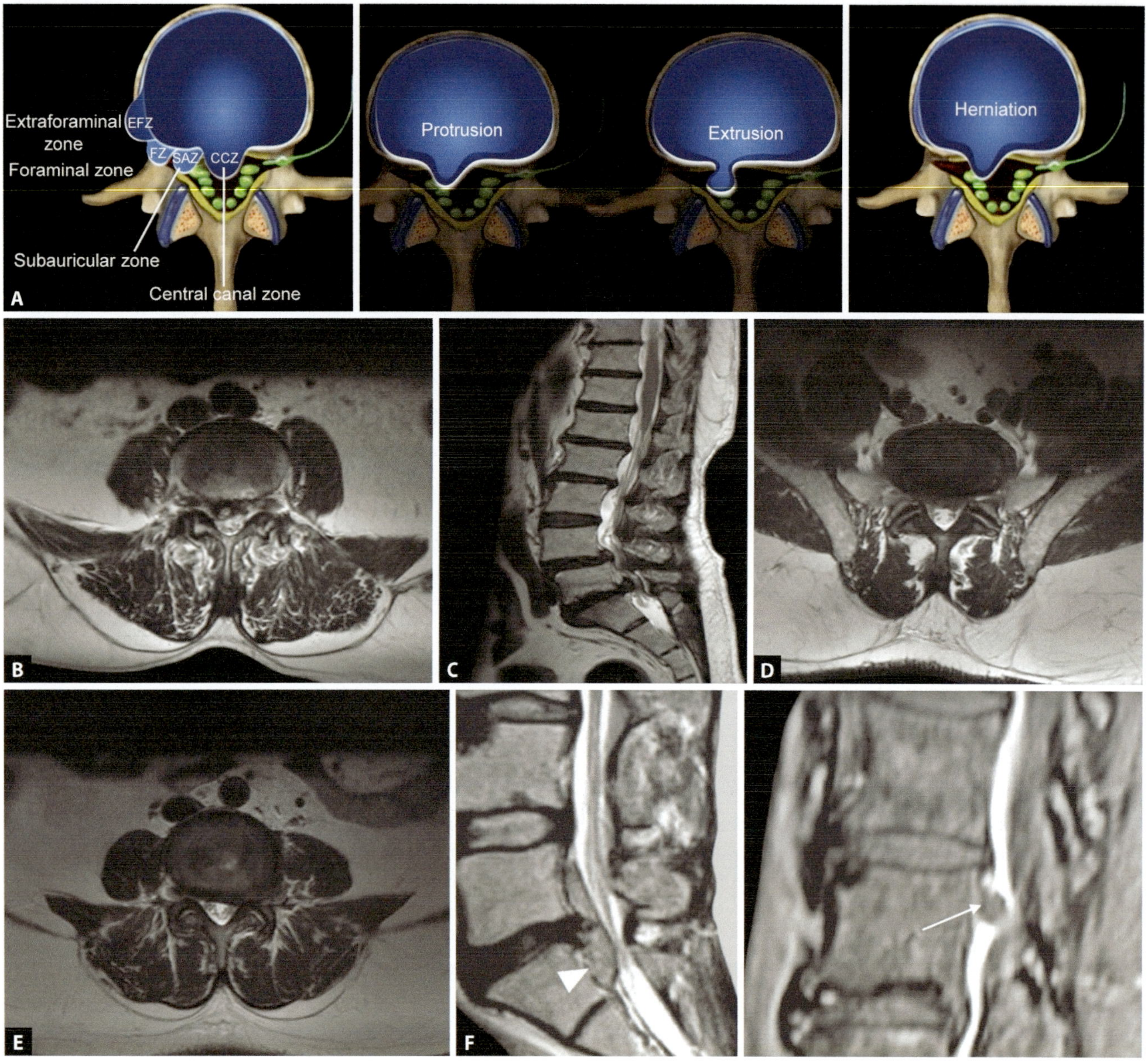

Figs. 2A to F: (A) Pictorial nomenclature of disks; (B) Paracentral protrusion; (C) Sagittal images with disk extrusion at L5-S1 and L4-L5 disk levels; (D) Left paracentral extrusion; (E) Left paracentral herniation; (F) Extrusion and inferior migration (white arrowhead) and sequestration (white arrow).[1]

intensity on T2-weighted images in the center with low-signal intensity in the periphery of annulus fibrosus.

The desiccated disk shows a hypointense signal on T2-weighted images with loss of internuclear cleft. The outer annular fibers of the disk are innervated by free nerve endings. The disruption of the fibers, known as annular tear, can be a source of back pain. The annular tear is seen as a high-signal intensity zone on T2-weighted images in the posterior annulus of the bulging disk.

The lumbar disk herniation is a focal extension of the nucleus pulposus beyond the margins of the disk. Posterior disk herniation can cause compression of the nerve roots and severe radicular pain. There are various terminologies of disk herniations including disk bulge, protrusion, and extrusion. The disk bulge is symmetrical, circumferential disk extension beyond the interspace. Protrusion indicates focal or asymmetrical disk extension beyond the interspace with broad base against the parent disk. Extrusion refers to

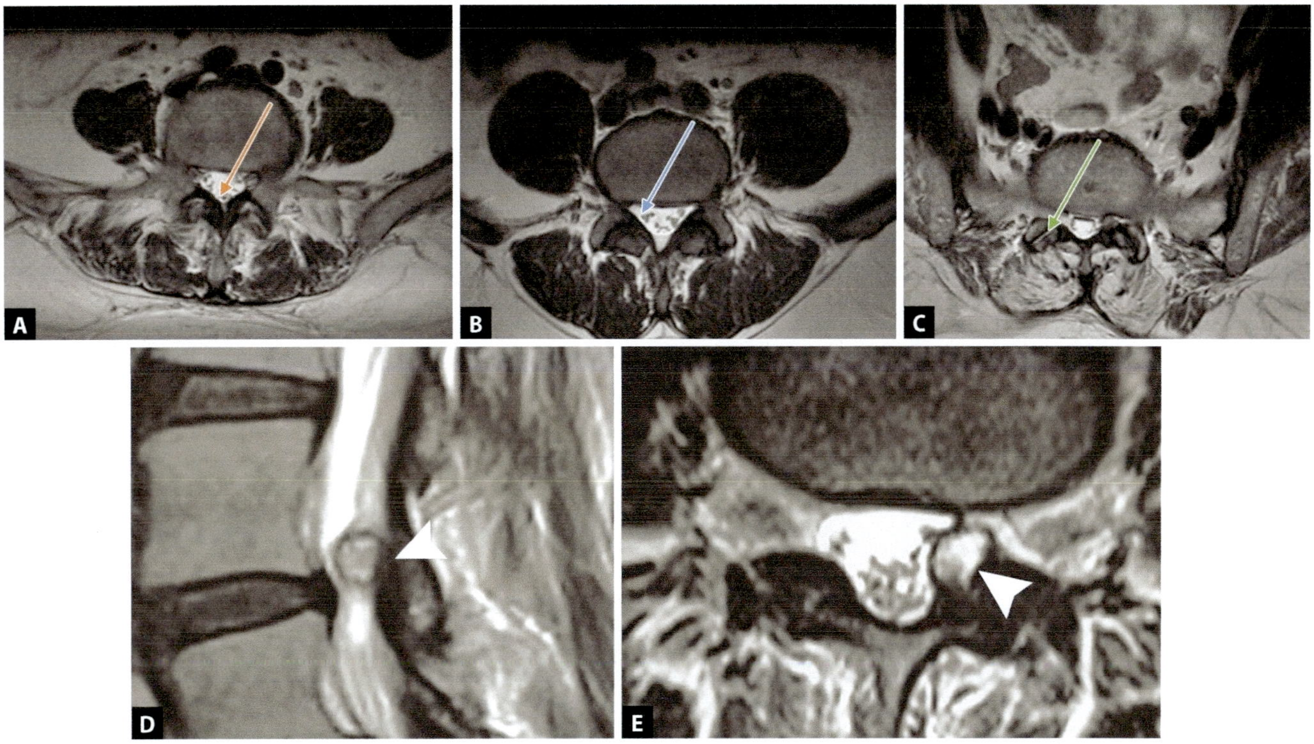

Figs. 3A to E: T2W axial images showing (A) ligamentum flavum thickening (orange arrow) and (B and C) facet arthropathy (blue and green arrows).[2] (D and E) Synovial cyst in T2W sagittal and axial images indenting nerve fiber (arrowhead).

focal extension beyond the interspace with a narrow neck against parent disk. The location of the disk herniation is also important which can be well assessed on MRI. On the axial images, the location of disk herniation can be characterized as central, paracentral (sub-auricular), foraminal and extraforaminal zones.

Facet Joints (Figs. 3A to E)

The facet joints comprise the posterior elements of the "three-joint complex" (with the intervertebral disk forming the anterior element) that describes a spinal segment. Facet joint degeneration occurs as part of this complex, and as the disk degenerates more load, it will shift posteriorly and facet joint osteoarthritis will subsequently develop.

Bulging/thickening of the ligamentum flavum can be associated with facet joint subluxation and may lead to severe spinal canal stenosis and radiculopathy.

Sacroiliitis (Figs. 4A to C)

Most common cause of chronic back pain. Intra-articular causes—arthritis, metabolic diseases, spondyloarthropathies.

MRI findings include:[3]

- *Marrow edema (first to appear):* High signal on water-sensitive sequences
- *Synovitis and capsulitis:* Thickening and contrast enhancement of the synovium and joint capsule
- *Enthesitis:* Thickening and contrast enhancement of ligaments and tendons at their attachments to bone.

Vertebral Body Collapse[4]

There are various causes of solitary vertebral collapse including trauma, tumor, and infection. In an old patient, it is often a diagnostic problem between osteoporotic[5] and malignant compression on a plain X-ray. MRI can help in differentiating between the various causes of vertebral body collapse.

Benign Compression Fractures[5] (Figs. 5A to C)

- No bony destruction
- Preserved normal fatty bone marrow T1WI signal
- Low signal intensity band on T1WI and T2WI indicating a fracture line
- Fluid sign

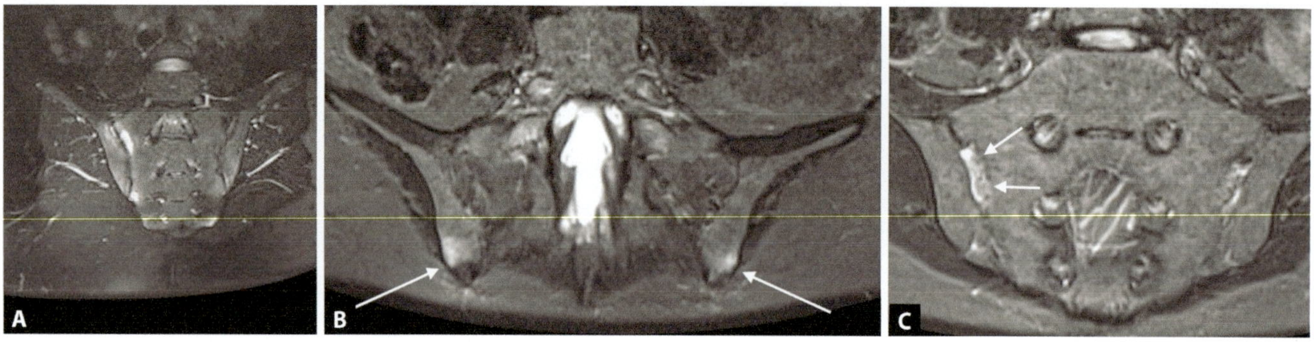

Figs. 4A to C: (A) T2 coronal short tau inversion recovery (STIR) image shows hyperintense signal in sacroiliac (SI) joint; (B) Axial STIR shows hyperintense signal in posterolateral ilium suggesting enthesitis (arrows); (C) Enthesitis.[3]

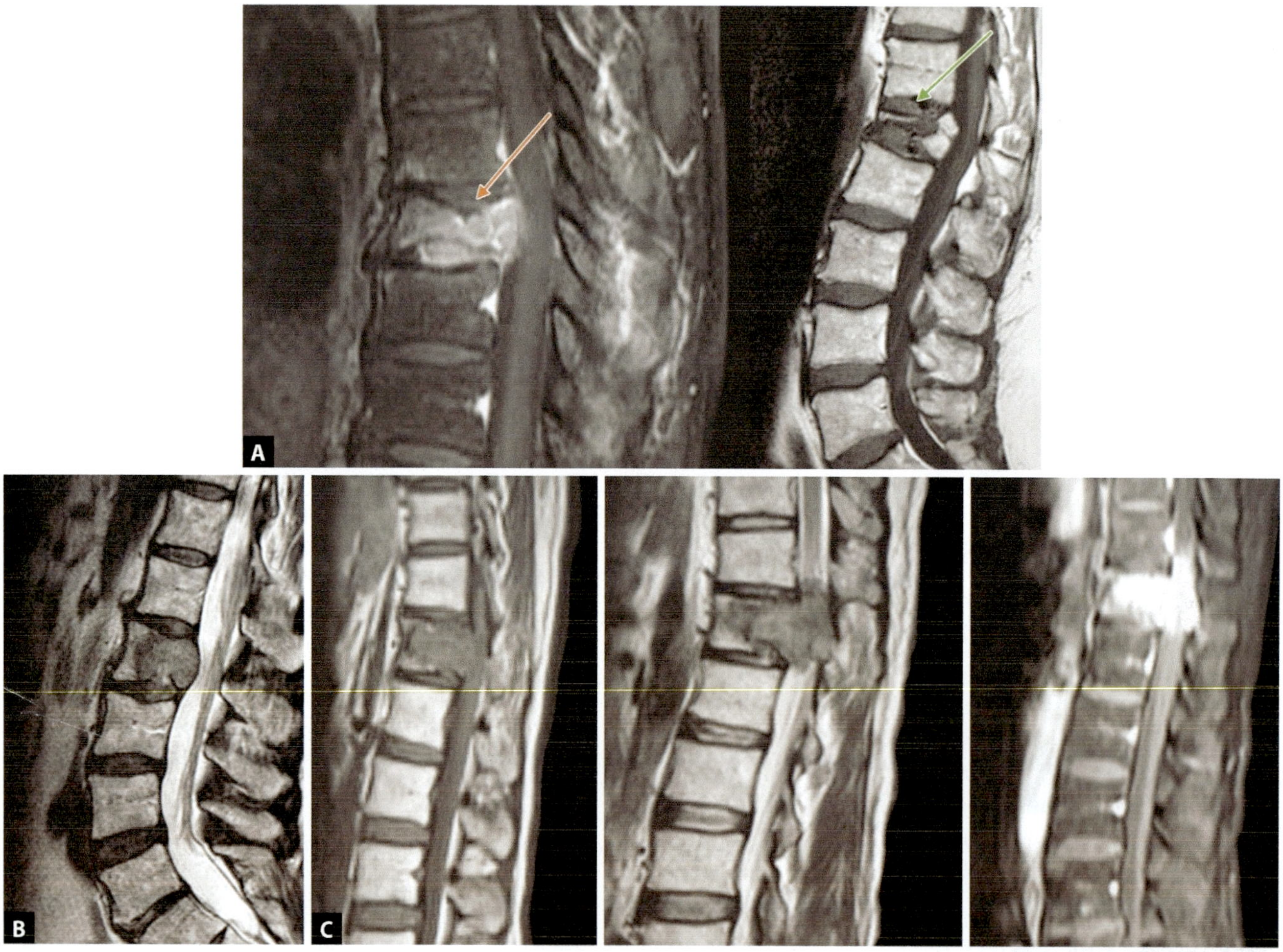

Figs. 5A to C: T2W short tau inversion recovery (STIR) hyperintense signal represents acute traumatic fracture (red arrow) and wedge compression collapse of vertebra in left (green arrow).[5] (B) T2 hypointense metastatic deposits. (C) T2 hypointense metastatic deposits invading spinal canal with STIR hyperintensity (left end).[4,6]

- Retropulsion (not posterior bulging) of the posterosuperior cortex of the vertebral body
- No epidural mass
- Multiple compression fractures.

Pathological Compression Fractures[4,6]

- Fracture with bony destruction
- Replaced signal of the vertebral body, especially extending into the pedicles or posterior elements
- Convex bulging (not retropulsion) of the posterior vertebral cortex into the spinal canal
- Epidural or paraspinal mass
- Other vertebral metastases.

Spinal Tumors

Spinal tumors are classified as intramedullary, intradural extramedullary (IDEM), and extradural **(Figs. 6 and 7)**.

- *Spinal cord (intramedullary):*[7] Spinal ependymoma, spinal astrocytoma (diffuse), spinal cord metastasis (intramedullary), spinal lymphoma/leukemia, and spinal ganglioglioma
- *IDEM:*[8] Spinal meningioma, spinal nerve sheath tumors, spinal schwannoma, spinal neurofibroma, spinal leptomeningeal metastases
- *Extradural:*[9] Epidural metastasis, epidural abscess, herniated nucleus pulposus, epidural angiolipoma, epidural lipomatosis, extramedullary hematopoiesis,

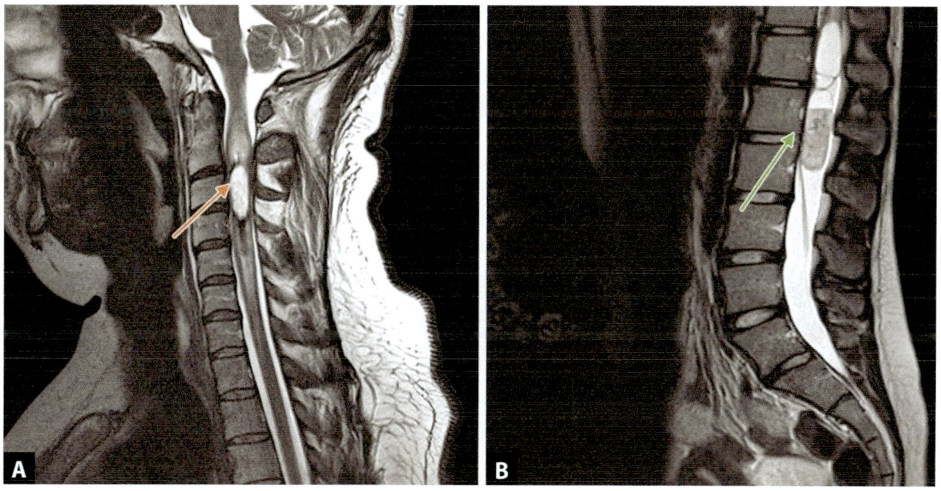

Figs. 6A and B: (A) T2 sagittal image with hyperintense intramedullary mass distends spinal cord (orange arrow); (B) T2 sagittal lumbar spine intramedullary mass at conus represents myxopapillary ependymoma (green arrow).[7]

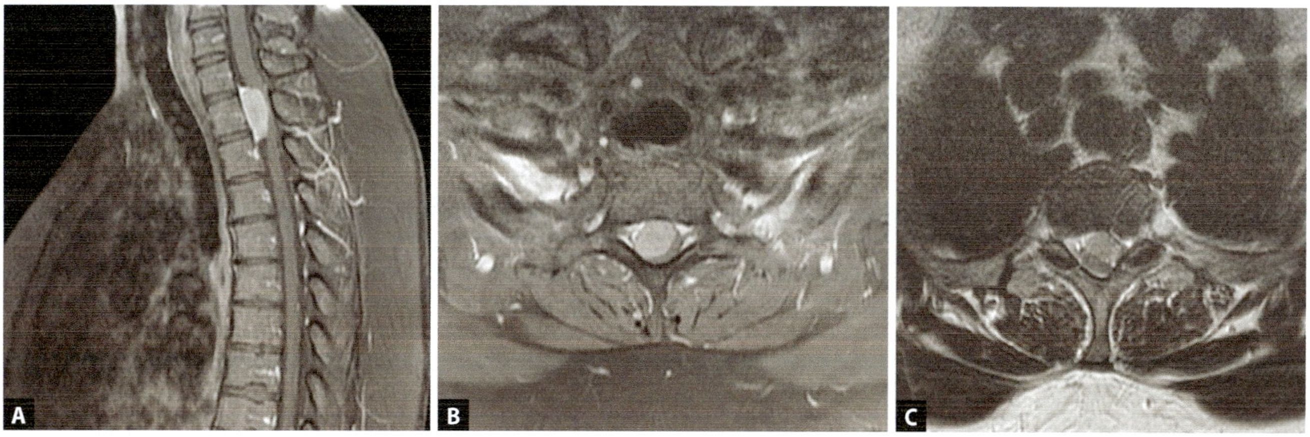

Figs. 7A to C: (A and B) Sagittal and axial postcontrast cervical spine shows enhancing intradural extramedullary (IDEM) mass; (C) Axial T2W images depicts the mass.[8]

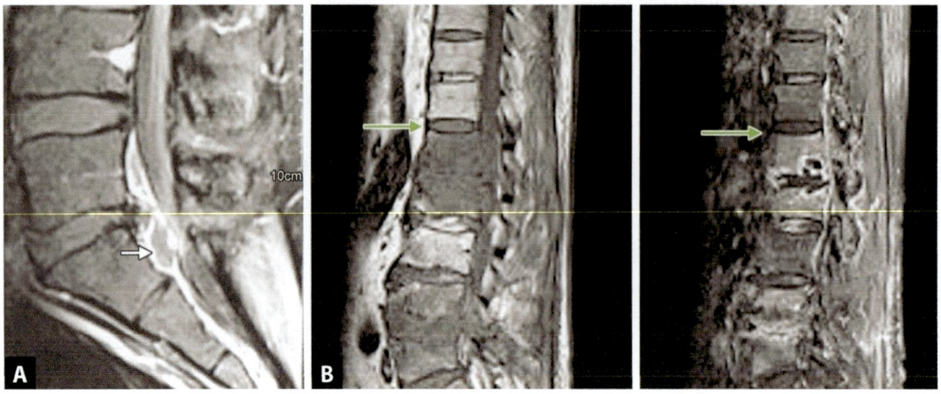

Figs. 8A and B: (A) Epidural phlegmon as altered signal intensity at S1 shows peripheral enhancement on postcontrast images; (B) T1 hypointensity and T2 short tau inversion recovery (STIR) hyperintensity with disk destruction (green arrow).[11]

local spread of primary bone or soft-tissue tumor, extradural spinal cavernous malformation.

Infective Spondylodiskitis[10] (Figs. 8A and B)

It is acquired by direct inoculation or hematogenous spread. The most common organism is *Staphylococcus aureus.*

- *Disk-endplate complex:* Producing diskitis-osteomyelitis
- *Facet joints:* Producing septic arthritis
- *Epidural space:* Producing an epidural abscess.

Vertebral infection commonly originates in the anterior endplate (due to its rich arterial supply) and therefore affects the psoas muscle before affecting paraspinous soft tissue including the epidural space.

MRI findings:

- Vertebral body T1 hypointensity
- Vertebral body and disk T2 hyperintensity
- Endplate destruction
- Psoas sign: Nonenhanced T2 hyperintensity in iliopsoas muscle—considered a key sign of early spondylodiskitis
- Epidural phlegmon.

Extravertebral Causes

Cholecystitis (Figs. 9A and B)

The development of acute calculous cholecystitis follows a sequence of events:

- Gallstone obstruction of the gallbladder neck or cystic duct
- Inflammation from chemical injury of the mucosa by bile salts

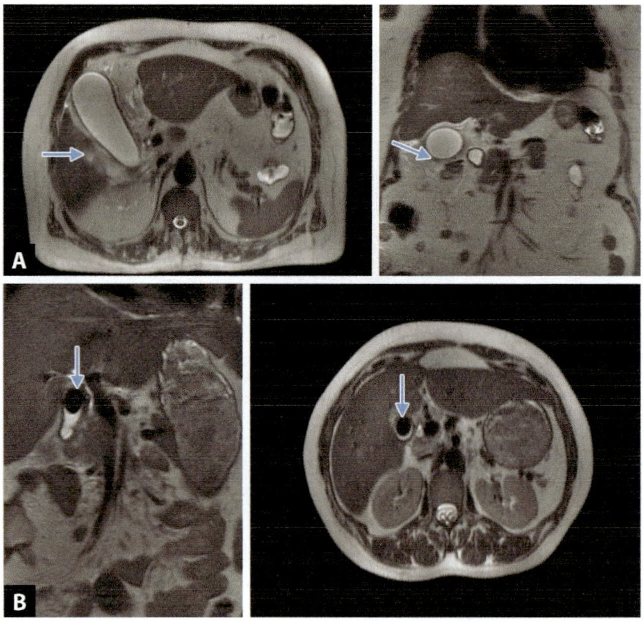

Figs. 9A and B: (A) T2W axial and coronal images showing distended gallbladder with thickened walls and surrounding fat stranding; (B) Signal void foci at neck of gall bladder represent calculus.

- Reactive production of mucus, leading to increased intraluminal pressure and distention
- Increased luminal distention restricting blood flow to the gallbladder wall (gallbladder hydrops)
- Increasing wall thickness from edema and inflammatory changes.

Pancreatitis (Figs. 10A to C)

Obstruction of biliary tree by calculi causes activation of pancreatic enzymes within the pancreas, disruption of small pancreatic ducts, and leakage of pancreatic

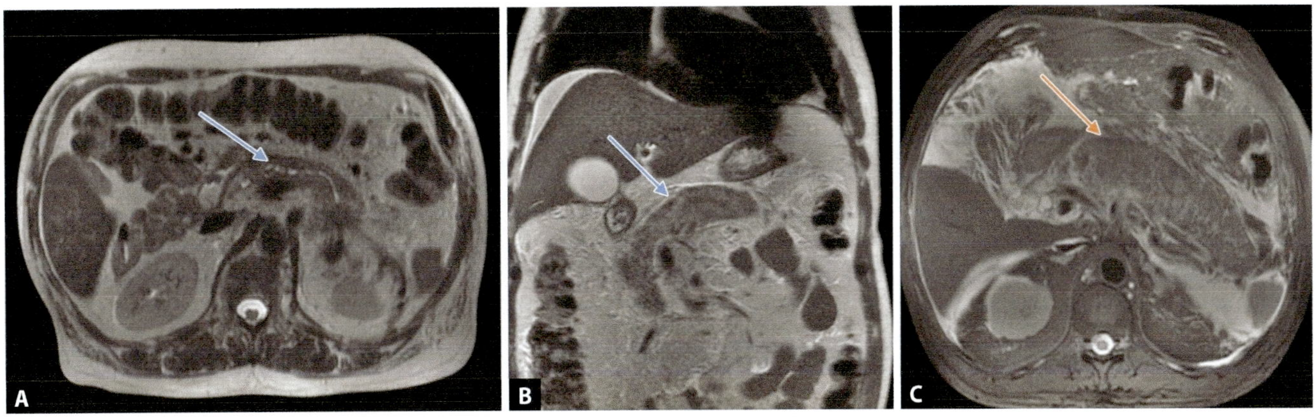

Figs. 10A to C: (A and B) Axial and coronal T2W images showing prominent pancreatic duct and atrophied pancreas in chronic pancreatitis (blue arrow); (C) Bulky inflamed pancreas with surrounding fat stranding (orange arrow).

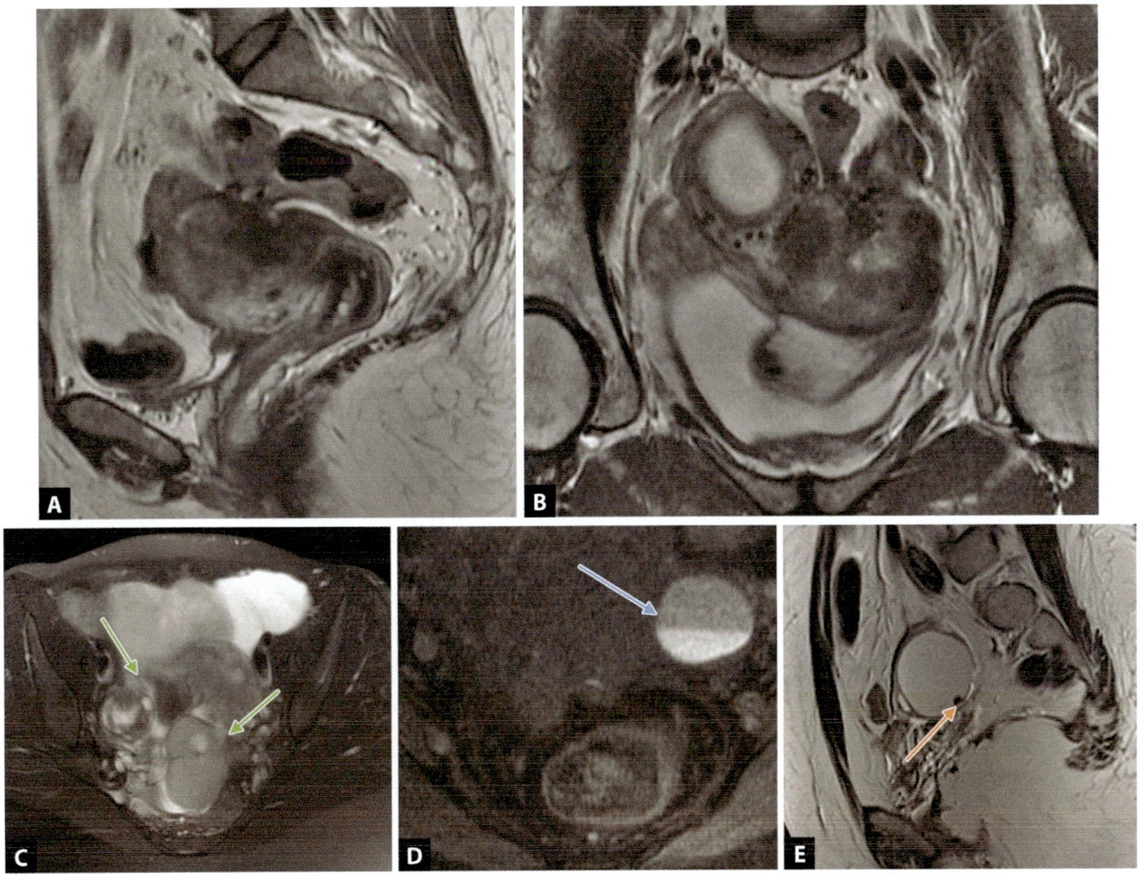

Figs. 11A to E: (A) T2 sagittal image shows adhesion of posterior wall of uterus with anterior rectal wall due to deep pelvic deposit (blue arrow); (B) T2W coronal image shows adhesion of ovary to uterus (red arrow)[12]; (C) Kissing ovaries due to adhesions (green arrow); (D) Shading sign of chocolate cyst (blue arrow); (E) T2 dark spot sign of endometrioma (orange arrow).

secretions. Because the pancreas lacks a capsule, the pancreatic juices have ready access to surrounding tissues. Pancreatic enzymes digest fascial layers, spreading the inflammatory process to multiple anatomic compartments.

Endometriosis (Figs. 11 A to E)

Endometriosis[12] is a common, chronic gynecological condition defined as the presence of functional endometrial glands and stroma-like lesions outside the uterus.

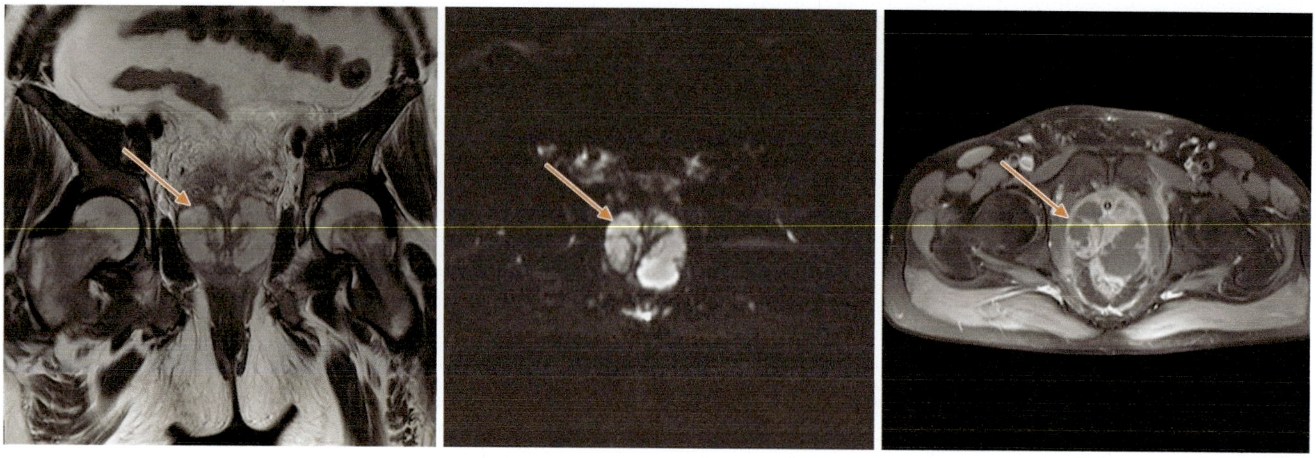

Fig. 12: T2W coronal, diffusion-weighted imaging (DWI) and postcontrast images of prostate show prostatitis with abscess formation (orange arrow).[13]

MRI has greater specificity for the diagnosis of endometriomas:

- *Hemorrhagic "powder burn"*:
  - Lesions appear bright on T1 fat-saturated sequences
- *Small solid deep lesions* **(Fig. 11A)**:
  - May be hyperintense on T1 and hypointense on T2
- *Adhesions and fibrosis:*
  - Isointense to pelvic muscle on both T1- and T2-weighted images
  - Spiculated low-signal intensity stranding that obscures organ interfaces
  - Distortion of normal anatomy
    - Posterior displacement of the uterus
    - Kissing Ovaries Sign and cloverleaf sign **(Figs. 11B and C)**: Seen in the severe forms of the disease
    - Angulation of bowel loops
    - Elevation of the posterior vaginal fornix
  - Loculated fluid collections
  - Hydrosalpinx
- *Endometriomas*:
  - Shading sign **(Fig. 11D)**
  - T2 dark spot sign **(Fig. 11E)**.

Prostatits (Fig. 12)

Prostatitis[13] refers to an infection or inflammation of the prostate gland that presents as several syndromes with varying clinical features. It is a clinical diagnosis and imaging is useful to evaluate abscess formation.

The prostate will be diffusely enlarged, often with associated inflammatory changes of periprostatic fat and of the seminal vesicles.

Acute prostatitis:

- *T1:* Peripheral zone iso- or hypointense to transition zone
- *T2:* Hyperintense
- *T1+C (Gd):* Diffusely enhancing.

Pelvic Inflammatory Disease (Figs. 13 and 14)

Pelvic inflammatory disease[14] is a broad term that encompasses a spectrum of infection and inflammation of the upper female genital tract, resulting in a range of abnormalities.

MRI may show an ill-defined adnexal mass containing fluid with various signal intensities:

- *T1:* If there is proteinaceous debris in a dilated tube, then it may have an increased T1 signal.
- *T1+ C (Gd):* Wall and surrounding tissues may enhance.

CONCLUSION

MRI has a good technical capacity to provide high-resolution images that contrast soft tissues. It is an excellent tool for detecting the presence of anatomic impairment. In the absence of serious disease, reasonable evidence exists to support an association between disk extrusion, free fragments of disk, and major nerve compression with low back pain (LBP). Disk degeneration, bulging, and small herniations are common in both individuals with and individuals without low back symptoms.

MRI, with its evolving invention of sequences and high sensitivity, is becoming a significant part of an investigation in the emergency room. Manipulating signal intensities,

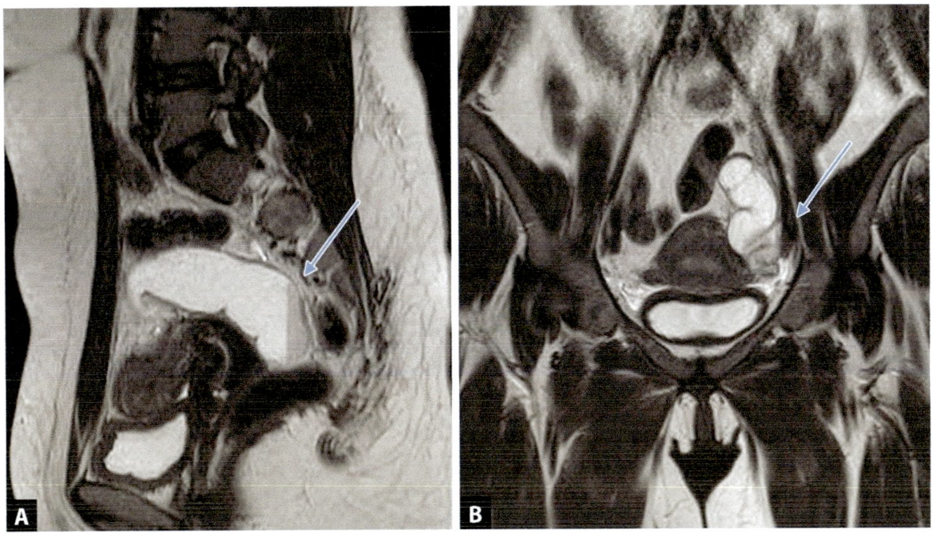

Figs. 13A and B: T2W sagittal and coronal images show retort-shaped T2 hyperintense hydrosalpinx with hypointense proteinaceous content within.[14]

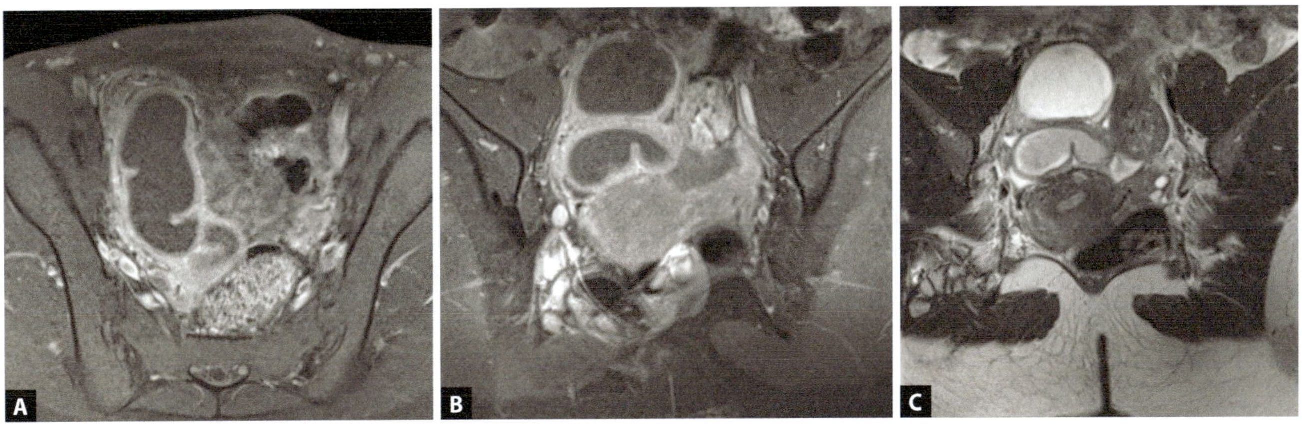

Figs. 14A to C: Postcontrast axial and coronal images show peripherally enhancing pyosalpinx. T2W axial image shows the same with hypointense debris suggesting pus within.

large imaging area, and soft-tissue contrast resolution provide functional and prognostic information. It also helps to find the subtle findings as in endometriosis, PID, etc.

Although it is cost-ineffective and time-consuming, it is the best noninvasive way to diagnose findings in spine and pelvis with evolving resolution of images and technologies associated with it.

REFERENCES

1. Fardon DF, Williams AL, Dohring EJ, Murtagh FR, Rothman SL, Sze GK. Lumbar disc nomenclature: version 2.0: Recommendations of the combined task forces of the North American Spine Society, the American Society of Spine Radiology and the American Society of Neuroradiology. Spine J. 2014;14:2525-45.
2. Degenerative diseases of the spine https://radiologykey.com/degenerative-diseases-of-thespine/.
3. Yu Jin T, Knipe H, Di Muzio B, et al. (2024). Sacroiliitis. [online] Available from https://radiopaedia.org/articles/sacroiliitis [Last accessed July, 2024].
4. https://radiopaedia.org/articles/osteoporotic-vs-pathologicalvertebral-fractures?lang=us [Last accessed July, 2024].
5. Wang G, Luk KD, Li Y, Zhang C, Sun J. Clinical and radiological outcomes of selective fusion for rotatory olisthesis in degenerative lumbar scoliosis: a retrospective cohort study. Asian Spine J. 2024;18:346-53.

6. https:www.researchgate.net/figure/Malignant-vertebralmetastasis-a-b-c-Magnetic-resonance-images-of-thoracicspine-of_fig1_24176344.
7. https://radiopaedia. org/articles/intramedullary-spinal-tumors.
8. Shih RY, Koeller KK. Intramedullary masses of the spinal cord: radiologic-pathologic correlation. Radiographics. 2020;40:1125-45.
9. Cugati G, Singh M, Pande A, Ramamurthi R, Balasubramanyam M, Sethi SK, et al. Primary spinal epidural lymphomas. J Craniovertebr Junction Spine. 2011; 2:3-11.
10. radiopaedia.org%2Farticles%2Fspondylodiscitis&psig=AOvVaw38-1v2w6M1NJ5gIzmDRBYh&ust=1719763768785000&source=images&cd=vfe&opi=89978449&ved=0CBQQjhxqFwoTCOC-4rSZgYcDFQAAAAAdAAAAABAg.
11. https:// radiopaedia.org/articles/spondylodiscitis.
12. Endometriosis-https://radiopaedia.org/articles/endometriosis.
13. Sah VK, Wang L, Min X, Feng Z, Rizal R, Li L, et al. Multiparametric MR imaging in diagnosis of chronic prostatitis and its differentiation from prostate cancer. Radiol Infect Dis. 2015;1:70-7.
14. https://radiopaedia.org/ articles/pelvic-inflammatory-disease.

2 CHAPTER

Radiological Anatomy of Spine

Amit Bharath, Harun Gupta

ABSTRACT

Magnetic resonance imaging (MRI) is the diagnostic tool of choice for spinal imaging, and computed tomography (CT) is increasingly being used for spinal intervention. Selective nerve blocks require an excellent understanding of spinal anatomy to ensure that the correct nerve root is targeted. This chapter reviews the salient anatomical features of different imaging modalities used to image the spine.

INTRODUCTION

There have been tremendous advancements in the quality and diagnostic yield of spinal imaging. In the past, X-rays and myelography were commonplace but now MRI is the diagnostic tool of choice, and CT is increasingly being used for spinal intervention. Spinal intervention requires an excellent understanding of spinal anatomy to ensure a safe approach and correct anatomical area to be targeted. Plain radiography, fluoroscopy, and CT are all forms of ionizing radiation; these imaging modalities provide excellent visualization of osseous structures, but they should be used with some caution as they can increase the long-term risk of cancer. MRI uses magnetic field and no nonionizing radiation and is superior to CT for assessing spinal soft-tissue and marrow abnormalities. An in-depth analysis of the flaws and benefits and the technical aspects of the different imaging modalities has not been done and is well covered in the radiology literature. The chapter covers the merits of particular modalities to illustrate the relevant spinal anatomy.

The vertebral column (or spine) forms the central axis of the skeleton. It has a great structural strength as well as considerable flexibility. These two properties of the spine arise from the number, morphology and articulations of its constituent bony elements, the vertebrae. The spine is normally made up of 33 vertebrae, divided into 5 distinct anatomical groups such as cervical, thoracic, lumbar, sacral, and coccygeal. In the adult spine, there are four curvatures in the anteroposterior plane. There is anterior flexion or concavity in the thoracic and sacrococcygeal parts of the spine, which is known as kyphosis, and anterior extension or convexity in the cervical and lumbar regions, which is known as lordosis. There are eight pairs of cervical nerve root; all cervical nerves except C8 emerge above their corresponding vertebrae, while the C8 nerve emerges below the C7 vertebra. Elsewhere in the spine, the nerve emerges below the vertebra with the same name (i.e., the L4 nerve root will exit at the level of L4/5 disk).[1-3]

Vertebrae are typically composed of a ventral body and a dorsal vertebral or neural arch. These two structures enclose the vertebral foramen; the foramen of vertebrae form the vertebral canal **(Figs. 1A to C)**. The contents of the vertebral canal include the dorsal root ganglia, epidural fat, spinal nerves, and blood vessels. Three osseous processes emerge from the vertebral arch—a posterior midline process known as the spinous process and two lateral processes known as the transverse processes. The part of the neural arch between the spinous process and the transverse processes is known as the lamina and the part between the transverse process and the vertebral body is called the pedicle. The root of the transverse process is formed at the junction of the pedicle and the lamina; it is here where the articular facets of the neural arch lie.

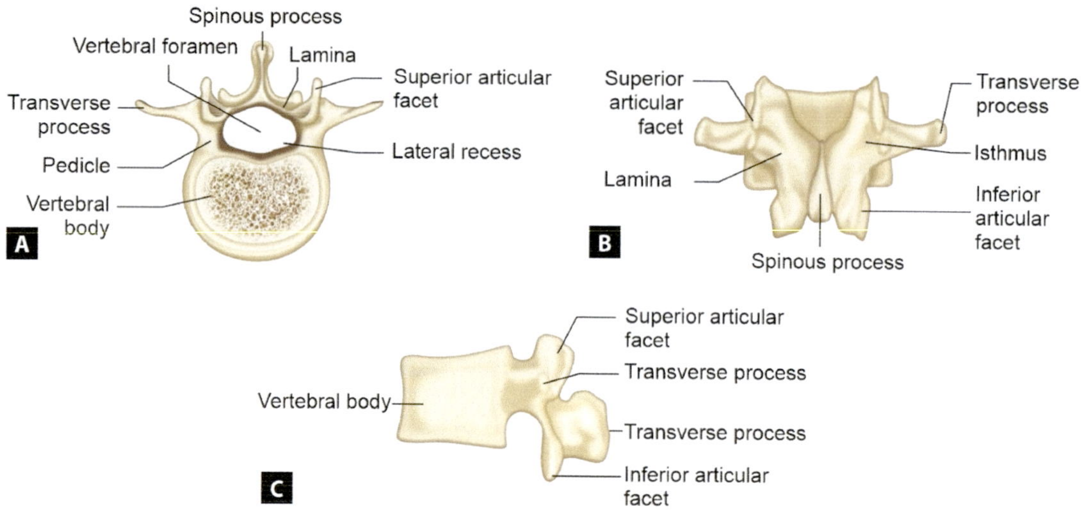

Figs. 1A to C: Line diagrams of typical lumbar vertebra with (A) superior, (B) posterior, and (C) lateral views.

There are two superior and two inferior articular facets in each neural arch, one pair of superior and inferior facets on either side.

FACET JOINTS

The joints between the superior articular facet of one vertebra and the inferior articular facet of the vertebra above are known as the zygapophyseal joints or more simply the facet joints. The facet joints are true synovial joints. The articular surfaces are covered by hyaline cartilage, which allows a sliding motion to occur in the posterior arch of the spinal column. The articular capsules are thin and have an inner synovial and an outer fibrous membrane. The anterior aspect of the facet joints and the lamina are covered by strong bands of fibrous tissue, called the ligamenta flava. They are attached above to the front of the upper lamina and below to the back of the lower lamina. They extend from the facet joints to the midline where they partially fuse. Cartilage loss from degenerative disease within the facet joint, in conjunction with disk height loss from degeneration, leads to inward buckling of the ligamentum flavum, which may cause central canal, lateral recess or exit foraminal stenosis.

The intervertebral foramen is the space formed between pedicles of two adjacent vertebrae; this is where the spinal nerve exits the vertebral canal. The facet joints themselves have a nerve supply from the nerve of their own segmental level and from the nerve of the segment above. One nerve thus supplies two joints, and this may be important when considering nerve root pain, which can be referred from facet joints.

INTERVERTEBRAL DISKS

The main structural articulation through which most of the weight is transferred between the spine occurs via the vertebral bodies and the intervening disks. The intervertebral disk is a secondary cartilaginous joint or symphysis. The vertebral bodies and disk are bounded anteriorly by the anterior longitudinal ligament, which extends from the basiocciput of the skull to the upper part of the sacrum. The anterior longitudinal ligament has strong attachments to the periosteum of the anterior aspects of the vertebral bodies but is less strongly attached to the disks. The posterior longitudinal ligament extends from the posterior aspect of the body of the axis to the anterior wall of the upper sacral canal. Intervertebral disks consist of a central gelatinous substance, composed of water and proteoglycans, called the nucleus pulposus.

This is surrounded by a ring called the annulus fibrosus, which has a narrow outer collagenous zone, and a wider inner fibrocartilaginous zone. The nucleus pulposus accounts for 15% of the whole disk. At birth, it is 90% water and this decreases to 70% in old age. Although CT scans delineate intervertebral disks and disk disease, MRI is far superior. It can be used to assess the disk structure and accurately evaluate spinal stenosis. MRI physics is a complicated and vast topic in itself; there are many different sequences which can now be used to assess the different spinal conditions. Essentially, there are two main sequences: T1 and T2, which can be distinguished by the color of the cerebrospinal fluid (CSF). CSF is low signal (dark) on T1 and high signal (bright) on T2. Fat, protein, and blood are bright on T1 and fluid is bright on T2. On MRI, a normal disk has a lower signal (darker) than normal adjacent bone marrow on T1-weighted (T1W) images. On T2-weighted (T2W) images, the nucleus pulposus is bright as it is filled with fluid and proteoglycans, and the outer fibrocartilaginous annulus fibrosis is dark. With age and degeneration, the disk loses its fluid and proteoglycans; in doing so, it becomes darker on T2W imaging whilst also losing its height and disrupting its internal architecture.

CERVICAL VERTEBRAE

The cervical spine consists of seven vertebrae **(Figs. 2 to 8)**. It is the most flexible part of the spine and the most complex. The cervical spine's range of motion is approximately 80–90° of flexion, 70° of extension, 20–45° of lateral flexion, and up to 90° of rotation to both sides. The cervical vertebrae have a lateral process, which is perforated by a foramen. The vertebral artery, accompanying sympathetic fibers, and the vertebral venous plexus lie in the foramen. The spinous processes are usually bifid with the exception of the C7 vertebrae. The vertebrae of C3-C7 have a similar morphology. A typical cervical vertebral body is kidney-shaped. On each side, it is projected up into a posterolateral lip (the uncus), and its lower margin is beveled reciprocally with this. The C3-C7 vertebral bodies articulate with one another at this point. This articulation is known as the uncovertebral joint or joint of Luschka.

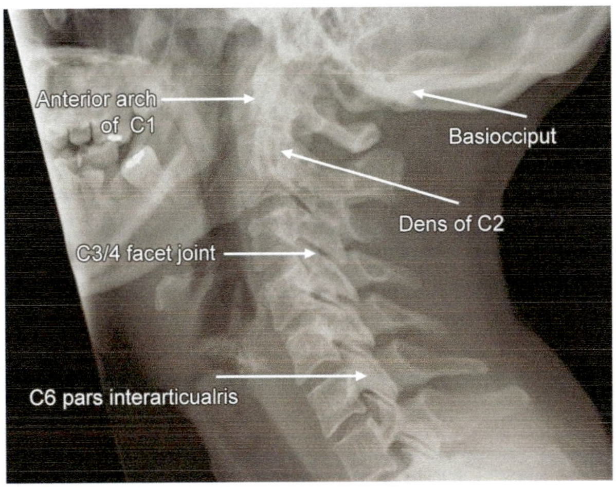

Fig. 2: Plain radiograph of cervical spine (lateral view).

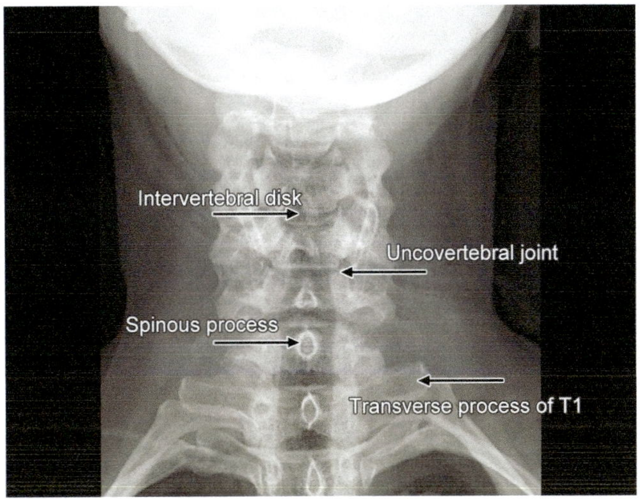

Fig. 3: Plain radiograph of cervical spine (anteroposterior view).

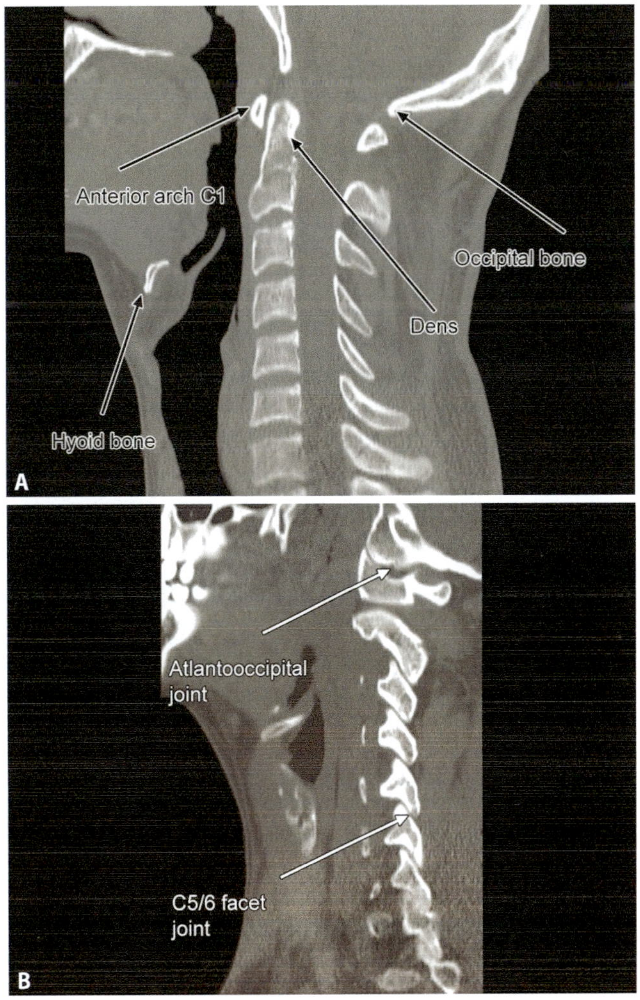

Figs. 4A and B: CT scan of cervical spine (sagittal reformat image).

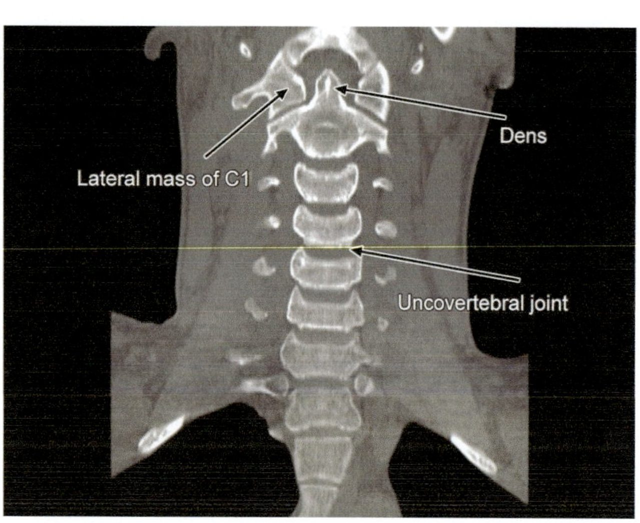

Fig. 5: CT scan of cervical spine (coronal reformat image).

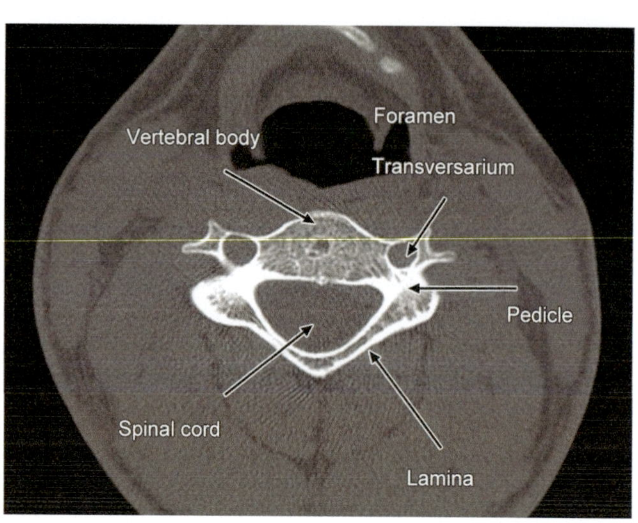

Fig. 6: CT scan of cervical spine (axial image).

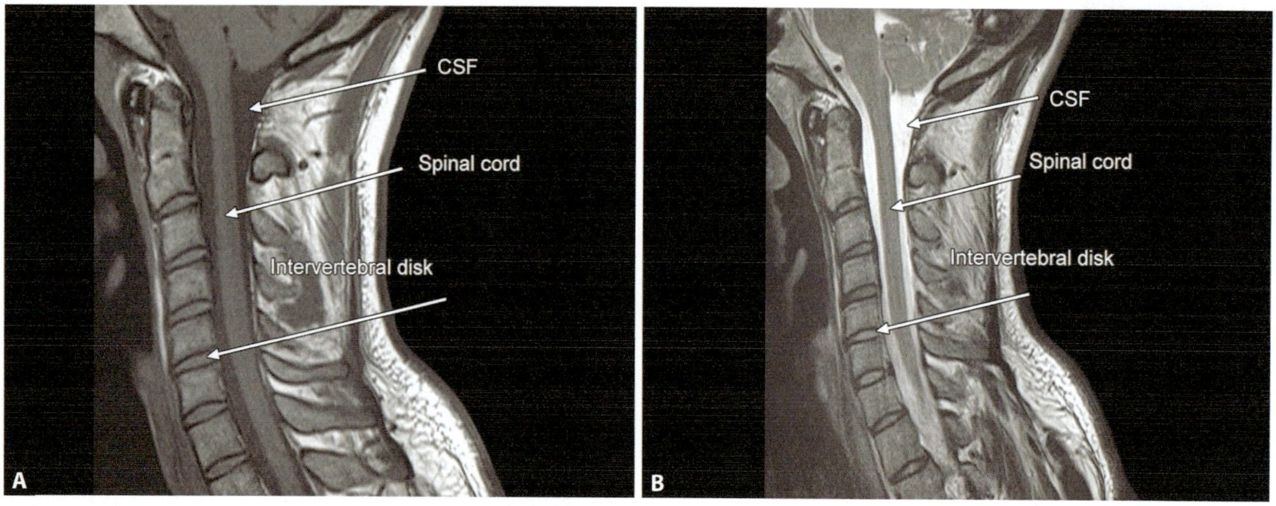

Figs. 7A and B: (A) MRI scan of cervical spine (sagittal T1 sequence image); (B) MRI scan of cervical spine (sagittal T2 sequence image). (CSF: cerebrospinal fluid)

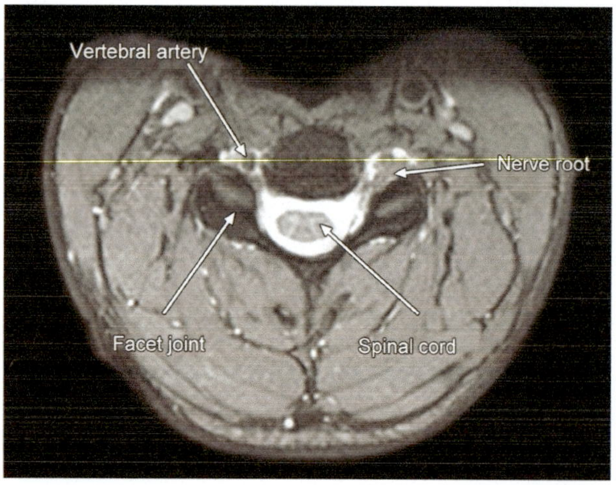

Fig. 8: MRI scan of cervical spine (axial T2 sequence image).

The first cervical vertebra is called the atlas. It is an atypical vertebra, which looks more like a ring; the vertebral body of C1 has been replaced by a small anterior tubercle to allow space for the dens of C2. The vertebral arches and articular facets are also modified to form lateral masses. The upper surface of the lateral mass is kidney-shaped and concave to articulate with the occipital condyle, while the lower surface is round and almost flat to accommodate the lateral atlantoaxial joint. The lateral masses of C1 and C2 lie anterior, compared with the facet joints of the other cervical vertebrae.[1-3]

The second cervical vertebra is also atypical. It is characterized by the odontoid process or dens, which is a large vertical spinous process arising from the body of

C2. The dens is nonweight bearing and articulates with the back of the arch of C1 at the median atlantoaxial joint allowing rotation. The axis articulation with C3 is the same as the other normal cervical vertebrae consisting of the vertebral body disk articulation, the uncovertebral and the facet joints. The facet joints are oriented approximately 45° superiorly from the transverse plane in the upper cervical spine, and they assume a more vertical orientation toward C7.

THORACIC VERTEBRAE

There are 12 thoracic vertebrae **(Figs. 9 to 15)**. The unique feature of thoracic vertebrae is the presence of a pair of semicircular demifacets on each side of the vertebral body, where the ribs articulate. The ribs articulate with the inferior demifacet and the transverse process of the associated vertebral body and the superior demifacet of the vertebra below (i.e., the 5th rib articulates with the inferior demifacet and transverse process of the 5th thoracic vertebra and the superior demifacet of the 6th thoracic vertebra). The upper demifacet is larger and lies at the junction of the vertebral body and the upper border of its pedicle. The smaller lower facet is at the lower border of the body. The thoracic vertebral body is heart-shaped and the vertebral foramen is almost round. The 10th, 11th, and 12th ribs have only single demifacets on each side of their bodies for articulation with the ribs.

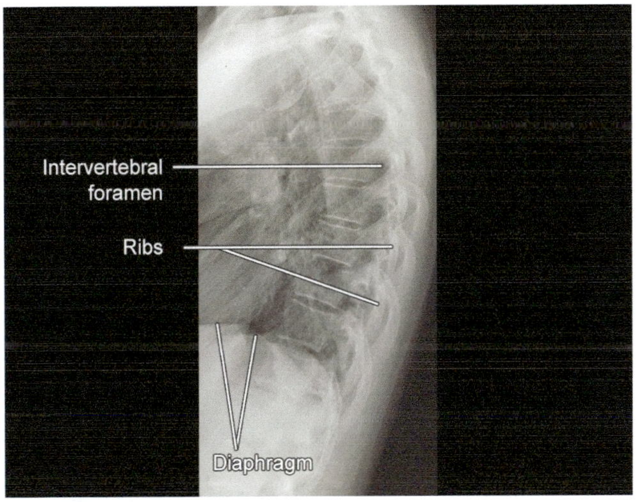

Fig. 9: Plain radiograph of thoracic spine (lateral view).

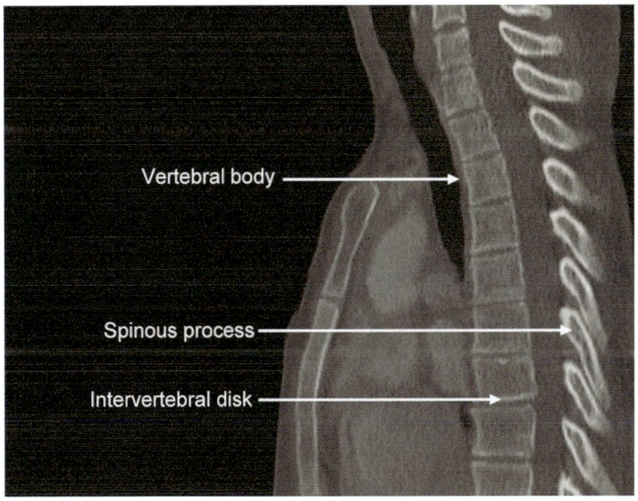

Fig. 11: CT scan of thoracic spine (sagittal reformat image).

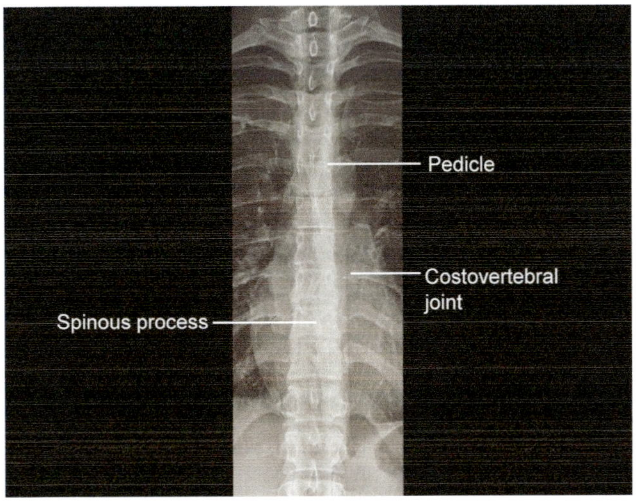

Fig. 10: Plain radiograph of thoracic spine (anteroposterior view).

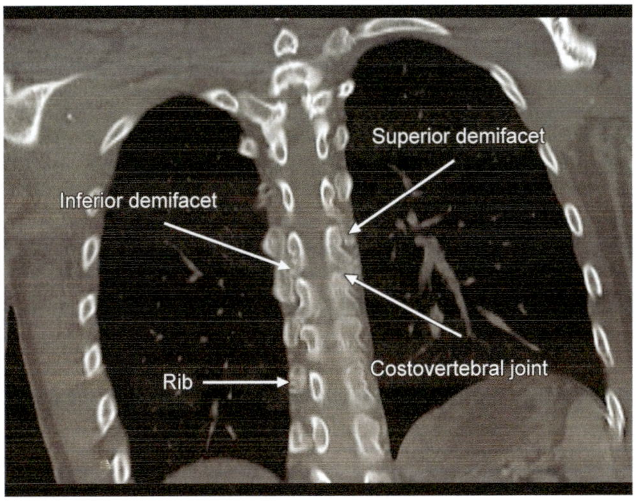

Fig. 12: CT scan of thoracic spine (coronal reformat image).

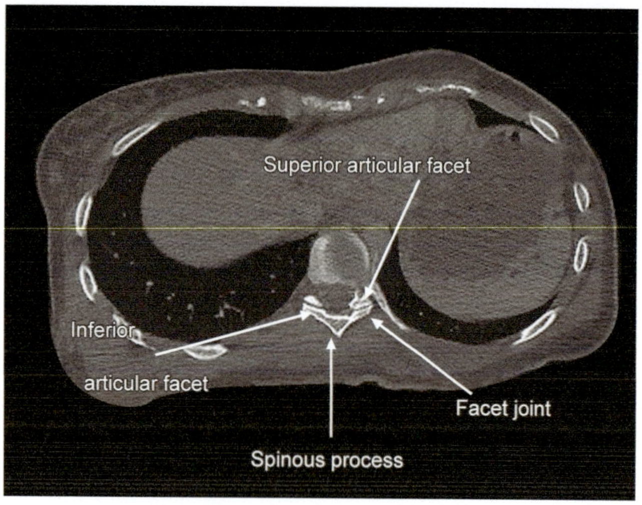

Fig. 13: CT scan of thoracic spine (axial image).

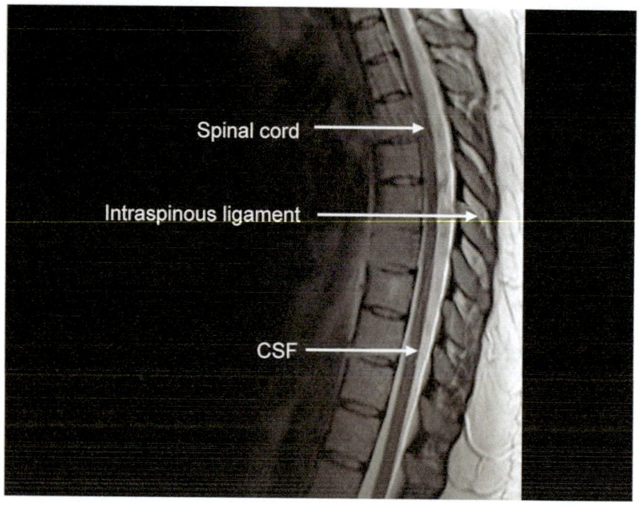

Fig. 15: MRI scan of thoracic spine (axial T2 sequence view). (CSF: cerebrospinal fluid)

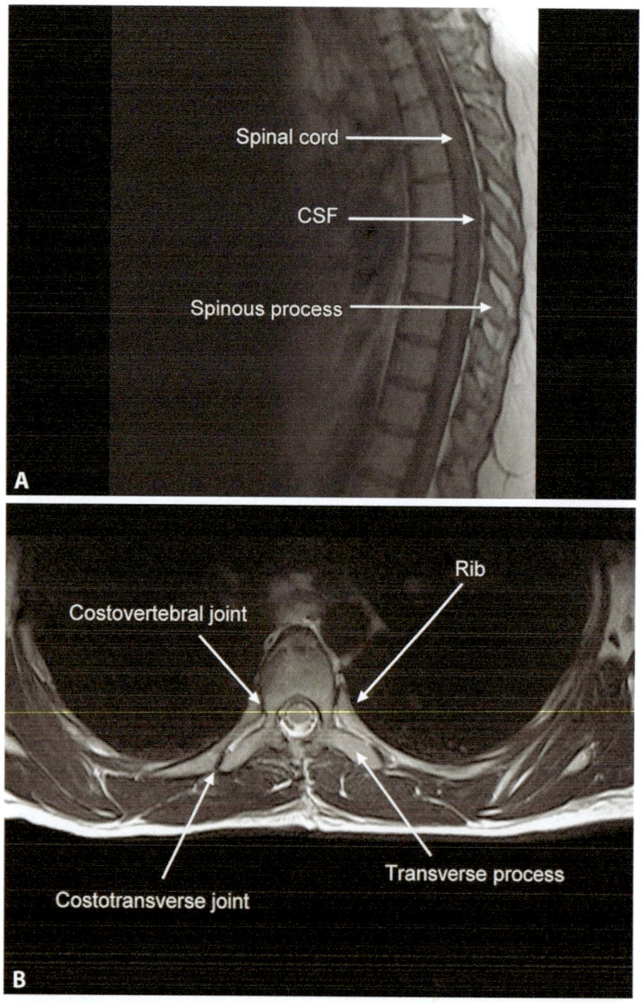

Figs. 14A and B: (A) MRI scan of thoracic spine (sagittal T1 sequence image); (B) MRI scan of thoracic spine (sagittal T2 sequence image). (CSF: cerebrospinal fluid)

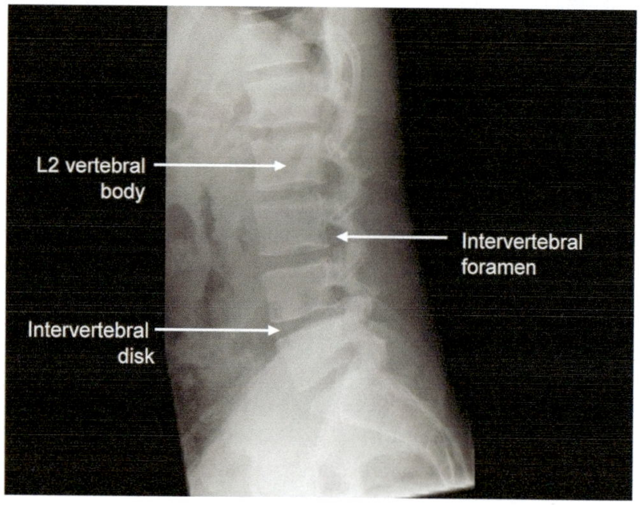

Fig. 16: Plain radiograph of lumbar spine (lateral view).

The superior articular facets of the thoracic vertebrae project up from the junction of the pedicle and the lamina. They face posteriorly and slightly laterally. The inferior articular facets face anteriorly and slightly medially. This arrangement permits some rotation between adjacent bodies.

LUMBAR VERTEBRAE

The normal appearance of the lumbar spine includes a gradual widening of interpedicle distance and an increase in disk height from the L1/2 to the L4/5 disk. The L5/S1 disk is usually slightly narrower. The lumbar vertebrae are characterized by large kidney-shaped vertebral bodies. The transverse and spinous processes are relatively short **(Figs. 16 to 22)**.

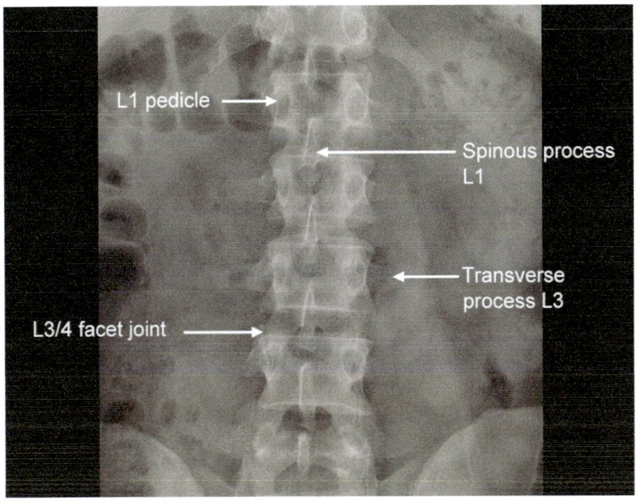

Fig. 17: Plain radiograph of lumbar spine (anteroposterior view).

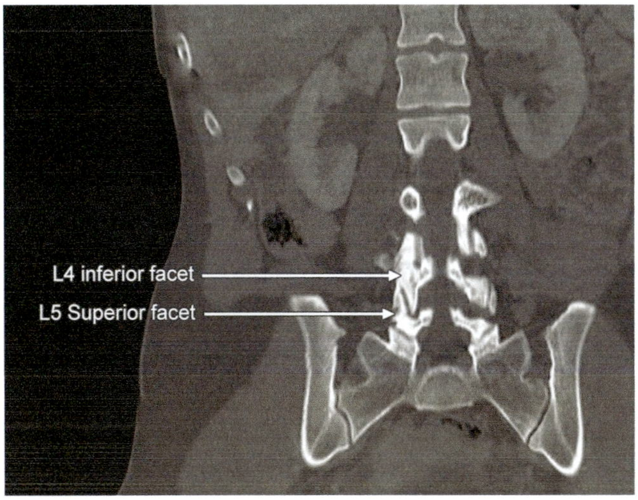

Fig. 19: CT scan of lumbar spine (coronal reformat image).

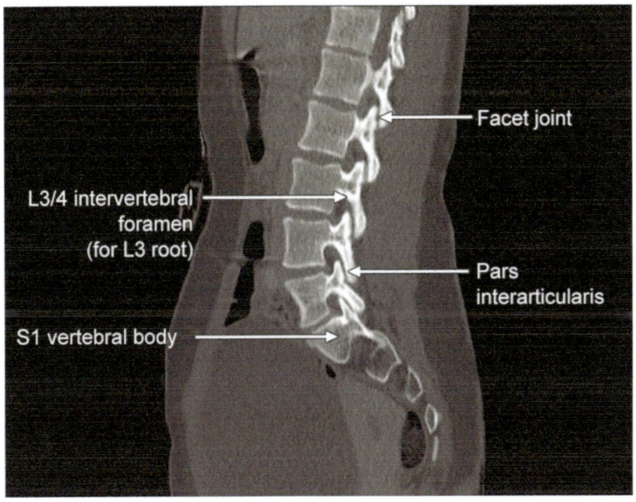

Fig. 18: CT scan of lumbar spine (sagittal reformat image).

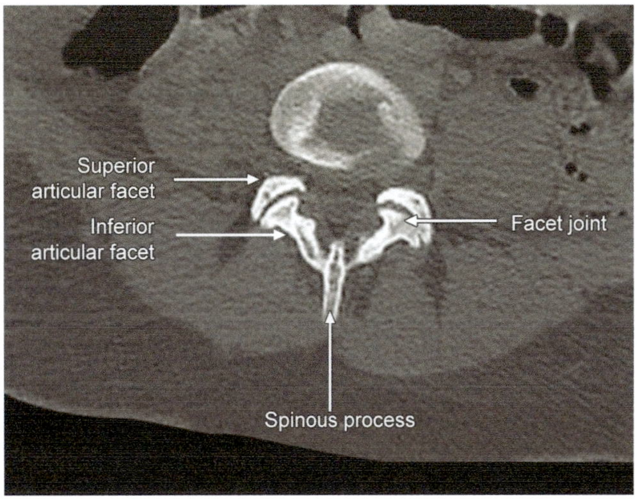

Fig. 20: CT scan of lumbar spine (axial image).

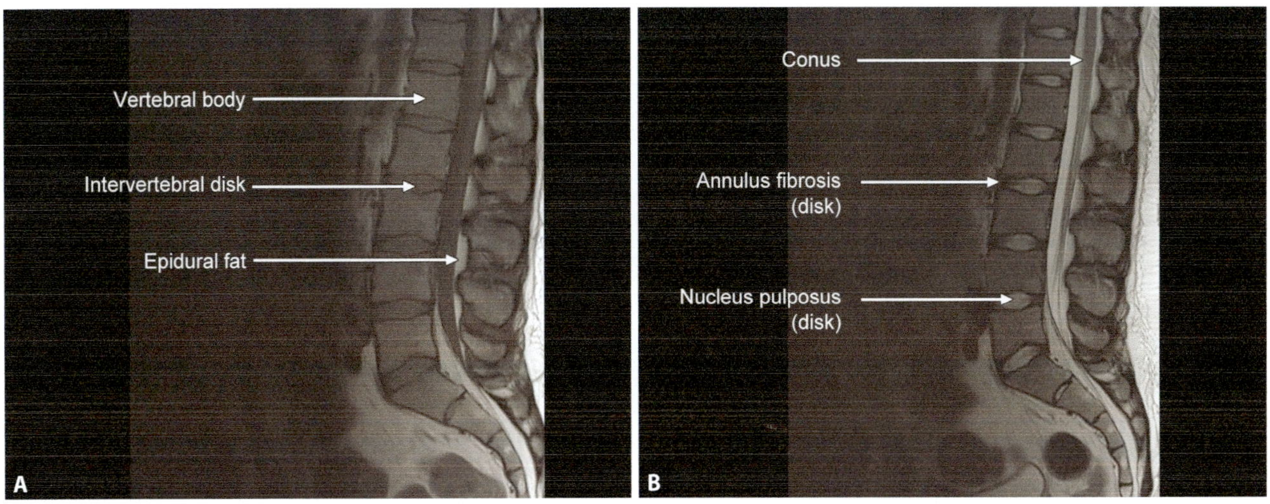

Figs. 21A and B: (A) MRI scan of lumbar spine (sagittal T1 sequence image); (B) MRI scan of lumbar spine (sagittal T2 sequence image).

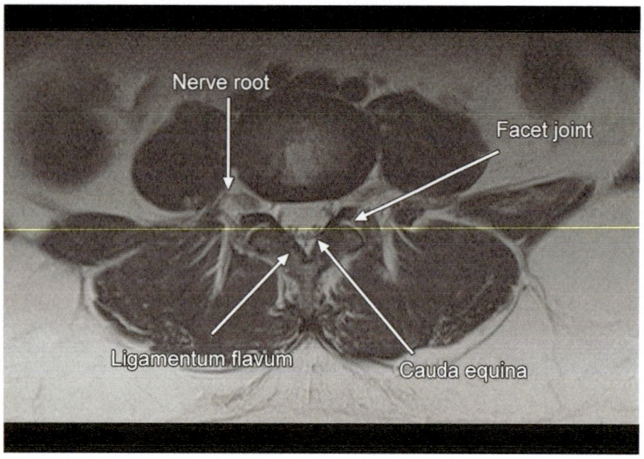

Fig. 22: MRI scan of lumbar spine (axial T2 sequence image).

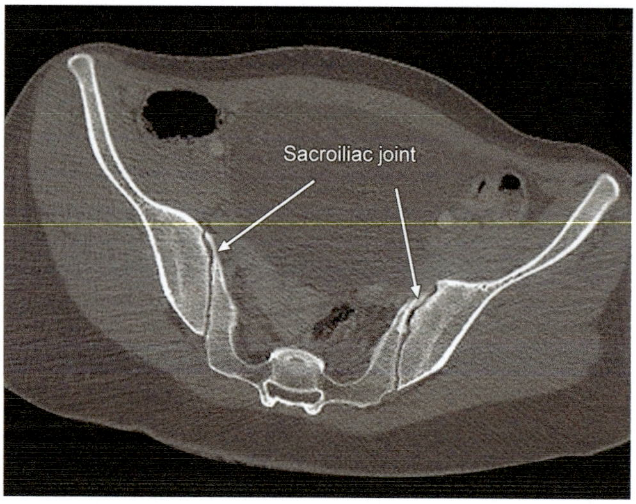

Fig. 24: CT scan of sacroiliac joint (axial image).

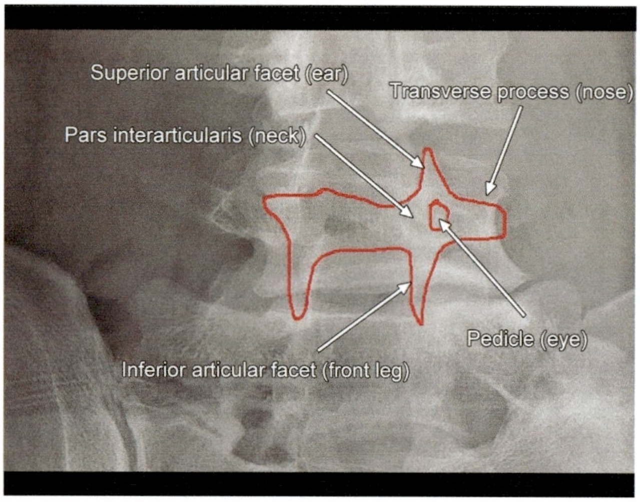

Fig. 23: Plain radiograph of lumbar spine (oblique "Scottie dog" view).

The articular processes are characteristic. The upper pair rises up and carries the articular facets, which face dorsomedial and are concave in the anteroposterior direction. The lower pair of articular processes project down; they face ventrolateral and are convex in the anteroposterior direction. This configuration is accentuated between L5 and S1, where the inferior articular process of L5 faces well forward and is received by the backward-facing facet of S1. This locks L5 in place and prevents it from sliding forward on S1.

On oblique radiographs, the posterior elements form the appearance of a "Scottie dog" **(Fig. 23)**.

Nose is the transverse process, eye is the pedicle, ear is the superior articular process, neck is pars interarticularis, and front leg is inferior articular process.

Lumbosacral transitional vertebrae are congenital anomalies defined as either sacralization of the lowest lumbar segment or lumbarization of the most superior sacral segment of the spine. Lumbosacral transitional vertebrae are common in the general population, with a reported prevalence of 4–30%. Correctly identifying a transitional vertebra is essential because there are important clinical implications. Inaccurate identification may lead to surgical and procedural errors and poor correlation with clinical symptoms. Additionally, some clinicians believe that low back pain is caused by transitional vertebrae; this is termed "Bertolotti syndrome".[4]

SACRUM AND SACROILIAC JOINT

The sacrum is a triangular bone made up of five fused sacral vertebrae. It is curved with a concavity toward the pelvis. The body of S1 is wide, and it articulates with L5 above; it tapers to an apex to articulate with the coccyx. It articulates with the body of the ileum on its lateral aspect to form the posterior wall of the pelvis. In addition to its characteristic shape, it contains anterior and posterior foramina through which the respective anterior and posterior rami of the spinal nerves pass. MRI is the fastest, cheapest, and most specific way in making the diagnosis of sacral insufficiency fractures, which are usually imperceptible on plain film and subtle on CT **(Figs. 24 and 25)**.

The sacroiliac joint is a synovial joint. With age, fibrous adhesions and gradual joint space narrowing occur. The joint is very stable permitting very little movement;

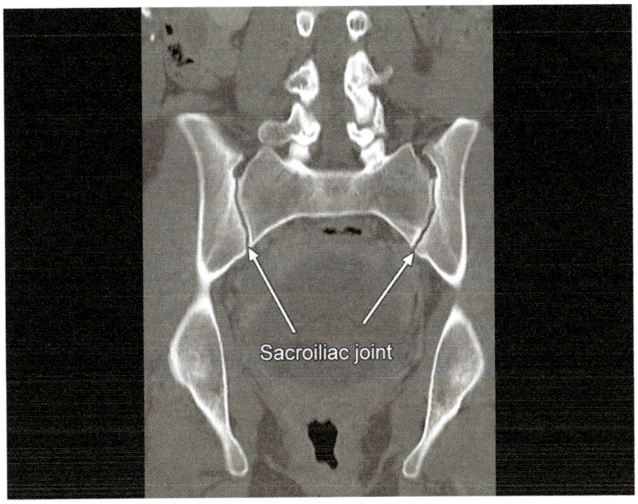

Fig. 25: CT scan of sacroiliac joint (coronal reformat image).

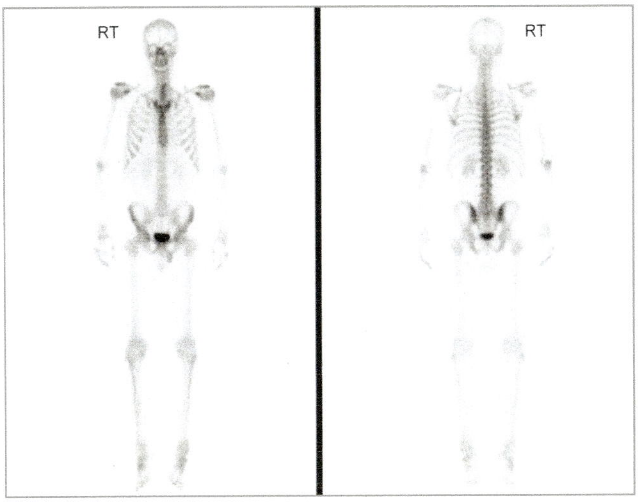

Fig. 26: Isotope bone scan.

the stability of the sacroiliac joint depends entirely on the sacroiliac ligaments.

SPINAL CORD

The spinal cord proper extends from the level of the foramen magnum in the skull to the level of L1/2 in the adult where it tapers in a cone-shaped ending called the conus medullaris. A stalk of pia mater, the filum terminale attaches from the conus medullaris to the dura mater at S2. The spinal nerve roots of the lumbar and sacral segments slope steeply downward forming the cauda equina. The space below the L2 vertebra, typically at L4, is considered safe to sample CSF since only nerve roots and not spinal cord are found there. Similarly, a lower lumbar posterior disk herniation can impinge upon individual nerve roots or the entire cauda equina to cause radiculopathy or cauda equina syndrome.[2,3]

RADIONUCLIDE IMAGING

The spine is also often imaged with gamma cameras, using radioactive technetium-99m-labeled diphosphonates. There is symmetric distribution of activity throughout the skeletal system in healthy adults **(Fig. 26)**. Urinary bladder activity, faint renal activity, and minimal soft-tissue activity are also normally present. In the neck, activity in the facet joints of the cervical vertebrae in patients with asymptomatic degenerative changes is frequently seen. Bone scintigraphy scans, as they are known, are not specific but they are extremely sensitive for picking up many pathologic conditions, such as metastatic disease, trauma, and infection as well as Paget disease and spondylolysis. Abnormalities that extend beyond the vertebral body are invariably due to osteophytes, whereas abnormalities that are confined to the articular facets are nearly always benign in origin. Radiotracer accumulation in both the vertebral body and pedicles usually indicates metastatic disease, whereas abnormalities that involve the vertebral body and facets, but spare the pedicles, are usually benign.

CONCLUSION

Interventional pain management requires the ability to interpret various different imaging modalities, including plain radiography, fluoroscopy, CT, and MRI. This chapter has given an overview of the basic radiological anatomy, which is required by the interventional pain physician. By actively studying the anatomical imaging in a clinical context, the pain physicians will increase the efficacy and accuracy of their interventions, which in turn will further help with the interpretation of imaging studies.

REFERENCES

1. Baheti DK, Bakshi S, Gupta S, Gehdoo RP. Interventional Pain Management: A Practical Approach. New Delhi: Jaypee Brothers Medical Publishers (P) Ltd.; 2009.
2. Stoller DW. Magnetic Resonance Imaging in Orthopaedics and Sports Medicine, 3rd edition. New York: Lippincott Williams and Wilkins; 2006.
3. Sinnatamby CS, Last RJ. Last's Anatomy: Regional and Applied, 12th edition. New York: Churchill Livingstone; 2011.
4. Jain A, Agarwal A, Jain S, Shamshery C. Bertolotti syndrome: a diagnostic and management dilemma for pain physicians. Korean J Pain. 2013;26(4):368-73.

3 CHAPTER

Understanding of Radiological–Spinal Imaging for Pain Physicians

Sarath Bethapudi, Harun Gupta

ABSTRACT

Spinal intervention is mainstay in a multimodal approach to spinal pain management. Perfect understanding of radiological imaging of the spine is key to performing successful interventional spinal blocks and guiding pain physician in the treatment of spinal disorders.

INTRODUCTION

Radiological investigations are routinely performed to diagnose spinal pathology. Imaging-guided spinal intervention is being increasingly used to achieve symptomatic pain relief in various spinal disorders. This chapter is an overview of imaging modalities, commonly occurring spinal disorders, and spinal interventional techniques.

IMAGING TECHNIQUES

Radiography

X-rays are commonly used as first-line investigations in spinal trauma, osteoporotic fractures, and for the evaluation of developmental disorders such as scoliosis and Scheuermann's disease. Despite increasing use of magnetic resonance imaging (MRI), some centers still use X-rays as screening tools for excluding pathological fractures, in patients with known malignancies. Frontal- and lateral-view X-rays are generally obtained for the evaluation of spinal pathology. In cervical spine trauma, an additional open-mouth peg view is obtained along with frontal and lateral projections as part of trauma series. Additional views such as Swimmer's view are performed in cervical spine trauma where the C7/T1 junction is not adequately seen on the standard lateral view. Oblique Scotty dog view of the lumbar spine is useful for assessment of pars interarticularis fractures.

Magnetic Resonance Imaging

Magnetic resonance imaging is an extremely useful radiological investigation for the evaluation of both acute and chronic spinal pathologies. The most common chronic indication is the investigation of chronic back pain with neurological symptoms. In acute setting, MRI is useful for the assessment of spinal trauma and for the evaluation of new-onset neurology, including suspected acute cord compression and cauda equina syndromes. Demyelination, spinal tumor, infections, inflammatory spondyloarthropathy, and spondylolisthesis are some of the other common indications for performing an MRI examination of the spine.

It is important to note that MRI gives better soft-tissue and vertebral bone marrow detail, compared to radiography and computed tomography (CT), which are better at showing trabecular and cortical bone detail.

Computed Tomography

One of the main indications for use of CT imaging in spine is acute trauma. Thin slice spiral CT acquisition also allows multiplanar reconstruction of images in all three planes, thereby providing vital information on spinal injuries and alignment and aiding decisions on management.

Computed tomography is also useful for the evaluation of postoperative spines to identify complications such as loosening and fatigue fractures of metal work. CT can also be used as an alternative to MRI in diagnosing disk herniations and central canal stenosis in patients, unable to have MRI due to contraindications such as aneurysm clips and permanent pacemakers. Assessment of morphology and degree of bony healing in pars stress fractures and evaluation of spinal tumors are among other indications for performing CT examination. CT fluoroscopy has major applications in performing imaging-guided intervention of the spine, and this is discussed separately in the intervention section of this chapter.

Other Imaging Modalities

The use of technetium 99m methylene diphosphonate (Tc99m-MDP) bone scintigraphy in spine is largely limited to the evaluation of primary and secondary tumors of the spine and used in conjunction with other imaging modalities.

Computed tomography and magnetic resonance (MR) myelography involve the performing of CT/MRI examinations with intrathecal contrast. Myelography offers the advantage of clearly discerning spinal cord and nerve roots within the thecal sac. The invasive nature of these examinations, risks of complications from injecting contrast into the thecal sac, and ever-improving quality of nonmyelographic CT and MRI examinations have resulted in a rapid decline in the number of myelographic examinations, performed over the recent years.

Bone mineral density is a test used for assessing strength and mineralization of the bones, to identify patients at risk of osteoporotic fractures.

IMAGE-GUIDED INTERVENTIONAL TECHNIQUES FOR CHRONIC PAIN MANAGEMENT

Chronic spinal pain is a common problem and can have functionally debilitating consequences. Image-guided interventional techniques are an integral part of pain-management strategy in patients with chronic symptomatic spinal problems. These procedures are generally reserved for nonsurgical patients who do not respond to conservative management, including physiotherapy, oral analgesics, and muscle relaxants. It is important to note that findings on imaging do not always correlate with the patients' symptoms.[1-4] Therefore, spinal injections are not only used for therapeutic purposes but can often be of diagnostic value to confirm the origin of symptoms, especially in patients being considered for surgical treatment.

Currently, there is controversy over increased efficacy of image-guided targeted spinal intervention over blind injections. Double-blind randomized controlled studies are required to settle the existing debate and arguments over this topic. However, increased accuracy of needle tip placement and reduced procedural complication rates for procedures performed under image guidance make this a preferred technique over blind procedures.[1] Most spinal injections are performed either under conventional or CT fluoroscopy. Low-dose CT fluoroscopy enables accurate visualization of needle tip and path in relation to the neighboring structures with reduced procedural times, compared to conventional fluoroscopy. Given these advantages, CT fluoroscopy is increasingly being used for spinal interventional procedures.[5] Commonly performed image-guided spinal interventional procedures for pain management include:

- Facet joint injection
- Spinal epidural injection
- Selective nerve root block
- Sacroiliac joint injection
- Injection of pars interarticularis defects.

These procedures are generally performed as outpatient procedures. Standard principles of patients' consent, asepsis, and guidance for patients on oral anticoagulants apply like any other needle procedure.

Computed Tomography-Guided Injection Technique

For spinal injections, performed under CT guidance, the patient lies flat in a prone position. Standard limited axial CT imaging is obtained through the region of interest with skin markers (e.g., paper clips, stuck to surgical dressing tape) placed on side of injection. The slice for injection is selected, and the table is moved to the position of the selected slice. Using laser beam and skin markers guidance, the injection site is marked on the skin. Using an aseptic technique, the skin and subcutaneous soft tissues are then injected with 1% or 2% lidocaine local anesthetic. Spinal needle (usually 22G) is angled roughly in the direction of target. The position of needle tip and track can be checked using step pedal, which obtains a stack of images (usually 3–6) along the placed needle. The needle tip position at the target site is confirmed using CT fluoroscopy and the injectant, which is a mixture of corticosteroid and local anesthetic, is injected and the needle is then withdrawn.

For spinal epidural injection, it is important to perform a final check of the needle tip position within the epidural space by injection of contrast **(Fig. 1)**. This ensures 100% accuracy and avoids inadvertent injection into thecal sac.

Use of contrast is not routinely recommended for confirming the intra-articular position of needle tips during facet and sacroiliac joint injections, when these procedures are performed under CT fluoroscopic guidance. Direct visualization of needle tip within the joint, prior to administration of medication, avoids needless exposure to extra radiation. In cases where osteophytes prevent entry into the joints, periarticular injections may be performed.

Conventional Fluoroscopic-Guided Spinal Injections Technique

Spinal injections are also routinely carried out under conventional fluoroscopic guidance. These procedures are generally performed with patients in prone position. The C-arm is angled to position the image intensifier in line with target for injection. Patients can also be turned into a semiprone position, with side of injection, facing up to achieve optimal visualization of the target. In some cases, a combination of C-arm and patient rotation has to be used to achieve a direct line of target. The skin for site of injection is marked and using aseptic technique, the skin and subcutaneous soft tissues are injected with 1% or 2% lidocaine local anesthetic. A spinal needle (usually 22G) is then introduced in the plane of the image intensifier. The needle can be held with long forceps to achieve the right plane of needle track. This maneuver helps performers avoid exposure to radiation field, during direct fluoroscopic screening. The final position of the needle tip is confirmed using a small volume of contrast. Once the targeted position of the needle tip is confirmed, the injectant, which is a combination of local anesthetic and corticosteroid, is injected and the needle is withdrawn.

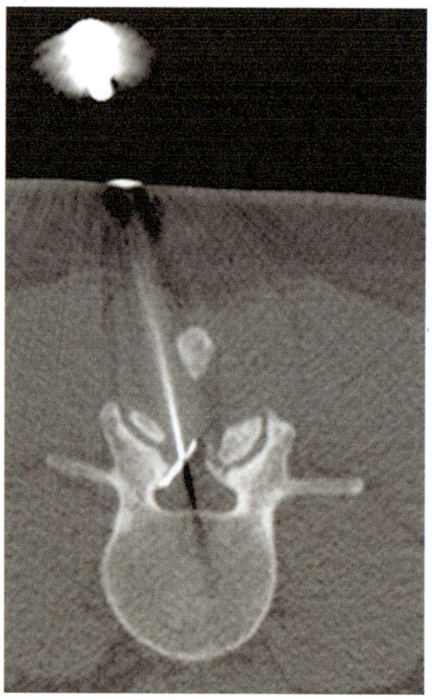

Fig. 1: CT lumbar epidural injection using a translaminar approach. Note needle tip in the posterior epidural space with adjoining epidural space contrast opacification.

COMMON SPINAL PATHOLOGIES

Disk Herniation

Disk herniation is a commonly encountered spinal pathology and involves extension of disk material beyond the margins of the vertebra. Acute disk herniations are spontaneous and can be associated with an episode of trauma. Chronic disk herniations usually occur as part of degenerate disk disease. Disk herniations are described as diffuse bulges, protrusions, extrusions, and sequestration **(Figs. 2 to 5)**.

The herniated disk material can encroach the exit foramen, lateral recesses, or both causing neural impingement **(Figs. 3, 6, and 7)**. Fissuring of the annulus fibrosus without actual disk herniation can cause localized symptomatic pain, without radiation. Postoperative

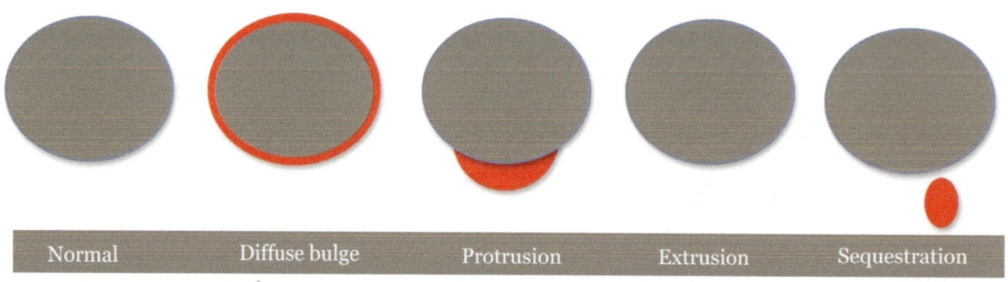

Fig. 2: Standard nomenclature used to describe the morphology of disk herniation.

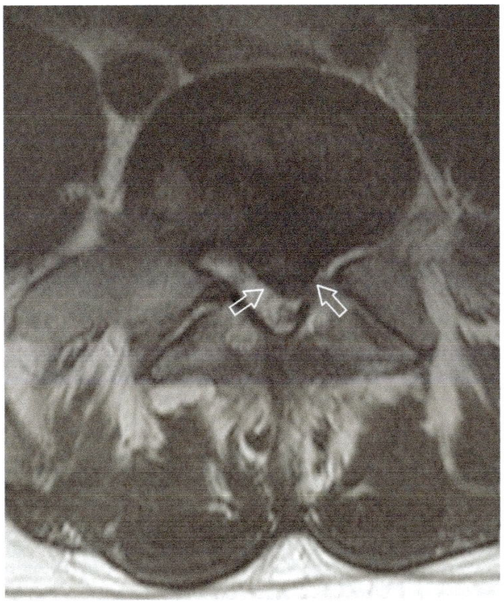

Fig. 3: MRI lumbar spine, axial T2 image demonstrating central and left paracentral disk protrusion (arrows), encroaching central canal, and left lateral recess causing transiting nerve roots impingement.

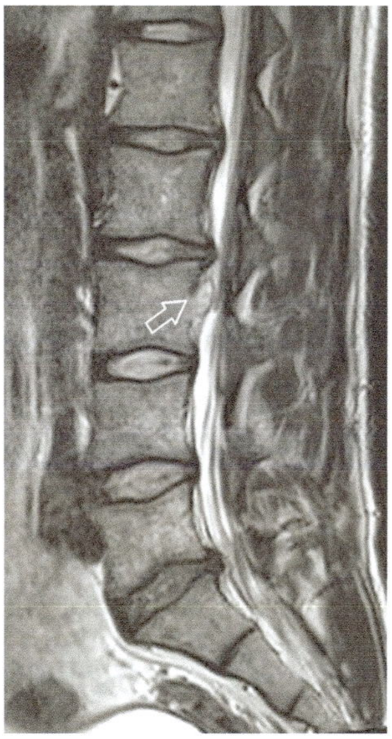

Fig. 5: MRI lumbar spine, sagittal T2 image demonstrating sequestrated disk (arrow).

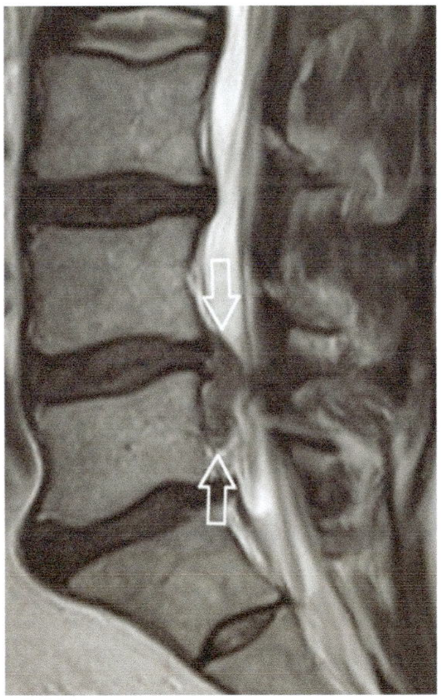

Fig. 4: MRI lumbar spine, sagittal T2 image demonstrating disk extrusion (arrows) at L4/5 level.

scarring and fibrosis can also cause symptoms from neural irritation **(Figs. 8A and B)**.

Disk herniations are best diagnosed with MRI. Patients who cannot have MRI due to metal in body or claustrophobia can undergo CT as an alternative test, with reliable diagnostic accuracy.

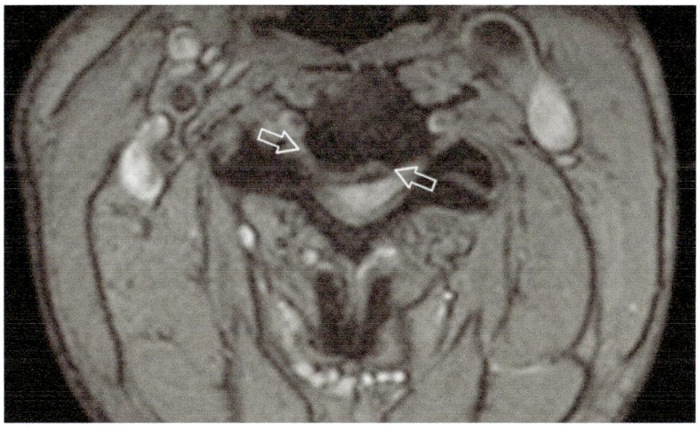

Fig. 6: MRI cervical spine, axial T2 image demonstrating posterior disk-osteophyte complex causing right exit foraminal narrowing with cervical nerve roots impingement (arrows).

Facet Joints Arthropathy

Facet joints arthropathy involves mechanical degeneration of the facet joints. These are associated with joint space loss, subarticular bony changes, and ligamentum flavum hypertrophy. Facet joints arthropathy with or without disks herniation can cause nerve roots impingement.

Active synovitis and inflammation within facet joints can produce facet joints synovial cysts, which can encroach the spinal canal causing neural impingement **(Figs. 9A to C)**. Facet joints arthropathy can be seen on X-rays, MRI, and

CT examinations, although soft-tissue changes such as ligamentum flavum thickening and associated synovial cysts are best appreciated on MRI.

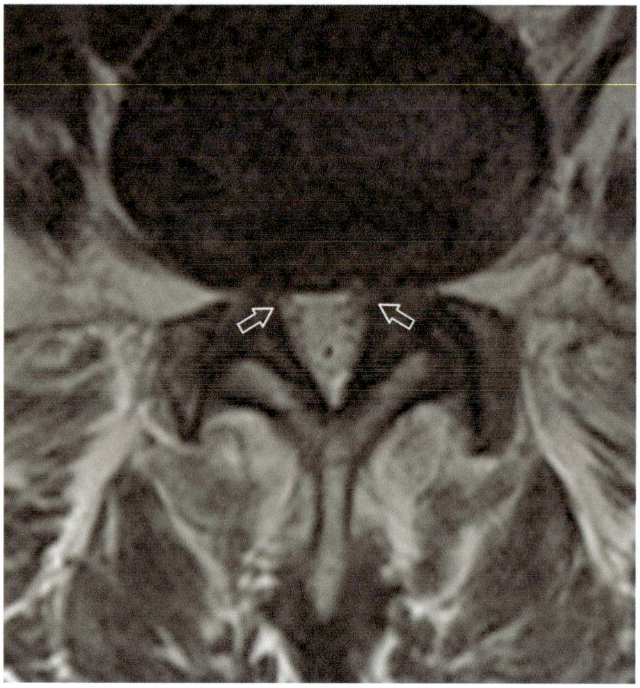

Fig. 7: MRI lumbar spine, axial T2 sequence demonstrating combination of disk disease and facet joints arthropathy with ligamentum flavum thickening, causing bilateral lateral recesses stenosis with transiting nerve roots impingement (arrows).

Spinal Canal Stenosis

Spinal canal stenosis is narrowing of spinal canal diameter and occurs due to disk herniation, facet joints arthropathy with ligamentum flavum thickening, or more commonly due to a combination of both **(Figs. 10A and B)**. Central canal stenosis can cause nerve roots impingement with or without cord/thecal sac compression. Central canal stenosis is graded visually on MRI as mild, moderate, and severe. The degree of spinal canal stenosis seen on imaging does not always reflect the severity of symptoms and, therefore, surgery is not considered in all patients with spinal stenosis.

Spondylolisthesis

Spondylolisthesis is loss of normal spinal alignment, resulting in slippage of a vertebral body in relation to the vertebral body below. Such slips when associated with fractures or defects of the pars interarticularis are referred to as spondylolytic spondylolisthesis **(Fig. 11)**.

Alternatively, the slip can be degenerative in etiology **(Figs. 10A and B)**. Meyerding classification is used to grade spondylolisthesis with grade I suggesting up to 25% slip, grade II up to 50%, grade III up to 75%, and grade IV up to 100%.[6]

Spondylolisthesis can cause central canal and exit foraminal narrowing with nerve roots impingement and cord or thecal sac compression **(Fig. 12)**.

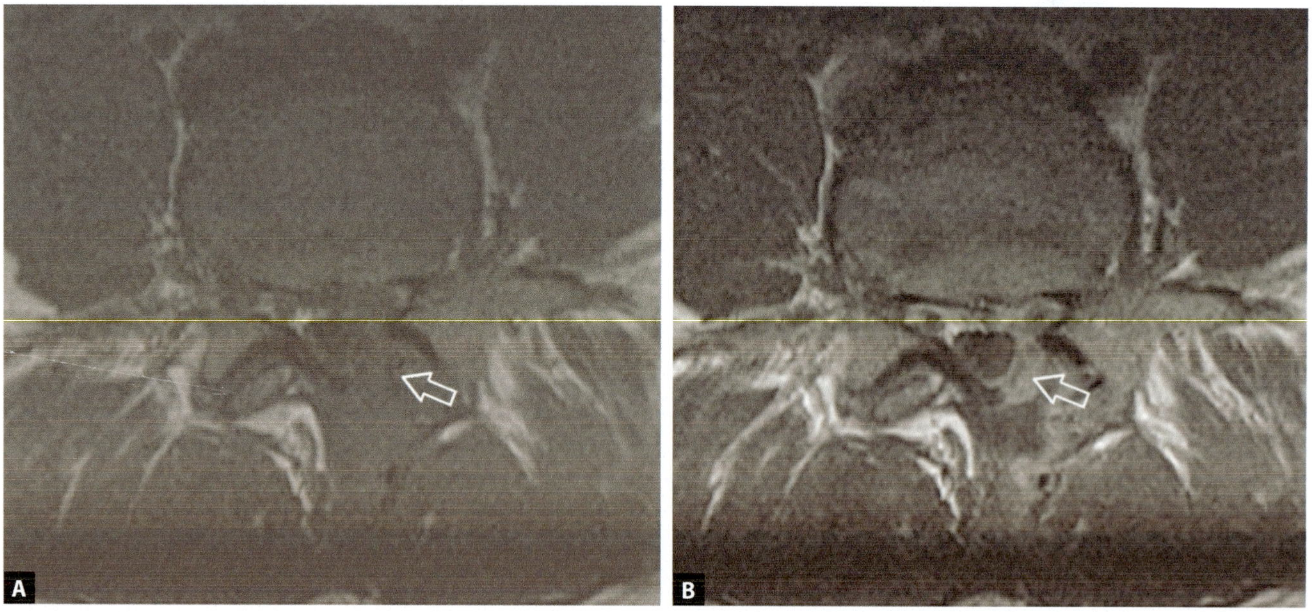

Figs. 8A and B: MRI lumbar spine, axial T1 (A) pre- and (B) postcontrast images in patient with microdiscectomy and left laminectomy demonstrating enhancing scar tissue within left epidural space and lateral recess (arrows).

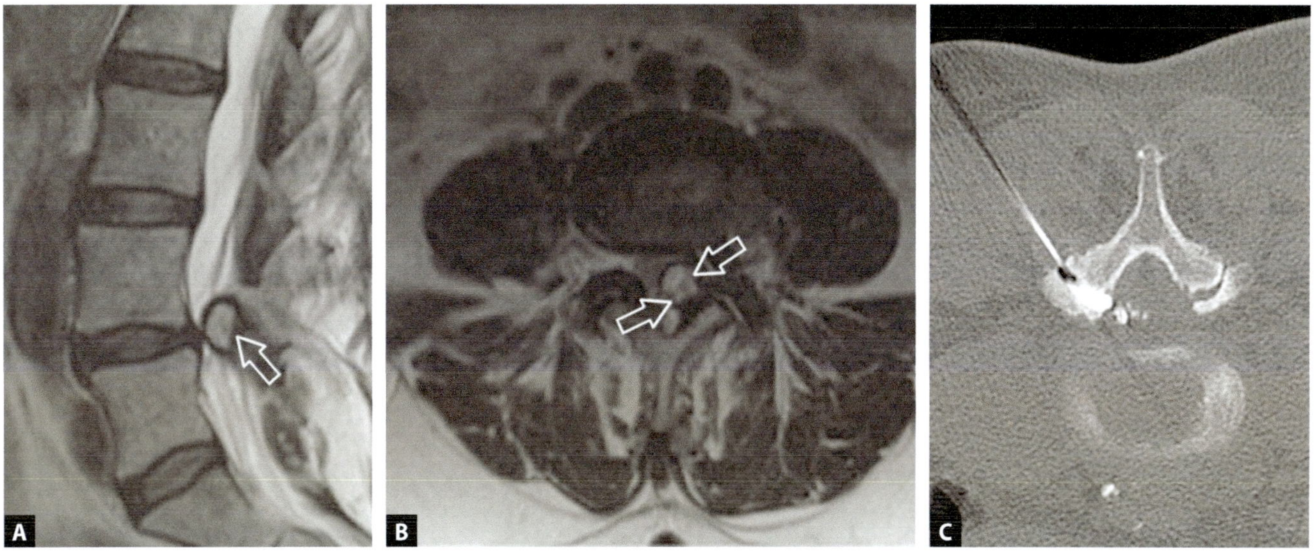

Figs. 9A to C: MRI lumbar spine. (A) Sagittal and (B) axial T2 images demonstrating facet joints arthropathy and intracanalicular left facet joint cyst (arrows) causing neural impingement. (C) Axial CT image demonstrating injection of facet joint cyst.

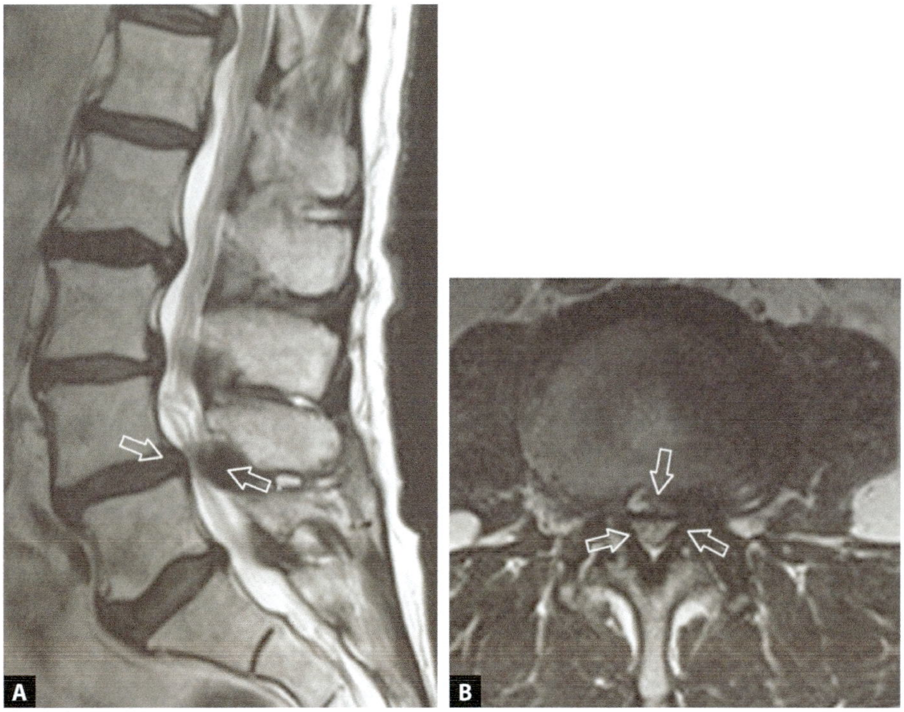

Figs. 10A and B: MRI lumbar spine. (A) Sagittal and (B) axial T2 images demonstrating combination of disk herniation, facet joints arthropathy, and grade I degenerative spondylolisthesis at L4/5 (arrows) causing central stenosis.

Spondylolisthesis can be diagnosed on X-rays, MRI, and CT. MRI offers the advantage of identifying active bone marrow edema in pars stress response and fractures and in assessment of neural impingement **(Fig. 13)**. CT is useful for the evaluation of fracture morphology and bony healing. Sometimes, weight-bearing X-rays are performed to identify accentuation of slip, which may be an indication for surgical management.

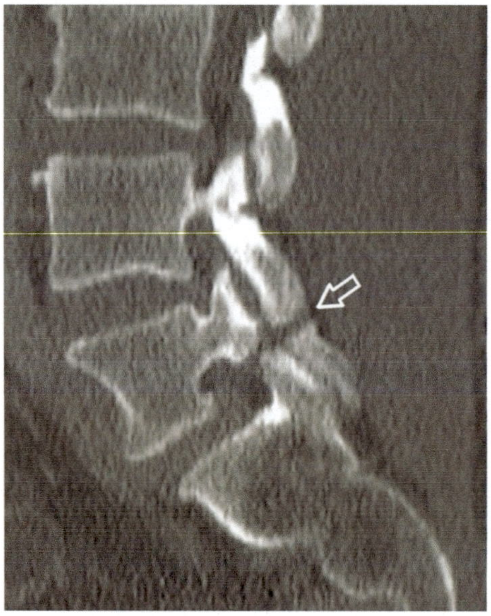

Fig. 11: CT lumbar spine sagittal reformat image demonstrating L5 pars defect (arrow) with grade I spondylolisthesis.

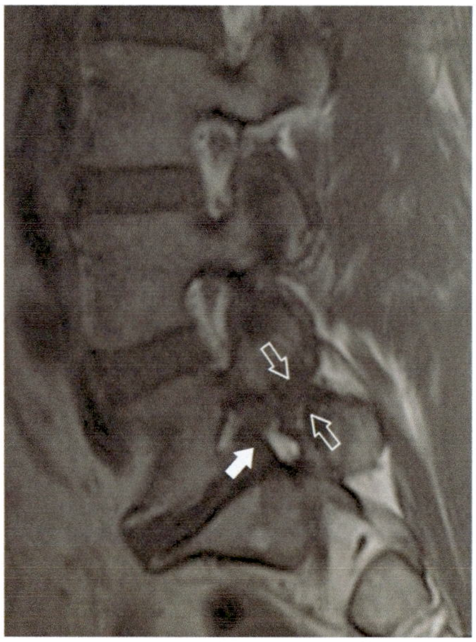

Fig. 12: MRI lumbar spine, sagittal T1 image, demonstrating L5 pars defect (hollow arrows) and grade I spondylolisthesis. Combination of disk herniation and spondylolisthesis also causes L5 exit foraminal narrowing with nerve roots impingement (white arrow).

INFECTED SPONDYLODISCITIS AND VERTEBRAL OSTEOMYELITIS

Infected spondylodiscitis and vertebral osteomyelitis affect single or multiple spinal levels. Fulminant spinal infections can cause pathological fractures with vertebral collapse and paravertebral and spinal epidural abscesses.[7] Both epidural abscesses and pathological vertebral fractures resulting from infection can cause cord compression or cauda equine, requiring urgent spinal surgical input. Spinal infections and abscesses are best diagnosed with MRI **(Figs. 14A and B)**. Initial MRI can be equivocal in early vertebral osteomyelitis, and such cases warrant treatment with follow-up MRI.[8]

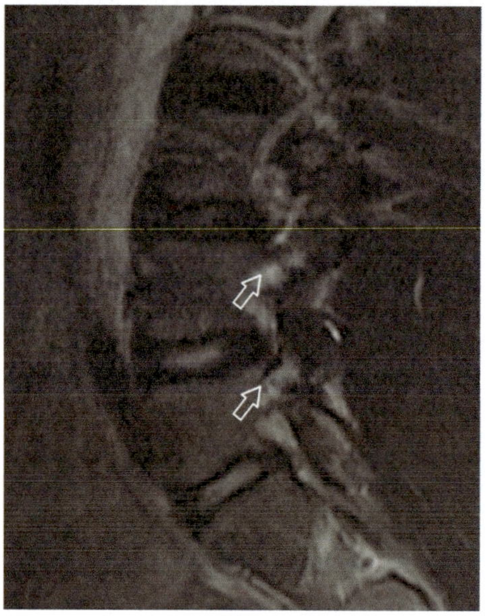

Fig. 13: MRI Lumbar spine, sagittal T2 fat-saturated image, demonstrating edema in L4 and L5 pars (arrows) in keeping with pars stress response.

INFLAMMATORY SPONDYLOARTHROPATHIES

Inflammatory spondyloarthropathies, especially seronegative arthropathies such as ankylosing spondylitis, can affect the axial skeleton, including the spine and sacroiliac joints **(Fig. 15)**. These inflammatory changes manifest as edema within the endplate corners on MRI and as sclerotic shiny corners on X-rays (Romano's lesions). Other changes include diskovertebral changes, which are seen as endplate erosions and aseptic spondylodiscitis (Andersson lesions). Inflammation of zygapophyseal joint and costotransverse joints can also be seen in inflammatory spondyloarthropathies. Chronic and more advanced cases cause ligamentous ossification, squaring of vertebral body with ankylosis, and fusion of the spine (Bamboo spine). Inflammatory spondyloarthropathy can be associated with active sacroiliitis, which manifest as inflammatory bone marrow edema and

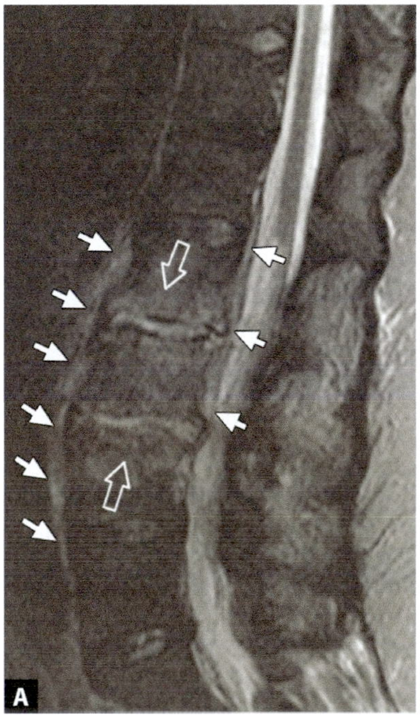

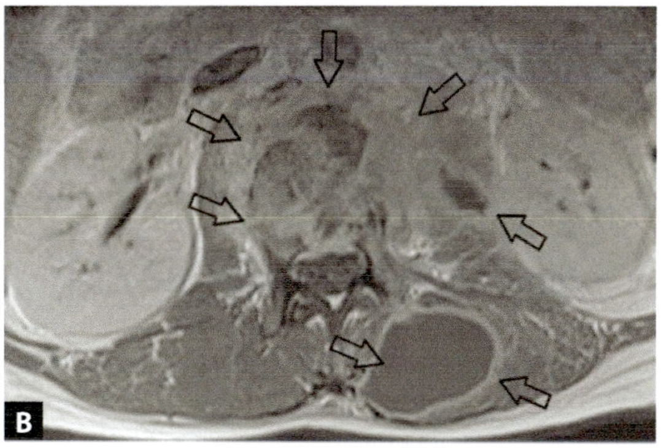

Figs. 14A and B: (A) Lumbar spine MRI sagittal fluid sensitive short tau inversion recovery (STIR) image demonstrating infected spondylodiscitis at L1/2 and L2/3 with intradiskal fluid and florid endplate edematous changes (hollow arrows). Note prevertebral and spinal epidural inflammatory soft tissue (white arrows) associated with infection. (B) Lumbar spine MRI, axial T1 postcontrast image in a different patient demonstrating extensive retroperitoneal and left paraspinal abscess formation (hollow black arrows) secondary to infected spondylodiscitis.

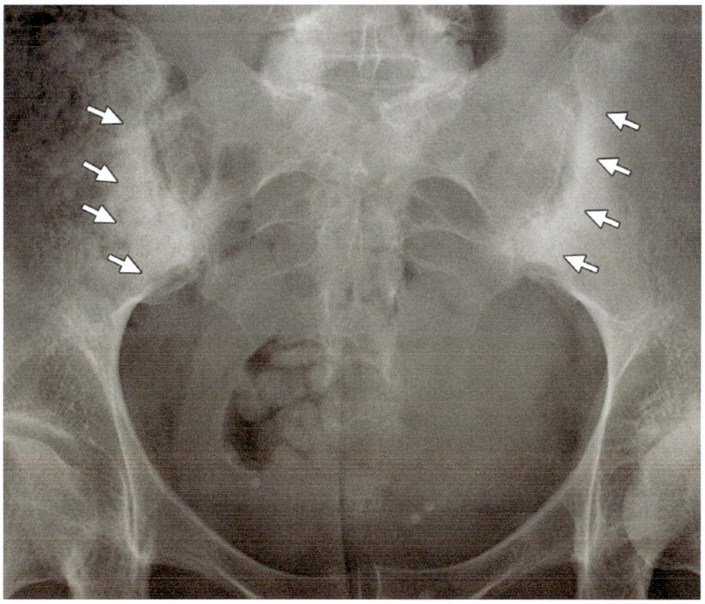

Fig. 15: Frontal pelvis radiograph demonstrating bilateral subarticular sclerosis at the sacroiliac joints, secondary to sacroiliitis (arrows).

articular erosions of sacroiliac joints. Concomitant imaging of sacroiliac joints is therefore performed along with spinal imaging for diagnosis and for assessment of disease activity in inflammatory spondyloarthropathies.[9] Active inflammation within spine and sacroiliac joints is best assessed on MRI **(Figs. 16A and B)**.

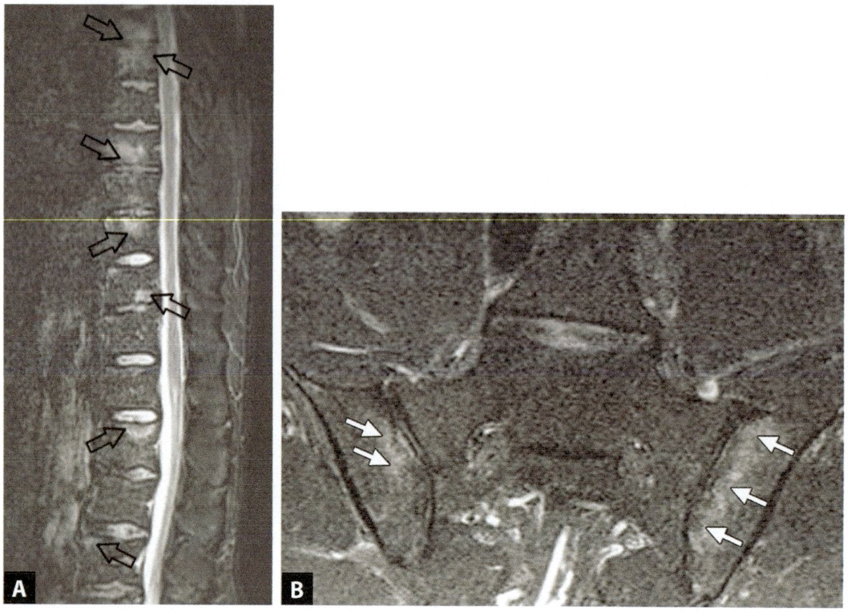

Figs. 16A and B: MRI (A) sagittal fluid-sensitive STIR image of spine and (B) coronal fluid-sensitive STIR image of sacroiliac joints, demonstrating edema and active inflammation within spine (black arrows) and sacroiliac joints (white arrows) in a patient with known ankylosing spondylitis. (STIR: short tau inversion recovery)

CONCLUSION

Imaging plays an important role in diagnosis and assessment of various spinal pathologies. Acute and chronic neurological symptoms, trauma, tumor, infection, osteoporotic and pathological vertebral fractures, pars fractures, inflammatory spondyloarthropathies, and chronic degenerate disease are some of the indications for performing spinal imaging. Image-guided spinal intervention is increasingly being used for the management of chronic symptomatic spinal problems, not responding to conservative management.

REFERENCES

1. Silbergleit R, Mehta BA, Sanders WP, Talati SJ. Imaging-guided injection techniques with fluoroscopy and CT for spinal pain management. Radiographics. 2001;21:927-42.
2. Haldeman S. North American Spine Society: failure of pathology model to predict back pain. Spine (Phila Pa 1976). 1990;15:718-24.
3. Wiesel SW, Tsourmas N, Feffer HL, Citrin CM, Patronas N. A study of computer-assisted tomography. I. The incidence of positive CAT scans in an asymptomatic group of patients. Spine (Phila Pa 1976). 1984;9:549-51.
4. Boden SD, Davis DO, Dina TS, Patronas NJ, Wiesel SW. Abnormal magnetic-resonance scans of the lumbar spine in asymptomatic subjects. A prospective investigation. J Bone Joint Surg Am. 1990;72:403-8.
5. Quek LH, Pua U, Chua GC, Tsou IY. Computed tomography fluoroscopic-guided percutaneous spinal interventions in the management of spinal pain. Ann Acad Med Singap. 2009;38(11):980-8.
6. Meyerding HW. Spondylolisthesis. Surg Gynecol Obstet. 1932;54:371-7.
7. Hong SH, Choi JY, Lee JW, Kim NR, Choi JA, Kang HS. MR imaging assessment of the spine: infection or an imitation? Radiographics. 2009;29(2):599-612.
8. Dunbar JA, Sandoe JA, Rao AS, Crimmins DW, Baig W, Rankine JJ. The MRI appearances of early vertebral osteomyelitis and discitis. Clin Radiol. 2010;65(12):974-81.
9. Hermann KG, Althoff CE, Schneider U, Zühlsdorf S, Lembcke A, Hamm B, et al. Spinal changes in patients with spondyloarthritis: comparison of MR imaging and radiographic appearances. Radiographics. 2005;25(3):559-70.

4 CHAPTER

Role of Electrodiagnosis in the Management of Pain

Khushnuma Mansukhani

ABSTRACT

Electrodiagnosis (EDX) of neuromuscular disorders, better defined as "electroneuromyography (ENMG)" and often inappropriately called electromyography (EMG), is a procedure conducted by trained doctors. It consists of a series of tests done to localize the site of lesion along the neural pathway. In the diagnosis of etiology of pain, it is a useful test to confirm or rule out involvement at nerve, plexus, root, or muscle level. However, it should be judiciously used as an extension rather than a replacement of the clinical neurological examination.

INTRODUCTION

Electrodiagnosis (EDX), more correctly called electroneuromyography (ENMG),[1] is a tool for the diagnosis and localization of neuromuscular diseases. It consists of a series of tests done to assess the function of the peripheral nerve, plexus, root, anterior horn cell, neuromuscular junction, and muscle.[2]

Pain generated in response to damage to the sensory nervous tissue is called neuropathic pain. Causes of neuropathic pain could be at nerve level, presenting as primary painful polyneuropathies, or could be polyneuropathies associated with pain. At the root level, pain could be due to compressive or noncompressive pathology. EDX, if correctly and adequately performed, could provide a clue to the referring physician regarding the source of the pain.

This chapter gives a very basic outline of EDX and its utility and limitations in the management of neuropathic pain with focus on diagnosis of peripheral neuropathies and radiculopathies. For more detailed description of techniques, other books and articles should be referred to.[3-8]

HOW DOES ELECTRONEUROMYOGRAPHY HELP?

- Localization
- Objective record, documentation, and later comparison
- Predominant pathology determined: Axonal, demyelinating, or combined
- Extent of lesion
- Distribution of abnormalities
- Predominant fibers involved sensory or motor
- *Temporal profile:* Acute, chronic, old, and progressive
- Severity of lesion
- Other disorders
- Assess progress.

WHY ELECTRONEUROMYOGRAPHY?

- To know whether there is a neural deficit responsible for the pain
- If there is a deficit, to objectively document it
- To narrow down the differential diagnosis to a few conditions that seem to be the most likely to be the cause of the peripheral neuropathy.
- In some cases to give the exact etiology
- To know whether the deficit is pure sensory or is there subclinical motor axon loss
- How severe is the damage?
- Is it due to focal demyelination, axon loss, or a combination of the two?
- Is it focal or diffuse, unilateral, or bilateral?
- Is the involvement acute or chronic?
- Is the finding on the magnetic resonance imaging (MRI) correlating with the deficit?

- Is the presenting neurodeficit a manifestation of noncompressive radiculitis?
- For assessing the progress of the deficit
- For diagnosing the presence of other conditions—motor neuron disease (MND), entrapment and generalized neuropathies, noncompressive radiculopathy, and cervical myelopathy.
- Postoperative follow-up.

PROTOCOL

- History is a must.
- Clinical examination
- Plan the ENMG study
- Interpret the report and correlate it with presenting symptoms.

It must be borne in mind that ENMG is an extension of the clinical examination and not a replacement; hence, a good history and clinical examinations are prerequisites to the test. A good referral letter from the referring physician is useful to customize the procedure for each patient. A sound technique, knowledge of neuromuscular disorders, and interpretation of results with the presenting problem provide a good ENMG study.

EQUIPMENT

Electromyograph is the machine used for the study. It picks up undistorted biological signals evoked from nerves and muscles with minimal noise disturbance. It is basically a computer with facilities of a headbox, stimulator, display screen, amplifiers, and filters. Since needle electromyography (EMG) is an audiovisual test, a loudspeaker is also fitted **(Fig. 1)**:

- Nerve conduction studies (NCS)
- Sympathetic skin response (SSR)
- Needle EMG
- Late responses: F waves and H reflex
- Somatosensory-evoked potential (SSEP) study: For conduction along the posterior columns of the spinal cord.

ELECTRONEUROMYOGRAPHY TESTS

Nerve Conduction Studies

This is a method of measuring changes in a peripheral nerve by stimulating it electrically and recording the action potential generated. There are two types of studies done: (1) Sensory NCS and (2) motor NCS.

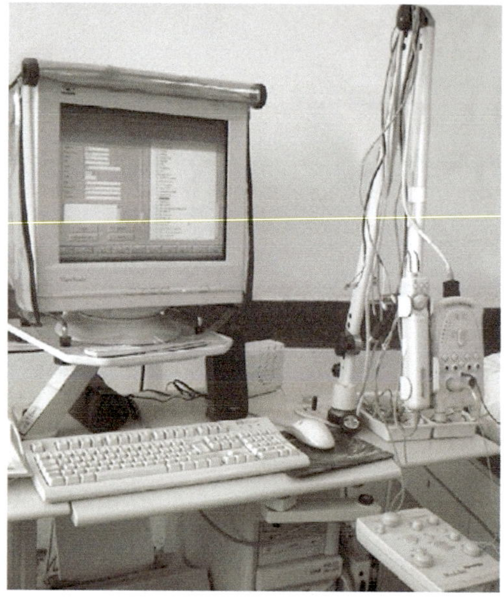

Fig. 1: Electromyograph.

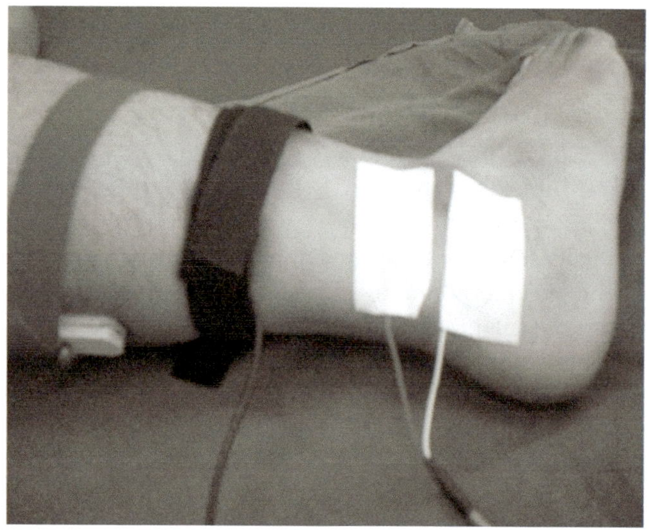

Fig. 2: Technique for recording sural sensory nerve action potential (SNAP).

Sensory Nerve Action Potential

The potential obtained from recording electrodes placed over a sensory nerve, while stimulating it at a point some distance away, is called a sensory nerve action potential (SNAP or SAP) **(Figs. 2 and 3)**. The SAP assesses integrity of the postganglionic sensory fibers and is a sensitive and specific test to localize the site of the lesion to the peripheral nerve, especially for the large myelinated fibers. This test cannot assess the small unmyelinated fibers and hence, NCS are normal when there is a pure small fiber peripheral neuropathy.

A lesion proximal to the dorsal root ganglion, i.e., at the root's level, will cause clinical sensory loss, but on NCS the relevant SAP will be normal. Hence, the relevant SAP will be normal in root lesions in spite of clinical sensory affection; for example, in an L5 radiculopathy, there will be sensory affection over the dorsum of the foot, but the superficial peroneal SAP recorded will be normal. Rarely, when there is a far lateral/foraminal disk prolapse, the SNAP may be affected due to involvement of the dorsal root ganglion, especially the L5 dorsal root ganglion.[9-11]

Motor Nerve Conduction (Figs. 4 and 5)

Motor NCS is a technique of stimulating a motor nerve at two sites serially and picking up the summated muscle action potential using surface electrodes from the relevant muscle. The amplitude of the compound muscle action potential (CMAP) indicates the number of functioning axons and muscle fibers and reflects the amount of axon loss and, hence, is absent or low amplitude in severe peripheral neuropathies. The CMAP in most root lesions is not affected, as 50% of the motor fibers need to be lost to show a significant drop in the amplitude and this is not often the case and also there is an overlap in the myotomes.[12]

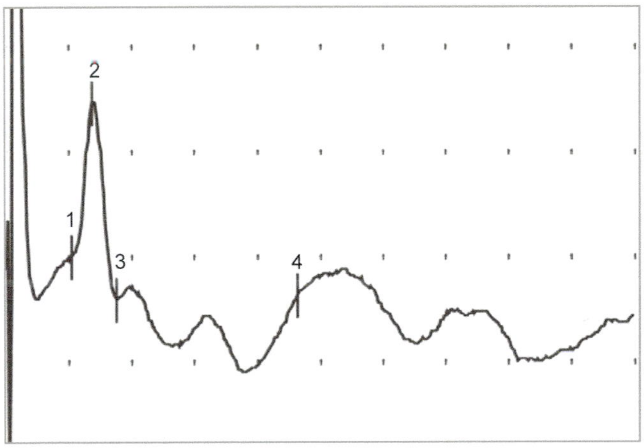

Fig. 3: Normal sural sensory nerve action potential (SNAP).

Sympathetic Skin Response

This is a method to evaluate the small fiber function (unmyelinated C fibers) in the peripheral nerves, by studying the changes in the resistance of skin to electric conduction. However, its presence does not rule out a small fiber peripheral neuropathy and other tests such as quantitative sensory testing, quantitative sudomotor axon reflex testing (QSART), and skin biopsy with intraepidermal nerve fiber (IENF) counting may be required.[13]

Needle Electromyography Examination or Electromyography (Fig. 6)

It is a method of studying the electrical activity of a muscle, by placing a needle electrode within it and observing the following:

- Spontaneous activity in the muscle at rest
- Action potentials [motor unit action potentials (MUAPs)] generated by voluntary contraction of the muscle by the patient.

This is an audiovisual diagnosis, and both the configuration and sound of the potentials are used. This test is the most important one for the diagnosis of

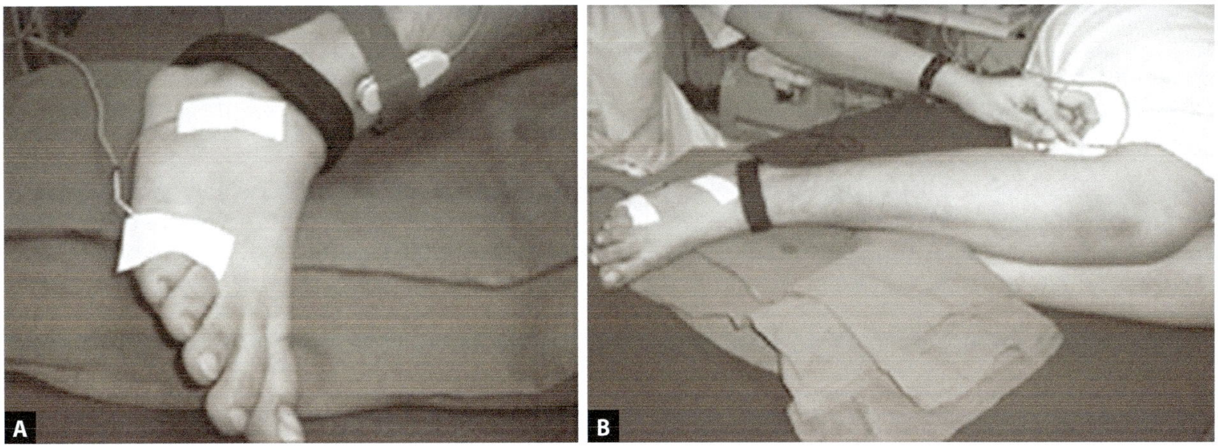

Figs. 4A and B: Motor conduction in common peroneal nerve.

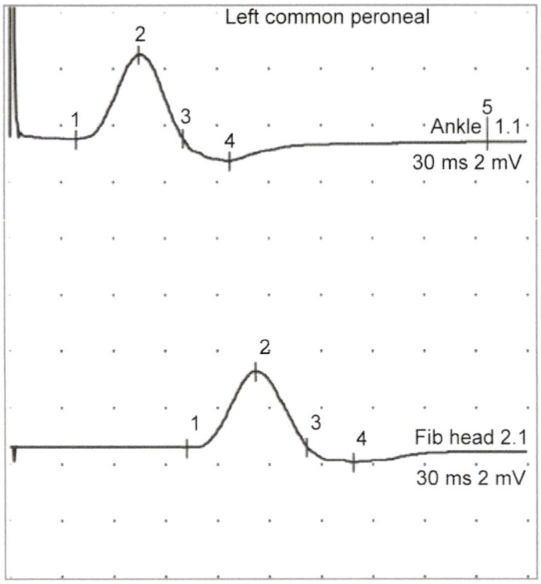

Fig. 5: Normal compound muscle action potential (CMAP) from common peroneal nerve.

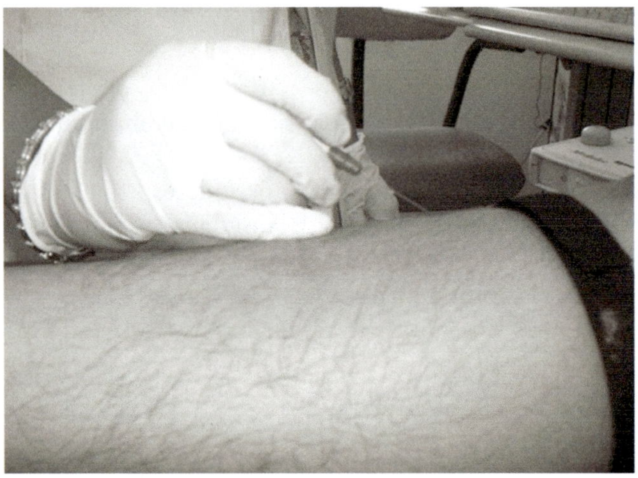

Fig. 6: Needle electromyography (EMG) examination.

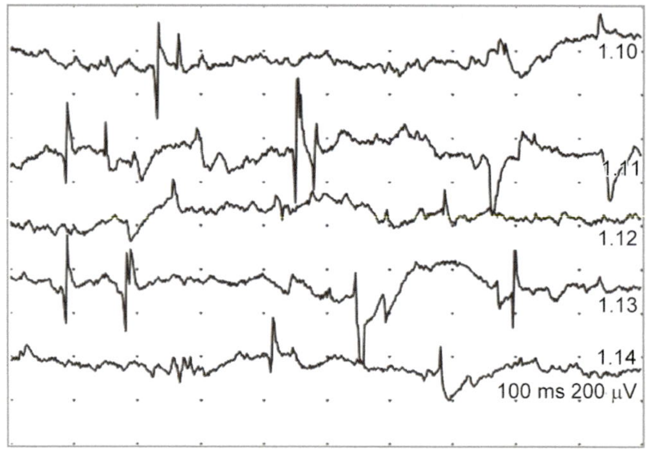

Fig. 7: Fibrillation potentials.

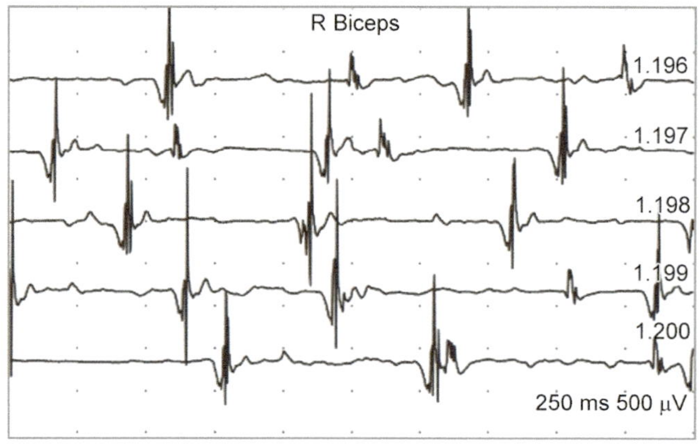

Fig. 8: Polyphasic units.

root lesions, as it is most sensitive and specific for the identification of axon loss motor radiculopathy. It detects the level and extent of root involvement, degree of axon loss, and whether the lesion is active or chronic. Paraspinal muscle EMG in root lesions adds support, if abnormal, but does not rule out root lesion, if normal.

Spontaneous activity on EMG in the form of fibrillation potentials is detected with the muscle at rest. It is a sign of acute/ongoing axon loss, especially when detected in proximal muscles or in distal muscles with recent-onset symptoms. In acute root lesions, spontaneous activity is seen in the paraspinal muscles after 7 days and limb muscles after 14–21 days **(Fig. 7)**.

The MUAP is the activity seen with mild-to-moderate voluntary effort; the configuration, size, and duration of the MUAP localize the site of the lesion and its chronicity. The small jagged polyphasics MUAPs **(Fig. 8)** suggest ongoing involvement, and large and wide triphasic MUAPs **(Fig. 9)** suggest that the lesion is chronic. Once the MUAPs become abnormal, they do not return to normal configuration and the abnormalities would be evident even when the patient becomes asymptomatic. The abnormalities should be present in at least two muscles of the same myotome and innervated by different peripheral nerves. The muscles of one myotome above and below the lesion should also be examined.[14]

To summarize, the abnormalities on needle EMG, which predict a root lesion, are:

- Spontaneous activity—fibrillations **(Fig. 7)**
- Reduced recruitment of motor units
- Increase in polyphasics **(Fig. 8)**
- Increased duration and amplitude of motor units **(Fig. 9)**.

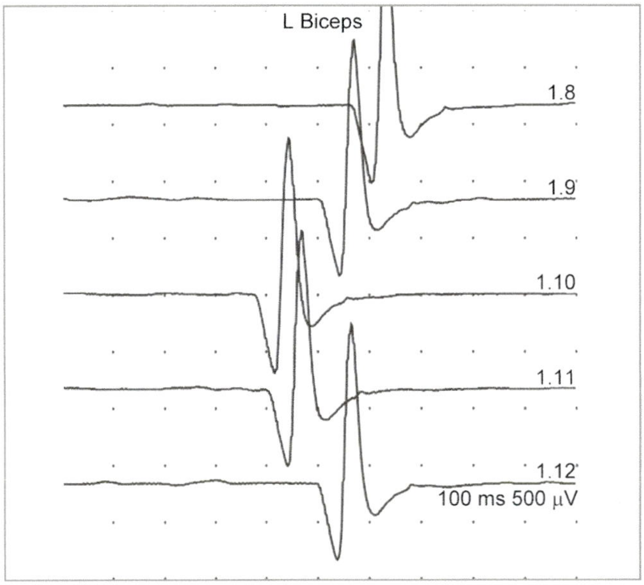

Fig. 9: Large wide triphasic units.

Late Responses F Waves

These are waves that occur after the direct motor response and were first described by McDougal and Magladery in 1950. They were first evoked from the small muscles of the foot, hence the name. They arise from the motor neurons, which fire impulses when activated by an antidromic volley from the nerve being examined; hence, they represent proximal conduction in motor fibers, which are not accessible to direct stimulation, when distal conduction is normal. However, they are not sensitive for demonstrating root lesions, as the segment being examined (roots) is very short and the abnormality gets diluted with the normal distal segment. Also, all the fibers may not be affected and even few preserved fast-conducting fibers would give normal F-wave latencies.[15] They do not assess the sensory pathway at all. The F-waves are more sensitive to abnormalities in the peripheral nerve and are useful for the diagnosis of demyelinating motor peripheral neuropathies.[16]

H Reflex Study

H reflex, also called Hoffman reflex, is the electrically elicited ankle jerk in the lower limbs and is abnormal in S1 radicular lesions and in length-dependent peripheral neuropathies. Unilateral absence and delay of the reflex elicited from the rested gastrocnemius: Soleus group of muscles, stimulating the tibial nerve at the knee, is an important finding to localize the root lesion to the sensory S1 fibers in the absence of motor involvement. The use of nomograms increases the diagnostic yield.[17] In the upper limbs, the flexor carpi radialis H reflex is useful to localize the lesion to the sensory C6 or C7 root when needle EMG is normal.[18]

Somatosensory-evoked Potential Study

This is a study to assess the conduction along the posterior columns of the spinal cord and is indicated when a cord compression is suspected. It is not useful for detecting root lesions. Electrical stimulus is given to mixed nerves distally, and the responses are picked up from the lumbar spine and the cortex in lower limbs and from the neck, cervical spine, and opposite cortex in the upper limbs.[15] Dermatomal SSEPs were used initially, where instead of stimulating a cutaneous or mixed nerve as in routine SSEPs, a dermatome was stimulated and the evoked response was recorded from the opposite cortex.[19] However, their usefulness over the routine tests has not been established and they are no longer used for the diagnosis of radiculopathies.[20]

Neural Deficits Associated with Back or Neck Pain

- *Acute nerve root compression due to an acutely prolapsed disk:* This causes initially a conduction block in the fibers, which are compressed, and later acute axon loss. It presents with back/neck and radicular pain in the limb with or without sensory ± motor loss.
- *Chronic nerve root compression due to degenerative changes:* This reduces the dimensions of the central or lateral canal. This causes slowly progressive chronic axon degeneration. The patient presents with back/neck pain and neurogenic claudication pain in the lower limbs; sensori-motor deficits may be present. In the upper limb, when the central canal is compromised, the presentation would be of a cord compression with upper motor signs in lower limbs, bladder bowel symptoms, posterior column involvement in lower limbs, and radicular involvement in upper limbs.
- *Acute on chronic compression shows a combination of lesions:* Chronic axon loss with conduction block initially and acute axon loss as well. It presents with acute recent-onset pain with sensory-motor deficit and previous history of such attacks or chronic pain.
- *Predominantly sensory or only sensory nerve root compression:* There is involvement of only sensory fibers. It presents with pain with or without sensory loss.
- *Multiple root lesions:* These are commonly seen with central disk lesions and lumbar canal stenosis and are usually bilateral even if symptoms are unilateral.

Electroneuromyography in Root Lesions Correlated with Pathophysiology

- Recent acute involvement is detected by noting fibrillations in proximal muscles of the same myotome.
- Chronic root compression is detected by noting large and wide triphasic or polyphasic units in muscles of the same myotome.
- Acute on chronic radicular lesions are detected by noting fibrillations and small wide polyphasic units in the proximal muscles of the myotome.
- Conduction block is detected by noting a good-amplitude motor response from a clinically weak muscle (on NCS) and fast firing but normal configuration motor unit potentials (MUPs) with a reduced interference pattern on needle EMG examination (NEE).
- When there is a cord compression, the SSEP shows delayed cortical responses.

Electroneuromyography in Peripheral Neuropathy

- Length-dependent sensory-motor axon loss with attenuated/absent SAP/SNAPs and attenuated motor responses in axonal peripheral neuropathies
- Focal conduction blocks, with motor slowing and dispersion in acquired demyelinating peripheral neuropathies, which is not length-dependent
- Abnormal SAP/SNAPs in pure sensory neuropathies
- Normal conductions in small fiber neuropathy.

Limitations of Electroneuromyography

- It identifies the root involved and not the vertebral level.
- Timing of study is important.
- All meaningful postoperative studies require preoperative evaluation.
- It can be normal even with a prolapsed intervertebral disk, which causes no neural compression (falsenegative).
- ENMG findings do not always correlate with the symptoms.
- Severity of "sensory involvement" cannot be assessed.
- Etiology is not determined.
- It does not diagnose abnormalities in small fiber peripheral neuropathies.

It can be false-positive, if:

- The examiner is not experienced
- Diagnosis criteria are not followed
- Inadequate study without clinical correlation
- Biased examiner.

Electroneuromyography in Postoperative Care

- Postoperative evaluation has value if a preoperative study has been done.
- EMG cannot answer the question, "whether adequate decompression has been achieved"?

Electroneuromyography versus Imaging

Over the years, MRI localization has reduced the importance of ENMG; however, it is the ONLY test for the function of the nervous tissue and is abnormal in noncompressive lesions, where an MRI without contrast would be normal. It detects additional lesions, which may be contributing to the symptoms. Since ENMG tests the functional integrity and MRI the anatomical lesion, both tests must be done as they complement each other.[21]

What Should Your Patient Expect?

- *NCS:*
  - NCS are done with surface electrodes.
  - The shocks given are in milliamperes and are quite bearable.
  - The stimulus is local and does not travel all over the body.
  - NCS are ALWAYS required.
  - NCS can be done very safely even in the newborn.
  - The motor conduction stimulus feels like a tap and moves the muscle.
  - The NCS may be contraindicated in patients with pacemakers.
- *EMG:*
  - The needle EMG examination is done using fine disposable electrodes, which are solid pins but thin and very sharp.
  - No shocks are given.
  - The needle is inserted just into the muscle for few seconds.
  - The patient is asked to contract the muscle and the activity is picked up by the electrode and displayed on the monitor and through a loudspeaker, audiovisual diagnosis is made online.
  - The number of muscles examined depends upon the working diagnosis.
  - Needle EMG should be avoided in patients with bleeding disorders, on anticoagulants, and in local infection.

How Can the Referring Doctor Help?

- The working diagnosis or differential diagnosis should be stated in the referral note.
- Relevant reports and supportive radiography should be sent with the patient.
- If the patient is hepatitis B surface antigen or human immunodeficiency virus-positive, has a pacemaker, or is on anticoagulants, the electromyographer must be alerted.
- Remember the limitations of the test before asking for it.

In conclusion, ENMG is a useful test in the management of pain related to peripheral nerves or roots.

CONCLUSION

Electroneuromyography in root lesions would show active or chronic motor axon degeneration in a myotomal distribution with/without proximal muscle involvement and normal relevant SNAPs with clinical evidence of sensory involvement.

The findings depend on the exact root involved, whether compression involves motor/sensory fibers, percentage of fibers compressed, type of pathophysiology, duration of lesion, completeness of study, and skill of the examiner.

REFERENCES

1. Katirji B. The clinical electromyography examination. An overview. Neurol Clin. 2002;20:291-303.
2. Aminoff MJ. Clinical electromyography. In: Aminoff MJ (Ed). Aminoff's Electrodiagnosis in Clinical Neurology, 6th edition. Philadelphia: Elsevier Saunders; 2012. p. 233.
3. Wilbourn AJ, Aminoff MJ. Radiculopathies. In: Brown WF, Bolton CF (Eds). Clinical Electromyography, 2nd edition. Boston, USA: Butterworth-Heinemann; 1993. pp. 177-209.
4. Wilbourn AJ, Aminoff MJ. AAEE minimonograph #32: the electrophysiologic examination in patients with radiculopathies. Muscle Nerve. 1988;11(11):1099-114.
5. Levin KH. Electrodiagnostic approach to the patient with suspected radiculopathy. Neurol Clin. 2002;20(2):397-421.
6. Claremont AC. Evaluation of the patient with possible radiculopathy. In: Johnson EW, Pease WS (Eds). Practical Electromyography, 3rd edition. Baltimore, USA: Williams and Wilkins; 1997. pp. 115-30.
7. Lower cervical nerve roots and spinal nerves. In: Stewart JD (Ed). Focal Peripheral Neuropathies, 3rd edition. Philadelphia, PA, USA: Lippincott Williams and Wilkins; 2000. pp. 97-116.
8. Aminoff MJ. Cauda equina: lumbar and sacral nerve roots and spinal nerves. In: Stewart JD (Ed). Focal Peripheral Neuropathies, 3rd edition. Philadelphia, PA, USA: Lippincott Williams and Wilkins; 2000. pp. 315-54.
9. Levin KH. Neurological manifestations of compressive radiculopathy of the first thoracic root. Neurology. 1999;53(5):1149-51.
10. Wiltse LL, Guyer RD, Spencer CW, Glenn WV, Porter IS. Alar transverse process impingement of the L5 spinal nerve: the far-out syndrome. Spine (Phila Pa 1976). 1984;9(1):31-41.
11. Levin KH. L5 radiculopathy with reduced superficial peroneal sensory responses: intraspinal and extraspinal causes. Muscle Nerve. 1998;21(1):3-7.
12. Berger AR, Sharma K, Lipton RB. Comparison of motor conduction abnormalities in lumbosacral radiculopathy and axonal polyneuropathy. Muscle Nerve. 1999;22(8):1053-7.
13. Singleton JR. Evaluation and treatment of painful peripheral polyneuropathy. Semin Neurol. 2005;25(2):185-95.
14. Levin KH, Maggiano HJ, Wilbourn AJ. Cervical radiculopathies: comparison of surgical and EMG localization of single-root lesions. Neurology. 1996;46(4):1022-5.
15. Aminoff MJ, Goodin DS, Parry GJ, Barbaro NM, Weinstein PR, Rosenblum ML. Electrophysiologic evaluation of lumbosacral radiculopathies: electromyography, late responses, and somatosensory evoked potentials. Neurology. 1985;35(10):1514-8.
16. Toyokura M, Murakami K. F-wave study in patients with lumbosacral radiculopathies. Electromyogr Clin Neurophysiol. 1997;37(1):19-26.
17. Braddom RI, Johnson EW. Standardization of H reflex and diagnostic use in S1 radiculopathy. Arch Phys Med Rehabil. 1974;55(4):161-6.
18. Schimsheimer RJ, de Visser BW, Kemp B. The flexor carpi radialis H-reflex in lesions of the sixth and seventh cervical nerve roots. J Neurol Neurosurg Psychiatry. 1985;48(5):445-9.
19. Aminoff MJ, Goodin DS, Barbaro NM, Weinstein PR, Rosenblum ML. Dermatomal somatosensory evoked potentials in unilateral lumbosacral radiculopathy. Ann Neurol. 1985;17(2):171-6.
20. Dubinsky RM, Miyasaki J. Assessment: efficacy of transcutaneous electric nerve stimulation in the treatment of pain in neurologic disorders (an evidence-based review): report of the Therapeutics and Technology Assessment Subcommittee of the American Academy of Neurology. Neurology. 2010;74(2):173-6.
21. Nardin RA, Patel MR, Gudas TF, Rutkove SB, Raynor EM. Electromyography and magnetic resonance imaging in the evaluation of radiculopathy. Muscle Nerve. 1999;22(2):151-5.

5

CHAPTER

Pharmacotherapy of Drugs Used in Interventional Pain Treatment Procedures

Raghbir Singh P Gehdoo

ABSTRACT

Interventional pain treatment procedures are mainstay in a multimodal approach for relief of chronic pain. However, one has to be very choosy in selecting the type of neurolytic procedure and must take patient and relatives in full confidence before performing. As liquid takes the route of spread by its viscosity and baricity, it may lead to untoward side effects and complications, which, at times, are difficult to explain.

INTRODUCTION

The neurolytic agents to destroy nerves and interrupt pain pathways are extensively used, while interventional pain treatment procedures to achieve "permanent" or long-term analgesia in patients with advanced chronic pain are being used for the last few decades. These techniques have effect, which is usually seen for only 3–6 months. Schloesser, in 1903,[1] used alcohol for the first time for trigeminal neuralgia. Swetlow,[2] in 1926, used neurolytic sympathetic block for providing the anginal and abdominal pain relief, and Dogliotti,[3] in 1933, reported intrathecal alcohol neurolysis for the intractable pain relief. The advances in spinal analgesia and increased life expectancy have decreased the use of neurolysis in malignancy.

Arnott,[4] in 1951, reported the application of cold in relieving cancer pain. In 1939, Smith and Fay[5] reported finding regression of tumor following localized freezing. But still, neurolysis remains to be a useful and effective option for pain control in cancer patients. Neurolysis is indicated in patients with severe intractable pain, in whom less aggressive maneuvers are ineffective or intolerable, because of either poor physical condition or the development of side effects.

The type of chemical agents used for neurolysis are alcohol, phenol, glycerol, chlorocresol, ammonium salts, and hypertonic saline. For neurodestruction cryoablation and radiofrequency (RF) lesioning is promising and efffective opitons in present clinical pain practice.

MECHANISM OF ACTION

Neurolytic agents such as alcohol or phenol act immediately after coming into contact with the nerve fiber and there is a rise in the endoneurial fluid pressure, secondary to the mast cell degranulation and release of vasoactive substances. This elevated pressure causes stretching of the perineurium and compression of the perineurial vessels, which leads to ischemia of nerve fiber and interruption of nerve impulses. The adequate amount of Wallerian degeneration should be accompanied to get good results.

TYPES OF NEURODESTRUCTIVE TECHNIQUES AND NEUROLYTIC AGENTS

Types of neurodestructive techniques and neurolytic agents are as follows:

- Chemical neurolysis; chemical neurolytic agents—alcohol, phenol, glycerol, ammonium salts, and hypertonic saline
- Cryoablation
- RF lesioning.

Chemical Neurolysis

Commonly Used Neurolytic Agents

The neurolytic agents commonly used for chemical neurolysis include ethyl alcohol, phenol, chlorocresol, ammonium salts, hypertonic saline, etc.

- *Ethyl alcohol:* It is a clear, colorless solution, stable at room temperature, hypobaric to cerebrospinal fluid (CSF), and absorbs water on exposure to air. It spreads quite rapidly from the injection site and it takes 12–24 hours to assess the effect. About 90–98% of injected alcohol is rapidly metabolized by oxidation in the liver principally, by the enzyme alcohol dehydrogenase. 50–100% of alcohol is used for neurolysis in clinical practice, as minimum concentration required for neurolysis has not been established. Labat,[6] in 1933, reported use of 33.3% alcohol for adequate pain relief in the treatment of painful disorders.

  Its mechanism of nerve destruction is similar to that of phenol. It extracts cholesterol, phospholipids, and cerebrosides from the nervous tissue and causes precipitation of lipoproteins and mucoproteins.[7] It initiates Wallerian degeneration and neurolysis as intrathecal alcohol produces similar changes in the nerve rootlets. There can be a minimal focal inflammation of meninges and patchy areas of demyelination in the dorsal column, Lissauer's tract, and dorsal root.[8] The ganglion cells get destroyed, when alcohol encounters sympathetic chain.[9-11] This blocks all postganglionic fibers to all effector organs.

  The patient complains of severe burning pain along the nerve's distribution following injection, which may last for few minutes and is subsequently replaced by a warm and numb sensation. The common practice is to add a local anesthetic agent prior and following the alcohol, which will reduce these symptoms. The alcohol is indicated for neurolysis of cranial nerves, intrathecal injection, sympathetic chain, and chemical hypophysectomy. The volume and concentration advised during fluoroscopy is a dose of 20–25 mL of 50% alcohol on either side, while during computed tomography guidance, 10 mL on either side in upper abdominal malignancies and 0.25–2 mL of absolute (97%) alcohol are advised for cranial and sympathetic nerves or ganglions.
- *Phenol:* This is a chemical composite containing carbolic acid, phenic acid, phenylic acid, phenyl hydroxide, hydroxybenzene, and oxybenzene. In its pure state, it is colorless, poorly soluble, and the shelf life exceeds 1 year when the solution is refrigerated and not exposed to light. Phenol turns red on exposure to sunlight and air because of oxidation. It is available as a sterile solution and can be prepared as a 6.7% solution in water and is available in concentrations from 4% to 10%. As phenol is hyperbaric, it will settle if injected into a liquid medium, such as the CSF-containing subarachnoid space. It is highly soluble in organic solvents, such as alcohol and glycerine. The addition of small amounts of glycerol or water-soluble radiopaque contrast material may increase the concentration to 15%. The solution can be diluted with saline and is compatible when mixed with radiocontrast dyes. The glycerin-mixed phenol is a thick solution and needs to be injected through a needle not <20 GHz. When mixed with glycerin, it slowly diffuses from the solution. This property of phenol can be taken into advantages, when injected intrathecally, because it allows for limited spread and is localized in the area that needs to be destroyed. When mixed with water, it has a wider spread, causing a bigger area of nerve destruction. Aqueous solution of phenol is more potent than the glycerin solution. The choice of diluents depends upon the extent of neurolysis desired. The use of higher concentrations of phenol might predispose to a higher incidence of vascular injury. It is metabolized in the liver by conjugation to glucuronides and oxidation to quinol compounds or to carbon dioxide and water. Excretion of metabolites is via kidneys. Phenol causes nonselective neurolysis by denaturing proteins of axons and perineural blood vessels.[12] The action is loss of cellular fatty elements, separation of the myelin sheath from the axon, and axonal edema.[13] The degeneration after contact with solution takes about 14 days and regeneration is completed in about 14 weeks.

  However, phenol is not as effective as alcohol at destroying the nerve cell body and its blocking effect tends to be less profound and of shorter duration than alcohol. At a concentration of 2–3% in saline, phenol seems to spare motor function. The efficacy of 3% phenol in saline is comparable to that of 40% alcohol. It acts as a local anesthetic in lower concentrations and as a neurolytic in higher concentrations. The effects of the block cannot be evaluated until after 24–48 hours, to allow time for the local anesthetic effect to dissipate. The neurolytic effect may be clinically evident only after 3–7 days. If inadequate pain relief is obtained after 2 weeks, this may indicate incomplete neurolysis and require repetition of the procedure. The subsequent fibrosis that occurs following phenol injection makes nerve regeneration more difficult but not impossible. Nerve regeneration can occur as long as the nerve cell body is intact, at a rate of 1–3 mm/day. Nerve arborization and neuroma formation can occur at the site of nerve disruption and can be a focus of a neuropathic type of pain. Phenol can be injected intrathecally and epidurally. Phenol in glycerin is hyperbaric compared to the CSF. It can also be used for paravertebral somatic block, peripheral nerve blocks, epidural blocks, peripheral nerve roots, intrathecal and cranial nerves, and sympathetic blocks. Phenol has systemic side effects, including central nervous system (CNS) stimulation, cardiovascular depression, nausea, and vomiting. Systemic doses of >5 g can cause convulsive seizures and CNS depression. Doses <100 mg are less likely to cause serious side effects.

- *Glycerol:* It is a mild neurolytic agent used preferably for the gasserian ganglion block, as it was found to preserve the facial sensations in most of the cases. It is usually used as 100% solution in 0.5–2 mL dose and due to a poor control of spread in the area close to the subarachnoid space, it is not used in the intrathecal injection. The mechanism of action is not completely understood. However, it appears to affect primarily damaged myelinated axons. Injection in the vicinity of the nerve causes perineural damage, while intraneural injection results in Schwann cell edema, axonolysis, and Wallerian degeneration. Intraneural injection destroys all the fibers.
- *Ammonium salts:* These are used for long-term pain relief. They are usually available in a concentration of 10%. At this concentration, a neuronal degeneration, including C-fibers neurolysis, appears with a success of 40%. Interestingly, it has been found that a 10% solution provides adequate analgesia without a significant motor block. These salts produce an acute degenerative neuropathy with obliteration of C-fibers and with a very small effect on A-fibers. However, the degeneration is nonselective and may affect all types of fibers. Complications due to ammonium salt injection are transient and include nausea and headache. Paresthesia and burning sensation may occur in 30% of patients at a dose of 500 mg of ammonium salts, lasting 2–14 days.
- *Hypertonic saline or normal saline:* Hitchcock,[14] in 1967, first reported the use of hypertonic saline by intrathecal injection to treat intractable pain. It is 10% aqueous solution and is used intrathecally as 40–60 mL of normal saline injection, after withdrawing an equal amount of CSF (a very distressing procedure). Its mechanism of action is not well elaborated. However, normal saline is thought to act specifically on C-fibers, sparing larger fibers of sensory, motor, and autonomic functions. The cold hypertonic saline produces C-fiber neurolysis with a success of 30%. It causes severe pain on injection, and local anesthetic is first injected before the saline solution. When injected intrathecally, it seems to produce its action by an intrathecal shift of water with extracellular change in osmolarity. Intrathecal injection of hypertonic saline can cause an increase in intracranial pressure, blood pressure, heart rate, and respiratory rate.

The duration of the pain relief is normally short-lived, may be from 10 to 25 days. The complications seen during and after saline include tachycardia, premature ventricular contractions and myocardial infarction, and localized paresis for many hours; paresthesia may last for many weeks, hemiplegia, pulmonary edema, pain in the ear, vestibular disturbances, and loss of sphincter control with sacral anesthesia.

Indications for Chemical Neurolysis

Chemical neurolysis is indicated in the following:
- Chronic, intractable, and nonterminal pain, not responsive to other modalities
- Pain patients who have short life expectancy (less than a year)
- Spasticity patients to improve balance, gait, self-care, and overall rehabilitation.

Complications of Chemical Neurolysis

Complications of chemical neurolysis include the following:
- *Skin and other tissues:* Necrosis and sloughing of the skin and other nontarget tissues, mainly due to damage of the vascular supply, and subsequent chronic trauma to denervated tissue.
- *Neuritis:* The incidence of neuritis is up to 10% and is caused by partial destruction of somatic nerve

and subsequent regeneration. At times, clinically manifested hyperesthesia and dysesthesia are worse than the original pain problem and are limiting factors in the use of chemical neurolysis.

- *Anesthesia dolorosa:* It is a poorly understood condition, whereby the patient complains of distressing numbness caused by an imbalance in afferent input. It is caused by long-term loss of afferent input and the resultant CNS changes. The treatment is a combination of tricyclic antidepressants, major antipsychotic tranquilizers, and anticonvulsants.
- *Prolonged motor paralysis:* This can be a major complication that occurs infrequently and is usually temporary.
- *Perineal and sexual dysfunction:* This is another fear-some complication that can occur temporarily. About 1.4% and 0.2% of patients will have bowel or bladder dysfunction at 1 week and 1 month, respectively.
- *Systemic complications:* These include hypotension secondary to sympathetic block; systemic toxic reactions; heart rate, rhythm disturbances, and blood pressure changes; and CNS excitation and depression.

Cryoablation/Cryoanalgesia

Cryoablation/cryoanalgesia is defined as pain relief due to the destruction of nerves, following exposure to extreme cold. Smith and Fay,[15] in 1939, reported a tumor regression following localized freezing. Lloyd and coworkers,[16] in 1976, used this method for pain relief and coined the term "cryoanalgesia". The absence of neuritis or neuroma formation, and prolonged analgesia with reversible effect unlike chemical neurolysis are main advantages[17] and to a certain extent RF lesioning.[18,19] It has no systemic side effects and produces minimal tissue damage. It can be performed as an outpatient procedure. The pain relief might last from 2 weeks to 5 months.

Cryoablation/cryoanalgesia involves inducing profound hypothermia over nerve fiber (at the contact point). A prolongation of action potential is seen, when nerve is cooled to 5°C. Unmyelinated fibers require a lower temperature. Cryolesioning is done by freezing of a small nerve segment with a 2-mm probe cooled at -60°C by rapid expansion of pressurized nitrous oxide from its tip. The probe is left in contact with the nervous tissue for 60–90 seconds and then allowed to thaw for another 45–60 seconds before being removed. An ice ball of 2–4 mm diameter is formed that freezes the nerve and completely damages the nerve fiber. The endoneurial fluid pressure is elevated up to 20 mm Hg within 90 minutes. It reduces over next 24 hours and then increases again, to reach a plateau after 6 days secondary to changes of Wallerian degeneration. It has a special N_2O delivery system that allows safe delivery of the gas up to 850 psi to the gas expansion orifice in the tip of the cryoprobe (14, 16, and 18G). Generally, the gas is delivered at an operating pressure of 600 psi. The minimum temperature at the tip of the probe can rapidly reach–60°C. The commonly encountered complications are frostbite and depigmentation of skin, sensory and motor damage, and damage to the adjacent structures due to movements or malpositioning of the probe.

It is particularly useful in the management of chronic pain syndromes such as neuralgias (facial, intercostal, post-therapeutic, post-traumatic), myofascial trigger point pain, postsurgical pain, cancer pain and neuroma, phantom limb pain, cervicogenic headache, and cervicalgia, thoracic, lumbar, and coccygeal pain. It is done as an outpatient procedure, is readily acceptable to patients, has minimal complications, and is an effective alternative to pharmacologic painkillers.

Radiofrequency Lesioning

Radiofrequency lesioning is the application of electric current to promote the thermocoagulation, leading ultimately to the nerve destruction. It is used to ablate pain pathways in the trigeminal ganglion, spinal cord, dorsal root entry zone, dorsal root ganglion, sympathetic chain, facet joints, failed back pain syndrome, and peripheral nerves.[20-24] Fluoroscopic guidance is required for proper needle placement. The patient should also be informed of the risks and benefits of the procedure and a written informed consent must be signed in front of a witness.

Mechanism of Action

Frictional heat is generated by molecular movement in a field of alternating electric current at RF. An electromagnetic field is created around an active electrode, when the frequency is set above 250 kHz. The active electrode is placed at the site for lesioning, and an indifferent electrode is placed to minimize passage of current through the myocardium. Heat is generated in the tissues, which conducts to the active electrode as current flows through a probe with a built-in thermocouple needle. The heat is not emitted from the probe itself but from the current movement that generates the heat as it passes through the tissues. The lesion is formed once the neural temperature exceeds 45°C, but temperature above 90°C can cause boiling and tissue tearing with electrode removal. The temperature is monitored and watt is adjusted to the desired level, which in turn determines the size of the lesion. Lesion plateaus with time. After 60 seconds at a certain temperature, lesion growth is minimal. The lesion is spheroidal and may extend several millimeters beyond the active electrode tip, but the majority of the lesion volume surrounds the axis of the active electrode. Pain is first replicated using higher frequencies and lower voltages prior to lesioning and the target tissue is localized; it is then only that thermocoagulation is instituted.

Technique Proper

Once the needle or cannula position is perfectly placed at the desired site and level, the RF electrode is introduced via the cannula. With older systems, the electrode itself needed to be touching the bone, but with newer systems, utilizing a cannula sheathed with plastic or Teflon with an exposed metal tip of varying lengths, the electrode need not actually touch the bone, although the exposed tip must. Stimulation is then carried out, using a frequency of 50 Hz and a current up to 1 mA for sensory detection and a frequency of 2 Hz with current between 3 and 5 mA for motor stimulation. A positive stimulation is that which reproduces the patient's pain, without producing other sensory or motor findings in the lower extremity or buttocks. Negative stimulation may be failure to produce the patient's pain or obvious stimulation of motor and sensory structures arising from the spinal nerve. In such cases, denervation should not be performed, and the cannula should be repositioned, followed by repeat stimulation. Once the stimulation pattern is acceptable, an RF lesion is created by passing current through the electrode to raise the tissue temperature to 60–80°C for 60–90 seconds. This portion of the procedure may be quite uncomfortable and judicious use of sedation and analgesics may be appropriate. Once the lesion is completed, the next level(s) can be treated in a similar fashion.

Complications

The usual complications encountered are as follows:

- Neuritis/neuralgia (incidence 10%). Pain may be worse than the original pain.
- Numbness and motor paralysis
- Pneumothorax and Horner syndrome
- Incomplete pain relief.

CONCLUSION

Chemical neurolysis or destruction of nerves by chemical neurolytic agents plays a vital role in providing relief in the chronic intractable pain patients. The newer techniques such as RF lesioning and cryoprobe have taken a front seat in the patient care recently and these are getting further improvised to produce effective prolonged analgesia for chronic pain syndromes. As a word of caution, these techniques require specialized training, in-depth knowledge of neural anatomy, and understanding of chronic pain physiology. So, their application should be limited only in painful conditions, where conventional conservative pain management fails.

REFERENCES

1. Scholoesse. Heilung peripharer reizzustande sensibler and motorischer nerven klin Monatsbl Augenhilkd. 1903; 41:244.
2. Swetlow GI. Paravertebral alcohol block in cardiac pain. Am Heart J. 1926;1:393.
3. Dogliotti AM. A new method of block anesthesia: segmental peridural spinal anesthesia. Am J Surg. 1933;20:107-18.
4. Arnott J. On the Treatment of Cancer by the Regulated Application of an Anesthetic Temperature. London: Churchill; 1851.
5. Smith LW, Fay T. Temperature factors in cancer and embryonal cell growth. JAMA. 1939;113:653-60.
6. Labat G. Effect of alcohol on the living nerve. Curr Res Anesth Analg. 1933;12:190.
7. Myers RR, Powell HC. Galactose neuropathy: impact of chronic endoneurial edema on nerve blood flow. Ann Neurol. 1984;16(5):587-94.
8. Gallager HS, Yonezawa T, Hay RC, Derrick WS. Subarachnoid alcohol block. II. Histological changes in the central nervous system. Am J Pathol. 1961;38:679-93.
9. May O. The functional and histological effects of intraneural and intraganglionic injections of alcohol. Br Med J. 1912;2:465-70.
10. Rumbsy MG, Finean JB. The action of organic solvents on the myelin sheath of peripheral nerve tissue. II. Short-chain aliphatic alcohols. J Neurochem. 1966;13:1509-11.
11. Myers RR, Katz J. Neural pathology of neurolytic and semidestructive agents. In: Cousins MJ, Bridenbaugh PO (Eds). Neural Blockade in Clinical Anesthesia and Management of Pain, 2nd edition. Philadelphia: JB Lippincott; 1988. pp. 1031-51.
12. Felsenthal G. Pharmacology of phenol in peripheral nerve blocks: a review. Arch Phys Med Rehabil. 1974;55:13-6.

13. Smith MC. Histological findings following intrathecal injections of phenol solutions for relief of pain. Br J Anaesth. 1964;36:387-406.
14. Hitchcock E, Prandini MN. Hypertonic saline in management of intractable pain. Lancet. 1973;1(7798):310-2.
15. Smith LW, Fay T. Temperature factors in cancer and embryonal cell growth. JAMA.1939;113:653-60.
16. Lloyd JW, Barnard JD, Glynn CJ. Cryoanalgesia. A new approach to pain relief. Lancet. 1976;2:932-4.
17. Swerdlow M. Intrathecal neurolysis. Anaesthesia. 1978;33:733-40.
18. Paintal AS. Block of conduction in mammalian myelinated nerve fibers by low temperatures. J Physiol. 1965; 180:1-19.
19. Myers RR, Powell HC, Heckman HM, Costello ML, Katz J. Biophysical and pathologic effects of cryogenic nerve lesion. Ann neurol. 1981;10(5):478-85.
20. Koning HM, Mackie DP. Percutaneous radiofrequency facet denervation in low back pain. Pain Clinic. 1994;7(3):199-204.
21. Sluijter ME. The use of radiofrequency lesions for pain relief in failed back patients. Int Disabil Stud. 1988;10(1):37-43.
22. Wilkinson HA. Stereotactic radiofrequency sympathectomy. Pain Clinic. 1995;8(1):107-15.
23. Shealy CN. Percutaneous radiofrequency denervation of spinal facets. Treatment for chronic back pain and sciatica. J Neurosurg. 1975;43:448-51.
24. Shealy CN. Facet denervation in the management of back and sciatic pain. Clin Orthop Relat Res. 1976;115:157-64.

6 CHAPTER

Radiofrequency Lesioning in Pain Management: Principles and Clinical Applications

Kailash Kothari

ABSTRACT

In comparison to available neurodestructive modalities, radiofrequency (RF) lesioning (RFL) has come long way. It has proved to be a useful tool, with refined techniques and advanced probes, and provides long-term pain relief in a variety of chronic pain conditions. This chapter will discuss principles and mechanisms of RF along with various applications of RF in treating pain.

INTRODUCTION

Radiofrequency lesioning is one of the very popular and well-established techniques to treat many painful conditions. With pain management becoming popular, use of RF has increased. RFL is a very precise and safe method to be used in ablating nerves in many painful conditions, e.g., trigeminal neuralgia, facet joint pain, and sympathetic pain.

Surgical techniques are usually more involved and serve as a last resort. Surgical transection of peripheral nerves may cause neuroma formation and deafferentation pain. After surgical lesioning of sympathetic nerves, symptoms may recur and surgical re-exploration may be difficult or impossible. Such considerations lead to a search for nonsurgical nerve destruction techniques.

OBJECTIVE

The objective is to deposit enough RF heating power into the tissue to raise the temperature of the targeted tissue above 45–50°C. This is referred to as the "lethal temperature range" as cell structures exposed to these temperatures for 20 seconds or more are known to be destroyed by the heat.

Three methods of nerve destruction are generally accepted:

1. Injection of neurolytic substances, such as absolute alcohol, phenol, or glycerin, is done under X-ray and is suitable for the destruction of larger units such as celiac plexus. The size of the lesion is difficult to predict, and the spread of neurolytic substance may cause unwanted side effects that will also be permanent.
2. Cryoanalgesia (freezing of a peripheral nerve) is more accurate but has the disadvantage of being short term, usually 3–6 months.
3. RFL is a more refined technique based on the thermocoagulation of selected nerves using an electrode, capable of accurate temperature generation.

The available RF generators have similar functions:

- Precise power control
- Impedance monitoring
- Ability to electrically stimulate
- Temperature monitoring.

PHYSICS

Radiofrequency neurotomy achieves its effect by alternating a high-frequency electrical current between a large surface area on ground plate and a small area on the surface of the uninsulated tip of the electrode. When the current approaches the electrode tip, its electric field becomes more dense and, therefore, stronger and as the current alternates, it causes charged molecules, notably proteins, to oscillate. Where the current is strong enough, this oscillation heats the tissues sufficiently to coagulate them. This occurs near the tip of the electrode, where the

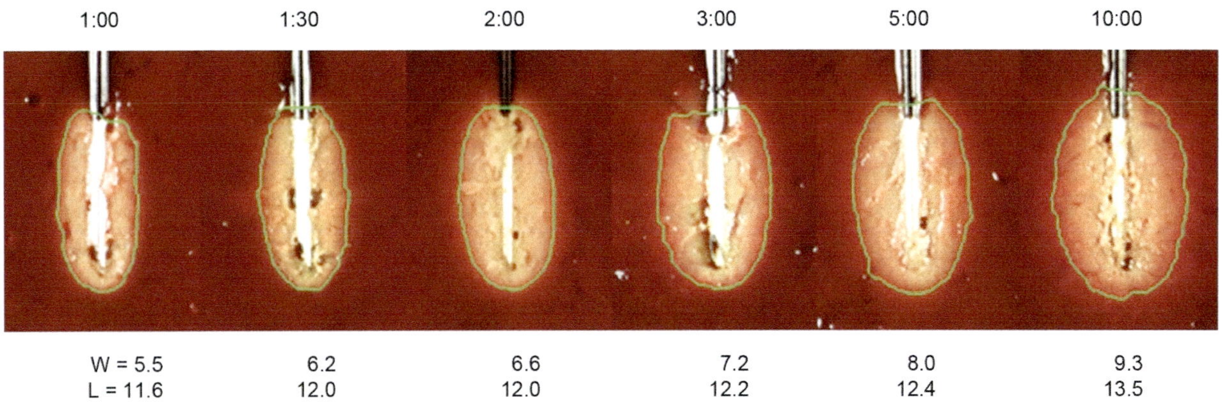

Fig. 1: Different types of tips of needles. (W: width of lesioning; L: length of lesioning)

electric field is most dense. The volume of coagulated tissue assumes the shape of a prolate spheroid, whose a long axis is formed by the uninsulated tip of the electrode.

- RF machine generates RF current.
- Utilizes a Teflon-coated needle with an uninsulated distal tip (2–15 mm): Normal and curved tip **(Fig. 1)**
- RF is applied through an electrode inserted in this needle.
- Need >45°C to destroy nerves
- Two events around the tip are important:
    - Formation of heat
    - Exposure of target tissue (nerve) to the electric field.

TYPES OF RADIOFREQUENCY LESIONING

Continuous Radiofrequency Lesioning

- RF is a high-frequency current, produced by an RF generator that passes from the electrode to the grounding pad through the body tissues to complete the circuit.
- The difference between the electrode and the receptive electrode is the voltage.[1,2]
- The electromagnetic field around the tip of the electrode causes the tissues to heat up and a lesion is formed, if the temperature within the neuronal tissues exceeds 40°C.[3]
- The electrode absorbs this heat and equilibrium is reached between 30 and 60 seconds; the temperature monitored is that of the electrode that has the highest temperature.
- The lesion size correlates with the electrode size, temperature generated, duration of RF application, local tissue characteristics, and configuration. The lesion is oval-shaped parallel to the needle that usually does not exceed the tip of the needle, so ideally the needle should be parallel to the targeted nerve a 15° curve may allow better targeting.[4]
- Tissue characteristics, such as the fluid content, specifically blood supply or cerebrospinal fluid, which acts as a heat sink, can affect the lesion size.
- Following the lesion, the tissues demonstrate scar formation; first coagulation, followed by acute inflammatory reaction, necrosis, and collagen deposition.
- The process takes 3 weeks.
- The basal lamina is often preserved allowing nerve regeneration. It was widely published that RFA is selective to C and Aδ fibers; however, this is debatable and was revoked in multiple histological studies.[5]
- It has been suggested that the electric field, rather than temperature, has neuromodulatory effects on pain-processing mechanisms at the dorsal root ganglion (DRG), dorsal horn, and molecular levels by changing gene expression in pain-processing neurons.[6,7]

Pulsed Radiofrequency Lesioning

A more recent RF method for the treatment of pain applies short pulses of RF signals from an RF generator to the neural tissue through the RF electrode[8] and is called "pulsed RFL (PRFL)":

- Commercially available RF lesion generators provide PRFL signals with pulse durations ranging from 10 to 30 ms and pulse repetition rates ranging from 1 to 8 Hz (pulses per second).
- The underlying RF frequency within each pulse is typically about 500 kHz, which is the same as for

continuous radiofrequency lesioning (CRFL). The heat generated is minimal and minimally destructive.

- The heat generated is dissipated between pulses. Because the RF pulse duration is only a small percentage of the time between pulses in PRFL, the average tissue temperature rise for the same RF voltage on the same electrode is less for PRFL than for CRFL. For the same reason, higher RF voltages can be applied to the electrode in PRFL than are commonly used in CRFL without raising the average tissue temperature near the electrode into the "lethal temperature range", i.e., at or above 45–50°C. This has been the approach used by most clinicians performing PRFL.[8]
- PRFL produces a transient inhibition of evoked synaptic activity and classic thermal RF (TRF) produces a lasting inhibition.
- Both CRFL and PRFL treatments induce distance-dependent tissue destruction under the stimulating needle, but the effect is more pronounced with CRFL.
- These findings suggest that the acute effects of PRFL are more reversible and less neurodestructive in nature than the CRFL mode, even in normothermia conditions. Proposed pulsing is 20 ms, temperature should be <42°C, and voltage <60 kHz.[9]
- It has led to PRFL being loosely described by some as a "nonthermal lesion" or as a "nondestructive" process. The implied assumption is that heat is not causing any clinical effect or any destructive effect in PRFL; rather, there are some other nondestructive agents that account for all effects seen from PRFL.
- Underlying physics are the same for both CRFL and PRFL.
- There are following variables which can be measured during lesioning: Tip temperatures, time dependencies, and impedances.

Pulsed Radiofrequency Waveform

- The RF signal on an electrode produces two types of basic fields in the tissue: Electrical fields and magnetic fields.
- It is the electric field (E) that is the origin of all effects we see in RFL, in both CRFL and PRFL:
    - *Continuous radiofrequency lesioning:* The E-field produces forces on ions and other charged structures. This produces movement of ions in electrolytes, current densities, and stresses on cellular substructures and membranes. Currents J, in turn, produce ionic friction and heat, and this then produces the increase in temperature seen in CRFL and PRFL. All of these mechanisms, not just temperature rise, have the potential of producing modifications of neural structures and neuronal behavior when the E-field becomes high enough. All of these mechanisms might be relevant in understanding how RFL produces its effects in pain relief therapy. Brodkey et al.[10] have shown that "reversible heat lesions" occur between temperatures 42.5 and 44°C in which range temporary cessation of neural activity occurs in brain tissue. Dieckmann et al.[11] have studied experimentally the morphology of heat lesions in the living brain of animals. They observed progressive layers of charring, coagulative necrosis, liquefaction necrosis, demyelinization, etc., as *T* decreases as a function of distance from the innermost lesion core to an outermost margin, which is probably near the 45–50°C margin.
    - *Pulsed radiofrequency lesioning (PRFL):* PRFL and CRFL originate from the same underlying physical laws, but differ in space, time, and strength of resultant fields. PRFL typically has much stronger E-fields than CRFL, and also as having temperature spikes above the average and can extend to the 45–50°C levels. In a frequently adopted practice of holding the average temperature background at or somewhat below about 42°C, PRFL also differs from CRFL in that the spatial extent of continuously elevated temperatures is much less than the CRFL. The effect on the neurons of a sustained stream of short heat bursts above 45–50°C is unknown. If the effect in PRFL of such a "thermal dose" is significant, then it is likely to be dependent on the heat spike amplitudes, durations, pulse rates, total number of heat spikes, and total exposure time. The mere existence of *T*-spikes with peak temperatures well above the "lethal temperature level" of 45°C does not necessarily mean that they will destroy cell structures in the same way as CRFL heat lesions. However, the existence of hot flashes indicates that temperature effects must be considered as a potentially significant neurolytic agent in PRFL and that PRFL cannot be described as a "nonthermal lesion". The high E-fields encountered in PRFL can have significant effects on neurons because of the transmembrane potentials that they induce.

Physical evidence has also shown that the PRFL is destructive and disruptive to neurons. Cahana et al.[12] performed PRFL on hippocampal cell cultures using an SMK electrode, T_{avg} = 38–42°C, D = 20 ms, N = 2 Hz, V_{peak} typically at 35–45 V, and t = 120 seconds. At distances of 0.5 mm from the electrode tip point, there was complete destruction of all neurons. Erdine et al.[13] performed PRFL on the DRG of rabbits, using the SMK electrode with T_{avg} = 42–43°C, V_{peak} = 45 V (and was adjusted to hold 42–43°C), D = 20 ms, N = 2 Hz, and t = 120 seconds. Neural tissue appeared normal under light microscopic analysis. Under electron microscopic analysis, the DRG cells showed microscopic disruption of cell substructures, less extensive than that for the 67°C CRFL. In both the PRFL case and the 67°C CRFL, there was microscopic destruction of the normal order of the neurons.

- There is indirect clinical evidence of injury to tissue from CRFL and PRFL. In the case of CRFL of the medial branch or the DRG, patients often experience a period of irritative symptoms lasting weeks or months. In the case of PRFL, Sluijter,[14] WE Cohen (private communication) and KE Vogel (private communication) describe that for a significant proportion of patients having a PRFL of the DRG, using typically $V_{peak} \cong 45$ V and $T_{avg} \cong 42$°C, there is a three-phase period of recovery. In phase I, pain relief is often immediate and lasts for a day or so. In phase II, there are irritative symptoms and a waxing and waning of relief lasting up to 4–6 weeks. In phase III, the irritation subsides, and there is pain relief for an extended time, often years. Both the irritation period of CRFL and the irritation (phase II) period of PRFL may be indications of healing of tissue following RF damage to cells. Discomfort from healing of injured tissue often follows a similar pattern, beginning within hours after the insult and lasting for weeks as inflammation, scarring, and neural reactions run their course. The most likely agents of RF neural destruction and injury are heat, high electric fields, and high current fields. It is plausible that the kind of damage to tissue by a CRFL at 55°C, say, and a PRFL heat spike at 55°C are the same. Tissue disruption by high E-fields would be more specific than by heat. The E-field induces charges on tissue and produces forces on charged molecular structures, causing them to distort and dislocate. E-field gradients produce dielectrophoretic forces on charged objects, causing stress, distortion, and movement. All such effects can happen at subcellular and biomolecular levels without substantially elevating temperature. They all could disrupt cell function; for example, any change in ion channel conductances across the neuron membrane would change its function. Ion channels and pumps are known to be delicate composites of charge proteins that control the conduction of Na^+, K^+, Ca^{2+}, Cl^-, and other ions vital to cell function. It is conceivable that violent 500 kHz agitation of structures by large PRFL E-fields could disrupt or modify them. Any temporary or permanent changes in the ion channels would alter Nernst concentration gradients and thus could alter resting and threshold potentials of neurons that mediate pain sensation.
- *Electroporation:* There is evidence that induced transmembrane potentials of U_m = 0.1–1 V cause nonlinear effects on cell membranes capable of deforming, creating pores in, and rupturing the membrane.[15] This process, known as electroporation, has been studied for pulsed, high E-field situations. It is possible that electroporation may occur in PRFL, particularly at the electrode's point and for larger Aδ- and A-motor fibers.
- *PRFL membrane rectification, long-term depression of nociception, and a connection to conditioning stimulation:* The action of PRFL transmembrane potentials U_m at lower E may produce additional effects and may induce synaptic plasticity and long-term depression (LTD) of synaptic transmission. The probable mechanism may be presynaptic depolarization by membrane rectification.[16,17]
- *Magnetic field effects:* Magnetic effects induced by E-field-generated currents at 500 kHz are biologically negligible, and these may not be significant.

VARIABLES FACTORS AFFECTING LESION SIZE (FIG. 2)

- Temperature (measured at tip) typical: 80°C
- Active tip, length (linear relationship) typical: 3, 4, 5, 10, and 15 mm exposure
- Electrode diameter (proportional to square of radius)
- Typical: 20 or 22G.

ADVANTAGES OF RADIOFREQUENCY LESIONING

- Lesion size can be accurately controlled, allowing lesioning of small nerves without damaging nearby motor and other sensory nerves.

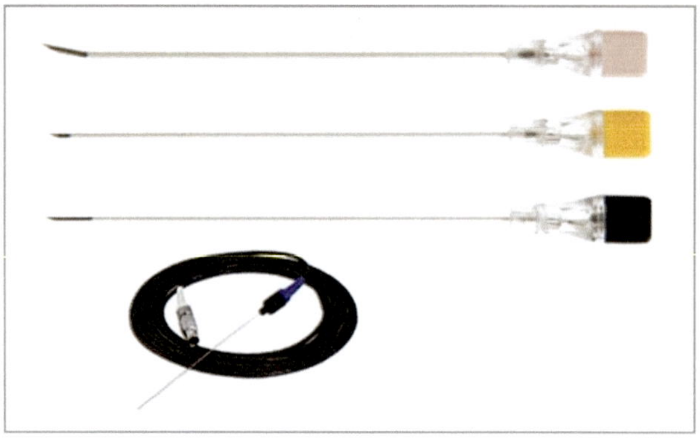

Fig. 2: Variables factors affecting lesion size at 80°.

- Recovery is rapid and usually uneventful, allowing the patient to return to work or normal daily activity more quickly.
- The nerve lesion is usually long-lasting. An accurately done lesion may give pain relief for years.
- Nerve lesion heals without neuroma formation.
- The rate of side effects and complications is low.
- When pain recurs, nerve lesion can be repeated as necessary.

CLINICAL USE OF RADIOFREQUENCY LESIONING IN PAIN MANAGEMENT

Since the pioneering work of White and Sweet in 1969,[18] RF neurotomy has been used successfully for the treatment of trigeminal neuralgia.[19] This success has inspired its application for the treatment of spinal pain. Its use for lumbar spinal pain was promoted first by Shealy[20-23] between 1974 and 1976.

Bogduk in 1979, in an anatomical study,[24] pointed out that the technique described by Shealy was inaccurate—that the electrode was being placed remote from the target nerve. Anatomically correct target points were defined, and a modified technique was described,[25] which had good results but others persisted with the Shealy method despite its errors.

Bogduk[26] in 1987, in a laboratory study, revealed a misconception that had been associated with RF neurotomy. The lesion made by the electrode did not extend distal to the tip of the electrode, but instead spread radially about the long axis of the electrode. This meant that electrodes placed perpendicular to the target would fail to coagulate the nerve adequately, even though they might be correctly placed directly on the nerve. A more appropriate placement required that the electrode lie parallel to the nerve.[27]

Since then, the following conditions were treated with CRFL lesioning:

- Gasserian ganglion RFA for trigeminal neuralgia
- Medial branch block for facet joint pain—cervical/thoracic/lumbar
- Sacroiliac joint (SIJ): L_5 medial branch and S_{1-3} lateral branches
- Sympathetic chains/ganglion lesioning: Sphenopalatine ganglion, stellate/T_{2-3} sympathetic ganglion/splanchnic/lumbar/superior hypogastric plexus/ganglion impar.

APPLICATION OF PULSED RADIOFREQUENCY LESIONING

- PRFL application to DRG: Cervical, thoracic, or lumbar
- Peripheral nerves pulsed RFA, e.g., ilioinguinal, intercostals
- Greater occipital nerve
- Facet joints PRFL
- Trigeminal PRFL (V_1)
- Intra-articular PRFL application, e.g., SIJ, knee, shoulder
- Splanchnic nerves
- Joints PRFL: Shoulder, knee, SI, etc.

ADVANCES IN RADIOFREQUENCY TECHNIQUES IN PAIN MANAGEMENT

Water-cooled Radiofrequency[28,29]

Although water-cooled radiofrequency (WCRF) ablation has been used in cardiac electrophysiology and tumor ablation for some time, its use in the treatment of pain is fairly recent. The basic principle of pain relief during WCRF application is similar to that of CRFL—a thermal lesion is created by the application of RF energy through an electrode placed in the vicinity of the target neural structure. However, WCRF is applied by using a specialized multichannel electrode that is actively cooled by the continuous flow of water at ambient temperature. The active cooling prevents the electrode from acquiring the high surrounding tissue temperatures and allows the continued flow of the RF current, with the consequent heating of a larger tissue volume and the creation of a larger thermal lesion. The resulting WCRF lesion is consequently comprised of a few millimeters of cooled tissue immediately surrounding the electrode, which is surrounded by spherical isotherms of increasing tissue temperature, which in turn are surrounded by lower temperature isotherms at an increasing distance from the electrode. Similar to CRFL, the size of the WCRF lesion is dependent on the probe size, the electrode temperature, and the duration of RF current applied. If a 50°C isotherm is used as a criterion for the lesion's edge while using an 18G electrode with a 6-mm active tip with the electrode temperature raised to 55–60°C and RF currents applied for 150 seconds, the lesion created would be 8–10 mm in diameter.

The review of the literature on the clinical use of WCRF identified two distinct forms of WCRF techniques: Monopolar and bipolar WCRF lesioning. These WCRF lesioning techniques were applied exclusively for the treatment of SIJ dysfunction (SJD) and diskogenic pain (DP), respectively. The unipolar WCRF in the treatment of SJD was applied to S_1, S_2, and S_3 lateral branches; either two or three monopolar lesions were created lateral to each sacral foramen. These lesions were created by using an 18G specialized electrode with a 4-mm active tip. The RF current was applied for 150 seconds, and the electrode temperature was raised to 60°C. Due to the larger anticipated lesion size, the introducer needle was kept at a "safe distance" from the sacral nerve roots: 8–10 mm from the lateral edge of posterior sacral foramen. To avoid injury to the segmental spinal nerve, WCRF was not applied to the L_4 and L_5 dorsal rami, and CRFL was used instead. For the treatment of DP, bipolar WCRF was applied to the posterolateral disk annulus by placing two 17G introducer needles and specialized RF electrodes. The electrode temperature was raised to 55°C over 11 minutes, and this temperature was maintained for an additional 4 minutes.

Currently, the use of WCRF is confined to pain syndromes, in which the pain generator is considered to have numerous and variable sources of innervation. The reported clinical use of WCRF is currently limited to four recently published articles in peer-reviewed journals. In two of these studies, WCRF was used for the treatment of SIJ, and the remaining two pertained to the treatment of DP. However, due to its ability to precisely deliver thermal energy to larger tissue volumes, WCRF may be effective, where more traditional forms of neuroablation have failed, and its use may be extended to other pain syndromes.

CONCLUSION

In the management of chronic pain, the value of permanent nerve blocks has long been recognized. To this end, several surgical and nonsurgical methods have been devised. RFL is a more refined technique based on the thermocoagulation of selected nerves using an electrode capable of accurate temperature generation. Newer RF like PRFL and WCRF lesioning is directed toward lesser tissue destruction and larger legions.

REFERENCES

1. Aronow S. The use of radio-frequency power in marking lesions in the brain. J Neurosurg. 1960;17:431-8.
2. Kapural L, Mekhail N. Radiofrequency ablation for chronic pain control. Curr Pain Headache Rep. 2001;5(6):517-25.
3. Slappendel R, Crul BJ, Braak GJ, Geurts JW, Booij LH, Voerman VF, et al. The efficacy of radiofrequency lesioning of the cervical spinal dorsal root ganglion in a double blinded randomized study: no difference between 40°C and 67°C treatments. Pain. 1997;73(2):159-63.
4. Finch PM. A curved approach to nerve blocks and radiofrequency lesioning. Pain Digest. 1997;7:251-7.
5. Smith HP, McWhorter JM, Challa VR. Radiofrequency neurolysis in a clinical model. Neuropathological correlation. J Neurosurg. 1981;55(2):246-53.
6. Uematsu S. Percutaneous electrothermocoagulation of spinal nerve trunk, ganglion, and rootlet. In: Schmidek HH, Sweet WH (Eds). Current Techniques in Operative Neurosurgery, 2nd edition. MA, USA: Grune and Stratton; 1977. pp. 469-90.
7. Letcher FS, Goldring S. The effect of radiofrequency current and heat on peripheral nerve action potential in the cat. J Neurosurg. 1968;29(1):42-7.
8. Cosman ER Jr, Cosman ER Sr. Electric and thermal field effects in tissue around radiofrequency electrodes. Pain Med. 2005;6(6):405-24.
9. Vaisman J. Pulse radiofrequency: a new and ingenious modality for pain management. N Engl Pain Assoc Newslett. 1999;4(2):4.
10. Brodkey JS, Miyazaki Y, Ervin FR, Mark VH. Reversible heat lesions with radiofrequency current. A method of stereotactic localization. J Neurosurg. 1964;21:49-53.
11. Dieckmann G, Gabriel E, Hassler R. Size, form and structural peculiarities of experimental brain lesions obtained by thermocontrolled radiofrequency. Confin Neural. 1965;26(3):134-42.
12. Cahana A, Vutskits L, Muller D. Acute differential modulation of synaptic transmission and cell survival during exposure to pulsed and continuous radiofrequency energy. J Pain. 2003;4(4):197-202.
13. Erdine S, Yucel A, Cunen A, Aydin S, Sav A, Bilir A. Effects of pulsed versus conventional radiofrequency current on rabbit dorsal root ganglion morphology. Eur J Pain. 2005;9(3):251-6.
14. Sluijter ME. Radiofrequency. Meggen, Switzerland: Flivo Press SA; 2001.

15. Weaver JC. Electroporation: a general phenomenon for manipulating cells and tissue. J Cell Biochem. 1993; 51(4):426-35.
16. Bear MF. Bidirectional synaptic plasticity: from theory to reality. Phil Trans R Soc Lond B Biol Sci. 2003; 358(1432):649-55.
17. Sandkühler J, Chen JG, Cheng G, Randić M. Low-frequency stimulation of afferent Aδ-fibers induces long-term depression at primary afferent synapses with substantia gelatinosa neurons in the rat. J Neurosci. 1997;17(16):6483-91.
18. Taha JM. Percutaneous radiofrequency trigeminal ganglionolysis. In: Burchiel K (Ed). Surgical Management of Pain. New York: Thieme Medical Publishers; 2002. pp. 841-48.
19. White JC, Sweet WH. Pain and the Neurosurgeon. Springfield, IL: CC Thomas; 1969. pp. 193-7.
20. Shealy CN. Facets in back and sciatic pain. A new approach to a major pain syndrome. Minn Med. 1974;57(3):199-203.
21. Shealy CN. The role of the spinal facets in back and sciatic pain. Headache. 1974;14(2):101-4.
22. Shealy CN. Percutaneous radiofrequency denervation of spinal facets. Treatment for chronic back pain and sciatica. J Neurosurg. 1975;43(4):448-51.
23. Shealy CN. Facet denervation in the management of back and sciatic pain. Clin Orthop Relat Res. 1976;(115):157-64.
24. Bogduk N, Long DM. The anatomy of the so-called "articular nerves" and their relationship to facet denervation in the treatment of low-back pain. J Neurosurg. 1979;51(2):172-7.
25. Bogduk N, Long DM. Percutaneous lumbar medial branch neurotomy: a modification of facet denervation. Spine (Phila Pa 1976). 1980;5(2):193-200.
26. Bogduk N, Macintosh J, Marsland A. Technical limitations to the efficacy of radiofrequency neurotomy for spinal pain. Neurosurgery. 1987;20(4):529-35.
27. Rashbaum RF. Radiofrequency facet denervation. A treatment alternative in refractory low back pain with or without leg pain. Orthop Clin North Am. 1983;14(3): 569-75.
28. Ho KY, Hadi MA, Pasutharnchat K, Tan KH. Cooled radiofrequency denervation for treatment of sacroiliac joint pain: two-year results from 20 cases. J Pain Res. 2013;6:505-11.
29. Kapural L, Vrooman B, Sarwar S, Krizanac-Bengez L, Rauck R, Gilmore C, et al. A randomized, placebo-controlled trial of transdiscal radiofrequency, biacuplasty for treatment of discogenic lower back pain. Pain Med. 2013;14(3): 362-73.

7 CHAPTER

Metaphors and Analogies for Patients and Healthcare Professionals

Sanjeeva Gupta, Risha Gupta, Manohar L Sharma, Prit Anand Singh, Dwarkadas K Baheti

INTRODUCTION

A metaphor is a figure of speech which compares one thing to another to create an image or resemblance. Metaphors are used in medicine to educate patients on their conditions and treatment plan, to improve understanding and compliance. In patients with persistent/chronic pain, metaphors can promote an understanding of the mechanism of chronic pain and available management options, including tools for self-management strategies to help improve engagement and compliance thereafter. Metaphors are a great way to help understand complex ideas by relating them to something more familiar and to add more depth and color to help language, either while speaking or writing; thus, they can be used in a consultation or even in leaflets.

Language is extremely important when it comes to explaining pain and doctors should understand that we need to construct and convey metaphors carefully, otherwise they can have a harmful effect on the patient. We should not use metaphors that have a negative effect on the patient as they can end up conveying the wrong information and may prevent patients from adhering to their treatment, therefore having the opposite effect of the intended metaphor. For example, chronic pain management is a journey that with time and different treatments can be helped and decreased; instead of using the metaphor "fighting pain", doctors should use "navigating pain". This metaphor has more positive connotations as it suggests a more mindful and adaptive approach to dealing with pain which portrays a comprehensive approach, compared to fighting which suggests you can either win or lose against the pain.

We believe that if the patients understand their pain condition and the rationale of the proposed treatment plan, they are more likely to comply with their treatment plan with the possibility of a better outcome and a greater satisfaction to the treating physician. We also believe that if the treating healthcare professionals communicate with the patients better, the engagement with and outcome of the treatments offered are likely to be better. The Faculty of Pain Medicine of the Royal College of Anaesthetists, London, considers that using metaphors in pain clinical practice can be a useful tool to improve chronic pain consultation's quality and impact.

We have included in this chapter some of the metaphors used in pain medicine and divided them into different sections. Some sections have more than one metaphor and analogies to explain the same topic and one may choose one or more of these to educate or empower the patients. The readers are encouraged to adopt them in daily practice as feasible. Please also refer to **Table 1** which summarises some commonly used metaphors and analogies in clinical practice. We have also included at the end of the chapter how various metaphors and analogies can be used in common conditions seen in the pain clinic.

MULTIMODAL PAIN MANAGEMENT

Metaphor 1: Vegetable Curry (Curry) (Figs. 1A and B)

This metaphor is used regularly by Dr Sanjeeva Gupta (SG) in his clinical practice.

We educate and support the patients to consider each modality of treatment in the metaphor as elucidated.

Metaphor 2: SOUP

SOUP analogy can be used with the dish being a Soup. When a soup is prepared, multiple ingredients are used and the soup tastes better than when each ingredient is

TABLE 1: Summary of some commonly used metaphors and analogies in clinical practice.

Multimodal management: • *SOUP:* Similar to the vegetable CURRY, a SOUP analogy can be used • *Buffet meal:* This metaphor is constructed as a personalized pain management tool for the patient • *Jigsaw puzzle:* Each component is equally important to complete the jigsaw puzzle. Until the last part falls into place the jigsaw puzzle is not complete • *Four legs of a chair:* Four legs of a Chair are required to stabilize the base for someone to sits on it *Diagnostic blocks:* • "Like going to the dentist" • "Electrical fuse in specific rooms". May be likened to a Coeliac plexus block, etc. • "Finding a thief and putting them in prison". Diagnostic block (finding a thief) and putting them in the prison (radiofrequency denervation)	*Regular physiotherapy:* • "You will not get better at playing a Piano by practicing the Trumpet". Patients should do appropriate physiotherapy exercises on a regular basis in addition to being active by other means • "Knife gets sharper by grinding". Regular physiotherapy exercises can sharpen the muscles in our back and improve the strength of these muscles • "Lack of physiotherapy is likened to an immobilized joint in the plaster cast – weakening of muscles and stiffening of the joint". Hence regular physiotherapy is important *Referred pain:* Chest pain and pain in the left arm with heart conditions

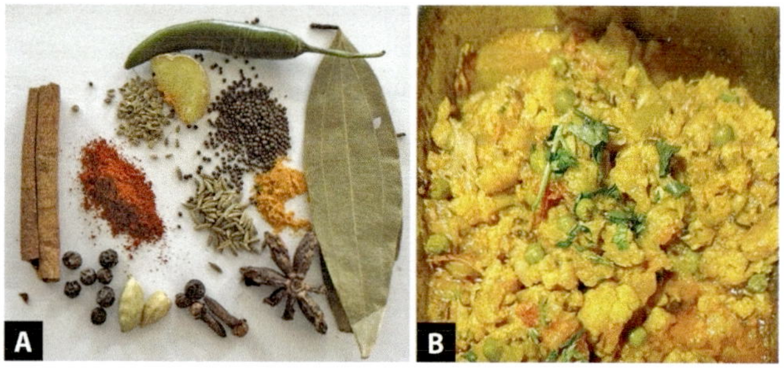

Figs. 1A and B: Multimodal pain management: Metaphor: CURRY. Various options are used for management of chronic pain (physiotherapy, pharmacotherapy, psychology, procedures, complementary and alternative therapy, etc.) and are likened to a spice/ingredient for the curry, e.g., chili, pepper, cinnamon, garlic, etc. If several spices are used we create a vegetable CURRY which tastes better than when only one spice is used. In a CURRY, each spice, in addition to having its effectlflavor also enhances the effect of other spices (synergism) and hence the vegetable CURRY with multiple spices in a specific combination/proportion is tastier than when a single spice is used. Similarly, when multiple modalities are used to manage chronic pain they can help each other with enhanced positive effect (synergism) and fewer side effects.

consumed on its own. Similarly, when multiple modalities of treatments (physiotherapy, pharmacotherapy, psychology, procedures, complementary and alternative therapies, etc.) are used to manage chronic pain they can help each other with enhanced effect (synergism) and fewer side effects.

Metaphor 3: Buffet Meal

This metaphor is constructed as a personalized pain management tool for the patient, so the offerings are changed as per the patient-specific issues. Patients are told to consider the treatment options as dishes in a buffet meal and the metaphor goes as described.

When we have a buffet meal, we choose what we like most from a variety of dishes available. Similarly, for the treatment of a given pain condition when multiple treatment modalities are available the pain physician can guide and coach the patients to choose/mix and match (like in a buffet meal) from the available treatments to cater for their own needs leading to maximum pain relief with fewer side effects.

Metaphor 4: Finger and fist—Gripping/Controlling the Pain

In this metaphor, each modality of treating chronic pain is considered as a finger of the hand. The patient is explained as follows: We cannot hold anything with one finger, but we can grip something when all the fingers are brought together to make a fist. Similarly, one modality of treatment (one finger) may not be effective to manage chronic pain but when multiple modalities of treatments (physiotherapy, pharmacotherapy, psychology, procedures, complementary and alternative therapies, etc.) are used (like making a fist to grip something), then this can hold/control the pain better.

Similarly, we may also say that if we want to hit an object (pain), then hitting with one finger will have less impact when compared to hitting the object (pain) with a fist. Using multiple treatment modalities is like making a fist to hit the object (controlling the pain).

Metaphor 5: Jigsaw Puzzle

The jigsaw puzzle is used frequently. Each component is equally important to complete the jigsaw puzzle. Until the last part falls into place, the jigsaw puzzle is not complete. Similarly, it is suggested that for pain management to be effective, all parts are needed (physiotherapy, pharmacotherapy, psychology, procedures, complementary and alternative therapies, etc.) to work together to control pain optimally with the least side effects. It is also suggested that a single modality of treatment is less likely to be enough to manage pain in the long term.

Metaphor 6: Four Legs of a Chair

This metaphor has been used in the complex regional pain syndrome (CRPS) guidelines published by the Royal College of Physicians and is based on a chair and is as follows: A chair has four legs, and each leg is required to stabilize the base when someone sits on it. Imagine different modalities (pillars) of treating pain as each leg of the chair (physiotherapy, pharmacotherapy, psychology, procedures, complementary and alternative therapies, etc.) Like the four legs of a chair are needed to support someone sitting on it, we will need different modalities of treatment to support/manage pain optimally. Like each leg of the chair is important, similarly each modality of treatment is equally important to manage pain.

Metaphor 7: Umbrella use

Like using an umbrella when it rains, modalities for pain management are likened to it and explained as follows: If patients have chronic pain, they may need some regular painkillers, do regular physiotherapy exercises, and use other modalities for pain control. This is like using an umbrella when there is rain. The umbrella does not stop the rain but does allow the individual to go out and do things, therefore stopping pain from being a barrier. Similarly, in chronic pain conditions, the pain medications and other modalities used to manage pain may not cure the pain but enable one to lead a better quality of life.

ANALOGIES TO HELP IMPROVE PATIENT ENGAGEMENT

Analogy: Balancing the Side Effects of Pain and Side Effects of the Treatments Advised

We come across some patients who are reluctant to take medications, do regular physiotherapy exercises, and pace their activities when needed as they are understandably worried about the side effects of medications and pain worsening after activities. In such patients, it would be reasonable to ask them to think about the side effects of pain (suffering, decreased mobility, inability to go out, etc., and the impact of all these on their mental health). These patients are then asked to consider the adverse effects of pain and then balance them with possible side effects of the treatment modalities suggested by the physician and decide for themselves to choose as they feel appropriate. Once the patient understands that the impact of pain on their lives outweighs the side effects of the management offered, they are more likely to engage with the pain physician and consider the advice given.

Another way to explain about the side effect of medications can be that there is nothing without side effects; for example, even drinking excessive water can be harmful or the fact that nature has allowed us only 21% oxygen because 100% oxygen is harmful.

As an example: Some patients may be reluctant to take pain medications when rightfully indicated as they are worried about the side effects. In such patients we can ask them to consider the side effects of pain (suffering, decreased mobility, the impact of pain on other organ functions of our body, e.g., increased heart rate) and the side effects of pain medications and ask them to strike a balance between them. Patients should also be informed that once their pain is better and their function improved/restored, the pain medications can be reduced gradually and stopped. It is important to note that if patients are taking regular medications, their side effects, including their impact on different organs, should be monitored.

CHRONIC PAIN AS A LONG-TERM CONDITION

Analogy: Compare Chronic Pain with the Other Chronic Conditions

Some patients have difficulty understanding the concept of chronic pain. For such patients, we can explain what other patients do when they have other chronic conditions such as asthma, hypertension, and diabetes. Patients with such chronic conditions manage their condition/symptoms with multiple modalities (lifestyle modification, weight management, relaxation techniques to reduce stress, medications, complementary and alternative therapies, etc.). Similarly, when pain becomes chronic, they are told that this also must be managed with multiple modalities for optimal outcome and improved quality of life. It may be reasonable to ask some patients to accept chronic pain as a disease that has to be managed with multiple modalities. Once they understand this concept, patients are more likely to engage with the advice given and live a better quality of life with improved function. They can also be encouraged to discuss with other patients with chronic pain or be associated with chronic pain groups as this may enable them to cope with their pain better.

ANALOGIES USED TO EXPLAIN REFERRED PAIN

Patients who have low back pain can also get pain in their buttocks, groin, anterolateral thigh and/or posterior thigh, and sometimes their calf muscles also. They often call this sciatica. We see that the spreading of the pain to the different areas occurs when the low back pain gets worse, implying that this is a referred pain and not a radicular pain which has a neuropathic character.

Analogy 1: Referred Pain: Candle Flame (Joints) and the Heat Above the Flame (Referred Pain) (Figs. 2A and B)—This Analogy is used Regularly by SG in his Clinical Practice

Patients who have low back pain often also complain that the pain can go to their groin, buttocks, and thighs. However, the pain in the groin, buttocks, and thighs is not shooting but travels down as the low back pain gets worse. This pain is likely to be a referred pain from the structures in the lower back (e.g., from the disk and/or facet joint and/or sacroiliac joints). Patients normally say that they have sciatica. We use the analogy, candle flame and the heat above the flame, to explain referred pain. We can feel the heat from a candle flame several inches above it in real life. Similarly, pain from the different structures (flame) in the lower back can gradually spread to the groin, buttocks, and thighs as the back pain worsens (like heat several inches above the candle flame). If we treat the main source of the pain in the lower back (dim or put out the flame) the pain in the groin, buttocks, and thighs will also be relieved (if the flame of the candle is taken off, the heat above also will disappear).

Similarly, when patients have neck pain, it can gradually get referred to the suprascapular area, lateral part of the upper arm, and/or interscapular area when the neck pain gets worse. The candle flame (joints) and the heat above the flame (referred pain) analogy can also be used to explain the concept of referred pain in this condition.

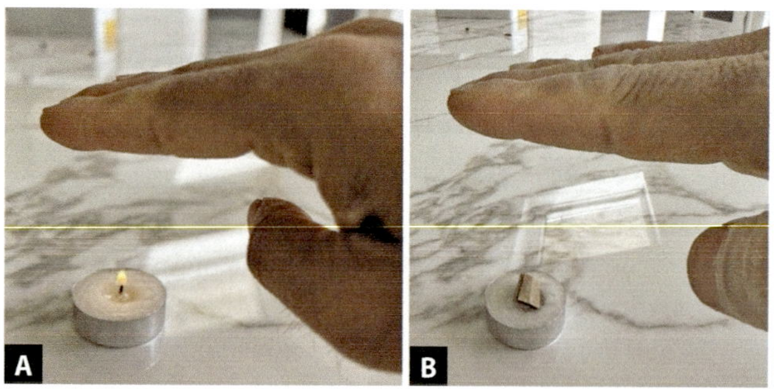

Figs. 2A and B: Metaphor: Referred Pain: Candle flame (joints) and the heat above the flame (referred pain).
Pain from the different structures (flame) in the lower back can gradually spread to the groin, buttocks, and thighs as the back pain worsens (like heat several inches above the candle flame). If we treat the main source of the pain in the lower back (dim or put out the flame) the pain in the groin, buttocks, and thighs will also be relieved.

Analogy 2: Chest Pain and Pain in the Left Arm with Heart Conditions

If a patient had a heart attack, they would get pain in their left arm in addition to chest pain. If the patient gets treated for a heart attack, the pain over the left arm disappears. The pain originating from the lower lumbar spine can travel to the buttocks, groin, and thighs. Like the heart attack analogy, if we treat the low back pain, the pain in the buttock, groin, and thigh will also get better. This metaphor is commonly used to allude to referred pain due to various reasons.

ANALOGIES USED TO EXPLAIN THE IMPORTANCE OF REGULAR PHYSIOTHERAPY EXERCISES

Analogy 1: Brick Wall as Spine—Plastering the Wall and/or Applying Scaffolding (Figs. 3A to E)—This Analogy is used Regularly by SG in his Clinical Practice

We ask patients what they would do if a brick wall (spine) is not strong enough. They would either replace the brick wall with a new one or support/strengthen the brick wall with further cement/plastering and/or apply scaffolding for support. Similarly, if our spine (brick wall) is not strong enough because of wear and tear we would strengthen the muscles around the spine and also the core muscles (similar to cement/plastering and/or apply scaffolding to support the brick wall) so that the muscles can hold the spine better as replacing the spine is not an option. This metaphor reinforces the importance of spine being a robust structure and the relevance of doing regular physiotherapy

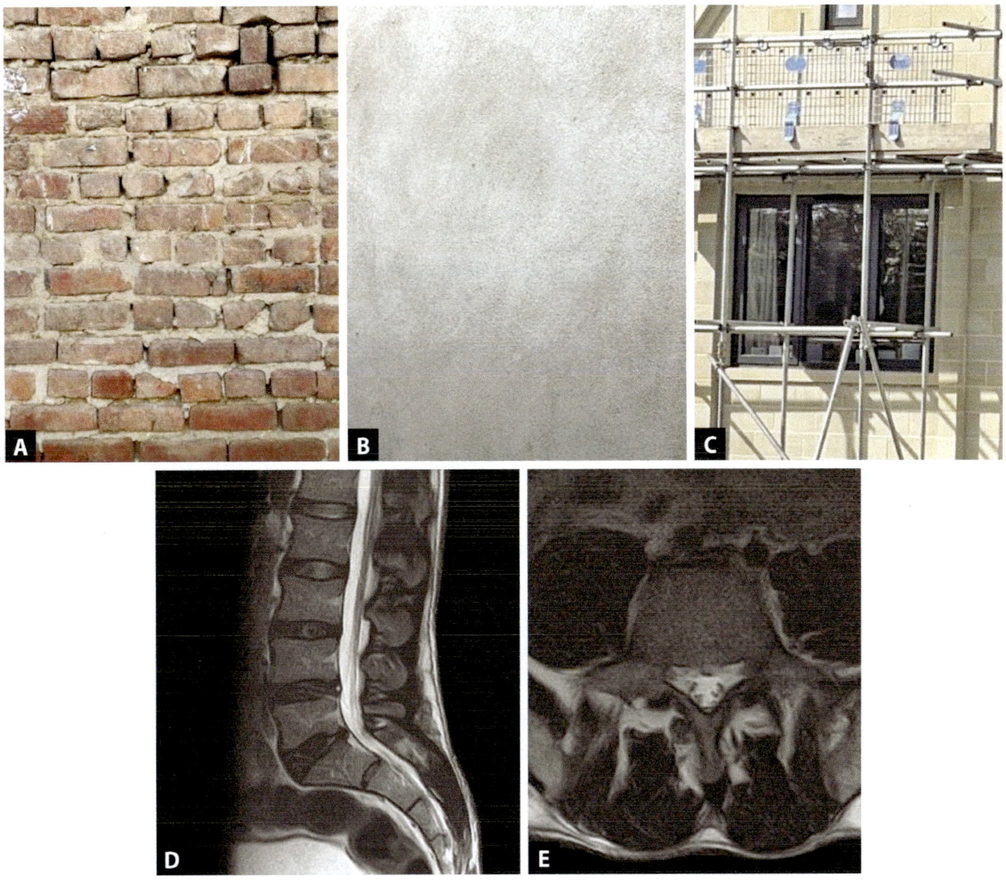

Figs. 3A to E: Importance of doing regular physiotherapy exercises: Analogy: Brick wall and spine.
If a brick wall is not strong enough, we would either replace the brick wall with a new one or support/strengthen the brick wall with further cement/plastering and/or apply scaffolding to support. Similarly, if our spine is not strong enough, we should strengthen the muscles around the spine and also the core muscles (similar to cement/plastering and/or applying scaffolding to support the brick wall) so that the muscles can hold the spine better as replacing the spine is not an option. This analogy will reinforce the importance of doing regular physiotherapy exercises and keep them active, thus avoiding deconditioning which is likely to help them in the long term and give them the confidence to manage back/neck pain or any other musculoskeletal pain.
(A) Weak Brick Wall; (B) Plastered Brick Wall; (C) Wall supported by Scaffolding; and (D and E) Sagittal and Axial MRI images showing changes in the paraspinal muscles.

exercises and keeping themselves active, thus avoiding deconditioning. This is likely to help them in the long term and give them the confidence to manage back/neck pain or pain from the joints (e.g., knee joint) better.

Analogy 2: You will not get Better at Playing a Piano by Practicing the Trumpet

Encouraging patients to do appropriate physiotherapy exercises on a regular basis in addition to being active by other means (e.g., walking) is important. Using this metaphor motivates patients to do regular physiotherapy exercises tailored to their condition alongside their routine activities.

Analogy 3: Knife Gets Sharper by Grinding

If we do regular physiotherapy exercises and are active, we sharpen the muscles in our back and the core muscles, improving the strength of these muscles. Strong muscles around the spine support the spine better and decrease the chances of injury and aid in a faster recovery if an injury is sustained.

Analogy 4: Joint Family and Physiotherapy

When living in a joint family if one brother has financial difficulties or has a health problem (like a problem with spine, e.g., disk disease, facet joint pain, sacroiliac joint pain) and if the other brother/relative has enough money and is healthy (paraspinal muscles and core muscles, etc.) then they can help the less fortunate brother and overcome the problems together. Similarly, regular physiotherapy exercise will increase the tone and strength of the muscles around the spine and the core muscles and support the spine better and assist in recovery.

Analogy 5: What Happens if Physiotherapy Exercises are not Done Regularly

In this metaphor, lack of physiotherapy is likened to an immobilized joint in the plaster cast and explained as follows: Patient is told that if his/her elbow joint is immobilized in a plaster cast, it will result in the muscles around the joint becoming weaker over time resulting in the joint becoming stiffer due to decreased movements. So, to avoid or overcome this problem, the patients should move/exercise the elbow joint regularly so that the function can be restored/maintained. Similarly, with back and neck pain, if regular exercises specific to the spine are done, they will be able to maintain the function and movements of the spine. The muscles around the spine will become stronger, thus holding the spine better and causing it to be less susceptible to injury.

As explained before, patients may also be informed that one of the immediate goals of regular physiotherapy exercises and activity is to keep the spine mobile with improved function as this can prevent deconditioning. The long-term goal is to keep the spine mobile which can be therapeutic.

Analogy 6: Rate of Improvement of Muscle Strength with Physiotherapy: Oil Tanker Turning

The speed of improvement of muscle strength with physiotherapy is usually slow and needs patience. This is like an oil tanker (ship) turning slowly and steadily. After turning the wheel, it takes a while before the ship starts turning, like how it takes time to improve with physiotherapy.

BACK OR NECK BRACES

Analogy: Natural Support Systems

Some patients ask about using neck or back support/braces for low back or neck pain. We can inform patients that the neck and lower back are designed to move and that they should be allowed to move, otherwise they will become stiff and the muscles will get weaker and deconditioned which can make their pain worse. They should strengthen the natural support system—the muscles in the back and neck and the abdominal core muscles which offer the benefit of strength and mobility.

DIAGNOSTIC BLOCKS AND RADIOFREQUENCY DENERVATION

Analogy 1: Electrical Light Switch (Facet Joint)–Electrical wire (Medial Branch)–Light Bulb (Brain) (Fig. 4)—This Analogy is used Regularly by SG in his Clinical Practice

When diagnostic spinal blocks are done (e.g., diagnostic medial branch block for lumbar or cervical facet joint pain), it is not easy to convey to the patient the concept of diagnostic block or test block. We ask the patient to consider the light switch as the joint that is being blocked/numbed, the wire that connects the light switch to the

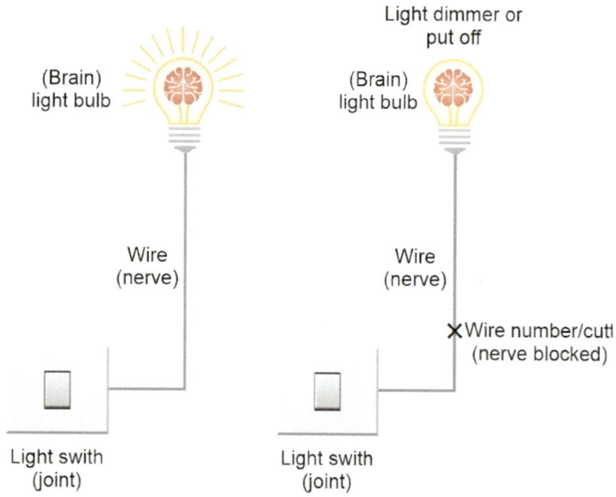

Fig. 4: Analogy: Diagnostic blocks: Electrical light switch (facet joint)–electrical wire (medial branch)–light bulb (brain).
We ask the patient to consider the light switch as the joint that is being blocked/numbed, the wire that connects the light switch to the light bulb as the nerve which carries the message from the joint to the brain, and the light bulb as the brain where the pain is experienced. The electricity/current has to travel from the light switch via the wire to the light bulb for it to light up. Similarly, the pain message has to travel from the joint that is the source of the pain via the nerves to the brain where the pain is experienced. If we numb or block the wire (nerve) and if the light bulb dims or shuts off (pain gets better) then as we know that the wire connects the light switch (joint) to the light bulb (brain), we can infer that the source of the pain could be the joint which is supplied by the nerve that was blocked. This can help us to identify the source of pain and plan further treatment.

light bulb as the nerve which carries the message from the joint to the brain, and the light bulb as the brain where the pain is experienced. The electricity/current must travel from the light switch via the wire to the light bulb for it to light up. Similarly, the pain message must travel from the joint that is the source of the pain via the nerves to the brain where the pain is experienced. If we numb or block the wire (nerve) and if the light bulb dims or shuts off (pain gets better) then as we know that the wire connects the light switch (joint) to the light bulb (brain), we can infer that the source of the pain could be the joint which is supplied by the nerve that was blocked. Similarly, if the tiny nerves that carry the message from the painful joints (light switch) to the brain (light bulb) are blocked with a local anesthesia and the pain decreases significantly, we can infer the joint as the source of the pain. This can help us to identify the source of pain and plan further treatment.

Analogy 2: Radiofrequency Denervation: Stopping the Pain Message from Reaching the Brain

Once the painful facet joints in the neck or lower back are identified by diagnostic block (electrical switch-wire-brain), we can cut (as we cannot replace the facet joints) the nerves that carry the pain message from the joints to the brain using radiofrequency denervation technique. This will stop telling the brain about the pain and allow patients to engage with physiotherapy, thus enabling them to strengthen the muscles around the spine and the core abdominal muscles which will hold the spine better and facilitate recovery.

Analogy 3: Diagnostic block: Like going to the Dentist

Patients are told the example of going to a dentist, where they do an injection to numb the nerves in the area before they do a procedure. Similarly, for diagnostic blocks the nerves are numbed to assess pain relief before they get a therapeutic intervention (e.g., radiofrequency ablation).

Analogy 4: Diagnostic and Therapeutic Block: Electrical Fuse in Specific Rooms

Celiac plexus block is done in some patients with abdominal pain. Similarly, other plexuses and ganglions are blocked for various pain conditions. The plexus and ganglions may be considered as a fuse in specific rooms in a building. Blocking the ganglion or plexus can be considered like switching off the fuse which stops electrical conduction in that specific room (e.g., celiac plexus block relieving abdominal pain). If the patient gets good pain relief for a short duration from the diagnostic block, then a therapeutic block with available modalities of treatment may be considered if appropriate.

Analogy 5: Diagnostic Block and Radiofrequency Denervation: Finding a Thief and Putting Him/Her in Prison

This is a common analogy that can be used as described: Finding the source of pain is like finding a thief. By blocking/numbing the nerves that supply the painful joints (thief) in the spine or other parts of the body, the source can be found out (thief). Once the thief (painful joint) is identified, we can punish the thief by putting him/her in prison/jail (like doing radiofrequency denervation procedure to ablate the nerve that is carrying the pain message from the joint to the brain).

EXPLAINING PACING TECHNIQUES

Analogy: Avoiding Overactivity and Underactivity Cycles: Changing the Color of the Wall

When patients have chronic pain, they should avoid overactivity and underactivity cycles. We can explain this to patients with chronic pain by describing how they would plan to change the color of the wall at their home. They can do this all in one go or in small sections. If they have chronic pain, it is likely that their pain will get worse if they paint the entire wall in a single day. This can also affect the following days (overactivity and underactivity cycles). However, if they paint the wall in portions every day, they are more likely to complete the task without much discomfort (pacing their activities). Therefore, it is important for the patient to know the desired outcome, i.e., change the color of the wall. Then how slowly or quickly this is achieved is not important to the outcome. When the task is completed, there is a degree of satisfaction and sense of achievement which can motivate the patient to do more activities in the future. Pacing can improve the number of activities of daily living performed despite being in chronic pain.

PSYCHOLOGICAL APPROACH TO MANAGING CHRONIC PAIN

Analogy 1: To Consider Psychology as Physiotherapy for the Mind/Emotions

It is discussed with the patient that it is well known that persistent pain can impact their mind and emotions, and this may also lead to increased pain perception and distress. If the patient indicates that chronic pain has impacted their quality of life, discuss the importance of consulting a psychologist. Some patients may express some degree of resistance to the psychological approach to manage their symptoms. However, if the above analogy (to consider psychology as physiotherapy for the mind/emotions) is explained to the patient, in our experience, they are more likely to accept psychological approaches and engage with a psychologist.

Analogy 2: Traffic Light System

A traffic light system metaphor is used in chronic pain, with sufferers told that in such conditions, our nervous system can go into overdrive mode, like the traffic light being amber or red all the time instead of being green. This can lead to increased pain perception and hypervigilance leading to adrenaline/cortisol response and giving rise to fatigue and other medical problems in addition to already being in pain. Psychological approaches can change the traffic light in our system from red to amber and from amber to green.

PSYCHOLOGY AND CENTRAL SENSITIZATION

Analogy: Rescue Dog Example to Retrain the Nervous System

We can use the concept of neuroplasticity to retrain our nervous system (alarm system) so that the pain experience can be decreased over time. In chronic pain conditions, we know that some of this is due to neuroplastic changes because of the way it behaves. We know many times it does not represent the damage it says. It is a bit like a rescue dog barking at a threatening situation. The example progresses by suggesting that the rescue dog was beaten on the nose with a newspaper when it was a puppy and made a mess in the house. Now, whenever it hears the paper rustle, it goes into defensive mode and changes its behavior—growls and barks and tenses up. We cannot retrain it by just getting hold of it by the collar and reaching for the paper. If we do this, we will only rewire the threat more and not help the dog in any way. It is important to show it some love, distract it with a tummy rub, and then rustle the paper-get its attention-distract it again and repeat this; if the dog does not get scared, it means that it is learning that this experience is safe (desensitizing). It will learn to trust and eventually accept the activity that in the past upset and threatened it. This can be used fruitfully when proceeding with graded exposure for routine back exercises in patients who are worried that they will damage their back by doing exercises. This will make the patients feel safe, increase their confidence, and allow them to engage in rehabilitation programs.

WILL MY SPINE GET WORSE AS I GET OLDER?

Analogy: Our Body is in a Constant State of Repair

Our body is always repairing. If we injure our skin, it heals in a few days. Similarly, the structures in the spine are also in a state of repair and any injury will repair itself but may take some time during which it is important that the pain is managed and the muscles around the spine are strengthened by regular pacing and physiotherapy exercises as this can decrease the chances of further injury.

MANAGING CHRONIC PAIN RATHER THAN LOOKING FOR A CURE

Analogy: Compare Chronic Pain with other Chronic/Long-term Conditions

In this analogy, even discussed previously, chronic pain is compared to other long-term conditions, and they are encouraged to manage these by multimodal approaches (lifestyle changes, weight reduction, exercises, pills, etc.) rather than looking for a cure per se. It is suggested that if each modality of treatment helps the patient's pain by 10–15% and if they use multiple modalities of treatment, a significant proportion of their pain can be managed with improved quality of life. Once the patient accepts this, it can reduce their distress and pain to a great extent. It is also informed to the patient that if someone has significant pain due to degenerative changes in the major joints (knee or the hip) and if they are old enough, these joints can be replaced but we cannot replace the spine; hence, spine pain has to be managed with multiple modalities unless there are specific conditions which may be amenable to operative/minimally invasive interventions. However, even in such conditions, the patients are counselled about the possibility of some pain persisting after the procedure.

MECHANISMS OF PAIN

Various metaphors are used for describing mechanisms of development and propagation of chronic painful conditions, as discussed in the following text.

Neuropathic Pain

Metaphor 1: Defectively Insulated Wire

An electric current wire is used as an example to explain neuropathic pain (e.g., trigeminal neuralgia, radicular pain). It is suggested that electricity flows through a wire which is insulated from one end to the other without any interruption. But when insulation is defective, a short circuit happens (ectopic current). Similarly, injury, ischemia, or inflammation of a nerve can produce breaches in nerve insulation or altered conduction which can lead to ectopic current generation. This can be experienced in neuropathic pain.

Metaphor 2: Touching a Live Electrical Wire

To explain radicular pain or neuropathic pain, we can discuss with the patient that this is like current-like sensation we experience when touching a bare electrical wire. Similarly, when the slipped disk or extruded disk material touches the spinal nerves, it can cause inflammation and excitation of the nerves resulting in nerve pain being felt which has a current-like sensation.

Central Sensitization

Analogy 1: Computer Hardware and Software Analogy

The concept of central sensitization may be explained by computer hardware and software examples. The computer may look fine (normal scan and other investigations), but the software is not functioning properly leading to chronic pain, e.g., chronic pain due to central sensitization. Desensitization as discussed under the analogy "Rescue dog example to retrain the nervous system" may be helpful in such situations.

Analogy 2: Faulty Car Alarm

Central sensitization is like a faulty car alarm which goes off without a reason. It is meant to detect a threat. However, in some situations, it goes off even when there is no threat. Desensitization as discussed under the analogy "Rescue dog example to retrain the nervous system" may be helpful in such situations.

Analogy 3: Like a Smoke Alarm in a Building

Discuss with the patient regarding pain sensitivity in terms of an alarm system. The smoke alarm in a building is very useful and should be triggered when the building is on fire. However, this can be incorrectly triggered (sensitized) by things such as cigarette smoke or burnt toast which is like the alarm going off when the building is not on fire.

Analogy 4: Signal Amplifier

When patients have chronic pain, they can at times feel excessive pain from a weak stimulus. The small biological signal is amplified by the brain/nervous system to be perceived as a more persistent or severe pain. Desensitization as discussed under the analogy "Rescue dog example to retrain the nervous system" may be helpful in gradually turning down the amplifier system, thus experiencing less pain from the same stimulus.

Phantom Pain

Analogy: Phantom Pain and Sleeping on Holidays

This is one way of explaining and reassuring patients regarding the presence of phantom pain, if they develop it. Knowing that their pain is real can help patients to accept their pain and consider options to manage this better. It is explained as follows:

At home, we sleep in our bed every day in a particular direction with, for example, a wall on the right side of the bed. However, when we are out of our home or on holiday, the direction of the bed in which we sleep and position of the wall may not be the same as when we were at home. When we are on holiday, if there is a wall on the left side of the bed, when we wake up in the morning and try to get out of bed, we are likely to get out of bed in the same direction as we would have done at home and may hit a wall! This is because our brain remembers our routine and tries to replicate this. Similarly, if patients have had pain in a given area (e.g. lower limb) and if that part is removed (amputation) then the brain can still remember this pain and feel it, despite the absence of the amputated area. However, with time the brain gets used to the loss of limb, subconsciously working at it (similar to the brain gradually adjusting to a changed morning routine) and thus this analogy should give patients the hope that their pain will resolve with time.

WILL MY PAIN GET BETTER?

Analogy: Wearing a Tight Clothing and Adaptation

Explaining to the patient with the help of this analogy the concept of repair and adaptation mechanism by our body can reassure them and encourage them to engage with the treatment modalities offered.

When we wear tight clothing that we like we feel that the clothing is tight for some time and then our body/mind gets adapted to this and we forget that the clothing is tight. Effectively, our body has adapted to the new circumstances. Similarly, changes are occurring in our joints/spine and the body is continuously trying to adapt to new circumstances. However, when there is an injury, the time to repair and adapt may take longer and the pain due to the injury may need to be managed by painkillers and other modalities of reducing pain. In addition, it is also helpful to support the injured area with regular physiotherapy exercises, etc., to improve the strength and tone of the muscles around the injured area as this can facilitate quicker recovery.

Spinal Stenosis with no Neurogenic Claudication

Analogy: Constant Adaptation and Sudden Change

The patient is explained that our body is in a continuous state to repair. As the changes are occurring in our spine, the body tries to adapt to the new circumstances and hence some patients may not complain of symptoms such as neurogenic claudication due to spinal stenosis. In such patients if surgery is not indicated it is important to inform them that the spinal stenosis has happened gradually, and the body has adapted to the change. However, if they have an injury to the spine (e.g., road traffic accident, fall), however small this may be, it may change the dynamics in the back and bring on symptoms of spinal stenosis/neurogenic claudication/cauda equina syndrome and that they should seek medical advice immediately.

When a patient understands his/her condition and the reasons for his/her symptoms, he/she will be able to manage his/her condition and seek appropriate help promptly when needed.

MISCELLANEOUS EXAMPLES

Normal MRI or X-ray but Still has Pain: Analogy: Beautiful House and People Living In It!

Some patients can have significant pain despite a normal MRI and other investigations. Discuss with the patient that this is like a beautiful well-maintained house with a large lawn with all the facilities for comfort. It looks lovely but there is no indication or prediction of whether it is a happy home inside. This correlates with a structurally sound spinal imaging that gives rise to pain.

If the MRI Scan of the Spine Shows Changes but the Patient does not have Pain: Used Car Analogy

This is like a used car. There will be changes as the car is used and gets older, but it is still running and should be fine. Inform the patient not to worry about the changes in the spine if there are no symptoms due to the changes.

Mechanisms of Pain in Other Parts of the Body when Patients have Low Back Pain Analogy: Four Tyres of a Car

When patients have back pain, they can sometimes develop pain in other parts of the body (e.g., pain in the buttock area or greater trochanter area). We can discuss with the patient that if one tyre in a car is not functioning properly this can have an impact on the other three tyres/body and the ride becomes bumpy, as all are connected to one another through the body of the car. Similarly, problems in one part of the body can affect other parts of the body.

USE OF METAPHORS AND ANALOGIES FOR CASE SCENARIOS

Some examples are illustrated here for common presentations in the pain clinic and readers are encouraged to use them freely from the text.

Metaphors and Analogies that can be used for Patients with Mechanical Neck Pain (Originating from the Facet Joints, Intervertebral Disks, or Sacroiliac Joints)

- Referred pain to the buttocks, groin, and thigh—candle and flame analogy
- Multimodal treatment—CURRY or SOUP metaphor

- Regular physiotherapy—brick wall and support analogy
- Diagnostic block—electrical switch-wire-light bulb analogy
- Radiofrequency denervation—cutting the wire connecting the electrical switch to the light bulb.

Metaphors and Analogies that can be used for Patients with Mechanical Neck Pain (Originating from the Facet Joints, Intervertebral Disks, or Other Areas of the Neck)

- Referred pain to the suprascapular area, interscapular area, and outer aspect of upper arm—candle and flame analogy
- Multimodal treatment—CURRY or SOUP metaphor
- Regular physiotherapy—brick wall and support analogy
- Diagnostic block for cervical facet joint pain—electrical switch-wire-light bulb analogy
- Radiofrequency denervation for facet joint pain—cutting the wire connecting the electrical switch to the light bulb.

Spinal Stenosis

- Spinal stenosis with no neurogenic claudication—wearing tight clothing and adaptation
- Neurogenic claudication symptoms in the lower limbs—candle and flame analogy
- Multimodal treatment—CURRY or SOUP metaphor.

Phantom Pain

- Understanding mechanisms—phantom pain and sleeping on holidays
- Regular physiotherapy—brick wall and support analogy
- Multimodal treatment—CURRY or SOUP metaphor.

Abdominal Pain

- Regular physiotherapy—brick wall and support analogy
- Multimodal treatment—CURRY or SOUP metaphor
- Celiac plexus block—electrical fuse in specific rooms.

Complex Regional Pain Syndrome

- Central sensitization—rescue dog example to retrain the nervous system; computer hardware and software analogy
- Normal investigations—beautiful house and people living in it
- Patients not engaging with multimodal pain management—balancing the side effects of pain and side effects of the treatments advised
- Multimodal treatment—CURRY or SOUP metaphor
- Pacing techniques—avoiding overactivity and underactivity cycles: Changing the color of the wall
- Psychological approach to managing chronic pain—to consider psychology as physiotherapy for the mind/emotions; traffic light system
- Desensitization—rescue dog example to retrain the nervous system.

ACKNOWLEDGMENT

We have included in this chapter some metaphors that were suggested by the respondents of the survey "Metaphors in Pain Management" conducted in 2024.

SUGGESTED READING

1. Darlow B, Dowell A, Baxter D, Mathieson F, Perry M, Dean S. The enduring impact of what clinicians say to people with low back pain. Ann Fam Med. 2013;11(6): 527-34.
2. Fatehi A, Table B, Peck S, Mackert M, Ring D. Medical Metaphors: Increasing Clarity but at What Cost? Arch Bone Jt Surg. 2022;10(8):721-28.
3. Goebel A, Barker CH, Turner-Stokes L, Atkins RM, Cameron H, Cossins L, et al. Complex Regional Pain Syndrome in Adults: UK Guidelines for Diagnosis, Referral and Management in Primary and Secondary Care. London: Royal College of Physicians; 2018. pp. 3-4.
4. Gupta, S. Sharma M. Top 5 abstracts from the 11th Annual North England pain medicine group meeting. British Journal of Pain. 2019;13(3 suppl):5-6.
5. Masukume G, Zumla A. Analogies and metaphors in clinical medicine. Clin Med (Lond)2012;12(1):55-6.
6. Mishra S. Using pictures and analogies to enhance the understanding of pain management principles. Transmitter. Spring. 2021:13-5.
7. Neilson S. Pain as metaphor: metaphor and medicine. Med Humanit. 2016;42:3-10.
8. Pena GP, de Souza Andrade-Filho J. Analogies in medicine: valuable for learning, reasoning, remembering and naming. Adv in Health Sci Educ. 2010;15:609-19.
9. Ring DC, Dobbs MB, Gioe TJ, Manner PA, Leopold SS. How the words we use affect the care we deliver. Clin Orthop Relat Res. 2016;474:2079-80.
10. Stilwell P, Stilwell C. Embracing metaphor in pain medicine. In: Bleakley A, Neilson S (Eds). Routledge Handbook of Medicine and Poetry. London: Taylor and Francis Group; 2024.
11. Wiggins NM. Stop using military metaphors for disease. BMJ. 2012;345:e4706.

2

SECTION

Documentation and Protocols

8 CHAPTER

Informed Consent Form for Pain Block (Interventional Pain Treatment Procedures)

Dwarkadas K Baheti

ABSTRACT

Written informed consent is of vital importance in day-to-day clinical practice. The present format of informed consent is redrafted in consideration of present medical practice. Obtaining informed consent is mandatory for all interventional pain treatment procedures (IPTPs).

INTRODUCTION

The interventional pain treatment procedure (IPTP) remains an important modality for relief of pain. It is the duty of the pain physician to make sure that he follows simple, safe, stress-free, devoid of complications, and on top of it cost-effective procedure. As any invasive procedure is as good as surgery, it may have unpredicted and unexpected complications. So it is advisable to follow a strict protocol for these procedures. Informed consent is part of this protocol.

The increase in medicolegal cases could be due to access of medical information via internet. Pain physician too is accountable. Due to the increasing awareness of patients and family about their right to information, it is mandatory to develop doctor-patient rapport for best results and patient care.

The pain physician must inform the patient and his relatives the factual condition of patient, procedure details, its outcome, and unforeseen complications if any.

The earlier informed consent[1] for IPTPs was used by the author in more than 5,000 patients, and the same was used by pain physicians in and around India.

The author has further modified the format of informed consent form as per change in scenario. Any pain physician is free to use the following format, but it is advised to obtain written consent from the author before using it. They should also check legal implications, if any of these informed consent forms are concerned with state or national authorities. The author is in no way liable for any consequences which may arise from the use of this informed consent. The revised format of informed consent is as follows.

INFORMED CONSENT FORM FOR INTERVENTIONAL PAIN TREATMENT PROCEDURES (IPTPs)
SAMPLE DRAFT

Name of Physician: ____________________ Date: ____________

Patient Name: ____________________

Age: ____________ Sex:____________ Male/Female:____________

Address: ____________________

____

I hereby authorize Dr. ____________ to perform an Interventional Pain Treatment Procedure known as ____________

____

This procedure has been explained to me by Dr. ________ and I completely understand the nature and consequences of the said procedure.

The following points have been made particularly clear.

1. These procedures are done under local anesthesia with anesthetist standby, may be with minimal sedation or anesthesia. I authorize Dr. ____________ to choose anesthetist of his choice for the above procedure. I understand the possible untoward reactions or complications of same.
2. The complications that may follow above procedure with/without pain relief are same as those that may follow any surgical procedure. The complications can be infection, hematoma formation, etc. These complications are enhanced in those cases, where the patient is old and infirm; those with diabetes and hypertension and in patients with history of previous cardiac ailments and decompensation.
3. The drugs that are being used in above procedure are generally used for relief of pain. However, a patient may be allergic/idiosyncratic to the drug used and may react in an unpredictable manner and rarely with unpredictable results.
4. Very rarely some procedures may be followed with paralysis of one or more limbs. These risks have been explained to me.
5. At times, specially prepared long needles needed to be used and these needles are known to break sometimes, though rarely. In this case, they become a foreign body and will require surgery to remove it. If surgery is required, then I authorize Dr. ____________ to get such surgery performed by a surgeon of his choice and blood transfusions may be required during or after surgery. Though the blood is fully tested, it may give rise to mismatch, B virus, malaria as well as AIDS.
6. I understand that the Dr. ________ relies on the qualified staff provided by the hospital or nominated by him for postoperative care of the patient. He personally may not be able to visit the patient every day.

I am aware that during the course of the procedure unforeseen condition may necessitate additional or different procedures than those set forth above. I, therefore, authorize and request that Dr. ________ to perform such procedures as are, in this professional judgment, necessary; these include but are not limited to, procedures stated above. The authority granted therein, shall extend to remedying conditions that were unknown before the start of the operation.

I understand the risks of local and general anesthesia and I consent to the administration of such anesthesia under the supervision of Dr. ________ or such anesthesiologist that he shall select, and to the use of such anesthesia as he may deem advisable.

The approximate recuperation time and the interval before I can return to work have been discussed with me. There is no guarantee when I shall be able to resume normal activities.

I consent to be photographed or filmed before, during, and after treatment, and that these pictures will be property of Dr. ____________ and may be published in scientific journals and/or shown for scientific purpose.

I am known/not known allergic to any drug.

I agree to keep Dr. ____________ informed of any change of address, so that he can notify me of any late findings, and I agree to cooperate with Dr. ____________ in the postoperative care until discharged.

I have read the above consent form/I have been explained the contents of this form in a language I understand ____________ and I understand the contents.

I have had sufficient opportunity to discuss my condition with Dr. ____________and all my questions have been answered to my satisfaction. I believe that I have adequate knowledge on which to base an informed consent to the proposed treatment.

____________ ____________

Witness Patient

I ____________ (Relation ________) of the patient ____________have understood and been explained the contents of the above form. The patient cannot be explained as he/she is minor/is tense is mentally disturbed and I would rather sign the form.

____________ ____________

Witness Relative

____

Name and Signature of pain physician

Date: ____________ Time: ____________

CONCLUSION

Obtaining an informed consent is an integral part of protocol for interventional pain treatment procedure for self-accountability, patient care, and medicolegal issues. This will safeguard a pain physician's interest and credibility.

REFERENCE

1. Baheti DK, Bakshi S, Gehdoo RP, Gupta S. Informed Consent for Pain Management Procedures. In: Interventional Pain Management: A Practical Approach. New Delhi: Jaypee Brothers Medical Publishers; 2010. pp. 39-41.

9 CHAPTER

Role of Investigations in Pain Block

Dwarkadas K Baheti

ABSTRACT

The investigations provide vital information about the overall health status of the patient while performing pain block or interventional pain treatment procedure. The dictum is to have normal investigations in order to reduce morbidity of pain block in chronic pain patients.

INTRODUCTION

To obtain history and other details of pain, clinical examination is of vital importance. This should be supported by relevant investigations, which help a pain physician to choose the type of pain block. All this will help in correct clinical judgment for total pain management in chronic pain patients.

Pain block is as good as any surgical procedure. That is why it should be performed with strict protocol to have minimum physiological and hemodynamic disturbances in body systems. So, it is mandatory to have utmost care and precautions to make it safe and, if needed, can be repeated safely.

The author has highlighted the role of investigations.[1] However, it needs to be revised in the present scenario keeping in mind the complex nature of chronic pain, use of multimodal approach, drug interactions, and investigations before pain block.

CLASSIFICATION OF INVESTIGATIONS

Investigations are classified as:

- Biochemical
- Diagnostic

Biochemical Investigations

Biochemical investigations are laboratory investigations such as:

- *Bleeding time, clotting time, and international normalized ratio (INR):* The status of coagulation is vital as pain block is a blind procedure, especially in patients on thrombolytic agents such as aspirin and clopidogrel. There will be an elevated risk of trauma to vessels or deeper structure, while the passage of needle through various planes may lead to bleeding and hematoma.
- *Human immunodeficiency virus (HIV) and Australia antigen:* To know the presence of these diseases which would help prevent the spread of HIV, Australia antigen, and other communicable diseases.
- *Complete blood count*—will give us information about any underlying infection and anemia.
- *Serum creatinine*—to know kidney function how safe is the use of NSAIDS and anti-inflammatory agents.

Diagnostic Investigations

The diagnostic investigations are imaging studies, electromyography (EMG), nerve conduction studies (NCS), diskography, and thermography.

Imaging Studies

The commonly done imaging studies are plain radiography, computed tomography (CT), magnetic resonance imaging (MRI), DEXA (dual-energy X-ray absorptiometry) scan, myelography, nuclear medicine scanning (bone scan), arthrography, diskography, and thermography.

The choice of imaging modality depends upon the site of pain, type of tissue involved, and diagnosis, such as CT scan is for bony structures in trauma and related diseases and MRI for soft-tissue structures that need more penetration.

Plain radiography ***(Figs. 1 and 2)****:* This is a commonly available, dependable, rapid, portable, and least expensive modality. It gives information about musculoskeletal disorders, including trauma, abnormality of joints, bony structures, and osteophytes.

Computed tomography: It will give us more information on the musculoskeletal system in comparison to plain radiography, especially in regard to bone and joint spaces. CT guidance allows exact needle positioning, reducing complications and improving the results in celiac plexus block, cervical spine injections, and cranial nerve blocks.

The help by interventional radiologists using an efficient, imaging-guided technique can increase the precision of the analgesic procedures, improving the results and reducing the complications.

Magnetic resonance imaging ***(Figs. 3 and 4)****:* It is the modality of choice for deeper structures, degree,

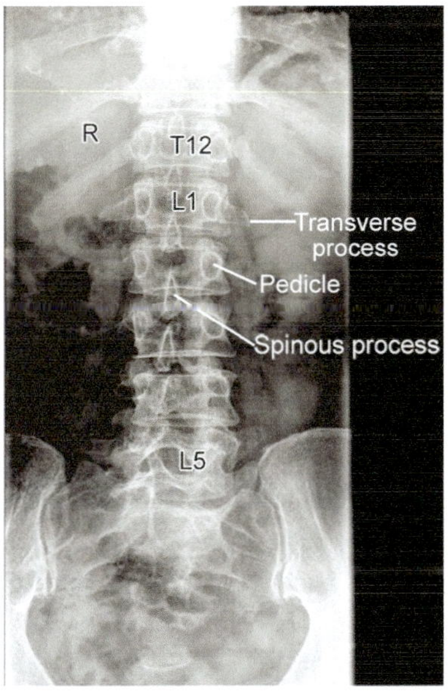

Fig. 1: Anteroposterior view of dorsolumbar spine.

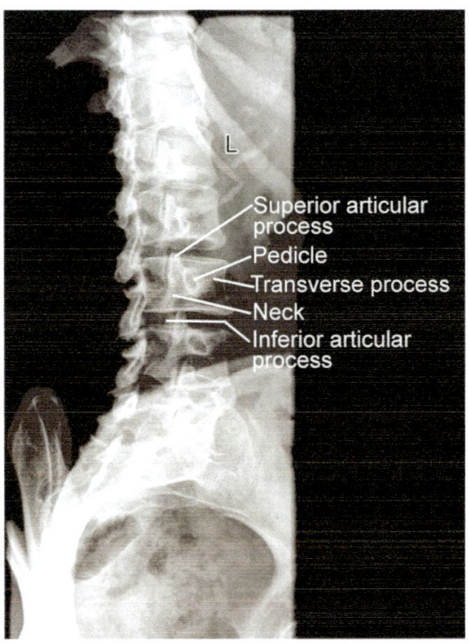

Fig. 2: Lateral view of lumbar spine.

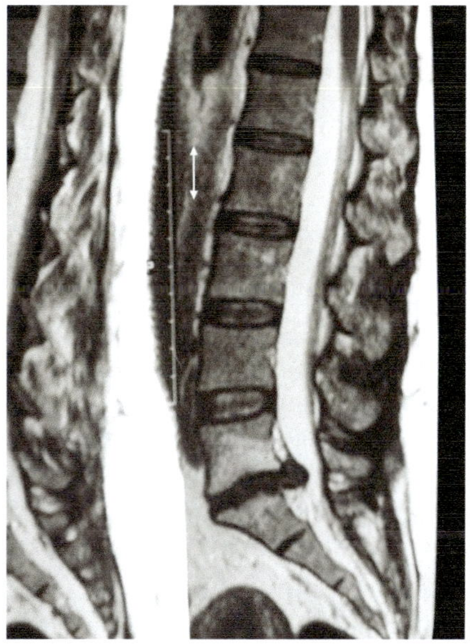

Fig. 3: Magnetic resonance imaging, showing disk protrusion at L5-S1.

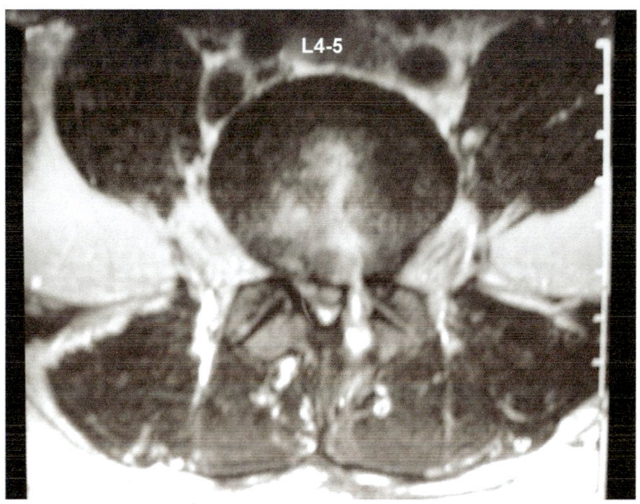

Fig. 4: Magnetic resonance imaging, showing root compression at L4-L5 nerve root.

position, and extension of spinal cord compression due to disk protrusion and musculoskeletal and intracranial structures.

The use of gadolinium contrast helps to find early inflammatory and infectious processes such as postprocedural diskitis and suspected intrathecal catheter tip granuloma. Gadolinium is iodine-free, so it scores over other agents in iodine allergy patients.

Magnetic resonance imaging is contraindicated in ferromagnetic implants such as cardiac pacemakers, intracranial clips, or claustrophobic patients. One must verify with the manufacturer for MRI compatibility while performing intrathecal implants.

DEXA: The condition and strength of bones is also a common cause of generalized body and musculoskeletal pain. DEXA scan will provide information about osteoporosis or osteopenia.[2] Radiographs have low sensitivity to the changes of osteoporosis and irrespective of cause, the appearances are the same.

Osteopenia is a nonspecific and descriptive term, used for rarefaction of the skeleton as seen on radiographs. Osteoporosis is the result of prolonged, slow bone loss, and the pattern of loss is different for trabecular and cortical bone. In postmenopausal women, the annual remodeling rate is 25% for trabecular bone and 3% for cortical bone.[3]

Hence, osteoporosis is more obvious in the axial skeletons and ends of long bones where trabecular bone is abundant. The structurally insufficient osteoporotic bone is predisposed to fractures.[4] Cancellous bone fractures the most, with spine being the most often affected site. The lifetime risk of osteoporotic fractures is estimated to be 40%, which is remarkably close to the risk of cardiovascular disease.[5]

Myelography: This is to visualize spinal canal and thecal sac. With the advent of MRI, myelography is done in selective patients. It is shown in the absence of MRI facility, where MRI does not correlate with clinical findings, and in a claustrophobic patient.

Nuclear medicine scanning (bone scan) ***(Figs. 5 and 6):*** This is bone scintigraphy with technetium (Tc)-99 phosphate. It shows bone turnover in bone metastases and other disorders involving bone metabolism.

Arthrography: It is an injection of dye into joint space. It is not very commonly done, as it has been replaced by MRI.

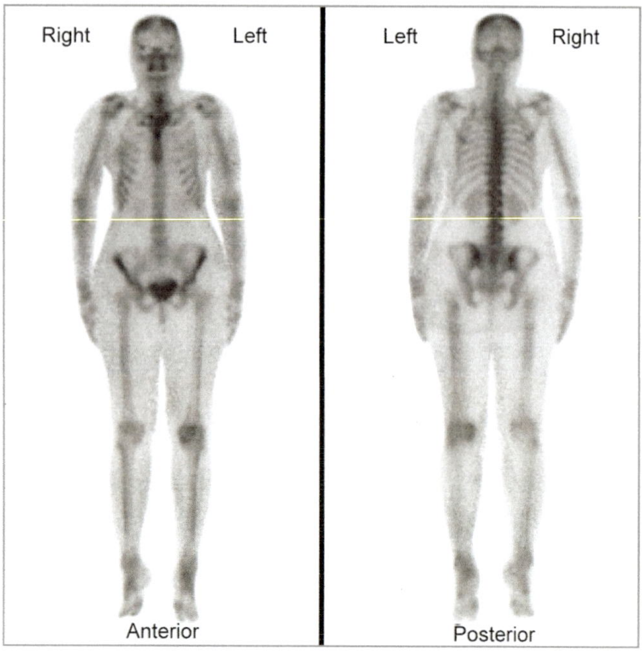

Fig. 5: Normal bone scan.

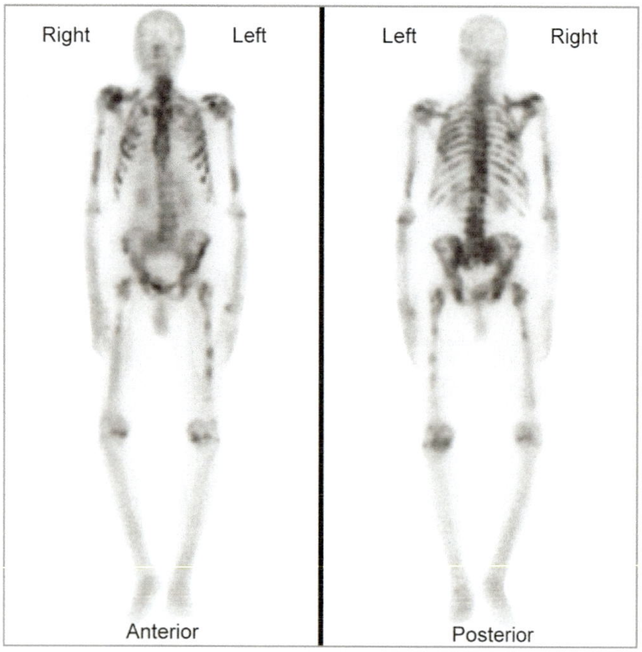

Fig. 6: Bone scan with secondaries.

Diskography ***(Fig. 7):*** This is done to confirm the diskogenic pain to localize the cause of pain due to disk herniation or degeneration. It can be done in conjunction with CT and MRI. Diskography is invasive and has a risk of infection and neural injury, so it should be used as a confirmatory and not initially diagnostic tool.

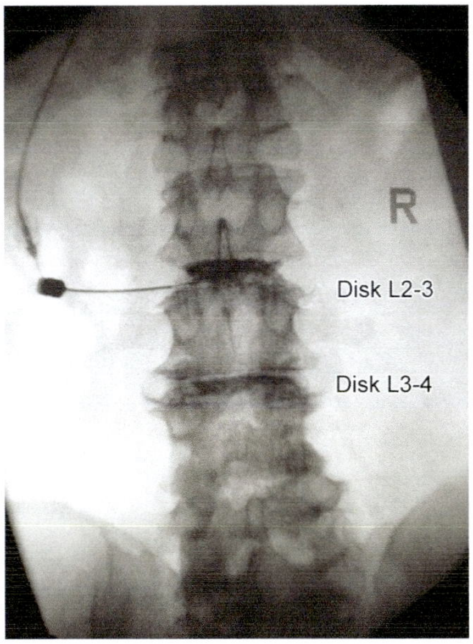

Fig. 7: Normal diskogram.

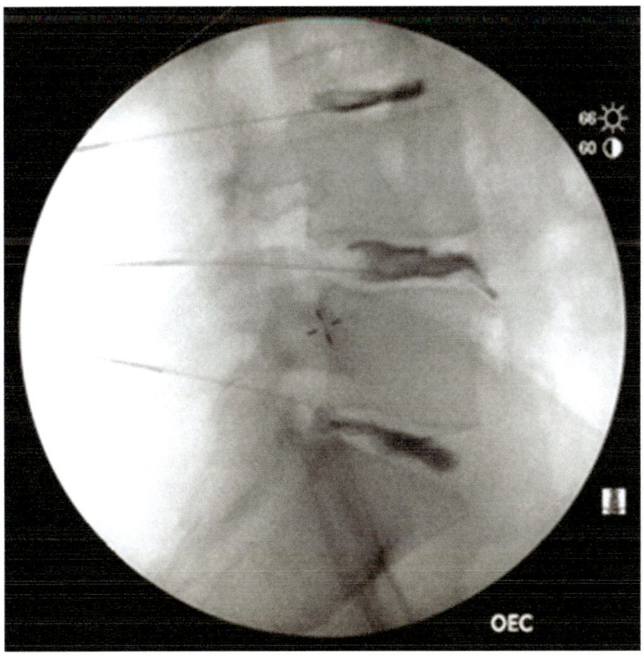

Fig. 8: Provocative diskogram.

Provocative diskogram: This is done for disk prolapse as seen in **Figure 8**. Dye leaking out confirms the disk prolapse as the possible cause of diskogenic pain.

Electromyography and Nerve Conduction Studies: Electrodiagnostic Studies (Figs. 9 and 10)

The electromyography (EMG) and nerve conduction studies (NCS) in a patient with neurological or muscular symptoms such as shooting or burning pain, numbness, or weakness are useful in the diagnosis of dorsal root ganglion lesion and its treatment.

In the case of neuropathy, electrodiagnostic studies (EDX) will show the type, whether axonal or demyelinating, severity, as well as muscle involvement that may be present as a result of denervation of the muscle. The severe neuropathies may cause weakness. The carpel tunnel syndrome may be bilateral, with only one hand clinically involved.

So, it is necessary to examine lower extremity as well to rule out generalized neuropathy. For suspected neuropathies in tibialis anterior, EMG needle examination is recommended as it may show enervation.

In order to confirm radiculopathies, both EMG and NCS are necessary. As NCS may be normal, the needle EMG is diagnostic.

The temperature of extremity will significantly alter the NCS. In myasthenia gravis, antibody assays are helpful to confirm the diagnosis.

Contraindications: The contraindications for EMG studies are:

- Uncooperative and unwilling patient
- Coagulopathies
- Lymph edema or anasarca
- Patient in whom muscle biopsy is to be performed.

Thermography (Figs. 11 and 12)

Thermography is a safe and noninvasive disease screening technique that can detect abnormalities/dysfunction for whole body health. Congestion, inflammation, and other conditions can be detected before any symptoms are given off by your body such as periodontal disease or infection that may go unnoticed by X-ray. It will guide the sympathetic part in sympathetically maintained pain (SMP). The qualitative data obtained reflect quantitative temperature difference up to 0.1°C.

The examination room's ambient temperature of 20°C, carpeted floor, and examination table in the center of the room will give more precise information. The patient should wear light clothing and has not recently exercised, smoked, or taken vasoconstrictor medicines.

The clinical application of thermography is a functional test of physiology to detect autonomic nervous system and blood flow responses to evaluate the dynamic physiological changes that reflect the underlying pathology. The changes in the pattern of temperature will help in differential diagnosis

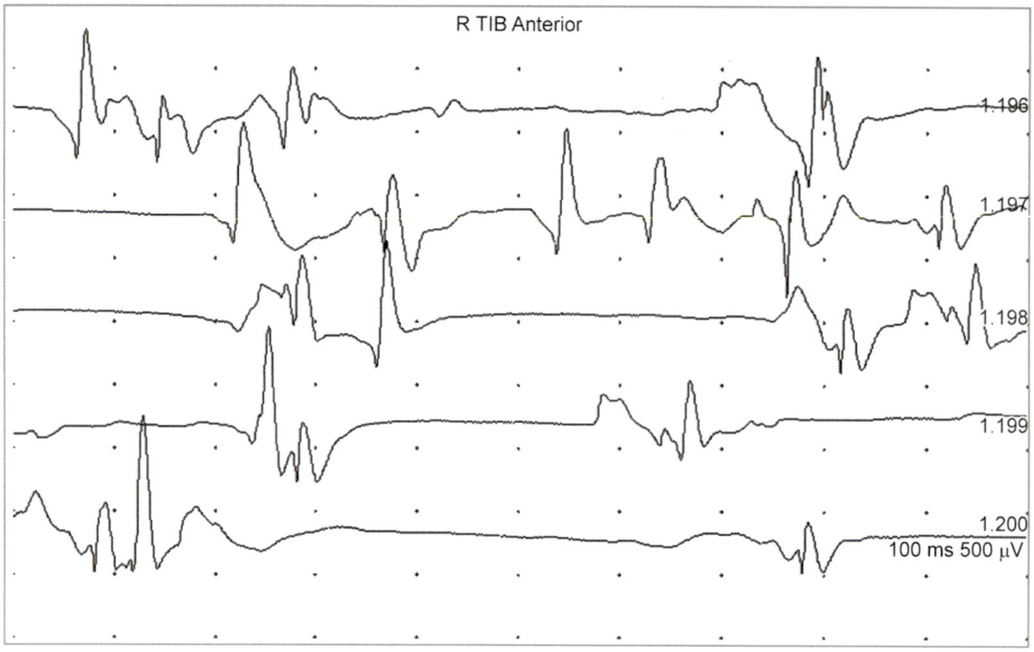

Fig. 9: Normal electromyography tracings.

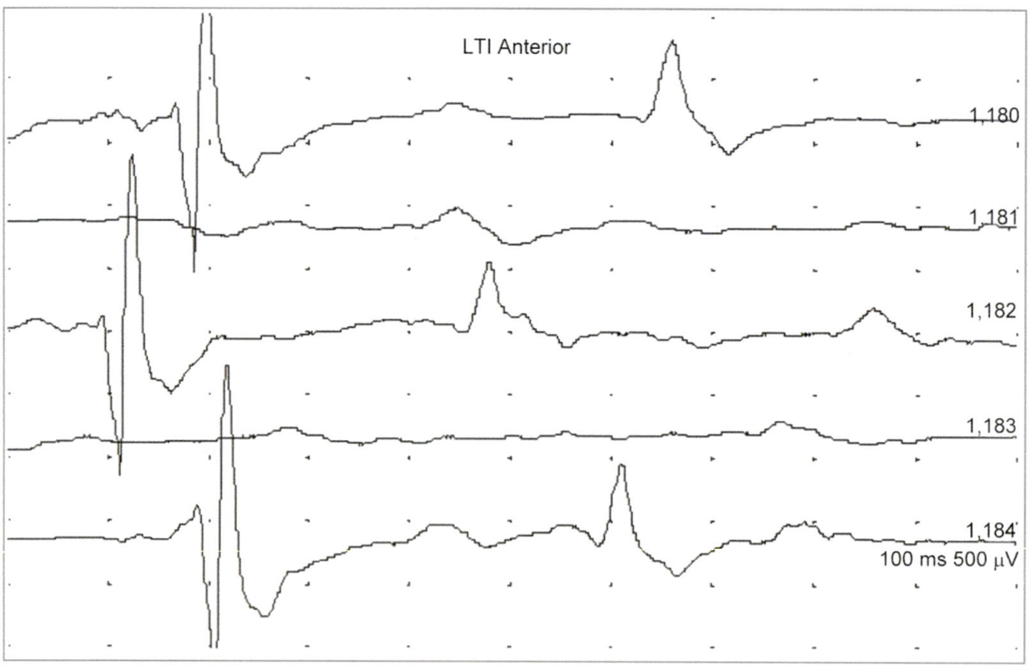

Fig. 10: Large wide triphasic units on needle electromyography of left tibialis anterior muscle in left L5 radiculopathy.

of pain due to peripheral nerve injury, spinal root pathology, and complex regional pain syndrome (CRPS). For example, increase in sympathetic activity causes vasoconstriction and resultant decrease in skin temperature, whereas decreased sympathetic flow causes an increase in regional blood flow that results in rise in skin temperature.

Normal thermogram **(Fig. 11)** displays temperature differentials in the entire area scanned. These images

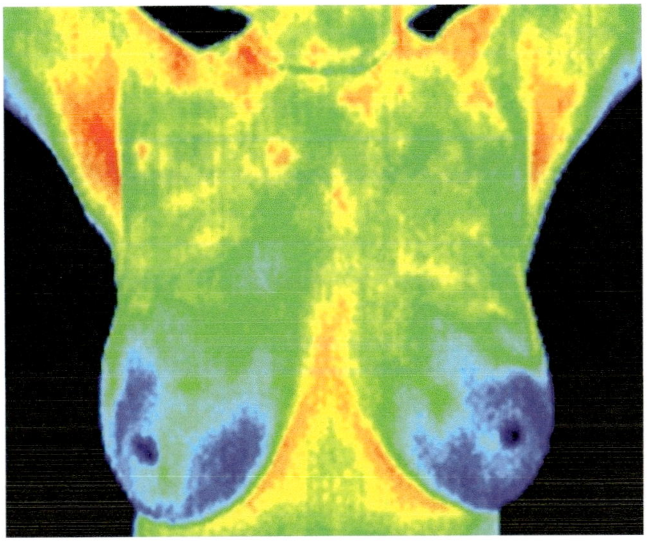

Fig. 11: Normal thermogram.

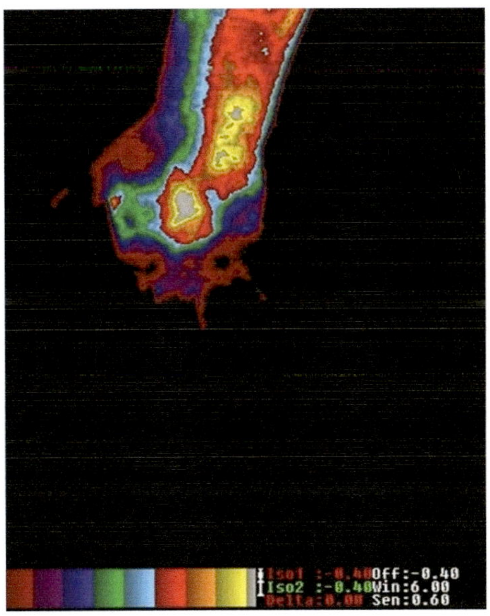

Fig. 12: Thermogram in complex regional pain syndrome.

reflect alterations in blood flow superficially or up to 27 mm deep.

Colder temperatures are reflected as blue-to-black hues and warmer temperatures as pink-to-red. The difference in temperature provides important diagnostic information.

The mean temperature differential in peripheral nerve injury is 1.5°C.

In sympathetic dysfunctions such as reflex sympathetic dystrophy (RSD), SMP, and CRPS **(Fig. 12)**, temperature differentials ranging from 1 to 10°C depending on severity are not uncommon. Rheumatologic processes appear as "hot areas" with increased temperature patterns. Pathology is an inflammatory process, i.e., synovitis of joints and tendon sheaths, epicondylitis, and capsular and muscle injuries.

Both hot and cold responses may coexist if the pain associated with an inflammatory focus excites an increase in sympathetic activity. Also, vascular conditions are readily proved by digital infrared thermal imaging (DITI), including Raynaud's disease, vasculitis, limb ischemia, and deep vein thrombosis (DVT).

CONCLUSION

Pain management is becoming a recognized specialty, so it has added more accountability for pain physicians. The awareness among patients, medical fraternity, and electronic media—every step in pain relief—is vital. That is why a pain physician's self-accountability should be a top priority looking at the complex nature of chronic pain to widen the horizon of safe pain practice.

Finally, thorough clinical examination supported by investigations does help to know the hematological and biochemical status of patients. In addition, the detailed study and understanding of the abovementioned investigations help in correct diagnosis and find the type of pain block to be performed. This, in turn, will decide the safe outcome of pain block for total pain relief.

REFERENCES

1. Baheti DK, Bakshi S, Gupta S, et al. Role of investigations in interventional procedures. In: Interventional Pain Management: A Practical Approach, 1st edition. New Delhi: Jaypee Brothers Medical Publishers (P) Ltd; 2010. pp. 42-9.
2. Queck ST, Peh WC. Radiology of osteoporosis. Semin Musculoskeletal Radiol. 2002;6:197-206.
3. Seeman E, Delmas PD. Bone quality—the material and structural basis of bone strength and fragility. N Engl J Med. 2006;354: 2250-61.
4. McKiernan FE. The broadening spectrum of osteoporotic vertebral fracture. Skeletal Radiol. 2009;38:303-8.
5. Kanis JA. Diagnosis of Osteoporosis and assessment of fracture risk. Lancet. 2002;359(9321):1929-36.

10 CHAPTER

Protocol for Pain Block: A Suggested Format

Dwarkadas K Baheti

ABSTRACT

This chapter suggests a protocol for performing pain block to provide maximum pain relief with minimum side effect and is cost-effective too.

INTRODUCTION

Pain block is still the mainstay in the multimodal approach for relief of chronic pain in order to have total pain relief.

In the era of Internet explosion, the pain physician is accountable for his deeds while performing an interventional pain treatment procedure (IPTP). The insurance agencies often have some queries about following necessary protocol before reimbursement of claims. Hence, it is mandatory for pain physicians to follow a strict protocol while performing any IPTP.

The author has changed the earlier protocol[1] to ensure safety; minimum or no morbidity; credibility of both the procedure and of the pain physician; and finally to make it cost-effective.

The suggested protocol for pain block is as follows:

- Document detailed history with symptoms and signs; physical and clinical examination; confirmation of clinical findings with investigations and evaluation with probable diagnosis.
- Explain to the patient and family members about the pain problem, medications needed, pain block details, side effects, and complications, if any.
- Obtain written informed consent: It must be explained in the language which the patient and the relatives understand, before signing.
- Hospital admission for a few hours to a few days as the case may be.
- Investigations such as bleeding time, clotting time, international normalized ratio (INR) (if the patient is on anticoagulants), human immunodeficiency virus (HIV), hepatitis C virus (HCV), and hepatitis B surface antigen (HBsAg).
- IPTP should be done either in the operating or in the procedure room equipped with monitoring and resuscitation facilities.
- Monitoring of pulse, noninvasive blood pressure (NIBP), and SaO_2.
- Secure intravenous (IV) line; the author prefers to have antibiotic cover.
- Anesthesiologist stands by
- Aseptic precautions such as wearing a gown and gloves
    - Radiological protection such as lead gown, thyroid shield, cervical lead collar, and radiation counter for all present in the procedure or the operating room. The author uses radiation gloves while performing the procedure.

PROCEDURE TIPS

- In order to alleviate the fear, keep talking to the patient while performing the procedure.
- Follow rule of three Ds, i.e. *D*irection, *D*epth, and *D*estination—aim for tunnel vision **(Fig. 1)**.
- Push the needle about 1 cm and confirm the three Ds at regular intervals to avoid accidental puncture of vital structure.
- Repeated negative aspiration before injection of dye, local anesthetic agent, steroid, and neurolytic agent.
- Confirm the spread of dye **(Fig. 2)**.

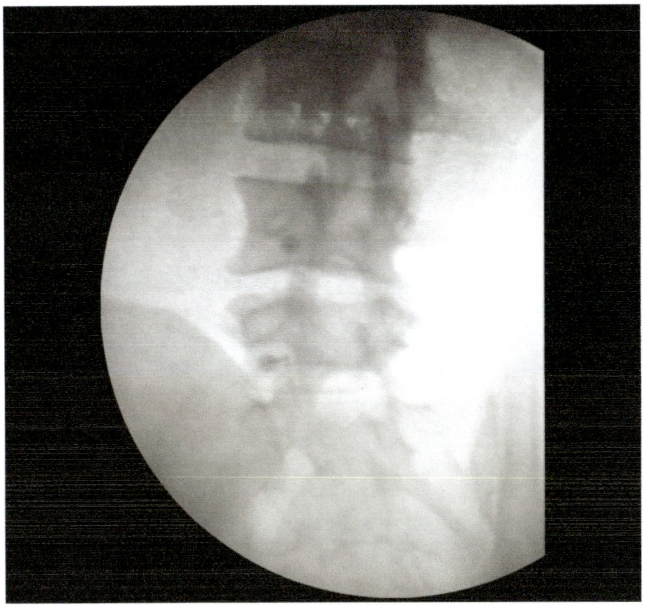

Fig. 1: Tunnel vision.

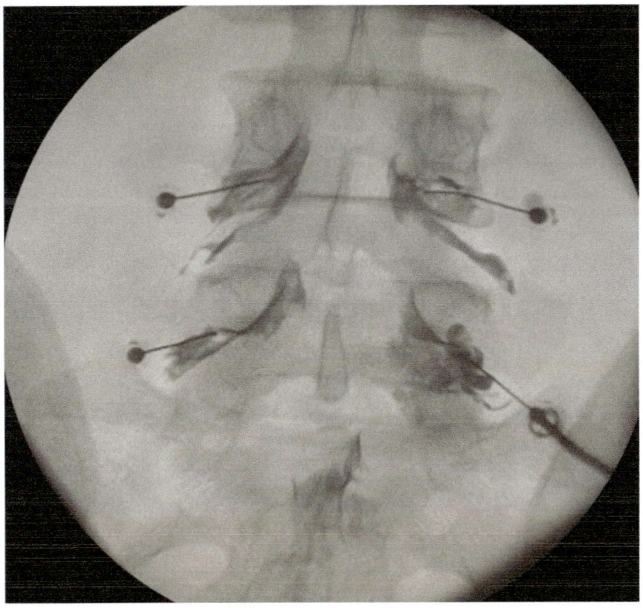

Fig. 2: Spread of dye—anteroposterior (AP) view—transforaminal lumbar epidural showing dye in epidural space with outlining of L4 nerve root sleeve.

Put the gauge or sponge before injecting a neurolytic agent around the needle to prevent spilling to avoid skin burns **(Fig. 3)**.

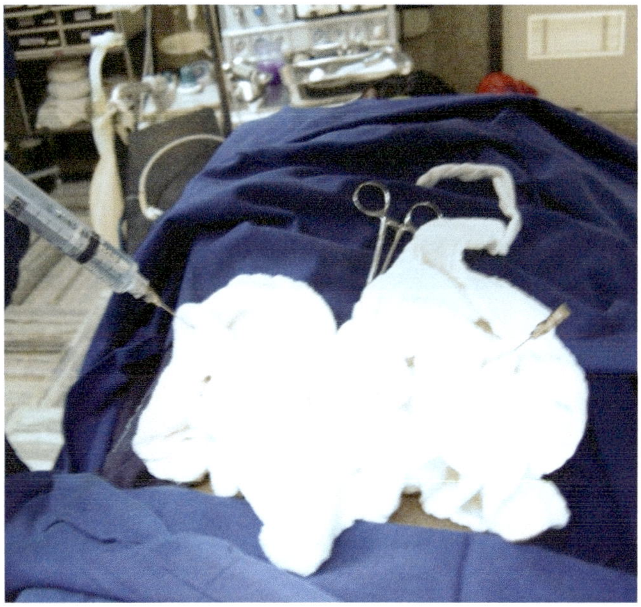

Fig. 3: Sponge around needles during celiac plexus block.

- While withdrawing, flush the needle with a local anesthetic agent into the track to reduce the postprocedure pain at the puncture site.
  - Keep one copy of a printout or CD for record purpose and give one to the patient.
  - Maintain record of postprocedure monitoring of vital signs.
  - Follow-up advice must be included.
- Dosage and schedule of medications
- Explain about the possible side effects of the drug.
- Date and time of the next visit
- Driving instruction to the patient if driving by himself.

CONCLUSION

The above protocol for pain block is for safety, to add credibility to the procedure and so to the pain physician.

The following protocol is necessary for self-accountability and for self-defense of any eventuality in medicolegal issues.

REFERENCE

1. Baheti DK. Protocol for Interventional Pain Procedures: A Suggested Format. In: Baheti DK, Bakshi S, Gupta S, Gehdoo RP (Eds). Interventional Pain Management: A Practical Approach. New Delhi: Jaypee Brothers Medical Publishers (P) Ltd; 2010. pp. 50-3.

11 CHAPTER

Evaluation of the Chronic Pain Patient

Evan C Grant, Julia M Webb, Pratik J Gandhi, Jacob R Peacock, Alex Moroz

ABSTRACT

Effective evaluation of the patient with chronic pain entails a thorough pain history, a focused physical examination, and imaging/diagnostic studies. The pain history is a tool in which the examiner methodically addresses the numerous characteristics of pain to formulate a preliminary differential diagnosis. Further inquiries are directed at evaluating the patient's comorbidities as well as establishing a perspective as to the interplay between the patient's social history and psychological state. The history, in turn, guides the focused physical examination, in which the physician obtains objective information to further his or her diagnostic suspicions. Lastly, imaging, laboratory tests, and electrodiagnostic studies serve to solidify the working diagnosis and to direct management.

INTRODUCTION

Effective management of the chronic pain patient begins with a comprehensive assessment, including specialized history, focused physical examination, and appropriate imaging or testing. The evolution of our understanding of chronic pain as a complicated disease entity with implications on a patient's physical, mental, and social well-being necessitates employing the biopsychosocial model.[1] Unlike many medical conditions, chronic pain offers the clinician few objectives and reliable clinical signs as pain, by definition, is a subjective experience. However, systematic assessment, consistent documentation, and focused physical examination provide the clinician with information to determine etiology, shape an appropriate treatment plan and monitor response to therapy.

THE PAIN HISTORY

The pain history emphasizes a problem-focused approach to systematically characterize pain using the "OPQRST" mnemonic that represents the following components:[2]

- Onset
- Provocation/palliation
- Quality
- Region/radiation
- Severity
- Temporality.

Onset

Assess the time and the circumstances under which the pain initially occurred. Pain that occurred spontaneously versus in the setting of a specific injury or activity, or the patient's perception of such, may have very different effects on the patient's attribution of pain and perceived self-efficacy.

Provocation and Palliation

Identify activities, treatments, movements, or situations that make the pain better or worse. This not only provides clues to etiology but also assists the patient and pain practitioner in creating a repertoire of management strategies. For example, back pain that is exacerbated with prolonged standing but improves with walking in a forward-flexed posture is classically associated with lumbar spinal stenosis. Back pain, which increases transiently when coughing or sneezing, suggests intervertebral disk bulge or herniation.

Quality

Ask the patient to describe the pain using a standard set of terms. Certain descriptors are reliably associated with distinct types of pain.[3,4] For example, "aching", "dull", and "throbbing" suggest somatic pain mediated by nociception.[5] "Burning", "tingling", and "electric" are more commonly associated with neuropathic pain.[6]

Region and Radiation

Assess the location of the pain, and the extent of radiation, if present. The patient can verbally describe the pain or draw the distribution of pain on a pain diagram.[7] Radiating pain is associated with, but not specific to, radicular pain. The perception of radiation can occur in other pain conditions such as trigger points or peripheral neuropathy. Pain diagrams have limited predictive value in determining the etiology of pain but do assist the patient and practitioner. Description of pain location has moderate reliability in predicting the etiology of pain.[8]

Severity

Pain is a subjective experience and intensity is based on a patient's self-report. The most widely accepted unidimensional rating scales for measuring pain intensity are the numeric rating scale (NRS-11), visual analog scales (VAS), and category rating scales. The NRS-11 assesses pain on an 11-point scale of 0–10 where "0" represents "no pain at all" and "10" represents "the worst pain imaginable". VAS employs a 10 cm line anchored at each pole by descriptors of each pain dimension assessed. The patient marks the severity of the dimension on the line, and the distance is measured by the examiner. Categorical rating scales use descriptors of discrete pain dimensions such as "mild, moderate, or severe".

The Wong-Baker FACES® Pain Rating Scale[9] combines numeric ratings from 0 to 10 in increments of 2 with corresponding verbal descriptors from "No Hurt" to "Worst Hurt", each of which is matched to faces depicting increasing levels of discomfort. Although it was initially developed for use in a pediatric population, it has been validated for use with a wide range of populations.

Regardless of the type of scale used, the same scale should be used to assess pain intensity at each visit as the scales are not interchangeable. Although these scales are meant to assess the somatosensory intensity of pain, the intensity rating is often influenced by other aspects of the pain experience, such as anxiety, catastrophizing and functional impairments.

Additional dimensions of pain are more adequately assessed with multidimensional pain questionnaires. The widely used McGill Pain Questionnaire is a checklist of 87 sensory and emotional descriptors related to the pain experience. It also includes a body map on which the patient marks the location of the pain.

Other multidimensional pain questionnaires include the initial pain assessment tool, which is administered at the first visit and assesses multiple dimensions of pain and the influence of pain on activities of daily living such as sleep, appetite, relationships, and emotions.[10]

The brief pain inventory measures the sensory component of pain in addition to quality-of-life indicators.[10] The Short-Form McGill Pain Questionnaire (SF-MPQ-2) is a validated assessment of pain using words to describe pain, and its various components, including sleep, appetite and activity, and accompanying symptoms.[11]

Temporality

The temporal patterns to assess pain include fluctuations or progression in pain intensity or quality over the course of a day or relapsing and remitting, progressive, or steady. Fluctuations in pain intensity over the course of a day correlate with certain pathologies and can help determine modifications to activity. Ascertain overall pain intensity not only at the time of initial evaluation but also ask the patient to recall intensity and function 2 weeks ago, 1 month ago, and 1 year ago to assess the pain symptoms as related to the time of day and if, in general, the pain is relapsing or remitting, steady, or steadily progressive. Use caution in interpreting patient recall of pain intensity as many factors, namely intensity of current pain, may inflate recall of pain intensity.

Associated Symptoms

Ask the patient if there are any symptoms associated with the pain such as numbness, tingling, or weakness. Be vigilant for the "Red Flag" symptoms associated with back pain which include thoracic pain, loss of bowel or bladder control, saddle anesthesia, fever or unexplained weight loss, progressive weakness, or gait disturbance as these are associated with infection, malignancy, or the surgical emergency cauda equina.

SOCIAL HISTORY

Almost no facet of life is spared from chronic pain. And develop a complete portrait of a patient's life including occupational history, social support, and substance use history.

A detailed and complete assessment of substance use is essential for safe and responsible prescribing of opioid pain medicine. Numerous scales and questionnaires can assist in this assessment. Substance dependence and abuse are associated with chronic pain but should not prevent patients from receiving adequate pain treatment.[12] Occupational history provides information about functional status, activity requirements at work, and potential exposure to injury. Among the important aspects to assess pain are time requirements for sitting or standing at a computer station and specific activity requirements.

Lower socioeconomic status is related to lower levels of function in chronic pain patients.[13] Social isolation or poor social support is also related to lower levels of function in chronic pain patients.

PSYCHOLOGICAL AND PSYCHIATRIC ASSESSMENT OF THE PAIN PATIENT

Pain catastrophizing and anxiety correlate with disability from pain.[14] Increasing evidence for pain-related disability and anxiety is directly related to a patient's perceived pain and also increases a patient's pain.[15]

FUNCTIONAL ASSESSMENT

The 18 items of the functional independence measure are each scored from 1 (complete dependence) to 7 (complete independence) and assess activities of daily living, including self-care, mobility, and bowel and bladder management. It provides an objective means to assess baseline functional status and subsequent progress. The Oswestry low back pain disability index[16] evaluates disability specifically related to back pain.

PHYSICAL EXAMINATION

Information obtained in the history guides the physical examination of the chronic pain patient. The examination serves as a useful tool for exploring suspicions generated by the patient's history and for narrowing the differential diagnosis. An examiner must systematically investigate the integrity of muscles, bones, tendons, ligaments, bursae, and other soft tissues. He or she must also seek peripheral or central neurological causes of pain. A comprehensive examination should, therefore, include a general examination, a detailed musculoskeletal examination, and a neurological examination, when appropriate.

General Examination

The goal of the general examination is to provide context meant to supplement findings from detailed musculoskeletal and neurological examinations. Vital signs, including blood pressure, heart rate, temperature, and respiratory rate, are recorded initially. Aberrations in vital signs may signal systemic inflammatory or infectious processes or may occur as a result of pain. The examiner can evaluate a patient's gait before he or she reaches the examination table. An antalgic gait results from an effort to offload a painful joint, while a Trendelenburg gait, recurvatum, or steppage gait suggests muscle weakness. The patient's dress, hygiene, and facial expression lend contextual clues regarding the patient's pain. A general systemic examination (cardiovascular, respiratory, abdominal, etc.) should be performed to explore the possibility of viscerally mediated pain.

Musculoskeletal Examination

It is imperative that the patient is gowned prior to the start of the musculoskeletal examination. An initial musculoskeletal survey comprises inspection, palpation, and range-of-motion maneuvers about the joint or structure in question.[17] The examiner inspects structures bilaterally in order to appreciate bodily asymmetries. Atrophy can be a subtle finding best illuminated when one side is compared to the other. Skin changes include Heberden's nodes seen in osteoarthritis, Bouchard's nodes in rheumatoid arthritis, and erythema, which suggest infection. Erythema over a joint suggests either septic or gouty arthritis, which accompanies inflammation of bone, tendon, or bursa. Displaced fractures often manifest with visible bone deformities. The curvatures of the cervical and thoracolumbar spines should be inspected individually, and in combination, as an abnormal curvature in the inferior spine can influence that of the cervical spine.[18] The peak iliac crest heights should be equal.[18] Valgus and varus deformities must be observed, if present.

Palpation, range of motion, and special maneuvers are performed in order to identify and reproduce pain. As such, the examiner must be gentle when performing the examination to avoid imposing unwarranted discomfort.

The caregiver begins palpation in a region slightly removed from the suspect source of tenderness and then palpates toward it. Palpation of the trapezius, including upper, middle, and lower fibers, as well as the scalenes and posterior cervical and capital musculature, is important for the detection of myofascial pain or muscle spasm. The paraspinal muscles, iliac crests, ischial tuberosities, and trochanteric bursae should also be palpated. Myofascial trigger points manifest as firm knots of tissue associated with tenderness, as well as radiation of pain. Palpation of a spinous process step-off accompanies vertebral compression fractures or spondylolisthesis.[18] Palpation of cervical facets is useful in the evaluation of neck dysfunction.[19]

As with palpation, range-of-motion maneuvers can be used to provoke pain. Flexion, extension, lateral bending, and rotation about the neck should be smooth and synchronized.[20] These motions reveal pathology about the atlantoaxial and facet joints. Similar maneuvers are performed with the lumbar spine, in addition to the oblique extension, to assess for zygapophyseal joint pain.

Special Maneuvers

Special maneuvers associated with each joint can reveal neurological causes for pain in addition to musculoskeletal ones. A Spurling's maneuver is performed by rotating the patient's head to one side while extending simultaneously.[21] The examiner provides an axial load by pressing inferiorly about the patient's head, narrowing cervical neuroforamina. This test has good diagnostic accuracy when used in combination with other provocative tests and examination items.[22] Lhermitte's test is performed with passive flexion of the neck with the patient in the seated position. Paresthesias or an electrical sensation traveling down the spine is thought to indicate cervical spinal cord pathology.[18] The straight-leg-raise maneuver has some diagnostic utility under circumstances in which the prevalence of lumbar disk herniation is high.[23] With the patient in the supine position, the hip is passively flexed to 30–70°.[24] This applies tension to lumbar nerve as it traverses the narrowed neuroforamina. Leg pain radiating beyond the knee is indicative of disk herniation.

When myelopathy is suspected, the examiner should attempt to elicit a Hoffmann's reflex. Findings of bilateral intrinsic hand muscle wasting, distal numbness and tingling, hyper-reflexia, and weakness should pique one's suspicion.[25] To perform the test, the examiner extends the patient's wrist and grasps the 3rd digit.[26] The distal phalanx is forcefully flicked. Subsequent flexion of the 1st and/or 2nd digits indicates a positive Hoffmann's test. The reliability of the test is considered poor in isolation[27] but may be useful when combined with other subjective and objective findings.

The sacroiliac (SI) joint does not produce motor, reflex, or sensory dysfunction and must therefore be tested using a variety of provocative tests.[18] The standing flexion test is performed with the patient in the standing position. The examiner places his or her thumbs on the patient's posterior superior iliac spine (PSIS) bilaterally, and the patient flexes forward with knees extended. An asymmetric anterior or superior tilt of one PSIS suggests hypomobility and indicates SI joint arthritis, tight hamstrings or quadratus lumborum, or hip joint restriction. To perform the pelvic compression test, the examiner applies a medially directed force to the patient positioned on his or her side. This stretches the posterior ligaments overlying the joint, eliciting pain if SI joint dysfunction is present.[28] The examiner can place a stretching force on the anterior SI ligaments by placing hands on bilateral anterior superior iliac spines with the patient in supine position and pressing posterolaterally.[29] This is called the distraction test and is considered positive if pain is reproduced. The Patrick test was originally described in 1917 as an indicator of hip arthritis if inguinal pain was elicited.[30] However, Kenna later reported that low back pain provoked by the same maneuver suggested SI joint dysfunction.[31] This test is performed with the patient in the supine position. The hip is flexed, and the ankle is placed and maintained over the patella. The hip is passively externally rotated with an inferiorly directed force at the medial knee. The Gaenslen maneuver is thought to induce pain by imparting a rotating force about the pelvis, resulting in abnormal motion about the SI joint.[32] To perform this maneuver, the patient lies supine and flexes the corresponding hip and knee. The patient hangs the contralateral leg over the table and the examiner gradually hyperextends this leg while stabilizing the flexed knee with the opposite. Low back pain suggests SI joint pathology, though lumbar nerve root lesions have also been implicated.[18]

Neurological Examination

The appeal of many of the eponymous special techniques stems from biomechanical basis they provide for various pain etiologies. However, the sensitivities and specificities of these tests are often inadequate for establishing a confident diagnosis. Further physical examination elements, such as motor, sensory, and reflex testing, must therefore be performed to strengthen one's suspicion. C7 radiculopathy may present with triceps weakness, a diminished triceps reflex, and loss of sensation in the C7 dermatomal distribution unilaterally. Myelopathy, on the other hand, may be present symmetrically and bilaterally, with weakness and numbness spanning multiple dermatomes and myotomes, in addition to hyper-reflexia. Asymmetric findings suggest radiculopathy, though the possibility of concurrent radiculopathy and myelopathy must be considered.

Nonorganic Signs

There exists a subset of patients for which subjective and objective data obtained during an evaluation do not fit commonly understood patterns of pain. In 1980, Waddell described a battery of signs, including tenderness, simulation, distraction, regional, and overreaction, to be used as a screen for "nonorganic" pain.[33] The battery includes maneuvers such as the seated versus supine straight leg raise, which serves as a means to determine if complaints of pain in both positions are consistent. The applicability of these tests during an office visit is uncertain, as their validity as a means of screening for malingering or underlying psychogenic contribution to pain has been questioned in recent years.[34] It may remain a reliable predictor of poor outcomes for treatment, both surgical and otherwise.

DIAGNOSTIC TESTING

Diagnostic testing provides additional support for pathology suspected from the pain history and physical examination. However, with few exceptions, treatment should be based primarily on clinical findings and not imaging or other testing.

Laboratory

Basic laboratory tests may identify common diagnoses and predispositions to pain etiologies such as vitamin deficiency, diabetes, thyroid dysfunction, or chronic inflammation.

Imaging

The history and physical examination should be used to formulate a clinical diagnosis and guide imaging. Computed tomography is most appropriate for imaging of bony structures, infection, or acute bleeding. Magnetic resonance imaging (MRI) is indicated for imaging of soft tissues such as the spinal cord, nerve roots, and intervertebral disks. It should be noted that the quantity of MRI findings does not necessarily correlate with the degree of disability.[35] If any red flags or alarm signs are present, imaging should be performed to evaluate for possible infection or malignancy. Ultrasound provides real-time imaging of superficial structures of soft tissues such as muscles, tendons, and ligaments without exposing the patient to radiation.

Neurophysiologic Testing

Nerve conduction studies and needle electromyography assist the clinician in localizing lesions that may cause weakness or pain.[36] In addition, the needle electromyography portion of this examination provides information about the degree of denervation and reinnervation.

CONCLUSION

The subjective and objective data obtained from taking a history and performing a physical examination on a patient with chronic pain serve many purposes. The value of a thorough history obtained with a systematic scheme of questioning cannot be overstated. Before the first physical examination element is performed, the examiner should have formulated a relatively narrow differential diagnosis. The history guides the physical examination, which serves to corroborate or dispel the suspicions previously formulated. The information thus obtained should guide further testing in the form of laboratory, radiographic, and neurophysiologic testing. In aggregate, the history, physical examination, and diagnostic testing results should posture the physician to impart therapies targeted at the patient's suspected/confirmed condition.

REFERENCES

1. Nielson WR, Weir R. Biopsychosocial approaches to the treatment of chronic pain. Clin J Pain. 2001;17(Suppl 4): S114-27.
2. Toth C, Moulin D. Neuropathic Pain: Causes, Management, and Understanding. New York: Cambridge University Press; 2013.
3. Jensen MP, Johnson LE, Gertz KJ, Galer BS, Gammaitoni AR. The words patients use to describe chronic pain: implications for measuring pain quality. Pain. 2013;154(12):2722-8.
4. Lin CP, Kupper AE, Gammaitoni AR, Galer BS, Jensen MP. Frequency of chronic pain descriptors: implications for assessment of pain quality. Eur J Pain. 2011;15(6):628-33.

5. Dworkin RH, Jensen MP, Gammaitoni AR, Olaleye DO, Galer BS. Symptom profiles differ in patients with neuropathic versus non-neuropathic pain. J Pain. 2007;8(2):118-26.
6. Galer BS, Jensen MP. Development and preliminary validation of a pain measure specific to neuropathic pain: the Neuropathic Pain Scale. Neurology. 1997;48(2):332-8.
7. Andersen T, Christensen FB, Høy KW, Helmig,P, Niedermann B, Hansen ES, et al. The predictive value of pain drawings in lumbar spinal fusion surgery. Spine J. 2010;10(5):372-9.
8. Depalma MJ, Ketchum JM, Trussell BS, Saullo TR, Slipman CW. Does the location of low back pain predict its source? PM R. 2011;3:33-9.
9. Baker C, Wong D. (2014). Wong-Baker FACES® Pain Rating Scale. [online] Available from http://wongbakerfaces.org/ [Last accessed June, 2015].
10. Cleeland CS, Ryan KM. Pain assessment: global use of the Brief Pain Inventory. Ann Acad Med Singapore. 1994;23(2):129-38.
11. Dworkin RH, Turk DC, Revicki DA, Harding G, Coyne KS, Peirce-Sandner S, et al. Development and initial validation of an expanded and revised version of the Short-form McGill Pain Questionnaire (SF-MPQ-2). Pain. 2009;144(1-2):35-42.
12. Egli M, Koob GF, Edwards S. Alcohol dependence as a chronic pain disorder. Neurosci Biobehav Rev. 2012; 36(10):2179-92.
13. Fitzcharles MA, Rampakakis E, Ste-Marie PA, Sampalis JS, Shir Y. The association of socioeconomic status and symptom severity in persons with fibromyalgia. J Rheumatol. 2014;41(7):1398-404.
14. Wong WS, Lam HM, Chow YF, Chen PP, Lim HS, Wong S, et al. The effects of anxiety sensitivity, pain hypervigilance, and pain catastrophizing on quality of life outcomes of patients with chronic pain: a preliminary, cross-sectional analysis. Qual Life Res. 2014;23(8):pp.2333-41.
15. Sternbach RA, Janowsky DS, Huey LY, Segal DS. Effects of altering brain serotonin activity on human chronic pain. In: Bonica JJ, Albe-Fessard D (Eds). Advances in Pain Research and Therapy. New York: Raven Press; 1976. pp. 601-5.
16. Changulani M, Shaju A. Evaluation of responsiveness of Oswestry low back pain disability index. Arch Orthop Trauma Surg. 2009;129(5):691-4.
17. Lynn S, Peter G. Bates' Guide to Physical Examination and History Taking. Philadelphia: Lippincott Williams & Wilkins; 2007.
18. Malanga GA, Nadler S. Musculoskeletal Physical Examination: An Evidence-Based Approach. Philadelphia: Elsevier Mosby; 2006. p. 353.
19. Sandmark H, Nisell R. Validity of five common manual neck pain provoking tests. Scand J Rehabil Med. 1995;27(3):131-6.
20. Waldman SD. Physical Diagnosis of Pain: An Atlas of Signs and Symptoms, 2nd edition. Philadelphia: Saunders/ Elsevier; 2010. p. 357.
21. Schneck JM. The unilateral Hoffmann reflex; clinical note. J Nerv Ment Dis. 1946;104(6):597.
22. Wainner RS, Fritz JM, Irrgang JJ, BoningerML, Delitto A, Allison S. Reliability and diagnostic accuracy of the clinical examination and patient self-report measures for cervical radiculopathy. Spine (Phila Pa 1976). 2003;28(1): 52-62.
23. van der Windt DA, Simons E, Riphagen II, Ammendolia C, Verhagen AP, Laslett M, et al. Physical examination for lumbar radiculopathy due to disc herniation in patients with low-back pain. Cochrane Database Syst Rev. 2010(2):CD007431.
24. Deyo RA, Rainville J, Kent DL. What can the history and physical examination tell us about low back pain? JAMA. 1992;268(6):760-5.
25. Yu YL, Woo E, Huang CY. Cervical spondylotic myelopathy and radiculopathy. Acta Neurol Scand. 1987;75(6): 367-73.
26. Echols DH. The Hoffmann sign: Its incidence in university students. J Nerv Ment Dis. 1936;84(4):427-31.
27. Glaser JA, Curé JK, Bailey KL, Morrow DL. Cervical spinal cord compression and the Hoffmann sign. Iowa Orthop J. 2001;21:49-52.
28. McCombe PF, Fairbank JC, Cockersole BC, Pynsent PB. 1989 Volvo Award in clinical sciences. Reproducibility of physical signs in low-back pain. Spine (Phila Pa 1976). 1989;14(9):908-18.
29. Thompson M, Newton DR, Grainger RG. Discussion of the clinical and radiological aspects of sacroiliac disease. Proc R Soc Med. 1957;50(10):847-58.
30. Patrick HT. Brachial neuritis and sciatica. JAMA. 1917;69:2176-9.
31. Kenna C, Murtagh J. Patrick or fabere test to test hip and sacroiliac joint disorders. Aust Fam Physician. 1989;18(4):375.
32. Gaenslen FJ. Sacroiliac arthrodesis: indicators, author's technique and end results. JAMA. 1927;89(24):2031-5.
33. Waddell G, McCulloch JA, Kummel E, Venner RM. Nonorganic physical signs in low-back pain. Spine (Phila Pa 1976). 1980;5(2):117-25.
34. Fishbain DA, Cole B, Cutler RB, Lewis J, Rosomoff Hl, Rosomoff RS. A structured evidence-based review on the meaning of nonorganic physical signs: Waddell signs. Pain Med. 2003;4(2):141-81.
35. Berg L, Hellum C, Gjertsen Ø, Neckelmann G, Johnsen LG, Storheim K, et al. Do more MRI findings imply worse disability or more intense low back pain? A cross-sectional study of candidates for lumbar disc prosthesis. Skeletal Radiol. 2013;42(11):1593-602.
36. Coster S, de Bruijn SF, Tavy DL. Diagnostic value of history, physical examination and needle electromyography in diagnosing lumbosacral radiculopathy. J Neurol. 2010;257(3):332-7.

12 CHAPTER

Stimulation-guided Pain Mapping

Sanjeeva Gupta

ABSTRACT

The nerve roots involved in carrying the nociceptive impulses can be identified either by looking at the pain dermatomal diagram or by injection of a small amount of local anesthetic along the nerve roots involved and assessing the patient's response. There is always a possibility that the injected local anesthetic can soak adjacent nerve roots, which can confuse the issue. Stimulation-guided stereotactic pain mapping allows us to identify the nerve root(s) involved in carrying the nociceptive impulses and provides us an anatomical diagnosis of the nerve root(s) involved. This can provide us and/or our surgical colleagues with information to target the site of pathology with available treatments precisely. This chapter explains the technique of stimulation-guided pain mapping.

INTRODUCTION

Pain is a subjective symptom, and expression of pain for the same degree of nociceptive input can vary between individuals. The nerve root(s) involved in carrying the nociceptive impulses can be identified either by looking at the pain dermatomal diagram or by injection of a small amount of local anesthetic along the nerve root(s) involved and assessing the patient's response. There is always a possibility that the injected local anesthetic can soak adjacent nerve roots, which can confuse the issue. Stimulation-guided stereotactic pain mapping allows us to identify the nerve root(s) involved in carrying the pain impulses and gives us an anatomical diagnosis of the nerve roots involved. This can provide us and/or our surgical colleagues with information to target the site of pathology with available treatments precisely.

Surgical teams at times ask pain medicine specialists to perform a diagnostic nerve root block to identify the nerve root involved in pain generation to aid surgical intervention. In these circumstances when a nerve root block or a transforaminal epidural injection is performed, it is more than likely that the injectate will spread beyond the nerve root in question. Sensory stimulation of the appropriate nerve(s) to reproduce the patient's pain before injecting the local anesthetic and steroid may assist in identifying the pathological nerve(s) and may also be therapeutic.

INDICATIONS

The procedure is indicated when patients have pain in a particular part of the body and the nerve root(s) involved in carrying the pain impulses need to be identified to plan further management.

CONTRAINDICATIONS

- *Absolute contraindications:* Systemic or localized bacterial infection in the region of the block to be performed, bleeding diathesis, patients on anticoagulants, and pregnancy.
- *Relative contraindications:* Allergy to contrast medium and local anesthetic

EQUIPMENT

- Fluoroscopy is mandatory. The procedure is performed under aseptic conditions. 25G and 23G hypodermic needles, and 2 and 5 mL syringes can be used.
- A 22G, 100-mm long straight or curved tip radiofrequency needle with 5- or 10-mm active tip is used. Intravenous solutions, sedation, or antibiotics are not required.
- Lignocaine 1% for local anesthesia

PROCEDURE

The patient is assessed for the suitability of the procedure, and an informed consent is obtained. The procedure is done under strict aseptic conditions and fluoroscopic guidance. A 22G, 100-mm long radiofrequency needle with a 5- or 10-mm active tip is placed along the dorsal root ganglion (DRG)/nerve root in question using a subpedicular technique[1-5] and sensory stimulation applied at 50 Hz **(Figs. 1 to 4)**. The stimulation is gradually increased, and the patient's response is assessed. The part of the body where the patient experiences pain and/or paresthesia on sensory stimulation is noted. The optimal stimulation at which the pain and/or paresthesia is reproduced should be between 0.3 and 0.6 V. The same procedure is carried out at the adjacent levels if appropriate until all the areas where the patient experiences pain are mapped. Once the procedure is complete, the information obtained is used to identify the DRG(s)/nerve root(s) involved in carrying the pain impulses from the painful area and further treatment is planned.

As an example, the author had a patient who had a degloving injury to his left lower limb. When the above technique was used, the author was able to reproduce the patient's pain in the left lower limb on stimulating the left L3, L4, and L5 DRG/nerve roots between 0.3 and 0.5 V.

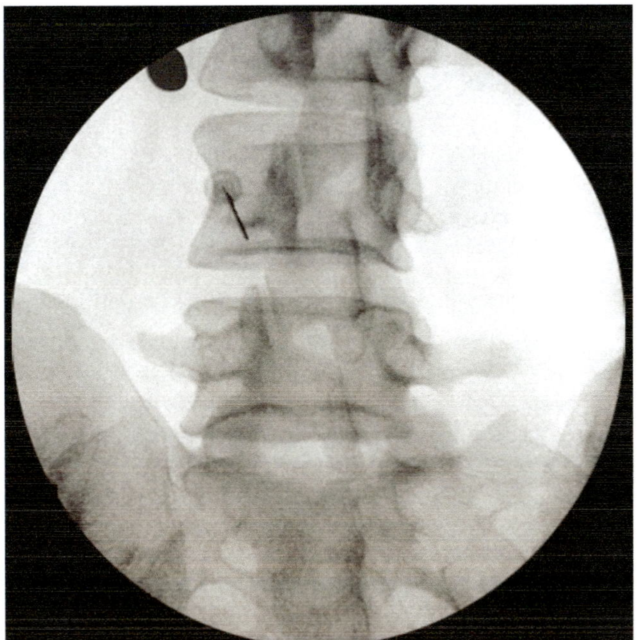

Fig. 1: Radiofrequency needle in position just below the left L4 pedicle in left oblique view.

This patient had a pulsed radiofrequency procedure of the respective DRG and obtained significant pain relief. Similar procedures to identify the DRGs/nerve roots

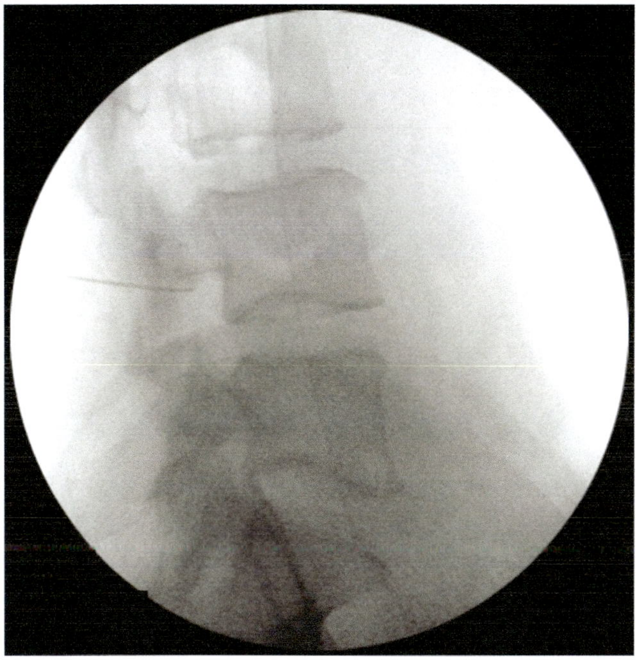

Fig. 2: Tip of the radiofrequency needle in the intervertebral foramen at L4 level in lateral view.

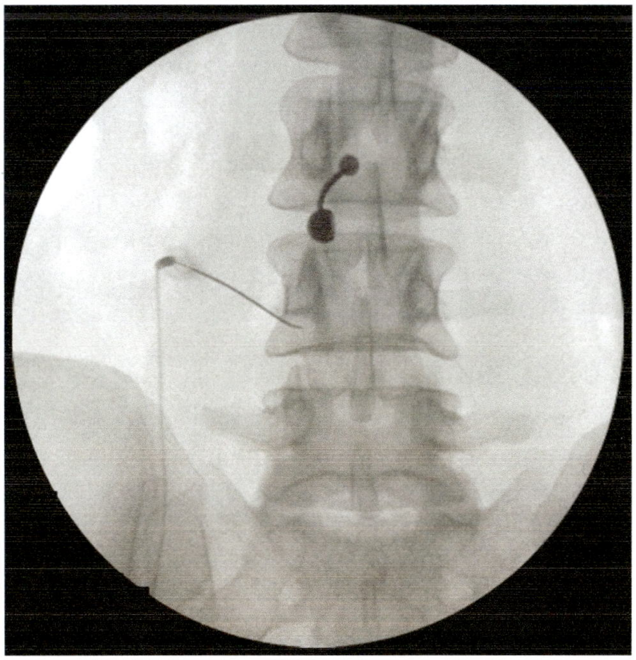

Fig. 3: Tip of the needle below the left L4 pedicle in anteroposterior (AP) view. Note that the tip of the needle is at about the 6 o'clock position of L4 pedicle. Sensory stimulation is carried out to find out if the patient's pain in the left lower limb is reproduced.

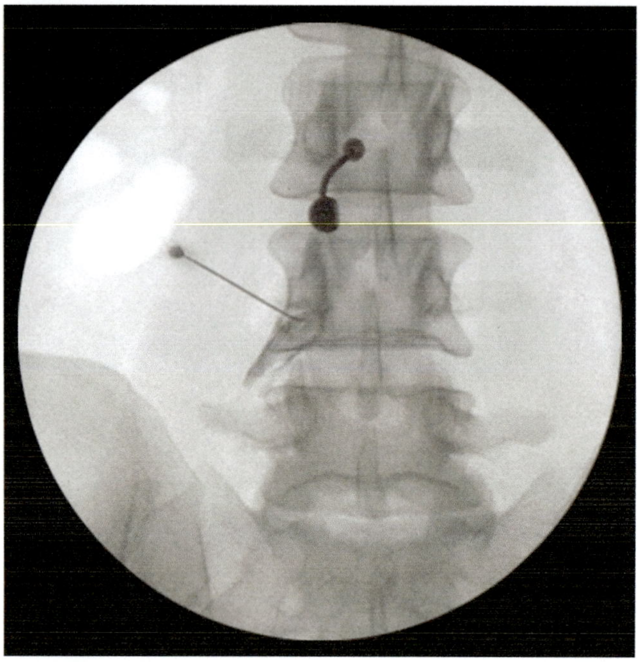

Fig. 4: Injection of contrast medium outlines the left L4 nerve root along with the dorsal root ganglion.

involved in nociceptive perception have been carried out at the thoracic levels for patients presenting with chronic chest pain due to various causes.

The author has also had instances where surgical colleagues have requested a nerve root block to be performed to diagnose if a particular nerve is involved in the pathology in the lumbar spine area giving rise to the neuropathic pain in the lower limb to facilitate surgical treatment. In such circumstances, the author has used the technique of stimulation-guided pain mapping to reproduce the patient's pain before injecting a mixture of local anesthesia and steroid.

DISCUSSION

If the needle is appropriately placed, pain and/or paresthesia is produced in a dermatomal distribution. If the patient experiences pain and/or paresthesia in the area where he/she normally experiences pain, this suggests that the DRG/nerve root(s) in question is involved in pain perception. One or several levels can be tested in a similar manner to assist with accurate diagnosis to plan further available treatments. As the stimulation-guided pain mapping is done before injecting local anesthesia and steroid, the possibility of local anesthetic spillage to adjacent DRG/nerve root(s) impacting our assessment is overcome.

In the case mentioned above, the patient's symptoms were reproduced on stimulating the left L3, L4, and L5 DRGs. The patient had DRG/nerve root(s) block which helped temporarily. Subsequently, the patient had a pulsed radiofrequency procedure at the same levels and benefited significantly. In another patient with chronic chest wall pain following rib fractures, clinical examination suggested that the pain could be in the area of T6, T7, and T8 distribution but on stimulation of the T7 DRG/nerve root the patient's entire pain symptoms were reproduced indicating the precise DRG/nerve root involved in carrying the pain impulse. This assisted in planning further treatment.

We can also assist our surgical colleagues in identifying or ruling out if a DRG/nerve root is responsible for the patient's pain by using the technique of stimulating-guided pain mapping before injecting the local anesthesia and steroid enabling them to plan further treatment if the local anesthetic and steroid injection do not help the patient significantly.

CONCLUSION

In the author's opinion, stimulation-guided pain mapping can be a very useful technique in selected groups of patients in identifying the DRG/nerve root(s) involved in the pathology and this can help target available treatments precisely.

REFERENCES

1. Baheti DK, Gupta S. Transforaminal lumbar epidural block. In: Baheti DK, Gupta S, Bakshi S, Gehdoo RP (Eds). Atlas of Interventional Pain Management Procedures: A Stepwise Approach. New Delhi: Jaypee Brothers Medical Publishers; 2023. pp. 111-20.
2. Gupta S, Baheti DK, Bakshi S. Lumbar transforaminal epidural steroid injection: technical chalanges. In: Baheti DK, Gupta S, Bakshi S, Gehdoo RP (Eds). Atlas of Interventional Pain Management Procedures: A Stepwise Approach. New Delhi: Jaypee Brothers Medical Publishers; 2023. pp. 121-31.
3. Bogduk N. Lumbar transforaminal access. In: Bogduk N (Ed). Practice Guidelines for Spinal Diagnostic and Treatment Procedures, 2nd edition. San Francisco, USA: Spinal Intervention Society; 2013. pp. 459-538.
4. Guarino AH, Staats PS. Diagnostic neural blockade in the management of pain. Pain Digest. 1997;7:194-9.
5. Levy BA. Diagnostic, prognostic, and therapeutic nerve blocks. Arch Surg. 1997;112:870-9.

3

SECTION

Head and Neck

13 CHAPTER

Trigeminal Nerve Block

Ramkumar Kalaiyarasan, Manohar L Sharma

ABSTRACT

Percutaneous trigeminal, as one-level interventions, are very effective and rewarding for medically refractory trigeminal neuralgia (TGN) as well as in cancer-related pain in trigeminal nerve distribution. Radiofrequency (RF), balloon microcompression, and glycerol injection around Gasserian ganglion are foramen ovale-based neuroablative procedures as covered in this chapter. It is helpful to have a very good understanding of radiological anatomy to safely conduct these techniques as otherwise there can be serious long-term complications. Provision of balanced information about risks and benefits of these techniques and letting patients decide their preferred option is very valuable as their perception of risks may not be the same as that of an operator. Following these procedures, patients usually have numbness in the trigeminal nerve distribution for variable periods. These should be offered for TGN rather than for atypical facial pain or any other facial pain in distribution of trigeminal nerve. In patients with atypical facial pain or atypical TGN, there is potential for further deterioration in pain if these neuroablative techniques are offered. If magnetic resonance imaging (MRI) scan shows neurovascular compression (conflict) at the trigeminal root entry zone on the affected side, microvascular decompression should be considered as it has excellent long-term outcome. Patients should be offered a clear explanation of the diagnosis and rationale of various treatment options, and they should be empowered to make a choice because of clear information and from the results of these techniques in your practice or hospital. It is recommended to offer written information on these procedures to help informed decision-making. Peripheral nerve blocks of trigeminal nerve with either local anesthetic, steroid, and neurolytic agents including cryotherapy have poorer long-term results along with higher incidence of neuritis-related complication, i.e., dysesthesia. Results of microvascular decompression surgery are poorer in patients with multiple sclerosis (MS) affected with TGN, and hence foramen ovale-based techniques are preferred over microvascular decompression in author's pain service. There are noninvasive techniques available to achieve similar pain relief for patients who may have contraindications to needle-based techniques or microvascular decompression, for example, gamma knife or radiosurgery. However, there is a limit as to how many times this treatment can be offered for fear of local tissue damage or tumor development in the treated area, though this is not confirmed or proven.

INTRODUCTION

The management for trigeminal neuralgia (TGN) can be either a surgical or pharmacological treatment.[1-3] Of the surgical treatment options, microvascular decompression is preferred option as it is almost curative and at 1–2 years, the incidence of complete pain relief is 75–80%. It is not a neuroablative procedure (hence, there are no problems related to deafferentation, i.e., unpleasant dysesthesia or anesthesia dolorosa).[4] If the etiology is at the level of Gasserian ganglion and there is no vascular compression or conflict at the trigeminal root entry zone as seen on imaging, then, the neuroablative procedures, which reduce the ectopic activity of neurons could possibly be used. The pharmacological treatment of TGN is mainly based on the antiepileptic drug carbamazepine, which will suppress the ectopic activity and is very effective, but, patients may have many side effects in short- and long-term.[1] For this reason in Liverpool, United Kingdom

(UK), it is a common practice in author's unit to offer microvascular decompression if magnetic resonance imaging (MRI) scan demonstrates vascular compression at the trigeminal nerve root entry zone.[1] However, 30% people do not get adequate pain relief after the surgical treatment (microvascular decompression) and pharmacological treatment with carbamazepine only helps about 70% people. Therefore, there is need of a service that can offer a range of foramen ovale-based neuroablative interventions. There is a large evidence base from multiple large studies to demonstrate a very good long-term outcome from these interventions.[4] Peripheral nerve blocks are not preferred as often the pain recurs soon and there is higher risk of neuritis-related neuropathic pain.

ANATOMICAL PERSPECTIVE

The trigeminal nerve is a mixed nerve that consists primarily of sensory neurons. It exits the brain on the lateral surface of the pons, entering the trigeminal ganglion within a few millimeters. The trigeminal ganglion corresponds to the dorsal root ganglion of a spinal nerve. Three major branches emerge from the trigeminal ganglion. Each branch innervates a different dermatome. Each branch exits the cranium through a different foramen. The first division (V1; ophthalmic nerve) exits the cranium through the superior orbital fissure, entering the orbit to innervate the globe and skin in the area above the eye and forehead. The second division (V2; maxillary nerve) exits through the foramen rotundum, into a space posterior to the orbit, the pterygopalatine fossa. It supplies the middle third of the face. The third division (V3; mandibular nerve) exits the cranium through an oval hole, the foramen ovale. It supplies the lower third of face. If the proposed needle trajectory is too posterior, it may enter foramen lacerum through which carotid artery passes. If the needle trajectory is too anterior, the needle may enter orbital cavity leading to retrobulbar hemorrhage. If the needle to too medial and deep, injury to cavernous sinus and cranial nerve supplying to eyeball may be encountered. To minimize the risk of complications related to suboptimal needle trajectory, it is preferred to undertake this procedure either in radiology suite with excellent imaging facilities **(Fig. 1)** or the operator should have excellent understanding of radiological anatomy of structures around foramen ovale **(Fig. 2)** and structures which may be along the path of needle trajectory to foramen ovale.

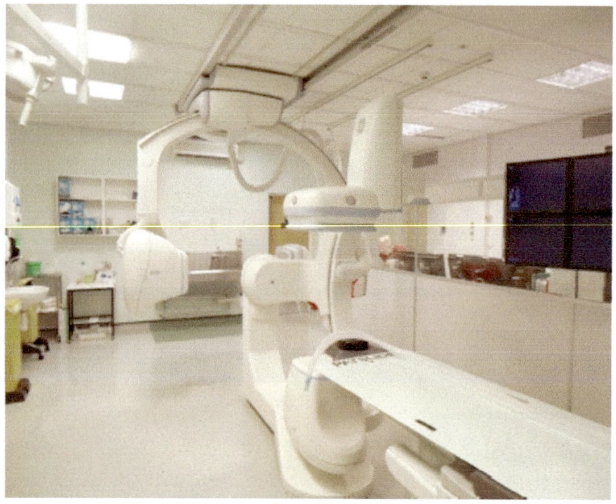

Fig. 1: Radiology biplane room as preferred by author for trigeminal interventions.

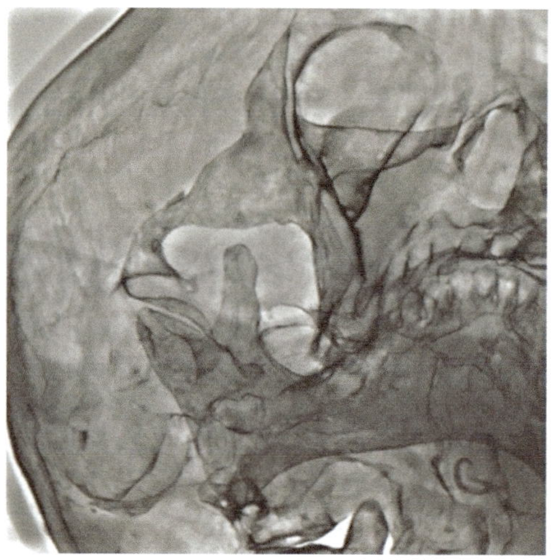

Fig. 2: Overview of radiological anatomy as seen imaging a manikin.

INDICATIONS FOR RADIOFREQUENCY/ BALLOON MICROCOMPRESSION/GLYCEROL INJECTION FOR TRIGEMINAL NEURALGIA

These interventions are indicated for medically refractory TGN and MRI scan not showing neurovascular compression.[5-7] It may be offered to patients with positive MRI scan, if the patient is not keen or fit to have surgery (microvascular decompression). It is very useful and effective for patients with multiple sclerosis (MS) suffering from TGN, as these patients do not respond well to microvascular decompression. Some patients may decide not to have microvascular decompression for fear of brain surgery, and they usually have very good outcomes with foramen ovale-based neuroablative techniques. Most patients who are offered these techniques can come of the medications (usually carbamazepine or other antiepileptic and strong pain killers including opioids) and these result in significant improvement in quality of life and help with severe anxiety for fear of neuralgia returning. There is not much difference in outcomes (pain relief and duration of effect) following various foramen ovale-based techniques, though some operators and patients will have a preference for one technique over other. Along with clinical discussion of pros and cons of various neuroablative options, written information on foramen ovale-based technique may help patients to choose their preferred option (*see* **Appendix 1** on patient information leaflet on balloon compression). There are some major differences as follows, which may decide which option is preferred.

SALIENT FEATURES RELATED TO EACH INTERVENTION AS RELEVANT IN PRACTICE

Radiofrequency Thermocoagulation of the Gasserian Ganglion

- In 1974, Sweet presented his method, which, by and large, is used today.[8]
- This needs the patient's cooperation with sensory stimulation and retesting after the radiofrequency (RF) lesion. It means that patient is awake, and this can be very painful to patient and distressing for the theater team, though this can be well managed by experienced anesthetist and theater team helping the operator.
- It is not preferred for first-division TGN (ophthalmic) for fear of causing irreversible deafferentation and consequences related to loss of corneal reflex and corneal damage.
- This technique is more likely to cause unpleasant dysesthesia including anesthesia dolorosa in comparison to other neuroablative techniques described in this chapter.
- The main advantage of this technique over other two techniques is the ability to control the degree of numbness and target the lesion based on sensory stimulation. However, there is a lot of debate in this area and some authors have published good results with this technique carried out under general anesthesia without the need of patient cooperation. This is outside the scope of this chapter.

Balloon Microcompression of the Gasserian Ganglion

- Balloon microcompression is preferred for first-division TGN (ophthalmic) in comparison with RF technique.
- Patient (operator) prefers to have the whole procedure under general anesthesia.
- Patients usually prefer this to RF in author's experience and the whole procedure is quicker and there is no difference in resource requirement in terms of anesthesia or theater team.
- Custom-made 14G (gauge) cannula and 4 FG Fogarty embolectomy catheter may be used to minimize the cost of the procedure. Author has access to Mullan percutaneous trigeminal balloon microcompression set available from Cook Medical **(Fig. 3)**. This set is more expensive but has many advantages, but these are outside the scope of this chapter.
- Cannula used for balloon compression is 14-G and radiological anatomy should be clearly displayed or there may be significant morbidity if the needle is introduced in the wrong foramen.

Trigeminal Glycerol Injection

- Håkansson introduced the method after a fortuitous discovery during the development of a stereotactic technique for gamma radiation that glycerol mixed

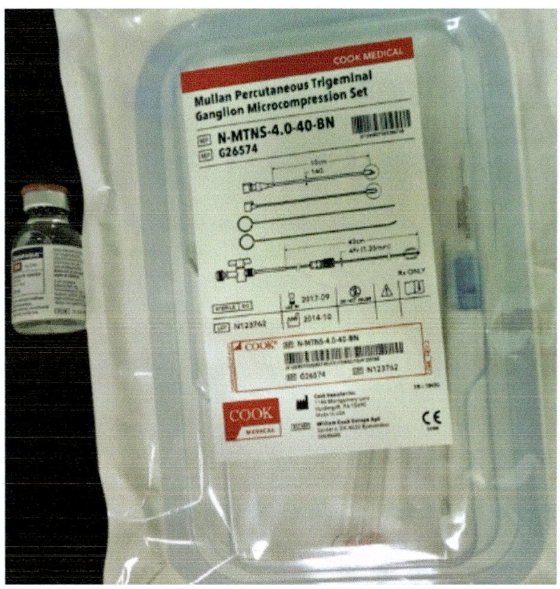

Fig. 3: Mullan percutaneous trigeminal microcompression set and water-soluble contrast (Omnipaque 300).

with tantalum powder not only visualized the trigeminal cistern but also abolished pain in patients with TGN. Technique and outcomes from over 2,500 patients have been described in this chapter.[9]

- This procedure may be carried out either under local anesthesia and sedation or under general anesthesia.
- Author has experience of carrying this for facial pain related to cancer in the distribution of trigeminal nerve.
- In experienced hands, the results of this technique are comparable to RF or balloon compression. Most of the technical considerations are as for RF and balloon compression.
- It is relatively inexpensive in comparison to the earlier mentioned techniques as glycerol is not very expensive.

CONTRAINDICATIONS TO RADIOFREQUENCY OR BALLOON MICROCOMPRESSION OR GLYCEROL INJECTION

The contraindications to RF, balloon microcompression, or glycerol injection are as follows:

- Local or systemic infection
- Bleeding diathesis or anticoagulation
- Numbness in painful area (trigeminal neuropathy)
- Lack of informed consent or patient not accepting of numbness in face
- Atypical TGN as results are not good
- Neuropathic pain in the distribution of trigeminal nerve but features not consistent with TGN.

RADIOFREQUENCY THERMOCOAGULATION OF GASSERIAN GANGLION

Preparation

The preparation includes the following:

- Consent includes discussion of likely success rate and potential complications. This is a potentially neuroablative and irreversible technique and side effects may last for long-term, and hence it is critical to have in-depth discussion of pros and cons of this procedure and need for patient to cooperate at certain stages of the procedure.
- All patients must be warned about the risks of numbness, treatment failure, and potential jaw weakness.
- All patients should have brain MRI to rule out neurovascular compression at the trigeminal root entry zone, tumor, MS, or any other central causes.
- Prepare the patient for general anesthesia and as per the local hospital policies and protocols.
- If taking aspirin, then it should be stopped for 7 days before the proposed date of the procedure.
- Position the patient supine on a radiolucent table with a thin pillow under the head. Thick pillow causes difficulties with visualization of foramen ovale by exaggerating neck flexion. Clear X-ray images are needed, as identification of foramen ovale is essential before inserting the needle.
- *Equipment needed:* RF lesion generator, 22G 100 mm, and RF needle with 5 mm active tip, thermocouple probe for sensory/motor stimulation and RF lesioning, local anesthetic, and simple equipment for sensory examination after the heat lesion or lesion titration.
- Strict asepsis is essential. It is usual to administer one dose of prophylactic antibiotic according to the local guidance.
- An anesthetist must be present to monitor the patient and administer general anesthesia as needed.

Technique

The technique is as follows:

- The C-arm should be positioned with around a 45° caudal tilt and a 15–30° ipsilateral oblique tilt to identify the foramen ovale **(Fig. 4)**. Minor adjustments may be needed to clearly define its margins. Usually, you need to increase caudal tilt to improve visualization of foramen ovale.
- Usually, the foramen ovale is visualized just medial to condyle of mandible **(Fig. 4)**. For beginners, it may be

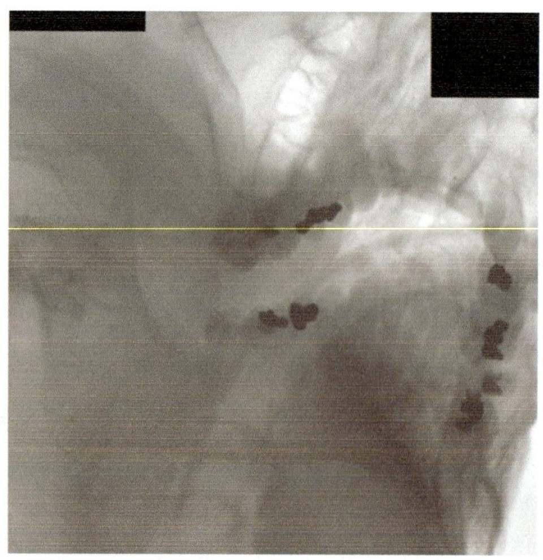

Fig. 4: Good view of foramen ovale with 38° caudal tilt and 24° oblique tilt.

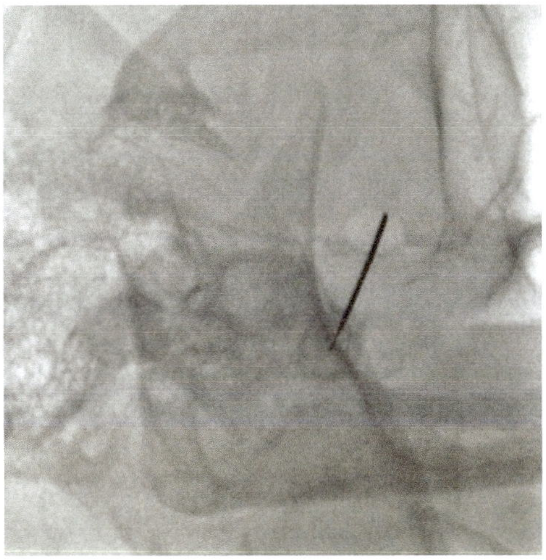

Fig. 5: Radiofrequency cannula through foramen ovale.

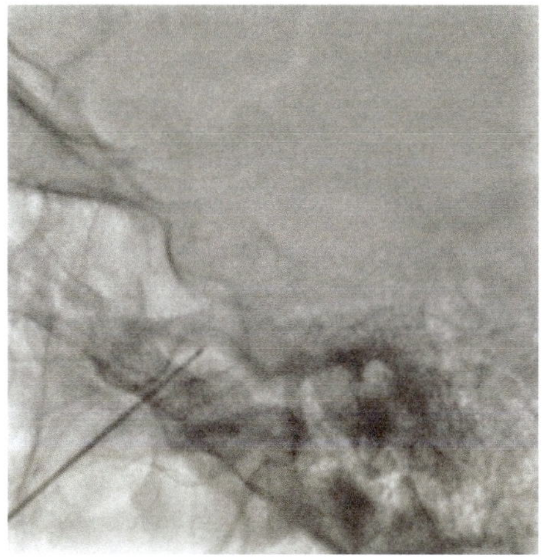

Fig. 6: Adequate insertion depth of radiofrequency cannula through foramen ovale ready for initial sensory stimulation and cannula can be inserted further by few millimeters, if needed.

beneficial to have experienced colleagues in theater or an experienced radiologist/radiographer.

- The entry point of needle is just lateral to the angle of the mouth (2–3 cm). The skin and subcutaneous tissues over this point are infiltrated with local anesthetic.
- An RF needle is advanced carefully toward foramen ovale **(Fig. 5)**. If targeting the second or third division, then enter at about 2 cm away from angle of the mouth aiming for the middle third of foramen ovale. If aiming for the first division, start about 3 cm away from angle of the mouth aiming to medial third of foramen ovale. Usually, it is possible to have tactile sensation while passing through foramen ovale. This can be very painful and general anesthesia or deep sedation may be needed at this stage.
- Perform motor stimulation at 2 Hz. If there are masseter movements at low sensory thresholds (<0.5 V), then advance the needle by couple of mm and retest, until these movements disappear **(Fig. 6)**. While sensory stimulation at the times of masseter movements seen with motor stimulation will produce paresthesia in the V3 distribution, the trigeminal ganglion will be spared of any heating effect of the procedure meaning shorter duration of pain relief. Check the needle position with a lateral X-ray view as well and the needle should not go deeper than an imaginary clival line. Stop anesthetic now, wake the patient, and perform sensory stimulation at 50 Hz. Try to produce paresthesia in the affected division of the trigeminal nerve at low thresholds (0.05–0.2 V). Cerebrospinal fluid (CSF) may drip through the needle, this is entirely acceptable. It is usual to check for impedance at this point, and essentially, if it is low then it may mean the needle tip is not in the ganglion and the trigeminal ganglion may be spared of full heating effect of RF.
- If paresthesia occurs in the correct division of the trigeminal nerve, then create an RF lesion at 75°C for 60 seconds. The patient will need to be anesthetized for this lesion, as it is very painful. After the lesion, check sensory testing in the affected area of face to see whether the patient has developed numbness. If not, the RF lesion will need to be repeated at 75°C and even up to 85°C, until there is objective evidence of numbness. Many patients find this process of repeat testing and RF inconvenient and painful but may not remember because of deep sedation or general anesthesia.

Important Technical Considerations

Some important technical considerations are as follows:

- After the RF needle has been inserted through the foramen ovale, check the depth of needle insertion with a lateral view. The needle should not be inserted beyond the imaginary clival line, as this can be very dangerous and fatal.
- Try to avoid inserting the RF needle through the buccal mucosa, as it can introduce infection. Prevent this by inserting one finger into the mouth when initially inserting the RF needle.
- It may be preferable to do this procedure in radiology suite with biplane imaging facilities to help with visualization of the needle trajectory in two planes as approaching the foramen ovale.

- One needs very cooperative patient, an experienced theater team, and anesthetist for this procedure.
- This procedure needs close cooperation between the operator and anesthetist, as the patient may need multiple sleep-awake cycles to produce numbness in the affected division of trigeminal nerve.

BALLOON MICROCOMPRESSION OF THE GASSERIAN GANGLION

The balloon microcompression of the Gasserian ganglion involves the following:

- This may be preferable in patients who cannot tolerate RF lesioning of the Gasserian ganglion as well as for the first division-related neuralgia.
- Consent, preparation, position, and image guidance to visualize the foramen ovale are the same as for the RF technique.
- *Equipment* includes 14G cannula, 4 FG Fogarty embolectomy catheter, and Omnipaque 300 contrast or Mullan percutaneous trigeminal balloon microcompression set available from Cook Medical. This kit has sharp and blunt trocars, which are helpful to minimize complications **(Fig. 7)**.
- The balloon should be de-aired to facilitate effective compression of the trigeminal ganglion. This means injecting radiopaque dye into the catheter while holding the catheter vertical and aspirating back as the air in balloon shifts above the dye **(Fig. 8)**.
- The procedure is carried out under general anesthesia, as the patient's cooperation is not needed.
- A 14G needle is passed under X-ray guidance up to the level of foramen ovale. The needle does not go as deep as in the RF technique as the balloon reaches the point of actual compression of the trigeminal ganglion **(Fig. 5)**. The author uses a sharp trocar until reaching the base of skull at the entrance of foramen ovale. He then replaces this with blunt trocar as available in Cook Medical Kit for balloon compression to avoid any injury to any structure deeper in the foramen ovale from sharper trocar.
- A 4 FG Fogarty embolectomy catheter or the one in the balloon compression kit is introduced through the 14G needle. The balloon is inflated **(Figs. 9 to 11)**

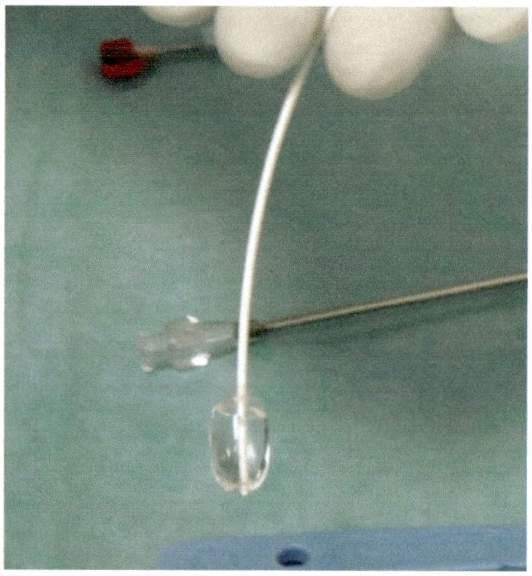

Fig. 8: Balloon being de-aired as it has air at the moment and if inflated with air the compression on ganglion is ineffective.

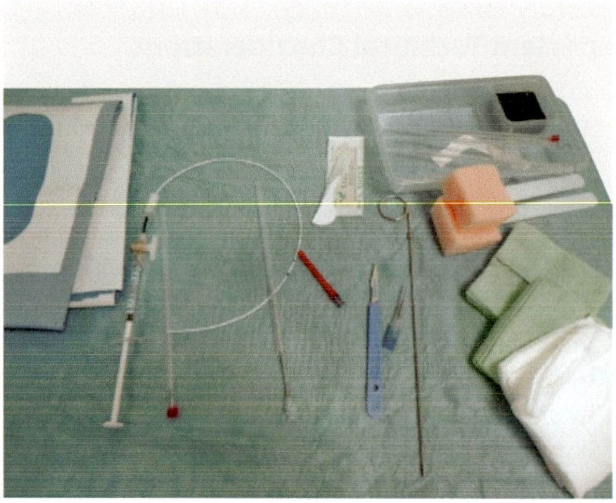

Fig. 7: Equipment setup for balloon microcompression (note a guard on the catheter).

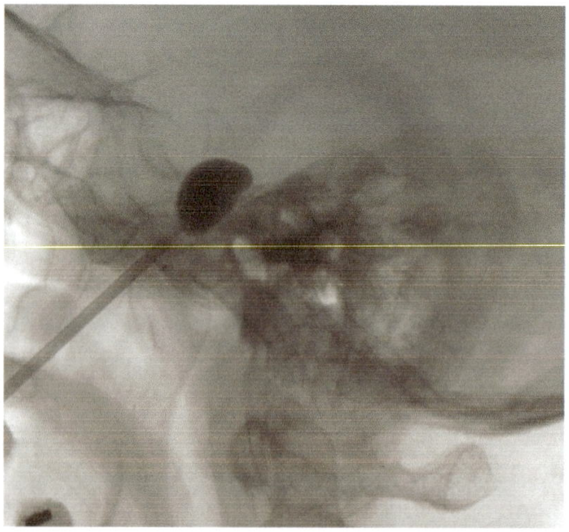

Fig. 9: Lateral view showing good pear shape of the inflated balloon compressing ganglion against petrous part of temporal bone.

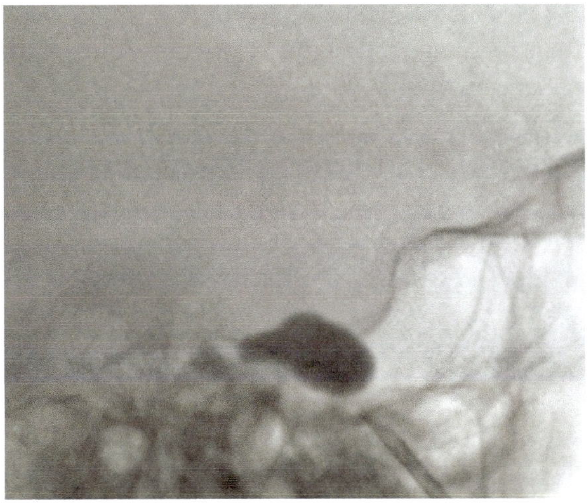

Fig. 10: Lateral view showing good pear shape of the inflated balloon compressing, but slightly excessive inflation.

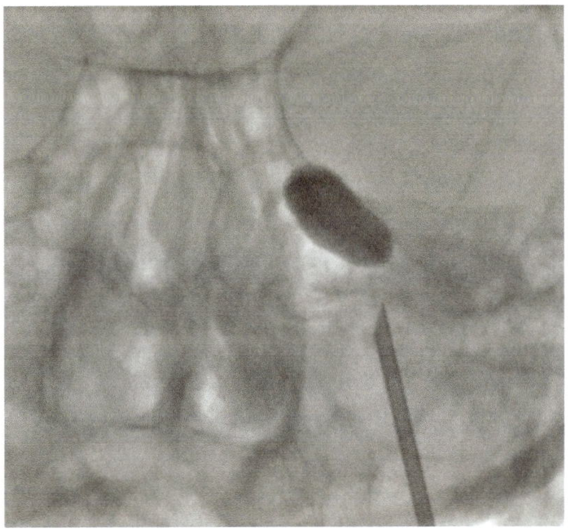

Fig. 11: Confirming good medial projection of inflated balloon in anteroposterior (AP) view.

with 0.6–0.8 mL of Omnipaque 300 or equivalent water-soluble contrast for 1 minute, and then deflated for 1 minute; two more cycles of inflation/deflation are repeated. There is no proven or recommended protocol for compression numbers and duration, but this is what author as well as his neurosurgical colleagues have practiced. On balance, it is preferred to be cautious rather than aggressive in duration of balloon compression as this may cause excessive deafferentation and associated risks. On the other hand, if there is limited response or pain recurs quickly, it is easier to repeat this procedure.

- A pear shape of inflated balloon reflects effective compression of Gasserian ganglion **(Fig. 9)**. It is reassuring to see medial projection of the inflated balloon on an anteroposterior (AP) view **(Fig. 11)**.
- At the end of procedure, the needle and the catheter with balloon are withdrawn together. Trying to remove the balloon catheter through the needle may result in shearing of bits of balloon and these may be left behind.

Important Technical Considerations

- The 14G needle should be introduced only up to the level of the foramen ovale and no further. However, needle may be introduced for about 5–8 mm using blunt trocar and then moved back up to the entrance of foramen ovale. Doing this helps in the insertion of catheter, as at times, otherwise, insertion of catheter may be difficult.
- It is important to either mark the catheter length in advance so as not to insert too deep through the cannula or the balloon may be inflated too deep within the brain. If the length introduced is not enough, then the balloon will not inflate as part of it may still be in the cannula. Cook Medical's Mullan balloon microcompression set has a mark on the catheter informing clinician of the length to be inserted and there is a guard, which can be tightened around the catheter to prevent overinsertion of catheter.
- Transient bradycardia or even asystole may be observed with balloon inflation or inserting the needle through the foramen ovale. This phenomenon of trigeminocardiac reflex has been reported with the incidence as high as 97% in literature.[10] Occasionally, author will request anesthetist to administer prophylactic glycopyrrolate to counter this.
- The author prefers to check the final shape and trajectory of the inflated balloon in both the planes, i.e., AP and lateral to ensure optimal positioning within Meckel's cave.
- Computed tomography (CT)-guided percutaneous balloon compression (PBC) might be a good option in patients with anatomical variants and difficulty in reaching foramen ovale.[11] Both 3D-CT and dyna-CT have been shown to assist foramen ovale puncture and improve the success rate of PBC procedures. From a technical aspect, CT imaging facilitates getting information regarding needle angulation, calculates balloon configuration and volume, reduces operative time, and avoids multiple punctures.

TRIGEMINAL GLYCEROL INJECTION

- Consent, preparation, position, and image guidance to visualize the foramen ovale is as for the RF or balloon-compression technique.
- *Equipment*: 20G needle, glycerol, and Luer lock syringe as otherwise it may be difficult to inject viscous glycerol through narrower gauge needle **(Fig. 12)**.

Technique

- Most of the technical aspects for visualization of foramen ovale and needle insertion are same as for RF or balloon microcompression. Once inside the foramen ovale, it is helpful to have free flow of CSF, and this may mean inserting the needle a bit further but not beyond the imaginary clival line.
- Once the 20G needle is in the correct place, by observing free flow of CSF and needle not beyond the imaginary clival line, the patient is asked to sit upright and needs to be supported by theater assistants. CSF is aspirated and 0.2–0.6 cc of glycerol is injected slowly, and patient is kept in upright position for about 45 minutes to allow glycerol to be taken up by neural tissue.
- The amount of glycerol injected depends on how many divisions of trigeminal nerve need to be covered by this technique.

Important Technical Considerations

- Ensure that you have the correct preparation to inject, otherwise, the aqueous phenol or alcohol may have excessive spread and outcome may be adverse, including serious catastrophe.

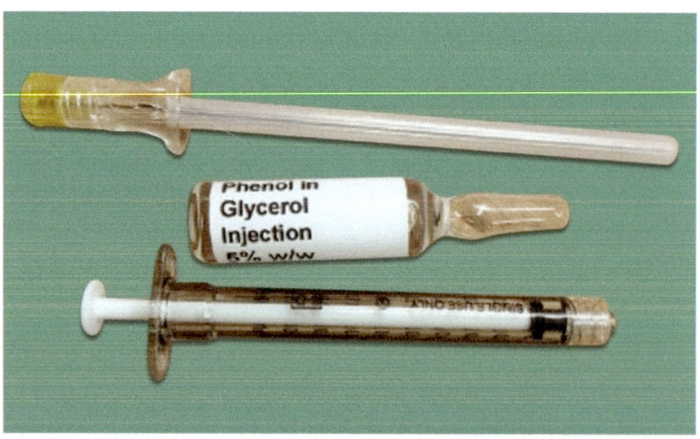

Fig. 12: Equipment needed for trigeminal glycerol injection.

- It is accepted to sit up the patient at the time of glycerol injection, but some studies claim this is not essential and affects safety.

POSTPROCEDURAL CARE FOLLOWING RADIOFREQUENCY/BALLOON MICROCOMPRESSION/GLYCEROL INJECTION

- The patient needs the usual postoperative care and can usually be discharged the next day. With careful planning, it can be performed as day case as well. They may need simple analgesics for postoperative pain.
- It is a good practice to do a neurological examination the day after and document any numbness, jaw weakness, and the presence or absence of a corneal reflex. It is useful to have documentation of these findings before the procedure as well.
- It is a good practice to collect outcome data in relation to pain scores, medications used for pain, and any complications related to procedure and have these documented at follow-up to reflect any changes regarding efficacy and safety of the technique. In the UK, it is becoming mandatory to have this data available to secure continued commissioning of services.

SIDE EFFECTS AND COMPLICATIONS OF RADIOFREQUENCY/BALLOON COMPRESSION/GLYCEROL INJECTION

- Temporary jaw weakness (more common with balloon microcompression) that usually resolves in 1–3 months
- Cheek hematoma related to needle injury (settles quickly)
- Headache for few days afterward, settles very quickly over a week or less
- Unpleasant dysesthesia (25% with RF with 8% requiring medical treatment) and this may take longer to settle and often may not settle, and some patients find it unpleasant and may need treatment as for pharmacological management of neuropathic pain.
- Anesthesia dolorosa (1–4%, more common and long-lasting with RF compared with balloon compression)
- Cranial nerves palsy, for example, diplopia,[12] is more likely related to too medial projection of balloon or excessive spread of glycerol or RF lesioning. Author has encountered couple of cases of diplopia post balloon

microcompression, and these settled within 3 months, and similar cases and recovery period are reported in literature.

- *Very rare complications:*
  - Corneal ulceration
  - Retrobulbar hemorrhage and loss of vision
  - Carotid artery puncture and caroticocavernous fistula
  - Intracranial hemorrhage
  - Meningitis
  - Facial nerve palsy (settles quickly)
  - Herpes simplex type-1 perioralis (settles quickly). There is some suggestion from literature regarding association between TGN and type-1 herpes virus being latent in Gasserian ganglion, though it is not widely accepted.
  - Death is very rarely reported.

PATIENT REPORTED OUTCOMES FROM AN AUDIT FROM AUTHOR'S UNIT

The author performed audit of trigeminal balloon compression in his unit. 43 patients were identified from theater records review. These patients were treated with balloon microcompression performed from June 2006 to June 2008. They were followed up telephonically till August 2009, allowing a follow-up of up to 38 months.

Out of total of 43 patients receiving this procedure over the 2 years period, 95% had immediate complete pain relief (also off medications used to treat TGN) with pain-relieving effect lasting in 60% patients (drug-free) with mean follow-up of 26 months. Allowing for repeat treatment and intake of medications, 41/43 patient's TGN-related pain was very well controlled.

In this audit there were 13/43 patients with MS-related TGN (30%). Immediate complete pain relief was seen in all the patients with MS and all were pain free in August 2009. However, five of these patients relapsed, but now, all were responsive to medication (they were unresponsive to these medications before offering balloon microcompression).

The author has observed large effect size on pain relief of this treatment, and it is life-changing because of excellent pain relief and the ability to reduce or come off medications used otherwise to control TGN.

In conclusion, this audit shows that 43 patients underwent 63 balloon microcompressions over 2 years period. 41/43 patients were pain-free. 27/43 patients were off medication, which they were using before the balloon microcompression to control pain. Side effects were minimal, and patients were very satisfied.

BILATERAL TRIGEMINAL NEURALGIA

It is extremely rare to have bilateral TGN and it is often seen in patients with MS-related TGN. It is unusual to have TGN-related pain on both side of the face at the same time. If this is suspected, then the diagnosis should be reviewed. Author has experience of offering balloon microcompression on both the sides of the face, but this is extremely rare and consequence of offering a neuroablative procedure on the both sides of the face should not be taken lightly and should be discussed in depth with the patient. Patients may find very hard to chew if they develop bilateral jaw weakness.

ALTERNATIVE OPTIONS

In patients who are not suitable for interventional techniques for variety of reasons or technical reasons, they may be considered for gamma knife or stereotactic radiosurgery to achieve similar effect as techniques described in this chapter. It is noninvasive, and hence avoids procedure-related complications, but the onset of effect is delayed by a few weeks and there is a limit on the amount of radiation dose that can be used. They usually cannot be offered this twice for fear of causing radiation-related complications in the trigeminal root entry zone region. Various neuromodulation techniques including transcutaneous electrical nerve stimulation (TENS), peripheral nerve stimulation, deep brain stimulation, and motor cortex stimulation have been tried with variable outcomes standards.[13] More robust studies with long-term data will be required to recommend these procedures in routine clinical settings. Apart from microvascular decompression (MVD), there are other alternate surgical options like internal neurolysis and intraoperative glycerin rhizotomy that are emerging with favorable results, especially in TGN patients without neurovascular conflict.[14,15] Partial sensory rhizotomy is the classical alternative surgical option used in the absence of neurovascular conflict.

CONCLUSION

In author's experience, earlier mentioned techniques are very effective to control intractable TGN, which otherwise is very distressing neuropathic pain condition. Good history taking is essential to diagnose TGN, and if in doubt assess patient at another time and take history again. This usually clarifies the diagnosis. A good understanding of local anatomy, good imaging facilities, theater setup, and theater team are essential for a good outcome. It is helpful to collect outcomes related to these interventions in a long term to justify going service, as there is increasing emphasis on commissioning services, which can demonstrate this in the UK. Author finds this part of his practice very rewarding, though it can be challenging in a small number of cases, which may turn out to be refractory to these interventions, and hence better to have access to a team with multidisciplinary approach including a neurologist, neurosurgeon, maxillofacial surgeon, and a psychologist with interest in complex facial pain.

APPENDIX 1

Balloon Compression for Trigeminal Neuralgia: Patient Information Leaflet.

What is balloon compression?

It is a procedure to selectively affect trigeminal ganglion (part of the nerve conveying pain signals to brain) in such a way as to disrupt pain signals from getting through to the brain. A balloon is inflated inside the skull to compress the ganglion and help with pain relief.

Where is it done?

The procedure is carried out in the radiology theater suite/ operating theater at Walton center.

How is it done?

The procedure is performed under brief general anesthesia.

X-ray pictures are taken throughout the procedure to help direct the needle to the correct place.

A needle is inserted through the cheek under X-ray until it just passes through the foramen ovale (a hole in the base of skull, through which the nerve comes out of skull). A catheter (with small balloon at the tip) is then advanced through the needle and the balloon is slowly inflated. The entire procedure takes only 30 minutes. The balloon is deflated and then withdrawn along with the needle. Dressing is then applied to the cheek.

How long will I be in hospital?

Although the procedure itself only takes 30 minutes, you may be asked for an overnight stay to make sure there are no problems.

Can I eat and drink?

Minimum of 6 hours of fasting is required before the procedure but clear instructions will be given to you with regards to this before your admission.

You will be offered a drink after the procedure when you have come back to the ward from recovery.

What can go wrong?

Usually a very safe procedure but is associated with very rare risks as any other invasive procedure.

The side effects which are common but not serious are:

- Mild discomfort at the site of the injection; this should last no longer than 48 hours. However, if the pain is severe or you feel unwell you should consult your own doctor [general physician (GP)] or us
- You will experience numbness of the face, tongue or throat which gradually diminishes. Your face may feel swollen to you but it will look normal in the mirror. Some patients do not like this numbness
- Jaw weakness is very common but rarely troublesome and usually settles in couple of months.

The side effects which are serious but not common are:

- Three out of 100 patients who have this procedure stand a chance of having infection of the brain (meningitis)
- One out of 50 patients who have this procedure stands a chance of having bleeding in the brain
- One out of 100 patients who have this procedure can have visual disturbance or dryness of the eye on same side
- Anesthesia dolorosa where you may be left with troublesome numbness of the face and continuous pain. It is a rare but reported complication
- Death and serious catastrophe has also been reported but are extremely rare.

Will it work?

The balloon compression is very effective but does not work for everyone. It works in 9 out of 10 patients.

What happens next?

We will ask you to reduce your medication gradually. You will be reviewed in the Outpatients Department in 4–6 weeks following your procedure.

Will my pain return?

It has been observed that in one out of five patients, the pain returns in 2 year's time. When it happens it is more manageable with medications. The procedure can be easily repeated, if needed.

What are the other options?

The one option is to do nothing and try to optimize your medications at their best. You may have already tried this or may not be able to tolerate the side effects.

Other options are other techniques, e.g. radiofrequency (RF) ablation techniques or Gamma knife surgery. You can discuss these options with your consultant. Gamma knife surgery is available in the Walton Center.

REFERENCES

1. Nurmikko TJ, Eldridge PR. Trigeminal neuralgia–Pathophysiology, diagnosis and current treatment. Br J Anaesth. 2001;87(1):117-32.
2. Devor M, Amir R, Rappaport ZH. Pathophysiology of trigeminal neuralgia: the ignition hypothesis. Clin J Pain. 2002;18(1):4-13.
3. Campbell FG, Graham JG, Zilkha KJ. Clinical trial of carbamazepine (tegretol) in trigeminal neuralgia. J Neurol Neurosurg Psychiatry. 1966;29(3):265-7.
4. Tatli M, Satici O, Kanpolat Y, Sindou M. Various surgical modalities for trigeminal neuralgia: literature study of respective long-term outcomes. Acta Neurochir (Wien). 2008;150(3):243-55.
5. Mullan S, Lichtor T. Percutaneous microcompression of the trigeminal ganglion for trigeminal neuralgia. J Neurosurg. 1983;59(6):1007-12.
6. Lichtor T, Mullan JF. A 10-year follow-up review of percutaneous microcompression of the trigeminal ganglion. J Neurosurg. 1990;72(1):49-54.
7. Skirving DJ, Dan NG. A 20-year review of percutaneous balloon compression of the trigeminal ganglion. J Neurosurg. 2001;94(6):913-7.
8. Sweet WH, Wepsic JG. Controlled thermocoagulation of trigeminal ganglion and rootlets for differential destruction of pain fibers. Part 1: Trigeminal neuralgia. J Neurosurg. 1974;40(2):143-56.
9. Zakrewska JM. Trigeminal Neuralgia. London, UK: WB Saunders; 1995.
10. Lv W, Hu W, Chi L, Zhang L. Factors that may affect recurrence of trigeminal neuralgia after percutaneous balloon compression. J Clin Neurosci. 2022;99: 248-52.
11. Xiao X, Wei Z, Ren H, Sun H, Luo F. Comparison of Effectiveness and Safety between Intraoperative 3D-CT-Guided and C-Arm-Guided Percutaneous Balloon Compression for Idiopathic Trigeminal Neuralgia: A Multi-Center Retrospective Study. Pain Res Manag. 2021;2021: 9306532.
12. Bergenheim AT, Linderoth B. Diplopia after balloon compression of retrogasserian ganglion rootlets for trigeminal neuralgia: Technical case report. Neurosurgery. 2008;62(2):E533-4.
13. Xu R, Xie ME, Jackson CM. Trigeminal neuralgia: current approaches and emerging interventions. J Pain Res. 2021;14:3437-63.
14. Durnford AJ, Gaastra B, Akarca D, Lodge A, Ewbank FG, Noorani I, et al. Internal neurolysis: 'Nerve combing' for trigeminal neuralgia without neurovascular conflict—early UK outcomes. Br J Neurosurg. 2022;36(2):175-8.
15. Xu R, Materi J, Raj D, Alomari S, Xia Y, Nair SK, et al. Internal neurolysis versus intraoperative glycerin rhizotomy for trigeminal neuralgia. J Neurosurg. 2022;138(1):270-5.

14 CHAPTER

Maxillary Nerve Block

Kristina Natan

ABSTRACT

Regional anesthesia of the maxillary nerve is used to relieve pain from various types of dental and maxillary surgical procedures as well as extraoral facial surgeries. It can also be used in the diagnosis of trigeminal neuralgia. These techniques, in turn, can be used to treat this condition by injecting neurolytic solutions. The trigeminal nerve is the largest of all cranial nerves that carries major sensory branches, one of which is maxillary nerve. The maxillary nerve exits the brain through the foramen rotundum and enters pterygopalatine fossa, through which it exits to provide several terminal branches that can be used to anesthetize various facial and dental areas. As it passes through pterygopalatine fossa, it then enters through inferior orbital fissure into the orbit to become infraorbital nerve. It also gives off terminal branches that are used to provide facial anesthesia. This chapter will focus on describing several branches of maxillary nerve and the different ways that are used to anesthetize them to provide anesthesia and pain relief to different locations.

INTRODUCTION

Regional anesthesia of the head and neck has many applications in postoperative and chronic pain settings. It becomes very important to know about the trigeminal nerve (5th cranial nerve) and its branches to be able to utilize this knowledge effectively when selecting various types of blocks to treat a certain chronic pain condition, such as carcinoma of maxilla and buccal mucosa.

There are three types of injection techniques that one should be aware of, which are local infiltration, field block, and nerve block.[1,2] Local infiltration anesthetizes individual nerve endings and is used for a specific small area, such as an individual tooth. The field block provides anesthesia to nerve branches and covers a larger area as compared to local infiltration. The area injected in the field block may be proximal to the area anesthetized, unlike infiltration. The nerve block covers the largest area as it anesthetizes the main branch of a specific nerve. An example of this would be a maxillary nerve block anesthetized within pterygopalatine fossa as described later in this chapter.

ANATOMY OF TRIGEMINAL NERVE

Trigeminal nerve is the largest of all cranial nerves that has motor and sensory components **(Fig. 1)**.[1] The small motor nucleus originates within the pons and medulla oblongata. It provides innervation to masticatory muscles, such as masseter, temporalis, medial and lateral pterygoids, mylohyoid muscle, anterior belly of the digastric muscle, tensor tympani, and tensor veli palatini. The sensory root of trigeminal nerve is the largest root and gives rise to three main branches: (1) Ophthalmic (V1), (2) maxillary (V2), and (3) mandibular nerve (V3).[1-4] In the middle cranial fossa, the nerve travels from the posterior cranial fossa to the petrous part of the temporal bone. It forms the trigeminal ganglion originating within Meckel's cavity within the temporal bone.[1,5] The motor root travels along with the sensory root but in separate routes. This motor nerve exits middle cranial fossa along with mandibular sensory nerve through foramen ovale. It unites with the mandibular nerve to form a single nerve trunk after exiting the skull to innervate the abovementioned muscles. The sensory maxillary nerve exits cranium

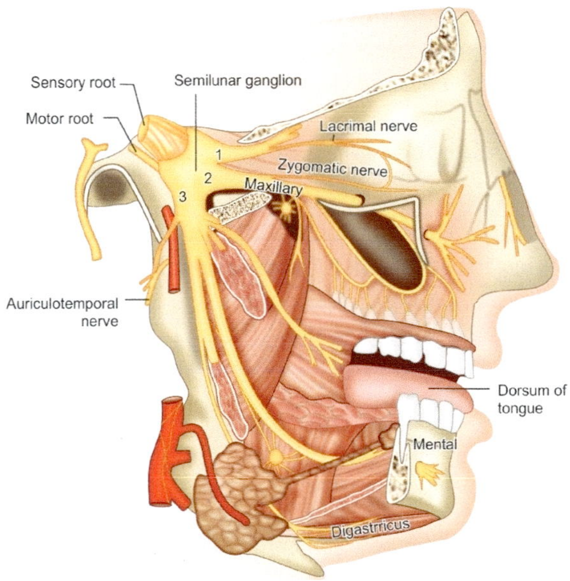

Fig. 1: Anatomy of trigeminal nerve and its three divisions: Ophthalmic (V1), maxillary (V2), and mandibular (V3). It also shows the sensory and motor components of the maxillary nerve that travel in separate trajectories.[6]

through foramen rotundum that later further divides into several branches to supply different parts of the face and oral cavity.[1-4] This chapter will focus on the maxillary nerve, its divisions, and blocks.

Maxillary Nerve

The maxillary nerve is a pure sensory nerve that arises from the trigeminal ganglion. It exits the cranium through foramen rotundum which is located in a greater wing of sphenoid bone. It gives off five branches: (1) Middle meningeal, (2) pterygopalatine nerves, (3) zygomatic nerves, (4) posterior superior alveolar (PSA) nerve, and (5) infraorbital nerves **(Fig. 2)**.[1-4]

Middle Meningeal Nerve

Middle meningeal nerve branch is given off within the cranium before the maxillary nerve exits. This nerve gives sensory innervation to dura that covers the middle cranial fossa **(Table 1)**.[1]

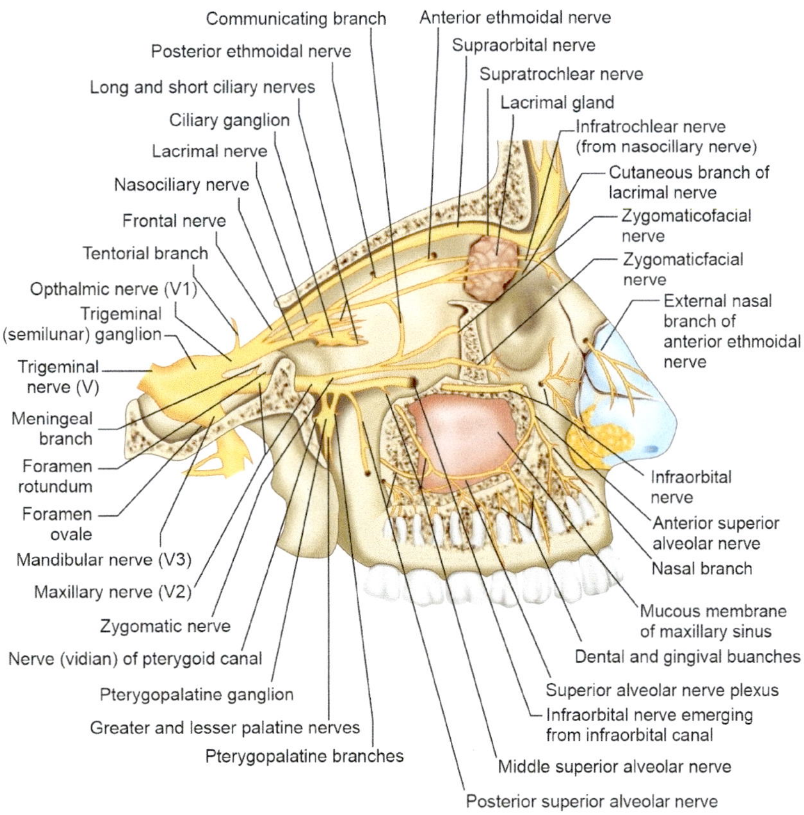

Fig. 2: This picture demonstrates different branches of maxillary nerve and the routes they travel. Maxillary nerve (V2) gives off several branches, such as middle meningeal nerve, pterygopalatine nerves, zygomatic nerves, posterior superior alveolar nerve, and infraorbital nerves.[7]

TABLE 1: Branches of the maxillary nerve.

1.	Middle meningeal nerve	
2.	Pterygopalatine nerves	• Sensory fibers to the orbit • Nasal branches • Nasopalatine nerve • Greater palatine nerve • Lesser palatine nerve • Pharyngeal branch
3.	Zygomatic nerve	• Zygomaticofacial nerve • Zygomaticotemporal nerve
4.	Posterior superior alveolar nerve	
5.	Infraorbital nerve	• Middle superior alveolar • Anterior superior alveolar • Inferior palpebral • Lateral nasal • Superior labial

Pterygopalatine Nerves

Pterygopalatine nerves are located within pterygopalatine fossa behind and below the orbital cavity, as maxillary nerve enters its right after it comes out from the cranium.[1-4] There are several branches within this fossa:

- Sensory fibers to the orbit innervate orbital periosteum.
- Nasal branches innervate posterior nasal septum, mucous membrane of the superior and middle conchae, and the posterior ethmoid sinus.
- Nasopalatine nerve travels across the roof of nasal cavity innervating anterior nasal septum and floor of the nose. It enters incisive foramen and provides palatal gingival innervation to the premaxilla.
- Greater palatine nerve travels through pterygopalatine canal and enters the palate through greater palatine foramen. It innervates palatal tissue from premolars to soft palate. It lies 1 cm medial from the second molar region
- Lesser palatine nerves come out from lesser palatine foramen and innervate the mucous membranes of the soft palate and parts of the tonsillar region.
- Pharyngeal branch exits pterygopalatine ganglion and travels through the pharyngeal canal where it provides sensation to nasal pharynx.

Zygomatic Nerve

Zygomatic nerve divides into zygomaticofacial and zygomaticotemporal nerves after the nerve travels through the inferior orbital fissure. It supplies skin over the malar prominence and the side of the forehead. It carries postganglionic secretomotor fibers through the zygomatic branch to the lacrimal gland via ophthalmic division.[1]

Posterior Superior Alveolar Nerve

Posterior superior alveolar nerve branches off prior to maxillary nerve entrance into infraorbital groove. It provides innervation to posterior maxillary alveolus, periodontal ligament, buccal gingiva, and pulpal tissue (only 1st, 2nd, and 3rd molars).[1]

Infraorbital Nerve

Infraorbital nerve arises within the infraorbital canal and gives rise to several branches:[1,2]

- *Middle superior alveolar nerve:* It innervates 1st and 2nd premolar teeth. It provides sensation to the periodontal ligament, pulpal tissues for the premolars, gingiva, and maxillary alveolus.
- *Anterior superior alveolar nerve:* It innervates maxillary alveolus, buccal gingiva, periodontal ligament, and pulpal tissue for the canines, lateral, and central incisors. A small terminal branch may also communicate with the middle superior alveolar nerve to innervate lateral wall and floor of the nose.

  The abovementioned three superior alveolar nerves form dental plexus which is composed of terminal branches coming off the larger nerve trunks. These terminal branches, such as dental, interdental, and interradicular nerves, provide further sensation to individual teeth. The dental nerve innervates each maxillary tooth pulp. Interdental and inter-radicular nerves innervate periodontal ligaments, interdental papillae, and buccal gingiva of adjacent teeth.
- *Inferior palpebral nerve:* It innervates skin on lower eyelid.
- *Lateral nasal:* It provides sensation to the lateral portion of the nose.
- *Superior labial:* It innervates mucous membranes of the upper lip.

TECHNIQUES OF MAXILLARY BLOCK

There are several areas where the maxillary nerve block can be performed which includes supraperiosteal local infiltration, periodontal ligament anesthesia, PSA nerve block, middle superior alveolar nerve block, anterior superior alveolar block, greater palatine nerve block, nasopalatine nerve block, local infiltration of the palate, and intrapulpal injection. Additionally, intraseptal injection and maxillary nerve block can be performed.

The volume of local anesthetics that can be used in the mouth is usually very small and maximum up to 4 mL with most injections of 0.5–2 mL. Such a small amount of volume is usually effective and avoids complications of intravascular injections that occur in 10–15% of intraoral injections. The usual length of needle is about 1.25–3.80 cm and varies between 25 and 27 g. The depth of the needle insertion averages to 15 mm.[1,4]

Topical local anesthetic can be applied prior to needle injection. Commonly used anesthetics include benzocaine 20% (one has to be cautious with the development of methemoglobinemia) and topical lidocaine 5%. For infiltration, lidocaine 2% and bupivacaine 0.25% are commonly applied. These blocks are often used with addition of epinephrine 1:100,000 or 1:200,000. Epinephrine is known to improve hemostasis and increase the duration of block and therapeutic index of anesthetic solution.[1,4,5]

It is also important to be familiar with the side effects of accidental intravascular local anesthetic infiltration or from the administration of a larger volume of anesthetic. These include systemic toxicity of a specific drug which often can include anxiety, numbness, dizziness, and central nervous system or cardiovascular collapse. Other side effects can also include allergic reactions which often occur due to preservatives or usage of an ester type of local anesthetic.[5]

Complications related to the procedure itself can also occur. These may include persistent paresthesia and numbness of the anesthetized area related to nerve trauma or the formation of a hematoma.[1,4,5,8] Rare complications can also include needle track infection, blockage of other nerves, retrobulbar nerve block, optic nerve block, facial nerve block, 6th cranial nerve block, retrobulbar hematoma, penetration of nasal cavity, edema, and sloughing of tissues from necrosis.[1,4-6,9]

Supraperiosteal Injection

This type of technique is performed to anesthetize individual tooth or soft tissue **(Fig. 3)**. This is an example of field block. The provider should first retract the lip and identify the mucobuccal fold. Insert a 25- or 27G needle with bevel facing bone above the center of the tooth to a depth of a few millimeters at the height of mucobuccal fold.[1,10] Aspirate and check for blood prior to injecting about 0.6–1.2 mL. The anesthesia of the tooth and associated tissue usually occurs within 2–4 minutes. Repeat this procedure if the patient does not feel adequate numbness. One of the contraindications to this procedure is acute infection over the required anesthetized area. Also, if there is a need to anesthetize multiple teeth at the same time adjacent to each other, then a nerve block would be a better method to achieve this. One of the contraindications to this block is infection or inflammation over the desired area.[1,9,10]

Periodontal Ligament Injection

This local infiltration technique is used to supplement supraperiosteal or a nerve block injection where individual teeth or soft-tissue numbness is desired **(Fig. 4)**.[1] To perform this block, a groove between the gingiva and selected tooth is identified as a site of injection of local anesthetic. The lip is retracted and a 25- or 27G needle is inserted to the depth of the gingival sulcus until resistance is met. The position of the needle should be parallel to the long axis of the tooth. Inject about 0.2 mL of local anesthetic solution over a few seconds. This technique is often used by dentists to achieve pulpal and soft-tissue numbness of desired teeth.[1,10]

Posterior Superior Alveolar Nerve block

Posterior superior alveolar nerve block anesthetizes maxillary molar teeth up to the 1st molar (1st, 2nd, and 3rd molars) with the exception of the mesiobuccal root of the 1st molar in some cases **(Figs. 5 and 6)**.[1,10,11] In cases where the 1st molar is not completely anesthetized, supraperiosteal injection of the middle superior alveolar nerve can be performed. PSA block provides a greater and longer anesthesia than supraperiosteal injection alone, and multiple teeth can be anesthetized with fewer needle injections. Unlike previously described infiltration techniques, PSA nerve block can be used to anesthetize areas where infection or inflammation is present.

One of the possible complications of this block is the possibility of hematoma formation if the needle is inserted and anesthetic is injected into the pterygoid plexus of veins or maxillary artery. Therefore, prior to injection, aspiration in two planes is performed to avoid this complication.

The procedure is initialized by localizing 2nd molar tooth while retracting the lip. A short 25- or 27G needle is inserted at the height of mucobuccal fold between the 1st and 2nd maxillary molar teeth to a depth of about

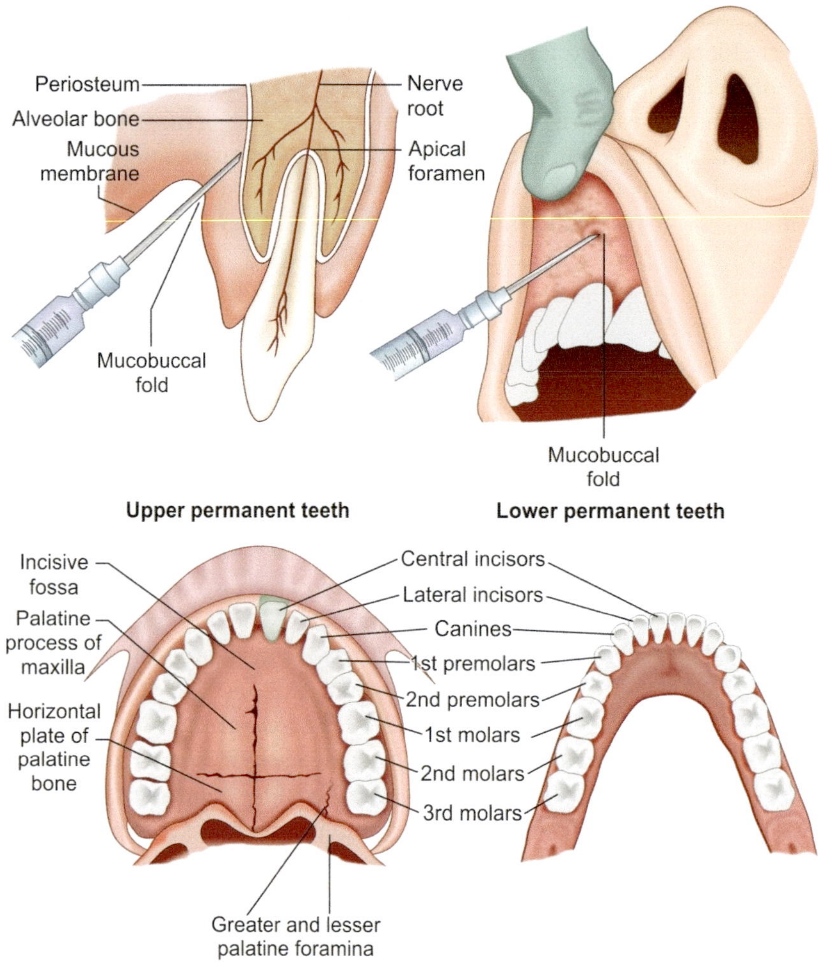

Fig. 3: This photograph demonstrates the height of the mucobuccal fold right where the needle is about to be inserted to anesthetize maxillary incisors (highlighted in green is the area to be anesthetized). It illustrates the supraperiosteal nerve block that is used to numb individual tooth. It also shows the anatomy of maxillary and mandibular teeth.[12]

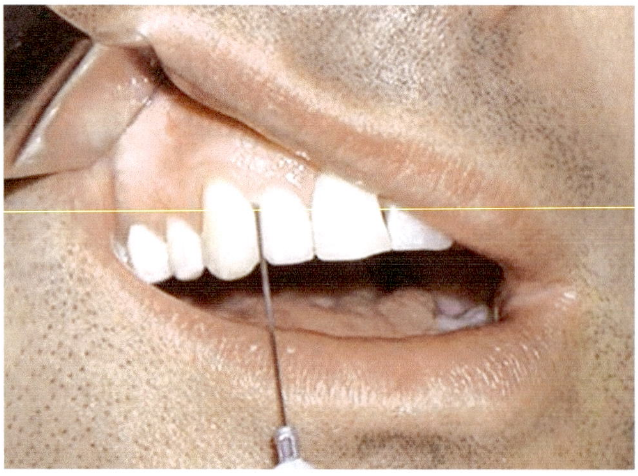

Fig. 4: This photograph illustrates the groove between the teeth where intraligamentary injection can be made to achieve better anesthesia of individual teeth.[13]

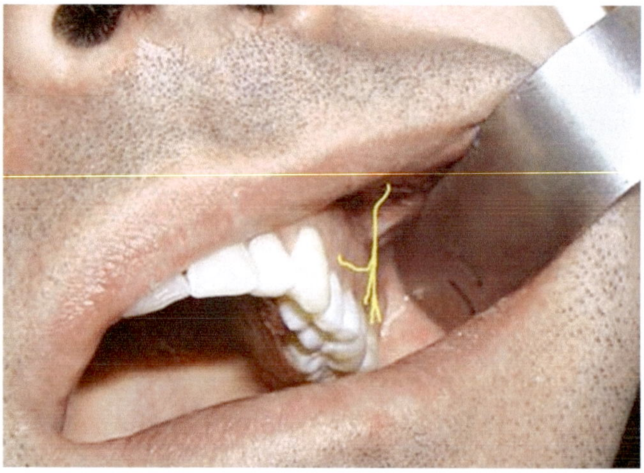

Fig. 5: This image depicts the location of the posterior superior alveolar nerve.[13]

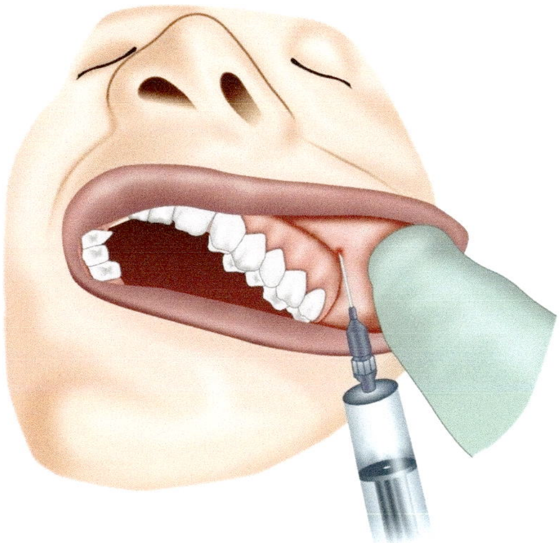

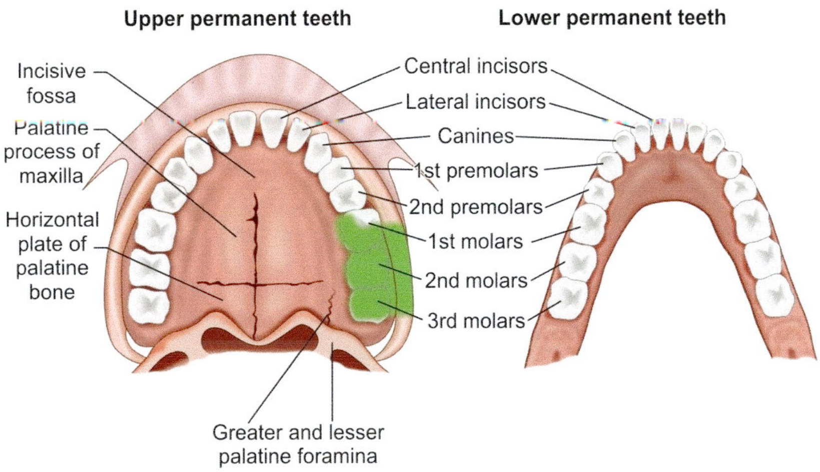

Fig. 6: These images show the location of injection to anesthetize the posterior superior alveolar nerve, which is located between 1st and 2nd molar teeth at the height of the mucobuccal fold. The needle is aimed at 45° superiorly, medially, and posteriorly. The area highlighted in green shows the distribution of anesthetics such as 1st, 2nd, and 3rd molar teeth.[12]

2–2.5 cm. The needle is directed at 45° superiorly, medially, and posteriorly and advanced until no resistance is felt while it traverses soft tissues.[1,10,11,14] If contact with the bone is made, retract the needle and direct it more lateral to the posterior aspect of the maxilla, and after negative aspiration inject local anesthetic by a rotating needle.

Middle Superior Alveolar Nerve block

This block is performed to anesthetize maxillary premolar teeth, pulp, surrounding soft tissue, or the mesiobuccal root of the 1st molar tooth.[1,10,11] It is present in about 28% of the population and in these cases can be substituted by PSA block or anterior superior alveolar block **(Fig. 7)**.[10] It can often be used to supplement

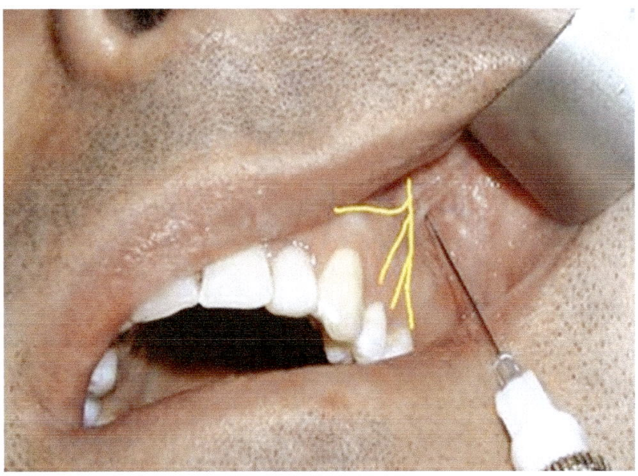

Fig. 7: Location of middle superior alveolar nerve.[13]

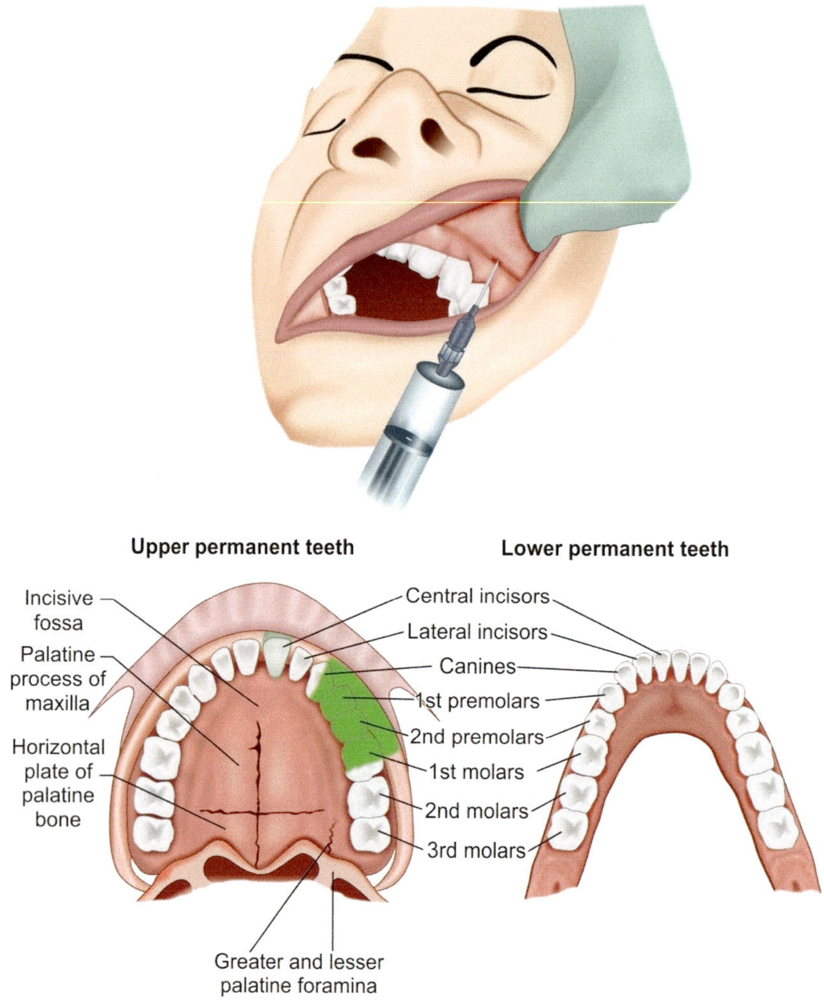

Fig. 8: This image demonstrates the insertion of the needle at the location of maxillary 2nd premolar tooth for middle superior alveolar block. The bottom image highlights the area that is anesthetized by the middle superior alveolar block.[12]

posterior and anterior superior alveolar nerve block or supraperiosteal infiltration if they did not; these cases can be substituted by PSA block at 2nd premolar tooth **(Fig. 8)**. Insert 25- or 27G needle into the apex of the 2nd premolar tooth at the mucobuccal fold to about 1–1.5 cm. Aspirate and slowly inject 0.9–1.2 mL over a minute. One of the contraindications to this block is infection or inflammation in the area to be anesthetized.

Anterior Superior Alveolar Nerve Block/Infraorbital Nerve Block

The anterior superior alveolar nerve block, also known as infraorbital block, is used to anesthetize maxillary central teeth, lateral incisors, and canine teeth along with the surrounding soft tissue.[1,10,11] It can supplement middle superior alveolar nerve block in patients who lack this nerve and may supply innervation to premolar teeth and mesiobuccal root of the 1st molar tooth. This block covers multiple teeth and is used if inadequate anesthesia is achieved by prior blocks. There are two approaches to performing this block, one is intraoral and the other is extraoral. The extraoral block is used to diagnose patients with trigeminal neuralgia as it anesthetizes lower eyelid, lateral part of nasal skin, upper lip, and skin of the cheek.

The infraorbital nerve is located by identifying infraorbital notch on the inferior orbital rim **(Fig. 9)**.[1,10] The notch indicates the location of infraorbital foramen, located beneath the notch, from which the infraorbital nerve is coming out. The infraorbital foramen usually lies

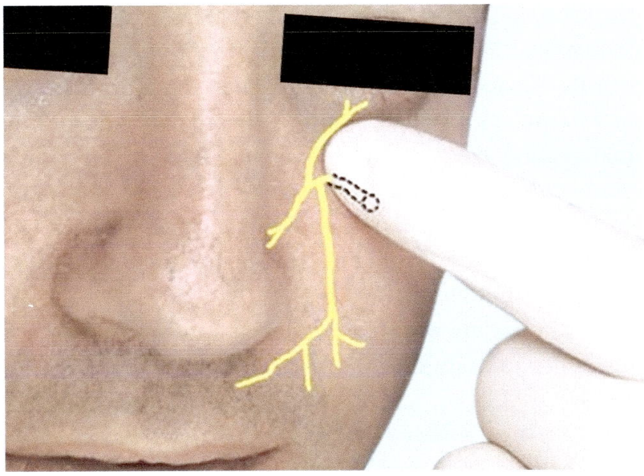

Fig. 9: Location of infraorbital nerve.[13]

in line with 2nd premolar maxillary tooth. It terminates with three branches: (1) Lateral nasal, (2) superior labial, and (3) inferior palpebral.

The procedure is performed by locating the 2nd premolar maxillary tooth and inserting a 25G long needle into the intersection of mucobuccal fold and the center of canine at 45° angle aiming toward the infraorbital notch **(Fig. 10)**.[1,10]

Advance the needle to about 1–1.5 cm. Once the bone over the roof of the foramen is palpated, aspirate and insert 0.9–1.2 mL of anesthetic solution over 1 minute. It is recommended to keep pressure over the site of injection to facilitate the spread of anesthetic into the foramen. Successful injection may anesthetize the lower eyelid, lateral aspect of the nose, and upper lip.

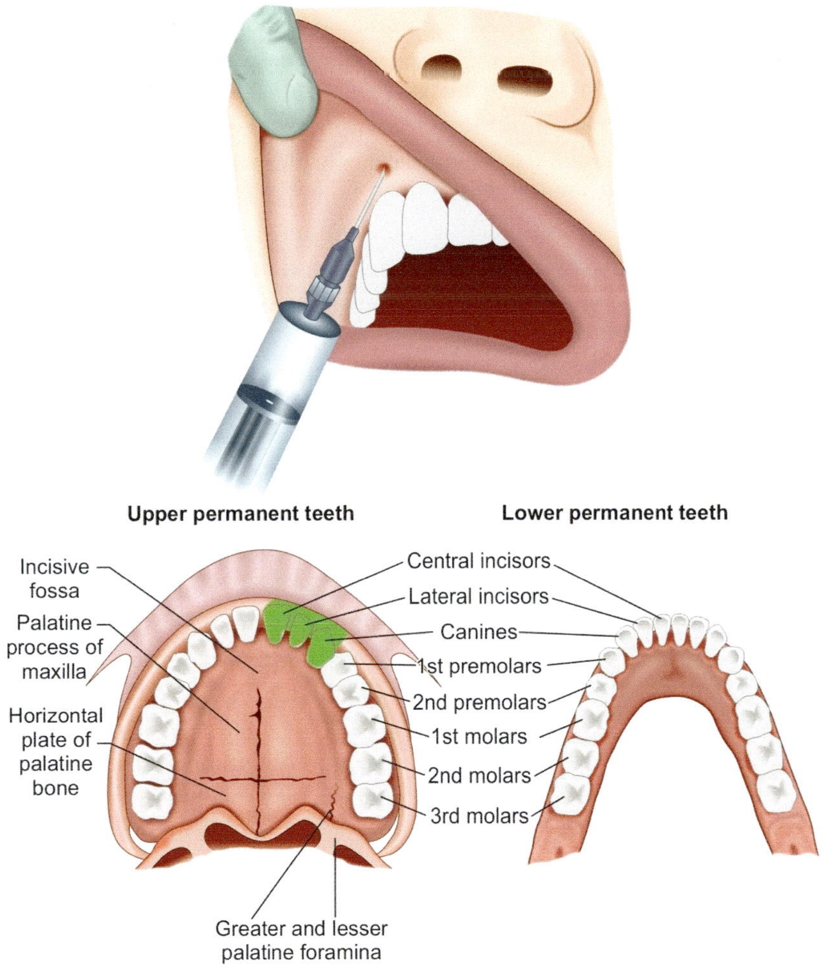

Fig. 10: This image demonstrates anterior superior alveolar/infraorbital block. The needle is inserted at the height of mucobuccal fold and the 1st premolar maxillary tooth. The image below shows the teeth that are anesthetized by this block, such as central and lateral incisors as well as canines.[12]

As was mentioned previously, extraoral injection of the infraorbital nerve is used for diagnoses or treatment of neuralgia as well as orbital surgical procedures.[3,15] The canal is identified just inferior to orbit at the mid-pupillary line. Palpation of the infraorbital canal can sometimes elicit paresthesia. Inject a few drops of local anesthetic for skin infiltration using a 22- or 25G needle. Then, advance the needle at a 30° angle to about 1–3 cm. If paresthesia is achieved at the point of insertion, one might be directly touching the nerve and the needle should then be withdrawn. Aspirate before injection and insert 2–5 mL of local anesthetic or neurolytic solution.[3]

Greater vigilance should be taken to look for hematoma or ecchymosis formation as the needle can damage the infraorbital artery on its way.[1,9,10] Therefore, negative aspiration is needed for confirmation prior to injection of the solution.

Greater Palatine Nerve Block

Greater palatine nerve block is used for paranasal sinus anesthesia and vasoconstriction with endoscopic sinus surgery. It anesthetizes palatal mucosa and hard palate from the 1st premolar and molar teeth. Greater palatine nerve exits to the hard palate through a greater palatine canal located about 1 cm medial to the 2nd and 3rd premolar **(Figs. 11 and 12)**.[1,10,11]

The patient is placed in a supine position with the face facing upward. To locate the greater palatine canal, use a cotton swab. A depression will be felt when the canal is identified **(Fig. 12)**. Some studies showed that foramen may be located in various places, such as medial to anterior half of the 3rd molar in 50% of cases, medial to the posterior half of the 2nd molar in 39% of cases, and medial to the posterior half of the 3rd molar in 9% of cases.[16] Once localized, leave the cotton swab in place and insert needle next to the cotton swab. Aim the needle perpendicular to the injection site and advance the needle until the bone is contacted about a few millimeters from the initial point. Once this point is reached, aspirate and inject 0.45 mL of anesthetic solution. Some resistance may be met once the injection is initiated.[1,10]

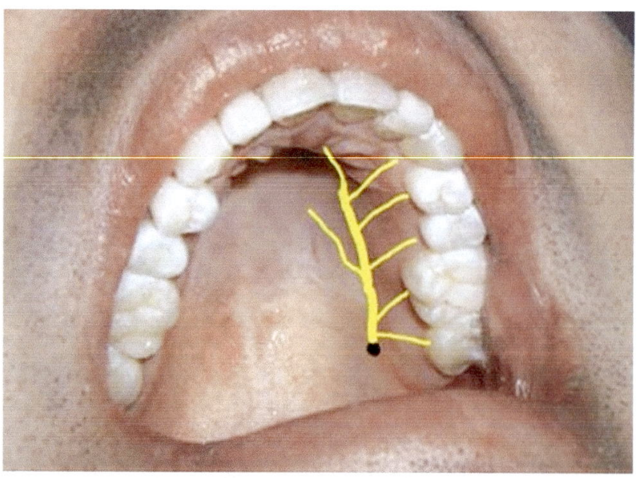

Fig. 11: Location of a greater palatine nerve.[13]

Inflammation or infection of the anesthetized area is one of the contraindications to this block.

Nasopalatine Nerve Block

Nasopalatine nerve block, also known as incisive block or sphenopalatine nerve block, is done to block nasopalatine nerves bilaterally **(Fig. 13)**.[1,10,11] It anesthetizes multiple incisive teeth bilaterally from one side of canine to the other side of the canine teeth as well as surrounding soft and hard tissues of the anterior incisive teeth.

The block is performed by placing the patient in a supine position with chin facing upward for better visualization of the block area **(Fig. 14)**. The incisive papilla is identified and a cotton swab is placed. It is located in the midline about 0.5 cm behind the central incisors.[1,10] The site of injection is lateral to incisive papilla, which is marked by slight soft elevation overlying incisive foramen. A short 25–27G needle is inserted until it contacts the bone, and with negative aspiration 0.25–0.45 mL of anesthetic solution is injected into the area over 30 seconds.[1,10]

Local Palatal Infiltration

Local palatal block is used to provide anesthesia to one or two teeth adjacent to the site of injection. A 25–27G short needle is used to inject local anesthesia. This block is done in a supine position and area that is anesthetized about 10 mm away from the center of the crown on the palatal side **(Fig. 15)**.[1,10] Direct the needle at a 45° angle toward the soft tissue facing the tooth. Aspirate and slowly inject 0.2–0.4 mL of anesthetic solution. Once the block is performed, blanching of the tissue is seen indicating a successful anesthetic procedure. This type of anesthesia can also provide hemostasis to the surrounding tissue around the injected area.

Intrapulpal Injection

This type of anesthesia is solely used for dental procedures and is done when all other blocks could not achieve

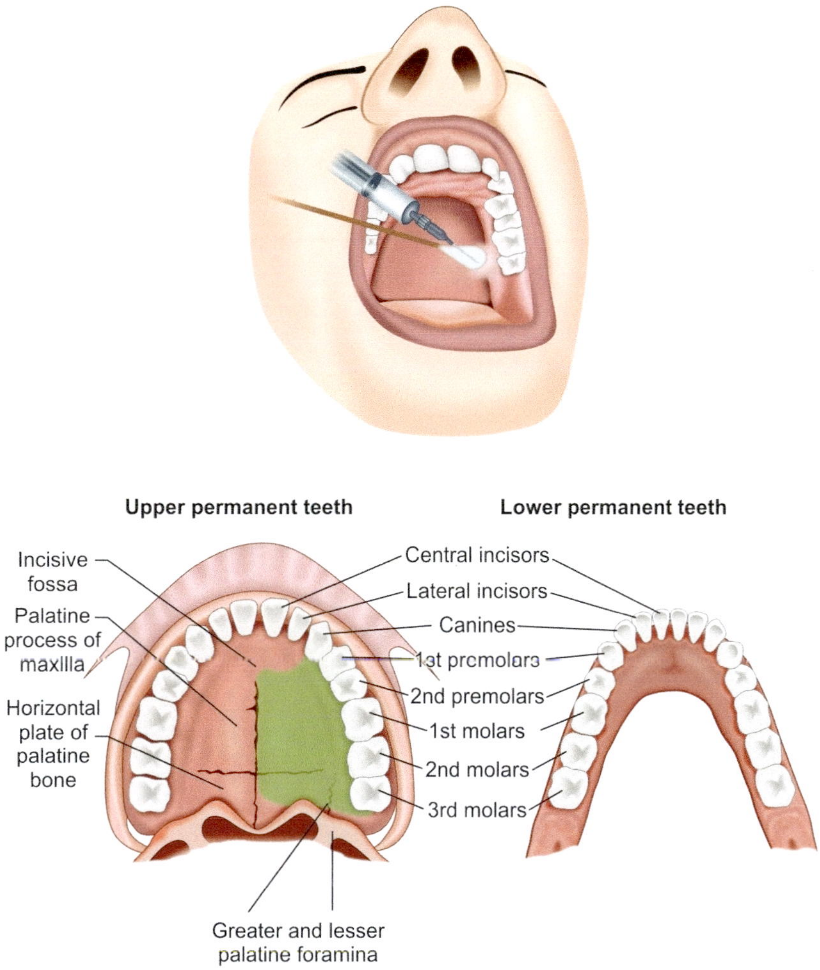

Fig. 12: The top image demonstrates the insertion of the needle around greater palatine foramen to block greater palatine nerve. The location of the block is about 1 cm away medial to the junction of the maxillary 2nd and 3rd molars. The bottom picture demonstrates the location of the foramen as well as the area in green that is anesthetized by this block.[12]

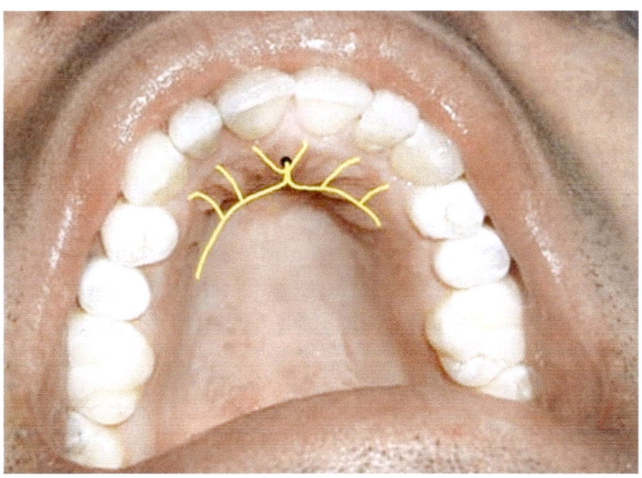

Fig. 13: Location and distribution of nasopalatine nerve.[13]

adequate anesthesia of the desired individual tooth.[1,10] To perform this block, a dentist should expose the pulp channel if it was not exposed prior. A needle is placed inside the pulp and a small amount of anesthetic solution, about one drop, is deposited within the pulp of individual tooth. The needle can be advanced a bit further and another dose of anesthetic can be administered. The patient will feel a brief intense pain followed by immediate relief of pain.

Maxillary Nerve Block

This block provides anesthesia to unilateral hemimaxilla, such as teeth, hard and soft palates, and buccal and lingual tissues. It anesthetizes multiple teeth with the surrounding tissues. The contraindication to this block as for any other previously described blocks is infection

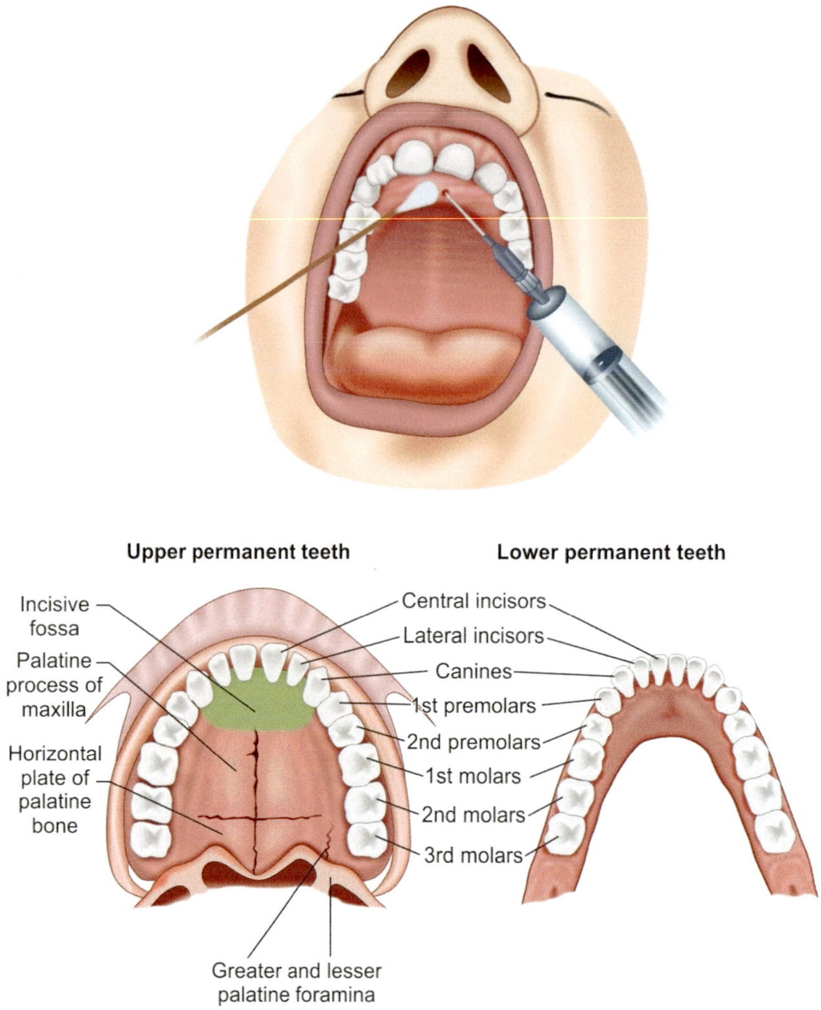

Fig. 14: Location of the needle insertion to perform nasopalatine nerve block. The upper picture demonstrates that the needle is inserted lateral to incisive papilla, which is located behind central incisors. The bottom drawing shows the green area that is anesthetized after this block is performed. It also shows the location of incisive papilla and anatomy of maxillary teeth.[12]

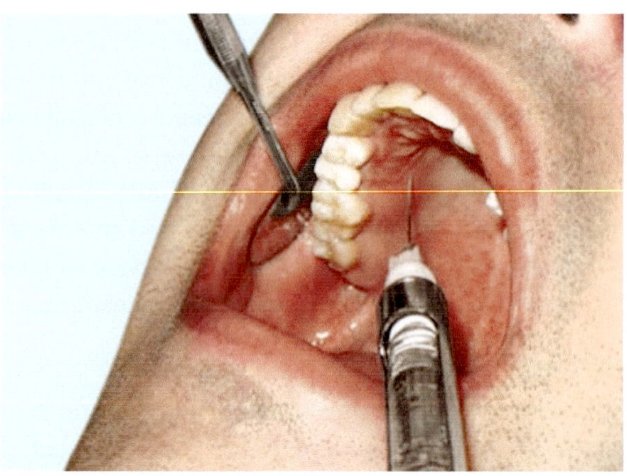

Fig. 15: Local palatal infiltration of the maxillary 1st premolar tooth. The needle is inserted about 5–10 mm away from the center of the crown on the palatal aspect of the maxilla.[13]

or inflammation at the injection site.[1,9,10] There are two approaches to performing this block: High-tuberosity and greater palatine canal approaches. This type of block can have several adverse effects, such as exophthalmos, anesthesia of ophthalmic nerve, paralysis of abducens nerve by accidental intraorbital injection, and intracranial and subarachnoid injection. These complications require recognition of apnea and other associated signs and prompt administration of assisted ventilation or administration of drugs to support the patient's vitals.

High-Tuberosity Approach

This block was named for the location of injection that is lateral to the tuberosity of the maxilla and posterior to its zygomatic process **(Fig. 16)**.[1,10,17] This block is performed

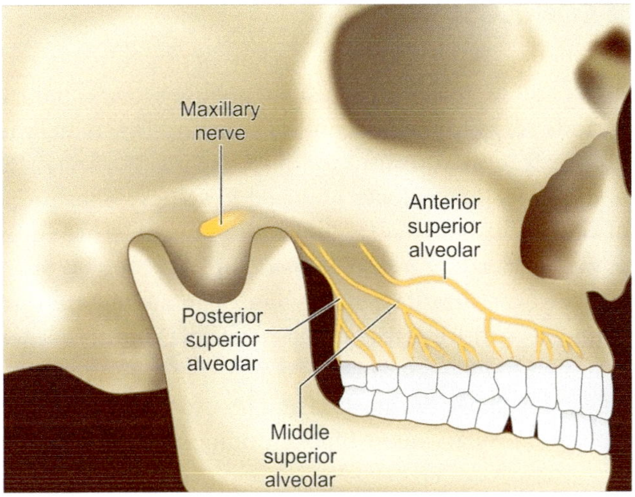

Fig. 16: Location of maxillary nerve within the pterygopalatine fossa.[18]

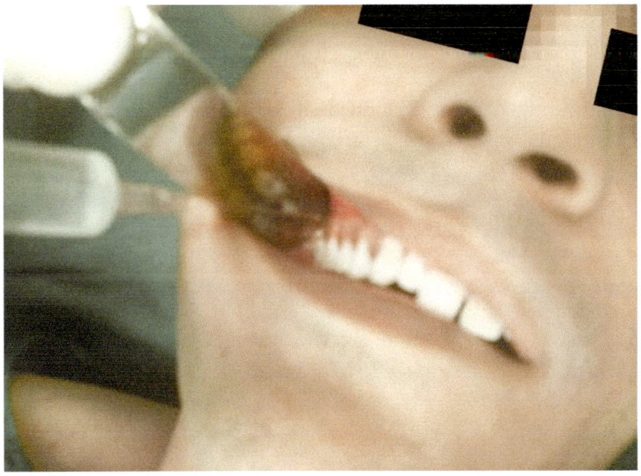

Fig. 17: This image shows the location of the needle insertion to anesthetize maxillary nerve using high-tuberosity approach. The needle is inserted at the height of mucobuccal fold above the maxillary 2nd molar tooth. Aim 45° posteriorly, superiorly, and medially. The needle is bent to better access the area.[19]

by placing the patient in a supine position with head and chin facing up to better access the area. Retract the cheek with a finger to access the zygomatic process. A 25G long needle is used to penetrate the area.[1,10] Maxillary nerve is anesthetized as it passes through pterygopalatine fossa. The needle is inserted at the height of mucobuccal fold distal to the maxillary 2nd molar. This injection site is located behind the zygoma. To reach the nerve within the pterygopalatine fossa, aim 45° posteriorly, superiorly, and medially **(Fig. 17)**.[1,10,17] The needle is advanced about 3 cm and may be slightly bent to 30° angle. Double

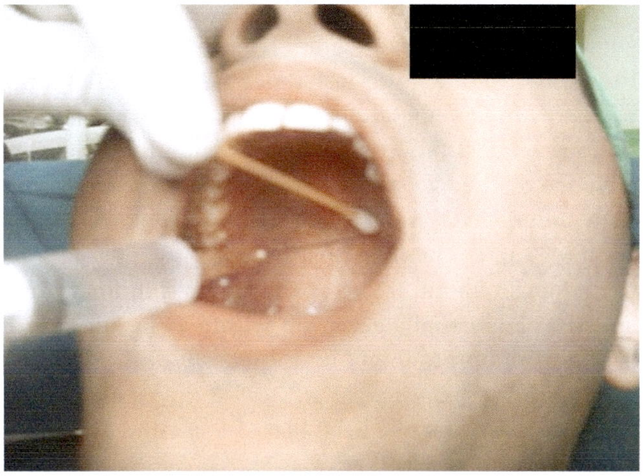

Fig. 18: This picture describes the needle insertion to anesthetize maxillary nerve via greater palatine canal approach to reach the nerve within the pterygopalatine fossa. Use a cotton swab to find a depression caused by greater palatine canal which is located about 1 cm lateral to the 2nd molar tooth. Advance the needle to a depth of 3 cm without resistance and deposit local anesthetic.[19]

aspiration is performed to avoid the risk of hematoma formation (the second aspiration is done by turning the needle one quarter of a turn). About 4 mL of anesthetic solution is deposited slowly. This block can also cause the spread of the local anesthetic to the optic nerve and cause temporary blindness. One of the treatment options is close observation and reassurance. Other concerns may also include orbital swelling due to the spread of anesthetic in orbital issues, ophthalmoplegia, and diplopia.[1,9,10]

Greater Palatine Canal Approach

This block is performed through greater palatine foramen to anesthetize the maxillary nerve as it travels within pterygopalatine fossa via greater palatine canal. This block is more frequently performed with high success rates. The foramen is located adjacent to the distal half of the 2nd maxillary molar tooth at the union of the alveolar process of the maxilla and the lateral border of the hard palate. It is about 1 cm lateral to the 2nd maxillary molar tooth;[1,10] however, as described before, the location may vary. A cotton swab is used to identify the area of depression created by the greater palatine foramen **(Fig. 18)**. A 25G long needle is inserted perpendicular, next to the cotton swab, and aimed posteriorly until contact with bone is made. Several studies indicated that the majority of canals were located at a 45–50° angle.[1,10] Once the foramen is located, the needle is advanced to about 30 mm. If the resistance is met at any point, withdraw the needle and redirect it at a different angle. If, however, resistance is met earlier with the inability to advance the needle, abort the procedure and perform a high-tuberosity approach block. Once the correct place for injection is identified, aspirate it in two planes and then deposit about 2–3 cc of anesthetic solution.[1,10] The anesthesia is usually achieved within 5–15 minutes. It is very common to inject into the surrounding mucosa instead of the palatine canal. One of the ways to avoid this is to insert the needle at least 1.5 cm and direct it at more acute angle.

Intraseptal Injection

This type of block is performed to supplement all the previously mentioned blocks, such as supraperiosteal, PSA block, middle superior alveolar block, and anterior superior alveolar block.[1] It helps to achieve greater hemostasis around the injection site. Inflammation and infection are among the contraindications to this block.

Use 27G short needle and identify interdental papillae located 2–3 cm above the apex of the papillary triangle **(Fig. 19)**. Advance the needle at a 45° angle into the soft tissue around the root until the bone is contacted.[1,10] The needle is then advanced into interdental septum where 0.2 mL of anesthetic solution is deposited. Resistance upon injection will be met and the block will anesthetize the surrounding tissue.

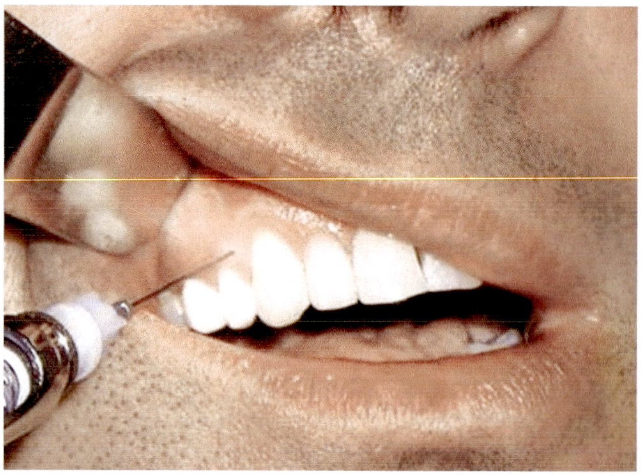

Fig. 19: Intraseptal injection of local anesthetic at the apex papillary triangle.[13]

CONCLUSION

Maxillary nerve is a second division of trigeminal nerve. It gives off multiple branches that are used to anesthetize various areas of the face and oral cavity. These include both extraoral and intraoral approaches. For majority of the time, these blocks are used to achieve anesthesia of oral cavity for dental and oral surgical procedures as well as facial surgeries **(Tables 2 and 3)**.

However, maxillary nerve block can also be used to diagnose and treat trigeminal neuralgia due to herpes zoster and malignancy. Upon conclusion, one should be able to recognize the location and how to perform various types of maxillary nerve blocks. Additionally, one should

TABLE 2: Techniques of anesthesia for the treatment of a localized area or one or two teeth.

Technique	*Area anesthetized*
Supraperiosteal injection	Individual teeth and buccal soft tissue
Periodontal ligament injection	Individual teeth and buccal soft tissue
Intraseptal injection	Localized soft tissue
Intrapulpal injection	Individual tooth

TABLE 3: Techniques of anesthesia for the treatment of a quadrant or multiple teeth.

Technique	*Anesthetized area*
Maxillary	
Posterior superior alveolar nerve block	Maxillary molars (except the mesiobuccal root of maxillary 1st molar in some cases), soft and hard tissues on buccal aspect
Middle superior alveolar nerve block	Mesiobuccal root of maxillary 1st molar (in some cases), premolars, and surrounding hard and soft tissues on buccal aspect
Anterior superior alveolar nerve block/infraorbital nerve block	Central and lateral incisors and canine, surrounding hard and soft tissues on buccal aspect, mesiobuccal root of maxillary 1st molar (in some cases)
Greater palatine nerve block	Palatal mucosa and hard plate from 1st premolar anteriorly to the posterior aspect of the hard plate and midline medially
Nasopalatine nerve block	Hard and soft tissue of the lingual aspect of maxillary anterior teeth from distal of canine on one side to distal of canine on the contralateral side
Maxillary nerve block	Hemimaxilla on side of the injection (teeth, hard and soft, buccal and lingual tissues)

be vigilant and be able to recognize various side effects of local anesthetics or complications of the procedure performed.

REFERENCES

1. Dubash BD, Hershkin AT, Seider PJ, Casey GM. Oral and maxillofacial regional anesthesia. In: Hadzic A (Ed). Regional Anesthesia and Acute Pain Management. New York, USA: McGraw Hill Publishers; 2007.
2. Wedel DJ, Terese TH. Nerve blocks. In: Miller RD (Ed). Miller's Anesthesia, 6th edition. Philadelphia, PA, USA: Elsevier; 2005.
3. Romanoff M. Somatic nerve blocks of the head and neck. In: Raj PP (Ed). Practical Management of Pain, 3rd edition. St. Louis, USA: Mosby; 2000.
4. Yagiela JA. Anesthesia and pain management. Emerg Med Clin North Am. 2000;18(3):449-70.
5. Morgan EJ, Mikhail MS, Murray MJ (Eds). Pain management. In: Clinical Anesthesiology, 4th edition. New York, USA: McGraw Hill Publishers; 2006. pp. 375-77.
6. Tewfik TL, Meyers AD. (2013). Trigeminal nerve anatomy. [online]. Available from emedicine.medscape.com/article/1873373-overview#showall [Last accessed July, 2024].
7. Netter FH. Atlas of Human Anatomy, 4th edition. Philadelphia, PA, USA: Elsevier Health Sciences; 2006.
8. Mahoney PM. Maxillary nerve block. Anesth Prog. 1977;24:47-9.
9. Stanley FM. Local complications. In: Malamed SF (Ed). Handbook of Local Anesthesia, 5th edition. St. Louis, USA: Mosby; 2004. pp. 285-303.
10. Stanley FM. Maxillary nerve block. In: Malamed SF (Ed). Handbook of Local Anesthesia, 5th edition. St. Louis, USA: Mosby; 2004. pp. 189-225.
11. Blanton PL, Jeske AH; ADA Council on Scientific Affairs; ADA Division of Science. The key to profound local anesthesia: neuroanatomy. J Am Dent Assoc. 2003;134(6):753-60.
12. Van Meter MW, Dave AK. (2013) Oral nerve block. [online]. Available from emedicine.medscape.com/article/82850-overview#showall. [Last accessed July, 2024].
13. Dubash BD, Hershkin AT, Seider PJ, Casey GM. (2013). Oral and maxillofacial regional anesthesia. [online]. Available from www.nysora.com/techniques/nerve-stimulator-and-surface-based-ra-techniques/head-and-neck-blocka/3420-oral-and-maxillofacial-regional-anesthesia.html [Last accessed July, 2024].
14. Padhye M, Gupta S, Chandiramani G, Bali R. PSA block for maxillary molar's anesthesia - an obsolete technique? Oral Surg Oral Med Oral Pathol Oral Radiol Endod. 2011;112(6):e39-43.
15. Spinelli G, Rocchetta D, Carnevali G, Valente D, Conti M, Agostini T. Infraorbital nerve block for isolated orbital floor fractures repair: review of 135 consecutive cases. Plast Reconstr Surg Glob Open. 2014;2(1):e97.
16. Malamed SF, Trieger N. Intraoral maxillary nerve block: an anatomical and clinical study. Anesth Prog. 1983;30(2):44-8.
17. Stajcić LS, Gacić B, Popović N, Stajcić Z. Anatomical study of the pterygopalatine fossa pertinent to the maxillary nerve block at the foramen rotundum. Int J Oral Maxillofac Surg. 2010;39(5):493-6.
18. Thomsen TW, Setnik GS. (2014). Dental nerve blocks. [online]. Available from www.proceduresconsult.jp/Home/ProcedureListing/ProcedureDetails/tabid/74/c/505/language/en-US/Default.aspx. [Last accessed July, 2024].
19. Cherian A, Raghavendra M. (2014). Maxillary nerve block technique. [online]. Available from emedicine.medscape.com/article/2040617-technique. [Last accessed July, 2024].

15 CHAPTER

Mandibular Nerve Block

Yashwant L Nankar

ABSTRACT

A mandibular nerve block is a useful procedure for a patient with lower jaw (mandible), part of the mouth, and tongue pain. It can give patients a very good relief from chronic pain conditions such as mandibular neuralgia, postherpetic neuralgia, atypical facial pain, and cancer pain in that region. This procedure can be performed under peripheral nerve stimulator guidance with imaging techniques such as C-arm, CT Scan, ultrasound or with landmark guidance, or even blind. Long-term relief can be obtained with radiofrequency (RF) ablation, use of neurolytics, or use of continuous catheter technique.

INTRODUCTION

Mandibular nerve is the branch of trigeminal nerve and supplies sensation to lower jaw and tongue along with motor supply to jaw muscles. Mandibular nerve block is useful for managing acute, chronic, and cancer pain of intraoral areas such as lower jaw, tongue, or oral mucosa.[1-4]

ANATOMY

Mandibular nerve that is the 3rd division of trigeminal nerve emerges from the floor of middle cranial fossa. It comes out of the foramen ovale into the infratemporal fossa **(Figs. 1 and 2)**.

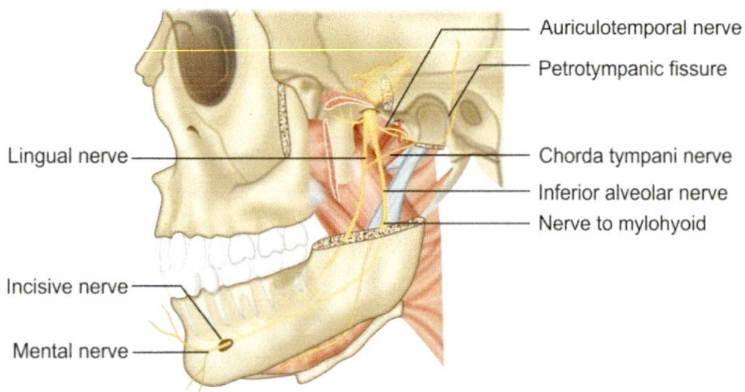

Fig. 1: Mandibular nerve out of the foramen ovale and its divisions.

Here it is surrounded by important structures. Posteriorly, it is bound by the carotid sheath and styloid apparatus. Anteriorly is the posterior wall of the maxillary sinus, laterally is the ramus of mandible, and medially, it is bound by the lateral plate of pterygoid which is the posterior extension of the sphenoid bone. It then divides into small anterior and large posterior trunks. The small anterior trunk gives off branch to masseter, the muscle of

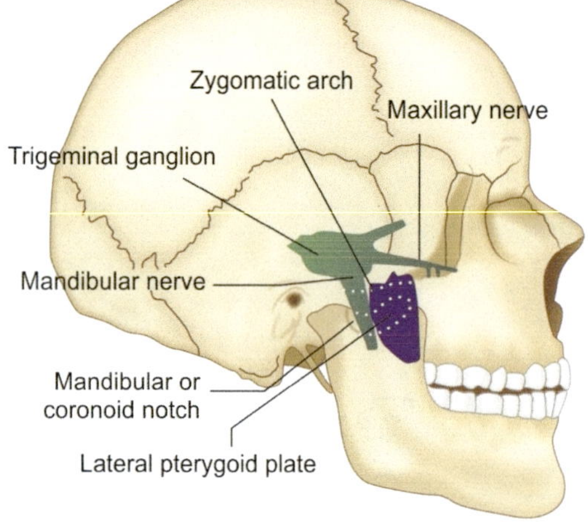

Fig. 2: Mandibular nerve coming out of trigeminal nerve just posterior to the lateral pterygoid plate. Also shown in the diagram is the approach to the needle through the "coronoid notch".

mastication, and a sensory branch covering the sensory area overlying the muscle, namely buccinators intraorally and over the skin. The large posterior trunk divides into auriculotemporal, lingual, and inferior alveolar nerves. It covers the anterior and external ear, temporomandibular joint, parotid gland, and temporal area. Intraorally, it takes sensory sensation from the anterior two-thirds of tongue, lower jaw, and mucosa of the cheek.

INDICATIONS

- Pain of malignant origin—tongue, floor of mouth, and lower jaw
- Acute herpes zoster
- Breakthrough pain of trigeminal neuralgia mandibular division
- Acute pain secondary to trauma, mandibular fracture
- Postsurgical pain
- Dental pain
- Atypical facial pain
- Trismus
- Postherpetic neuralgia.

CONTRAINDICATIONS

- Local infection
- Coagulopathies
- Distorted anatomy.

EQUIPMENT AND DRUGS

Needles

- 25G ¾-inch needle, for local infiltration
- 22G spinal needle
- Peripheral nerve stimulator needle >8 cm (Stimuplex)
- RF (radiofrequency) needle—10 cm needle with 5 mm active tip.

Syringes: 1 mL, 2 mL, 5 mL,10 mL—2 each

Equipment:

- RF lesion generator
- Peripheral nerve stimulator

Imaging modalities:

- C-arm
- Computed tomography (CT)
- Ultrasound

Drugs:

- Lignocaine 2%
- Bupivacaine 0.5%
- Normal saline
- *Depot steroids:* Triamcinolone or alpha-methyl prednisolone 40 mg
- Alcohol 99%
- Phenol 6% for neurolysis.

PREPARATION

History and physical examination of the local area before the procedure.

Laboratory investigation: Preoperative blood investigation, and coagulation profile (PT/INR).

Preoperative patient explanation and consent:

- He or she might feel numbness or current-like sensation on the jaw during the procedure.
- There might be slight numbness over the jaw area after the procedure.
- If neurolysis is planned, then there might be weakness in chewing from that side of the jaw along with loss of sensation in mandibular division.

Sedation

- It is usually not necessary for a block with local anesthetics.
- It may require for RF thermocoagulation.

POSITION

Supine position **Figure 3**.

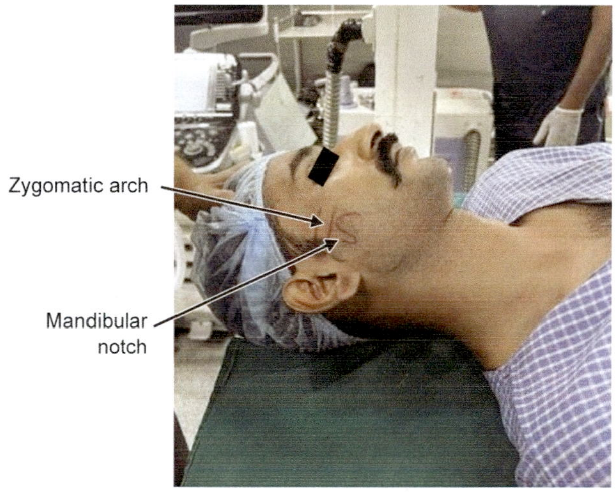

Fig. 3: Supine position of head with surface marking for bony landmarks—zygomatic arch and mandibular or coronoid notch.

PROCEDURE

- Preoperative antibiotic might be given depending on the institutional practice.
- Mandibular or coronoid notch is identified by asking the patient to open and close his mouth.
- Bite Block is placed in between teeth
- Needle entry point is from the center of the mandibular notch or coronoid notch, i.e., mandibular or coronoid notch of the mandibular bone and just below the zygomatic arch.
- Entry point is confirmed by placing a metal marker at the entry point and anterioposterior (AP) view **(Fig. 4)**.
- First antiseptic is applied.
- Local anesthetic using 1% lignocaine is given along the skin **(Fig. 5)**.

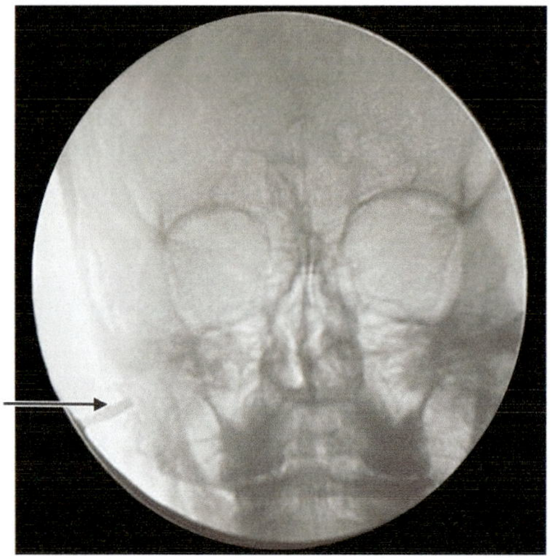

Fig. 4: Tip of the metal marker placed at the entry point as seen on anteroposterior (AP) view.

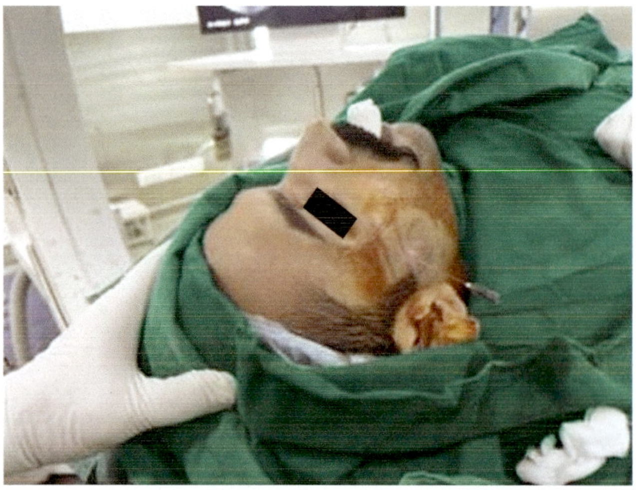

Fig. 5: Needle entry for local anesthesia (Bite block in mouth).

- Block needle, 3.5-inch spinal needle, or Stimuplex needle is inserted just below the zygomatic arch directly in the middle of the coronoid notch.
- The needle is advanced in a plane perpendicular to the skull until contact is made with the pterygoid plate.
- This can be confirmed by AP view of fluoroscopy **(Fig. 6)**.
- The needle is then redirected posteriorly and advanced a few millimeters medially and cephalad to target the mandibular nerve maintaining the same depth at the same level.
- Patient might encounter paresthesia at this point or complain radiating pain in the lower lip and tongue apex.
- Use of peripheral nerve stimulator would be strongly recommended to place the needle as close to the nerve as possible. Contractions of the masseter will confirm the needle tip near nerve **(Fig. 7)**.
- Intravascular spread could also be used to rule out by injecting contrast with fluoroscopy.

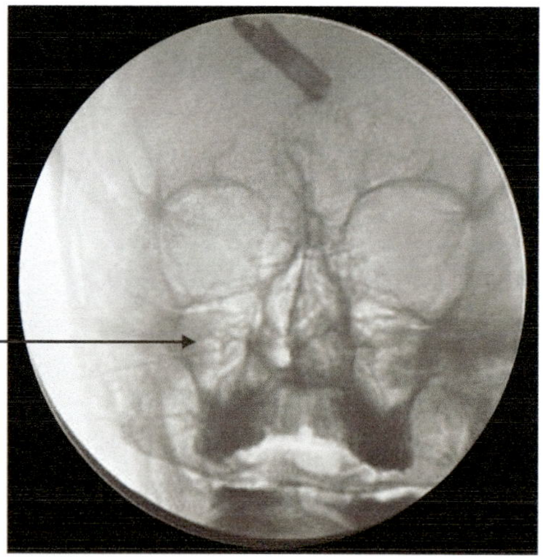

Fig. 6: Needle at foramen under fluoroscopy.

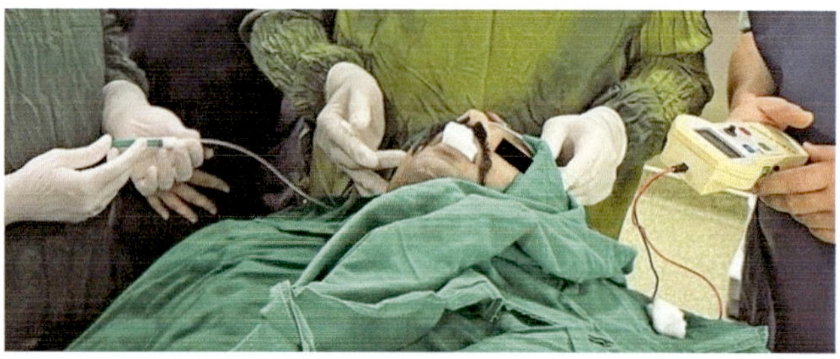

Fig. 7: Stimulation under process (Mandibular nerve block—PNS needle, stimulator and injection.

- Once the placement is confirmed, 2–4 mL of local anesthetic is injected.
- Continuous catheter could also be placed once the placement is confirmed.[5]

NEUROLYSIS

Persistent severe cancer pain in this region can be managed by neurolysis, although it is not done very commonly. Phenol 6% or alcohol 50–60% can be used in incremental doses of 0.1–0.2 mL so as to prevent any form of accidental intravascular or intracranial injection.

RADIOFREQUENCY ABLATION

- Both conventional and pulsed RF can be done for long-term pain relief.[6,7]
- For conventional RF, sensory stimulation of 50 Hz at 0.4–0.6 V and RF is used at 80°C for 90 seconds.
- For pulsed RF- Lesioning is done at 42°C for 120 seconds. At least 2–3 lesions are required to get good pulsed RF lesioning.
- Pulsed RF is strongly recommended instead of conventional.
- Immediate postprocedure, there might be weakness of the jaw along with numbness. Patients should be warned about these in advance.

POSSIBLE COMPLICATIONS

- Bleeding—injury to middle meningeal artery in the infratemporal fossa—so careful aspiration of blood should always be done to prevent any accidental vascular injection[8]
- Hematoma of the cheek
- Infection
- Intracranial spread of medicines
- Pharyngeal puncture
- Side effects with relation to local anesthetic, alcohol, or phenol.

CONCLUSION

Usually, mandibular nerve block is a very useful procedure. It should be performed carefully to avoid major complications. It should be commonly used by pain physicians for helping patients suffering from acute, neuralgic, chronic, and cancer pain.

REFERENCES

1. Raj PP, Lou L, Erdine S, Staats PS, Waldman SD. Radiographic Imaging for Regional Anesthesia and Pain Management, 1st edition. Philadelphia: Churchill Livingstone; 2003.
2. Waldman SD. Atlas of Interventional Pain Management, 2nd edition. Philadelphia: WB Saunders; 2004.
3. Romanoff M. Somatic nerve blocks of the head and neck. In: Raj PP (Ed). Practical Management of Pain, 3rd edition. St Louis: Mosby; 2000.
4. Ohseto K, Uchino H, Iida H. Nerve blockade and interventional therapy. Japan: Springer; 2019.
5. Kohase H, Umino M, Shibaji T, Suzuki N. Application of a mandibular nerve block using an indwelling catheter for intractable cancer pain. Acta Anaesthesiol Scand. 2004;48:382-3.
6. Koizuka S, Saito S, Kubo K, Tomioka A, Takazawa T, Sakurazawa S, et al. Percutaneous radio-frequency mandibular nerve rhizotomy guided by CT fluoroscopy. Am J Neuroradiol. 2006;27:1647-8.
7. Koizuka S, Saito S, Tobe M, Sekimoto K, Obata H, Koyama Y. Technical communication: percutaneous radiofrequency mandibular nerve rhizotomy guided by high-speed real-time computed tomography fluoroscopy. Anesth Analg. 2010;111:763-7.
8. Wilkie GJ. Temporary uniocular blindness and ophthalmoplegia associated with a mandibular block injection: a case report. Aust Dent J. 2000;45(2):131-3.

16 CHAPTER

Sphenopalatine Ganglion Block

Yashwant L Nankar

ABSTRACT

Sphenopalatine ganglion (SPG) block is a very useful procedure for patients with headache and facial pain. It can give patients very good relief from chronic pain conditions such as cluster headache, migraine, postherpetic neuralgia, atypical facial pain, and cancer pain in that region. This procedure can be performed with guidance of imaging techniques like C-arm or CT guidance. Long-term relief can be obtained with radiofrequency (RF) ablation.

INTRODUCTION

Sphenopalatine ganglion (SPG) is one of the four ganglia in head and neck area; situated in pterygopalatine fossa found outside the cranium is an important facial ganglion having sympathetic and parasympathetic fibers with related functions along with somatic sensory nerves to the orofacial region. Sphenopalatine ganglion block (SPGB) provides excellent analgesia in various types of acute and chronic orofacial pain.[1-3] It can be approached externally through the nares by using cotton pledgets soaked with local anesthetic to anesthetize this region. This simple approach can be used by headache sufferers to manage their own pain control at home.[4,5] In this chapter, we will focus mainly on the technical aspect of fluoroscopic-guided nerve block from a pain physician's point of view.

ANATOMY

Sphenopalatine ganglion is located in the pterygopalatine fossa. The pterygopalatine fossa is a small, upside-down pyramidal space about 2 cm high and 1 cm wide and is located behind the posterior wall of the maxillary sinus. It is bordered posteriorly by the medial plate of the pterygoid process, superiorly by the sphenoid sinus, and medially by the perpendicular plate of the palatine bone, and laterally it opens into the infratemporal fossa. Superolaterally, the foramen rotundum with the exiting maxillary nerve is located, and inferomedially, there is the vidian nerve (greater petrosal and deep petrosal nerves) within the pterygoid canal. The pterygopalatine fossa contains the internal maxillary artery and its branches, the maxillary nerve, and the SPG and its afferent and efferent branches. The ganglion is "suspended" from the maxillary nerve by the pterygopalatine nerves and is medial to the maxillary nerve **(Fig. 1)**.

Posteriorly the ganglion is connected to the vidian nerve, which is formed by the deep petrosal (sympathetic from the

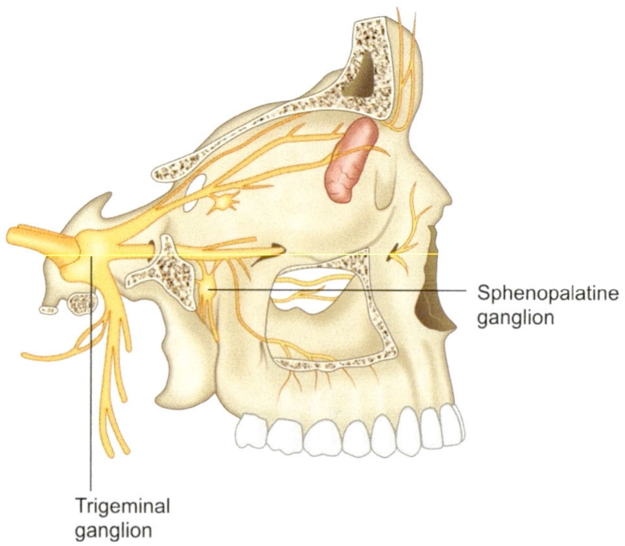

Fig. 1: Sphenopalatine ganglion in pterygopalatine fossa suspended from maxillary nerve via sphenopalatine nerves.

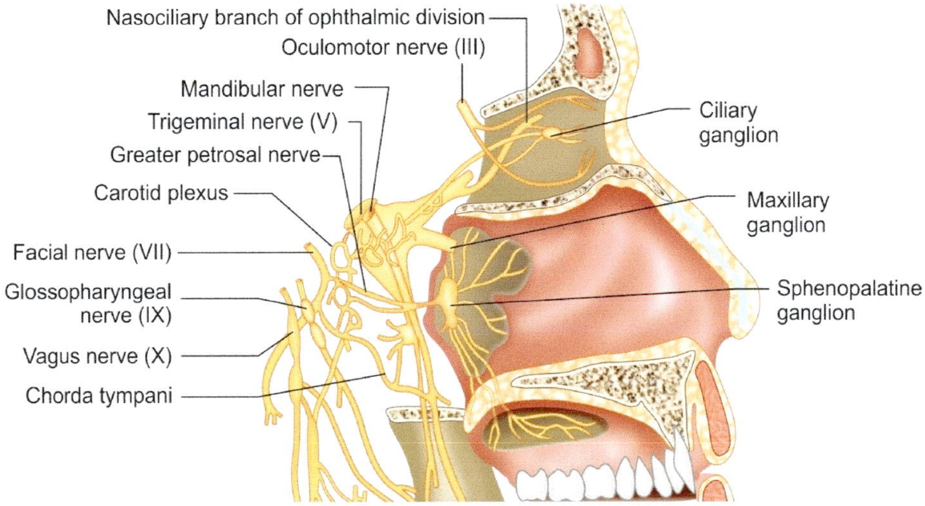

Fig. 2: Sphenopalatine ganglion with its neural connections.

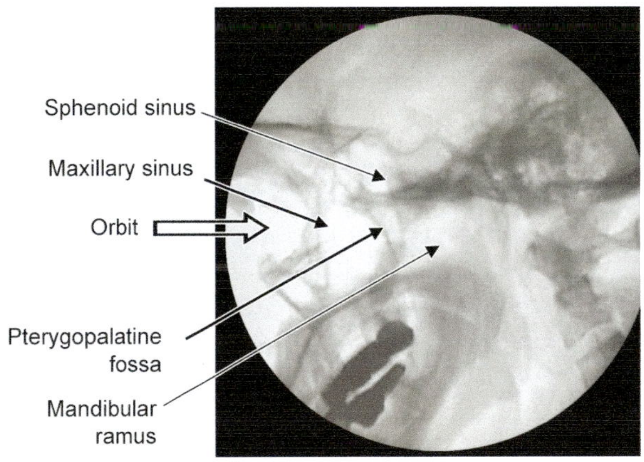

Fig. 3: Fluroanatomy lateral view of pterygopalatine fossa.

upper thoracic spinal cord) and greater petrosal (parasympathetic from the superior salivatory nucleus) nerves.

The ganglion has efferent branches and forms the superoposterior lateral nasal and pharyngeal nerves. Caudally, the greater and lesser palatine nerves exit the ganglion. Sensory fibers arise from the maxillary nerve, pass through the SPG, and innervate the upper teeth, nasal membranes, soft palate, and some parts of the pharynx **(Fig. 2)**. Sympathetic and postganglionic parasympathetic neurons pass through ganglion and innervate lacrimal glands, inferior and posterior septum, lateral wall of nasal cavity, and nasal glands.

The pterygopalatine fossa resembles a V-shaped vase on a lateral fluoroscopic image[1] **(Fig. 3)**. The pterygomaxillary fissure allows passage of a needle into the fossa.

INDICATIONS

- Cluster headache[6-8]
- Migraine
- Trigeminal neuralgia[9]
- Paroxysmal hemicrania
- Facial pain that is atypical
- Postherpetic neuralgia[10,11]
- Complex regional pain syndrome (CRPS)
- Temporomandibular disorder
- Unexplained intraoral pain
- Nasal contact point headache
- Vasomotor rhinitis
- Cancer of the head or neck region arising from buccal mucosa, tongue, alveolus, larynx, pharynx, floor of mouth, etc.[12]

CONTRAINDICATIONS

- Local infection
- Coagulopathy

EQUIPMENT AND DRUGS

Needles

- 25 G ¾-inch needle, for local infiltration
- 22 G spinal needle
- RF ("Radiofrequency" needle—10 cm needle with 5 mm active tip)

Syringes: 1 mL, 2 mL, 5 mL, 10 mL—2 each

Equipment:

Same as in Chapter 15.

Imaging modalities:

- C-arm
- Computed tomography (CT)

Drugs:

- Lignocaine 2%
- Bupivacaine 0.5%
- Normal saline
- Depot steroids: Triamcinolone or alpha methylprednisolone 40 mg
- Alcohol 99%
- Phenol 6% for neurolysis.

PREPARATION

Same as in Chapter 15.

POSITION

Position of the patient is supine **(Fig. 4)**.

Zygomatic arch and mandibular or coronoid notch marked on patients face (**Fig. 3** Chapter 15)

C-arm is placed in lateral position **(Fig. 5)** so that temporomandibular joint and external auditory meatus of both sides overlap each other. Pterygopalatine fossa should be visible as "inverted vas" posterior to maxillary sinus and just anterior to the anterior end of the petrous part of temporal bone.

PROCEDURE

Preoperative antibiotic might be given depending on the institutional practice.

Coronoid notch is identified by asking the patient to open and close his mouth.

Needle entry point is from the center of the coronoid notch, i.e., mandibular notch of the mandibular bone and just below the zygomatic arch.

First antiseptic is applied.

Local anesthetic using 1% lignocaine is given along the skin.

With the patient in the supine position and the head inside the C-arm, a lateral view is obtained, and either the C-arm or the head of the patient is rotated until both pterygoid plates are superimposed on each other to precisely visualize the ipsilateral pterygopalatine fossa.

The needle is first introduced in the lateral view and advanced medially and superiorly toward the pterygopalatine fossa that is inverted vas using intermittent fluoroscopy is slightly superior, medial and anterior **(Fig. 6A)**.

This can be confirmed by the AP view of fluoroscopy **(Fig. 6B)**.

It should not cross the lateral border of nose and should rest at the superior-medial end of the maxillary sinus on C-arm. At this point, some patients might complain of nasal or palatal sensation and even upper teeth pain.

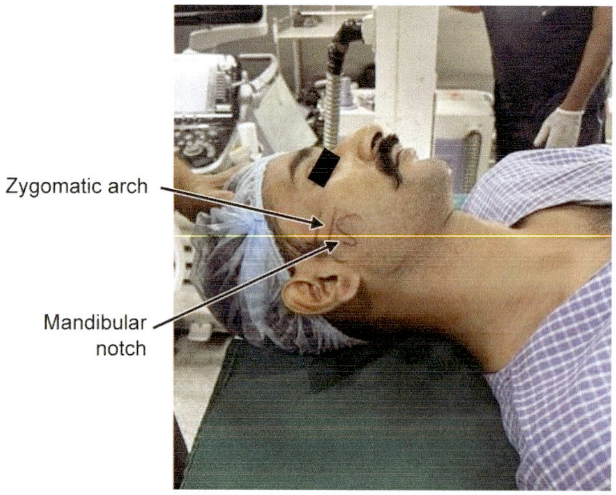

Fig. 4: Patient position—supine. Surface marking—zygomatic arch and mandibular or coronoid notch.

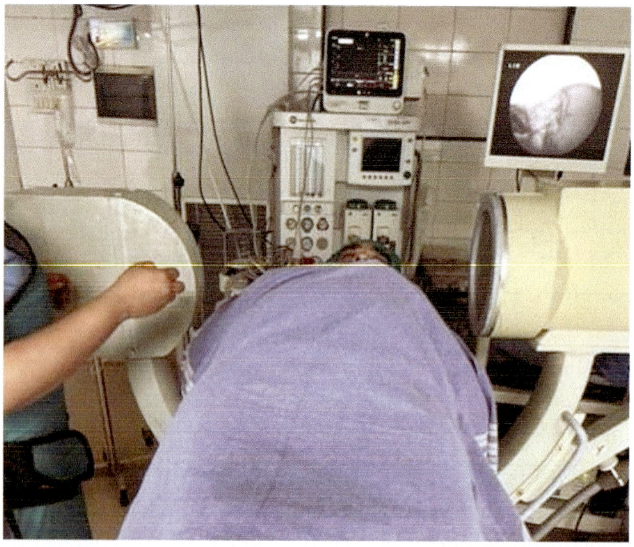

Fig. 5: Patient position, supine C-arm for lateral view.

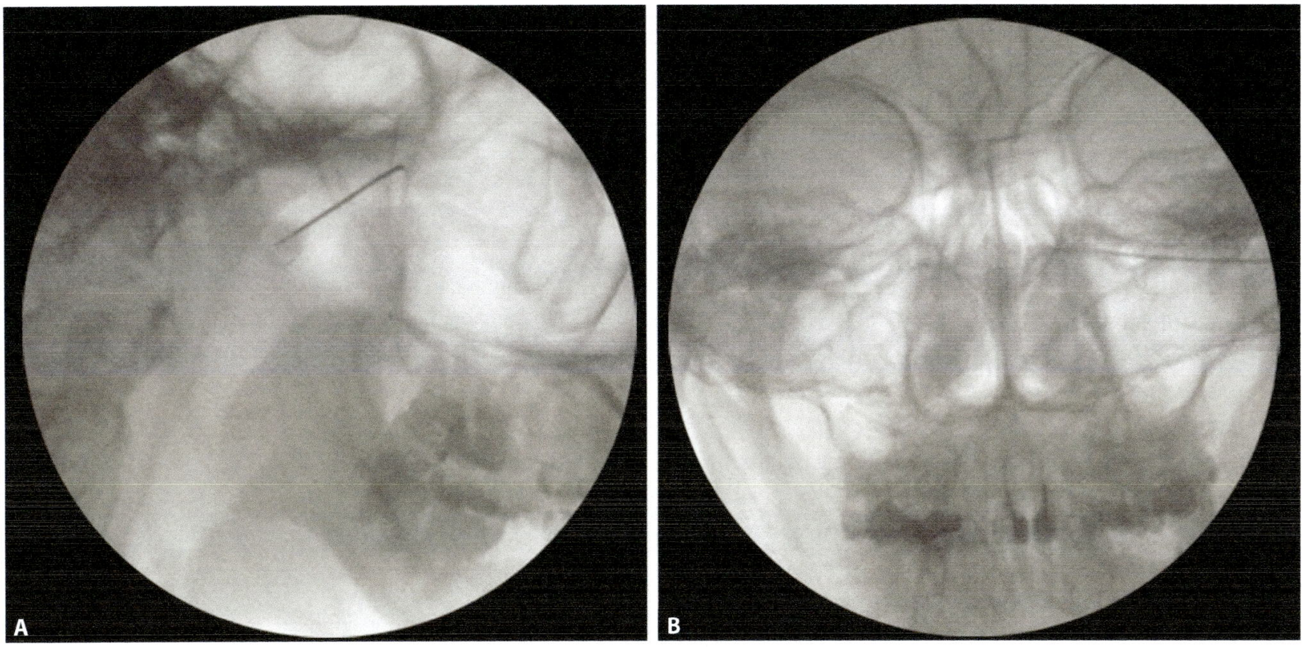

Figs. 6A and B: Final needle position: (A) Lateral and (B) anteroposterior (AP) views.

Negative aspiration is a must for blood, air (if the needle tip is advanced into the nasal cavity or the maxillary sinus), or clear fluid which could even be cerebrospinal fluid. Intravascular spread could also be ruled out by injecting nonionic, water soluble, radiopaque contrast media with fluoroscopy.

Once the placement is confirmed, 2–2.5 mL of local anesthetic is injected slowly with or without steroid.

Volume usually should not be >2 mL, so if one is injecting contrast then one must be sure about the volume.

The patient should be monitored in the recovery room for 40–60 minutes for any signs of bleeding or unexpected neurological symptoms/signs.

This would mainly work as a diagnostic-cum-therapeutic block. If it is positive, then "radiofrequency" of the same could be planned at a later date.

This procedure can be performed with CT guidance.[13]

RADIOFREQUENCY ABLATION[7,14]

Both conventional and pulsed RF can be done for long-term pain relief. For conventional RF sensory stimulation, the response of the patient is important. Stimulation is performed with 50 Hz at 0.4–0.6 V. The best stimulation felt is in the nose or at the base of the nose. Also, there might be stimulation of the painful area.

If stimulation or tingling sensation occurs at upper teeth then needle might be near superior alveolar nerve, a branch of maxillary nerve, then the needle should be redirected slight posteriorly to avoid damage to this nerve. If stimulation or tingling sensation occurs at hard or soft pallet then needle might be near palatine nerve, then the needle should be redirected slight cranially to avoid damage to this nerve. If one is having numbness or stimulation of the hard or soft palate, then it might be that the needle is inferior. Once the stimulatory parameters are met, then "conventional radiofrequency" is used at 80°C for 90 seconds after injecting local anesthetic drug 1 mL with 2% lignocaine or 0.5% bupivacaine. 5 mg of triamcinolone (or 2–4 mg of dexamethasone) is injected with the aim to prevent postprocedure neuritis.

For pulsed RF lesion is done at 42°C for 120 seconds. At least 2–3 lesions should be done for a good pulsed RF lesion.[15]

POSSIBLE COMPLICATIONS

- Bleeding: As nose is rich in vasculature, it usually respond to pressure.
- Hematoma of the cheek can occur after maxillary artery or branch injury, which is located within the pterygopalatine fossa.

- Infection: If nasal mucosa is breached at the lateral border of nose
- Intracranial spread of medicines
- Bradycardia, while performing RF ablation (RFA). Atropine should be kept ready.
- Pharyngeal puncture
- Radiofrequency lesioning of the SPG can result in permanent or, more commonly, temporary hypesthesia or dysesthesia in the palate, maxilla, or posterior pharynx.
- Dryness of the eye as a result of interruption of the parasympathetic supply is also common; however, it is usually only temporary.
- Temporary diplopia, which is more common after local anesthetic injections rather than RFA, can be explained by the spread of the injectate from the pterygopalatine fossa to the inferior orbital fissure containing the abducent nerve.[8] This is the reason why we limit the injectate volume to only 1–2 mL.
- Side effects with relation to local anesthetic, alcohol, or phenol

CONCLUSION

The SPGB is used for a variety of headache and facial pain syndromes and has variable efficacy depending on the disease process treated. Significant reduction in pain is meaningful when followed by an increase in functional capacity and reduction in use of analgesics. If the SPGB works for a short duration of time, it can be followed by RFA to increase the duration of pain relief. It should be judicially used by pain physicians for helping patients suffering from neuralgic, chronic, and cancer pain in head and face region.

REFERENCES

1. Raj PP, Leland L, Serdar E, Staats PS. Radiographic Imaging for Regional Anesthesia and Pain Management, 1st edition. Philadelphia: Churchill Livingstone; 2003.
2. Waldman SD. Atlas of Interventional Pain Management, 2nd edition. Philadelphia: WB Saunders; 2004.
3. Leong MS, Gjolaj MP, Gaeta RR. Sphenopalatine ganglion block. In: Deer TR, Leong MS, Buvanendran A, Kim PS, Panchal SJ (Eds). Treatment of Chronic Pain by Interventional Approaches: The American Academy of Pain Medicine Textbook on Patient Management. Springer; 2014. pp. 93-7.
4. Saade E, Paige GB. Patient-administered sphenopalatine ganglion block. Reg Anesth. 1996;21:68-70. 15.
5. Sanghavi PR, Shah BC, Joshi GM. Home-based application of sphenopalatine ganglion block for head and neck cancer pain management. Indian J Palliat Care. 2017;23:282-6.
6. Sanders M, Zuurmond WW. Efficacy of sphenopalatine ganglion blockade in 66 patients suffering from cluster headache: a 12- to 70-month follow-up evaluation. J Neurosurg. 1997:87:876-80.
7. Narouze S, Kapural L, Casanova J, Mekhail N. Sphenopalatine ganglion radiofrequency ablation for the management of chronic cluster headache. Headache. 2009;49:571-7.
8. Narouze SN. Role of sphenopalatine ganglion neuroablation in the management of cluster headache. Curr Pain Headache Rep. 2010;14:160-3.
9. Manahan AP, Malesker MA, Malone PM. Sphenopalatine ganglion block relieves symptoms of trigeminal neuralgia: a case report. Nebr Med J. 199681:306-9.
10. Saberski L, Ahmad M, Wiske P. Sphenopalatine ganglion block for treatment of sinus arrest in postherpetic neuralgia. Headache. 1999;39:42-4.
11. Prasanna A, Murthy PS. Sphenopalatine ganglion block and pain of cancer. J Pain Symptom Manage.1993;8:125.
12. Prasanna A, Murthy PS. Combined stellate ganglion and sphenopalatine ganglion block in acute herpes infection. Clin J Pain. 1993;9:135-7.
13. Fang L, Jingjing L, Ying S, Lan M, Tao W, Nan J. Computerized tomography-guided sphenopalatine ganglion pulsed radiofrequency treatment in 16 patients with refractory cluster headaches: Twelve- to 30-month follow-up evaluations. Cephalalgia. 2016;36:106-12.
14. Salar G, Ori C, Iob I, Fiore D. Percutaneous thermocoagulation for sphenopalatine ganglion neuralgia. Acta Neurochir (Wien).1987;84:24-8.
15. Shah RV, Racz GB. Long-term relief of posttraumatic headache by sphenopalatine ganglion pulsed radiofrequency lesioning: a case report. Arch Phys Med Rehabil. 2004;85:1013-6.

17 CHAPTER

Glossopharyngeal Nerve Block

George C Chang Chien, Jianguo Cheng

ABSTRACT

Glossopharyngeal neuralgia (GPN) is characterized by unilateral paroxysmal pain in the oropharynx, nasopharynx, larynx, base of the tongue, lower jaw, and ear. These attacks are typically excruciating and described as sharp, stabbing, "shocks of electricity", that can last from seconds to minutes. The diagnosis is primarily based on the description of the location and pattern of the pain. A block of the glossopharyngeal nerve with hours of pain relief during a flareup is a useful tool to confirm the diagnosis. Magnetic resonance imaging (MRI) is routinely performed to rule out a tumor, other mass lesions, or blood vessels that may be compressing the glossopharyngeal nerve. Antiepileptic drugs and tricyclic antidepressants may be used to ameliorate the pain of GPN. Blocks with a local anesthetic with or without a corticosteroid, chemical neurolysis, and radiofrequency ablation are all options in the management of GPN. When a blood vessel is identified as compressing the glossopharyngeal nerve, surgery may be performed to move the vessel or to position a Teflon pad between the blood vessel and the nerve, in order to mitigate any pressure on the nerve. In severe cases that are refractory to other treatments, surgery that severs the glossopharyngeal nerve may be the only treatment to relieve the pain. Here, we will focus on the techniques of glossopharyngeal nerve block.

INTRODUCTION

Although uncommon as an etiology of head and neck pain (0.57–1.3% of cases of facial pain),[1-3] impingement or injury to the glossopharyngeal nerve (cranial nerve IX) can lead to glossopharyngeal neuralgia (GPN), a potentially life-threatening disease.[4,5] Pain management specialists should learn to recognize it and become facile with techniques of providing analgesia to this disorder.

Glossopharyngeal neuralgia, or Weisenburg–Sicard–Robineau Syndrome, was first described by the American neurologist TH Weisenburg in 1910 in a case of facial pain misdiagnosed as tic douloureux (trigeminal neuralgia) secondary to a cerebellopontine tumor.[6] Although the French neurologists Jean-Anathase Sicard and Maurice Robineau also published cases in 1920 where they treated cases of atypical facial pain by dissection of the ninth cranial nerve,[7] it was the British neurologist Wilfred Harris who coined the term "glossopharyngeal neuralgia" in 1921.[3,4]

Glossopharyngeal neuralgia is characterized by unilateral paroxysmal pain in the oropharynx, nasopharynx, larynx, base of the tongue, tonsillar region, and lower jaw. It can also radiate to the ipsilateral ear. These attacks are excruciatingly painful and typically described as sharp, stabbing, "shocks of electricity", which can last from seconds to minutes.[2,3,8] These painful attacks are triggered by stimulation to the oropharynx such as mechanical swallowing, yawning, coughing, laughing, and chewing, and sensory stimulation such as cold, salty, acidic, or bitter foods.[2,3]

The incidence of GPN increases with age and most often affects persons older than 50 years; however, in patients with multiple sclerosis, GPN tends to occur at a younger age.[9,10] In 217 cases of GPN seen at the Mayo Clinic,[11] 57% of the cases were in patients >50 years old, while 43% were between the ages of 18 and 50 years. About 12% of these patients had bilateral involvement, but a frequency as high as 25% has been reported.[11,12] Additionally,

12% of the patients exhibited both glossopharyngeal and trigeminal neuralgia.[11] A greater prevalence in males has also been reported by some authors,[2] while others have reported no difference in prevalence by gender.

Cardiovascular symptoms such as bradycardia, hypotension, and even cardiac arrest may accompany the attacks in 1-2% of the cases.[4,5,13] The close association between the glossopharyngeal nerve and the vagus nerve (cranial nerve X) may underlie, in part, the etiology between GPN and the cardiac symptoms.[14] Seizures have also been associated with episodes of GPN.[5,15,16]

Although most cases are categorized as "idiopathic", the majority of cases are believed to be caused by vascular compression of the glossopharyngeal nerve.[13,17] Kawashima studied 14 cases of idiopathic GPN. In all of the cases, vascular compression on the glossopharyngeal nerve was found.[18] Most commonly, it is the posterior inferior cerebellar artery (PICA), followed by the anterior inferior cerebellar artery (AICA) that compresses the glossopharyngeal nerve.[13,18-20] Other causes for GPN include tumors with local invasion,[21] parapharyngeal abscess,[22] trauma,[23] multiple sclerosis,[9,10,24] carotid puncture,[25] styloid carotid artery syndrome (Eagle syndrome),[17,26,27] adhesive arachnoiditis,[28] and C1 Jefferson fracture.[29]

Glossopharyngeal neuralgia may mimic trigeminal neuralgia. Both may present with facial/jaw pain, elicited by the same mechanical and sensory mechanisms. Cases may be difficult to differentiate in patients with pain in the region of the tragus or deep to the angle of the jaw.[2] However, compared to trigeminal neuralgia, GPN is relatively rare,[1-3] although dual diagnosis has been reported.[11] A diagnostic interventional block may be useful in differentiating the two neuralgias and indeed may be the only way to definitively establish the diagnosis of GPN.[30]

ANATOMY

The glossopharyngeal nerve (cranial nerve IX) is a mixed-function nerve with motor, sensory, and special sensory fibers. The rootlets originate in the upper part of the postolivary sulcus, between the olive and the inferior peduncle of the medulla oblongata, and exit the cranium with parasympathetic nerve fibers from the salivatory nucleus, the vagus, and spinal accessory nerves (cranial nerves X and XI) via the jugular foramen **(Fig. 1)**. All three cranial nerves lie between the internal jugular vein and the internal carotid artery.

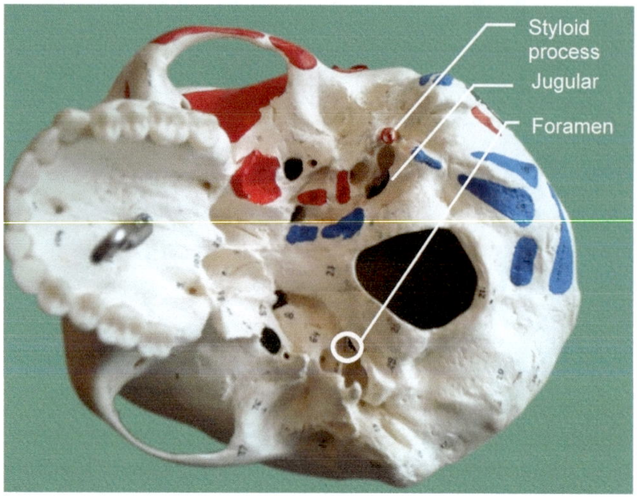

Fig. 1: Base of the skull—the jugular foramen is where the glossopharyngeal, vagus, and accessory nerves exit the cranium. *Courtesy:* Kenneth D Candido, MD.

The glossopharyngeal nerve has many branches, including tympanic, carotid, pharyngeal, muscular, tonsillar, and lingual. The tympanic branch innervates the tympanic membrane. The carotid branch innervates the carotid sinus and the carotid body. Damage to this branch may lead to deregulation of blood pressure, pulse, and respiration. The pharyngeal branch carries sensory nerve from the walls of the pharynx. The tonsillar branch transmits sensory nerves from the tonsils. The lingual branch innervates the anterior surface of the epiglottis, the posterior third of the tongue, and the vallecula. The motor component innervates the stylopharyngeus muscle, which elevates the pharynx during talking and swallowing. The sensory portion innervates the palatine tonsils, the posterior third of the tongue, and the mucous membranes of the oropharynx. Special sensory afferent fibers transmit information for taste from the posterior third of the tongue.

DIAGNOSIS

Diagnosis is typically based on clinical presentation, physical examination, imaging studies, and diagnostic blocks.

Imaging

High-resolution magnetic resonance imaging (MRI)[31,32] or computed tomography scan of the head may reveal tumor, bony erosion, multiple sclerosis plaques, abscess, or infection. Three-dimensional visualizations of the brainstem or magnetic resonance angiography may identify neurovascular compression or arteriovenous malformation. Visualization of the offending vessel was better in cases of compression from the PICA compared to the AICA.[32]

Balloon Test Occlusion

Hasegawa et al. reported a case, where MRI suggested that the right vertebral artery (VA) was pressing on the glossopharyngeal nerve.[33] Balloon test occlusion of the VA was used to confirm the cause of the neuralgia. The neuralgia disappeared and reappeared with balloon inflation and deflation. Balloon test occlusion may be useful in the diagnosis of GPN and the selection of the most appropriate surgical treatment.[33,34]

MEDICAL TREATMENT

Medical treatment of GPN is similar to the treatment for other forms of neuropathic pain, including trigeminal neuralgia. Antiepileptic drugs (AEDs) and tricyclic antidepressants, alone or in combination, have been studied with variable efficacy.[35] There is also a case report of GPN refractory to AEDs that responded well to opioids.[36] AEDs that have been used include carbamazepine, lamotrigine, diazepam, and gabapentin; tricyclic antidepressants such as amitriptyline and nortriptyline have been used.[37-41]

INTERVENTIONAL TECHNIQUES

The following are the indications for glossopharyngeal nerve block (GNB) or neurolysis:

- Glossopharyngeal neuralgia (GPN)
- Post-tonsillectomy pain control
- Cancer pain
- To reduce gag reflex for awake endotracheal intubation
- Singultus (hiccups)
- Carotid sinus syndrome
- Patients who are poor candidates for microvascular decompression.

Techniques for extraoral, intraoral, fluoroscopic, or ultrasound-assisted procedures have been described. Compared to ultrasound-assisted intervention,[42] the use of fluoroscopy allows real-time imaging of the contrast media and helps minimize intravascular injection, in case the needle tip has penetrated either the carotid or jugular vessels. Injections of local anesthetic (LA) and/or steroids, or chemical neurolysis,[43] and radiofrequency ablation[44,45] are all options in the management of glossopharyngeal nerve dysfunction.

Patients need to be monitored for a minimum of 30 minutes following the block to verify that there has been no systemic response to the injected LA solution. Even taking these precautions and using fluoroscopy or ultrasound guidance does not completely eliminate the possibility of LA spillover onto the vagus nerve (with resultant ipsilateral vocal cord paralysis) or onto the spinal accessory nerve (weakness of the trapezius muscle). An obtunded gag reflex is an indicator of successful GNB.

Extraoral (Peristyloid) Technique with Fluoroscopy

The patient is placed supine with the head rotated slightly opposite from the affected side. The styloid process is used to identify the course of the GPN. Once identification of the mastoid process and the ipsilateral angle of the mandible is performed, the styloid process can be found equidistant between these structures **(Figs. 2A to D)**.

The skin overlying the styloid process should be prepped and draped in sterile fashion. A small skin wheal is made over the styloid process using a 25 g, 1.5-inch needle and 3–4 mL of 1% plain lidocaine. A 22 g, 1.5–2-inch blunt-tipped needle may be advanced perpendicular to the skin toward the process, aiming for its posterior aspect. The styloid process should be met at a depth approximating 1.5–4 cm. Once the styloid process is encountered, the needle is slightly withdrawn and "walked off" posteriorly. Aspiration should be performed to ensure that there is no blood or cerebrospinal fluid. About 1 mL of water-soluble, iodinated contrast media is incrementally injected under live continuous fluoroscopy. Then, barring any intravascular spread, a short-acting, preservative-free anesthetic (3–5 mL lidocaine or mepivacaine at 1% concentration) is incrementally injected in divided doses. Nonparticulate corticosteroid (dexamethasone, betamethasone) may be added to the injectate.

The styloid process (yellow oval) is typically found equidistant between the mastoid process (red line) and the ipsilateral angle of the mandible (blue line). This surface anatomy is important for the extraoral approach for GNB.

The spatial relationship between the styloid process (red arrow), the angle of the mandible, and the mastoid process is shown. Note the depth of the styloid process in relation to these structures.

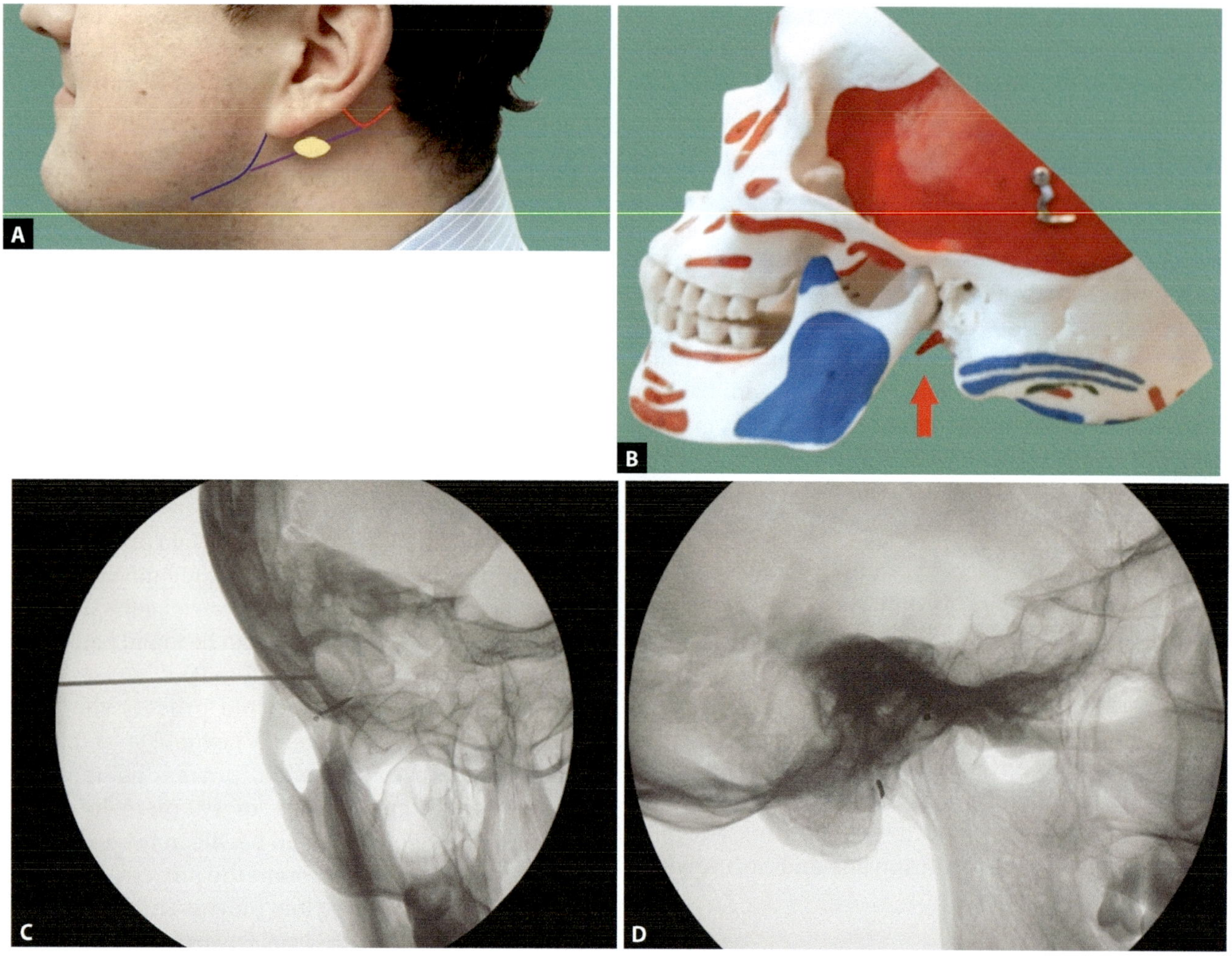

Figs. 2A to D: (A) Surface anatomy—glossopharyngeal nerve block; (B) Osseous anatomy—glossopharyngeal nerve block; (C) Anteroposterior fluoroscopic image of the right glossopharyngeal nerve block; (D) Lateral fluoroscopic image of the right glossopharyngeal nerve block.
Courtesy: (A and B) George C Chang Chien, DO; (C and D) Steven D Waldman, MD, JD.

Intraoral Technique

Anterior Tonsillar Pillar Method[46]

The patient is asked to open the mouth widely. The anatomical landmarks for intraoral GNB are shown **(Fig. 3)**. The operator may choose to anesthetize the tongue to facilitate the procedure. The tongue is swept to the opposite side with a tongue depressor, laryngoscope blade, or gloved fingers. A 25 g, 3.5-inch spinal needle is inserted 0.5 cm deep, just lateral to the base of the anterior tonsillar pillar (ATP). Use of a spinal needle is advantageous for visualization of the tonsillar pillars by keeping the syringe out of the patient's mouth. After careful aspiration for blood or cerebrospinal fluid, 2 mL of LA or LA plus nonparticulate steroid is injected. The advantages of this

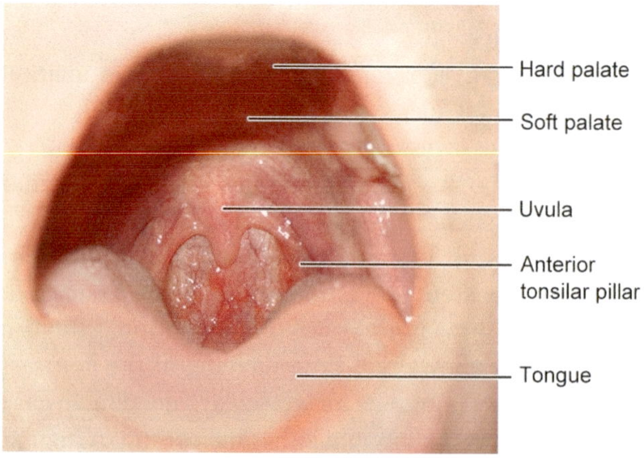

Fig. 3: Anatomy for intraoral glossopharyngeal nerve block.
Courtesy: George C Chang Chien, DO.

method are that the ATP is easily identified and exposed, and the tongue movement does not trigger the gag reflex.

Posterior Tonsillar Pillar Method[47]

The patient is asked to open the mouth widely. The tongue is depressed down with a laryngoscope blade (if done in the OR) or a tongue blade. A 22 g, 3.5-inch spinal needle bent 1 cm from the distal end is directed laterally into the submucosa along the caudal aspect of the palatopharyngeal fold (PTP). After careful aspiration for blood and cerebrospinal fluid, 2 mL of LA and/or steroid is injected. The PTP method becomes more difficult in patients with large tongues or small oral opening and may cause greater gag reflex.

POTENTIAL COMPLICATIONS/SIDE EFFECTS

Potential side effects of GNB may include:

- Dysphagia secondary to weakness of the stylopharyngeus muscle
- Upper airway obstruction/loss of protective reflexes secondary to bilateral nerve block
- *Ecchymoses/hematoma:* Trauma to internal carotid artery and/or internal carotid vein
- Infection
- Trauma to the nerve
- Toxicity due to intravascular injection of LA
- Tachycardia from vagus nerve block
- Hoarseness/dysphonia secondary to vagus nerve block, and paralysis of the ipsilateral vocal cord
- Postprocedure dysesthesias or anesthesia dolorosa
- Cardiovascular complications resulting in acute-onset hypotension with right bundle branch block secondary to dissection of the uppermost rootlets of the vagus nerve
- Block of the hypoglossal nerve with resultant tongue weakness (cranial nerve XII)
- Trapezius muscle weakness secondary to inadvertent block of the spinal accessory nerve (cranial nerve XI).

CONCLUSION

Orofacial pain can be difficult to diagnose and treat. The intricate anatomical relationships between the glossopharyngeal nerve and other cranial structures, neural as well as osseous, ligamentous, and vascular, impose a challenge for even seasoned interventional pain management physicians. The use of GNB is part of a multidisciplinary and multimodal approach to pain control.

REFERENCES

1. Harris W. Persistent pain in lesions of the peripheral and central nervous system. Brain (Lond). 1921;44:557.
2. Chawla JC, Falconer MA. Glossopharyngeal and vagal neuralgia. Br Med J. 1967;3:529-31.
3. Fraioli B, Esposito V, Ferrante L, Trubiani L, Lunardi P. Microsurgical treatment of glossopharyngeal neuralgia: case reports. Neurosurgery. 1989;25:630-2.
4. Weinstein RE, Herec D, Friedman JH. Hypotension due to glossopharyngeal neuralgia. Arch Neurol. 1986;43(1):90-2.
5. Kong Y, Heyman A, Entman ML, McIntosh HD. Glossopharyngeal neuralgia associated with bradycardia, syncope, and seizures. Circulation. 1964;30:109-13.
6. Weisenburg TH. Cerebello-pontine tumor diagnosed for six years as a tic douloureux: the symptoms of irritation of the ninth and twelfth cranial nerves. JAMA. 1910;54:1600-4.
7. Sicard R, Robineau J. Communications et presentations: I Algie Velo-pharyngeal essentielle. Traitement chirurgical. Rev Neurol. 1920;36:256-7.
8. Dandy WE. Glossopharyngeal neuralgia (tic douloureux). Arch Surg. 1927;15:198.
9. Minagar A, Sheremata WA. Glossopharyngeal neuralgia and MS. Neurology. 2000;54:1368-70.
10. Gaitour E, Nick ST, Roberts C, Gonzalez-Toledo E, Munjampalli S, Minagar A, et al. Glossopharyngeal neuralgia secondary to vascular compression in a patient with multiple sclerosis: a case report. J Med Case Rep. 2012;6:213.
11. Rushton JG, Stevens JC, Miller RH. Glossopharyngeal (vagoglossopharyngeal) neuralgia: a study of 217 cases. Arch Neurol. 1981;38:201-5.
12. Katusic S, Williams DB, Beard CM, Bergstralh E, Kurland LT. Incidence and clinical features of glossopharyngeal neuralgia, Rochester, Minnesota, 1945-1984. Neuroepidemiology. 1991;10:266-75.
13. Ferrante L, Artico M, Nardacci B, Fraioli B, Consentino F, Fortuna A. Glossopharyngeal neuralgia with cardiac syncope. Neurosurgery. 1995;36(1):58-63.
14. Karnosh LJ, Gardner WJ, Stowell A. Glossopharyngeal neuralgia: physiological consideration of the role of ninth and tenth cranial nerves: report of cases. Trans Am Neurol Assoc. 1947;72:205-7.
15. Takaya N, Sumiyoshi M, Nakata Y. Prolonged cardiac arrest caused by glossopharyngeal neuralgia. Heart. 2003;89(4):381.
16. Varrasi C, Strigaro G, Prandi P, Comi C, Mula M, Monaco F, et al. Complex pattern of convulsive syncope in glossopharyngeal neuralgia: video/EEG report and short review. Epilepsy Behav. 2011;20(2):407-9.
17. Soh KB. The glossopharyngeal nerve, glossopharyngeal neuralgia and the Eagle's syndrome—current concepts and management. Singapore Med J. 1999;40(10):659-65.
18. Kawashima M, Matsushima T, Inoue T, Mineta T, Masuoka J, Hirakawa N. Microvascular decompression

for glossopharyngeal neuralgia through the transcondylar fossa (supracondylar transjugular tubercle) approach. Neurosurgery. 2010;66(6 Suppl Operative):275-80.
19. Resnick DK, Jannetta PJ, Bissonnette D, Jho HD, Lanzino G. Microvascular decompression for glossopharyngeal neuralgia. Neurosurgery. 1995;36(1):64-9.
20. Kondo A. Follow-up results of using microvascular decompression for treatment of glossopharyngeal neuralgia. J Neurosurg. 1998;88(2):221-5.
21. Dykman TR, Montgomery EB Jr, Gerstenberger PD, Zeiger HE, Clutter WE, Cryer PE. Glossopharyngeal neuralgia with syncope secondary to tumor. Treatment and pathophysiology. Am J Med. 1981;71(1):165-70.
22. Sobol SM, Wood BG, Conoyer JM. Glossopharyngeal neuralgia-asystole syndrome secondary to parapharyngeal space lesions. Otolaryngol Head Neck Surg. 1982;90(1):16-9.
23. Waga S, Kojima T. Glossopharyngeal neuralgia of traumatic origin. Surg Neurol. 1982;17(1):77-9.
24. Kahana E, Leibowitz U, Alter M. Brainstem and cranial nerve involvement in multiple sclerosis. Acta Neurol Scand. 1973;49(3):269-79.
25. Weinstein RE, Herec D, Friedman JH. Hypotension due to glossopharyngeal neuralgia. Arch Neurol. 1986;43(1):90-2.
26. Carrieri PB, Montella S, Petracca M. Glossopharyngeal neuralgia as onset of multiple sclerosis. Clin J Pain. 2009;25(8):737-9.
27. Shin JH, Herrera SR, Eboli P, Aydin S, Eskandar EH, Slavin KV. Entrapment of the glossopharyngeal nerve in patients with Eagle syndrome: surgical technique and outcomes in a series of 5 patients. J Neurosurg. 2009;111(6):1226-30.
28. Fukuda H, Ishikawa M, Yamazoe N. Glossopharyngeal neuralgia caused by adhesive arachnoid. Acta Neurochir (Wien). 2002;144(10):1057-8.
29. Dettling SD, Morscher MA, Masin JS, Adamczyk MJ. Cranial nerve IX and X impairment after a sports-related Jefferson (C1) fracture in a 16-year-old male: a case report. J Pediatr Orthop. 2013;33(3):e23-7.
30. Aicardi J. Disorders of the peripheral nerves. In: Aicardi J (Ed). Diseases of the Nervous System in Childhood, 2nd edition. London: MacKeith Press; 1998. p. 733.
31. Hiwatashi A, Matsushima T, Yoshiura T, Tanaka A, Noguchi T, Togao O, et al. MRI of glossopharyngeal neuralgia caused by neurovascular compression. Am J Roentgenol. 2008;191:578-81.
32. Gaul C, Hastreiter P, Duncker A, Naraghi R. Diagnosis and neurosurgical treatment of glossopharyngeal neuralgia: clinical findings and 3-D visualization of neurovascular compression in 19 consecutive patients. J Headache Pain. 2011;12(5):527-34.
33. Hasegawa S, Morioka M, Kai Y, Kuratsu J. Usefulness of balloon test occlusion in the diagnosis of glossopharyngeal neuralgia. Case report. Neurol Med Chir (Tokyo). 2008;48(4):163-6.
34. Matsushima T, Goto Y, Ishioka H, Mihara F, Fukui M. Possible role of an endovascular provocative test in the diagnosis of glossopharyngeal neuralgia as a vascular compression syndrome. Acta Neurochir (Wien). 1999;141(11): 1229-32.
35. Dworkin RH, Backonja M, Rowbotham MC, Allen RR, Argoff CR, Bennett GJ, et al. Advances in neuropathic pain: diagnosis, mechanisms, and treatment recommendations. Arch Neurol. 2003;60(11):1524-34.
36. Kouzaki Y, Takita T, Tawara S, Otsuka T, Hirano T, Uchino M. Opioid effectiveness for neuropathic pain in a patient with glossopharyngeal neuralgia. Rinsho Shinkeigaku. 2009;49(6):364-9.
37. Finnerup NB, Otto M, McQuay HK, Jensen TS, Sindrup SH. Algorithm for neuropathic pain treatment. An evidence-based proposal. Pain. 2005;118:289-305.
38. Cheshire WP Jr. Defining the role for gabapentin in the treatment of trigeminal neuralgia: a retrospective study. J Pain. 2002;3(2):137-42.
39. Titlic M, Jukic I, Tonkic A, Grani P, Jukic J. Use of lamotrigine in glossopharyngeal neuralgia: a case report. Headache. 2006;46(1):167-9.
40. Saviolo R, Fiascanoro G. Treatment of glossopharyngeal neuralgia by carbamazepine. Br Heart J. 1987;58(3): 291-2.
41. Ekbom KA, Westerberg CE. Carbamazepine in glossopharyngeal neuralgia. Arch Neurol. 1966;14(6):595-6.
42. Funasaka S, Kodera K. Intraoral nerve block for glossopharyngeal neuralgia. Arch Otorhinolaryngol. 1977; 215(3-4):311-5.
43. Bedder MD, Lindsay D. Glossopharyngeal nerve block using ultrasound guidance: a case report of a new technique. Reg Anesth. 1989;14(6):304-7.
44. Isamat F, Ferrán E, Acebes JJ. Selective percutaneous thermocoagulation rhizotomy in essential glossopharyngeal neuralgia. J Neurosurg. 1981;55(4):575-80.
45. Tew JM Jr. Treatment of pain of glossopharyngeal and vagus nerves by percutaneous rhizotomy. In: Youmans JR (Ed). Neurological Surgery. Philadelphia: WB Saunders Co. 1982. pp. 3609-12.
46. Isbir CA. Treatment of a patient with glossopharyngeal neuralgia by the anterior tonsillar pillar method. Case Rep Neurol. 2011;3:27-31.
47. Katz J. Glossopharyngeal nerve block. In: Katz J (Ed). Atlas of Regional Anesthesia. Norwalk: CT. Appleton and Lange; 1994. p. 54.

18 CHAPTER

Stellate Ganglion Block

Preeti P Doshi

ABSTRACT

Sympathetic blocks in the cervical and upper thoracic regions are commonly used techniques for a variety of diagnostic, therapeutic, and prognostic purposes.[1] Stellate ganglion is formed by the fusion of the inferior cervical ganglia, located on the transverse process of the C7 vertebrae, with the first thoracic ganglia situated in front of the neck of the first rib. Although stellate ganglion block is common nomenclature utilized, it is present in only 80% of the population, and in the remaining 20%, as the ganglia are not fused, either lower cervical sympathetic block or upper thoracic sympathetic block may seem a more appropriate term.

Stellate ganglion block is used in a variety of chronic pain conditions such as complex regional pain syndrome 1 and 2 (CRPS 1 and 2), herpes zoster affecting the face and neck, refractory chest pain or angina, and phantom limb pain besides pain due to vascular diseases such as Raynaud's phenomenon. There are varieties of techniques used for performing stellate ganglion block, but in view of several vital structures in the vicinity of the ganglion and potential serious complications, it is essential to perform this block under image guidance. Fluoroscopy-guided technique is most often used by the pain physician, but there is a change in paradigm nowadays to greater use of ultrasound guidance for the same. The details of practical considerations while performing this useful intervention are discussed.

INTRODUCTION

Sympathetic blocks in the cervical and upper thoracic regions are commonly used techniques for diagnostic, therapeutic, and/or prognostic purposes for a variety of chronic pain conditions involving head, face, neck, and upper extremity when pharmacotherapy and other conservative methods fail to produce adequate pain relief.

Selective sympathetic block was first described by Sellheim, followed shortly by Kappis in 1923 who described the use of sympathetic block in the paravertebral region for the treatment of severe visceral pain syndromes. Shortly thereafter, Mandl in 1924 introduced percutaneous interruption of sympathetic chain to treat pain of vascular insufficiency of lower extremities, which has been the mainstay of treatment thereafter to treat the ischemic pain.

Autonomic or sympathetic nervous system is directly involved in homeostatic activities and has a major role in vascular, visceral, and neuropathic pain. Sympathetically maintained pain occurs in a multitude of vascular pathologies such as occlusive arterial diseases, diabetes mellitus, or venous ulceration and neuropathic conditions such as CRPS, postherpetic neuralgia, and after peripheral nerve lesion. The complexity of vascular (ischemic) pain can be traced to a dysfunctional microcirculation. Neuropathic pain can be due to neural ischemia with resultant neurogenic inflammation.[2] The exact pathophysiological mechanism for CRPS is unknown, but there is a possibility of abnormal coupling between sympathetic and somatosensory nervous system occurring either at dorsal root ganglion or at peripheral nerve level. CRPS is associated with cortical, sensory, and motor dysfunction along with peripheral inflammatory changes.

It has been proposed that a temporary sympathetic block can be useful in the discrimination of sympathetically maintained and sympathetically independent pain; however, the role of these blocks in providing effective therapeutic analgesia is undetermined with evidence coming from very few placebo-controlled, blinded studies.[3]

INDICATIONS

Stellate ganglion block or cervical sympathetic block is typically considered for diagnostic, therapeutic, and prognostic purposes in the following conditions:

- Pain which has failed to respond to conservative measures as in:
  - CRPS I and CRPS II
  - Acute herpes zoster or postherpetic neuralgia involving head, face, neck, or upper arm
  - Neuropathic pain in neoplastic encroachment of the brachial plexus
  - Lymphedema and local edema of the upper extremity following mastectomy
  - Neuropathic pain as in Bell's palsy or post trigeminal ganglion radiofrequency (RF) ablation
  - Post amputation or phantom limb pain in upper extremity
- Vascular disorders such as Raynaud's disease or phenomenon, vasculitis, scleroderma, traumatic or embolic occlusion, accidental intra-arterial injection of α-adrenergic drugs (e.g., thiopentone) causing vasospasm.
- *Miscellaneous:* Refractory angina, hyperhidrosis, Ménière's disease, frostbite, quinidine poisoning, anosmia, long COVID, chronic fatigue syndrome, refractory ventricular tachyarrhythmias.
- Emerging use in hallucinations in schizophrenia, climacteric psychosis, and post-traumatic stress disorder (PTSD).[4] A right-sided stellate ganglion block (SGB) is necessary because right-sided blocks affect right hemisphere structures that are pertinent to PTSD since the right hemisphere is responsible for producing autonomic responses to emotional stimuli and the right amygdala is critically linked to unconscious emotional memories.[5]

CONTRAINDICATIONS FOR PERFORMING STELLATE GANGLION BLOCK

Absolute:

- Patient refusal
- Local infection or sepsis
- Allergic reaction to local anesthetic drug
- Primary and secondary coagulopathy.

Relative:

- Recent myocardial infarction or a severe cardiac conduction defect
- Glaucoma
- Contralateral pneumonectomy or pneumothorax.

APPLIED ANATOMY

It is essential to have a thorough knowledge of anatomical position and relations of the stellate ganglion for carrying out its block in a safe and effective manner. Stellate word is derived from its Latin equivalent, which implies "star shaped".

Four cervical sympathetic ganglia are anatomically identified bilaterally in most individuals. The upper three cervical sympathetic ganglia will not be discussed here, as they contribute very little to the practice of chronic pain management. The inferior cervical ganglion is fused with the first thoracic ganglion in 70–80% individuals to be labeled as stellate ganglion, but since may be separate in 20–30%, it may be more appropriate to label it as either lower cervical sympathetic or upper thoracic sympathetic block or cervicothoracic sympathetic block.[6]

Sympathetic nerves to the upper extremity exit T2–T8 through ventral spinal roots, travel as white communicating rami to the sympathetic chain, then pass cephalad to synapse at the T2 ganglion, first thoracic or the inferior cervical ganglion, and occasionally middle cervical ganglion. Most postganglionic nerves leave the chain as gray communicating rami to join the anterior divisions at C5-T1 nerves that form the brachial plexus. Some postganglionic nerves pass directly from the chain to form the subclavian perivascular plexus and innervate the subclavian, axillary, and upper parts of the brachial arteries.

Stellate ganglion is either star-shaped or an oval ganglion, which measures approximately 2.5 cm long, 1.0 cm wide, and 0.5 cm thick **(Fig. 1)**. The shape and the position, however, vary even in the same subject[7] It usually lies in front of the neck of the first rib and extends to the interspace between C7 and T1. When elongated, it may overlie the anterior tubercle of C7.

The relevant anatomical relations in most individuals are noted as follows:

- *Anterior:* Skin, subcutaneous tissue, carotid sheath, subclavian artery with origin of vertebral artery at C7 level.
- *Posterior:* Transverse process of C6 or C7 with prevertebral fascia, head of first rib, longus colli muscle **(Fig. 2)**.
- *Medial:* Esophagus, recurrent laryngeal nerve, thoracic duct, C7 vertebral body.

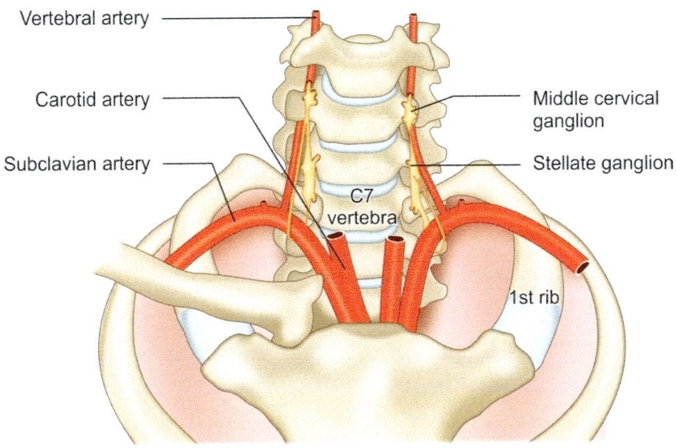

Fig. 1: Anatomy of stellate ganglion.

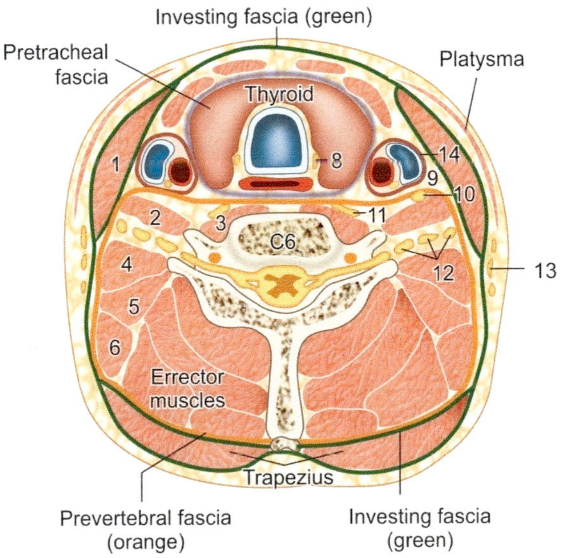

Fig. 2: Relations in axial section.
1. Sternocleidomastoid muscle; 2. Anterior scalene muscle; 3. Longus colli; 4. Middle scalene muscle; 5. Posterior scalene muscle; 6. Levator scapulae muscle; 7. See in **Fig. 1**; 8. Recurrent laryngeal nerve; 9. Vagus nerve; 10. Phrenic nerve; 11. Sympathetic ganglion; 12. Brachial plexus; 13. Superficial cervical plexus; 14. Carotid sheath.

- *Lateral:* Anterior scalene muscle, origin of brachial plexus, superior intercostal vein, superior intercostal artery, ventral ramus of first thoracic nerve.
- *Inferior:* Posterior part of apical pleura.

It is important to bear in mind that there are a significant number of individuals in whom the intrathoracic somatic branches from the second thoracic spinal nerve join the first thoracic spinal nerve. This intrathoracic branch is joined by the gray rami communicans carrying the sympathetic fibers that arise from the second thoracic sympathetic ganglia and possibly the T3 ganglia as well. These fibers join the lower part of the brachial plexus without passing through the stellate ganglia. This explains the incomplete sympathetic blockade of the upper extremity in a pure stellate ganglion block. These anomalous pathways are referred to as Kuntz's nerves. They bypass the stellate ganglia and so a pure stellate ganglion block will not produce complete sympathetic denervation of the upper extremity in these patients.

It is very important to understand the anatomical structure of the sympathetic ganglia, as failure to do so can contribute to either false-positive or false-negative test results during sympathetic blockade. This can also contribute to the failure of some neuroablative procedures following what was considered to be a successful diagnostic stellate ganglion block.[8]

TECHNIQUES FOR STELLATE GANGLION BLOCK

After ensuring suitability of the patient to undergo the procedure, one should examine for the following before proceeding:

- Anatomical variation
- Neck mobility/extension
- Prior radical neck surgery/thyroid surgery scar
- Any infection at the site of injection.

It is important to explain the patient about immediate reversible effects, possible complications, and discharge instructions. If the cause of pain is unclear and block is diagnostic, a clear understanding may allow the patient to record valuable information vital for diagnosis. The goals of blockade and the number of blocks given vary with each individual patient and each pain condition.

The preparation for this intervention is identical to other pain interventions such as:

- Consent after full explanation
- Blood tests as necessary
- Fasting for 4–6 hours
- Withholding medications such as antiplatelet/anticoagulant agents as appropriate
- Optimizing any comorbidity for safe practice.

Although it is a fairly simple block in skilled hands, standard resuscitation equipment, drugs, suction, oxygen delivery systems, cardiac defibrillator, and equipment for endotracheal intubation should be readily available, no matter which imaging guidance is utilized.

Intravenous line is secured for sedation or administration of emergency drugs if necessary. This is a precaution, which the author strongly recommends considering potential for complications such as convulsions or respiratory arrest. Monitored anesthesia care which includes pulse oximeter, ECG, and noninvasive blood pressure is advocated to monitor any hemodynamic alterations. A surface thermometry probe is positioned on the ipsilateral upper extremity to record the baseline temperature and observe any rise in the temperature of the affected extremity following the intervention. If possible, two probes can be used on either side for comparison of baseline.

EQUIPMENT

- 22 G spinal needle or 1.5″ long hypodermic needle (for lean patients)
- 10 cm extension tube with a three-way
- 25 G hypodermic needle for local infiltration

Optional: If RF lesion to be done,

- RF needle, 10 cm long needle with 5-mm tip
- Radiofrequency lesion generator and accessories
- Surface thermometry device
- Imaging equipment as necessary.

DRUGS

- *Local anesthetic:* 1% lignocaine or 0.25% bupivacaine or 0.5% ropivacaine.
- *Steroids (optional):* Inj methylprednisolone 40 mg or Dexamethasone 4 mg.
- *Nonionic contrast:* Iohexol 240 or 300
- *Neurolytic drug:* 6% phenol or 100% alcohol (used at very few centers).

To ensure safe and accurate administration of drugs, image guidance is strongly recommended. The choice depends on the availability and skills of the operator. The following approaches are commonly advocated in clinical practice.

Fluoroscopy-assisted Technique

Fluoroscopy-assisted technique is most frequently practiced by pain physicians at present time although many are switching to ultrasound guidance for its claimed superior safety profile.

The two methods used most widely to block the stellate ganglion are as follows:

1. At the level of the C6 transverse process (Chassaignac's tubercle) without or with the use of using anteroposterior and lateral fluoroscopy.
2. At the level of C7, the more medial approach at the anterolateral aspect of the vertebral body as the target.[9]

Even though both the techniques may adequately block the stellate ganglion, inadvertent placement of the needle into the vertebral artery, adjacent disk, neural tissue, esophagus, or intrathecal space can have serious consequences.

Patient is positioned supine with head straight with a small support under the head to stabilize it and a pad beneath the shoulder on a radiolucent table **(Fig. 3)**. This facilitates extension of the neck and accentuates the landmarks. Hyperextension also moves the esophagus out of the way to the target. The jaw may be kept slightly open to relax the neck muscles. The patient should refrain from speaking as this can move the muscle and dislodge the needle. The patient should also be instructed not to swallow once the needle is in situ as it can lead to esophageal injury in case of an erroneous placement on the right side. The patient should be instructed to raise his hand to indicate any difficulty.

The skin over the target is aseptically prepared and draped. The index finger of the nondominant hand should be used for palpation of the landmarks. Retraction of the carotid sheath laterally with the nondominant hand assists in avoiding vascular injury. After making a skin wheal, a 22 G preferably short-bevel needle is introduced with the dominant hand directly posterior and perpendicular to the table in all directions. The needle passes through

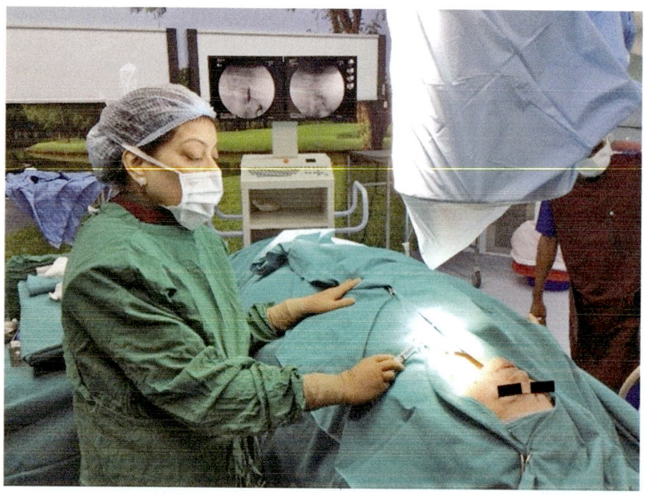

Fig. 3: Positioning for fluoroscopy-guided stellate ganglion block.

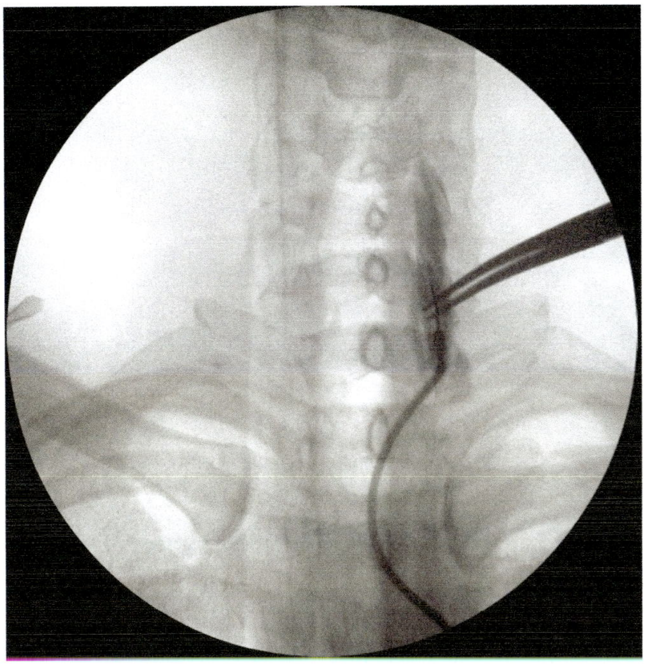

Fig. 4: Anteroposterior view during fluoroscopy.

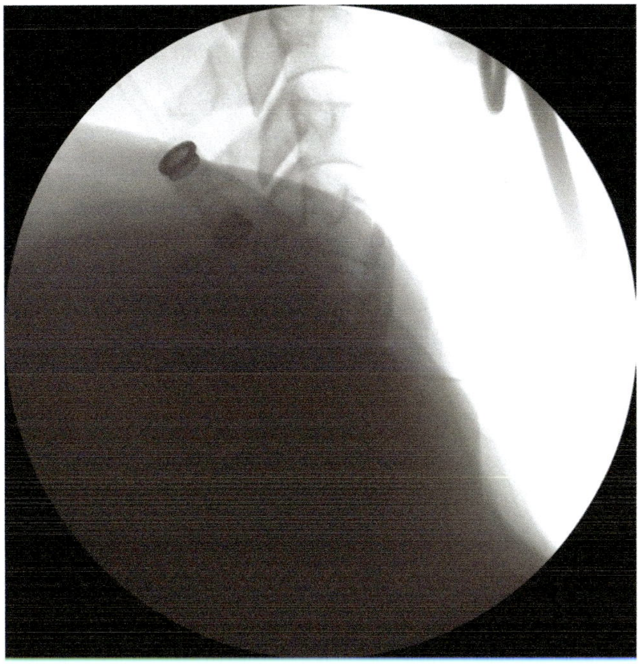

Fig. 5: Lateral view during fluoroscopy.

the underlying tissues till it contacts the bone at the C6 tubercle on the transverse process or its junction with the vertebral body. Once the bone is encountered, the needle is withdrawn 2–3 mm to avoid injecting into the longus colli muscle. The needle should preferably be attached to the extension tubing with the three-way to avoid chances of displacement while switching the syringes. One can also release the dominant hand to aspirate and/or inject while grasping the needle with an artery forceps.

After negative aspiration tests for blood and cerebrospinal fluid (CSF), 1–2 mL of Iohexol (nonionic contrast) should be injected with real-time fluoroscopy to exclude intravascular or neuraxial spread **(Figs. 4 and 5)**. Injection into the longus colli muscle is indicated by the inability of the contrast medium to spread in between the tissue planes while instantaneous disappearance indicates the presence of the needle in a vessel.

If dye spread is satisfactory, 1 mL of the local anesthetic agent should be injected to observe any adverse effect such as convulsion or effect on respiration or sensorium. After this, the remaining volume is slowly injected with intermittent aspiration and ensuring the tip remains in same position. An artery forceps to hold needle steady at the skin entry point and an extension with three-way can be of help here. At our center, a total volume of 10 mL is used. A modification of this technique includes needle placement at the C7 level, which is preferable to improve success of the outcome. This is impossible without imaging as there is no tubercle, and the transverse process is not as well developed as at C6 level in addition to which there is a likelihood of injury to the pleura and vertebral artery. The advantage is that one can use a minimal amount of the drug like 1–2 mL for sympathetic block of the head, face, and neck, and 5–7 mL of local anesthetic is required to reach a level of T2/T3 to block.

Another approach described by Abdi et al.[10] claimed to be easy and more effective is by oblique angulation using fluoroscopic guidance to visualize the junction of the uncinate process with the vertebral body. The needle is introduced directly to the junction and drug is injected after satisfactory spread of the contrast.

Ultrasound-guided Technique

Ultrasound-guided block may improve patient safety by avoiding the soft-tissue structures in the needle path that cannot be readily seen by fluoroscopy. Ultrasound-guided stellate ganglion block may improve the safety of the procedure by direct visualization of the related anatomical structures by which the risk of injury to the thyroid gland and vessels, vertebral artery, or esophagus may be minimized **(Fig. 6)**. Also, ultrasound guidance will allow direct monitoring of the spread of the local anesthetics in

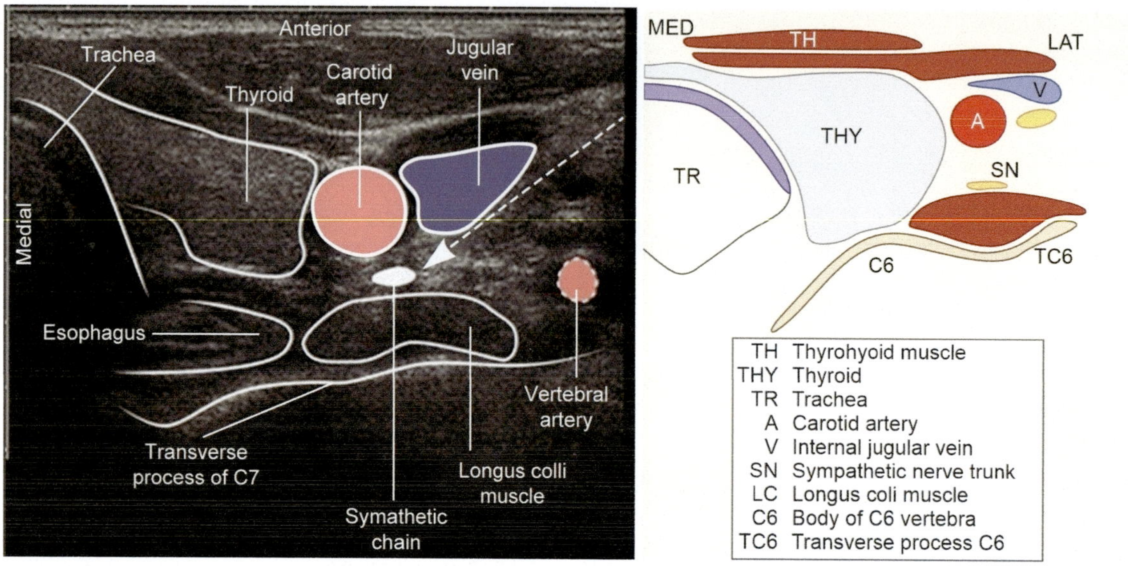

Fig. 6: Sonoanatomy for stellate ganglion block.

real time and hence complications like recurrent laryngeal nerve palsy, intrathecal, epidural, or intravascular spread may be minimized as well.[11]

Ultrasound imaging can easily identify the esophagus on the left, which is a very important tool, as it avoids esophageal penetration and prevents the potential development of mediastinal infection and/or mediastinal emphysema. This may be particularly useful in a patient with asymptomatic pharyngoesophageal diverticulum (Zenker diverticulum).

Another advantage is that the volume of local anesthetic, which can be potentially toxic, can be reduced by almost 50% enhancing safety of the procedure. This is a technique becoming more popular in recent time, especially in centers with availability of the necessary equipment and expertise.

Positioning is similar to the fluoroscopic approach, but an ultrasound machine with a 3–12 MHz linear array probe is necessary.

CT-Guided Approach

The patient is supine with the chin turned away from the injection site. The head of the first rib, adjacent vertebral artery, and vein are identified and a 25 G spinal needle is directed onto the head of the first rib, as close to the vertebral body as possible.

Blind Landmark-based Approach

This approach was widely practiced earlier but is no longer recommended. In this, positioning is same, i.e., supine with extended neck to move the esophagus medially. It is important to feel the Chassaignac tubercle and cricoid cartilage, which coincide with C6 vertebral level. The sternocleidomastoid muscle is retracted laterally with nondominant finger to move the carotid artery and internal jugular vein out of the path and a needle is advanced straight perpendicular through skin and deeper tissues to reach the bone. It is then withdrawn by 2 mm to position the needle tip anterior to the longus colli muscle before the drug is injected. If the patient gets paresthesia or pain in the upper extremity, the needle insertion is lateral and deep and should be redirected medially.

POSTPROCEDURE INSTRUCTIONS

The patient should be explained beforehand as to what the procedure involves and also be reassured about the signs of Horner syndrome, which disappears by about 2 hours in most patients. The patient should be given a 15° head-up position for about 10–15 minutes, especially if the procedure is performed for the upper extremity. Patients often have a lumpy feeling in the throat and should be kept nil by mouth for at least 4 hours.

Once good pain relief ensues, the patient has to be initiated on good physiotherapy and rehabilitation to restore normal function of the affected extremity.

HOW TO EVALUATE RESPONSE TO CERVICAL SYMPATHETIC/STELLATE GANGLION BLOCK

Presence of Horner syndrome is observed after a correctly performed block, which indicates the right target but it does not confirm sympathetic block to the upper extremity. The patient needs to be explained about the features to avoid distress when these occur. These are ptosis, meiosis, enophthalmos, anhidrosis, and conjunctival and/or nasal congestion.

To confirm the sympathetic blockade of upper extremity, the following features should be noted:

- Dilatation of the veins, which is not consistent
- Temperature measurement of the surface and preferably comparison with the other extremity are most reliable. Elevation of the temperature by 1–3° is typically indicative of sympathetic blockade[12] and should be monitored with thermography or thermometry. It may be absent if the temperature is already elevated.
- Sympathetic blockade causes increase in skin resistance, monitoring of which is available at select centers and can indicate completeness of the block.
- Microneurography, which is a direct but invasive test (requiring elaborate equipment and experience), can be used.[13]
- The sweat test (ninhydrin, cobalt blue, and iodine-starch test) which indicates change in color due to sweating is cumbersome and time-consuming and not well accepted by a fair number of patients and therefore not widely used.

Other methods used to measure blood flow include plethysmography (muscle and skin), xenon-133, and sodium-24 clearance (by the skin and muscle).

Malamqvist suggested the following criteria to indicate successful sympathetic blockade:

- Horner syndrome in 5 minutes
- 1–3°C temperature increase
- An increase in blood flow by 50% or more from the preblock status
- Abolition of skin-resistant response on the radial and ulnar sides following the block
- An increase in the skin-resistant response amounting to 13% or more of the preblock value on the radial and ulnar sides of the blocked extremity.[14]

HOW TO PRODUCE PERMANENT OR LONG-TERM BLOCKADE OF STELLATE GANGLION

In spite of using long-acting local anesthetic drug, the duration of effect of stellate ganglion block is generally short-lasting and hence various techniques have been described and adopted in an effort to prolong the effect.

Repeat Blocks

Repeat blocks at regular interval are shown to sequentially reduce the pain intensity, and when combined with good physical therapy, complete restoration of function is often noted in the author's clinical practice. The frequency and intervals between blocks vary from center to center and as often as every alternate day and as many as 40 injections have been used at some centers. By and large, it may be prudent to repeat once every week for three injections if there is a progressive benefit. If one is properly performed, block does not yield any improvement in symptoms; it does not make sense to repeat it further.

Continuous Block

In patients with vascular insufficiency or postherpetic neuralgia, a continuous stellate ganglion block may be considered to avoid doing frequent repeat blocks. An epidural catheter can be introduced through an introducer at C6 or C7 using a similar anterior paratracheal technique under imaging guidance. There however can be a risk of migration into dural cuff, vertebral artery, or adjoining structures. Hence, a test dose should be given prior to each dose, or ideally, fluoroscopic guidance should be used.

Chemical Sympathectomy

Although not used personally in my the author's practice, the use of neurolytic agents to produce a long-term blockade is practiced at few centers, especially due to economic considerations or unavailability of equipment or skills for safer techniques.

An injection of 1 mL of 6% aqueous phenol or 10% phenol at the level of C7 or C6 has been used to produce neurolysis. This technique is not commonly practiced because of the proximity of the somatic nerves as inadvertent spread can result in neuritis. The dural sheath may also be entered during the injection. Injection of a solution into the epidural space may lead to a devastating condition, and a case of paraplegia has been reported following upper thoracic sympathectomy using a neurolytic agent. Racz[15] has described a relatively safe technique using both phenol 3% and a mixture of 6% phenol with 0.5% plain bupivacaine.

Surgical Neurolysis

Open or endoscopic surgical neurolysis from T2 to T4 can be used for long-term relief, but T1 should be avoided to prevent Horner syndrome. Incomplete pain relief and recurrence are known with the surgical technique also.

Radiofrequency Ablation

This modality was used first in 1988 to target stellate ganglion and is the safest and effective technique in present time. It can produce a circumscribed lesion of desired size and avoid side effects like Horner syndrome.

The patient is explained the procedure and positioned similar to the standard paratracheal anterior approach. A prior positive diagnostic block is essential preferably with a small 2 mL volume of local anesthetic drug.

A special RF machine and insulated needles are required to produce the lesions. Under fluoroscopic guidance, the following three points are targeted to create a triangular lesion **(Fig. 7)**:

1. A point on the anterolateral aspect of C7
2. A point at the medial aspect of C7 transverse process
3. A point 1 cm caudal to the first point on C7 body.

Cepeda[18] has also advocated an additional fourth lesion in such a way that the RF cannula is directed caudally to the groove where the head of the first rib meets the ventral lateral aspect of the body of T1 vertebra. At this ventrolateral position, a fourth lesion can be made to interrupt some of the thoracic sympathetic fibers. This can provide a much wider sympathetic blockade, especially to the upper extremity. This is about 1 cm caudal to the third point.

A 10 cm long, 5 mm active tip needle is introduced to hit the first point as described above. A sensory stimulation (50 Hz) and motor (2 Hz) stimulation are carried out to ensure proper positioning of the needle. The patient is asked to say E...E...E...at 2 Hz and if he is unable to say the needle is presumed to be close to the recurrent laryngeal nerve and repositioned laterally. If the diaphragm is seen to contract, the needle is lateral and close to the phrenic nerve and needs medial repositioning. After satisfactory placement, 1 mL of 2% lignocaine can be injected. Few seconds later, the RF lesion is started at 80°C for 60 seconds at each point.

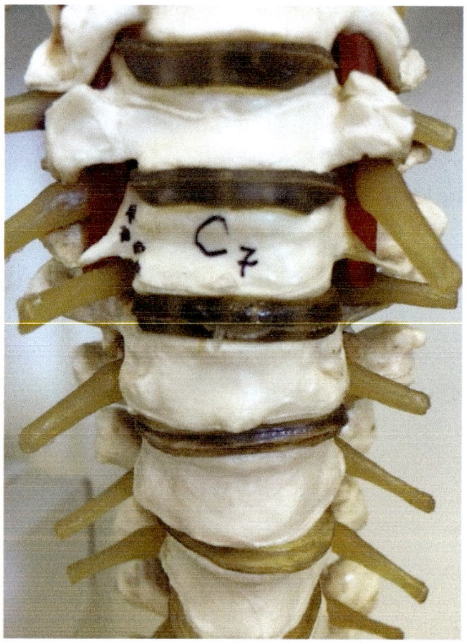

Fig. 7: Target points for radiofrequency ablation of stellate ganglion.

Complications of these techniques are similar to those produced by local anesthetic sympathetic ganglia block, with the exception of a longer-lasting block and potential neuritis.

COMPLICATIONS AND SIDE EFFECTS

Side effects should be differentiated from complications as features of Horner syndrome are common, and in fact help to establish precise targeting. Complications can be broadly categorized into pharmacological (drug-related), technical, and infectious complications.

Pharmacological Complications

Due to the spread of the local anesthetic to the adjoining structures like recurrent laryngeal nerve, there may be hoarseness, lump in the throat, and shortness of breath.

Phrenic nerve involvement can result in respiratory distress in already compromised patients.

Spread to cardioaccelerator fibers can result in bradycardia and/or hypotension.

Deep placement of needle can result in brachial plexus palsy. These generally recover once the effect of local anesthetic wears off, but can be catastrophic if a neurolytic drug has been injected.

Technical Complications

Technical complications result due to a misplaced needle during the block. The most dangerous complications are from intravascular and intrathecal injection. Intra-arterial injection into the vertebral artery or the carotid artery can produce a high concentration of a local anesthetic agent in the central nervous system (CNS), leading to seizures. Intravenous injection can lead to seizure, but this is unlikely due to a small volume of local anesthetic. Intrathecal injection of the local anesthetic producing high spinal blockade has been reported with respiratory arrest. Hematoma formation and air embolism are other potential complications.

Infectious Complications

Infectious complications are possible such as cellulitis, local abscess, and osteitis of the vertebral body and transverse process. There can be mediastinitis due to esophageal puncture.

POSTSYMPATHECTOMY SYNDROME

Postsympathectomy syndrome is an ill-understood condition found in 50% subjects after sympathectomy and is shown to occur in patients after stellate and cervical or thoracic sympathetic block. It can start few days to few weeks after the chemical or surgical sympathectomy with deep, dull aching pain associated with burning and hyperalgesia. It is also thought to be sympathetically maintained. Postsympathectomy neuralgia is proposed to be a complex neuropathic and central reafferentation and deafferentation syndrome. Postsympathectomy neuralgia is usually localized to the proximal region of the sympathectomized limb and to the trunk. The incidence is reported higher in CRPS patients.

Treatment of postsympathectomy neuralgia depends on the symptoms. If it is due to firing and spontaneous pain, then phenytoin, carbamazepine, or gabapentin can be helpful. Mexiletine or lidocaine given intravenously can also be helpful in cases where there is spontaneous pain or allodynia.

Tricyclic antidepressants can also be helpful to reduce the incidence of postsympathectomy neuralgia. Repeat sympathetic block or more complete sympathectomy can be used in some patients who do not respond to drugs. Use of pre-emptive analgesia can help to reduce the incidence of this syndrome.

Stellate ganglion block application using light irradiation effectively relieves pain of various etiologies and successfully induces a sympatholytic response. Stellate ganglion block application using light irradiation may be a valuable addition to the contemporary pain management armamentarium useful in certain patients like cardiac patients, anticoagulated where it may be challenging to do a percutaneous intervention.

EFFICACY AND CURRENT EVIDENCE

Stellate ganglion block is found to be more effective if performed in a timely manner, ideally within the first 16 weeks from the onset of pain and other symptoms, especially in patients with CRPS. A study also showed that a reduction in perfusion of more than 22% between normal and affected limbs adversely affect the effect of stellate ganglion block.[16]

A literature search of 11 studies revealed an evidence of 1C (strong recommendation, low-quality, or very-low-quality evidence) for stellate ganglion block.[17]

A 2010 systematic review on local anesthetic sympathetic blockade for CRPS revealed the scarcity of published evidence to support the use of sympathetic blockade as the "gold standard" treatment for CRPS and raises questions as to its efficacy.[18] Stellate ganglion block continues to be used as a treatment modality in the management of CRPS, but further randomized controlled trials would be required to more confidently validate its usefulness.

CONCLUSION

When conservative therapy fails, the pain practitioner needs to move forward in the treatment algorithm to control pain with interventional procedures. Stellate ganglion or cervical sympathetic block is the most commonly performed procedure for diagnostic, therapeutic, or prognostic purpose in the management of sympathetically maintained pain of head, face, neck, and upper extremities. In addition, it is also used for vascular pathologies resulting in reduced perfusion and pain. It is recommended to use monitoring and imaging guidance for better efficacy and safety considering its proximity to many vital structures and potential for serious complications. Ultrasound-guided stellate ganglion block may improve the safety of the procedure by direct visualization of the related anatomical structures and accordingly, the risk of thyroid gland and vessels, vertebral artery, or esophagus injury may be minimized. Depending on the response to the first block, a series of blocks or techniques for permanent blockade, such as RF ablation, may be offered. Besides the standard indications, there is an emerging potential of this technique to be used in newer indications, which are complex and difficult to treat in a conservative manner.

REFERENCES

1. Elias M. Cervical sympathetic and stellate ganglion blocks. Pain Physician. 2000;3:294-304.
2. Schattschneider J, Binder A, Siebrecht D, Wasner G, Baron R. Complex regional pain syndromes: the influence of cutaneous and deep somatic sympathetic innervation on pain. Clin J Pain. 2006;22:240-4.
3. Boas RA. Sympathetic nerve blocks: in search of a role. Reg Anesth Pain Med. 1998;23:292-305.

4. Navaie M, Keefe MS, Hickey AH, McLay RN, Ritchie EC, Abdi S. Use of stellate ganglion block for refractory post-traumatic stress disorder: a review of published cases. J Anesth Clin Res. 2014;5:403.
5. Gainotti G. Unconscious processing of emotions and the right hemisphere. Neuropsychologia. 2012;50:205-18.
6. Elias M. The anterior approach for thoracic sympathetic ganglion block using a curved needle. Pain Clinic. 2000;12:17-24.
7. Hogan QH, Erickson SJ. MR imaging of the stellate ganglion: normal appearance. AJR Am J Roentgenol. 1992;158:655-9.
8. Christie JM, Martinez CR. Computerized axial tomography to define the distribution of solution after stellate ganglion nerve block. J Clin Anesth. 1995;7:306-11.
9. Anterior (paratracheal) approach for block of the stellate ganglion. In: Moore DC (Ed). Regional Block: A Handbook for Use in the Clinical Practice of Medicine and Surgery. Springfield, IL: Charles C Thomas; 1975. pp. 123-37.
10. Abdi S, Zhou Y, Patel N, Saini B, Nelson J. A new and easy technique to block the stellate ganglion. Pain Physician. 2004;7:327-31.
11. Narouze S, Vydyanathan A, Patel N. Ultrasound-guided stellate ganglion block successfully prevented esophageal puncture. Pain Physician. 2007;10:747-52.
12. Malmqvist EL, Bengtsson M, Sörensen J. Efficacy of stellate ganglion block: a clinical study with bupivacaine. Reg Anesth. 1992;17:340-7.
13. Lidberg L, Wallin BG. Sympathetic skin nerve discharges in relation to amplitude of skin resistance responses. Psychophysiology. 1981;18:268-70.
14. lofstrom B, Michael J. Sympathetic neural blockade of the upper and lower extremity. In: Cousins MJ, Bridenbaugh PO (Eds). Neural Blockade in Clinical Anesthesia and Management of Pain. Philadelphia: Lippincott Williams and Wilkins; 1988.
15. Stevens RA, Stotz A, Kao TC, Powar M, Burgess S, Kleinman B. The relative increase in skin temperature after stellate ganglion block is predictive of a complete sympathectomy of the hand. Reg Anesth Pain Med. 1998;23:266-70.
16. Ackerman WE, Zhang JM. Efficacy of stellate ganglion blockade for the management of type 1 complex regional pain syndrome. South Med J. 2006;99:1084-8.
17. Day M. Sympathetic blocks: the evidence. Pain Pract. 2008;8:98-109.
18. Cepeda MS, Carr DB, Lau J. Local anesthetic sympathetic blockade for complex regional pain syndrome. Cochrane Database Syst Rev. 2005;CD004598.

19 CHAPTER

Occipital Nerve Stimulation

Vijay B Bandikatla, Chaitanya Veera, Nikhitha Peechera

ABSTRACT

Occipital nerve stimulation (ONS) emerges as a viable therapeutic strategy for the management of chronic refractory headaches, such as occipital neuralgia and migraine, particularly when conventional medical and interventional measures have proven ineffective. The occipital region is innervated by the greater, lesser, and third occipital nerves (TONs), which converge at the trigeminocervical complex (TCC). This complex is characterized by an anatomical and functional overlap of trigeminal and higher cervical afferents. ONS serves to modulate the TCC through the stimulation of the cervical afferent nerves. The procedure can be executed via two distinct approaches: Midline cervical approach and retromastoid approach. Prior to implantation, meticulous patient selection is of paramount importance to ensure the efficacy of the treatment and the well-being of the patient.

INTRODUCTION

Headache, a symptom frequently encountered in clinical practice, encompasses a spectrum of chronic pain conditions, including trigeminal autonomic cephalgia (TAC), chronic daily headaches, and cervicogenic headaches.[1] These conditions significantly impinge on the quality of life, presenting severe manifestations that can be debilitating and, in extreme cases, may even precipitate suicidal tendencies in patients.

While numerous guidelines have been established for the management of primary headaches, the treatment of occipital headaches continues to pose a formidable challenge. This chapter focuses on occipital nerve stimulation (ONS), exploring its potential as a viable treatment modality for chronic refractory headaches such as migraine and occipital neuralgia.

APPLIED ANATOMY

The occipital region is innervated by three nerves: Greater, lesser, and third occipital nerves (TONs). The medial branch of the dorsal ramus of the C2 nerve is the greater occipital nerve (GON) **(Fig. 1)**. After emerging from the suboccipital triangle, it passes beneath and posterior to the obliquus capitis inferior muscle. It, then, passes between the obliquus capitis inferior and the semispinalis capitis muscles in a superomedial fashion at the level of C1-C2 vertebrae. The nerve can be blocked here under ultrasound guidance **(Figs. 2A and B)**. The nerve, then, crosses over the rectus capitis posterior major muscle and arises medial to the semispinalis capitis muscle, which it occasionally pierces.[2,3] Along with the occipital artery, it pierces the trapezius muscle and ascends to innervate the occipitoparietal part of the scalp to the vertex. The GON provides innervations to an occipitoparietal area 6–8 cm wide, ascending paramedially from the subocciput to the vertex.[4] The traditional landmark technique for GON block involves palpating the occipital artery and injecting the drug medially.

The lesser occipital nerve is composed of branches of the C2 and C3 spinal roots. It runs laterally to the GON, crosses over the sternocleidomastoid muscle, and courses superolaterally toward the region behind and above the ear **(Fig. 1)**.

The TON has a unique course, the medial branches of the C3 dorsal rami. It has a unique course compared

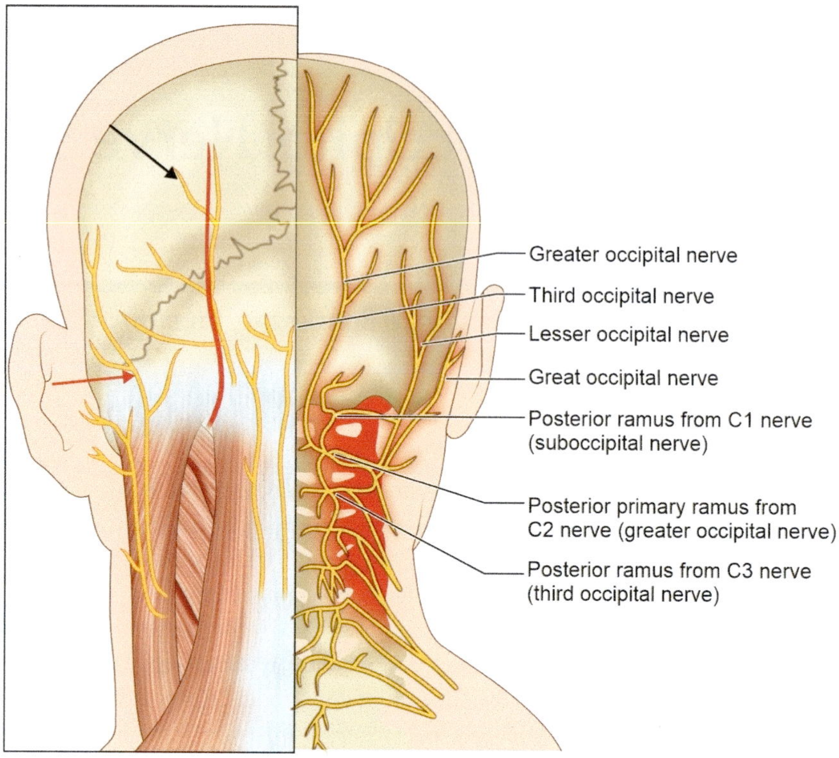

Fig. 1: Distribution of occipital nerves.

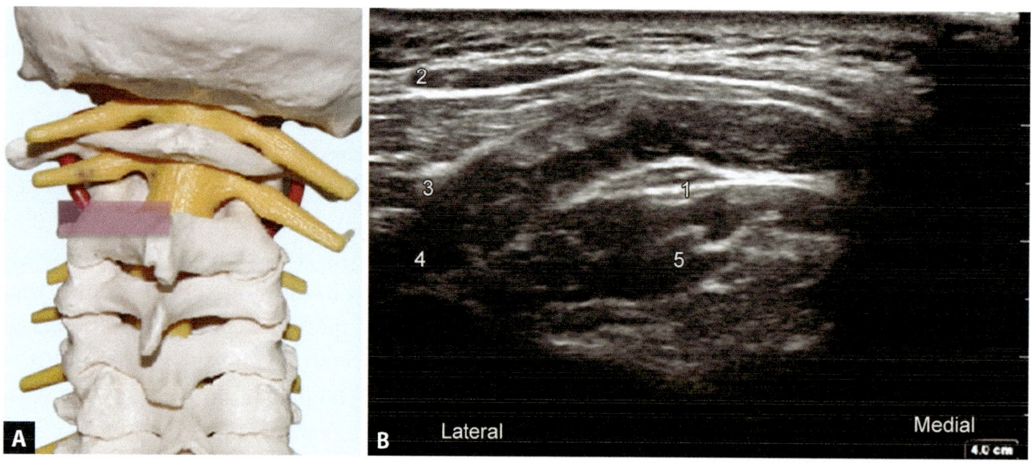

Figs. 2A and B: (A) Transducer position—transverse at C2. (B) Ultrasonographic image of the left greater occipital nerve. 1. Greater occipital nerve; 2. Trapezius muscle; 3. Splenius capitis muscle; 4. Semispinalis capitis muscle; 5. Obliquus capitis inferior muscle; 6. Spinous process; and 7. Lamina.

to the other cervical medial branches. After emerging from the C2-C3 intervertebral foramen, the dorsal ramus divides into two branches **(Fig. 3)**. The deep medial branch passes around the waist of the C3 articular pillar, similar to other cervical medial branches, and supplies the C3-C4 zygapophysial joint. The larger superficial medial branch of C3 is also known as the TON. This nerve runs close to the C2-C3 zygapophysial joint, giving articular branches to the joints. Continuing further, the TON provides cutaneous innervation to the suboccipital region. This branch of the C3 nerve has been implicated in cervicogenic headaches. It lies medial to the GON and communicates with it **(Fig. 1)**.

From here, these nerves terminate into the trigemino-cervical complex (TCC) **(Fig. 4)**. There is an anatomical

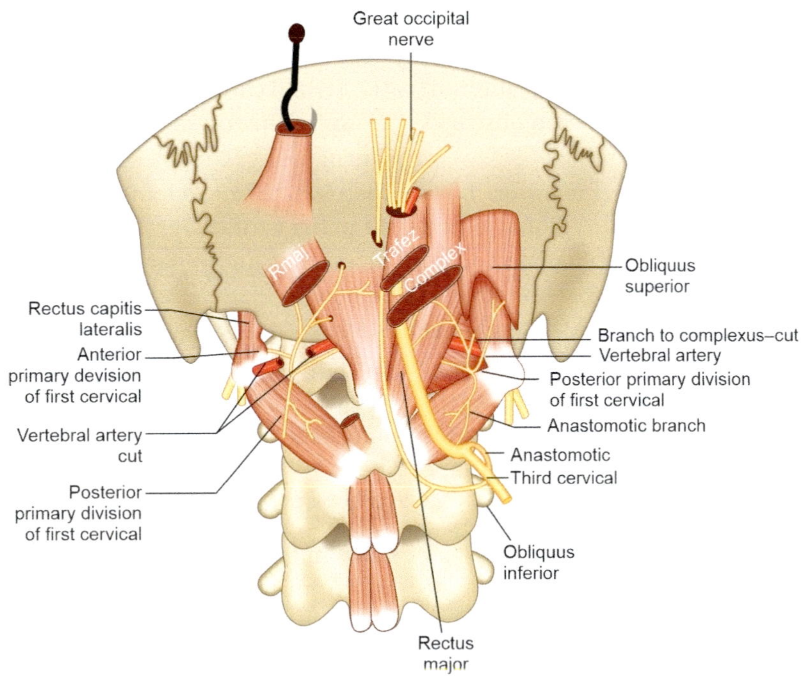

Fig. 3: Third occipital nerve: Note that the larger superficial and medial branch of C3 is the TON. (TON: third occipital nerve; VA: vertebral artery)

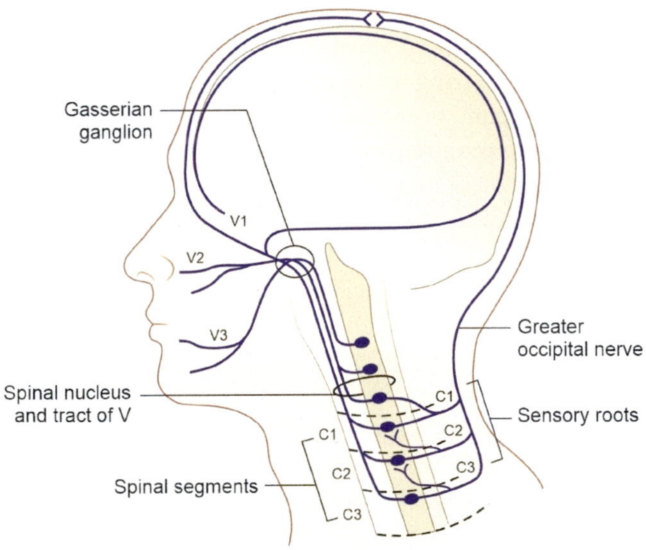

Fig. 4: Trigeminocervical complex (TCC): The trigeminal and cervical nerve fibers enter the trigeminal and cervical nuclei, respectively.
Notice the overlap of the fibers, making it a combined TCC.

and functional overlap of trigeminal and cervical afferents throughout the TCC, from the level of the caudal trigeminal nucleus to at least the C2 segment.[5] This convergence explains how nociceptive activation at either end of this structure can result in pain in both the trigeminal and the cervical distributions.

MECHANISMS OF ACTION

The technique of ONS capitalizes on the "functional overlap" of the higher cervical nerve roots and the trigeminal nerve nucleus to modulate the TCC **(Fig. 3)**.[6,7] It is a plausible assumption that the application of electrical pulses directly onto the dorsal columns at the level of the C2-C3 vertebrae would yield a neuromodulatory effect on the TCC comparable to, if not exceeding, that of peripheral ONS.[8] Both the antidromic activity of the dorsal column and the supraspinal sensory pathways, including the periaqueductal gray and thalamus, play a role in the perception of pain.[9-12] Consequently, cervicomedullary spinal cord stimulation (SCS) has been employed over the past 30 years to alleviate intractable head and facial pain, albeit at the cost of a complex, time-consuming, and expensive neurosurgical procedure.

The mechanisms through which peripheral neurostimulation mediates its antinociceptive effect remain elusive. Several sites of action within the peripheral and central nervous systems have been proposed, encompassing the peripheral nerve, spinal segmental level, and supraspinal levels. The widely accepted gate control theory of pain posits that the activation of large-diameter afferent nerve fibers in the spinal dorsal horn inhibits onward transmission in small-diameter primary afferent nociceptive fibers, thereby preventing nociceptive signals from reaching the higher neural centers where they are interpreted as pain.[13,14] Indeed, numerous physiological studies have corroborated that afferent activity induced by peripheral neurostimulation obstructs nociceptive transmission in the spinal cord.

Positron emission tomography (PET) studies have demonstrated significant alterations in regional blood flow in the dorsal rostral pons, anterior cingulate cortex, and cuneus, correlating with pain scores. The changes observed in the anterior cingulate cortex and left pulvinar are correlated with stimulation-induced paranesthesia scores when the ONS is activated.[15] The activation pattern in the dorsal and rostral pons in this study strongly suggests a role for this structure in the pathophysiology of chronic migraine.

INDICATIONS

Occipital nerve stimulation is considered as a treatment for various refractory primary and secondary headache disorders.

Primary headaches:[16]

Occipital neuralgia:

- Chronic refractory migraine
- Cluster headache
- Hemicrania continua
- Short-lasting unilateral neuralgiform headache attacks with cranial autonomic symptoms (SUNA)
- Short-lasting unilateral neuralgiform headache attacks with conjunctival injection and tearing (SUNCT)
- Hypnic headache

Secondary headaches:

- Post-traumatic occipital headache
- Cervicogenic headache.

EFFICACY

As chronic refractory headaches are difficult to manage, the enthusiasm for ONS as a treatment modality is growing. The most common condition studied so far that has shown positive overall efficacy is chronic refractory migraine. Pooled results from three multi-centered randomized controlled trials (RCTs) showed that ONS was associated with a mean reduction of 2.59 days [95% confidence interval (CI) 0.91–4.27, I2 = 0%] of prolonged, moderate-to-severe headaches per month at 3 months compared with a sham control.[17] Open-label follow-up of RCTs and case series suggests that long-term effectiveness can be maintained.

Occipital nerve stimulation was considered effective in various TACs, particularly with chronic cluster headache (CCH) and chronic refractory migraine.[1,2] Burns et al.[18] first recorded the role of ONS in CCH in a series of 14 patients. Out of these, 10 reported benefits, 3 with a benefit of more than 90%, and 3 with more than 40%. Magis et al. followed 14 patients of CCH treated with ONS over an average of 37 months and reported 11 to be receiving at least 90% reduction in attacks.[19] In a series of nine cases of SUNA/SUNCT, ONS was effective in eight and four of them had freedom from pain.[20] Successful treatment of refractory occipital neuralgia with an occipital nerve stimulator has long been reported.[16,21-23]

ASSESSMENT

The implementation of ONS necessitates the collaboration of a multidisciplinary team encompassing pain specialists, neurologists, surgeons, physiotherapists, and psychologists. A preliminary assessment by a neurologist is crucial to confirm the clinical diagnosis of headache, establish the failure of conservative treatments, and rule out other surgical options prior to considering ONS.

It is essential to ensure that primary psychiatric conditions, barring anxious-depressive symptoms as a reaction to pain, do not influence the clinical outcomes. Patients are required to demonstrate good compliance with the instructions pertaining to the operation of the stimulator and maintain realistic expectations of the treatment.

The collection of baseline and ongoing data serves to enhance physician–patient communication and monitor progress. As a research tool, it aids in the identification of suitable patients and the measurement of headache-related disability. Commonly used scores include the Migraine Disability Assessment Scale score exceeding 21, the Headache Impact Test-6 (HIT-6) score more than 50, and the Numeric Rating Scale score surpassing 5.

SURGICAL EQUIPMENT

The procedure of ONS for chronic refractory headaches is typically conducted in two stages, although a single-stage procedure may occasionally be employed. This procedure is performed using equipment conventionally used for SCS.[21] In the future, perineural catheter placement of an extremely small, insulated electrical lead can be inserted adjacent to the peripheral nerve through a 14G Tuohy needle and under ultrasound guidance. Power is provided to the implanted wireless leads by an external pulse generator that is wearable in belts, fabrics, jewelry, etc. This technique eliminates the need for an implantable pulse generator (IPG) and tunneling of the electrodes to the IPG, thereby reducing the expense and morbidities.

The requisite equipment for the current technique includes electrodes, lead anchors to secure the leads to connective tissue, lead extensions, a tunneler, and the IPG. Two types of electrodes can be used: Thin cylindrical-style electrodes that can be inserted through a needle or flat and broad paddle-style electrodes. Owing to their shape, paddle electrodes are inherently more stable and associated with a lower incidence of lead migration. However, their placement requires more extensive surgical dissection.[24-26] Paddle leads are generally considered for patients who have previously had implanted cylindrical leads that migrated multiple times, necessitating several revisions.

There are a multitude of variations pertaining to needle insertion, electrode placement, and anchoring techniques. The procedure delineated in this chapter employs standard cylindrical electrodes with two, four, or eight contacts, akin to those used for the implantation of a spinal cord stimulator. Broadly, there are two predominant approaches for implantation: Midline cervical and retromastoid techniques.[27] The retromastoid approach is frequently employed for unilateral lead placement. However, for bilateral lead placement, our preference leans toward the midline cervical approach.

Midline Cervical Approach

In authors' clinical experience, a significant majority of patients derive benefit from a tunneled trial. The procedure commences with the patient being positioned in a prone orientation, followed by the administration of appropriate intravenous (IV) antibiotics. Sedation is meticulously titrated to maintain a level that allows for verbal communication with the patient during testing, subsequent to the insertion of the leads.

TUNNELED TRIAL

Patient Preparation

The patient is positioned in a prone orientation, with the head maintained in a neutral position. Pillows are strategically placed under the chest, and a head ring is used to support the forehead. This arrangement ensures both adequate access to the nuchal region and patient comfort. The skin is prepared by shaving the hair from the lower hairline up to an inch above the occiput. The skin is then meticulously cleaned twice with a 0.5% chlorhexidine or povidone-iodine solution. The patient is carefully draped from the occiput down to the mid-thoracic region to facilitate tunneling.

Procedure

Following skin marking under fluoroscopic guidance, a midline craniocaudal posterior nuchal skin incision, measuring 3–4 cm in length, is made corresponding to the C1-C2 spinous processes. Subsequent to blunt dissection, a subcutaneous pocket is bilaterally created to securely accommodate the redundant coil of leads. A 16 g, curved Tuohy needle is introduced from the upper end of the incision, leaving space at the lower end for the placement of anchors **(Fig. 5)**. The needle is passed above the cervicodorsal fascial layer, directed toward the medial side of the mastoid process, and positioned close to the lateral edge of the occipital bone **(Figs. 6A and B)**. This placement ensures proper stimulation, even in the event of mild-to-moderate migration. While deeper needle placement may reduce the risk of erosion, it could potentially increase the risk of direct muscle stimulation.[20] Two standard quadripolar or octopolar leads are positioned prior to the withdrawal of the needle **(Figs. 7A and B)**.

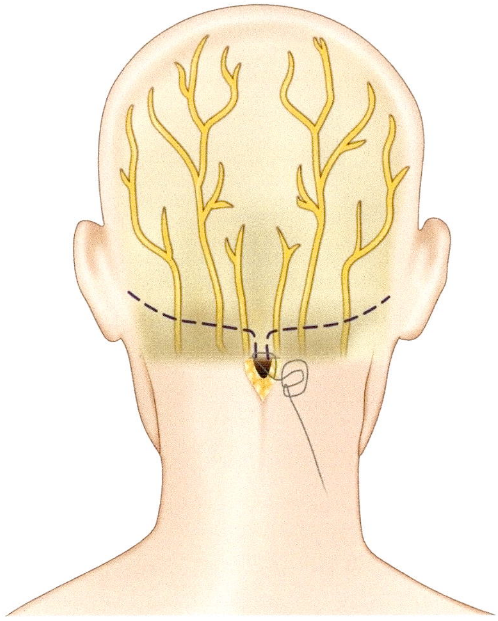

Fig. 5: Occipital nerve stimulation—midline cervical approach, tunneled trial with two octopolar leads.

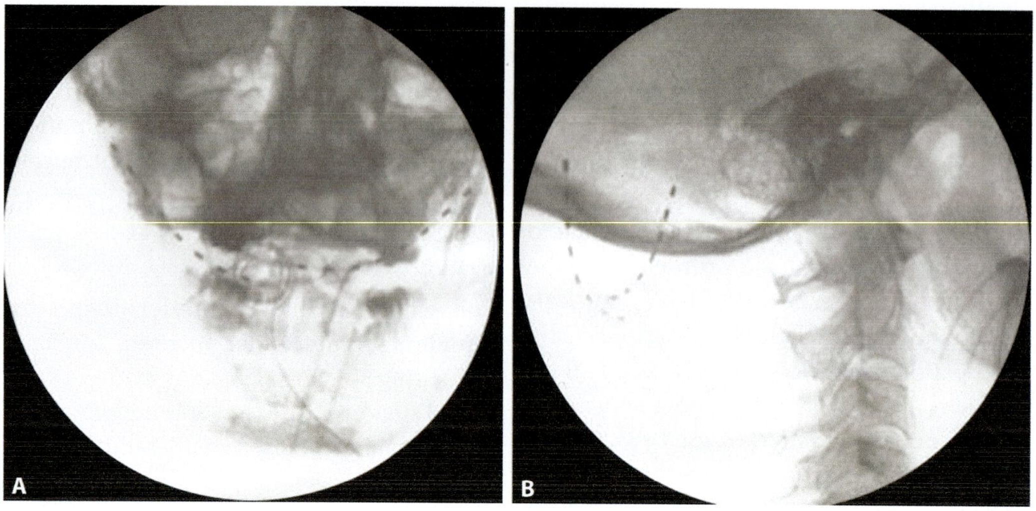

Figs. 6A and B: Fluoroscopic images showing the optimal position of electrodes on the medial side of the mastoid process and positioned close to the lateral edge of the occipital bone.

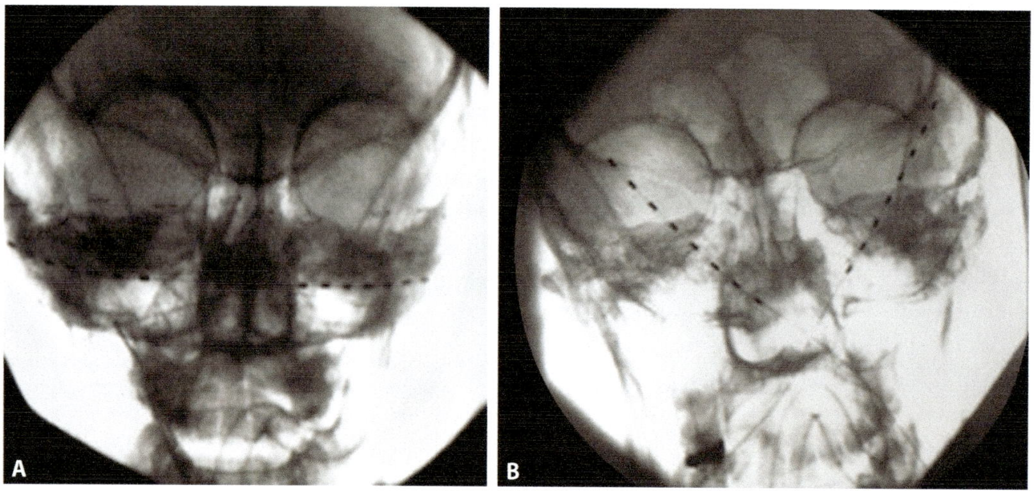

Figs. 7A and B: Fluoroscopic images showing the optimal position of electrodes for bilateral occipital nerve stimulation.

Upon confirmation of the lead position on fluoroscopy, the patient is awakened for intraoperative testing. Once satisfactory thresholds are achieved, the guidewires are removed, and the leads are secured in place using appropriate anchors and strong, braided, nonabsorbable, polyester sutures on a curved needle. It is crucial to ensure that the knots and coils of leads are not too superficial to avoid lead erosion.

The electrodes are connected to the extensions and tunneled away from the preferred site of final implant placement. The extra length of the lead is positioned as coils into the preformed pocket, and the lead junctions are tucked away from the midline prior to closure. Skin clips or nonabsorbable sutures can be used. The lead extensions are connected to the external trialing system and battery unit.

Education on the usage of the patient programmer and providing at least some flexibility with amplitude adjustment is crucial to the success of the procedure. Prior to discharge, we routinely prescribe a 5-day course of oral antibiotics, along with analgesics.

Successful trial: A successful trial that proceeds to a second phase of implanting should fulfill the following criteria:

- A reduction in the number of migraine attacks or headache days by more than 40%.

- A reduction in the intensity of the crisis by more than 40%.
- An adequate functional recovery and a reduction of perceived discomfort in everyday life.[28]
- Tolerable paresthesia, patient compliance, and realistic expectations.[29,30]

Second stage:

Following a favorable response to the ONS trial phase over a period of 1–2 weeks, the patient is readmitted for the implantation of the pulse generator. The preferred sites for IPG placement are the abdomen or the infraclavicular areas, as these locations are associated with the least change in electrode pathway length during patient movements compared to the buttocks.[31] The chosen site is marked, and the patient is positioned laterally with the implanting side facing upward.

This procedure can be performed under general anesthesia or continuous IV sedation. To prevent contamination of the skin incision, the external battery system is first disconnected, and the lead extension is carefully secured to prevent its retraction under the skin. The skin incision site is opened under fully aseptic conditions. The junction between the lead and extension is located and disconnected using a screwdriver. The proximal end of the lead is identified and secured. Using scissors, the extension leads are cut close to the "distal end" that connects the lead to the extension, and the remaining extension lead is removed through the skin.

A pouch is created in the subcutaneous tissue to accommodate the IPG, and a tunneler is used to reach the electrode in the incision. The lead extension is threaded through this tunnel and securely connected to the lead.

The junction of the lead and extension is secured away from the incision. Subsequently, the proximal lead extension is connected to the battery after cleaning the electrode of any organic material with water.

A povidone-iodine and saline wash is used before positioning the IPG into the pocket. After checking for impedance, the pocket is closed with nonabsorbable sutures. Similarly, the lead insertion site is also closed in layers. The patient is monitored in the postanesthetic recovery for the adequacy of coverage.

Retromastoid Technique

This technique encompasses a percutaneous trial, subsequent removal of electrodes after a duration of 1–2 weeks, and a comprehensive implantation procedure following a successful percutaneous trial. This method is particularly popular for unilateral headaches that necessitate the placement of a single lead. The procedure can be effectively performed in a lateral decubitus position **(Fig. 8)**.

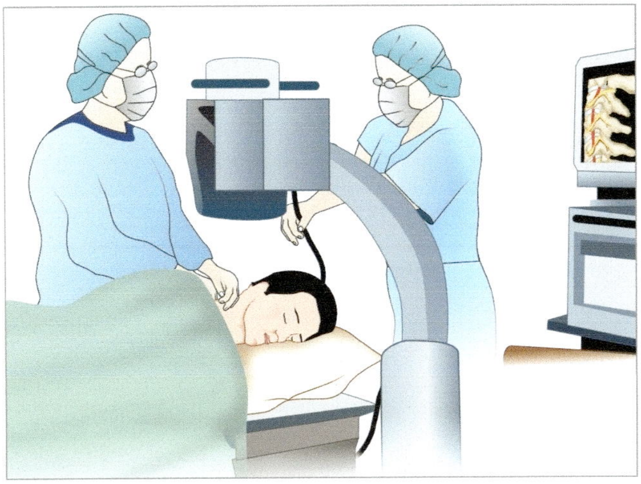

Fig. 8: Retromastoid approach—percutaneous lead positioning can be achieved when the patient is positioned laterally.

PERCUTANEOUS TRIAL

This procedure is undertaken with the objective of refining patient selection. This relatively straightforward technique necessitates IV sedation and local anesthetic infiltration. The procedure commences with the insertion of the needle, 1 cm caudal and medial, to the tip of the mastoid, advancing horizontally at the craniovertebral junction along the contour of the C1 lamina or arcus vertebralis. Contralateral ONS can be achieved from the same insertion point by further advancing the needle, crossing the midline **(Fig. 9)**. In this position, the needle superficially crosses over the anatomical course of the occipital nerves.

Upon satisfactory positioning of the needle, standard eight-contact electrodes are advanced through the needle. The electrode is placed near the greater and lesser occipital nerves. The correct positioning of the electrode is verified by intraoperative test stimulation of the patient, who is awake during this process. Once adequate coverage has been achieved, the electrode is secured in place using the manufacturer-provided anchors and nonabsorbable sutures. A sterile dressing is applied over the insertion sites upon completion of the procedure.

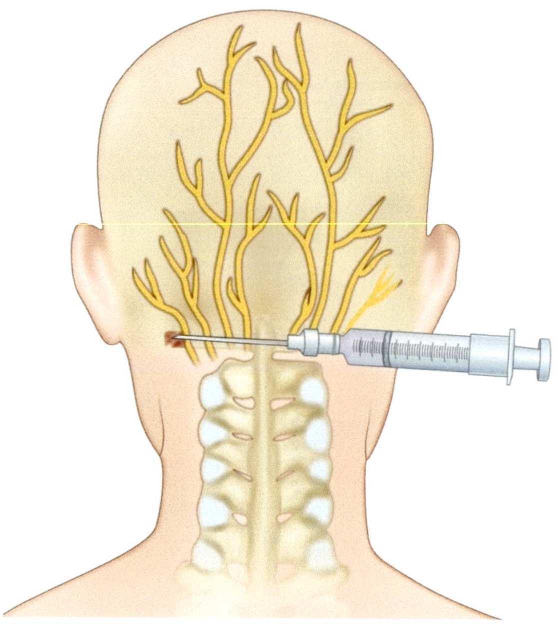

Fig. 9: Retromastoid approach: In a percutaneous trial, needles and leads are advanced horizontally over the C1 lamina.

Full Implant Stage: Retromastoid Approach

Following a successful trial, the full implant procedure is initiated. A skin incision is made along the retromastoid area in a vertical direction. The soft tissues are meticulously dissected down to the fascia, and a small pocket is created above the fascial layer. Once the permanent lead is positioned in the appropriate and satisfactory position, mirroring the percutaneous trial, the needle is removed. The lead is anchored to the occipital fascia using nonabsorbable sutures and an anchor.

A subcutaneous pocket is created to accommodate the neurostimulator at the chosen site, which could be the infraclavicular region, infra axillary, or abdominal wall. Extension leads are advanced through a subcutaneous tunnel, establishing a connection between the electrode and the neurostimulator. After ensuring that impedances are within the acceptable range, all incisions are closed, cleaned, and covered with sterile dressings.

Upon completion of the procedure, the patient is discharged home. Prior to discharge, a demonstration of the use of the remote control is provided, along with instructions for skin suture removal.

PARAMETERS

The most optimal stimulation patterns are obtained with an amplitude of 0.5–4.0 V, a pulse width of 90–200 μs, and a frequency varying between 20 and 200 Hz.

Safety

While no serious adverse events have been reported, there was a single instance of hemicrania continua, which was successfully managed with indomethacin.[32] The most commonly encountered adverse events associated with ONS include lead erosion, lead migration, pain at the lead site, neck stiffness, discharged battery, pain at the battery site, and contact dermatitis.[33]

Lead migration appears to occur more frequently with percutaneous cylindrical leads, with incidences ranging between 9% and 33%,[34,35] but only in 6% of patients implanted with paddle-type leads. Symptoms such as muscle contractions, often described as a "grabbing sensation" or a burning sensation typically indicate that the electrodes or the permanent lead are positioned too deep (anterior) in the subcutaneous tissue.

Future

As a relatively simple technique to treat some of the more complex and chronic refractory headaches, ONS holds promise. The bigger challenge for the manufacturers is lead migration and erosion. Manufacturing custom-made leads that reduce the risk of migration and erosion could improve compliance and reduce surgical revision. Perineural catheter placement of an extremely small, insulated electrical lead that can be inserted adjacent to the peripheral nerve through a 14G Tuohy needle and under ultrasound guidance. Power is provided to the implanted wireless leads by an external pulse generator that is wearable in belts, fabrics, jewelry, etc. This technique eliminates the need for an IPG and tunneling of the electrodes to the IPG, thereby reducing the expense and morbidities.

Larger randomized controlled trials (RCTs) are also needed to establish the safety and efficacy of ONS in refractory headaches, but the problem with a bona fide placebo group with a placebo stimulus that is not in itself therapeutically effective is difficult. Newer targets that are now explored include supraorbital nerve stimulation as a standalone procedure or in combination with ONS in view of the frequent occurrence of pain in the first branch of the trigeminal nerve, percutaneous stimulation of the sphenopalatine ganglion due to its connections with the TCC, and also vagal nerve stimulation.

CONCLUSION

Occipital nerve stimulation is rapidly gaining recognition as a promising therapeutic modality for medically intractable primary headache syndromes. This includes refractory migraine, cluster headache, hemicrania continua (HC), SUNCT/SUNA, as well as occipital neuralgia.

With the availability of recent results from RCTs for ONS, it appears prudent to cautiously proceed with the open-label use of this procedure, ideally within tertiary referral settings.[36] A successful trial phase, preceding a full implant, presents an opportunity to refine patient selection, thereby enhancing the overall efficacy of the treatment.

There is a pressing need for improvements in the equipment to mitigate the risk of lead erosion and issues related to the IPG.

REFERENCES

1. Headache Classification Committee of the International Headache Society (IHS). The International Classification of Headache Disorders, 3rd edition. Cephalalgia. 2018; 38:1-211.
2. Tubbs RS, Watanabe K, Loukas M, Cohen-Gadol AA. The intramuscular course of the greater occipital nerve: novel findings with potential implications for operative interventions and occipital neuralgia. Surg Neurol Int. 2014;5:155.
3. Natsis K, Baraliakos X, Appell HJ, Tsikaras P, Gigis I, Koebke J. The course of the greater occipital nerve in the suboccipital region: a proposal for setting landmarks for local anesthesia in patients with occipital neuralgia. Clin Anat. 2006;19:332-6.
4. Poletti CE. C2 and C3 pain dermatomes in man. Cephalalgia. 1991;11:155-9.
5. Kerr FW, Olafson RA. Trigeminal and cervical volleys. Convergence on single units in the spinal gray at C-1 and C-2. Arch Neurol. 1961;5:171-8.
6. Ellens DJ, Levy RM. Peripheral neuromodulation for migraine headache. Prog Neurol Surg. 2011;24:109-17.
7. Goadsby PJ, Charbit AR, Andreou AP, Akerman S, Holland PR. Neurobiology of migraine. Neuroscience. 2009;161:327-41.
8. Tomycz ND, Deibert CP, Moossy JJ. Cervicomedullary junction spinal cord stimulation for head and facial pain. Headache. 2011;51(3):418-25.
9. Stiller CO, Linderoth B, O'Connor WT, Franck J, Falkenberg T, Ungerstedt U, et al. Repeated spinal cord stimulation decreases the extracellular level of gamma-aminobutyric acid in the periaqueductal gray matter of freely moving rats. Brain Res. 1995;699(2):231-41.
10. Nyquist JK, Greenhoot JH. Responses evoked from the thalamic centrum medianum by painful input: suppression by dorsal funiculus conditioning. Exp Neurol. 1973;39(2):215-22.
11. Linderoth B, Meyerson BA. Spinal cord stimulation: mechanism of action. In: Burchiel K (Ed). Surgical Management of Pain. New York: Thieme; 2002. pp. 505-26.
12. Hansson P, Lundeberg T. Transcutaneous electrical nerve stimulation, vibration, and acupuncture are pain-relieving measures. In: Melzack R, Wall PD (Eds). Textbook of Pain. New York: Churchill Livingstone; 1999. pp. 1341-51.
13. Stanton-Hicks M. Peripheral nerve stimulation for pain: peripheral neuralgia and complex regional pain syndrome. In: Krames ES, Peckham H, Rezai AR (Eds). Neuromodulation. San Diego: Academic Press; 2009. pp. 397-407.
14. Melzack R, Wall PD. Pain mechanisms: a new theory. Science. 1965;150(3699):971-9.
15. Matharu MS, Bartsch T, Ward N, Frackowiak RS, Weiner R, Goadsby PJ. Central neuromodulation in chronic migraine patients with suboccipital stimulators: a PET study. Brain. 2004;127(Pt 1):220-30.
16. Martelletti P, Jensen RH, Antal A, Arcioni R, Brighina F, de Tommaso M, et al.; European Headache Federation. Neuromodulation of chronic headaches: a position statement from the European Headache Federation. J Headache Pain. 2013;14:86.
17. Chen YF, Bramley G, Unwin G, Hanu-Cernat D, Dretzke J, Moore D, et al. Occipital nerve stimulation for chronic migraine—a systematic review and meta-analysis. PLoS One. 2015;10(3):e0116786.
18. Burns B, Watkins L, Goadsby PJ. Treatment of intractable chronic cluster headache by occipital nerve stimulation in 14 patients. Neurology. 2009;72(4):341-5.
19. Magis D, Gerardy PY, Remacle JM, Schoenen J. Sustained effectiveness of occipital nerve stimulation in drug-resistant chronic cluster headache. Headache. 2011;51(8):1191-201.
20. Lambru G, Shanahan P, Watkins L, Matharu MS. Occipital nerve stimulation in the treatment of medically intractable SUNCT and SUNA. Pain Physician. 2014;17(1):29-41.
21. Weiner RL, Reed KL. Peripheral neurostimulation for control of intractable occipital neuralgia. Neuromodulation. 1999;2(3):217-21.
22. Chaiban G, Tolba R, Eissa H, Lirette LS, Almualim M, Malaty A, et al. Successful treatment of occipital neuralgia with implantable peripheral nerve stimulation in a pacemaker-dependent patient. Ochsner J. 2014;14(1):119-22.
23. Skaribas I, Calvillo O, Delikanaki-Skaribas E. Occipital peripheral nerve stimulation in the management of chronic intractable occipital neuralgia in a patient with neurofibromatosis type 1: a case report. J Med Case Rep. 2011;5:174.
24. Oh MY, Ortega J, Bellotte JB, Whiting DM, Aló K. Peripheral nerve stimulation for the treatment of occipital neuralgia and transformed migraine using a C1-2-3 subcutaneous paddle style electrode: a technical report. Neuromodulation. 2004;7:103-12.
25. Burchiel KJ. Effects of electrical and mechanical stimulation on two foci of spontaneous activity which develop in

primary afferent neurons after peripheral axotomy. Pain. 1984;18:249-65.

26. Hayek SM, Jasper JF, Deer TR, Narouze SN. Occipital neurostimulation-induced muscle spasms: implications for lead placement. Pain Physician. 2009;12:867-76.
27. Trentman TL, Slavin KV, Freeman JA, Zimmerman RS. Occipital nerve stimulator placement via a retromastoid-to-infraclavicular approach: a technical report. Stereotact Funct Neurosurg. 2010;88:121-5.
28. Cady R, Farmner K, Dexter JK, Screiber C. Cosensitization of pain and psychiatric comorbidity in chronic daily headache. Curr Pain Headache Rep. 2005;9(1):47-52.
29. Trentman TL, Zimmerman RS, Dodick DW. Occipital nerve stimulation: technical and surgical aspects of implantation. Prog Neurol Surg. 2011;24:96-108.
30. Pompili M, Di Cosimo D, Innamorati M, Lester D, Tatarelli R, Martelletti P. Psychiatric comorbidity in patients with chronic daily headache and psychiatric migraine: a selective overview including personality traits and suicide risk. J Headache Pain. 2009;10:283-90.
31. Henderson JM, Schade CM, Sasaki J, Caraway DL, Oakley JC. Prevention of mechanical failures in implanted spinal cord stimulation systems. Neuromodulation. 2006;9:183-91.
32. Shanahan P, Watkins L, Matharu MS. Treatment of medically intractable short-lasting unilateral neuralgiform headache attacks with conjunctival injection and tearing (SUNCT) and short-lasting unilateral neuralgiform headache attacks with autonomic symptoms (SUNA) with occipital nerve stimulation (ONS) in 6 patients. Cephalalgia. 2009;29 (Suppl 1):150.
33. Jasper JF, Hayek SM. Implanted occipital nerve stimulators. Pain Physician. 2008;11:187-200.
34. Melvin EA Jr, Jordan FR, Weiner RL, Primm D. Using peripheral stimulation to reduce the pain of C2-mediated occipital headaches: a preliminary report. Pain Physician. 2007;10:453-60.
35. Schwedt TJ, Dodick DW, Hentz J, Trentman TL, Zimmerman RS. Occipital nerve stimulation for chronic headache—long-term safety and efficacy. Cephalalgia. 2007;27:153-7.
36. Dodick DW, Silberstein SD, Reed KL, Deer TR, Slavin KV, Huh B, et al. Safety and efficacy of peripheral nerve stimulation of the occipital nerves for the management of chronic migraine: long-term results from a randomized, multicenter, double-blinded, controlled study. Cephalalgia. 2015;35(4):344-58.

4

SECTION

Chest and Thorax

20 CHAPTER

Suprascapular Nerve Block

Vijay B Bandikatla, Chaitanya Veera, Nikhitha Peechera

ABSTRACT

Suprascapular nerve (SSN) block is a safe and effective pain management technique for chronic and refractory shoulder pain. Up to 70% of sensory nerve supply to the shoulder joint and overlying skin is by the SSN. The entrapment of SSN in the suprascapular notch and rotator cuff muscle tendinopathy can contribute to shoulder pain. Pain or weakness on top or back of the shoulder preventing lifting of the arm above the shoulder with a painful arc between 60° and 120° movement helps in making a diagnosis. SSN block can be used both for diagnostic and therapeutic purposes. It can be performed using anatomical landmarks, nerve stimulator, ultrasound, or fluoroscopic guidance.

INTRODUCTION

Shoulder pain leads to significant functional disability with a decrease in quality of life, especially in the elderly. It has an overall prevalence of approximately 20% in the general population.[1] The suprascapular nerve (SSN) can be specifically targeted to provide shoulder analgesia while potentially sparing blockade of the phrenic nerve.[2-5] Role of SSN block as a regional anesthetic choice for intraoperative and postoperative pain management has been well established.[4-6] SSN block is used as a safe and effective chronic pain management technique for treating shoulder pain.[7-11] Due to the SSN passing through an irregularly shaped bone called "scapula", a clear understanding of its anatomical course, innervation, and the involved mechanisms of injury lead to greater success with the blockade. Use of imaging or electrophysiological guidance improves the effectiveness of the block.[12]

ANATOMY

Suprascapular Nerve

The SSN comprises motor and sensory fibers originating from the 5th and 6th cervical spinal nerves; occasionally, fibers from the 4th cervical spine also contribute.[6,7] The fibers are contained within the upper trunk of the brachial plexus and course across the posterior triangle of the neck laterally and parallel to the inferior belly of the omohyoid muscle. SSN passes deep and posterolateraly under the trapezius muscle toward the suprascapular notch of the scapula. Here, it traverses through an opening created by the superior transverse scapular ligament (STSL), which is the most common site for entrapment injury to the nerve **(Fig. 1)**.[13]

The SSN is a mixed nerve, providing motor supply to the rotator cuff muscles. In the supraspinatus fossa it gives off two branches, one to the supraspinatus muscle with minor branch to teres minor muscle and one to the shoulder joint as an articular branch. This in the infraspinatus fossa terminates as two branches in the infraspinatus muscle after passing underneath the inferior transverse ligament in the spinoglenoid notch **(Fig. 2)**.

The sensory fibers of the SSN provide up to 70% of the shoulder joint, including the superior and posterosuperior regions of the shoulder joint, the capsule, and the overlying skin.[14,15] It also innervates the glenoid, acromion, and posterior surface of scapula bones. The sensory innervation to the remaining part of the shoulder joint is provided by the axillary nerve and lateral pectoral nerves.

Rotator Cuff

The rotator cuff is formed by the supraspinatus, infraspinatus, subscapularis, and teres minor muscles

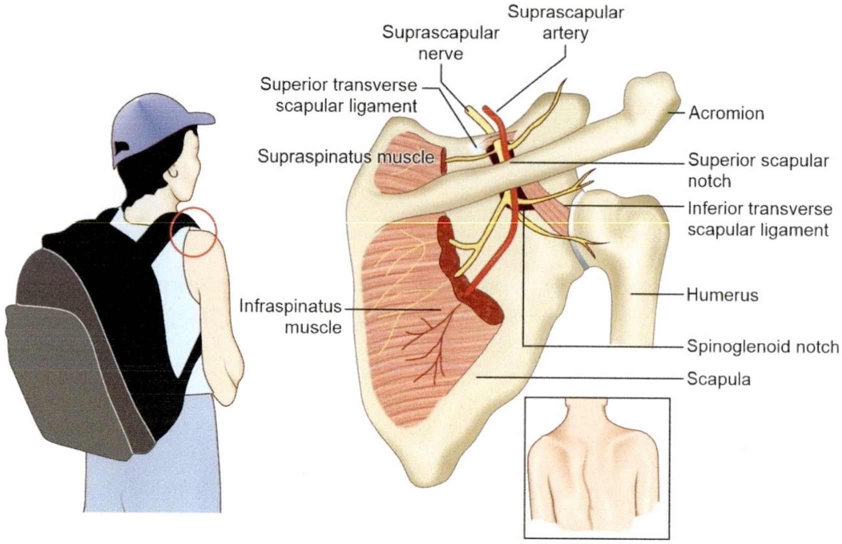

Fig. 1: Course of the suprascapular nerve after traversing the suprascapular notch and its innervation of supraspinatus and infraspinatus muscle. Sensory branches are to the shoulder. Damage to the nerve occurs due to carrying loads on the shoulder.

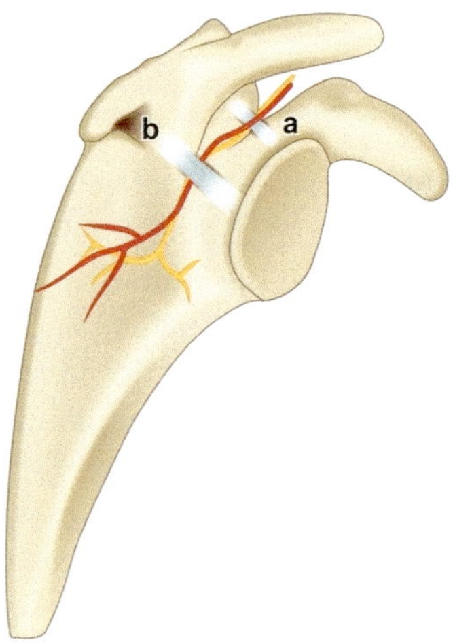

Fig. 2: Sites of entrapment of suprascapular nerve—(a) suprascapular notch and (b) spinoglenoid notch. Note the relation of the suprascapular artery near the suprascapular notch to the superior transverse scapular ligament.

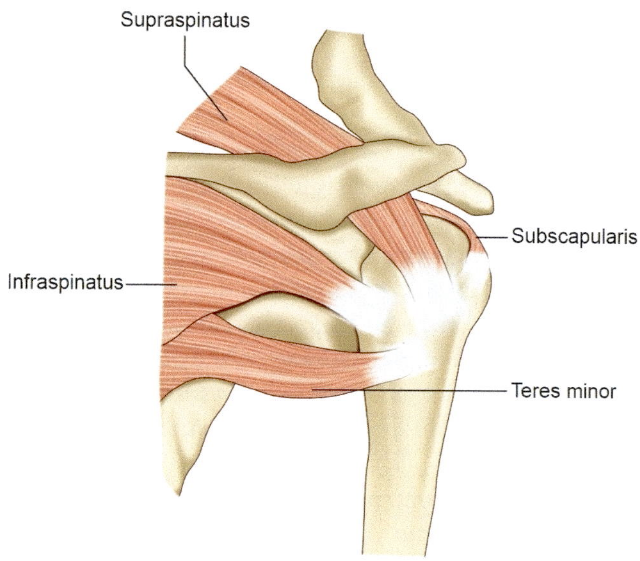

Fig. 3: Shoulder rotator cuff muscles.

(Fig. 3). Their essential functions are to function as dynamic stabilizer and also facilitate shoulder movements. When the rotator cuff is damaged, the fine movements provided by the muscles to enable smooth movement of the head of humerus are lost leading to pain.

SHOULDER PAIN AMENABLE TO SUPRASCAPULAR NERVE BLOCK

Entrapment of the SSN occurs within the suprascapular notch or in the spinoglenoid notch **(Fig. 2)**. However, the notch is absent in up to 8% cadavers.[8] This occurs due to the thickening and/or bony ossification of the overlying STSL or inferior transverse scapular ligament, respectively. Compression of the nerve by a paralabral ganglion cyst at these vulnerable points can also lead to entrapment neuropathy.[16-18]

Suprascapular nerve entrapment can result in secondary neuropathy due to compression of the nerve in the bony suprascapular notch.[19] Suprascapular notches are found to have different shapes. The most common variant

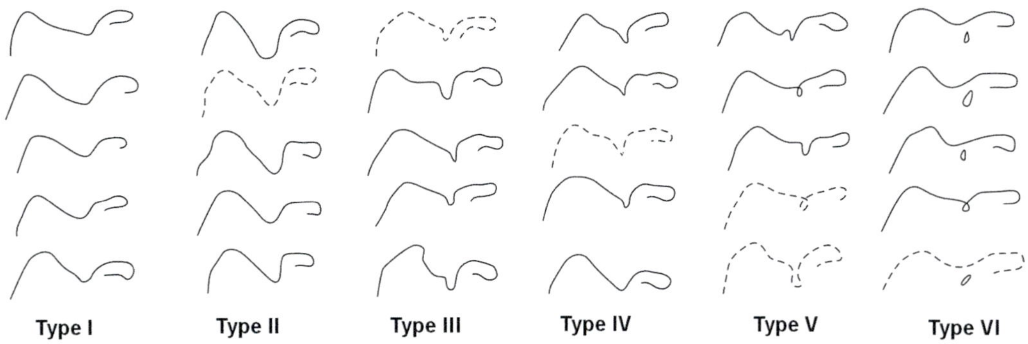

Fig. 4: Rengachary's classification of suprascapular notch.

is J-shaped, accounting for about 22%. V and U shapes are the other variations encountered, while some scapulae do not have an identifiable notch.[18,20] A narrow and V-shaped notch predisposes to entrapment of the nerve.[21,22] The entrapment syndrome is more likely to be associated with a type III notch on Rengachary's classification because of its specific features **(Fig. 4)**.

Muscle Injury and Tendinopathy of the Rotator Cuff Muscles

It can occur in young patients due to violent or repetitive trauma. Frequent overhead lifting of weights can lead to rotator cuff tear, fractured scapula, or even shoulder arthrodesis causing inflammation and pain. This is seen in sports, such as cricket, tennis, weightlifting, boxing, or swimming. It can also be implicated in certain professionals, such as painters, operative camera operators, pressing and assembling workers.[23]

Frozen Shoulder

Frozen shoulder is a nonspecific chronic pain condition that restricts shoulder motion more often in the elderly. This has a higher incidence of 10–36% among diabetic patients.[24]

Neuralgic Amyotrophy

Neuralgic amyotrophy is an uncommon condition characterized by an acute-onset shoulder pain followed by motor weakness without loss of sensation. The etiology of the condition is not very well understood but is thought that it may be due to a viral infection, such as cytomegalovirus, or may follow the administration of certain vaccines.[25,26]

Presentation

In practice, suprascapular neuropathy is a clinical diagnosis made after excluding other sources of pain. Unless the treating physician is aware and vigilant about this treatable condition, it can easily be overlooked.

Typical patients are those involved in overhead loading, athletes involved in contact sports or someone with poor physical conditioning. They present with pain and/or reduced muscle bulk in the suprascapular and sometimes even in the infrascapular fossa, depending on the location of the compression of the SSN. Although bilateral involvement is possible, it occurs in the dominant arm. This condition does not show sexual preponderance.[27]

Symptoms

The pain is described as a deep, dull, aching discomfort, exacerbated by overhead or rotational activity of the shoulder. There can be a burning sensation and weakness on raising the arm, often at the top or back of the shoulder that worsens toward the end of the day, occurring due to nerve incarceration.

Signs

Painful arc syndrome is characterized by pain in the shoulder, specifically over the bulk of deltoid, occurring on lateral abduction from 60° to 120° movement. The restriction happens due to SSN impingement in the suprascapular notch or subacromial impingement of supraspinatus. Tenderness and occasionally allodynia are demonstrated on the superior or posterior aspect of the shoulder. Other signs of neuropathic pain are rarely seen. The weakness on overhead abduction and outward rotation of the shoulder and arm are also found due to supraspinatus and infraspinatus involvement, respectively. Atrophy of the supraspinatus or infraspinatus muscle is occasionally seen.

INVESTIGATIONS

Traditionally, a diagnosis of SSN entrapment was only considered after development of marked weakness and atrophy of the supraspinatus or infraspinatus muscles.[28] Earlier diagnosis after a magnetic resonance imaging (MRI) scan is now possible in nonspecific shoulder pain.[29] MRI scan may also be helpful to identify the surgically amenable tears of the rotator cuff or a cystic ganglion in the notch causing SSN entrapment. Among the other imaging techniques that assist in making a diagnosis include X-ray and computed tomography arthrography.

Electromyography or nerve conduction studies help confirm the site of nerve impingement and also determine the status of the nerve function. Fluoroscopy(X-ray)-guided or ultrasound-guided diagnostic injection may also be used.

TREATMENT OPTIONS

A multidisciplinary and multimodal treatment is recommended for this chronic and often disabling pain. SSN has a long course in the neck and shoulder. During its path, there are multiple points where it can get implicated. The rotator cuff formed by the supraspinatus, infraspinatus, and subscapularis muscles can also be damaged. Depending on the pathology and the severity of symptoms, various treatment strategies can be undertaken.

Conservative Approach

Rest from the offending activity, gentle stretching, and gradual strengthening exercises of the involved shoulder muscles are useful. Expert guidance of a physical therapist is recommended. Further treatments including acupuncture, ultrasound, and other modalities can be tried.

Pharmacological Approach

Paracetamol, nonsteroidal anti-inflammatory drugs (NSAIDs) may help to reduce inflammation and pain in the short term and for acute flare-ups. Antineuropathic agents can also be used if neuropathic pain is suspected.

Surgical Approach

Traditionally, an open surgical decompression of the suprascapular notch was performed.[30,31] Recently, an arthroscopic decompression of the SSN, while passing through the suprascapular notch and spinoglenoid notch, through the subacromial space is performed with good success.[32-34]

Interventional Techniques

Suprascapular nerve block can be used both for diagnostic and therapeutic purposes.[35] Depending on the clinical condition, operator preference, and access to equipment, it can be performed under landmarks, nerve stimulator, ultrasound, or fluoroscopic guidance. After excluding contraindications and obtaining informed patient consent, the procedure is performed under full aseptic precautions.

Blockade of the SSN in the notch is considered more appropriate for entrapment of the nerve under the STSL. The commonly performed Meier's landmark technique for providing surgical analgesia is associated with less risk of pneumothorax.[36] But, this is less helpful in chronic pain conditions since the blockade of the SSN is done in lateral part of the supraspinous groove along its course from the suprascapular notch to the spinoglenoid notch, but not precisely targeting the supraspinous notch where the entrapment occurs. A total volume of 5–10 mL is prepared.[1]

Contraindications

Contraindications for the interventional techniques include:

- *Absolute contraindications:*
  - Patient refusal
  - Systemic sepsis
  - Infection at injection site.
- *Relative contraindications:*
  - Allergy to local anesthetic (LA)
  - Coagulopathy due to anticoagulation or hematological disease.

Landmark Technique

Equipment: A 100 mm long, 22G needle with LA for skin infiltration and a 5–10 mL of a chosen mixture containing steroid and long-acting LA are prepared.

Procedure: With patient in sitting position and arm relaxed in adducted position, a linear line is drawn over the superior border of the spine of scapula connecting the medial end of the scapular spine to the acromion. An intersecting vertical line is drawn, passing through the inferior angle of the scapula. Entry point is marked about 2.5 cm in the upper outer quadrant from this point. This is usually felt as a depression on the skin to deep palpation **(Fig. 5)**.[9]

After skin infiltration with LA, a 100 mm needle is introduced perpendicular to all the planes. The needle is

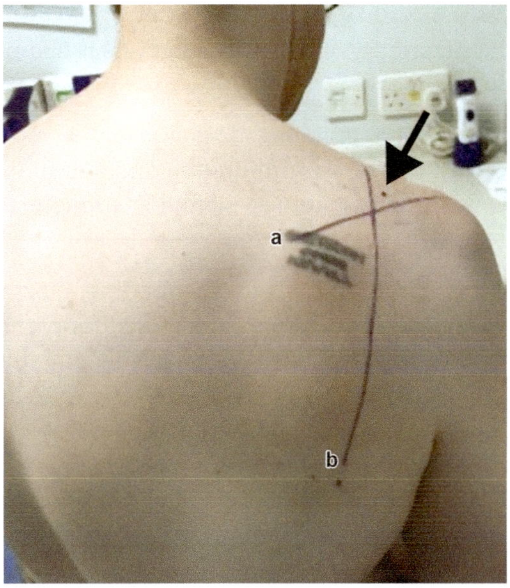

Fig. 5: Landmark and nerve stimulator-guided techniques for suprascapular nerve block. Note the entry point from the point of intersection of the supraspinous line (a) to the vertical line passing through the inferior angle of the scapula (b).

pointed caudally, medially, and anteriorly until it touches the supraspinous groove. After injecting 5 mL of the drug, withdraw the needle and redirect the needle to walk off the supraspinous notch with gentle advancement past the free edge of the bone to inject the remaining 5 mL of the mixture. Sometimes, mild pain felt in the shoulder radiating down the arm confirms accurate placement.

Complications: Pneumothorax can occur in <1% of cases with landmark technique. This serious complication occurs more likely with poor anatomical landmarking or due to advancing the needle too deep into the notch. Intravascular injection of LA mixture can occur due to the close proximity of the suprascapular artery and vein.

Peripheral Nerve Stimulation-guided Technique

Equipment: A 100 mm, 22 g, short beveled, insulated needle with LA for skin infiltration and a 5–10 mL of a chosen mixture containing a steroid and long-acting LA drugs are prepared.

Procedure: With patient in sitting position and arm relaxed in adducted position, a linear line is drawn over the superior border of the spine of scapula connecting the medial end of the scapular spine to the acromion. An intersecting vertical line is drawn, passing through the inferior angle of the scapula. Entry point is marked about 2.5 cm in the upper outer quadrant from this point. This is usually felt as a depression on the skin to deep palpation.

After skin infiltration with LA, a 100 mm insulated needle is introduced perpendicular to all the planes. The needle is pointed in a caudal, medial, and anterior direction to touch the suprascapular fossa. Sensory stimulation at 50 Hz frequency starting with 1 mA current amplitude is performed to obtain reproducible paresthesia in the shoulder joint. Advance the needle closer to the nerve to reach minimum threshold amplitude between 0.3 and 0.5 mA. Motor stimulation is checked with 2 Hz frequency and a minimum current threshold ranging between 0.3 and 0.5 mA. This causes contractions of the supraspinatus and infraspinatus muscles leading to minor abduction and external rotation of the arm. 10 mL of chosen drug mixture is deposited after aspiration.

Complications: Pneumothorax can occur in <1% of cases. This serious complication occurs more likely with poor anatomical landmarking or due to advancing the needle too deep into the notch. Intravascular injection of LA mixture can occur due to the close proximity of the suprascapular artery and vein.

Fluoroscopy-guided Technique

Equipment: A 100 mm long, 22 g needle, with LA for skin infiltration and a 5–10 mL of a chosen mixture containing steroid and long-acting LA are prepared.

Procedure: Patient is positioned in prone position with arms by the side. Using a C-arm fluoroscopic guidance, locate the suprascapular notch medial to the base of the coracoid process and lateral to the rib margins. An approximate 16°–18° tilt in craniocaudal and ipsilateral oblique rotation is necessary.[37] A 100 mm needle is advanced into the outer half of the notch **(Fig. 6)**. After the needle touching the coracoid bone, a Neer's or lateral view of the scapula is obtained to ascertain the final needle position midway over the base of the coracoid. 1 mL contrast agent is injected to note the spread before depositing 5–10 mL of chosen LA and steroid mixture.

Complications: Pneumothorax can occur in <1% of cases. This serious complication occurs more likely with poor anatomical landmarking or due to advancing the needle too deep into the notch. Intravascular injection of LA mixture can occur due to the close proximity of the suprascapular artery and vein.

Ultrasound-Guided Technique

Ultrasound-guided technique helps in increasing the safety and efficiency of the SSN block, because the nerve can be visualized in the notch and also in close proximity of the suprascapular artery.[38-41] The debate over the superiority of the ultrasound versus fluoroscopic techniques is ongoing.[42]

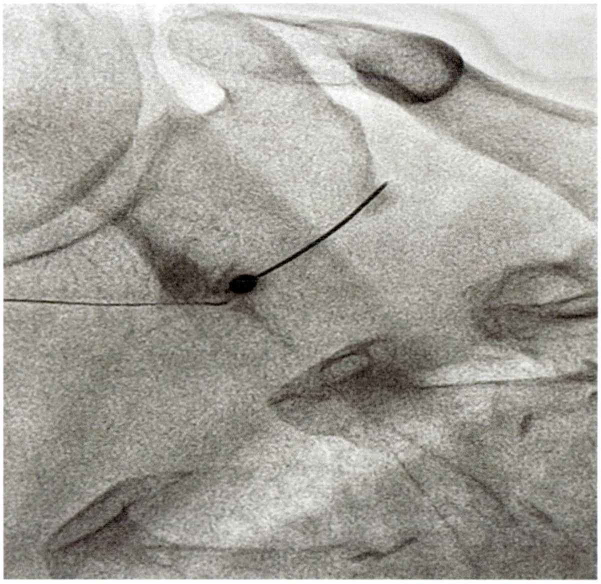

Fig. 6: Fluoroscopic image of the suprascapular notch. Needle placed close to the floor of the notch. Here, the nerve lies beneath the ligament, separated from the artery.

Equipment: A 100 mm long, 22 g ultrasound compatible needle with LA for skin infiltration and a 5–10 mL of a chosen mixture containing a steroid and long-acting LA are prepared.

Procedure: Either a high-frequency linear or a low-frequency curvilinear probe can be used for performing the block depending on the patient body habitus. The ultrasound technique can be more easily done in sitting or prone positions with the shoulder in full adduction.

With transducer placed vertically over the fossa, first locate the spine of the scapula. After locating the supraspinatus muscle in the fossa, turn the probe to image the floor of the supraspinous fossa along its long axis **(Figs. 7A and B)**.

Identify the point at which the scapular bone becomes discontinuous due to the suprascapular notch **(Figs. 8A and B)**. Bridging the notch in its base is the STSL. The SSN is found under the STSL.

Overlying the ligament is the suprascapular artery, which is to be avoided during needle insertion, can be seen **(Fig. 9)**. Covering the notch are the supraspinatus and the trapezius muscles. The needle is advanced in plane into its final position in the notch and LA and steroid mixture is injected after safety checks.

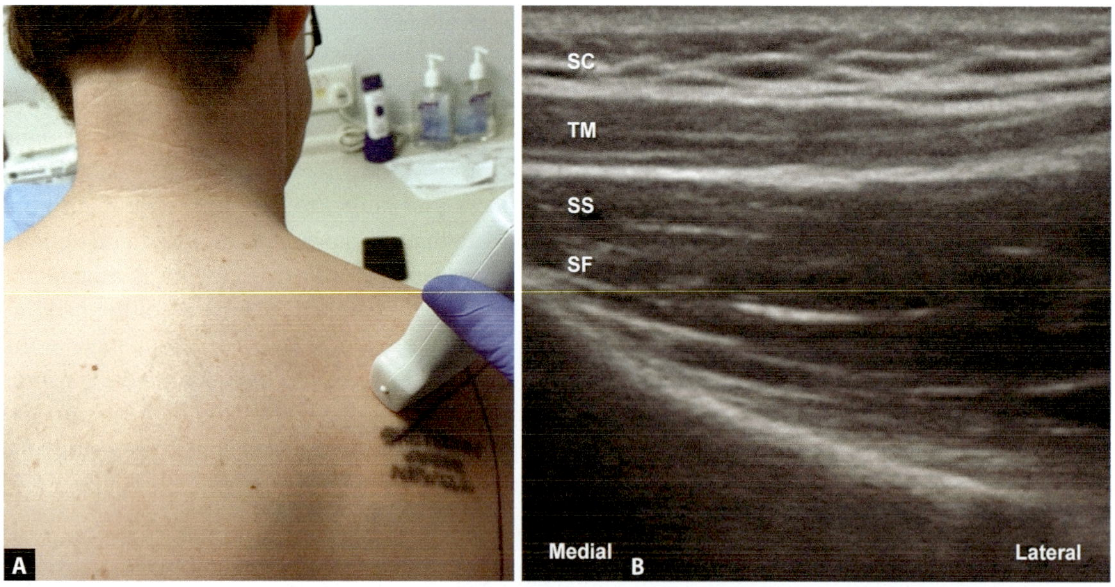

Figs. 7A and B: Suprascapular fossa: (A) Transducer over the medial side of the fossa and (B) ultrasonographic image of medial fossa. (SC: subcutaneous tissue; SF: supraspinous fossa; SS: supraspinatus muscle; TM: trapezius muscle)

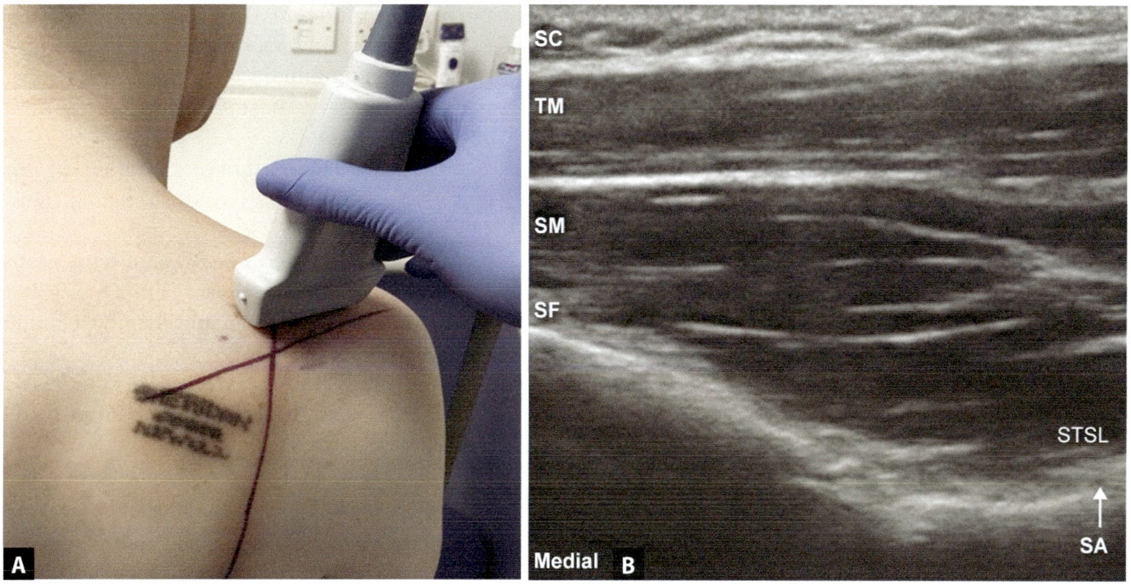

Figs. 8A and B: Suprascapular notch: (A) Transducer over the lateral end of the fossa and (B) ultrasonographic image of lateral fossa. (SC: subcutaneous tissue; SF: supraspinous fossa; SS: supraspinatus muscle; STSL: superior transverse scapular ligament; TM: trapezius)

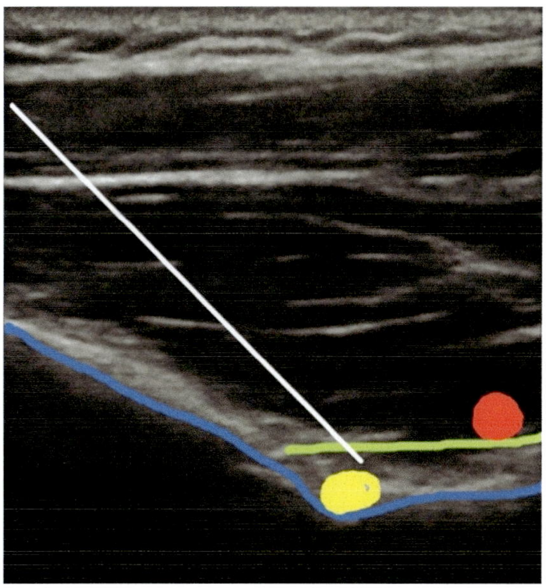

Fig. 9: Illustration of the suprascapular notch and suprascapular nerve (yellow) in relation to the suprascapular artery (red). The green line is the superior transverse scapular ligament.

An out-of-plane approach of needle advancement is possible, but visualizing the needle tip can be difficult.

Complications: Pneumothorax is a rare complication with ultrasound-guided SSN blocks. This serious complication occurs due to poor anatomical landmarking or due to advancing the needle too deep into the notch. Intravascular injection of LA mixture can occur due to the close proximity of the suprascapular artery and vein to the nerve.[43]

Pulsed Radiofrequency of the Suprascapular Nerve

Pulsed radiofrequency (PRF) is a non-neurolytic neuromodulatory technique, which can be effective in alleviation of neuropathic pain. There is growing evidence for longer lasting effectiveness of the technique lasting for up to 9 months. It provides pain control and reduces disability while improving functioning.[44-47]

Equipment: A 20G, 100 mm long radiofrequency (RF) needle with a 10 mm active tip, RF probe, RF pulse generator with LA for skin infiltration, and a 5–10 mL of a chosen mixture containing steroid and long-acting LA are prepared.[40]

Procedure: Use of either fluoroscopy or ultrasound guidance ensures accurate needle placement. After appropriate positioning of the needle into the suprascapular notch, the RF probe is inserted and checked for stimulation. Gentle adjustment of needle with sensory stimulation at 50 Hz, 0.2 ms pulse width is used to elicit reproducible paresthesias in the shoulder joint between 0.3 and 0.5 V.

Motor stimulation at 2 Hz frequency and 0.2 ms pulse width triggers contractions of the infraspinatus and supraspinatus muscles between 0.3 and 0.5 V.

Three cycles of 120 seconds pulsed mode RF lesioning is performed keeping the temperature constant at 42°C, at a frequency of 2 Hz and pulse width of 20 ms.[48] The chosen LA and steroid mixture is deposited near the nerve at the end of the procedure. PRF can accept up to 6 weeks to provide sustained pain relief.

Though RF denervation has been documented in literature, the risk of neuropathic pain due to damage to a mixed nerve like the SSN warrants caution. Recently, implanted peripheral nerve stimulators have also been utilized successfully to manage refractory cases.

Complications: Pneumothorax can occur in <1% of cases. This serious complication occurs more likely with poor anatomical landmarking or due to advancing the needle too deep into the notch. Intravascular injection of LA mixture can occur due to the close proximity of the suprascapular artery and vein to the nerve location in the notch.

CONCLUSION

Suprascapular nerve block, when utilized effectively and performed safely could be a useful tool in reducing pain, not only in acute stages but also in chronic pain states. It facilitates mobilization of the arm and allows engagement with physiotherapy and strengthening exercises. The unique anatomy of the scapula allows various approaches to block the SSN. The choice of the technique is determined by the demands of the clinical situation, availability of equipment, and skill of the physician. PRF could potentially increase the duration of pain relief. Though RF denervation of SSN nerve has been documented, the risk of neuropathic pain due to damage to a mixed nerve like the SSN warrants caution. Recently, implanted peripheral nerve stimulators have been utilized successfully to manage refractory cases.

REFERENCES

1. Taskaynatan MA, Yilmaz B, Ozgul A, Yazicioglu K, Kalyon TA. Suprascapular nerve block versus steroid injection for non-specific shoulder pain. Tohoku J Exp Med. 2005;205(1):19-25.
2. Tran DQ, Elgueta MF, Aliste J, Finlayson RJ. Diaphragm-Sparing Nerve Blocks for Shoulder Surgery. Reg Anesth Pain Med. 2017;42(1):32-8.
3. Bergmann L, Martini S, Kesselmeier M, Armbruster W, Notheisen T, Adamzik M, et al. Phrenic nerve block caused by interscalene brachial plexus block: breathing effects of different sites of injection. BMC Anesthesiol. 2016;16(1):45.
4. Borgeat A, Ekatodramis G. Anaesthesia for shoulder surgery. Best Pract Res Clin Anaesthesiol. 2002;16(2):211-25.
5. Boezaart AP. Continuous interscalene block for ambulatory shoulder surgery. Best Pract Res Clin Anaesthesiol. 2002;16(2):295-310.
6. Ajmani ML. The cutaneous branch of the human suprascapular nerve. J Anat. 1994;185 (Pt 2) (Pt 2) 439-42.
7. Vorster W, Lange CP, Briët RJ, Labuschagne BC, du Toit DF, Muller CJ, et al. The sensory branch distribution of the suprascapular nerve: an anatomic study. J Shoulder Elbow Surg. 2008;17(3):500-2.
8. Natsis K, Totlis T, Tsikaras P, Appell HJ, Skandalakis P, Koebke J. Proposal for classification of the suprascapular notch: a study on 423 dried scapulas. Clin Anat. 2007;20:135-9.
9. Price DJ. The shoulder block: a new alternative to interscalene brachial plexus blockade for the control of postoperative shoulder pain. Anaesth Intensive Care. 2007;35(4):575-81.
10. Allen ZA, Shanahan EM, Crotty M. Does suprascapular nerve block reduce shoulder pain following stroke: a double-blind randomised controlled trial with masked outcome assessment. BMC Neurol. 2010;10:83-7.
11. Shanahan EM, Ahern M, Smith M, Wetherall M, Bresnihan B, FitzGerald O. Suprascapular nerve block (using bupivacaine and methylprednisolone acetate) in chronic shoulder pain. Ann Rheum Dis. 2003;62(5):400-6.
12. Fernandes MR, Fernandes RJ. Artroscopia no tratamento da tendinite calcária refratária do ombro. Rev Bras Ortop. 2010;45:53-60.
13. Chan CW, Peng PW. Suprascapular nerve block: a narrative review. Reg Anesth Pain Med. 2011;36(4):358-73.
14. Ko SH, Kang BS, Hwang CH. Ultrasonography- or electrophysiology-guided suprascapular nerve block in arthroscopic acromioplasty: a prospective, double-blind, parallel-group, randomized controlled study of efficacy. Arthroscopy. 2013;29(5):794-801.
15. Arad E, Li Z, Sitzman TJ, Agur AM, Clarke HM. Anatomic sites of origin of the suprascapular and lateral pectoral nerves within the brachial plexus. Plast Reconstr Surg. 2014;133(1):20e-27e.
16. Brown DE, James DC, Roy S. Pain relief by suprascapular nerve block in gleno-humeral arthritis. Scand J Rheumatol. 1988;17(5):411-5.
17. Akboru IM, Solmaz I, Secer HI, Izci Y, Daneyemez M. The surgical anatomy of the brachial plexus. Turk Neurosurg. 2010;20(2):142-50.
18. Tan BY, Lee K. SLAP lesion with supraglenoid labral cyst causing suprascapular nerve compression: a case report. Malays Orthop J. 2012;6(Suppl A):46-8.
19. Rizzello G, Longo UG, Trovato U, Fumo C, Khan WS, Maffulli N, et al. Bilateral suprascapular nerve entrapment by ganglion cyst associated with superior labral lesion. Open Orthop J. 2013;7:129-32.

20. Kumar A, Sharma A, Singh P. Anatomical study of the suprascapular notch: quantitative analysis and clinical considerations for suprascapular nerve entrapment. Singapore Med J. 2014;55(1):41-4.
21. Rengachary S, Neff JP, Singer PA, Brackett CF. Suprascapular entrapment neuropathy: a clinical, anatomical, and comparative study, Part 1: clinical Study. Neurosurgery. 1979;5:441-6.
22. Iqbal K, Iqbal R, Khan SG. Anatomical variations in shape of suprascapular notch of scapula. J Morphol Sci. 2010; 27:1-2.
23. Antoniadis G, Richter HP, Rath S, Braun V, Moese G. Suprascapular nerve entrapment: experience with 28 cases. J Neurosurg. 1996;85(6):1020-5.
24. Rengachary SS, Burr D, Lucas S, Hassanein KM, Mohn MP, Matzke H. Suprascapular entrapment neuropathy: a clinical, anatomical, and comparative study, Part 2: anatomical study. Neurosurgery. 1979;5(4):447-51.
25. Karataş GK, Gögüş F. Suprascapular nerve entrapment in newsreel camera. Am J Phys Med Rehabil. 2003;82(3): 192-6.
26. Ozkan K, Ozcekic AN, Sarar S, Cift H, Ozkan FU, Unay K. Suprascapular nerve block for the treatment of frozen shoulder. Saudi J Anaesth. 2012;6(1):52-5.
27. Feinberg JH, Radecki J. Parsonage-Turner Syndrome. HSS J. 2010;6(2):199-205.
28. Fransz DP, Schönhuth CP, Postma TJ, van Royen BJ. Parsonage-Turner syndrome following post-exposure prophylaxis. BMC Musculoskelet Disord. 2014;15:265.
29. Ferretti A, De Carli A, Fontana M. Injury of the suprascapular nerve at the spinoglenoid notch. The natural history of infraspinatus atrophy in volleyball players. Am J Sports Med. 1998;26(6):759-63.
30. Liveson JA, Bronson MJ, Pollack MA. Suprascapular nerve lesions at the spinoglenoid notch: report of three cases and review of the literature. J Neurol Neurosurg Psychiatry. 1991;54(3):241-3.
31. Fritz RC, Helms CA, Steinbach LS, Genant HK. Suprascapular nerve entrapment: evaluation with MR imaging. Radiology. 1992;182(2):437-44.
32. Kim DH, Murovic JA, Tiel RL, Kline DG. Management and outcomes of 42 surgical suprascapular nerve injuries and entrapments. Neurosurgery. 2005;57(1):120-7; discussion 120-7.
33. Fabre T, Piton C, Leclouerec G, Gervais-Delion F, Durandeau A. Entrapment of the suprascapular nerve. J Bone Joint Surg Br. 1999;81(3):414-9.
34. Lafosse L, Tomasi A, Corbett S, Baier G, Willems K, Gobezie R. Arthroscopic release of suprascapular nerve entrapment at the suprascapular notch: technique and preliminary results. Arthroscopy. 2007;23(1):34-42.
35. Bhatia DN, de Beer JF, van Rooyen KS, du Toit DF. Arthroscopic suprascapular nerve decompression at the suprascapular notch. Arthroscopy. 2006;22(9):1009-13.
36. Shah AA, Butler RB, Sung SY, Wells JH, Higgins LD, Warner JJ. Clinical outcomes of suprascapular nerve decompression. J Shoulder Elbow Surg. 2011;20(6):975-82.
37. Moore DC. Regional Block: A Handbook for Use in the Clinical Practice of Medicine and Surgery. 4th edition. Springfield (IL): Charles C. Thomas; 1965. pp. 300-3.
38. Feigl GC, Anderhuber F, Dorn C, Pipam W, Rosmarin W, Likar R. Modified lateral block of the suprascapular nerve: a safe approach and how much to inject? A morphological study. Reg Anesth Pain Med. 2007;32(6):488-94.
39. Gorthi V, Moon YL, Kang JH. The effectiveness of ultrasonography-guided suprascapular nerve block for perishoulder pain. Orthopedics. 2010;33(4).
40. Choi S, Brull R. Is ultrasound guidance advantageous for interventional pain management? A review of acute pain outcomes. Anesth Analg. 2011;113(3):596-604.
41. Lotero MAA, Díaz RCR, Escobar DC, Aguila MAM, Ramírez SAM. Efficacy and safety of ultrasound-guided suprascapular nerve block in patients with chronic shoulder pain. Rev Colomb Anestesiol. 2013;41(2):104-8.
42. Shim JH. Is fluoroscopy-guided suprascapular nerve block better than other techniques? Korean J Pain. 2013;26(1):102-3.
43. Standring S, Borley NR, Collins P, Crossman AR, Gatzoulis MA, Healy JC, et al. Gray's Anatomy: The Anatomical Basis of Clinical Practice, 40th edition. Edinburgh: Elsevier; 2008. pp. 449-50.
44. Wu YT, Ho CW, Chen YL, Li TY, Lee KC, Chen LC. Ultrasound-guided pulsed radiofrequency stimulation of the suprascapular nerve for adhesive capsulitis: a prospective, randomized, controlled trial. Anesth Analg. 2014;119(3):686-92.
45. Liliang PC, Lu K, Liang CL, Tsai YD, Hsieh CH, Chen HJ. Pulsed radiofrequency lesioning of the suprascapular nerve for chronic shoulder pain: a preliminary report. Pain Med. 2009;10(1):70-5.
46. Jang JS, Choi HJ, Kang SH, Yang JS, Lee JJ, Hwang SM. Effect of pulsed radiofrequency neuromodulation on clinical improvements in the patients of chronic intractable shoulder pain. J Korean Neurosurg Soc. 2013;54(6):507-10.
47. Wu YT, Ho CW, Chen YL, Li TY, Lee KC, Chen LC. Ultrasound-guided pulsed radiofrequency stimulation of the suprascapular nerve for adhesive capsulitis: a prospective, randomized, controlled trial. Anesth Analg. 2014;119(3):686-92.
48. Shah RV, Racz GB. Pulsed mode radiofrequency lesioning of the suprascapular nerve for the treatment of chronic shoulder pain. Pain Physician. 2003;6(4):503-6.

21 CHAPTER

Intercostal Nerve Block

Gerard DeGregoris III

ABSTRACT

Pain management physicians have found a wide variety of applications for the intercostal nerve block (INB) to treat a variety of acute, chronic, and cancer pain syndromes. The intercostal nerves arise from the ventral rami of nerve roots T1 through T11. Each ramus exits from the spinal foramen and enters the paravertebral space as the intercostal nerve at that level. Classically, this block is performed without the aid of advanced imaging techniques. In this manner, the physician locates the angle of the rib approximately 8 cm lateral to the spine. A 22-gauge, short-bevel needle is inserted to contact the inferior portion of the rib. After contact, the needle is redirected and translated inferiorly to "walk off" the inferior margin of the rib. The needle is then advanced approximately 3 mm deep to the lower margin and aspirated. Assuming negative aspiration, the anesthetic modality of choice (local anesthetic, steroid, radiofrequency, or cryoablation) is then utilized at that location. Absolute contraindications include patient refusal, allergy to the injectate, and infection at the injection site. Complications are rare, but the most often reported is pneumothorax. The incidence of pneumothorax after individual INB for postoperative pain reportedly varies from 0.073 to 19%

INTRODUCTION

The intercostal nerve block (INB) is a valuable tool for a pain management physician for the management of acute, chronic, and cancer pain syndromes.[1-4] It has been described as an adjunct to general anesthesia, as well as a primary treatment for acute and chronic pain.[1] When accompanying general anesthesia, the goal is to decrease the amount of volatile anesthetic required in open surgery including thoracic[2-5] and general surgical procedures. The technique has also been used with an indwelling peripheral catheter with good results for postoperative thoracotomy pain.[6,7] It can be performed for the treatment of acute rib fracture pain with local anesthetic[8] and cancer-related pain with local anesthetic[9] and/or neurolytic agents. Additionally, enterprising physicians have shown that post-thoracotomy pain syndrome can be treated with this technique.[10] The technique has been used to deliver various pain-abating modalities to the intercostal neurovascular bundle including local anesthetic, neurolytic agents, steroid, radiofrequency, and cryoablation.[1-4]

MEDICATION CHOICE

The choice of medication depends upon the goals for pain management. If the block is to be performed for intraoperative or postoperative pain control, then local anesthetic is used, and steroid is usually not employed. If the goal of the block is sensory analgesia, then a lower concentration of local anesthetic is usually employed, such as 1% mepivacaine, 1% lidocaine, or 0.25% bupivacaine.[11] These agents would be appropriate if the indications for block were for an acute pain condition such as rib fracture. If, however, this block is being performed as an adjunct to general anesthesia (such as in the case of abdominal surgery), then a higher concentration of local anesthetic may be desirable. This higher concentration is more likely to provide somatic effects including muscle relaxation, which will facilitate surgical manipulation and visualization. In this case 1.5% mepivacaine, 1.5% lidocaine, or 0.5% bupivacaine would all be reasonable choices.[5]

OTHER USEFUL MODALITIES

Prolonged INB has also been described for postsurgical pain via an indwelling catheter technique.[12] A study of 124 patients found that similar pain control was achieved using either epidural anesthesia or a combined intercostal nerve catheter/patient-controlled anesthesia technique. The authors suggested that the latter had the advantage of saving time because the surgeon was able to place the nerve catheter intraoperatively obviating the need for an anesthesiologist to place an epidural catheter preoperatively or postoperatively.[6] Intercostal cryotherapy has been found to be a safe and effective way to provide relief for post-thoracotomy neuralgia and cancer pain.[4,13]

ANATOMY

Origin of Intercostal Nerves

The intercostal nerves arise from the ventral rami of nerve roots T1 through T11. Each ramus exits from the spinal foramen and enters the paravertebral space as the intercostal nerve at that level.[5] Each intercostal nerve may receive innervation from the sympathetic trunk by way of rami communicantes. Many of those nerve fibers originating from T1 will combine with those from the C8 nerve root to then form the lower trunk of the brachial plexus. Other fibers from nerve roots T2 and T3 will combine to form the intercostobrachial nerve.[14] This nerve along with other fibers from the brachial plexus will innervate the upper chest wall. Inferiorly, the intercostal nerves will supply the thoracoabdominal wall from the nipple line (T4 dermatome) down to below the umbilicus (T11 dermatome).

Branches of Intercostal Nerves

As each intercostal nerve travels distally, it enters the intercostal space lying inferior to the costal margin. The nerve lies between the innermost intercostal muscle and the pleura.[15] Anatomic studies of intercostal nerves have described five general branches. First, each intercostal nerve contributes preganglionic sympathetic fibers to the thoracic sympathetic chain via white rami communicantes. Second, these nerves also receive postganglionic neurons from the sympathetic via gray rami communicantes. Third, once the nerve has left the intervertebral foramina, the dorsal rami carry the posterior cutaneous and motor fibers branch to supply the skin and musculature in the paravertebral region. Fourth, a lateral cutaneous branch arises just before the nerve crosses the mid-axillary line. Lastly, the nerve terminates as the anterior cutaneous branch to innervate the anterior chest wall. Of note, a collateral branch of each intercostal nerve commonly branches inferiorly to join with the intercostal nerve at the upper border of the next inferior rib.[16] Muscular branches from each intercostal nerve are directed toward the intercostal muscles and multiple pleural sensory branches will be directed toward the pleura. Additionally, the seventh through eleventh intercostal nerves run parallel to the parietal peritoneum and give off sensory branches to that structure.

Variability in Anatomical Arrangement

Traditionally it was taught that the intercostal nerves lie in the intercostal groove caudad to the intercostal vein and artery, but more recent research has shown that this may not be the case.[17] Hardy showed in a 1998 paper that this commonly taught anatomical arrangement occurs only 17% of the time. More frequently, the intercostal nerve was found in a mid-costal location (73% of the time). The intercostal nerve was even found to lie superiorly to the vasculature in approximately 10% of cases. This anatomic variability demands utmost attention from the provider during the performance of this block.

T12 Ventral Ramus

The ventral ramus of T12 exits the paravertebral space to become the twelfth thoracic nerve. This nerve travels inferiorly to the twelfth rib and as such is only bounded on one side by rib. It is therefore not an intercostal nerve but a subcostal nerve. Each subcostal nerve may give off nerve fibers that join with the ilioinguinal and iliohypogastric nerves.

PROCEDURE

To perform INB, the patient is positioned prone. Placing a pillow under the abdomen and allowing both of the arms to hang over the sides of the table will maximize the anterior motion of the scapula and the surface of the upper ribs that is accessible from a posterior approach. This positioning technique will allow for the block to be performed bilaterally without a position change as well as allow access to the angles of the ribs which will enhance patient safety and the efficacy of the procedure.[9] If the physician intends to perform the block unilaterally, then the lateral decubitus position will be acceptable and may be more comfortable for the patient depending on the nature and location of his or her pain.

Classic Technique

Classically, this block is performed "blind", that is, without the aid of advanced imaging techniques such as fluoroscopy or ultrasound. In this manner, the physician will locate the angle of the rib approximately 8 cm lateral to the spine **(Fig. 1)**. This is the point at which most ribs make a sharp turn in direction from extending laterally to pointing anteriorly. Typical needle choice is a 22G, 1.25-inch needle attached to a 10 cc controller syringe. Once this landmark has been located the needle is inserted to contact the inferior portion of the rib. After contacting the rib, the needle is redirected and translated inferiorly to "walk off" the inferior margin of that rib. Once this is done, the needle is advanced approximately 3 mm deep to the lower margin and the syringe is aspirated to suggest (but not ensure) that a large vessel has not been inadvertently perforated. The anesthetic modality of choice (local anesthetic, steroid, radiofrequency, or cryoablation) is then deployed at that location.

While the classic technique has long been shown to be safe and efficacious, recently ultrasound-guided approaches have been employed and described for this and other nerve blocks in various sources.[9,18,19]

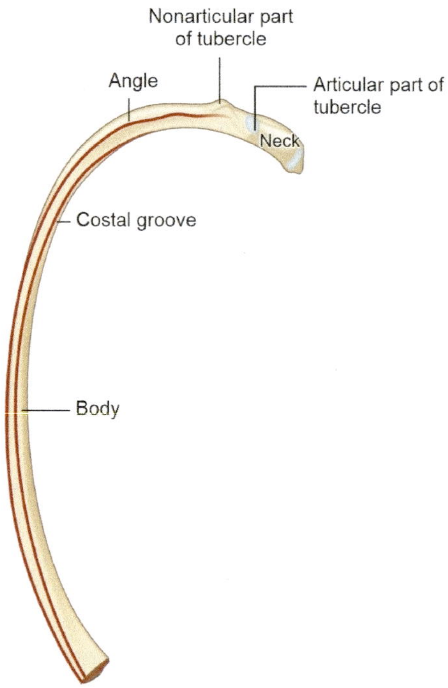

Fig. 1: Bony anatomy of a rib, as seen from below. Note the costal groove where the neurovascular structures are found.
Source: http://www.theodora.com/anatomy/the_ribs.html [Last accessed July, 2024].

Ultrasound-guided Technique

Ultrasound offers several distinct advantages for this block. First, it allows real-time appreciation of anatomical structures including the different layers of the intercostal muscles, as well as the pleura. Identification of this latter structure can be especially valuable since it can be avoided once identified. Ordinarily, the neurovascular bundle cannot be seen using ultrasound as it lies inferior to the bony rib, through which ultrasound waves cannot pass (i.e., within the "rib shadow").

For an ultrasound-guided approach, a high-resolution linear probe is preferred. The patient is placed in the prone position and the ultrasound probe is placed parallel to the spine 3–5 cm lateral to midline so that the ribs may be counted and labeled on the skin. Many physicians find it easiest to start with the twelfth rib and work cephalad as there are fewer structures interfering with sonography inferiorly. In contrast, if one begins from the superior ribs, the scapula may interfere with the sonographic identification of the upper thoracic ribs. As with the blind approach, the preferred site of injection is at the angle of each rib. The intercostal nerve has not yet branched into smaller divisions at this point. In most adults, this point is found approximately 6–8 cm lateral to the spinous process. This author prefers to place the ultrasound machine on the opposite side of the physician performing the block so that the physician has in one field of view both the operative field and the ultrasound video display. The ultrasound probe is generally held in the physician's nondominant hand and placed parallel to the spine over the angle of the rib such that the ultrasound image will reveal two consecutive ribs in cross section **(Fig. 2)**.

Once the rib of interest and the rib below are both visible on the ultrasound display screen in cross-section, depth and gain should be adjusted on the ultrasound console such that the view of the intercostal muscles and pleura is optimized. Next, a 22G 1.5-inch needle attached to a controller syringe may be inserted using the operator's dominant hand at the superior margin of the lower rib and advanced toward the upper (target) rob making a 45° angle to the skin **(Fig. 3)**. It is not necessary to contact the rib with the needle. Note that for the dominant hand to be able to conveniently approach the rib in this fashion, the right-handed operator will stand on the prone patient's left side and the left-handed operator will stand on the prone patient's right side. The needle should only be advanced if the entire needle including the needle tip is clearly visible in the ultrasound image. This is known as the "in plane approach". If only a portion

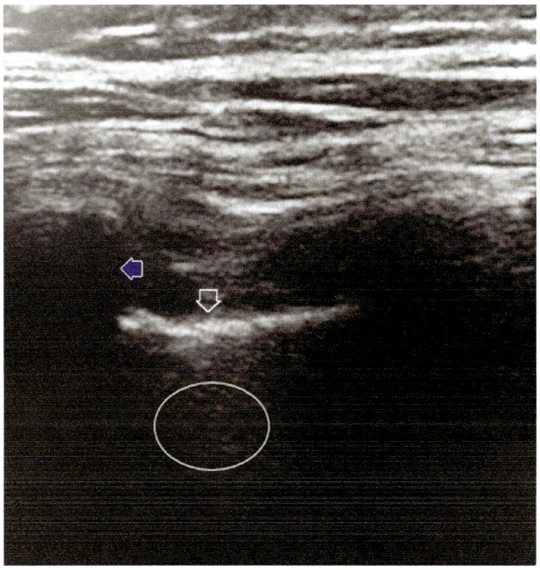

Fig. 2: Transverse ultrasound image of T8 and T9 ribs showing relevant ultrasonic landmarks. Note the hyperechoic pleura (white unfilled arrow), the inferior margin of the T8 rib (target for the INB) (filled blue arrow), and lung parenchyma (white oval).
Source: Ultrasound image with all patient identifiers removed from author's portfolio.

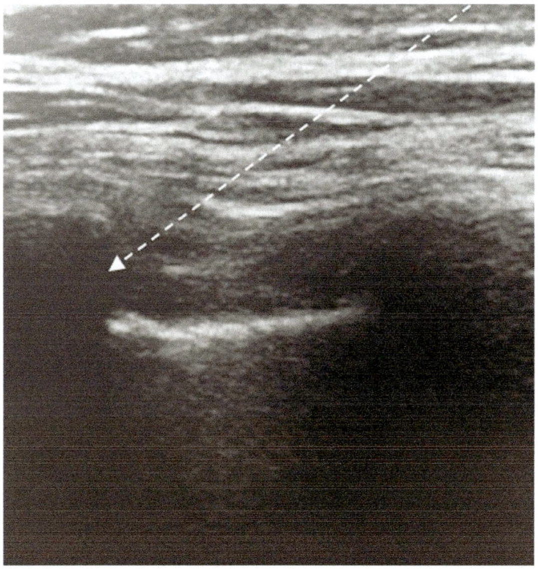

Fig. 3: Transverse ultrasound image of T8 and T9 ribs showing needle trajectory and endpoint for ultrasound-guided intercostal nerve block. Note that the needle is superficial to the hyperechoic pleura and does not violate the ultrasound shadow cast by the hyperechoic eighth rib.
Source: Ultrasound image with all patient identifiers removed from author's portfolio.

of the needle is visible in the ultrasound image, then most likely the ultrasound transducer and needle are not in the same sagittal plane. In this case, many times a slight change in the sagittal alignment of the ultrasound probe will restore the entire needle into view and the block may then proceed. If a large adjustment of the ultrasound probe is required, this may sacrifice the image quality of the ribs, intercostal muscles, and pleura. In this case the needle should be slowly withdrawn, the image optimized, and the needle reintroduced paying careful attention to ensure that the needle travels beneath the exact center of the ultrasound probe in the same sagittal plane. Once the needle has been advanced into the outermost intercostal layer, the physician should consider injecting a small amount of injectate which should appear as a dark (hypoechoic) area on the ultrasound image. This is known as "hydro dissection" and is helpful to verify the exact placement of the needle tip. It is critical that the needle tip does not violate the pleura as pneumothorax may be the result of such a violation. The pleura can be visualized as a bright echogenic horizontal line nearly tangentially contacting the inner borders of two adjacent ribs. Lung parenchyma may be visible beneath the pleura and can often be seen sliding superiorly and inferiorly with a period that matches the patient's respiratory rate. As the needle tip is advanced, the target should be just deep to the internal intercostal muscle immediately caudad to the point where the muscle becomes obscured by the rib shadow. Once the needle tip is confirmed to be deep to the intercostal muscle and superficial to the pleura, the physician may wish to aspirate the plunger to look for inadvertent vascular puncture. Next, the local anesthetic can be injected under live ultrasound guidance. Usually, 1–2 mL of local anesthetic is sufficient for each level to be blocked.[11]

CONTRAINDICATIONS

Contraindications to INB are similar to those for other percutaneous needle-based procedures.[20] Absolute contraindications include patient refusal, allergy to the injectate, and infection at the injection site. This block is relatively contraindicated in patients with significant coagulopathy or in patients who are currently anticoagulated. Other relative contraindications are few and include patients with cardiac disease who might be sensitive to the cardiac depressant effects of systemically absorbed local anesthetic.[21] Other conditions that may be considered relative contraindications include significant contralateral lung disease (including pneumothorax) or pneumonectomy (such that pneumothorax on the operative side would be poorly tolerated).

COMPLICATIONS

The most discussed side effect of INB is pneumothorax.[3,22] Less commonly discussed complications include local anesthetic systemic toxicity and neuropathic pain. The incidence of pneumothorax after individual INB for postoperative pain reportedly varies from 0.073 to 19%, but it is usually quoted around 0.5%. Some smaller studies report a rate of pneumothorax as low as 0%.[4] In a study published by Shanti, 161 patients received 249 intercostal nerve block procedures (INBPs). They defined an INBP as one session where a set of (one or more) intercostal nerves are blocked. In this study, a total of 1,020 individual intercostal nerves were blocked and there were 14 pneumothoraxes. The overall incidence of pneumothorax per patient was 8.7%, with an incidence of pneumothorax per INBP of 5.6%. The incidence of pneumothorax was 1.4% for each individual INB.[22]

There is some evidence that intercostal cryotherapy may increase the risk of long-term neuropathic pain when performed intraoperatively for postoperative pain control, but this has not yet been shown conclusively.[23] This possible risk must be considered and weighed against potential benefits.

CONCLUSION

The INB has a long history of providing safe and well-tolerated relief from a variety of pain syndromes. The block is routinely done without imaging, but ultrasound provides the theoretical advantage of tracking the needle tip in real time. The physician must be vigilant with appropriate needle placement to avoid pneumothorax, but the incidence of this is quite low.

REFERENCES

1. Dowling R, Thielmeier K, Ghaly A, Barber D, Boice T, Dine A. Improved pain control after cardiac surgery: results of a randomized, double-blind, clinical trial. J Thorac Cardiovasc Surg. 2003;126(5):1271-8.
2. Detterbeck FC. Efficacy of methods of intercostal nerve blockade for pain relief after thoracotomy. Ann Thorac Surg. 2005;80(4):1550-9.
3. Joshi GP, Bonnet F, Shah R, Wilkinson RC, Camu F, Fischer B, et al. A systematic review of randomized trials evaluating regional techniques for postthoracotomy analgesia. Anesth Analg. 2008;107:1026-40.
4. Eng J, Sabanathan S. Site of action of continuous extrapleural intercostal nerve block. Ann Thorac Surg. 1991;51(3):387-9.
5. Sabanathan S, Smith PJ, Pradhan GN, Hashimi H, Eng JB, Mearns AJ. Continuous intercostal nerve block for pain relief after thoracotomy. Ann Thorac Surg. 1988;46:425-6.
6. Luketich JD, Land SR, Sullivan EA, Alvelo-Rivera M, Ward J, Buenaventura PO, et al. Thoracic epidural versus intercostal nerve catheter plus patient-controlled analgesia: a randomized study. Ann Thorac Surg. 2005;79:1845-50.
7. Cousins MJ, Carr DB, Horlocker TT, Bridenbaugh PO. Intercostal, intrapleural, and peripheral blockade of the thorax and abdomen. In: Cousins MJ, Carr DB, Horlocker TT, Bridenbaugh PO (Eds). Cousins and Bridenbaugh's Neural Blockade in Clinical Anesthesia and Pain Medicine, 4th edition. Philadelphia, PA: Lippincott Williams and Wilkins; 2009. pp. 386-90.
8. Karmakar MK, Ho AM. Acute pain management of patients with multiple fractured ribs. J Trauma. 2003;54(3): 615-25.
9. Wong FC, Lee TW, Yuen KK, Lo Sh, Sze WK, Tung SY. Intercostal nerve blockade for cancer pain: effectiveness and selection of patients. Hong Kong Med J. 2007;13:226-70.
10. Moorjani N, Zhao F, Tian Y, Liang C, Kaluba J, Maiwand MO. Effects of cryoanalgesia on post-thoracotomy pain and on the structure of intercostal nerves: a human prospective randomized trial and a histological study. Eur J Cardiothor Surg. 2001;20(3):502-7.
11. Brown DL. Atlas of Regional Anesthesia, 3rd edition. Pennsylvania: Elsevier/Saunders; 2006.
12. Eng J, Sabanathan S. Site of action of continuous extrapleural intercostal nerve block. Ann Thorac Surg. 1991;51(3):387-9.
13. Byas-Smith MG, Gulati A. Ultrasound-guided intercostal nerve cryoablation. Anesth Analg. 2006;103(4):1033-5.
14. Henry G. Anatomy of the Human Body, 29th edition. Philadelphia, PA: Lea & Febiger; 1973. pp. 978-83.
15. Benzon H, Fishman S, Raja S, Cohen S, Liu S. Essentials of Pain Medicine, 3rd edition. Philadelphia: Elsevier/ Saunders; 2005. p. 590.
16. Fishman S, Ballantyne J, Rathmell J. Bonica's Management of Pain, 4th edition. Pennsylvania: Lippincott Williams & Wilkins; 2010. p. 1044.
17. Hardy PA. Anatomical variation in the position of the proximal intercostal nerve. Br J Anaesth. 1988;61(3): 338-9.
18. Curatolo M, Eichenberger U. Ultrasound in interventional pain management. Eur J Pain Suppl. 2008;2:78-83.
19. Peng PW, Narouze S. Ultrasound in pain medicine. Reg Anesth Pain Med. 2009;34(5):462-4.
20. Nielsen CH. Bleeding after intercostal nerve block in a patient anticoagulated with heparin. Anesthesiology. 1989;71(1):162-4.
21. Franco K, Putnam J. Advanced Therapy in Thoracic Surgery, 2nd edition. Hamilton, Ontario: BC Decker, Inc; 2005.
22. Shanti CM, Carlin AM, Tyburski JG. Incidence of pneumothorax from intercostal nerve block for analgesia in rib fractures. J Trauma. 2001;51(3):536-9.
23. Mustola ST, Lempinen J, Saimanen E, Vilkko P. Efficacy of thoracic epidural analgesia with or without intercostal nerve cryoanalgesia for postthoracotomy pain. Ann Thorac Surg. 2011;91(3):869-73.

22 CHAPTER

Intrapleural Block

Dwarkadas K Baheti

ABSTRACT

The intrapleural block (IPB) is a useful interventional pain treatment procedure for thoracic and upper back pain due to malignancy of lung, and cancer. This chapter describes a stepwise approach on how to perform IPB.

INTRODUCTION

Intrapleural block is known to provide safe, highly effective pain relief for unilateral surgical pain such as cholecystectomy, thoracotomy, and renal and breast surgery. IPB is also used for relief of nonsurgical pain such as multiple rib fractures, herpes zoster, complex regional pain syndrome, and carcinoma of lung.[1] IPB followed by pleurodesis mostly reduces pain.

ANATOMY

The lung is covered with two layers of pleura, one is parietal and the second is visceral. The cavity between these two layers is a pleural cavity as depicted in **Figure 1**. The nerve supply of pleura is by all the intercostal nerves.

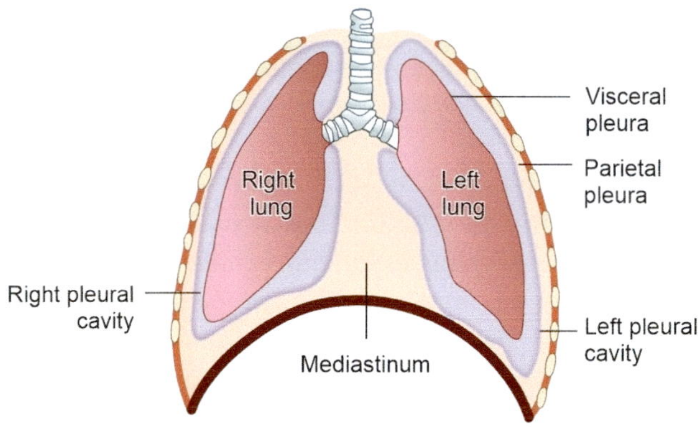

Fig. 1: Anatomy of pleural cavity.

PATHOPHYSIOLOGY OF PAIN

The etiology of pain is due to the friction between both the layers of pleura, and in pathological conditions, even normal breathing causes pain. This is a peculiar situation for a patient; that is, if he breathes normally, it causes pain and the intensity of pain increases if he tries to take a deep breath. This holding of breath for fear of pain may lead to CO_2 retention and hypoxia. There is retrograde diffusion of local anesthetic back toward intercostal nerves.

INDICATIONS

- Chest wall tumor[2]
- Herpes zoster postherpetic neuralgia
- Carcinoma of lung, lower end of esophagus, gallbladder
- Multiple rib fractures
- Post-thoracotomy[3] or cholecystectomy pain.

CONTRAINDICATIONS

Absolute

- Unwilling or uncooperative patient
- History of allergy to local anesthetic or contrast
- Skin infection.

Relative

- Patient with respiratory or cardiac compromise
- Immunosuppression
- Emphysema

- Bullous lung disease
- Recent pulmonary infection or empyema
- Pleural adhesions or pleurodesis
- Hemothorax
- Coagulopathy
- Contralateral phrenic nerve paralysis.

EQUIPMENTS

- Monitoring and resuscitation facility, C-arm fluoroscopy
- *Epidural set:* 16G Tuohy needle, catheter, and filter
- Luer lock syringes and needles for skin infiltration.

MEDICATIONS

- *Local anesthetic:* Inject lignocaine 2% (Xylocard, preservative-free), bupivacaine, ropivacaine
- *Dye:* Inject Iohexol (Omnipaque), a nonionic and water-soluble contrast
- *Agents for pleurodesis:* Inject phenol[4] in glycerin 6–10% or inject tetracycline

Another agent can be used:

- Opioids[5]
- Pethidine
- Clonidine.[6]

PREPROCEDURE VISIT PROTOCOL

- Obtain a written informed consent
- *Investigations:* Complete blood count, bleeding time, clotting time, human immunodeficiency virus (HIV), hepatitis C (HCV), hepatitis B surface antigen (HbsAg)
- Secure an intravenous line.
- Monitoring of vital signs
- A suitable antibiotic cover.

PROCEDURE DETAILS

The author always prefers an anesthetist to stand by and monitoring of vital signs and intravenous (IV) antibiotic.

Step 1: Keep the patient in sitting position with the arm rested on Mayo's trolley. After preparation of the site with suitable antiseptic solution, identify 8th, 9th, and 10th intercostal spaces and outline the surfacing marking of 8th, 9th, and 10th intercostal spaces as shown in **Figure 2**.

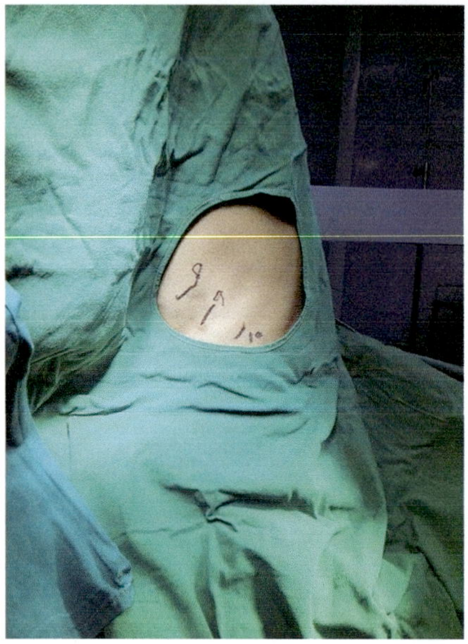

Fig. 2: Sitting position of patient with surface marking of 8th, 9th, and 10th intercostal space.

Step 2: Now inject xylocaine 2–3 cc in the 10th intercostal space at the midaxillary line **(Fig. 3)**.

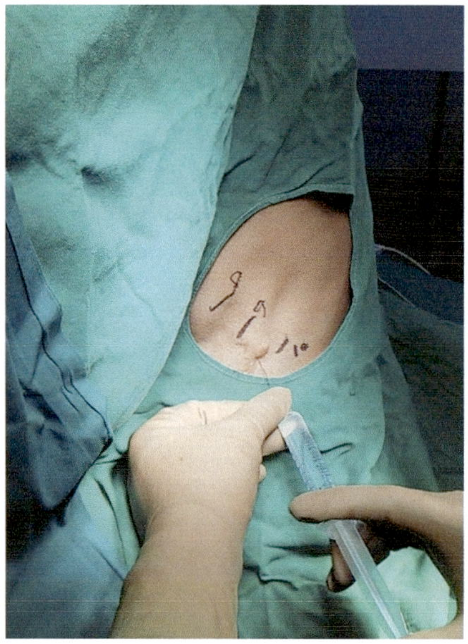

Fig. 3: Injecting local anesthesia into the space.

Step 3: Gently advance 16G Tuohy for about half a centimeter into the 10th intercostal spaces and put few drops of normal saline at the hub of needle for hanging drop technique. Now slowly advance Tuohy needle further; as the needle enters the interpleural space, the drop gets sucked in due to negative pressure **(Fig. 4)**.

Step 4: After repeated negative aspiration, inject nonionic, water-soluble dye Omnipaque 3–5 cc and confirm the spread of the dye under fluoroscopy **(Fig. 5)**.

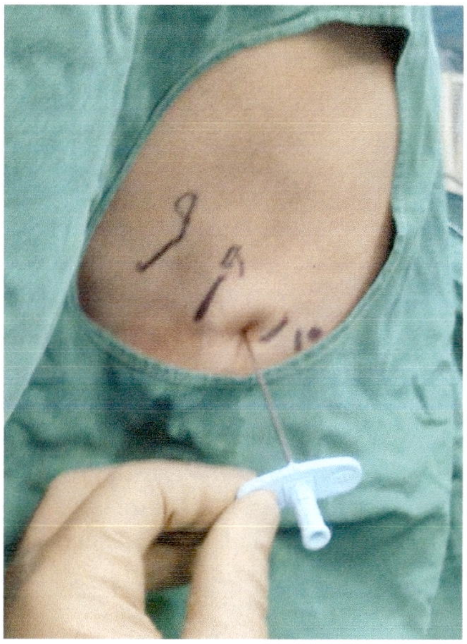

Fig. 4: Tuohy needle in 10th intercostal space.

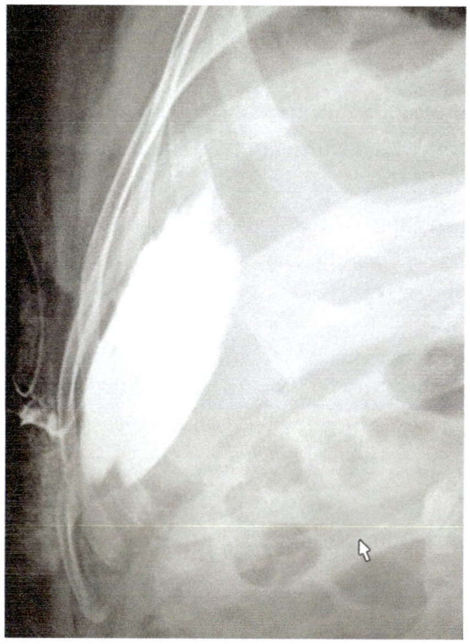

Fig. 6: Tunneled epidural catheter in intrapleural space.

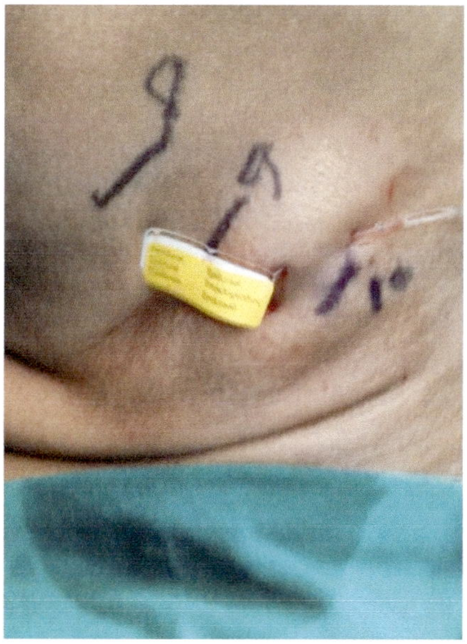

Fig. 5: Dye in interpleural space.

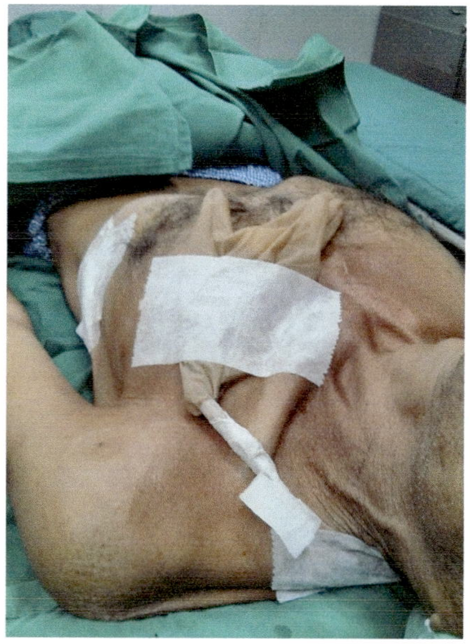

Fig. 7: Final dressing.

Now, inject 3–5 cc of Xylocard (preservative-free xylocaine) into the intrapleural space for pain relief.

Step 5: Gently introduce an epidural catheter via an epidural needle about 3–5 cm into the pleural space. Again, inject 2–3 cc Omnipaque into the epidural catheter and confirm the spread of dye under fluoroscopy in both anterior–posterior and lateral views.

Step 6: Under local anesthesia, tunnel the catheter under skin and fix as shown in **Figure 6**.

Step 7: Now, fix the catheter with Tegaderm or Micropore and tape it to the chest wall as shown in **Figure 7**.

Step 8: Tetracycline 8–10 cc is injected through the epidural catheter slowly followed by flushing of the epidural catheter with injection of bupivacaine 0.25% 1–2 cc.

Step 9: Shift to recovery area and monitor the vital parameters for 2–3 hours.

Complications

- Pneumothorax
- Allergic reaction to local anesthesia
- Possible toxic reactions of drugs, due to proximity to blood vessels
- Infection.

CONCLUSION

Intrapleural block is a simple, safe, and effective interventional pain treatment procedure for chronic pain patients for post cholecystectomy, thoracotomy, and renal and breast surgery. IPB is also used for relief of nonsurgical pain such as multiple rib fractures, herpes zoster, complex regional pain syndrome, and carcinoma lung. Pleurodesis caused by neurolytic or other drugs prevents brushing or rubbing of parietal and visceral pleura, and results in pain relief. The author has mainly used tetracycline for pleurodesis which resulted in pain relief. However, use of opioid, phenol, and clonidine is reported in literature.

REFERENCES

1. Baheti DK, Bakshi S, Gehdoo RP, Gupta S. Intrapleural Block: Interventional Pain Management: A Practical Approach. New Delhi: Jaypee Brothers Medical Publisher; 2010. pp.130-6.
2. David RM, Paur RE. Interpleural block: part 2. Anaesthesia, 2007;62:1143-53.
3. Bachman-Mennenga B, Biscoping J, Kuhn DF, Schürg R, Ryan B, Erkens U, et al. Intercostal nerve block, interpleural analgesia, thoracic epidural block or systemic opioid application for pain relief after thoracotomy? Eur J Cardiothorac Surg. 1993;7:12-8.
4. Lema MJ, Myers DP, De Leon-Casasola O, Penetrante R. Pleural phenol therapy for the treatment of chronic oesophageal cancer pain. Reg Anesth. 1992;17:166-70.
5. Welte M, Haimerl E, Groh J, Briegel J, Sunder-Plassmann L, Herz A, et al. Effect of interpleural morphine on postoperative pain and pulmonary function after thoracotomy. Br J Anaesth. 1992;69:637-9.
6. Canver C, Pilli G. The use of intrapleural clonidine for postoperative pain control. J Cardiovasc Surg (Torino). 1996;37:183-5.

23 CHAPTER

T2/T3 Sympathetic Block

Prakash Deshmukh

ABSTRACT

This research chapter delves into the T2/T3 sympathetic block, an intricate procedure for managing pain that targets the sympathetic nervous system. The chapter initiates with an examination of the technique, elucidating the utilization of anesthetics like 2% lidocaine for infiltration and 0.75% ropivacaine with Triamcinolone to establish the block. The procedure, guided by real-time C-arm fluoroscopy for visualization, entails precise needle insertion between the T2 and T3 vertebrae, meticulously avoiding potential complications such as pneumothorax. Neurolysis, accomplished through the administration of contrast, local anesthetic, and absolute alcohol, aims to offer prolonged pain relief. The chapter underscores a comprehensive approach, encompassing anesthetic administration, fluoroscopy-guided needle insertion, and postprocedure assessments to ensure both effectiveness and patient safety. The findings contribute valuable insights into the T2/T3 sympathetic block, laying groundwork for further advancements in pain management strategies.

INTRODUCTION

The sympathetic nervous system has been connected to several pain syndromes, including neuropathic, vascular, and visceral pain. Considering this, efforts have been undertaken to pinpoint the role played by the sympathetic nervous system in transmitting pain by blocking local anesthetics. Neurolysis with chemicals or heat has been employed to provide long-term relief if analgesia is attained by inhibiting a local anesthetic. While pain physicians commonly use neurolysis and minimally invasive sympathetic blocks, there is little data to support their efficacy in producing analgesia. There are comparatively few anonymous, placebo-controlled trials compared to many published case reports and case series.[1,2] There will be a review of previous studies on sympathetic blocks and a synopsis of the most recent results for each sympathetic block. Regardless of when they were trained, the goal is to provide pain specialists with current knowledge that will enable them to treat patients effectively.

The sympathetic nervous system has been connected to several pain syndromes, including neuropathic, vascular, and visceral pain. Its role in other painful conditions, such as musculoskeletal pain and headaches, has been studied occasionally. Today, one common pain management technique is the local anesthetic suppression of the sympathetic ganglia to identify and treat sympathetically associated pain.[1,2] Once the first block has reduced pain, attempts have been made to produce lasting analgesia using chemical neurolysis and heat. According to the most recent version of the "Current Procedural Terminology (CPT)" coding book, the following sympathetic blocks have codes. Many pain practitioners believe that the sympathetic fibers found in the sphenopalatine ganglion, hypogastric plexus, and celiac plexus/splanchnic nerves are involved in the transmission of pain, even though they are not strictly sympathetic ganglia or nerves. All blocks lacking a specific designation for the ganglion impar are given the CPT number 64999, which falls under the category of "unspecified, other". Even though the CPT code book already includes codes for the previously mentioned sympathetic blocks, it also includes two codes expressly for neurolysis of sympathetic nerves. It raises the question of why the other sympathetic blocks do not have their neurolysis codes, even if they are used frequently.

The thoracic sympathetic block is a targeted intervention within the sympathetic autonomic nerve system (SANS) to alleviate pain. By selectively disrupting sympathetic pathways in the prevertebral and paravertebral regions, this procedure effectively reduces pain without compromising somatic sensory awareness.[3] It is particularly useful for treating ischemia-related pain and can directly alleviate nociceptive pain transmission from internal organs. However, careful consideration is essential to prevent an imbalance in the homeostatic regulation, which may lead to physiological implications associated with parasympathetic predominance. Like complex regional pain syndrome (CRPS) or "sympathetically mediated pain", the SANS can pathologically worsen and become a major source of pain.[4] Ischemia pain, or pain generated by the sympathetic nervous system, can be effectively treated during intervention by blocking certain sympathetic pathways. Because of their structural differences from somatic nerves, most big sympathetic ganglia and plexi in prevertebral and paravertebral regions are easily accessible for percutaneous disruption. When utilized properly, sympathetic blocks can effectively reduce pain without impairing somatic sensory awareness.[5-8] However, if visceral sympathetic outflow is decreased, the target region's homeostatic balance will shift in favor of parasympathetic predominance, with associated physiological implications.[9-13]

INDICATIONS

Sympathetic blocks are versatile interventions employed for diagnostic, therapeutic, and prognostic purposes across various medical conditions. They are particularly considered when traditional treatments for persistent pain prove ineffective.

Pain which has failed to respond to conservative measures as in:

- CRPS 1 (old name, reflex sympathetic dystrophy) and CRPS 2 (old name, causalgia)
- Acute herpes zoster (HZ) or postherpetic neuralgia (PHN) involving head, face, neck, or upper arm
- Neuropathic pain in neoplastic encroachment of the brachial plexus
- Poor lymphatic drainage and local edema of the upper extremity following mastectomy or lymphedema
- Neuropathic pain as in Bell's palsy or patients who have undergone trigeminal ganglion radiofrequency (RF) ablation
- Post amputation or phantom limb pain (PLP) in upper extremity
- Vascular disorders such as Raynaud's disease or phenomenon, vasculitis, scleroderma, traumatic or embolic occlusion, accidental intra-arterial injection of α-adrenergic drugs (e.g., thiopentone) casing vasospasm
- *Miscellaneous:* Refractory angina, hyperhidrosis, Meniere's disease, frost bite, quinidine poisoning, certain types of cardiac arrhythmias.

Complex Regional Pain Syndrome

- CRPS presents a perplexing and painful clinical scenario, often emerging in the extremities following a traumatic event.
- The syndrome is stratified into two types based on the presence or absence of nerve injury, impacting the upper limb most frequently.
- Although the prevalence of CRPS may exhibit variability based on social and ethnic factors, middle-aged women appear to be more susceptible to its development.[14-18] As the predominant feature, pain is accompanied by a diverse clinical picture involving sensory, motor, autonomic, and trophic domains.[19-26]

Postherpetic Neuralgia (Early)

- PHN emerges as the most prevalent long-term complication following the reactivation of the varicella-zoster virus (VZV), also known as human herpesvirus-3 (HHV-3).
- This reactivation, termed herpes zoster or shingles, occurs when the dormant VZV, responsible for childhood chickenpox, becomes active.
- Before widespread vaccination in the late 1990s and early 2000s, up to 90% of American adults tested seropositive for VZV.
- Although this percentage may decrease with vaccinations, PHN remains clinically significant. PHN is characterized by lancinating/burning pain persisting for 3 or more months in a unilateral dermatomal pattern after the onset of HZ.[27-30]

Postradiation Arteritis

Postradiation arteritis is a constant problem for neuroradiologists and neuro-oncologists to discern between the effects of radiation therapy and the advancement of disease in the central nervous system. Common clinical signs and symptoms between the two entities may appear later in the disease or shortly after starting treatment. They are distinguished by a magnetic resonance imaging (MRI) by a higher contrast enhancement. Changes in imaging or clinical decline associated with radiation may be misinterpreted as an indication of an escalating disease, necessitating needless surgery or altering a patient's otherwise effective treatment regimen. Similarly, a potentially ineffective medication may be continued in the face of a worsening illness when the course of the disease is mistaken with the efficacy of the treatment.

Neuropathic Pain Associated with Central Nervous System Pathology

The term "neuropathic pain" describes discomfort resulting from anomalies in the nervous system. Neuropathic pain can be caused by nerve compression, diabetes, autoimmune illnesses, zoster infections, herpes simplex infections, trauma, and "channelopathies". Advances in pharmaceutical methods and animal models have led to more research on the underlying mechanisms. Neuropathic pain reflects both peripheral and central sensitization pathways. Anomalies may result from both intact nociceptors and damaged axons sharing the innervation zone of the injured nerve:[2,3]

- Widespread and unexplainable suffering
- Burning pain
- Skin sensitivity to mild touches
- Attacks of pain without provocation.[12-16]

Paget Disease

- Paget disease, a skeletal growth disorder, can lead to abnormal bone growth, causing widespread musculoskeletal discomfort.
- Characterized by elevated osteoblastic and osteoclastic activity, it is the second most common metabolic bone disease in the elderly. In severe cases, Paget's illness may result in pagetic sarcoma, a potentially fatal cancer.[31-35]

Phantom Limb Pain

There were 1.6 million (or 1 in 190) survivors of limb loss in the United States in 2005. The same study projects a startling rise in cases to 3.6 million by 2050. Reports that are available to the public show that between 60 and 85% of amputees have PLP.[29-31] Clinically, we consider the primary causes as listed below:

- French military surgeon Ambroise Pare (1510–1590) first documented the phantom limb phenomenon in the sixteenth century.
- The pathophysiology of this complicated phenomenon can be explained by several processes despite the lack of a comprehensive explanation. Theories are based on these mechanisms, which are not always mutually exclusive.
- The most prevalent vascular etiologies; trauma, cancer, or other malignancies; congenital disabilities.

Angina Pectoris

- Medical therapy can aid in the management of symptoms as well as slowing the progression of atherosclerosis and the risk of cardiac events. Antianginal medications can be used to classify angina symptoms according to how well they relieve them. Often, myocardial oxygen consumption is decreased to alleviate symptoms.
- Heart rate is the primary cause of most angina attacks since it is the primary measure of oxygen consumption.[36-42]
- Reduced symptoms, protection against myocardial damage, and a decrease in morbidity and mortality rates are the objectives of treating unstable angina.

CONTRAINDICATIONS

Sympathetic blocks are medical interventions considered for various conditions, yet their application requires careful evaluation of contraindications.

Absolute

- Patient refusal
- Local infection or sepsis
- Allergic reaction to local anesthetic drug
- Primary and secondary coagulopathy.

Relative

- Recent myocardial infarction or a severe cardiac conduction defect
- Glaucoma
- Contralateral pneumonectomy or pneumothorax.

APPLIED ANATOMY

The central sympathetic nuclei, housed in the intermediolateral nucleus of the lateral gray column of the spinal cord, have a geographic range spanning from T1 to L2-L3 levels. The axons emerging from these nuclei evolve into white rami shortly after the ventral ramus separates from the spinal nerve. Crucially, the paravertebral or prevertebral ganglia, specifically associated with T1-T4, receive these myelinated white rami. This intricate arrangement forms the sympathetic trunk, which aligns along the thoracic spinal column.

At the coccygeal level, approximately 20–24 paired ganglionic nodes join forces to establish the ultimate unpaired node of the sympathetic chain. This distinctive anatomy is particularly relevant to T1-T4, outlining the specific boundaries of the sympathetic and somatic nervous systems within this thoracic region. This precision in anatomy allows for targeted understanding and potential interventions related to the sympathetic nervous system in the T1-T4 segments of the spine.

In some situations, a stellate ganglion block (SGB) may be ineffective in diagnosing or treating sympathetically maintained pain in the upper extremity. The observation by Kuntz in 1927 that in 20% of people, nerves from the 2nd and 3rd thoracic sympathetic ganglia bypass the stellate ganglion and directly join the brachial plexus may explain the situation.[31] The nerves are appropriately called "Kuntz fibers". The sympathetic ganglion cell bodies that supply the upper limbs originate in the intermediolateral horn of the spinal cord from the T2 through T8 levels.[31] The preganglionic sympathetic fibers pass through the white rami communicantes and synapse with their postganglionic components primarily in the T2 ganglion. They also synapse in the T3, stellate, and middle cervical ganglia. Although many techniques existed for open, surgical sympathectomies, it was Wilkinson in 1979 who devised a percutaneous technique.[43]

TECHNIQUE AND TREATMENT

The T2/T3 sympathetic block is a meticulous procedure designed for effective pain management. The initial phase involves anesthetic administration, with 2% lidocaine utilized for infiltration, creating a localized numbness. Subsequently, a block is established using 0.75% ropivacaine, accompanied by the anti-inflammatory agent Triamcinolone to enhance therapeutic outcomes. The procedure unfolds under the guidance of a C-arm, a fluoroscopy device aiding real-time visualization **(Fig. 1)**.

Careful identification of thoracic vertebrae, specifically T1 to T4, is crucial. The skin is marked at corresponding spinous processes **(Figs. 2 and 3)**.

The C-arm is manipulated to an ipsilateral oblique angle of 20° until the spinous process reaches the opposite lateral vertebral border, optimizing visualization of the costovertebral junction during needle insertion **(Fig. 6)**.

The needle's entry point is strategically positioned between 3.5 and 3 cm to avoid pneumothorax. Local infiltration with a 30G hypodermic needle is performed at the junction of the transverse process and vertebral border approximately 3 cm from the midline **(Fig. 7)**.

Needle insertion is executed with a 23G 10 cm spinal needle featuring a curved tip **(Fig. 8)**.

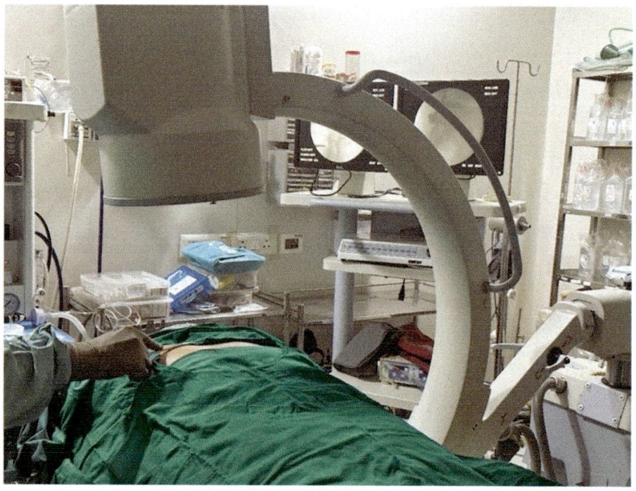

Fig. 1: Position of patient and fluoroscope and surgeon.

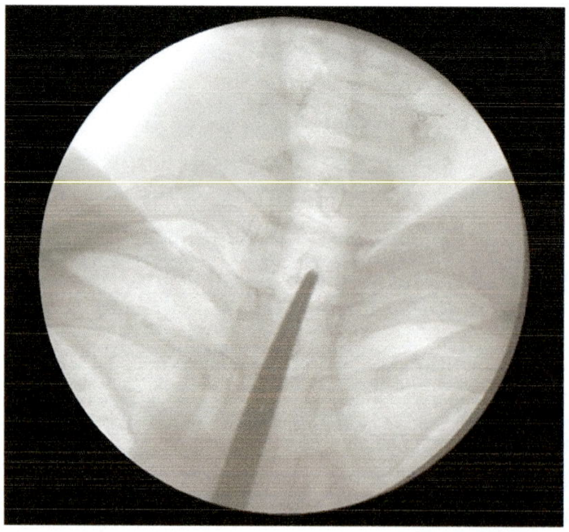

Fig. 2: Spinous process of T1.

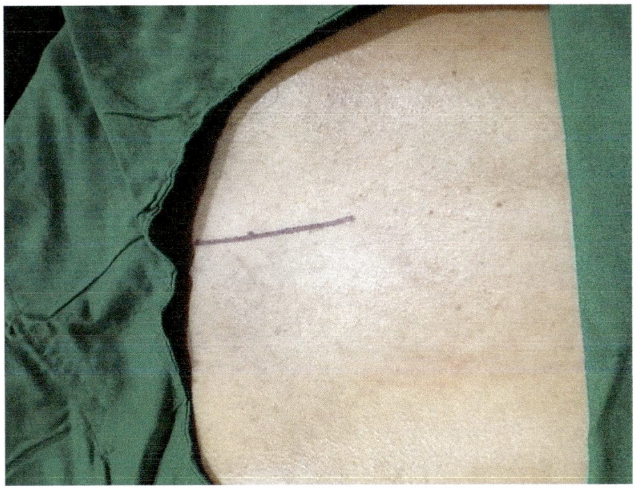

Fig. 3: A-line joint spinous process T1 to T4 and parallel lines are drawn at 2.5 and 4 cm.

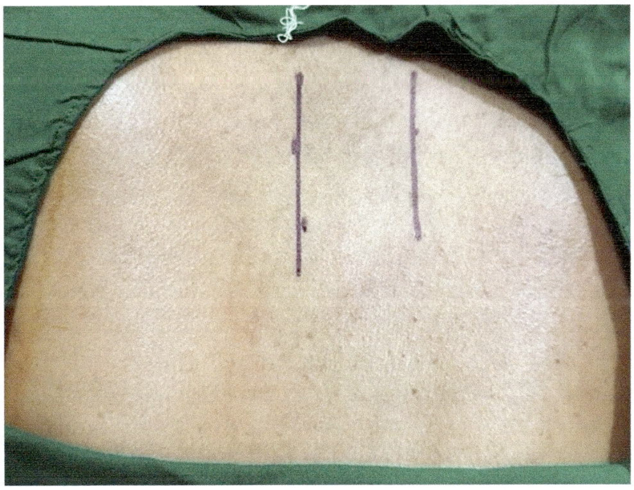

Fig. 4: Second line 4 cm to midline **(Figs. 4 and 5)**.

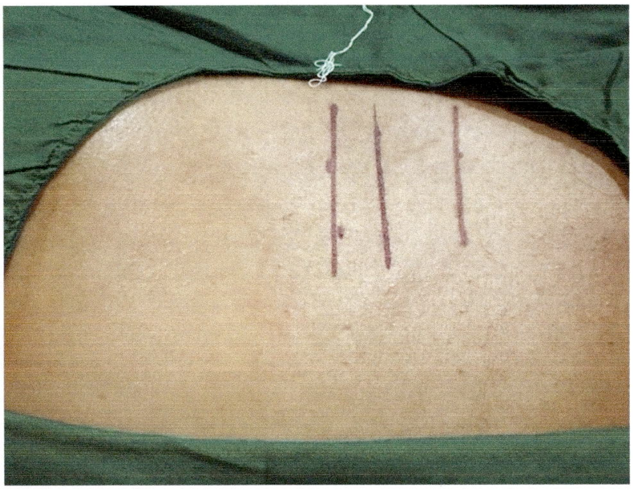

Fig. 5: Middle line 2.5 cm from the midline.

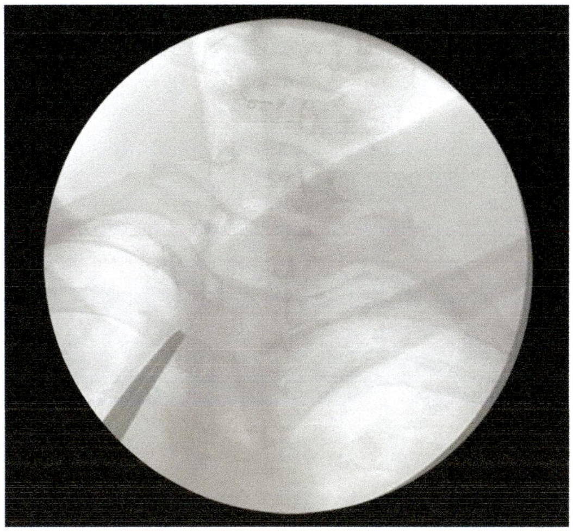

Fig. 6: C-arm made ipsilateral oblique till the spinous process reaches the opposite lateral vertebral border.

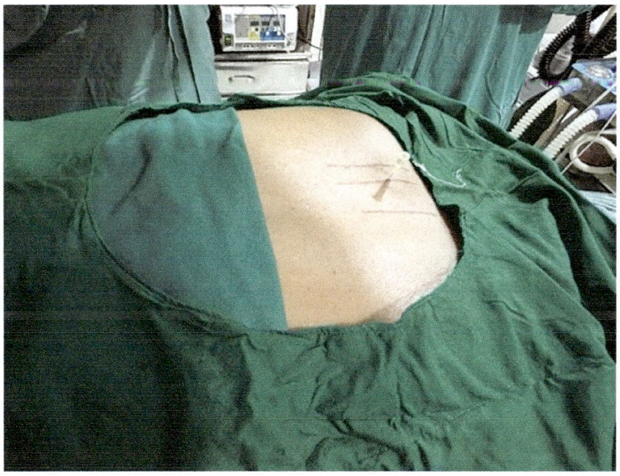

Fig. 7: Local infiltration with a 30G hypodermic needle at the junction of the transverse process and vertebral border approximately 3 cm from midline.

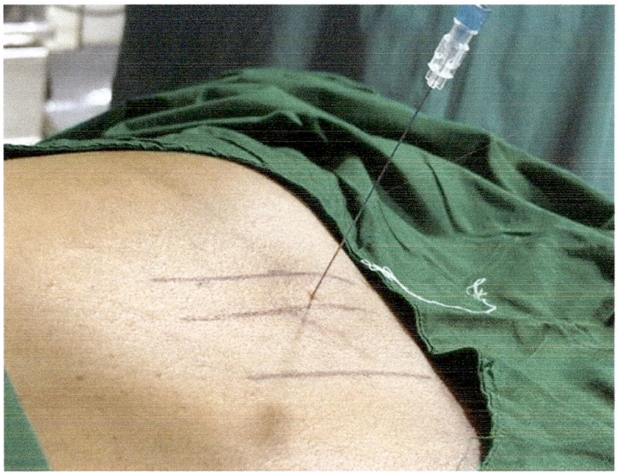

Fig. 8: Spinal needle at entry point.

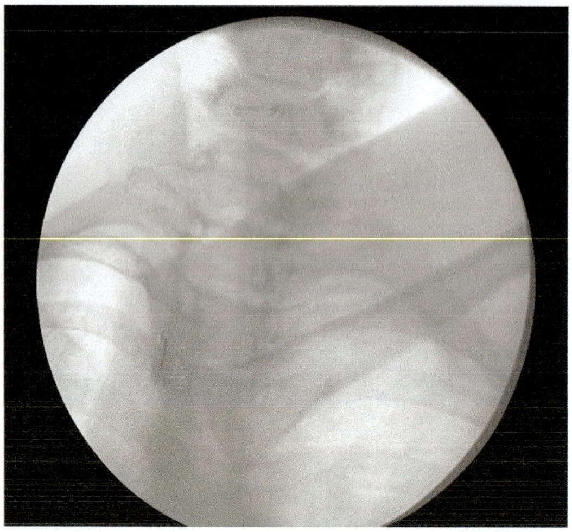

Fig. 9: Needle hugging the vertebral body.

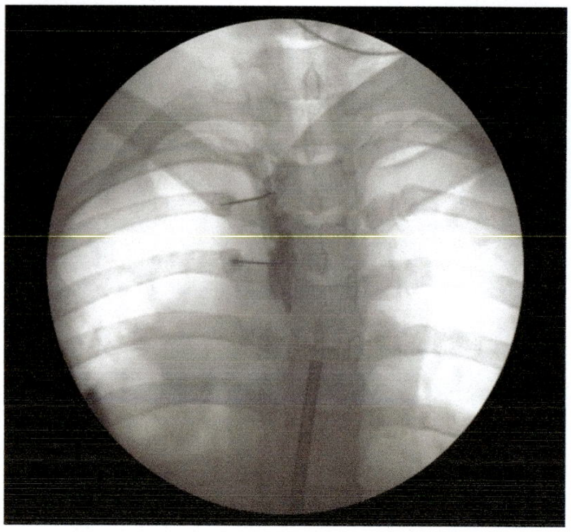

Fig. 11: Contrast in anteroposterior (AP) view.

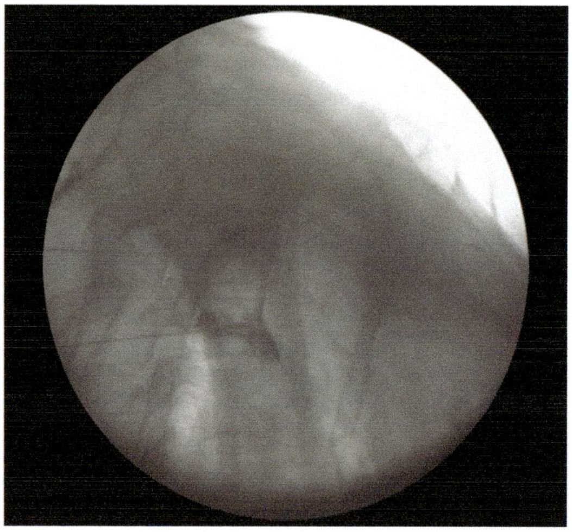

Fig. 10: Contrast in lateral view.

Commencing from the 3 cm mark, the needle is precisely guided to the point just above the head of the 3rd rib for T2 block **(Fig. 9)**.

As the needle advances, the C-arm is maneuvered to a lateral view to confirm crossing the foramen. The endpoint is the junction of the posterior 1/3rd and anterior 2/3rd in lateral view. In the anteroposterior (AP) view, the needle should hug the vertebral body closely.

Contrast is administered and visualized in both AP and lateral views to confirm proper placement and distribution **(Figs. 10 and 11)**.

For neurolysis, a combination of 1.5 mL contrast, 1.5 mL local anesthetic, and 3 mL absolute alcohol is administered, aiming to provide prolonged pain relief.

Postprocedure, the patient undergoes a chest X-ray to document the presence or absence of pneumothorax, a potential complication. Patients are informed in advance about the risk of pneumothorax and instructed to report immediately in case of respiratory distress, ensuring timely intervention in the event of complications.

In summary, the T2/T3 sympathetic block is a carefully orchestrated procedure, encompassing meticulous anesthetic administration, precise needle insertion guided by fluoroscopy, and a thorough postprocedure assessment. This multidimensional approach ensures the efficacy of pain management and the patient's safety throughout the intervention. Effective communication with patients about potential risks further enhances the procedural experience, fostering a collaborative and informed healthcare environment.

RADIOFREQUENCY TECHNIQUE

A 20G RF needle, 10 cm in length with a 1 cm active curved tip, was introduced (end-on) at the desired entry point, and then the C-arm was turned to the lateral view to check the needle depth; the final needle tip position was at the posterior third of the vertebral body shadow, just below the level of the pedicle, which is the common site of sympathetic ganglia sensory testing (at 50 Hz, up to 0.6 V). Motor test stimulation (at 2 Hz, up to 1.2 V) was performed to verify the location. If the patient experienced no dermatome-related sensation and had no intercostal muscle contractions, the needle positions were deemed satisfactory and at a safe distance from the thoracic nerve root.[22] Then 1 mL of radiopaque dye was injected to exclude an intravascular or intrapleural location **(Fig. 4)**. Finally, sympathetic denervation was accomplished by delivering the RF current for 120 seconds at 80°C. The needle hub was rotated 180° in a mediocaudal direction and another 120 seconds of RF current at 80°C was delivered.[44]

CONCLUSION

The T2/T3 sympathetic block, integral in pain management, demands precise coordination within the healthcare team. Effective communication and a closed-loop system are vital for success. Before the intervention, thorough communication about risks, benefits, and expectations is crucial, and obtaining documented informed consent is essential. A crucial step involves a timeout with the interprofessional team and the patient to confirm the accuracy of the procedure and anatomical location. For sedation, two timeouts are typically conducted. The block is commonly performed under direct visualization using fluoroscopy, ultrasound, or CT guidance for accuracy.

Healthcare providers must recognize potential complications promptly, establishing protocols and using pre-made supplies for efficient complication management. While new techniques emerge, evaluating their effectiveness is a gradual process. Providers assess whether a new approach suits the specific condition and patient anatomy, weighing potential advantages before incorporation. Continuous evaluation and adherence to best practices ensure the safety and success of T2/T3 sympathetic block procedures.

REFERENCES

1. Tsigos C, Chrousos GP. Hypothalamic-pituitary-adrenal axis, neuroendocrine factors and stress. J Psychosom Res. 2002;53(4):865-71.
2. Millan MJ. Descending control of pain. Prog Neurobiol. 2002;66(6):355-474.
3. Pongratz G, Straub RH. The sympathetic nervous response in inflammation. Arthritis Res Ther. 2014;16(6):504.
4. Chen SS, Zhang JM. Progress in sympathetically mediated pathological pain. J Anesth Perioper Med. 2015;2(4):216-25.
5. McCorry LK. Physiology of the autonomic nervous system. Am J Pharm Educ. 2007;71(4):78.
6. Blumberg H, Hoffmann U, Mohadjer M, Scheremet R. Sympathetic nervous system and pain: a clinical reappraisal. Behav Brain Sci. 1997;20(3):426-34; discussion 435-513.
7. Bussa M, Mascaro A, Cuffaro L, Rinaldi S. Adult complex regional pain syndrome type I: a narrative review. PM R. 2017;9:707-19.
8. Harden R, Bruehl S. Diagnostic criteria: the statistical derivation of the four criterion factors. In: Wilson PR, Stanton-Hicks M, Harden RN (Eds). CRPS: Current Diagnosis and Therapy. Seattle: IASP Press; 2005. pp. 45-58.
9. Harden RN, Bruehl SR. Diagnosis of complex regional pain syndrome: signs, symptoms, and new empirically derived diagnostic criteria. Clin J Pain. 2006;22:415-9.
10. Heineman TC, Cunningham A, Levin M. Understanding the immunology of Shingrix, a recombinant glycoprotein E adjuvanted herpes zoster vaccine. Curr Opin Immunol. 2019;59:42-8.
11. Watanabe D. [Cutaneous herpesvirus infection]. Brain Nerve. 2019;71(4):302-8.
12. Yu YH, Lin Y, Sun PJ. Segmental zoster abdominal paresis mimicking an abdominal hernia: a case report and literature review. Medicine (Baltimore). 2019;98(15):e15037.
13. Senderovich H, Grewal J, Mujtaba M. Herpes zoster vaccination efficacy in the long-term care facility population: a qualitative systematic review. Curr Med Res Opin. 2019;35(8):1451-62.
14. Warren-Gash C, Forbes HJ, Williamson E, Breuer J, Hayward AC, Mavrodaris A, et al. Human herpesvirus infections and dementia or mild cognitive impairment: a systematic review and meta-analysis. Sci Rep. 2019;9(1):4743.
15. Davis AR, Sheppard J. Herpes zoster ophthalmicus review and prevention. Eye Contact Lens. 2019;45(5):286-91.
16. Forstenpointner J, Rice AS, Finnerup NB, Baron R. Update on clinical management of postherpetic neuralgia and mechanism-based treatment: new options in therapy. J Infect Dis. 2018;218(Suppl 2):S120-6.
17. Lu WH, Lin CW, Wang CY, Chen LK, Hsiao FY. Epidemiology and long-term disease burden of herpes zoster and postherpetic neuralgia in Taiwan: a population-based, propensity score-matched cohort study. BMC Public Health. 2018;18(1):369.
18. Gabutti G, Valente N, Kuhdari P, Lupi S, Stefanati A. Prevention of herpes zoster and its complications: from the clinic to the real-life experience with the vaccine. J Med Microbiol. 2016;65(12):1363-9.
19. Zorzoli E, Pica F, Masetti G, Franco E, Volpi A, Gabutti G. Herpes zoster in frail elderly patients: prevalence, impact, management, and preventive strategies. Aging Clin Exp Res. 2018;30(7):693-702.
20. Schutzer-Weissmann J, Farquhar-Smith P. Post-herpetic neuralgia - a review of current management and future directions. Expert Opin Pharmacother. 2017;18(16): 1739-50.
21. Delaney A, Colvin LA, Fallon MT, Dalziel RG, Mitchell R, Fleetwood-Walker SM. Postherpetic neuralgia: from preclinical models to the clinic. Neurotherapeutics. 2009;6(4):630-7.
22. Hicks LD, Cook-Norris RH, Mendoza N, Madkan V, Arora A, Tyring SK. Family history as a risk factor for herpes zoster: a case-control study. Arch Dermatol. 2008;144(5):603-8.

23. Werner RN, Nikkels AF, Marinović B, Schäfer M, Czarnecka-Operacz M, Agius AM, et al. European consensus-based (S2k) Guideline on the Management of Herpes Zoster – guided by the European Dermatology Forum (EDF) in cooperation with the European Academy of Dermatology and Venereology (EADV), Part 1: Diagnosis. J Eur Acad Dermatol Venereol. 2017;31(1):9-19.
24. Koshy E, Mengting L, Kumar H, Jianbo W. Epidemiology, treatment and prevention of herpes zoster: a comprehensive review. Indian J Dermatol Venereol Leprol. 2018; 84(3):251-62.
25. Gilden D, Nagel MA, Mahalingam R, Mueller NH, Brazeau EA, Pugazhenthi S, et al. Clinical and molecular aspects of varicella zoster virus infection. Future Neurol. 2009;4(1):103-17.
26. Lawrence YR, Li XA, el Naqa I, Hahn CA, Marks LB, Merchant TE, et al. Radiation dose-volume effects in the brain. Int J Radiat Oncol Biol Phys. 2010;76(Suppl. 3):S20-7.
27. Freeman JE, Johnston PG, Voke JM. Somnolence after prophylactic cranial irradiation in children with acute lymphoblastic leukaemia. Br Med J. 1973;4(5891):523-5.
28. Sheline GE, Wara WM, Smith V. Therapeutic irradiation and brain injury. Int J Radiat Oncol Biol Phys. 1980;6(9):1215-28.
29. Brown MS, Stemmer SM, Simon JH, Stears JC, Jones RB, Cagnoni PJ, et al. White matter disease induced by high-dose chemotherapy: longitudinal study with MR imaging and proton spectroscopy. Am J Neuroradiol. 1998;19(2):217-21.
30. Lillemon JN, Nardos R, Kaul MP, Johnson AN, Choate A, Clark AL. Complex female pelvic pain: a case series from a multidisciplinary clinic in urogynecology and physiatry. Female Pelvic Med Reconstr Surg. 2019;25(2):e34-9.
31. Ralston SH, Corral-Gudino L, Cooper C, Francis RM, Fraser WD, Gennari L, et al. Diagnosis and management of Paget's disease of bone in adults: a clinical guideline. J Bone Miner Res. 2019;34(4):579-604.
32. McLaughlin MB, Awosika AO, Jialal I. Calcitonin. StatPearls [Internet]. Treasure Island (FL): StatPearls Publishing; 2023.
33. Mantovani G, Fagotti A, Franchi M, Scambia G, Garganese G. Reviewing vulvar Paget's disease molecular bases. Looking forward to personalized target therapies: a matter of CHANGE. Int J Gynecol Cancer. 2019:ijgc-2018-000080.
34. Choi YJ, Sohn YB, Chung YS. Updates on Paget's disease of bone. Endocrinol Metab (Seoul). 2022;37(5):732-43.
35. Gennari L, Rendina D, Merlotti D, Cavati G, Mingiano C, Cosso R, et al. Update on the pathogenesis and genetics of Paget's disease of bone. Front Cell Dev Biol. 2022;10: 932065.
36. Makaram NS, Ralston SH. Genetic determinants of Paget's disease of bone. Curr Osteoporos Rep. 2021;19(3):327-37.
37. Cuperus AA, Disco RT, Sligte IG, van der Kuil MN, Evers AW, van der Ham IJ. Memory-related perceptual illusions directly affect physical activity in humans. PLoS One. 2019;14(5):e0216988.
38. Wittkopf PG, Lloyd DM, Coe O, Yacoobali S, Billington J. The effect of interactive virtual reality on pain perception: a systematic review of clinical studies. Disabil Rehabil. 2020;42(26):3722-33.
39. He Y, Qiu D, Zhou D, Li L, Wang B, Wang L. Treatment of partial traumatic hemipelvectomy: a study of 21 cases. J Bone Joint Surg Am. 2019;101(9):e36.
40. Luza LP, Ferreira EG, Minsky RC, Pires GK, da Silva R. Psychosocial and physical adjustments and prosthesis satisfaction in amputees: a systematic review of observational studies. Disabil Rehabil Assist Technol. 2020;15(5):582-9.
41. Ephraim PL, Wegener ST, MacKenzie EJ, Dillingham TR, Pezzin LE. Phantom pain, residual limb pain, and back pain in amputees: results of a national survey. Arch Phys Med Rehabil. 2005;86(10):1910-9.
42. Balla C, Pavasini R, Ferrari R. Treatment of angina: where are we? Cardiology. 2018;140(1):52-67.
43. Wilkinson HA. Radiofrequency percutaneous upper-thoracic sympathectomy. Technique and review of indications. N Engl J Med. 1984;311:34-6.
44. Hetta DF, Mohamed AA, Hetta HF, Abd El-Hakeem EE, Boshra MM, El-Barody MM, et al. Radiofrequency thoracic sympathectomy for sympathetically maintained chronic post-mastectomy pain, a preliminary report: 6-month results. Pain Pract. 2021;21(1):54-63.

5 SECTION

Abdomen and Pelvis

24 CHAPTER

Celiac Plexus Block

Dwarkadas K Baheti

ABSTRACT

Many patients with upper abdominal cancer, i.e., pancreatic cancer, duodenal cancer, and stomach cancer with intractable pain prior to and after their diagnosis, chemotherapy, surgery, or radiation therapy, continue to experience pain. The pharmacological therapy is either not adequate to relieve the pain or the potential side effects affect the quality of life of the patient. A celiac plexus block (CPB) has been shown to benefit in reducing their pain and improving their quality of life. The CPB can be performed using proper preparation and various radiological techniques, such as fluoroscopy, transaortic, and transdiskal. The block can be achieved more precisely by using computed tomography (CT) guidance with an anterior approach to place the needle bilaterally at the celiac ganglion. In recent years, a sonographic technique has been used to perform a celiac plexus nerve block.

INTRODUCTION

One of the most satisfying procedures for relieving upper abdominal pain has received worldwide attention. The initial celiac plexus block (CPB), as recommended by Kappis in 1919, was performed using anatomical landmarks under fluoroscopy.[1,2] Moore has studied the spread of solutions following roentgenographic study and understanding the anatomical basis of CPB.[3] This technique continues to improve using various methods, including transaortic approach proposed by Ischia, anterior approach proposed by Liberman et al., and CPB during surgery proposed by Lillemore.[4] The technique was further modified by various authors, including Moore, Jain, and Brown.[5-7] The use of computed tomography (CT)-guided procedures has allowed physicians to visualize the precise location of tumors and determine the relationship with anatomical variation and variability of the location of the celiac axis as identified by the presence of the celiac artery and superior mesenteric artery.[6] Other techniques for performing a celiac block include the sonographic technique using ultrasound which has eliminated repeated exposure of radiation to the patient and the intradiskal approach proposed by a group in Japan.

INDICATIONS FOR CELIAC PLEXUS BLOCK

- *Upper abdominal malignancy:* Stomach cancer, pancreatic cancer, gallbladder cancer, duodenal cancer, distal esophageal malignancy, small bowel malignancy, proximal transverse colon, and ascending colon tumors
- *Retroperitoneal tumors:* Adrenal gland tumors and renal cell carcinoma
- Alcoholic pancreatitis
- Chronic pancreatitis
- Upper abdominal chronic pain of unknown origin.

CONTRAINDICATIONS

- Unwilling patient
- Bleeding disorders
- Local skin infection.

PREPARATION FOR CELIAC PLEXUS NERVE BLOCK

Prior to performing a celiac block, a thorough review of the patient's history and a physical examination must be performed. Recent laboratory work, scans, and chemotherapy or radiation therapy must be assessed.

A recent complete hematological profile, including complete blood count (CBC), prothrombin time (PT), partial thromboplastin time (PTT), and platelet count, must be reviewed. If a patient is receiving anticoagulant therapy, a hematologist must consult and review the patient's profile. Patients requiring an anticoagulant must be switched to a short-acting anticoagulant and discontinue it 12 hours prior to the procedure. A written informed consent must be obtained.

Once the procedure is planned, the patient is hydrated by the placement of an intravenous line. At least 750–1,000 mL of crystalloid fluid and balance salt solution is given in the past 8 hours. Prior to the procedure, the patient is encouraged to drink an adequate amount of fluids. If a patient has no contraindication for using contrast material, a baseline renal function, including blood urea nitrogen (BUN) creatinine, must be checked.

FLUOROSCOPICALLY GUIDED TECHNIQUE

This is the most common technique that is performed throughout the world.[5] This technique requires a fluoroscopic X-ray machine capable of providing anteroposterior (AP) and lateral views of the procedure. Once the patient is prepared following nothing by per oral route 6 hours prior to the procedure, the patient is placed on the fluoroscopic procedure table in a prone position. The American Society of Anesthesiologists (ASA) recommends all vital signs to be monitored and recorded, including pulse, blood pressure, oxygen saturation, and cardiac rate and rhythm.

Step 1: Following the placement of the patient on the fluoroscopic table, a pillow is placed under the abdomen to flex the thoracolumbar spine and the spine of L_1 vertebra. The surface marking includes, identifying of the inferior border of the12th rib on either side. A line is drawn approximately 6–7 cm from the midline of the L_1 spinous process and a second line is drawn to join both sides laterally to make a triangle as shown in **Figure 1**. The posterior part of the back from T_{10} to L_{4-5} level is prepared aseptically. Fenestrated drapes are placed in usual fashion.

Step 2: The second marker point at 6–7 cm from spine to the midline is anesthetized using 5 mL of 1% lidocaine bilaterally. Once the local anesthetic is effective, a 20–22 g 10–12 cm spinal needle is placed at the anesthetized point. The needle is directed toward the body of L_1 vertebrae. The tip of the needle should be moved slowly toward the anterior aspect of the L_1 vertebral body. The needle placement should be done similarly on the opposite site.

Step 3: The location of the tip of the needle must be confirmed in both the AP and the lateral views of the fluoroscopic images **(Figs. 2A and B)**. The needle tip is then confirmed for a negative aspiration of blood, lymph, and cerebrospinal fluid (CSF). Following a negative aspiration, a few cc of a water-soluble radiographic-contrast solution, i.e., Isovue or Omnipaque, should be injected to see the spread of contrast medication. Once the radiograph appears satisfactory in both the AP **(Fig. 3)** and the lateral views, 3–5 cc of a test dosage of 1% lidocaine should be given. If the patient feels no signs of the intravascular or intra-articular injection, then 15–20 mL of 50% absolute alcohol should be given at each injection site. To avoid unexpected spillage of a neurolytic agent on the skin, put a sponge around the needle.

In the past, a diagnostic nerve block was performed on patients who have advanced cancer, but it has been argued that there is no advantage of performing a diagnostic procedure on this type of patient population. Several factors are responsible for an ideal outcome of the procedure, including the size and type of tumor, primary versus secondary tumor, and how far the metastatic tumor has spread to the peritoneum and liver. The choice for neurolytic agents varies from center to center. Several authors recommend 50% alcohol as a safe and effective

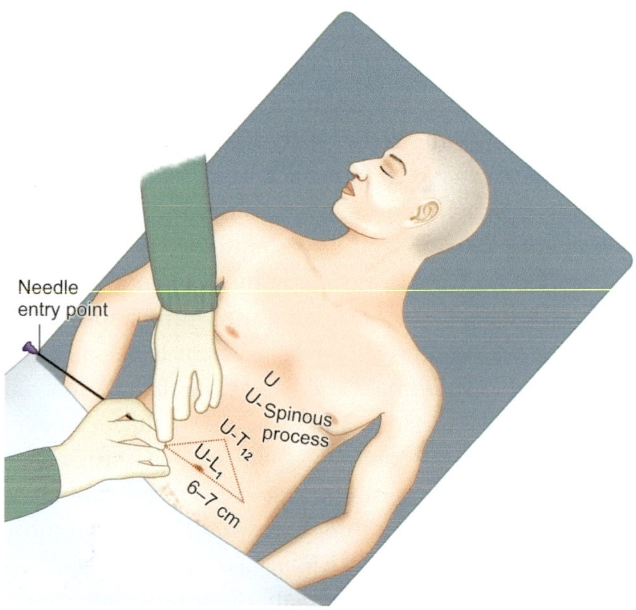

Fig. 1: Surface marking celiac plexus block (CPB).

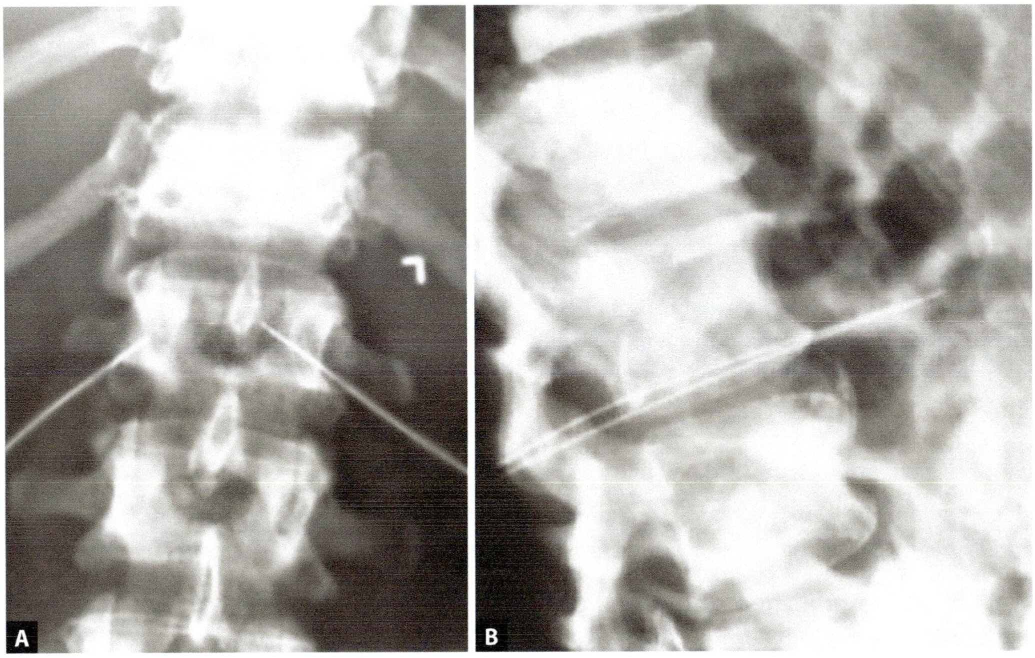

Figs. 2A and B: (A) Celiac plexus block (CPB) needle position in anteroposterior (AP) view; (B) CPB needle in lateral view.

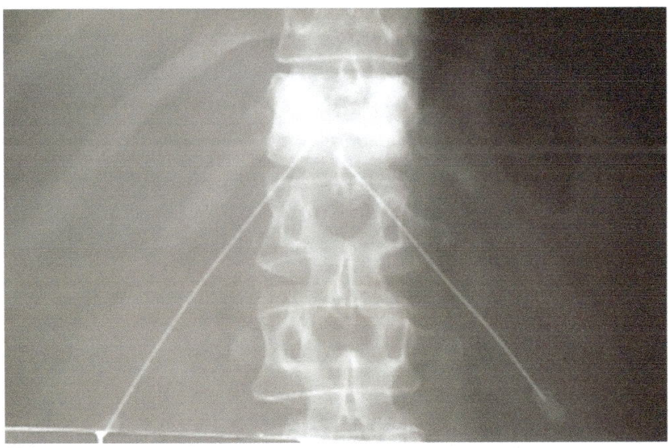

Fig. 3: Celiac plexus block (CPB) dye spread in anteroposterior (AP) view.

agent. The 6% phenol has been used if the cost of the agent and its availability become important factors. With phenol, an effective celiac plexus neurolysis can be performed using 5–6% of 8–10 mL of phenol at each site.

Moore and his coworkers have reported the spread of solution primarily by cephalad spread from the tip of the needle and only 3–5 cm caudally.[5] Singler reported that the spread is greater on the cephalic side, which has shown to provide pain relief.[8] In spite of performing this procedure successfully, the results are not predictable. The factors responsible for an unsuccessful block include the following—postoperative changes after previous surgical procedure, radiation therapy, and certain chemotherapeutic agents producing irregularities in the spread of neurolytic agents.

Computed-tomography-guided Celiac Plexus Block

Prior to performing a CT-guided CPB, recent scans of the patient must be taken and reviewed. The physician must view various anatomical organs in the scan. The size and location of tumor and the relationship to the celiac plexus must be reviewed. The tumor itself, surgery-related changes, or postradiation changes can distort normal anatomical locations of the celiac ganglion.

As we know, the celiac plexus is the largest ganglion of the sympathetic nervous system. Moore et al. have studied the location of the ganglion in the cadavers and reported various locations of the ganglion. As I mentioned earlier, tumor size, ascites, liver metastasis, and normal variation in human beings have a major impact on the injected solutions. The celiac ganglion varies in number, size, and location. There are two to five celiac ganglions, and the sizes could vary from 0.5 to 4.5 cm. The location of the left-sided ganglion is lower than the right-sided ganglion. The vertebral location varies between the body of L_1 and L_2 vertebrae. The left-sided ganglions are present in front of the aorta, while the right-sided ganglions are usually at the medial aspect of the inferior vena cava. The spread of the contrast media on the left is distributed in the front and lateral side of the aorta, and medial to the inferior vena cava on the right side. A butterfly-shaped spread is observed.

Computed-tomography-guided Technique

The patient is prepared similar to a fluoroscopic procedure. History, physical examinations, and anatomical location of the tumor type and size are reviewed. A hematological profile, including CBC, PT, PTT, bleeding time, and platelet count, is reviewed. Prior to starting the procedure, an intravenous line is secured to keep the patient hydrated; 700–800 mL of crystalloid solution, i.e., Ringer's lactate, is given to the patient.

Step 1: Once the patient is brought to the radiological CT suite, the patient is placed in a comfortable posture. A preliminary scout film from the lower border of the T_{10} vertebral body to the lower body of the L_4 lumbar vertebrae is marked. Initially, a 3 mm section is done, and a preliminary CT scan is also done, and various viscera and vessels are identified. The viscera include the liver, spleen, stomach, bilateral location of kidneys, and the extended lower part of the lungs that are also visualized. These structures and their extensions must be reviewed. If metastatic lesions are present, further evaluation needs to be done. A radiologist who has expertise in reviewing the CT scan must be consulted for entry points of both sides of the needles **(Fig. 4A)**. The vessels need very specific identifications, i.e., the aorta, inferior vena cava, superior mesenteric artery, renal, splanchnic vessels, adrenals, and celiac arteries. In most of the patients, the celiac ganglion lies just below the celiac artery between the celiac artery and the superior mesenteric artery.

Step 2: Following the identification of these structures, a 1–2 mm slice should be done just above and below the superior mesenteric artery. Using the cursor, one must select the path of the needle from the skin to the targeted area. This will allow you to know the angle and depth of the target location. The right side of the targeted tip of the needle must be at the medial aspect of the inferior vena cava, and on the left side of the needle the tip must be in front of the aorta **(Fig. 4B)**. Once the location of the needle tip is satisfactory, the needle with stylet (20–22G spinal needle) is withdrawn following a negative aspiration of blood, lymph and ascetic fluid, or urine. A few cc of water-soluble radiopaque dye, i.e., Isovue or Omnipaque, is injected slowly. The total volume of 5 mL is adequate on each side. This will allow to appreciate the distribution of contrast media at various structures **(Fig. 4C)**.

Once you are satisfied with the injection, a test dose of 3–4 mL of 1% lidocaine is injected on each site. This will allow you to observe any effect of the local anesthetic if it is intravascular. This will also help the patient to tolerate the neurolytic agent. The patient is given 20–25 mL of 50% absolute alcohol slowly. Vital signs are monitored every 3–5 minutes. Following the procedure, the patient will be placed in a supine position. Following a satisfactory hemodynamic monitoring of the patient, the patient will be transferred to a recovery area where they can be monitored and simultaneously be given oral fluids, etc. Patients can then be sent back to their bed if they are inpatient at a hospital or be discharged to go home.

Transaortic Technique

Ischia et al.[9] from Italy reported a new approach to perform a celiac plexus nerve block. The concept of this approach is under CT guidance using a single needle that can be placed on the left side at lumbar level L_1. The needle was pierced from the posterior aspect of the aorta to bring the tip of the needle anteriorly which is very close to the celiac plexus ganglion. Subsequently, Jain et al. performed and compared the advantages and the disadvantages of this technique. Initially, a single needle was ideal for bilateral use, and it was validated by the spread of radiographic solution on both sides of the ganglion. However, the factors that interfere with the spread of radiographic solution include distorted anatomy, postradiation changes, surgical clips in the celiac axis area, and organomegaly.

The transaortic approach requires a thorough preblock assessment of a recent CT scan. The location of tumors, periaortic nodes, and the position of the aorta in relation to the body of the vertebra must be reviewed. In our experience, >15% of cancer patients with various tumors or metastatic tumors had a disrupted anatomy. The landmarks and location of the celiac artery and the superior mesenteric artery must be reviewed. Routine physical examinations, and a recent hematological profile, including CBC, PT, PTT, bleeding time, and platelet count, must be reviewed. Prior to starting the procedure, an intravenous excess is secured to keep the patient hydrated; 700–800 cm^3 of crystalloid solution, i.e., Ringer's lactate, is given to the patient.

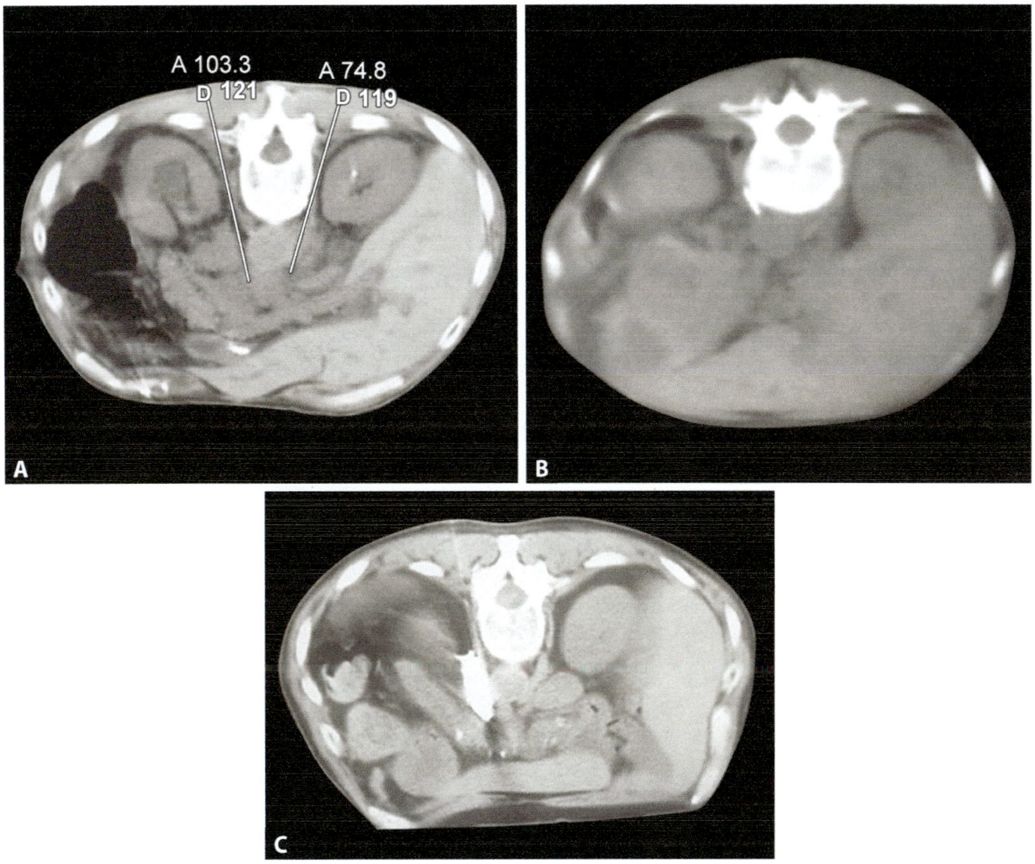

Figs. 4A to C: (A) Celiac plexus block (CPB) computed tomography (CT) entry point and depth of needle; (B) CPB CT needle position; (C) CPB CT dye spread.

The patient is placed in a prone position on the CT table. The patient's back at the lower thoracic region from T_{10} to the upper lumbar region up to L_3-L_4 level must be visualized. A scout film of the patient is taken to appreciate the bony landmarks and soft tissue. Then, the patient's spine from the lower thoracic region to L_1, L_2, and L_3 is identified, and a marker is placed at the level of vertebral body L_1. Initially, 5–10 mm CT cuts are done and reviewed. A marker is placed on the left side, and the path of the needle, including the angle and depth, is visualized on the CT scan. They are recorded and the patient is aseptically prepared. The patient is also attached to an ASA monitor in usual fashion. The surgical drapes are placed again at the needle's entry site and the angle of the needle is reassessed. At the point of entry, 4–5 mL of 1% lidocaine is injected locally to anesthetize the skin for needle placement using a 20–22G 7-inch spinal needle. A pillow is placed under the patient's abdomen to improve the spinal angle. The spinal needle is placed at the point of entry and pushed through slowly. The spinal needle is pushed in the direction of the aorta and gently toward the posterior aspect of the aorta. The needle will be pushed until arterial blood is aspirated. Following this, the needle is visualized until it has reached the anterior wall and then lies at least 0.5 cm in front of the aorta **(Fig. 5A)**. The needle tip is then confirmed for a negative aspiration of blood, lymph, and CSF. After the loss of resistance inject 3 mL of normal saline followed by 5–7 mL of injection Omnipaque and confirm the dye spread **(Fig. 5B)**. Again, multiple sections or cuts are done to the localized final position of the needle tip. For neurolysis of the celiac ganglion, 15–20 mL of 50% alcohol is given. During the procedure, the physician must be careful, for any possibility of disrupting calcified plaque in the aorta. Following the procedure, the patient is monitored for a few hours for any hemodynamic changes, and once cleared, the patient can be discharged to his/her room.

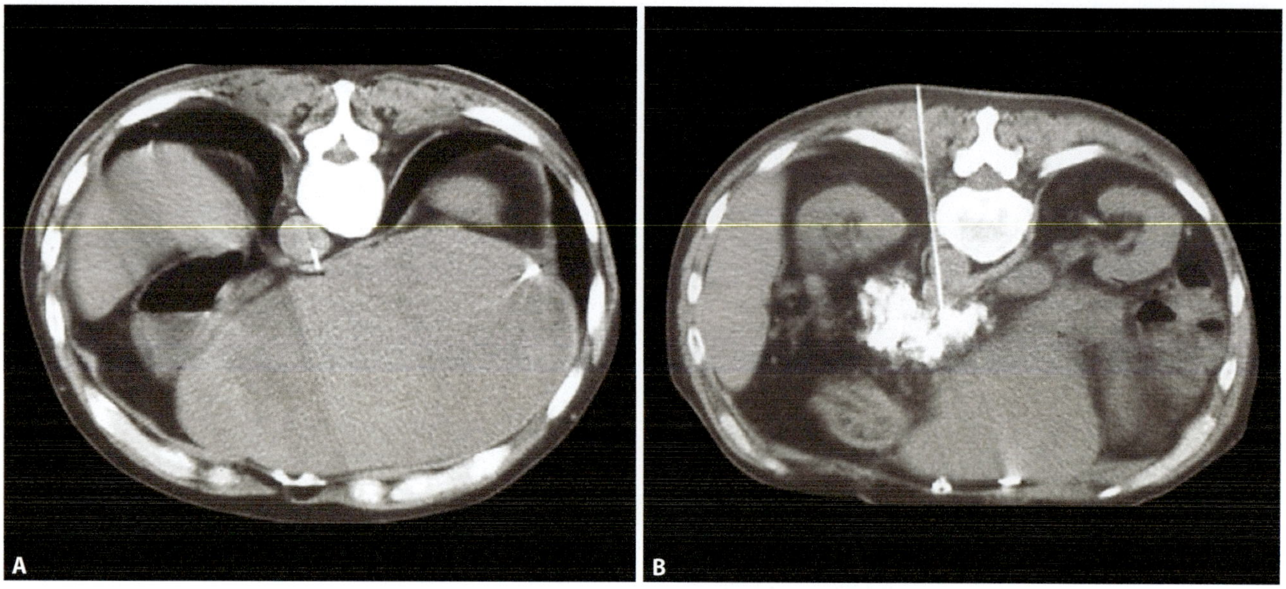

Figs. 5A and B: (A) Celiac plexus block (CPB) transaortic needle position; (B) CPB transaortic dye spread.

Celiac Plexus Block Using Single-needle Anterior Placement Technique

This anterior approach to achieve an effective block is used for the patient, who possibly has a distorted anatomy, distorted organs, and abdominal anasarca and is unable to lie in a prone position, or bilateral lungs are pushed down in the area where the block will be performed. Also, patients who have a surface ileostomy or colostomy would be appropriate candidates to have this procedure performed.

The patient's recent CT scan must be reviewed. A thorough physical examination and a recent hematological profile and coagulopathy must be assessed prior to the procedure. The patient is placed on a CT table and is attached to an ASA monitor. The patient is then placed in a supine position. A scout film is then taken and all the abdominal viscera, blood vessel, and the location of the tumor are assessed. As an extra precaution, the patient's bile ducts will be dilated prior to the drainage procedure, to prevent spillage of bile. A marker is placed close to the xiphoid point as a place of reference. On the CT scan, multiple images are taken from the lower border of the thoracic vertebrae to the upper portion of the lumbar vertebrae. Once the 5-mm scans are performed, they are reviewed and the following structures are identified—liver lobes, stomach, renal vessels, iliac vessel, superior mesenteric artery, kidneys, and abdominal aorta. Once the celiac artery and the superior mesenteric artery are identified, a marker is placed on the epigastric region where a path to reach below the celiac artery is visualized. The depth and distance are also measured. A 20–22G spinal needle is then placed from the skin to the targeted area. The needle is pushed in and the tip is identified in front of the anterior aspect of the aorta **(Fig. 6)**. Following a negative aspiration for blood, 2–3 mL of a water-soluble radiopaque contrast is injected. The distribution of

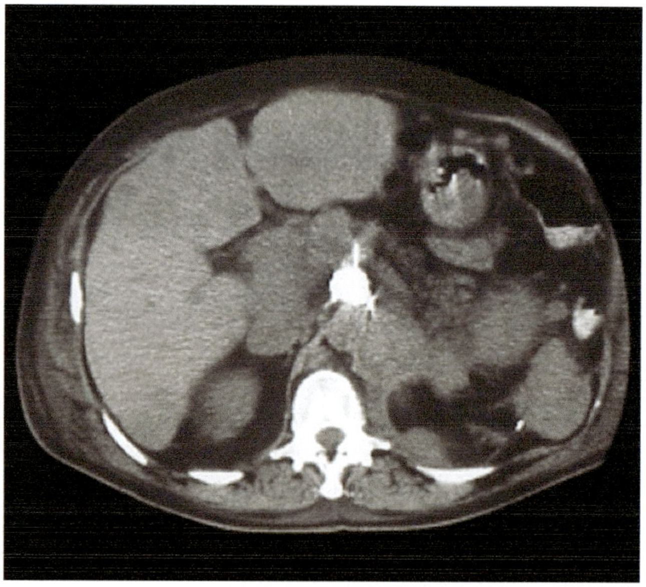

Fig. 6: Celiac plexus block computed tomography (CT) anterior approach.

the contrast media is assessed. Then a test dose of 1% lidocaine is injected to anesthetize prior to the injection of 50% absolute alcohol. A total of 15–25 mL of alcohol solution is injected. Following the injection, the patient is observed for a few hours. During the anterior approach, the best way to pierce the left lobe of the liver is to avoid the transverse colon.

Intra- or Transdiskal Technique

The CPB can be done via intra- or transdiskal approaches under either fluoroscopy or CT guidance.

Step 1: The standard position of the patient is to lie prone with a pillow under the iliac crests to increase the intradiskal space. The T_{12} and L_1 vertebrae are identified with C-arm rotated obliquely to the left at an angle of 15–20° and align the lower endplates in a cranial caudal projection.

Step 2: After draping and preparing, the needle entry point is 5–7 cm from the midline. The local anesthetic is injected, and needle is shifted by means of tunnel vision toward the inferior aspect of the facet joint. If an intervertebral disk is punctured, 0.5 mL contrast (Omnipaque) is injected to confirm needle position in the disk **(Fig. 7)**. Now the needle is advanced until there is a feeling of "loss of resistance"; this confirms that the needle is outside the Th_{12}/L_1 disk. After confirming the spread of contrast, inject 10 mL phenol in 10% sodium chloride (NaCl). At the end, inject 2–3 mL of saline to prevent leakage of the neurolytic solution into the disk.

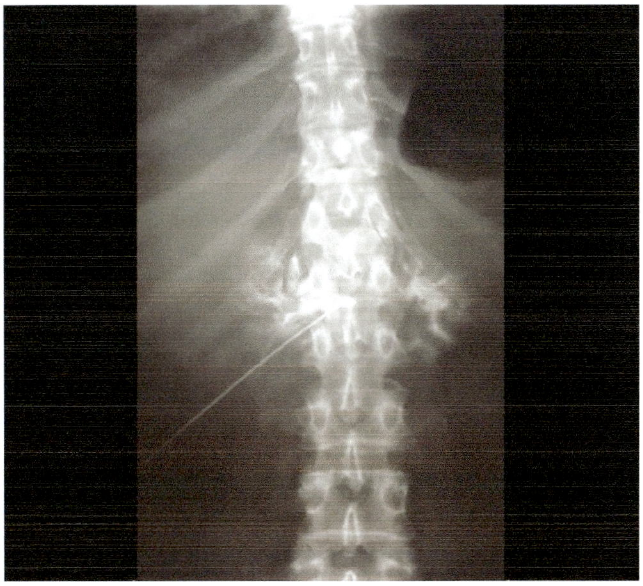

Fig. 7: Celiac plexus block transdiskal spread of contrast.

For diagnostic test blocks during retrocrural techniques, 2–15 mL lidocaine 1% or 0%, 25% ropivacaine is injected through both needles. During therapeutic blocks, after the injection of 10–16 mL local anesthetic, it is also advisable to inject 10–16 mL 96% ethyl alcohol or a 10% solution of phenol in Glycerin through both needles. Many researchers inject contrast dye simultaneously to check the spread of the medication. Before injecting the neurolytic solution, the area of the needles is covered by wet sterile gauze to prevent the neurolytic solution spreading into the adjacent structures. After the neurolytic solution has been injected, each needle should be flushed with normal saline to prevent pain in the track of the needle.

Ultrasound-guided Technique

In recent years, the ultrasound-guided celiac plexus has been performed using the anterior approach. The patient is placed in the supine position on the X-ray table. A patient's abdominal area from the xiphoid process to the midline of the umbilicus region is visualized using a low-frequency ultrasound transducer. The various structures, including the aorta, inferior vena cava, liver, stomach, and the vertebral body of L_1, are visualized. The celiac vessels are identified.

The aorta is identified by seeing the arterial pulsation on the left side. Using color-Doppler imaging can help in identifying the celiac axis. Once the location of the celiac axis is confirmed, by using a sonographic transducer, the transverse view both above and below the L_1 vertebra is visualized. The marker is placed a few millimeters below the celiac trunk area. The skin is anesthetized using a local anesthetic. A 20–22G needle is placed at a 90° angle and the tip is to be placed below the celiac axis area. The tip is reconfirmed and 1–2 cm^3 of lidocaine is injected. Following a negative aspiration, 15–20 mL of solution for neurolysis is injected. Tight pressure is placed at the point of entry. This technique is not indicated in a patient with coagulopathy, very low platelets, and abnormal PT and PTT.

SIDE EFFECTS AND COMPLICATIONS OF THE CELIAC PLEXUS BLOCK

Immediate Complications

- Hypotension
- Diarrhea
- Intravascular injection

- Intra-arterial injection
- Sedation
- Dural puncture
- Epidural
- Unilateral paresis, paraplegia
- *Puncture to viscera:*
    - Lung and pleura, i.e., pneumothorax
    - Kidney
    - Spleen
    - Transient hematuria
    - Injury to ureters
    - Renal pelvis injury
    - Chylothorax
    - Injury to somatic nerve roots
    - Seizure
- *Vascular injury:*
    - Bleeding, hematoma
    - Inferior vena cava
    - Renal artery
    - Splenic artery
    - Aortic subintimal injury
    - Aortic injury
    - Injury to artery of Adamkiewicz (nutrient artery of spinal cord).

Delayed Complications

- Paresis
- Paraplegia
- Hemiplegia
- Prolong diarrhea
- Orthostatic hypotension
- Alcoholic neuritis
- Neurogenic
- Lumbar plexus injury.

CONCLUSION

Neurolytic CPB is the best option in a multimodal approach for chronic upper abdominal pain of any cause. The advent of fluoroscopy, CT, and ultrasound along with the various approaches, such as posterior, transaortic, and transdiskal, has made a pain physician's life easy and provides safety for chronic pain patients.

REFERENCES

1. Kappis M. Die ansthesierung des nervus splanchnicus. Zentralbl. 1918;45:709.
2. Kappis M. Erfahrungen mit lokalansthesia bei bauch-operationen. Verh Dtsch Ges Circ. 1914;43:87-9.
3. Moore DC. Regional Block: A Handbook for Use in the Clinical Practice of Medicine and Surgery, 4th edition. Springfield, IL, USA: Charles C. Thomas; 1978.
4. Lieberman RP, Waldman SD. Celiac plexus neurolysis with the modified transaortic approach. Radiology. 1990; 175(1):274-6.
5. Moore DC, Bush WH, Scurlock JE. Intercostal nerve block: a roentgenographic anatomic study of technique and absorption in humans. Anesth Analg. 1980;59(11): 815-25.
6. Jain S. The role of celiac plexus block in intractable upper abdominal pain. In: Racz GB (Ed). Techniques of Neurolysis. Boston, USA: Kluwer Academic; 1989. pp. 161-70.
7. Brown DL, Moore DC. The use of neurolytic celiac plexus block for pancreatic cancer: anatomy and technique. J Pain Symptom Manage. 1988;3(4):206-9.
8. Singler RC. An improved technique for alcohol neurolysis of the celiac plexus. Anesthesiology. 1982;56(2): 137-41.
9. Ischia S, Luzzani A, Ischia A, Faggion S. A new approach to the neurolytic block of the celiac plexus: the transaortic technique. Pain. 1983;16(4):333-41.

25 CHAPTER

Splanchnic Nerve Block

Dhruv Bibra, GP Dureja

ABSTRACT

Splanchnic nerve block stands out as a highly effective and relatively straightforward interventional procedure designed to manage moderate-to-severe pain associated primarily with malignancies affecting various abdominal organs. These include the lower esophagus, liver, biliary system, stomach, pancreas, kidneys, adrenals, and the small intestine extending up to the right transverse colon. Notably, it serves as a valuable recourse for patients who have not achieved adequate pain relief through conventional means or in cases where celiac plexus block has proven ineffective.

Originating from the thoracic sympathetic trunk ganglia 5–12, splanchnic nerves traverse the crura of the diaphragm at the T11 and T12 levels to join the celiac ganglion, making them prime targets for neurolysis. This procedure can be conducted under various imaging modalities such as fluoroscopy, computed tomography (CT), magnetic resonance imaging (MRI), or ultrasonography, each offering unique advantages in terms of visualization and precision. The primary objective remains consistent across these techniques—to precisely place the needle along the anterolateral border of the T12 vertebra, retrocrurally, ensuring optimal delivery of therapeutic agents.

While the traditional approach involves fluoroscopy-guided posterolateral needle placement, the advent of CT guidance has revolutionized procedural accuracy by providing a comprehensive three-dimensional perspective. This facilitates meticulous planning to circumvent vital structures, achieve precise needle positioning, and visualize the spread of therapeutic agents effectively. Splanchnic nerve block may involve the administration of local anesthetic agents for diagnostic purposes, neurolytic agents such as alcohol or phenol, or the application of radiofrequency ablation.

Diagnostic blocks typically precede neurolytic procedures to ascertain efficacy and safety. Splanchnic nerve block has demonstrated equianalgesic efficacy compared to celiac plexus block, accompanied by reductions in opioid consumption, improvements in overall quality of life, and enhanced patient satisfaction. However, it is essential to note that postprocedural complications such as diarrhea and hypotension are common occurrences, necessitating vigilant monitoring and appropriate management strategies.

INTRODUCTION

The advancement in cancer diagnosis and therapeutic options has significantly prolonged the lifespan of patients.[1] However, pain management for these individuals remains a challenge. Thus, adopting a multidisciplinary approach is advocated, incorporating both interventional treatments like neurolysis [utilizing alcohol, phenol, or radiofrequency (RF)] and pharmacotherapy.[2] Neurolysis disrupts pain signals along neural pathways, offering relief, particularly to patients unresponsive to pharmacotherapy or experiencing medication-related side effects.[3]

Sympathetic blocks have been integral to acute and chronic pain management, especially in cancer patients, for nearly a century.[4] Although their precise mechanism is complex, they play a crucial role in alleviating cancer-related pain. Various sympathetic blocks, including stellate ganglion, celiac, splanchnic, superior hypogastric, and ganglion impar sympatholysis, have been employed for cancer pain management. For instance, the celiac plexus block is commonly administered to patients with pancreatic, gastric, or biliary cancer experiencing severe abdominal pain.[5]

Splanchnic nerve block emerges as a straightforward and repeatable interventional technique for moderate-to-severe pain management arising from malignancies affecting various abdominal organs.[6] Its origins trace back to Max Kappis's introduction of splanchnic nerve block in 1914[7] for surgical anesthesia, followed by the pioneering neurolytic splanchnic nerve block by Jones et al. in 1957.[8] Contemporary techniques utilize radiological imaging guidance such as fluoroscopy or computed tomography (CT) for precise needle placement. This method has gained traction due to enhanced accuracy and efficacy, particularly for patients unresponsive to celiac plexus block.[9]

Splanchnic nerves, originating from the thoracic sympathetic trunk ganglia, innervate abdominal structures and contribute to the formation of the celiac plexus. Early consideration of neurolytic blocks in cancer treatment aims to improve patients' quality of life and reduce reliance on opioids and nonsteroidal anti-inflammatory drugs (NSAIDs), thus potentially enhancing overall survival.

APPLIED ANATOMY[10,11]

The splanchnic nerves, comprising the greater (T5-T10 spinal roots), lesser (T10-T11), and least (T11-T12) pairs, play a crucial role in conveying preganglionic fibers to the celiac ganglia. These fibers exit the spinal cord through the ventral roots, join the white communicating rami of the sympathetic chain **(Fig. 1)**, and traverse the diaphragm to synapse on the celiac ganglia. Postganglionic fibers then follow the path of blood vessels, transmitting nociceptive signals from various abdominal organs, including the distal esophagus, stomach, duodenum, small intestine, ascending and proximal transverse colon, adrenal glands, pancreas, spleen, liver, and biliary system.

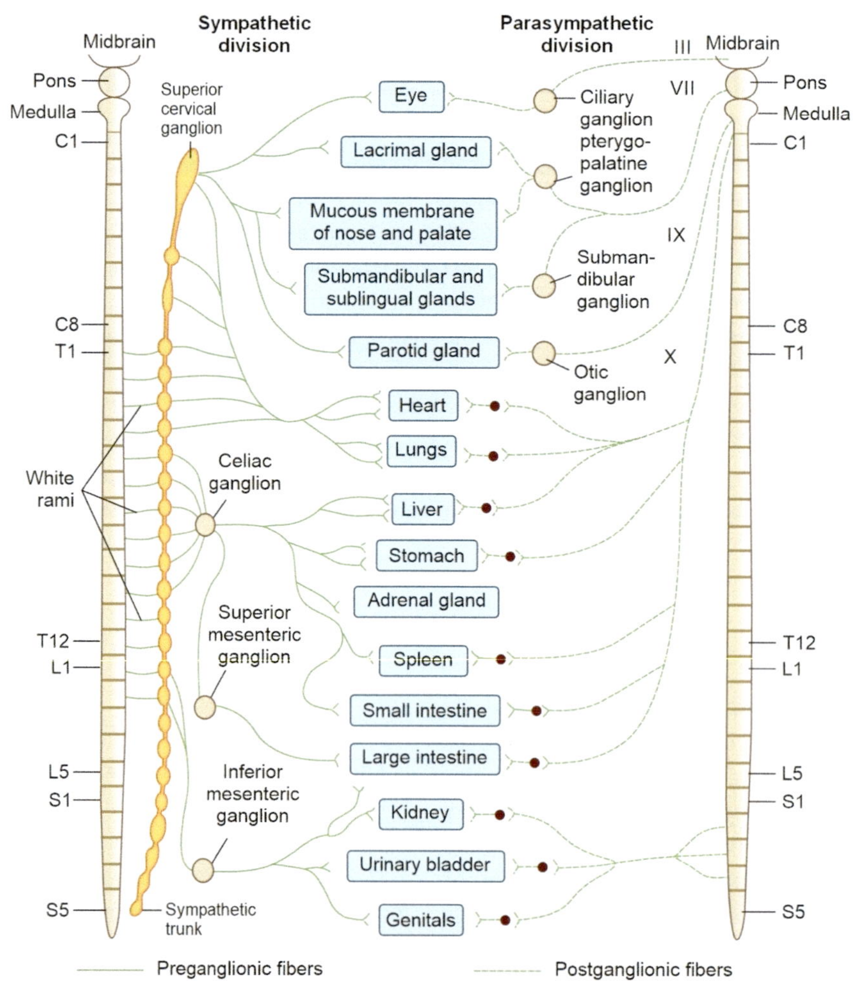

Fig. 1: Sympathetic system.
Source: Reprinted with permission from Ternopil State Medical University, Ukraine

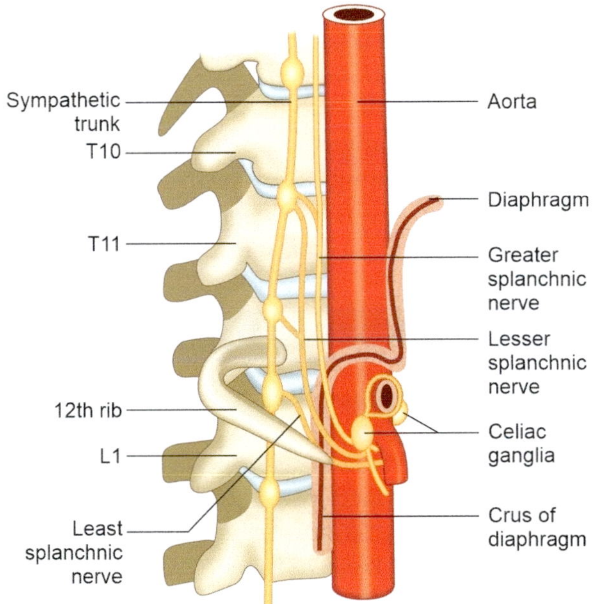

Fig. 2: Anatomic relations of splanchnic nerves.
Source: Reprinted with permission from http://bagherzadi.com. [Last accessed August, 2024].

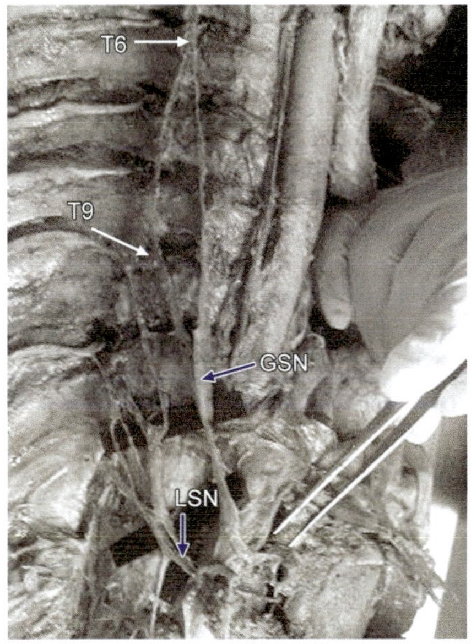

Fig. 3: Pattern of origin of greater splanchnic nerve from four ganglia (T6-T9). (GSN: greater splanchnic nerve; LSN: lesser splanchnic nerve)
Source: Reprinted with permission from Editor, International Journal of Anatomical Sciences[7]

Splanchnic nerves **(Figs. 2 and 3)** are situated within a confined space, bordered medially by the vertebral body, laterally by the pleura, ventrally by the posterior mediastinum, and dorsally by the pleural attachment to the vertebra. The crura of the diaphragm define the caudal boundary of this compartment. Studies, such as the one conducted by Swayam et al., have highlighted significant anatomical variability in the greater splanchnic nerve, with its origin observed to range from T4 to T11, most commonly arising from T6 to T9 ganglia.

Anatomical nuances and variations in the splanchnic nerves are essential considerations for interventional procedures targeting abdominal pain management, underscoring the importance of a comprehensive understanding of their applied anatomy.

TABLE 1: Indications and contraindications for splanchnic block.[12-14]

Indications	*Contraindications*
Severe abdominal pain refractory to pharmacotherapy	Coagulopathy or bleeding diathesis
Cancer-related abdominal pain	Local infection at the injection site
Pain due to intra-abdominal malignancies	Allergy to local anesthetics or contrast agents
Palliation of pain in pancreatic, gastric, or biliary cancer	Patient refusal or inability to cooperate
Relief of pain associated with abdominal visceral disorders	Unstable hemodynamic or severe cardiopulmonary compromise

PREPROCEDURAL PREPARATION FOR SPLANCHNIC NERVE BLOCK[15-17]

Indications and contraindications for splanchnic block depicted in **Table 1**.

- *Comprehensive patient assessment:*
  - Thoroughly review the patient's medical history, including any previous procedures and current medications.
  - Perform a focused physical examination, paying close attention to abdominal findings and assessing vital signs.
- *Informed consent process:*
  - Engage in a detailed discussion with the patient regarding the nature of the procedure, its potential risks, anticipated benefits, and available alternatives.
  - Provide ample opportunities for the patient to ask questions, express concerns, and ensure that they fully understand the procedure and its implications.
- *Laboratory investigations:*
  - Conduct a series of laboratory tests to evaluate the patient's baseline health status and assess for any

underlying medical conditions that may impact the procedure.

- Complete blood count (CBC) to screen for hematologic abnormalities
- Coagulation profile, including prothrombin time (PT), international normalized ratio (INR), and activated partial thromboplastin time (aPTT), to assess bleeding risk
- Renal function tests, such as serum creatinine and blood urea nitrogen (BUN), to ensure adequate renal function and clearance of contrast agents.

- *Medication management:*
  - Evaluate the patient's current medication regimen, with particular attention to anticoagulant or antiplatelet therapies.
  - Consider adjustments or temporary discontinuation of anticoagulation therapy, under the guidance of a healthcare provider, to minimize bleeding complications during the procedure.
- *Nil Per Os (NPO) status:*
  - Instruct the patient to refrain from eating or drinking for a specified period prior to the procedure, typically starting at midnight the night before, to reduce the risk of aspiration during sedation or anesthesia.
- *Hydration optimization:*
  - Encourage the patient to maintain adequate hydration in the hours leading up to the procedure to optimize intravascular volume and facilitate the clearance of contrast agents used during imaging guidance.
- *Patient education and counseling:*
  - Provide detailed instructions to the patient regarding preprocedural preparations, including fasting requirements, medication management, and any specific guidelines for postprocedure care.
  - Educate the patient about what to expect during the procedure, including potential sensations, the role of sedation or anesthesia, and strategies for managing anxiety or discomfort.
- *Premedication:*
  - *Sedation:* Mild sedation may be administered to alleviate anxiety. Commonly used agents include midazolam or fentanyl.
  - *Prophylactic antibiotics:* Administer prophylactic antibiotics if there is a significant risk of infection.
- *Review anatomy:* Review the patient's imaging studies to plan the needle trajectory.

CT-guided splanchnic nerve block: In the posterior approach utilizing two-needle techniques[22-24] **(Table 2 and Fig. 4)**, the patient is positioned in the prone position, and a screening CT scan of the T11-L1 area with a 2-mm slice thickness is obtained. The insertion point is marked using a laser on both sides, and the trajectory of

TABLE 2: Techniques.

Technique	***Description***	***Level of evidence***
CT-guided splanchnic nerve block[18]	Utilizes computed tomography (CT) imaging for precise visualization and needle guidance	II
Fluoroscopy-guided splanchnic nerve block[19]	Real-time fluoroscopic imaging guides needle placement for accurate nerve blockade	II
Ultrasound-guided splanchnic nerve block[20]	Employs ultrasound imaging for real-time visualization of anatomy and needle placement	II
MRI-guided splanchnic nerve block[21]	MRI provides precise visualization for needle guidance and injection	II

Note: Level II evidence indicates evidence obtained from well-designed cohort or case-control analytic studies, preferably from more than one center or research group.

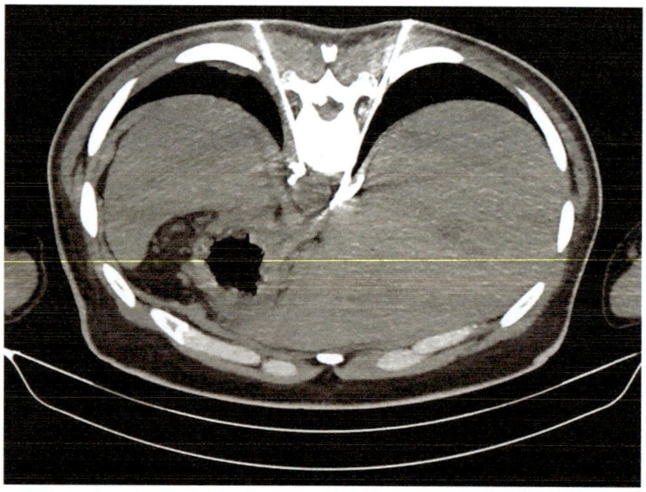

Fig. 4: Computed tomography image depicting splanchnic nerve block with posterior approach (two-needle technique). On the left side, dye spread is retrocrural, whereas on the right side dye spread is seen in both antecrural and retrocrural region.

the needle is estimated. Following skin preparation with an antiseptic solution and local anesthetic infiltration, a 20G, 15 cm needle with a stylet is inserted on each side. Confirmation of the needle tip placement is done in the retrocrural area above the level of the celiac artery. Subsequently, 2 mL of contrast dye is injected to observe the spread in the retrocrural area bilaterally. If the spread is observed in the antecrural space, the needle should be withdrawn.

For the anterior approach,[25-27] the patient is placed in the supine position, and a screening CT scan of the T11-L1 area with a 2-mm slice thickness is obtained. The insertion point is marked with the assistance of a laser, and the trajectory of the needle is estimated, taking care to avoid major organs and the periceliac mass. After skin preparation with an antiseptic solution and infiltration with local anesthesia, a 20G, 20 cm needle with a stylet is inserted. Confirmation of correct needle placement is achieved by injecting 2 mL of contrast dye to observe the spread in the retrocrural area bilaterally. If the spread is observed in the antecrural space or is unilateral, adjustments such as needle advancement or consideration of two-needle techniques may be necessary.

Fluoroscopy-guided splanchnic nerve block:[28,29] To perform a splanchnic nerve block, begin by identifying the T11 and T12 vertebral bodies with the 12th rib in a posteroanterior (PA) view. Using fluoroscopic C-arm, rotate it 5–10° obliquely toward the ipsilateral side and mark the entry site of the needle below the transverse process, along the pedicle **(Fig. 5)**. After preparing the injection site with antiseptic solution and infiltrating with 2% lignocaine, insert a 20G, 15 cm styleted needle directed medially toward the T12 vertebral body, avoiding the exiting nerve root. Establish a "tunnel" view of the needle, ensuring that it moves toward the target as a pinhead **(Fig. 6)**. Advance slowly in 0.5 cm thrusts under fluoroscopy guidance, feeling for the grating sensation along the lateral part of the T12 vertebral body. Confirm needle placement at the junction of the anterior one-third and posterior two-thirds of the vertebral body in lateral and PA views **(Figs. 7A and B)**. After negative aspiration, inject 1–2 mL of a nonionic water-soluble contrast agent to visualize a spread moving in a cephalocaudal direction along the anterolateral border of the T11 and T12 vertebrae before administering the desired drug. If the contrast fans out, it indicates pleural placement of the needle, requiring needle replacement.

Another technique involves viewing the T12-L1 vertebrae in the C-arm with the patient in the prone

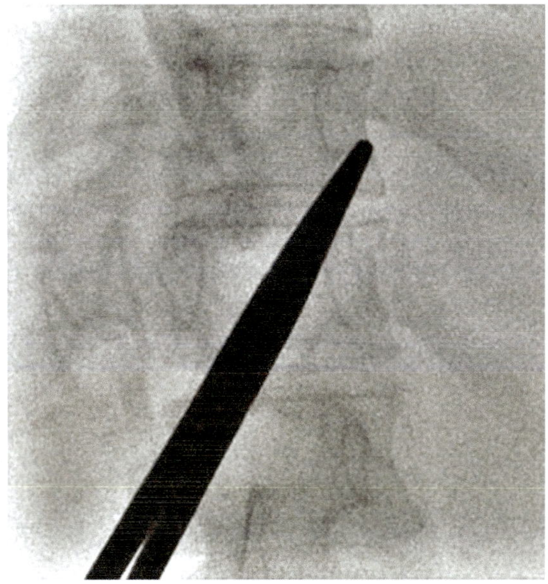

Fig. 5: Needle entry point below transverse process, along the pedicle.
Source: Reprinted with permission from Editor, Pain Physician Journal.[10]

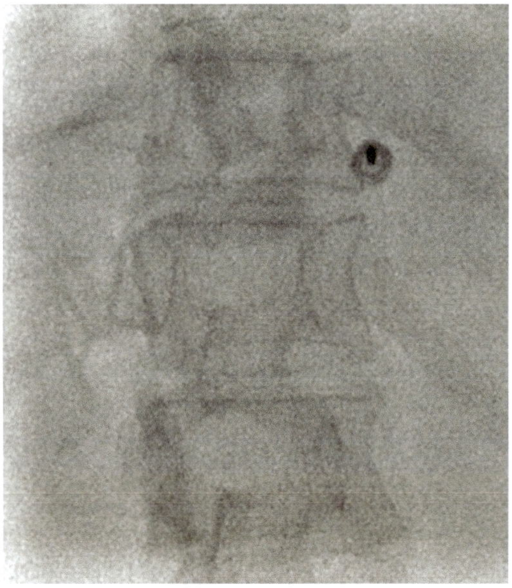

Fig. 6: Oblique fluoroscopic view: advancement of needle in tunnel view.
Source: Reprinted with permission from Editor, Pain Physician Journal.[10]

position. Mark a point 6 cm lateral to the spinous process of the L1 vertebra and infiltrate with 2% lignocaine. Insert a 20G, 15 cm long styleted needle from the entry point directed medially and cephalad toward the T12 vertebral body at an angle of 45–60°. Once bone contact is made, withdraw the needle and redirect it to walk off the lateral

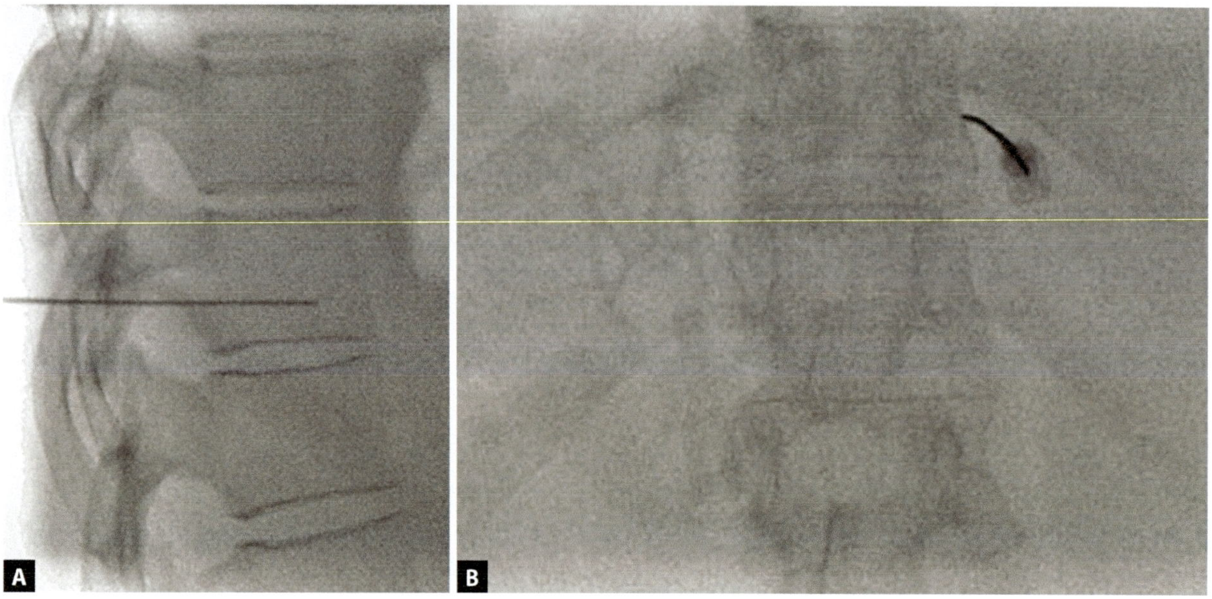

Figs. 7A and B: Confirming the needle placement in (A) lateral and (B) posteroanterior fluoroscopic views.
Source: Reprinted with permission from Editor, Pain Physician Journal.[10]

side of the T12 vertebral body, confirming its placement at the anterolateral part of the T12 vertebral body at the junction of the anterior one-third and posterior two-thirds. Use a contrast agent to visualize the spread as described above.

These techniques provide detailed steps for performing splanchnic nerve blocks, ensuring accurate needle placement and effective pain relief for patients with minimal risk of complications.

For RF ablation (RFA) of the splanchnic nerves,[30,31] needle placement follows a similar approach to that described earlier, with dye spread obtained in a corresponding pattern. After ensuring correct needle placement, an RF probe is applied to provide sensory stimulation at 50 Hz/1 V, eliciting an epigastric burning sensation. If intercostal paresthesia occurs, the needle is carefully advanced anteriorly. Motor stimulation at 2 Hz/3 V is performed to rule out any stimulation in the intercostal muscles. Once needle placement is confirmed, RF lesioning is conducted at 80°C for 90 seconds in the first cycle, followed by rotating the RF probe by 180° and providing the second cycle.

In the transdiskal technique, the patient is positioned prone with a pillow under the chest/abdomen to open the interdiskal space. Using fluoroscopy in a PA view, the T11-12 intervertebral disk is identified. The fluoroscope is then angled obliquely at 15–20° cephalocaudally to square the vertebrae. After cleaning, draping, and infiltrating with 2% lignocaine, a 20G, 15 cm styleted needle is inserted in a cephalocaudal direction, lateral to the inferior aspect of the facet joint, and advanced through the disk under lateral fluoroscopic view. Confirmation of needle placement outside the disk is achieved by injecting 1–2 mL of dye, followed by a diagnostic or neurolytic block. It is crucial to flush the needle with saline after performing a neurolytic block.

These techniques provide effective methods for performing RFA and transdiskal procedures for splanchnic nerve blocks, ensuring accurate needle placement and successful pain management for patients.

Ultrasound-guided splanchnic nerve block:[19,32] Ultrasound imaging provides real-time visualization of soft-tissue structures and vascular anatomy. Anatomical landmarks include the T12 vertebral body, aorta, superior mesenteric artery (SMA), and celiac artery. The transducer is placed longitudinally or transversely over the epigastric region to visualize the target structures. The celiac artery and aorta appear as hypoechoic structures, while the surrounding tissue exhibits echogenicity. The needle insertion point is identified lateral to the probe, guided by ultrasound imaging to ensure accurate placement adjacent to the celiac ganglia. Real-time ultrasound guidance allows for precise needle advancement and visualization of local anesthetic spread, enhancing the safety and efficacy of the procedure.

MRI-guided splanchnic nerve block:[33,34] MRI provides detailed soft-tissue visualization without ionizing radiation. Anatomical landmarks include the T12 vertebral body, aorta, SMA, and celiac artery. MRI sequences allow for precise localization of these structures in multiple planes. The needle insertion point is typically identified based on the relationship between the vertebral body and the target structures visualized on MRI images. The needle trajectory is guided by real-time MRI imaging to ensure accurate placement adjacent to the celiac ganglia. Injection of a neurolytic agent provides sustained pain relief by disrupting nociceptive signals transmitted via the splanchnic nerves.

Successful splanchnic neurolysis hinges on several critical factors, as underscored by the literature. Patient education emerges as a cornerstone, emphasizing that neurolysis is just one facet of a comprehensive treatment approach for cancer-related pain. It serves to diminish opioid requirements and mitigate associated side effects rather than entirely eradicating pain. Patients and their families must grasp that pain relief may not be absolute post procedure, necessitating the inclusion of psychotherapy and emotional support in pain management strategies.

The timing of neurolysis concerning the disease stage significantly influences its efficacy, with early intervention yielding superior and enduring pain control outcomes compared to late-stage procedures. Moreover, patients with shorter disease durations and lower opioid analgesic requirements tend to experience more comprehensive pain alleviation. Employing imaging guidance, particularly CT, during the procedure enhances precision and safety. Thorough preprocedural planning is imperative to delineate patient positioning, needle trajectory, site of neurolytic agent administration, and potential complications **(Table 3)**. Proper patient positioning ensures comfort and minimizes movement, facilitating the safest path to the splanchnic nerves. Notably, the extent of pain relief correlates with the degree of splanchnic nerve destruction.

When neurolysis fails to achieve pain relief, various factors merit consideration, including patient-related aspects (such as nonphysical pain components or hindered agent access due to disease), physician-related factors (e.g., diagnostic accuracy or procedural technique), and the neurolytic agent itself. Drugs for the block depicted in **Table 4**.

TABLE 3: Complications.[35,36]

Technique	*Complications*	*Nerves/Blood vessels at risk*
CT-guided splanchnic block	Hematoma	Aorta, inferior vena cava
	Pneumothorax	Pleura, lung tissue
	Infection	Surrounding tissues
	Neural injury	Splanchnic nerves, nearby nerves
Fluoroscopy-guided block	Retroperitoneal hemorrhage	Aorta, inferior vena cava
	Paralysis	Spinal nerves
	Inadvertent vascular injury	Renal arteries, other blood vessels
Ultrasound-guided block	Nerve injury	Splanchnic nerves, nearby nerves
	Postprocedural pain	Injection site
	Vascular puncture	Renal arteries, other blood vessels
MRI-guided block	Allergic reaction to contrast agent	Nearby blood vessels
	Contrast-induced nephropathy (CIN)	Renal arteries, other blood vessels

POSTPROCEDURAL CARE[43,44]

- *Immediate observation and monitoring:*
    - Patients should be closely monitored in a designated recovery area immediately after the procedure.
    - Vital signs, including blood pressure, heart rate, respiratory rate, and oxygen saturation, should be monitored regularly to detect any signs of distress or complications.
    - Assess the patient for immediate postprocedural pain relief or any adverse reactions, such as allergic reactions, bleeding, or neurologic deficits.
- *Pain management:*
    - Provide adequate pain management to alleviate discomfort at the injection site and any residual pain.
    - Nonopioid analgesics such as acetaminophen or NSAIDs may be prescribed to manage postprocedural pain.
    - Local anesthetics or ice packs applied to the injection site can help reduce swelling and discomfort.
- *Activity restrictions:*
    - Advise patients to avoid strenuous activities, heavy lifting, or driving for a specified period following the procedure.

TABLE 4: Drugs for the block.

Drug/technique	*Mechanism of action*	*Dosage and concentration*	*Level of recommendation*	*Advantages*	*Disadvantages*
Alcohol (ethanol)[37]	Alcohol causes neurolysis by denaturing proteins, cellular dehydration, and disruption of cellular membranes. This process leads to the destruction	*Concentration:* Typically, 50–100%	Level B	Effective neurolytic action	Potential for damage to surrounding structures
		Dosage: Varies based on patient and condition, often 10–20 mL per injection		Relatively simple procedure	Risk of alcohol leakage and spread to unintended areas
				Cost-effective	Potential for postprocedure pain and discomfort
Phenol[38]	Phenol induces neurolysis through protein coagulation, cellular degeneration, and disruption of nerve conduction. This results in the cessation of pain transmission along the affected nerves.	*Concentration:* Usually 5–10% for splanchnic nerve blocks	Level C	Effective neurolytic action	Potential for chemical neuritis and pain along the injection site
				Lower risk of systemic toxicity	Potential for inadvertent damage to adjacent structures
		Dosage: Varies based on patient and condition, often 5–10 mL per injection		Can be performed under imaging guidance	Risk of transient postprocedure hypotension
					Need for specialized equipment and expertise
Bupivacaine[39]	Bupivacaine is a local anesthetic that blocks nerve conduction by inhibiting sodium influx through cell membranes. This prevents the propagation of pain signals along the nerve fibers, leading to	*Concentration:* Usually 0.25–0.5% for splanchnic nerve blocks	Level C	Provides temporary pain relief	Limited duration of action
				Lower risk of systemic toxicity	Potential for local anesthetic toxicity
		Dosage: Varies based on patient and condition, often 10–20 mL per injection		Rapid onset of action	Risk of transient postprocedure hypotension
					Need for repeated injections to maintain pain relief

Contd...

Contd...

Drug/technique	***Mechanism of action***	***Dosage and concentration***	***Level of recommendation***	***Advantages***	***Disadvantages***
Lidocaine[40]	Lidocaine, another local anesthetic, exerts its action by blocking nerve conduction through inhibition of sodium influx. This blocks the transmission of pain signals along the nerves	*Concentration:* Usually 1–2% for splanchnic nerve blocks *Dosage:* Varies based on patient and condition, often 10–20 mL per injection	Level C	Rapid onset of action Lower risk of systemic toxicity Can be performed under imaging guidance	Limited duration of action Potential for local anesthetic toxicity Risk of transient postprocedure hypotension Need for repeated injections to maintain pain relief
Radiofrequency ablation[41]	Radiofrequency ablation uses heat generated by radiofrequency waves to disrupt nerve function and provide long-term pain relief. The heat generated by the probe damages the nerve tissue	*Temperature:* Typically, 60–80°C *Dosage:* Varies based on patient and condition, typically a single session	Level B	Provides long-term pain relief Minimally invasive procedure Reduced need for repeated procedures	Potential for thermal injury to adjacent structures Risk of transient postprocedure discomfort and pain Need for specialized equipment and expertise Potential for recurrence of pain in some cases
Coolief RFA[42]	Coolief RFA utilizes cooled radiofrequency energy to target and disrupt pain-transmitting nerves while minimizing the risk of tissue damage	*Temperature:* Typically, 45–55°C *Dosage:* Varies based on patient and condition	Level B	Provides long-term pain relief Reduced risk of tissue damage Minimally invasive procedure	Risk of thermal injury to adjacent structures Potential for transient postprocedure discomfort and pain Need for specialized equipment and expertise

  - Encourage gentle movements and walking to prevent stiffness and promote circulation without exacerbating pain.
- *Hydration and fluid intake:*
  - Ensure adequate hydration by encouraging the patient to drink plenty of fluids.
  - Hydration helps flush out contrast dye or residual neurolytic agents from the body and reduces the risk of dehydration, especially if the patient received intravenous sedation.
- *Follow-up appointment:*
  - Schedule a follow-up appointment within a specified timeframe to assess the patient's response to the procedure and monitor for any delayed complications.
  - Evaluate pain levels, functional status, and the need for additional interventions or adjustments to pain management strategies.
- *Patient education:*
  - Provide comprehensive postprocedural instructions to the patient and their caregivers, including:
    - Guidance on managing postprocedural pain and discomfort
    - Signs and symptoms of potential complications, such as infection, bleeding, or nerve injury, and when to seek medical attention
    - Medication instructions, including dosage, frequency, and potential side effects
    - Activity restrictions and gradual resumption of normal activities
- *Emotional support and counseling:*
  - Offer emotional support, reassurance, and counseling to address any anxiety, fear, or concerns the patient may have about the procedure, pain management, or recovery process.
  - Provide resources for psychological support or referral to a pain psychologist or counselor if needed.
- *Documentation:*
  - Thoroughly document the postprocedural care provided, including vital signs, pain assessment, medication administration, patient education, and any adverse events or complications encountered.
  - Document the patient's response to treatment and any changes in symptoms or functional status during follow-up visits.

DISCUSSIONS

There are various studies comparing imaging guidance for splanchnic nerve blocks but no large-sized randomized controlled trials. Each imaging modality has issues that need to be considered before selecting the modality of choice. Fluoroscopy and CT have associated radiation exposure, and transabdominal sonography has a learning curve. Additionally, the nonusage of radiocontrast dye associated with the procedure makes the results unpredictable. Though all three modalities have been used successfully for celiac plexus block, transabdominal sonography has not been described for splanchnic nerve block.

The classical splanchnic nerve block technique is a percutaneous posterior approach under fluoroscopy guidance. However, with the accessibility and availability of CT to the interventional pain physician, the anterior approach has gained popularity. The guiding landmarks differ with each radiological modality: T11/T12 vertebral body in fluoroscopy and celiac artery, crura of the diaphragm, and dye spread in the retrocrural region with CT guidance. The advantage of the CT-guided block is that it provides a three-dimensional view, which helps plan a convenient approach avoiding vital organs. Accurate needle position and dye spread can be seen in the retrocrural region, providing a theoretical edge to the technique. The advantage of the anterior approach is that the patient lies supine, a comfortable position, especially for patients with a colostomy bag in situ.

Disadvantages of using a CT suite for the pain procedure include higher radiation exposure and longer procedure times, which add to the cost. Although the evidence is limited for a head-to-head comparison of the two radiological techniques, the efficacy of splanchnic nerve block in pain relief, decreasing opioid consumption, and improving the quality of life of cancer patients is undisputed.

Keith et al.[45] found that intraoperative splanchnic neurolytic block not only provides pain relief and improves the quality of life but also significantly improves survival in patients with unresectable carcinoma of the pancreas who have preoperative pain. The effect of the block usually lasts around 4 months, and a percutaneous block can be repeated if needed.

A review of the literature comparing celiac and splanchnic neurolytic block shows conflicting reports. In a randomized controlled single-blind study, Özyalçın et al.[46] preferred fluoroscopic splanchnic nerve block over celiac plexus block due to equal efficacy in relieving pain and improving quality of life, with fewer complications such as severe pain at neurolysis, hypotension requiring inotropic treatment, and intractable diarrhea, which affected patient satisfaction and quality of life in the initial 2 weeks post neurolysis. Ischia et al.[47] compared fluoroscopic-guided transaortic celiac plexus blockade, retrocrural celiac plexus blockade, and bilateral splanchnic nerve blockade, finding all three techniques equally effective and carrying a low side-effect profile. Marra et al.[48] compared CT-guided neurolytic blocks, finding better results in terms of pain relief with the splanchnic block and suggesting its use as a rescue technique when inadequate dye spread is seen in the celiac plexus region under CT guidance.

It has been observed that splanchnic nerve block provides pain relief in patients where celiac plexus block has failed, likely because the celiac plexus region is invaded earlier by cancer. Although it is not possible to definitively state that splanchnic nerve block should be preferred over celiac plexus block, it can be used as a rescue option when celiac plexus block fails to provide pain relief. In their study, Cicco et al.[49] found that only complete dye spread in the celiac plexus block, observed in merely 8% (9/177) of patients, provided long-lasting analgesia.

Various newer techniques of neurolysis have been described apart from image-guided procedures, such as videoscopic splanchnicectomy. In one study, Stefaniak et al.[50] compared fluoroscopic-guided neurolytic celiac block with videoscopic splanchnic neurolysis, finding that the percutaneous block provided an equianalgesic effect and should be preferred over the more invasive procedure.

The efficacy and duration of pain relief by splanchnic nerve block are said to be equal to celiac neurolytic block. According to a meta-analysis, this provides pain relief with medication in about 70–80% of abdominal or pelvic cancer patients for >3 months or until death. Intraoperative splanchnic neurolysis should be considered, especially in patients with preoperative pain and unresectable tumor mass, as it significantly decreases postoperative opioid requirements and impacts the overall survival of the cancer patient.[51]

CONCLUSION

Pancreatic cancer poses a significant clinical challenge due to its aggressive nature and propensity to cause severe abdominal and/or back pain. Unfortunately, conventional analgesics and opioids often provide inadequate relief for these patients, impacting their quality of life substantially. Recognizing the crucial role of pain management within the realm of palliative care, particularly in conditions such as chronic pancreatitis and pancreatic malignancies, becomes paramount. In this context, thoracic splanchnic nerves emerge as pivotal conduits for transmitting nociceptive stimuli from the upper abdominal viscera. Comprising preganglionic fibers originating from the anterolateral horn of the spinal cord bilaterally, along with the T5-T12 ventral spinal roots, these nerves become targets for therapeutic interventions aimed at alleviating malignant abdominal pain.

Splanchnic nerve block assumes significance as a vital adjunct in managing such pain, demonstrating comparable efficacy to celiac plexus block. Notably, its utility becomes particularly pronounced in cases where the celiac axis presents challenges for drug dispersion. Under the guidance of experienced pain physicians and aided by imaging modalities such as fluoroscopy and CT, the procedure offers a lower incidence of serious side effects. The traditional technique for splanchnic nerve block involves a fluoroscopy-guided posterolateral approach, ensuring accurate needle placement and visualization of dye spread. However, the advent of CT guidance enhances procedural precision by providing a three-dimensional view, aiding in strategic planning to avoid vital structures and ensuring optimal needle positioning.

Despite the therapeutic benefits of splanchnic nerve block, postprocedural complications such as diarrhea and hypotension are common occurrences. However, with proper management strategies in place, these adverse events can be effectively addressed. Overall, the comprehensive understanding and technical proficiency in performing splanchnic nerve blocks serve as indispensable components in the multidisciplinary management of malignant abdominal pain, ultimately contributing to enhanced patient comfort and improved quality of life.

REFERENCES

1. Miller KD, Nogueira L, Mariotto AB, Rowland JH, Yabroff KR, Alfano CM, et al. Cancer treatment and survivorship statistics, 2019. CA Cancer J Clin. 2019;69(5):363-85.
2. Raphael J, Ahmedzai S, Hester J, Urch C, Barrie J, Williams J, et al. Cancer pain: part 1: Pathophysiology; oncological, pharmacological, and psychological treatments: a perspective from the British Pain Society endorsed by the UK Association of Palliative Medicine and the Royal College of General Practitioners. Pain Med. 2010;11:742-64.
3. Portenoy RK, Ahmed E. Interventional therapies for cancer pain management. Oncologist. 2018;23(5):495-507.

4. Brown DL, Bulley CK. Sympathetic blocks in the management of cancer pain. Cancer Control. 2000;7(2):149-57.
5. Mercadante S. Malignant abdominal pain: pathophysiology and treatment. Pain. 1997;69(1-2):1-18.
6. Sharma V, Fraser R, Kiser AC, et al. Efficacy and safety of splanchnic nerve blocks in the treatment of chronic abdominal pain: a retrospective study. Pain Med. 2015; 16(9):1690-5.
7. Kappis M. Erfahrungen mit lokalanästhesie bei bauchoperationen. Verhandl D Deutsch Gesellsch F Cir. 1914;43:87-9.
8. Jones RR. A technique for injection of the splanchnic nerves with alcohol. Anesth Analg. 1957;36(5):75-7.
9. Hoffmann VL, Vogl TJ, Klisch J, Mack MG, Muller PK. CT-guided neurolytic splanchnic nerve block in upper abdominal cancer pain. Pain. 1993;52(2):223-9.
10. Drake RL, Vogl AW, Mitchell AWM, Tibbitts RM, Richardson PE. Gray's Anatomy for Students, 4th edition. Philadelphia, PA: Elsevier; 2020.
11. Moore KL, Dalley AF, Agur AM. Clinically Oriented Anatomy, 8th edition. Philadelphia, PA: Wolters Kluwer; 2018.
12. Gress F, Schmitt C, Sherman S, Ikenberry S, Lehman G. A prospective randomized comparison of endoscopic ultrasound- and computed tomography-guided celiac plexus block for managing chronic pancreatitis pain. Am J Gastroenterol. 1999;94(4):900-5.
13. Benzon H, Raja SN, Fishman SM, Liu SS, Cohen SP. Treatment of cancer pain. In: Hurley RW (Ed). Essentials of Pain Medicine, 4th edition. Elsevier; 2017. pp. 385-92.
14. Manchikanti L, Singh V, Boswell MV. Interventional techniques in chronic spinal pain. Techn Regional Anesth Pain Manage. 2002;6(2):110-15.
15. Niv D, Gofeld M, Devor M. Splanchnic nerve block for visceral pain. J Pain Palliat Care Pharmacother. 2003;17(3-4):45-58.
16. Deer TR, Provenzano DA, Hanes M, Pope JE. The neuroanatomy of the splanchnic nerves and their role in visceral sensation and autonomic regulation. Pain Med. 2019;20(Suppl 1) doi:10.1093/pm/pny272.
17. Kambadakone A, Thabet A, Gervais DA, Mueller PR, Arellano RS. CT-guided celiac plexus neurolysis: a review of anatomy, indications, technique, and tips for successful treatment. Radiographics. 2011;31(6):1599-621.
18. Peng PW, Tumber PS. Ultrasound-guided interventional procedures in pain management: evidence-based medicine. Pain Physician. 2008;11(2):215-24.
19. Narouze SN. Ultrasound-guided interventional procedures in pain management: evidence-based medicine. Reg Anesth Pain Med. 2010;35(4 Suppl):S55-8.
20. Tsui BC, Dillane D, Pillay JJ. Ultrasound-guided splanchnic nerve radiofrequency thermocoagulation in a patient with severe chronic pancreatitis: a case report. J Pain Res. 2018;11:141-7.
21. Lim HY, Lee JH, Moon HS, Lee MK, Kim JH. Fluoroscopy guided thoracic splanchnic nerve block: a technical note. Korean J Pain. 2013;26(1):104-7.
22. Schroeder S, Koulousakis A, Kettler E, et al. CT-guided neurolytic splanchnic nerve block: technique, results, and complications. Cardiovasc Intervent Radiol. 2001; 24(6):356-61.
23. Moore DC, Bush WH. CT-guided splanchnic nerve block technique for the management of chronic upper abdominal pain. Clin Radiol. 1995;50(3):173-7.
24. Bhatia A, Brull R. Review of CT-guided blocks for abdominal pain. Reg Anesth Pain Med. 2008;33(5):452-61.
25. Nahas FX, Ferreira LM, Juliano Y. Anterior approach for CT-guided splanchnic nerve block. Pain Pract. 2001;1(3):228-31.
26. Talu GK, Erdine S. Neurolytic celiac plexus and splanchnic nerve blocks: the anterior approach. Tech Reg Anesth Pain Manag. 2002;6(4):196-201.
27. Polati E, Finco G, Gottin L, et al. The role of the anterior approach in CT-guided splanchnic nerve block for the management of abdominal cancer pain. Eur J Pain. 2002;6(5):379-85.
28. Sahin T, Togral G, Bacanli K, et al. Transpedicular approach for thoracic splanchnic nerve block: a cadaveric study. Reg Anesth Pain Med. 2015;40(5):470-4.
29. Prakash S, Rathore MA, Bharath KV, Vasudeva VS, Kumar S. Fluoroscopy guided thoracic splanchnic nerve block: a technical note. Korean J Pain. 2013;26(1):104-7.
30. Bhagat S, Raza A, Mahapatra AK, Verma AK, Agarwal A. Fluoroscopy guided percutaneous neurolysis of thoracic splanchnic nerves: a retrospective analysis of 30 cases. J Anaesthesiol Clin Pharmacol. 2013;29(4):507-11.
31. Amr YM. The long-term efficacy of thoracic splanchnic nerve radiofrequency ablation for the management of abdominal cancer pain. Indian J Palliat Care. 2012;18(2):126-30.
32. Chin KJ, Chan V. Ultrasound-guided interventional procedures for chronic pain management. Pain Manag. 2011;1(2):143-50.
33. Fichtel F, Leiser A, Carter GT, Chuang DC. The role of sympathetic nerve blocks in herpes zoster and postherpetic neuralgia. Pain Physician. 2010;13(1):17-26.
34. Inoue S, Kawaguchi M, Inoue S, et al. Cost-effectiveness of ultrasound-guided peripheral nerve blocks versus continuous epidural analgesia for pain relief after major abdominal surgery: a randomized controlled trial. Reg Anesth Pain Med. 2014;39(3):200-6.
35. Han KR, Kim MD, Kim JH, et al. Efficacy and safety of CT-guided percutaneous neurolytic celiac plexus block for managing pain in patients with unresectable pancreatic cancer. Radiology. 2019;291(3):678-84.
36. Cerci SS, Güleç S, Talas DU, Yıldız S, Cerci C. Efficacy and safety of ultrasound-guided splanchnic nerve block in patients with chronic pancreatitis and intractable abdominal pain. J Pain Res. 2016;9:1235-42.

37. Brennan TJ, Kehlet H. Preventive analgesia to reduce wound hyperalgesia and persistent postsurgical pain: not an easy path. Anesthesiology. 2005;103(3):681-3.
38. Agarwal-Kozlowski K, Lorke DE, Habermann CR, Laniado M, Eibenberger K, Gorzolla C. CT-guided splanchnic nerve block with alcohol for treating cancer pain: a retrospective analysis in 249 patients. Cardiovasc Intervent Radiol. 2009;32(1):38-45.
39. Anderson BA, Kaczynski KG, Anderson DR. Peripheral nerve blocks for palliative treatment of pain in a terminally ill patient. Ann Pharmacother. 2005;39(12):2116-9.
40. Moore DC, Bridenbaugh LD, Bridenbaugh PO. Nerve blocks in palliative care. J Palliat Med. 2008;11(9):1249-74.
41. Choi E, Nahm FS, Lee PB, et al. Ultrasound-guided splanchnic nerve radiofrequency thermocoagulation in a patient with severe chronic pancreatitis: a case report. Medicine (Baltimore). 2018;97(50).
42. Malhotra V, Singh S, Sood D. Coolief cooled radiofrequency for sacroiliac joint pain: two-year results from 20 cases. Indian J Orthop. 2018;52(2):168-74.
43. Manchikanti L, et al. Comprehensive review of therapeutic interventions in managing chronic spinal pain. Pain Physician. 2014;17(3).
44. Mercadante S, Nicosia F, Sapio M, et al. Celiac plexus block: a retrospective study of efficacy, safety, and predictors of outcome. Pain Med. 2011;12(3):435-9.
45. Keith W, et al. Intraoperative splanchnic neurolytic block and its impact on survival in unresectable carcinoma pancreas patients. Ann Surg. 2014.
46. Özyalçın NS, Dereli E, Talu GK, Kanpolat Y. Comparison of celiac plexus block and splanchnic nerve block in cancer pain management. Pain Pract. 2004;4(3):161-5.
47. Ischia S, Ischia A, Polati E, Finco G. Comparison of fluoroscopic guided transaortic celiac plexus blockade, retrocrural celiac plexus blockade, and bilateral splanchnic nerve blockade. Acta Anaesthesiol Scand. 1992;36(7):658-62.
48. Marra V, et al. CT-guided neurolytic blocks: a comparative study of celiac plexus and splanchnic nerve blocks. Pain Med. 2013;14(5):678-84.
49. Cicco J, et al. Dye spread and pain relief in celiac plexus block: a correlation study. Pain Physician. 2015;18(4):335-42.
50. Stefaniak T, Basinski A, Vingerhoets A, Makarewicz W, Connor S, Kaska L, et al. A comparison of two invasive techniques in the management of intractable pain due to inoperable pancreatic cancer: neurolytic celiac plexus block and videothoracoscopic splanchnicectomy. Eur J Surg Oncol. 2005;31(7):768-73.
51. Lillemoe KD, Cameron JL, Kaufman HS, Yeo CJ, Pitt HA, Sauter PK. Chemical splanchnicectomy in patients with unresectable pancreatic cancer. A prospective randomized trial. Ann Surg. 1993;217(5):447-57.

26 CHAPTER

Lumbar Sympathetic Block

Neel Mehta, Rajiv Shah, Sadiah Siddiqui

ABSTRACT

Lumbar sympathetic nerve blocks are used to evaluate and manage sympathetically mediated pain in the lower limbs.[1] The lumbar sympathetic ganglion is located along the anterolateral surface of the lumbar vertebral bodies.[2] During the procedure, patients are monitored with electrocardiogram, blood pressure cuff, and pulse oximetry. Temperature-sensing probes are placed on the patient's feet. A successful block includes vasodilation, rise in temperature of at least 2°C, and a decrease in pain on the ipsilateral lower limb.[3] Complications from the block include hypotension, back pain, intravascular injections, spinal/epidural injections, and genitofemoral neuralgia.[2]

INTRODUCTION

The lumbar sympathetic nerves are responsible for regulating various homeostatic mechanisms, including mediating the neuronal and hormonal stress responses for the lower extremities, and abdominal and pelvic viscera.[4] In certain conditions, these sympathetic nerves can transmit pain information from the peripheral tissues back to the spinal cord. Lumbar sympathetic nerve blocks are used to diagnose and treat sympathetically maintained pain.[2]

INDICATIONS

These blocks often are used to treat a variety of conditions involving the lower extremities, including neuropathic pain, claudication, complex regional pain syndromes, phantom limb syndrome, herpes neuralgia, recurrent bladder spasm, and lower limb lymphedema.[1,2,5]

CONTRAINDICATIONS

However, patients with any of the following conditions should not undergo a lumbar sympathetic block without further evaluation, including active bacterial infections, bleeding diathesis, allergy to injectants, steroid psychosis, local neoplasm, and local vascular anomalies.[1,6]

ANATOMICAL DESCRIPTION

The lumbar sympathetic chain is located along the anterolateral surface of the 1st through 4th lumbar vertebral bodies and anteromedial to the psoas muscle.[2,7] The vena cava lies just anterior to the right sympathetic chain, and the aorta lies anterior to the left sympathetic chain.[2] The lumbar sympathetic chain consists of two to six interconnected ganglia with the largest portion of ganglia located around the 2nd and 3rd lumbar vertebrae. Blocking the lumbar sympathetic chain with adequate medication spread at the L2 and L3 levels can provide an effective single-level block; however, L4 can also be utilized.[1]

DESCRIPTION OF PROCEDURE

Preparation

Intravenous access is recommended for the procedure. Physiologic monitoring is initiated, including electrocardiogram (ECG), pulse oximetry, and blood pressure monitoring. Sedation is avoided to prevent analgesic effect and to determine the effectiveness of the block at the end of the procedure. Skin is prepped and draped in a sterile manner. Each temperature probe is attached to the plantar aspect of the big toes on both sides.[3,7]

Technique

The patient is placed in a prone position with a pillow placed under the lower abdomen and iliac crest to reduce the normal lumbar lordosis. In the anteroposterior view, the L2 and L3 vertebral bodies are identified. The fluoroscope is rotated such that the facet line bisects the vertebral body, and the lateral border of the transverse process is in line of the lateral border of the vertebral body, at about 45° of rotation. Using 1% lidocaine, a skin wheal is raised over the lateral border of the vertebral body, just above or below the transverse process. At roughly a 45° angle, a 22G, 15 cm spinal needle is advanced along the vertebral body and until the vertebral body is contacted, at a depth confirmed with fluoroscopy **(Fig. 1)**.

After switching to the lateral view, the needle is advanced until reaching the anterior border of the vertebral body. Care must be taken, as advancing through the psoas muscle can be painful for the patient. After negative aspiration, the fluoroscopic image is observed as a 2–3 mL of nonionic radiocontrast medium is injected to rule out an intravascular or intraspinal needle tip placement. The correct placement of the needle is indicated by the presence of a layer of contrast medium in a thin line along the anterior border of the vertebral column **(Fig. 2)**.

On the anteroposterior view, the needle tip should not cross past the 6 o'clock mark of the pedicle. A test dose of 3 mL of lidocaine 1% is given and the patient is observed for metallic taste, tinnitus, and arm or hand numbness. After negative aspirations, 15 mL of 0.25% bupivacaine is slowly injected over the course of 15 minutes. The patient is questioned about pain relief, and observations of skin temperature are made. Sensory and motor functioning of the lower extremities is checked and the patient is observed for an additional 30 minutes.[3,6,7]

An alternative to the single-needle technique, which is described above, is the multiple-needle technique for lumbar sympathetic blockade. This initial "classic technique" was first described by Mandl and Kappis in the 1920s.[8,9] This technique involves the use of a total of three needles placed at the L2, L3, and L4 vertebral levels. First in the anteroposterior view, the L2, L3, and L4 vertebral bodies are identified. Using 1% lidocaine, three skin wheals are made 5–6 cm from midline at each vertebral level.[8] A 22G, 15 cm spinal needle is then placed at each vertebral level with the needle angled medially in order to contact the respective transverse process of the vertebral body.[8,10] Under fluoroscopic guidance, the needle is then directed toward the vertebral body by pointing inferiorly and medially to the transverse process.[8] In the lateral view, the needles are advanced until they reach the anterior border of the respective vertebral bodies. As with the single-needle technique, care must be taken

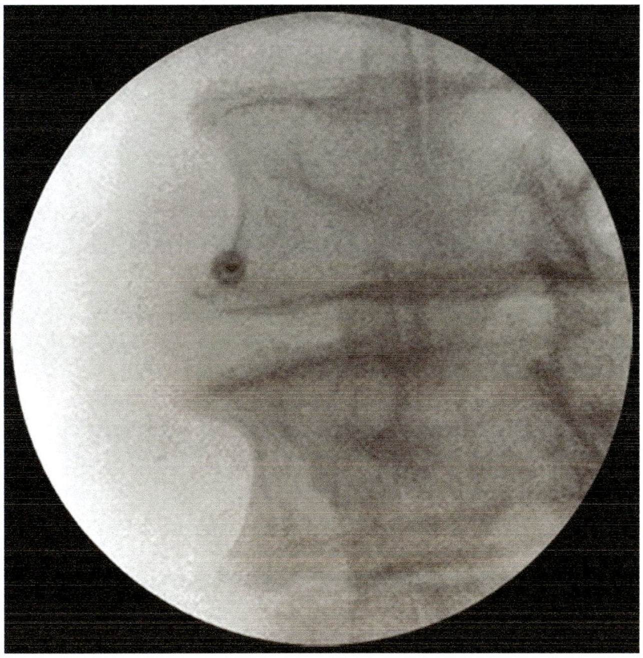

Fig. 1: Oblique view showing a facet line at halfway position of vertebral body.

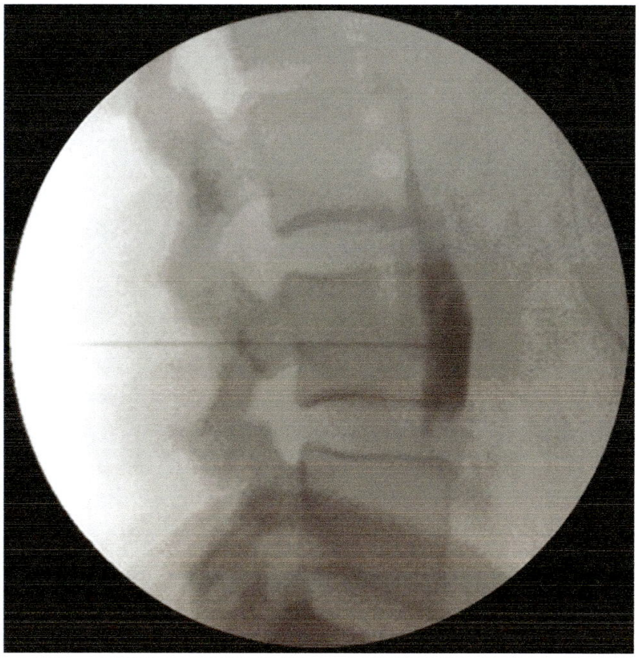

Fig. 2: Lateral view showing a thin contrast line at the anterior border of vertebral body.

with correct needle placement. After a negative test dose and aspiration, the solution of local anesthetic is divided equally among each of the levels. Of the two techniques, the multiple-needle technique has fallen out of favor since it is more time-consuming and causes more patient discomfort. Typically, there is no difference in outcome between the single- and multiple-needle techniques.[11] In addition, when the lumbar sympathetic block was performed at the L2 level, it showed the lowest incidence of psoas muscle injection of contrast in comparison to the L3 and L4 levels.[9,10]

Assessment of Block

There are numerous tests that can be used to assess the adequacy of the block and sympatholysis. Subjective tests of the lower limb on the injected side include vasodilatation, warmth, change in color, anhidrosis, and assessment of pain levels pre- and postprocedure.[12] Objective tests of the lower limb on the injected side include an increase in temperature by at least 2°C, increase in blood flow, provocative sweat tests, and depression of the psychogalvanic reflex that measures the electrical conductance of the skin.[7,13]

COMPLICATIONS

The complications from a lumbar sympathetic block include infection, backache, retroperitoneal bleed or hematoma, intravascular injection, intrathecal or epidural injection, sympathectomy-related hypotension, genitofemoral nerve injury-induced groin pain, and visceral perforation.[14,15]

CONCLUSION

The lumbar sympathetic nerve block is a safe procedure that can provide adequate relief for patients with sympathetically maintained pain. Due to the location of the lumbar sympathetic chain to key vascular structures, careful monitoring under fluoroscopy must be employed. The effects of the local anesthetic can provide immediate pain relief that can be assessed both subjectively and objectively. Although the complications of a lumbar sympathetic block are rare, when they occur, they can be catastrophic if not treated in a timely response.

REFERENCES

1. Stone JB, Gilhool JJ, Furman MB. Lumbar sympathetic block. In: Lee TS, Berkwits L, Furman MB (Eds). Atlas of Image-guided Spinal Procedures. Philadelphia, PA: Elsevier/Saunders; 2013.
2. Gulati A, Khelemsky Y, Loh J, Puttanniah V, Malhotra V, Cubert K. The use of lumbar sympathetic blockade at L4 for management of malignancy-related bladder spasms. Pain Physician. 2011;14(3):305-10.
3. Connor T, Abram SE. Lumbar nerve root block. In: O'Connor TC, Abram SE (Eds). Atlas of Pain Injection Techniques, 2nd edition. China: Churchill Livingstone; 2014.
4. Gray H, Clemente CD. The great plexuses of the sympathetic system. In: Gray's Anatomy of the Human Body. Philadelphia: Lea & Febiger; 1985.
5. Woo JH, Park HS, Kim SC, Kim YH. The effect of lumbar sympathetic ganglion block on gynecologic cancer-related lymphedema. Pain Physician. 2013;16(4):345-52.
6. Pauza KJ. (2014). Educational guidelines for interventional spinal procedures. Academy of Physical Medicine and Rehabilitation. [online] Available from http://www.aapmr.org/practice/guidelines/documents/edguidelines.pdf [Last accessed August, 2024].
7. University of Pittsburgh. (2014). Lumbar sympathetic block. [online] Available from http://www.pitt.edu/~regional/Lumbar%20Sympathetic%20Block/Lumbar%20Sympathetic%20Block.htm [Last Accessed June, 2015].
8. Montgomery KA, Hurley RW. Nerve destruction for the alleviation of visceral pain. In: Huntoon MA, Benzon HT, Narouze S, Deer TR (Eds). Spinal Injections and Peripheral Nerve Blocks: Interventional and Neuromodulatory Techniques for Pain Management. Philadelphia, PA: Elsevier/Saunders; 2011.
9. Narouze S, Graham S. Cervical and lumbar sympathetic blocks. In: Huntoon MA, Benzon HT, Narouze S, Deer TR (Eds). Spinal Injections and Peripheral Nerve Blocks: Interventional and Neuromodulatory Techniques for Pain Management. Philadelphia, PA: Elsevier Saunders; 2011.
10. Hong JH, OH MJ. Comparison of multilevel with single level injection during lumbar sympathetic ganglion block: efficacy of sympatholysis and incidence of psoas muscle injection. Korean J Pain. 2010;23(2):131-6.
11. Rastogi R, Agarwal S, Enany N, Munir M. Sympathetic blockade. In: Smith HS (Ed). Current Therapy in Pain. Philadelphia, PA: Elsevier Saunders; 2009.
12. Tran KM, Frank SM, Raja SN, El-Rahmany HK, Kim LJ, Vu B. Lumbar sympathetic block for sympathetically maintained pain: changes in cutaneous temperatures and pain perception. Anesth Analg. 2000;90:1396-401.
13. Werdehausen R, Braun S, Hermanns H, Freynhagen R, Lipfert P, Stevens MF. Uniform distribution of skin-temperature increase after different regional-anesthesia techniques of the lower extremity. Reg Anesth Pain Med. 2007;32:73-8.
14. Menon R, Swanepoel A. Sympathetic blocks. Contin Educ Anaesth Crit Care Pain. 2010;10(2):88-92.
15. Sayson SC, Ramamurthy S, Hoffman J. Incidence of genitofemoral nerve block during lumbar sympathetic block: comparison of two lumbar injection sites. Reg Anesth. 1997;22:569-74.

27

CHAPTER

Superior Hypogastric Plexus Block

Dwarkadas K Baheti

ABSTRACT

Lower pelvic, rectal, bladder, sigmoid, and anal pain is very difficult to treat and manage. The overall pharmacological management of patients suffering from these conditions has become inadequate, and their pain is difficult to manage. The superior hypogastric plexus nerve block is a procedure that can provide relief to the patient and improve their quality of life. The superior hypogastric plexus nerve block is indicated for various malignancy-related pains from pelvic organs, i.e., uterus, rectum, and cervix. The procedure can be safely performed under fluoroscopy or computed tomography (CT) guidance. Neurolysis is only indicated for tumor pain.

INTRODUCTION

The continuation of the lumbar sympathetic chain in the lumbosacral area has its origin in preganglionic fibers from the lower thoracic region and lumbar region. From the spinal cord, together with the fibers from the parasympathetic sacral ganglion, the postganglionic fibers exit the lumbar sympathetic chain. The ganglion lies in front of the sacral promontory at the L4-5 level and passes through the L5-S1 interspace.[1]

The superior hypogastric plexus block is an indication of painful nonmalignant and malignant conditions. These conditions include endometriosis, proctalgia, postradiation neuritis, palliation of malignancy, i.e., uterine cancer, rectal and sigmoid cancer, and bladder cancer.

INDICATIONS FOR SUPERIOR HYPOGASTRIC PLEXUS BLOCK

- Tumors of uterus
- Malignancy of cervix and uterus
- Metastatic tumors of colon
- Rectal malignancy
- Anal canal
- Bladder tumor
- Chronic pelvic pain
- Testicular tumor
- Penile cancer
- Prostate malignancy
- Seminal vesicle.

CONTRAINDICATIONS

- Unwilling patient
- Bleeding disorders
- Local skin infection.

SUPERIOR HYPOGASTRIC PLEXUS BLOCK UNDER FLUOROSCOPY

A detailed patient's history, physical examination, and routine blood work must be assessed. Any abnormalities in the hematological profile must be corrected prior to the procedure. Once the patient is cleared for the procedure, he/she is brought to the radiological suite. The patient is then placed on the X-ray table in a prone position.

Step 1: A pillow is placed underneath the lower abdomen. The spinous process of the lumbar vertebra is marked. The lower vertebral bodies of L3-L4, L4-L5, and L5-S1 are visualized. A marker is placed at the L4 level just above the iliac crest approximately 5 cm^3 lateral from the midline. The local area is anesthetized at the marker point and then a 20G 10 cm needle is pushed in the direction of the sacral promontory. At the same time,

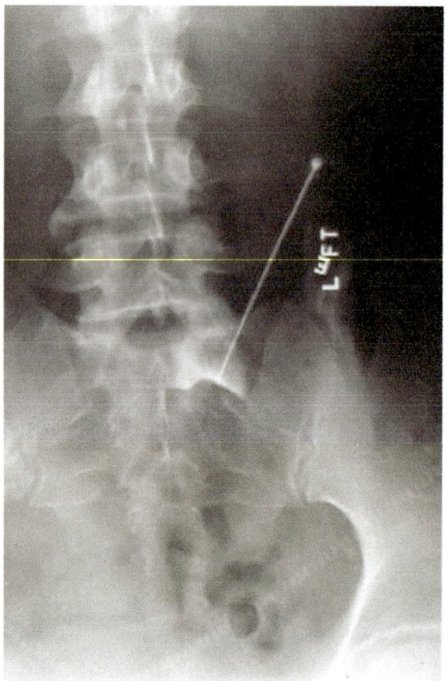

Fig. 1: Anteroposterior view of superior hypogastric plexus block.

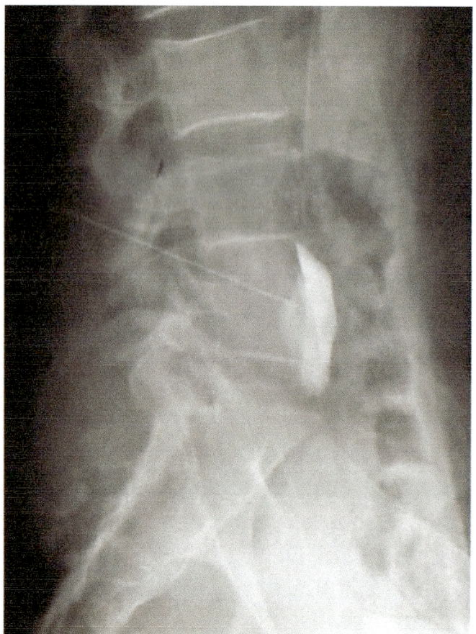

Fig. 2: Lateral view of superior hypogastric plexus block.

anteroposterior (AP) and lateral views should be taken. Once the tip is directed caudally and lies in front of the sacral promontory, the needle is aspirated for blood or *cerebrospinal fluid* (CSF).

Step 2: Following a negative aspiration, 3 mL of water-soluble radiopaque contrast media is injected. Similarly, the procedure is repeated in the same fashion on the opposite side. The spread of dye is confirmed in AP and lateral view **(Figs. 1 and 2)**.

Step 3: For the diagnostic block, 15 mL of 1% lidocaine is injected on both sides. If there is an indication of malignancy, then 10 mL of 50% alcohol is injected slowly on both sides.[1-3]

SUPERIOR HYPOGASTRIC PLEXUS BLOCK UNDER COMPUTED TOMOGRAPHY

Patients with malignancy from various tumors related to rectum, sigmoid colon, uterus, ovarian, tubal, and urinary bladder in advanced stages will require palliative care to improve their quality of life. A neurolytic procedure where the patient has a disrupted anatomy of viscera needs precise treatment.

Step 1: Patient is prepared in the same manner as described under X-ray control. Once the patient is cleared to proceed, the patient is placed on the computed tomography (CT) table. Once the patient is attached to an ASA (American Society of Anesthesiology) monitor, a scout film is taken from lumbar to sacral 3–4 level. Multiple 5-mm sections are cut at the L4-L5-S1 region. The sacral promontory, bifurcation of aorta (both iliac vessels), and the body of L5 vertebra are identified. A marker is placed at the outer border of the transverse process of L4 and L5 vertebrae.

Step 2: A possible path and angle of needle are prescanned using a laser path on the CT machine, followed by a 1% lidocaine injection at the marker point. A 20G 10–12 cm spinal needle is placed in the caudal direction until the needle tip is visualized at the bottom of the vertebral body of L5 and upper part of the sacral promontory. Similarly, the opposite side of the needle is placed in the same fashion. Both tips are visualized up to 2-mm cuts on the CT screen; once the tip is satisfactory, the aspiration of both needles are done.

Step 3: Following a negative aspiration for blood, urine, and CSF, 3–5 cc water-soluble contrast media is injected to visualize the distribution of solution. Once this is done, a test dose of 1–3 mL of 1% lidocaine is used to anesthetize the ganglion followed by 6–8 mL of 50% absolute alcohol injected slowly. A large volume injected on the inferior hypogastric plexus may cause adversary effects on nervi erigentes and parasympathetic fibers that cause an increased risk of affecting their bowel or bladder sphincter.

Ultrasound-guided Technique

In the last 5 years, ultrasound technology has been used to perform various diagnostic and therapeutic nerve blocks.

Most of these procedure applications were for nerve localization as well as nerve blocking for preoperative and postoperative anesthesia and analgesia. The superior hypogastric block is performed using the anterior approach.

Step 1: Patient is placed on the procedure table in a supine posture. The abdominal structures are visualized on the ultrasound machine. Multiple levels in the transverse ultrasound view are seen. The scans are done from the umbilicus to the suprapubic region. The L4, L5 body and sacral promontory are identified. The ultrasound transducer is placed in a transverse position. The abdomen is prepared aseptically with alcohol or betadine solution and a marker is placed at the area of the celiac vessels.

Step 2: A local anesthetic is produced by injecting 4–5 mL of 1% lidocaine. A 20–22G spinal needle with stylet is placed at the marker point and the needle is slowly pushed at the bifurcation of the aorta; following a negative aspiration, 8–10 mL of 1% lidocaine is slowly injected.

Step 3: If neurolysis is planned, then 10–15 mL of 50% absolute alcohol is slowly injected. The patient must be monitored using an ASA monitor, which records hemodynamics, blood pressure, ECG, and oxygen saturation. Once the patient is hemodynamically stable, he/she is transferred to the recovery area. The piercing of vessels or organs, including the bladder or colon, is possible. This technique is not widely used and should only be done with the help of a trained ultrasound radiologist.

Postprocedural Care

The postprocedural care remains the same for the use of fluoroscopy, ultrasound, and CT-guided procedures. After successful block, the patient is shifted to a recovery room for monitoring of vital signs for 1–2 hours. The necessary instructions are given to patients to contact for any untoward reactions.

COMPLICATIONS

- Injury to ureter and bladder
- Intravascular injection
- Intra-arterial injection
- Injury to inferior hypogastric plexus
- Impotence
- Loss of bowel or bladder function due to sphincter injury
- Intrathecal, epidural injection
- Unilateral or bilateral paraplegia.

CONCLUSION

The neurolytic superior hypogastric plexus block is an important modality in the multimodal treatment approach for chronic pelvic pain conditions. With the advent of imaging facilities such as fluoroscopy, ultrasound, and CT guidance, it provides long-term pain relief in these patients.

REFERENCES

1. Plancarte R, Amescua C, Patt RB, Aldrete JA. Superior hypogastric plexus block for pelvic cancer pain. Anesthesiology. 1990;73(2):236-9.
2. Waldman SD, Wilson WL, Kreps RD. Superior hypogastric plexus block using a single needle and computed tomography guidance: description of a modified technique. Reg Anesth. 1991;16(5):286-7.
3. Jain S, Kestenbaum A, Shah N, Khan Y. Hypogastric plexus block: a new technique for treatment of perineal pain. Anesth Analg. 1990;70:S175.

CHAPTER 28

Ganglion Impar Block

George C Chang Chien, Harpreet Singh, Bruce M Vrooman

ABSTRACT

The ganglion impar (ganglion of Walther) is the ganglion located most caudally in the sympathetic chain and is the only unpaired ganglion in this chain. It is a potential therapeutic target in patients with pelvic and perineal pain. Multiple approaches have been described to perform the ganglion impar block, including the trans-sacrococcygeal approach, anococcygeal ligament approach, and transcoccygeal and paracoccygeal corkscrew approaches. Although the ganglion impar block is a relatively low-risk procedure, there is a risk of bowel perforation, nerve injury, or bleeding into the retroperitoneal area. We describe the most straightforward and commonly utilized approaches to the ganglion impar block.

INTRODUCTION

The ganglion impar (ganglion of Walther) is the ganglion located most caudally in the sympathetic chain and mediates sympathetic and nociceptive pain arising from the perineum, distal rectum, anus, distal urethra, vulva, and distal third of the vagina. Anesthetic blockade of the ganglion impar can be both diagnostic and therapeutic and should be considered for the treatment of refractory cases of chronic pelvic and perineal pain.

Reported indications include coccygodynia, idiopathic perineal pain, pain from prostatitis, proctitis, vulvovaginitis, pelvic tumors, postherpetic neuralgia, spinal cord malformations, vaginal protrusion, failed back surgery syndrome, and testicular ablation **(Table 1)**.[1-5]

TABLE 1: Indications for ganglion impar block.

Pain originating from	*Pain secondary to*
Perineum	Metastatic cancer to the perineum
Distal rectum	Postherpetic neuralgia
Anus	Postsurgical thrombosis of perineal veins
Distal urethra	Spinal cord malformations
Vulva	Vaginal protrusion
Distal third of the vagina	Failed back surgery syndrome, metastatic cancer to the perineum

APPLIED ANATOMY

The ganglion impar is the only unpaired ganglion in the body and is formed by the union of the caudal ends of two sympathetic chains anterior to the coccyx. Although it lies within the pelvic cavity in close proximity to rectum **(Fig. 1)**,[6] the exact location of ganglion impar is variable. It can range from the anterior to the sacrococcygeal joint to the midpoint of the body of coccyx **(Fig. 2)**. This anatomical variation may contribute to the possible inefficacy of this nerve block in some patients. The branches from the ventral ramus of the sacral nerve were reported to be in proximity of the ganglion impar in 6% of the samples.[7] The close relationship between these structures raises the risk for the development of neuritis and neuralgia after chemical neurolysis of unintended targets.

The ganglionic impar receives visceral afferents from the distal rectum, anus, distal urethra, distal one-third of the vagina, vulva, and penis. It may also pass through postganglionic sympathetic fibers from the sympathetic chain via gray rami communicantes to innervate the pelvic viscera and the perineum.[8]

The most important bony landmark for the access of the ganglion impar is the coccyx. It is a small triangular

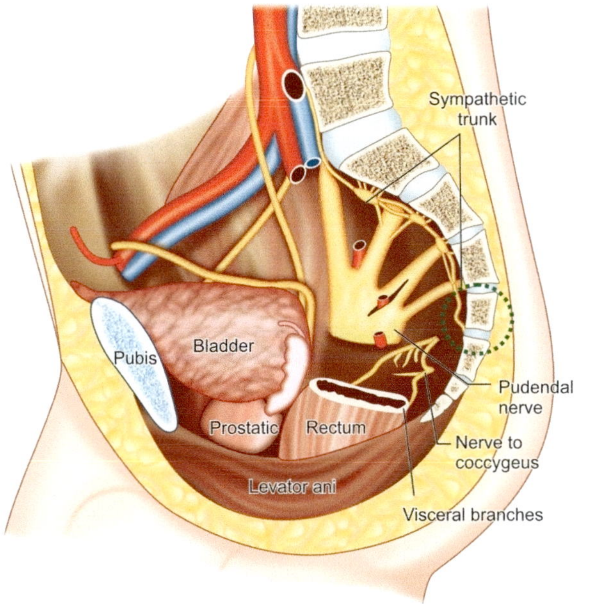

Fig. 1: Sagittal dissection depicting the location of the ganglion impar. Anatomy of the ganglion impar. Illustration shows the common location of the ganglion impar (dashed circle).
Source: Gray H, Lewis WH. Anatomy of the Human Body, 20th edition. New York: Bartleby.com; 2000.

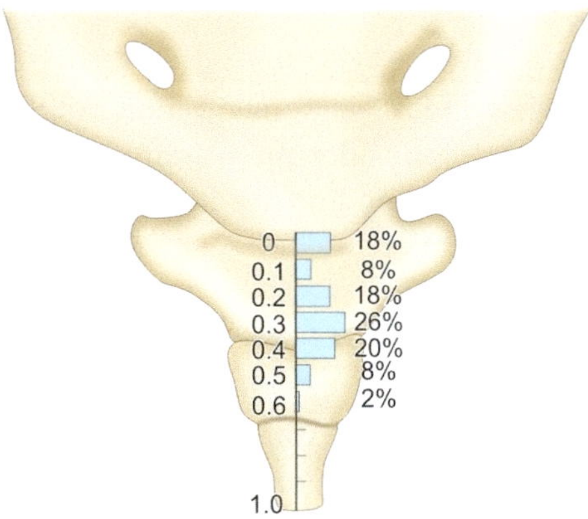

Fig. 2: Location of ganglion impar.
Source: Oh et al.[7]

bone formed by the fusion of four rudimentary vertebrae. The base of the coccyx articulates with the apex of the sacrum to form the sacrococcygeal joint which is usually a symphyseal joint; it is directed downward and anteriorly from the sacrococcygeal joint. As many as 51% of patients with coccygodynia may have fused sacrococcygeal joint making the trans-sacrococcygeal approach impossible. However, the first intercoccygeal joint is fused only in 12% of the cases, offering another window to approach the ganglion impar.[9]

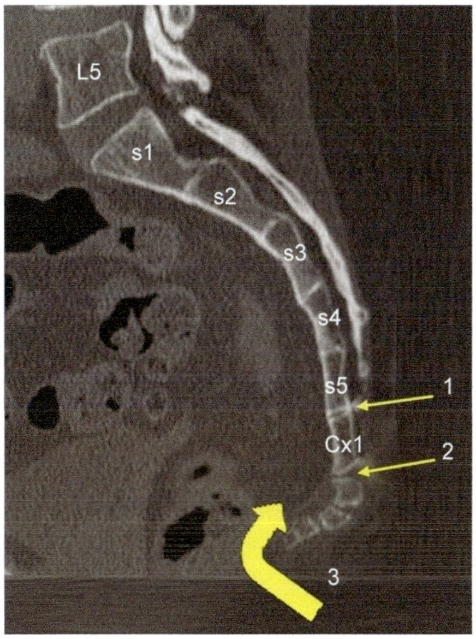

Fig. 3: Sagittal magnetic resonance imaging of the sacrum demonstrating different approaches to the ganglion impar block. Arrow 1: Trans-sacrococcygeal approach; Arrow 2: Transcoccygeal approach; Arrow 3: Anococcygeal approach.

APPROACHES TO THE GANGLION IMPAR

Multiple approaches have been described to perform the ganglion impar block, utilizing fluoroscopic, computerized tomography (CT), magnetic resonance imaging (MRI), or ultrasound guidance. Many techniques have been described including anococcygeal ligament, sacrococcygeal joint, transcoccygeal, paramedian, and paracoccygeal corkscrew approaches **(Fig. 3)**. The trans-sacrococcygeal approach through the intercoccygeal disk to the ganglion impar block is the most direct, simple, and commonly taught technique. A summary is given in **Table 2**. For the purposes of this chapter, we will focus on the two most direct approaches to the ganglion impar block.

TECHNIQUES

Trans-sacrococcygeal Approach

The patient is positioned prone on the fluoroscopy table. A large sterile preparation of the skin in the sacrococcygeal region is performed. Anteroposterior (AP) fluoroscopic imaging is used to identify the sacrum and coccygeal bone elements in a midline position. The most caudal coccygeal elements are identified, and a small skin mark is made to identify this at the midline. A lateral fluoroscopic image is

TABLE 2: Approaches to the ganglion impar block **(Fig. 3)**.

Approach	***Technique***	***Risks/benefits***
Anococcygeal ligament	• Bent or curved 22G spinal needle introduced through the anococcygeal ligament and directed under fluoroscopic guidance to lie with its tip retroperitoneally at the sacrococcygeal junction[1,10] • It is recommended that the operator place the index finger of the nondominant hand inside the rectum to monitor for pressure from the needle	• Rectal perforation • Tissue trauma along the plane of the needle • Needle-stick injury to the operator's intrarectal finger • Failure rate of 20–30% for this approach[11]
Paramedian	Introduce the needle below the transverse process of the coccyx and then alter its angulation to have the needle tip anterior to the sacrococcygeal joint[3,12]	• Rectal perforation • Tissue trauma along the plane of the needle
Trans-sacrococcygeal approach	• Introduce the needle through the sacrococcygeal joint and ligaments either using a single-needle[13] or • A needle-inside-needle technique[14]	• Penetration of the disk may lead to diskitis • Breakage of needle • Difficulty passing the needle due to joint ossification
Trans-sacrococcygeal approach	Needle introduced through the intercoccygeal space, most commonly between first and second coccygeal segments[15]	• Visualization not obstructed by sacral cornu[16] • Closer proximity to ganglion impar location[7] • Less likely to be ossified compared to sacrococcygeal joint[9]
Corkscrew paramedian approach[17]	Small bent-tip spinal needle used to walk of the lateral margin of coccyx than tip rotated medial to reach the target	Useful in patients with fused sacrococcygeal and intercoccygeal joints

utilized to identify the coccyx bones and the disks between them. A radiopaque pointer can be used to verify the appropriate level for needle entry. Once the needle entry site is confirmed, the skin is anesthetized with 3 mL of 1% lidocaine. A needle is advanced through the anesthetized skin under intermittent fluoroscopic guidance toward the radiolucent disk between the selected coccygeal bones. A 22- or 25G, 1.5-3.5-inch needle may be appropriate for most patients. Needle advancement primarily takes place in the lateral view. Care is made to align the initial entrance into the joint with a trajectory that is well aligned with the joint space to allow smooth travel through the sacrococcygeal disk. The final needle position is just at the anterior line of the coccyx bone **(Figs. 4A and B)**. Caution is made to ensure that the needle does not venture too far beyond the anterior coccygeal border as this could result in possible trespass into the bowel elements. Once negative aspiration is confirmed, 2 mL of contrast is injected to ensure appropriate placement of the needle tip. Contrast dye should flow along the anterior aspect of the coccygeal bones without vascular uptake **(Fig. 4C)**. Once appropriate contrast flow pattern is identified on the lateral view and AP view, medication can be injected. Practitioners can consider the use of extension tubing to reduce the likelihood of needle movement prior to injection of medication.

Paracoccygeal Corkscrew Approach

The patient is positioned prone on the fluoroscopy table. A large sterile preparation of the skin in the sacrococcygeal region is performed. AP fluoroscopic imaging is used to identify the sacrum and coccygeal bone elements in a midline position. The most caudal coccygeal elements are identified, and a small skin mark is made to identify this at the midline. A lateral fluoroscopic image is utilized to identify the coccyx bones and the disks between them **(Figs. 4A and B)**. A radiopaque pointer can be used to verify the appropriate level for needle entry. Once the needle entry site is confirmed, the skin is anesthetized with 3 mL of 1% lidocaine. A needle is advanced through the anesthetized skin under intermittent fluoroscopic guidance toward the lateral border of the selected coccygeal bones. A 22- or 25G, 1.5-3.5-inch needle with a curved tip will be appropriate for most patients. Needle advancement

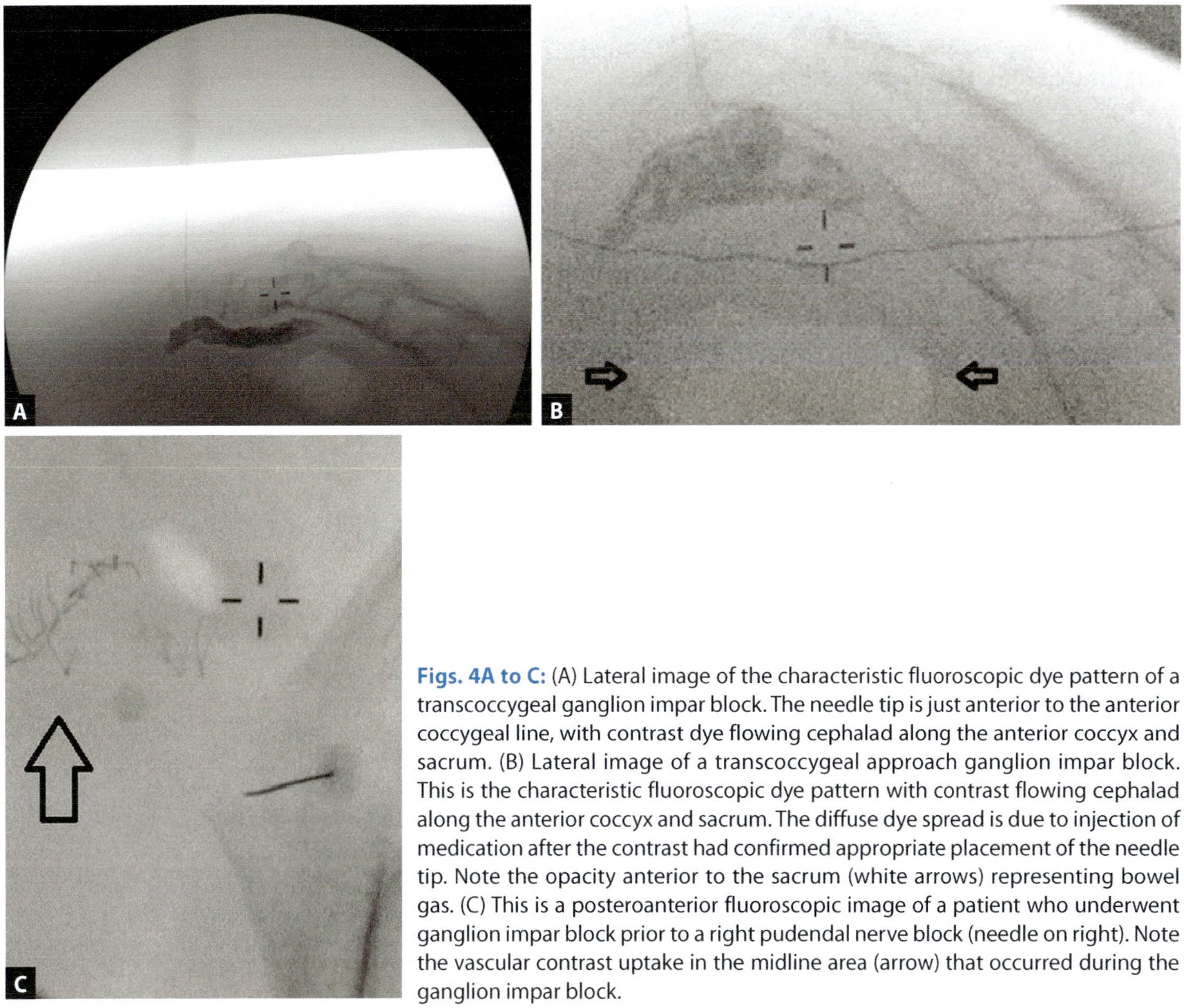

Figs. 4A to C: (A) Lateral image of the characteristic fluoroscopic dye pattern of a transcoccygeal ganglion impar block. The needle tip is just anterior to the anterior coccygeal line, with contrast dye flowing cephalad along the anterior coccyx and sacrum. (B) Lateral image of a transcoccygeal approach ganglion impar block. This is the characteristic fluoroscopic dye pattern with contrast flowing cephalad along the anterior coccyx and sacrum. The diffuse dye spread is due to injection of medication after the contrast had confirmed appropriate placement of the needle tip. Note the opacity anterior to the sacrum (white arrows) representing bowel gas. (C) This is a posteroanterior fluoroscopic image of a patient who underwent ganglion impar block prior to a right pudendal nerve block (needle on right). Note the vascular contrast uptake in the midline area (arrow) that occurred during the ganglion impar block.

primarily takes place in the lateral view. Once the needle tip makes contact with the osseous elements, the curve of the needle is rotated away from the bone such that the needle can be advanced beyond the edge of the bone. Once the tip is near the anterior coccygeal line, the needle tip is rotated medially such that injectate will emerge midline. Caution is made to ensure that the needle does not venture too far beyond the anterior coccygeal border as this could result in possible trespass into the bowel elements. Once negative aspiration is confirmed, 2 mL of contrast is injected to ensure appropriate placement of the needle tip. Contrast dye should flow along the anterior aspect of the coccygeal bones without vascular uptake **(Fig. 4C)**. Once an appropriate contrast flow pattern is identified on the lateral view and AP view, medication can be injected. Practitioners can consider the use of extension tubing to reduce the likelihood of needle movement prior to injection of medication.

RISKS

Risks involved in these procedures include bleeding, bruising, infection, and complications associated with bowel perforation. Improper positioning of the needle could potentially cause nerve injury, bleeding into the retroperitoneal area, paralysis or puncture of the rectum, surrounding organs, and adjacent blood vessels.

CONCLUSION

The ganglion impar (ganglion of Walther) is the ganglion located most caudally in the sympathetic chain and is the only unpaired ganglion in this chain. It is the putative target in the treatment of nociceptive pain arising from the perineum, distal rectum, anus, distal urethra, vulva, and distal third of the vagina. Anesthetic blockade of the ganglion impar can be both diagnostic and therapeutic and should be considered for the treatment of refractory cases of chronic pelvic and perineal pain.

Multiple approaches have been described to perform the ganglion impar block including transsacrococcygeal, anococcygeal ligament, transcoccygeal, and paracoccygeal corkscrew approaches. Although the ganglion impar block is a relatively low-risk procedure, there is a risk of bowel perforation, nerve injury, or bleeding into the retroperitoneal area. We describe the most straightforward and commonly utilized approaches to the ganglion impar block.

REFERENCES

1. Plancarte R, Amescua C, Patt RB, Allende S. Presacral blockade of the Ganglion of Walther (Ganglion Impar). Anesthesiology. 1990;73(3A):A751.
2. Agarwal-Kozlowski K, Lorke DE, Habermann CR, Am Esch JS, Beck H. CT-guided blocks and neuroablation of the ganglion impar (Walther) in perineal pain: anatomy, technique, safety, and efficacy. Clin J Pain. 2009;25(7): 570-6.
3. McAllister RK, Carpentier BW, Malkuch G. Sacral post-herpetic neuralgia and successful treatment using a paramedial approach to the ganglion impar. Anesthesiology. 2004;101(6):1472-4.
4. DeMedicis E, de Leon-Casasola O. Ganglion impar block: critical evaluation. Tech Reg Anesth Pain Manage. 2001;5:120-2.
5. Kabbara AI. Trans sacrococcygeal ganglion impar block for postherpetic neuralgia. Anesthesiology. 2005;103(1):211-2.
6. Susan S. Gray's Anatomy, 40th edition. London: Churchill Livingstone; 2009. pp. 1039-54.
7. Oh CS, Chung IH, Ji HJ, Yoon DM. Clinical implications of topographic anatomy on the ganglion impar. Anesthesiology. 2004;101:249-50.
8. Walters A, Muhleman M, Osiro S, Bubb K, Snosek M, Shoja MM, et al. One is the loneliest number: a review of the ganglion impar and its relation to pelvic pain syndromes. Clin Anat. 2013;26(7):855-61.
9. Postacchini F, Massobrio M. Idiopathic coccygodynia. Analysis of fifty-one operative cases and a radiographic study of the normal coccyx. J Bone Joint Surg Am. 1983;65(8):1116-24.
10. Nebab EG, Florence IM. An alternative needle geometry for interruption of the ganglion impar. Anesthesiology. 1997;86(5):1213-4.
11. Toshniwal GR, Dureja GP, Prashanth SM. Trans-sacrooccygeal approach to ganglion impar block for management of chronic perineal pain: a prospective observational study. Pain Physician. 2007;10(5):661-6.
12. Huang JJ. Another modified approach to the ganglion of Walther block (ganglion of Impar). J Clin Anesth. 2003;15(4):282-3.
13. Wemm K Jr, Saberski L. Modified approach to block the ganglion impar (Ganglion of Walther). Reg Anesth. 1995;20(6):544-5.
14. Munir MA, Zhang J, Ahmad M. A modified needle-inside-needle technique for the ganglion impar block. Can J Anaesth. 2004;51(9):915-7.
15. Foye PM. New approaches to ganglion impar blocks via coccygeal joints. Reg Anesth Pain Med. 2007;32(3):269.
16. Foye PM. Ganglion impar blocks via coccygeal versus sacrococcygeal joints. Reg Anesth Pain Med. 2008;33(3): 279-80.
17. Foye PM, Patel SI. Paracoccygeal corkscrew approach to ganglion impar injections for tailbone pain. Pain Pract. 2009;9(4):317-21.

6 SECTION

Spine and Back

29 CHAPTER

Cervical Epidural Block: Interlaminar Approach

Rishi Khanna, James Taylor

ABSTRACT

To perform a safe and efficacious interlaminar epidural in the cervical region, it is vital to understand the anatomy and radiological images, appreciate what are appropriate indications and contraindications, and practice a safe technique. This chapter will familiarize the reader with the anatomy, aid selection of appropriate patients, and provide a foundation for the technique which will then need to be developed under supervision before attempting the procedure independently.

INTRODUCTION

Cervical interlaminar epidural injections are primarily used to treat chronic upper limb radicular pain. In this chapter, we will describe the technique to perform this in a safe and effective manner. It is a procedure that requires care, attention, and experience in fluoroscopically guided spinal injections. Those embarking on this procedure for the first time are advised to do so under strict supervision.

ANATOMY

There are seven cervical vertebrae, three "atypical" and four "typical". The 1st, 2nd, and 7th cervical vertebrae are atypical in that they possess unique anatomical characteristics.

Typical cervical vertebrae, C3-C6, have a small broad body anterior to a relatively large triangular vertebral foramen. The spines of the vertebrae are small and bifid, and the transverse processes possess a transverse foramen for the passage of the vertebral artery and vein.

The 1st cervical vertebra C1 (the atlas) has no body or spinous process and instead is a ring-like structure with an anterior and a posterior arch.

The 2nd cervical vertebra, C2 (the axis), has a superior projection from the body called the odontoid peg, which forms a synovial joint with the anterior arch of C1.

The 7th cervical vertebra, C7, is of greater clinical significance and is illustrated in **Figure 1**.

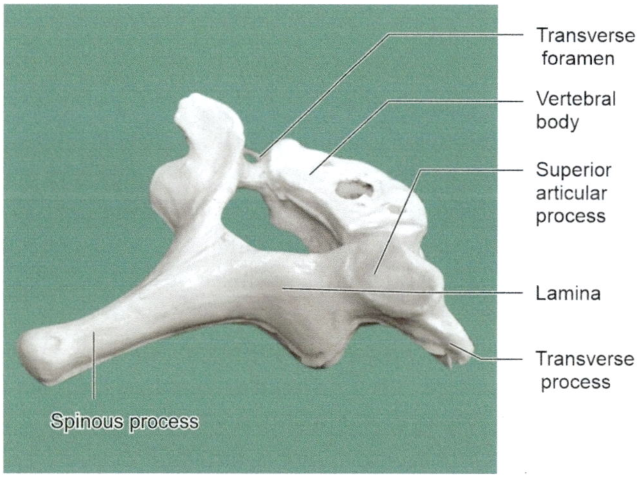

Fig. 1: Seventh cervical vertebra.

The C7 is also called the vertebra prominens because it has the longest spinous process. Unlike a typical cervical vertebra, the C7 spinous process is not bifid, and the transverse foramen is present but smaller and only contains the vertebral vein.

The atlantooccipital and atlantoaxial joints have a complex ligament arrangement beyond the scope of this chapter. For the remainder of the cervical vertebrae, the vertebral arches are joined in a manner consistent throughout the vertebral column with synovial facet joints and four ligaments, namely **(Fig. 2)**:

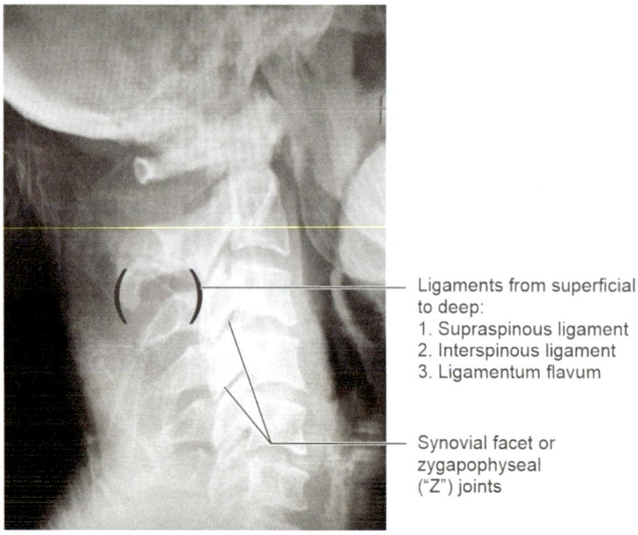

Fig. 2: X-ray with ligaments and zygapophyseal joint identified.

1. The supraspinous ligament joins the tips of the spinous processes.
2. The interspinous ligament runs between the spinous processes.
3. The intertransverse ligament runs between the transverse processes.
4. The ligamentum flavum joins the laminae. A midline Flavel gap is common in the cervical and high thoracic region, forming a triangle with its base lying caudally at the spinolaminar junction and apex at the superior vertebral level. In practice, this can lead to a less distinct loss of resistance and the risk of a dural tear.

In the cervical spine, the supraspinous and interspinous ligaments are thickened to form the ligament nuchae that run from the occipital protuberance to the spine of C7.

There are eight cervical nerves supplying motor and sensory nerves to the neck and upper limb. These emerge from the intervertebral foramen above their segmental vertebra except for C8 that emerges between C7 and T1.

At the C6/C7 and C7/T1 levels, the epidural space is 3-4 mm, increasing to 5-6 mm with neck flexion. More cephalad, the epidural space narrows especially at C5/C6 where it is only 1-2 mm due to the cervical enlargement of the cord. It is therefore recommended that interlaminar cervical epidurals are performed at either the C7/T1 or T1/T2 level to minimize the risk of injury to the cord.

Despite the proximity of the target site to the brain, the risk of supraspinal spread of drug is minimal. The dura and the endosteum fuse at the foramen magnum and so spread of epidural-administered drugs intracranially is not anatomically possible. Also, the risk of inadvertent intrathecal administration is reduced by a thick cervical dura, 2.5 mm as compared to 0.5 mm in the lumbar region making dural puncture relatively rare.

When performing a cervical epidural, the needle will pass through skin, subcutaneous tissue, ligament nuchae, interspinous ligament, and ligamentum flavum before reaching the epidural space. In the cervical region, there is a significant venous plexus that ultimately drains into the brachiocephalic veins and may be punctured leading to vascular spread or hematoma. As a rough guide, the depth of the epidural space may be between 4 and 6 cm.[1] However, there is a significant correlation between the depth and the weight, neck circumference, and body mass index of the patient.[2]

INDICATIONS

Chronic Pain

- Chronic cervical radicular pain
  - >50% pain relief in 68–77% of patients[3]
- Cervical postsurgery syndrome (a combination of neck and upper limb pain caused by pseudoarthrosis, adjacent segment degeneration, inadequate decompression, iatrogenic instability, and spinal stenosis)
  - >50% pain relief in 68% of patients[4]
- Cervical stenosis
  - >50% pain relief in 70% of patients.[5] Other upper limb neuropathic pains, including complex regional pain syndrome (CRPS), painful diabetic neuropathy, phantom limb pain, postherpetic neuralgia, and pain caused by neck or upper limb malignancy and its treatment (chemoradiotherapy or surgery)[6]
- Diskogenic neck pain
- >50% pain relief in 68–80% of patients[7-9]
- Nonspecific refractory upper limb pain.

Acute pain

- Temporary relief of upper limb vasospastic or vaso-occlusive disease while pharmacological, surgical, or radiological intervention is instigated[6]
- Acute cervical radicular pain triggered by trauma or pathological fractures (cancer-related)[6]
- Acute herpes zoster.[6]

CONTRAINDICATIONS

Systemic or Local Infection

There is a risk of homogenous spread of organisms, either from the skin and subcutaneous tissue or bacteremia, into the epidural space leading to abscess formation or meningitis. An epidural abscess may be present with a triad of symptoms—pain, fever, and neurological deficit—can be detected on magnetic resonance imaging (MRI). However, the onset may be insidious, and one should have a higher index of suspicion in high-risk groups, namely patients with diabetes mellitus, chronic renal failure, previous spinal surgery or trauma, malignancy, alcohol excess, and rheumatoid arthritis. If the initial MRI is negative, continuous reassessment should be made and it may be necessary to repeat imaging if there is further deterioration.

Congenital or Acquired Anatomical Anomalies

An epidural should not be attempted in patients with congenital or acquired anatomical anomalies that prevent accurate recognition of anatomical landmarks on fluoroscopy and potentially deform anatomy in such a way as to increase the likelihood of epidural puncture or spinal cord injury.

Coagulopathy and Anticoagulation

Performing epidurals in patients with coagulopathy or while receiving antithrombotic and antiplatelet medication can increase the risk of epidural hematoma leading to cord ischemia. An epidural hematoma may present with new-onset neck pain, radicular pain, and neurological deficit and can be detected on MRI. The severity of the neurological deficit and the delay between presentation, MRI diagnosis, and surgical evacuation has a key influence on outcome. The neurological outcome is likely to be more favorable if the hematoma can be removed within 8 hours of symptoms developing. It is therefore vital that patients are warned about the symptoms and encouraged to present early, and that imaging and surgical input is available in a timely fashion.

Consult with your patient's general practitioners and/or cardiologist to determine whether it is safe to omit antithrombotic and antiplatelet medication. **Table 1** is for guidance only and one should refer to one's local policy for more definitive recommendations.

TABLE 1: Medication and guidance for coagulopathy and anticoagulation.

Medication	*Guidance*[10]
Warfarin	• Stop for 5 days prior to epidural and check INR • Proceed if INR is <1.5 • Restart on evening following procedure
Clopidogrel	• Stop for 7 days • Restart on morning following procedure
Low-molecular weight-heparin (LMWH)	• Check platelets • Prophylactic dose. Perform epidural after 12 hours • Therapeutic dose. Perform epidural after 24 hours • Withhold for 6 hours after procedure
Unfractionated heparin infusion	• Check platelets • Stop for 6 hours and perform epidural if APTT ratio 1 • Infusion can be restarted 1 hour postprocedure
Rivaroxaban	• Stop for 24 hours. Caution: Action may be prolonged in renal failure. Check PT and APTT • Withhold for 6 hours postprocedure

(APTT: activated partial thromboplastin time; INR: international normalized ratio; PT: prothrombin time)

INFORMED CONSENT

To gain informed consent for a procedure, it is important to ensure that the patient has sufficient information about the benefits and risks of the procedure. They must be competent and have the time to consider this information and then be given an opportunity to ask questions if required.

The potential risks of a cervical epidural commonly quoted to a patient are:

- Failure to improve the pain
- Superficial infection (skin and subcutaneous tissues)
- Headache (caused by dural puncture)
- Direct or indirect injury to the spinal cord causing increased pain, pins and needles, numbness, weakness, or paralysis
  - Direct injury caused by contact with the needle. This may not be painful, although injection of air or fluid is and can be extremely detrimental.[11]
  - Indirect injury resulting from spinal ischemia caused by epidural abscess or hematoma or compromise to spinal circulation
- Meningitis

Other potential complications to be aware of include:

- High spinal blockade/subdural spread with rapid loss of consciousness, apnea, and refractory hypotension
- Intravascular injection causing local anesthetic toxicity or compromise to posterior circulation leading to cerebral ischemia (cerebrovascular accident)
- Pneumocephalus with headache, seizures, and loss of consciousness.[12] This can occur if air is used for the loss of resistance technique and a dural puncture occurs. Also, pneumocephalus, use of air is also associated with air embolism, an increased risk of dural puncture, and nerve root compression by air accumulation. Air myelopathy with upper and lower limb pain on injection and postinjection neurological deficit has also been reported.[13]
- Cerebral venous sinus thrombosis presents most commonly with headache but also visual disturbance, motor weakness, and seizures. It is postulated that a dural puncture causes a drop in cerebrospinal fluid pressure leading to compensatory venodilation and reduced flow.[14]
- Epidural lipomatosis, an accumulation of epidural fat caused mostly by exogenous steroid use. This can produce back pain and nerve root impingement producing radiculopathy.[15]

EQUIPMENT

- An intravenous (IV) cannula and sterile dressing. A cannula should be inserted using an aseptic technique prior to performing an epidural. This will allow rapid IV access in the event of complications requiring resuscitation. Note that cervical epidurals can trigger a vasovagal syncope, and a prophylactic dose of IV glycopyrrolate 200 μg may be helpful.
- Surgical hat, mask, sterile gown, and gloves. It is vital that this procedure is carried out in an aseptic manner.
- Skin preparation with povidone-iodine or chlorhexidine. This should be applied before opening equipment and drawing up drugs that will enter the epidural space, to avoid cross-contamination leading to neurotoxicity.
- Adequate sterile drapes for the patient and the image intensifier (X-ray machine) to prevent accidental desterilization of the operating field or equipment
- Sterile pointer to establish needle entry point
- 25G needle and 5 mL syringe for skin infiltration of local anesthetic
- 16–18G Tuohy needle and "Loss of Resistance" syringe
- 2 mL syringe and contrast medium (nonionic iodine-based agent)
- 5 mL syringe for administration of the epidural injectate.

EPIDURAL INJECTATE

For chronic pain indications, a combination of steroid and saline or a low dose of local anesthetic is used.

Administration of the steroid has a local anti-inflammatory role reducing the production of inflammatory mediators that trigger and perpetuate neural hypersensitivity and has actions that are not anti-inflammatory by producing membrane stabilization and nerve hyperpolarization.[16] It is common to use particulate steroids, either triamcinolone (40–80 mg) or methylprednisolone (40–80 mg); however, there are case reports attributing spinal and cerebral ischemia to embolization of the steroid particles. An alternative is preservative-free dexamethasone (4–8 mg), classified as nonparticulate and with no similar documented complications. However, it may be the case that dexamethasone offers a shorter duration of action.

Local anesthesia, usually bupivacaine or lignocaine, is used to reduce the pain and discomfort associated with administration of epidural steroid but may also have an anti-inflammatory effect. As with epidural injections, at all levels, it is important to minimize the amount of local anesthetic administered to reduce the blockade of motor and sympathetic outflow. The consequences of this at the cervical level are blockade of the phrenic and upper limb motor neurons and cardiac sympathetic stimulus leading to upper limb motor weakness, respiratory compromise, or apnea and bradycardia to full cardiac arrest.[17] It is advisable, therefore, to use concentrations of ≤0.125% bupivacaine and 0.5% lignocaine.

TECHNIQUE (INTERLAMINAR APPROACH)

The procedure should be performed on awake, cooperative patients. Sedation is a relative contraindication and has been associated with neurological sequelae.[18] If the patient is not fully compliant, then the procedure should be abandoned.

This is an interlaminar approach at C7/T1 or T1/T2. Poor positioning can lead to suboptimal fluoroscopic images and increase the risk of complications **(Fig. 3)**. Position the patient prone on the X-ray table with a pillow under their upper chest to encourage neck flexion that

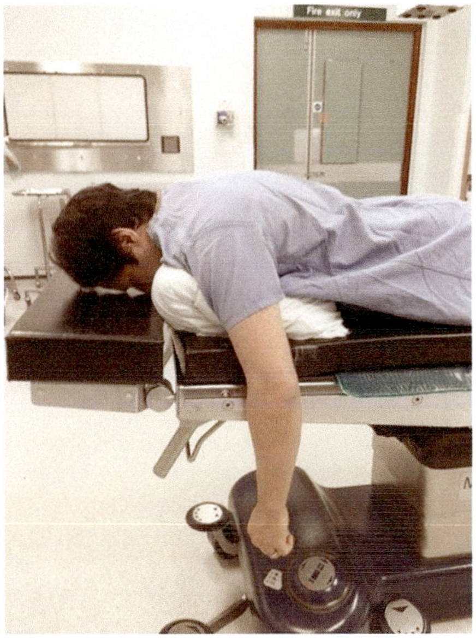

Fig. 3: Suboptimal neck flexion and shoulders obscuring C7/T1.

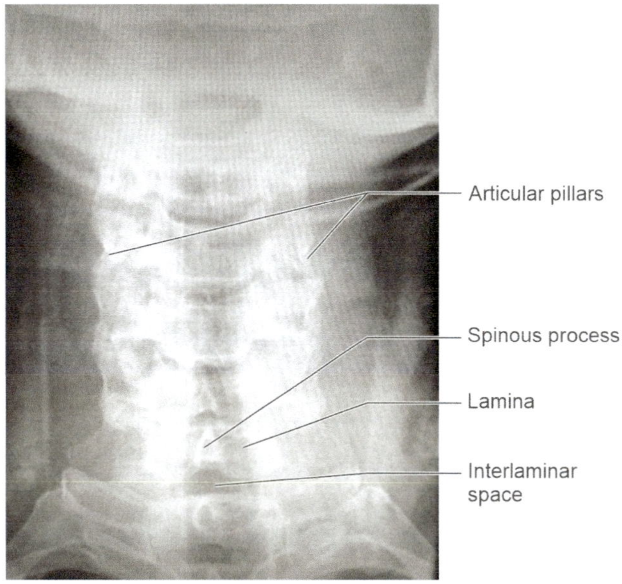

Fig. 5: Posterior–anterior (PA) cervical spine X-ray.

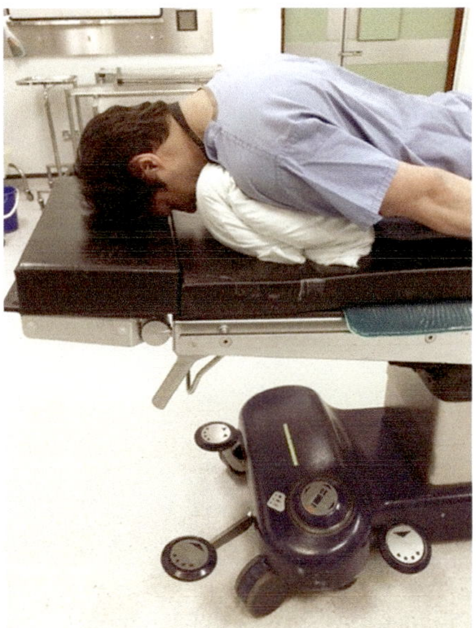

Fig. 4: Better neck flexion and shoulders extended to feet.

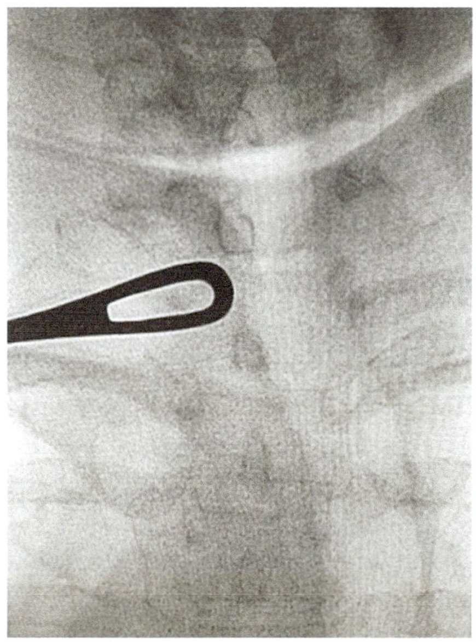

Fig. 6: Sterile pointer indicating needle entry point for interlaminar approach.

causes divergence of the spinous processes and increases the anteroposterior diameter of the epidural space. The arms should be by the patient's sides, and they should be encouraged to "reach for their trouser pockets" **(Fig. 4)** to lower the shoulders and improve the lateral view.

Be very clear to the patient that they cannot move during this procedure.

Prepare the skin and apply the drapes ensuring that the skin entry point over the lower half of the cervical spine is clean and accessible. Rotate the image intensifier laterally and cephalocaudally until an optimal image is obtained with the spinous processes in the midline and the vertebral endplates at the target level clear **(Fig. 5)**.

Use the sterile pointer to confirm the skin entry point with fluoroscopy **(Fig. 6)** and following local anesthetic skin infiltration, place the tip of the Tuohy needle at the interlaminar space **(Fig. 7)**.

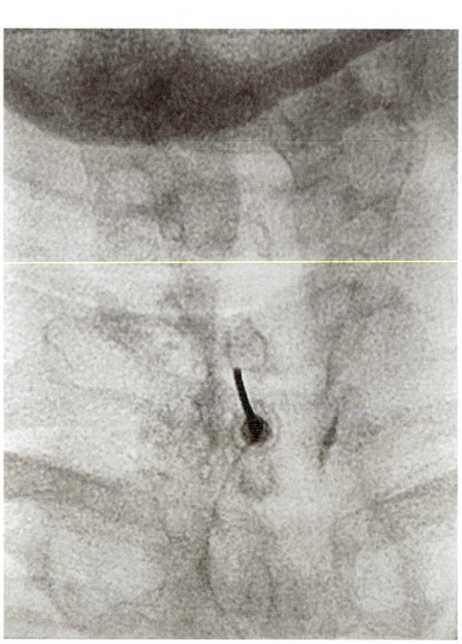

Fig. 7: Tuohy needle positioned between spinous processes.

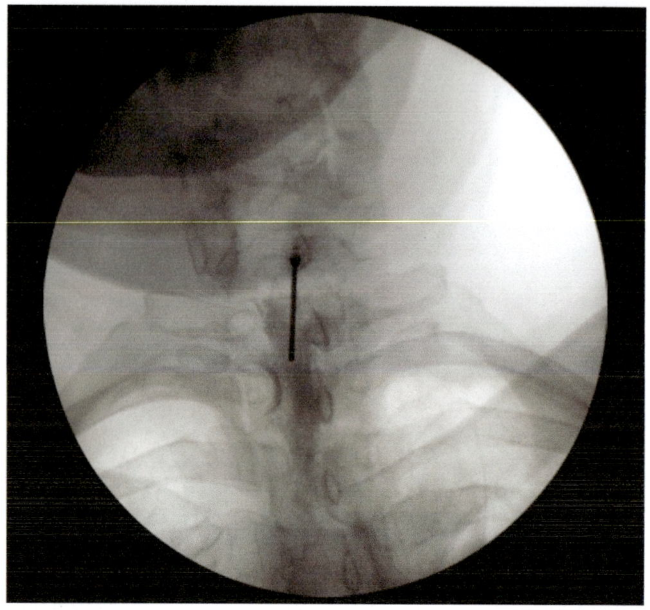

Fig. 8: Contrast spread into epidural and extraforaminal space, more on the left than on the right.

Aiming to contact the lamina first may reduce the risk of dural puncture, although it can be uncomfortable. Infiltrate the skin with local anesthetic.

Using tactile feedback and a loss of resistance to saline technique, advance the Tuohy needle toward the epidural space perpendicular to the skin. If you are uncertain about the needle trajectory and depth or the patient complains of pain, "stop and check". Use fluoroscopy in an anteroposterior and lateral views to ensure that the needle does not stray from the initial trajectory and to check depth. If radicular pain is precipitated by needle insertion, cord or root trauma may have occurred and contrast should not be injected to confirm position as this could potentiate further cord or root injury.

In the lateral view, loss of resistance should occur just anterior to the lamina and the tip of the needle should not advance beyond the posterior margin of the intervertebral foramen. Bear in mind that there may be no loss of resistance with midline placement, and great caution should be exercised when the needle tip is beyond the junction between spinous process and lamina (spinolaminar line). Try to avoid injecting more than a few milliliters of saline once in the epidural space as the resulting pressure may exacerbate radicular pains and cause the patient to move.

Confirm that the tip of the needle is in the epidural space by slowly injecting 1–2 mL of contrast and acquiring images in the anteroposterior **(Fig. 8)** and lateral **(Fig. 9)** views.

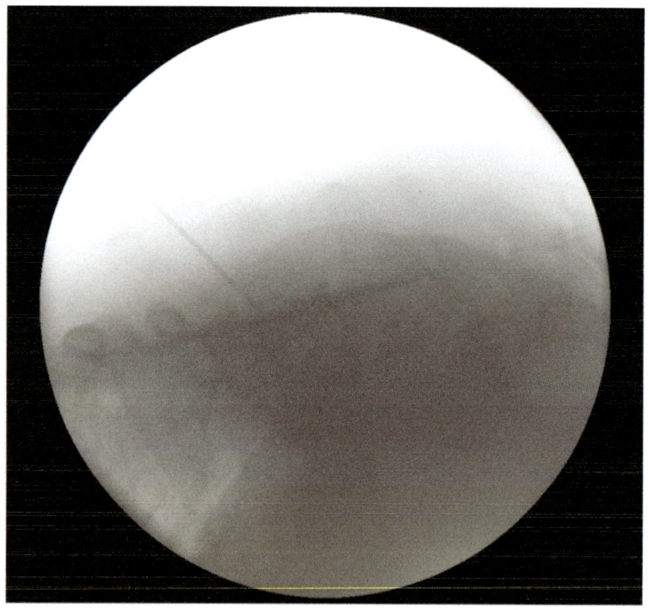

Fig. 9: Lateral view with contrast spreading cephalocaudal in the posterior epidural space. Tuohy needle near spinolaminar junction.

Continuous screening may provide additional reassurance, if vascular spread is suspected. Then, slowly inject 5 mL of the injectate in 1 mL aliquots stopping if the patient develops pain that does immediately resolve between each mL. 5 mL provides optimal distribution throughout the cervical spine.[19]

Remove the needle with stylet in situ and cover the entry point with a sterile dressing.

CONCLUSION

A cervical epidural steroid injection is a safe, effective, and ultimately rewarding treatment for upper limb radicular pain. However, patient selection, aseptic technique, and knowledge of fluoroscopic anatomy are essential in avoiding potentially catastrophic consequences.

REFERENCES

1. Zhao Q, Huang K, An J, Fang Q, Wen H, Qian X, et al. The distance from skin to cervical and high thoracic epidural space on chinese adults as read from MRI. Pain Physician. 2014;17(2):163-8.
2. Fujinaka MK, Lawson EF, Schulteis G, Wallace MS. Cervical epidural depth: correlation between needle angle, cervical anatomy and body surface area. Pain Med. 2012;13(5):665-9.
3. Manchikanti L, Cash KA, Pampati V, Wargo BW, Malla Y. Management of chronic pain of cervical disc herniation and radiculitis with fluoroscopic cervical interlaminar epidural injections. Int J Med Sci. 2012;9:424-34.
4. Manchikanti L, Malla Y, Cash KA, McManus CD, Pampati V. Fluoroscopic cervical interlaminar epidural injections in managing chronic pain of cervical postsurgery syndrome: preliminary results of a randomized, double-blind, active control trial. Pain Physician. 2012;15(1):13-25.
5. Manchikanti L, Malla Y, Cash KA, McManus CD, Pampati V. Fluoroscopic epidural injections in cervical spinal stenosis: Preliminary results of a randomized, double-blind, active control trial. Pain Physician. 2012;15(1):E59-70.
6. Simpson K, Baranidharan G, Gupta S. Spine Interventions in Pain Management, 1st edition. Oxford: Oxford University Press; 2012.
7. Manchikanti L, Cash KA, Pampati V, Wargo BW, Malla Y. A randomized, double-blind, active control trial of fluoroscopic cervical interlaminar epidural injections in chronic pain of cervical disc herniation: results of a 2-year follow-up. Pain Physician. 2013;16(5):465-78.
8. Manchikanti L, Cash KA, Pampati V, Malla Y. Fluoroscopic cervical epidural injections in chronic axial or disc-related neck pain without disk herniation, facet joint pain or radiculitis. J Pain Res. 2012;5:227-36.
9. Manchikanti L, Cash KA, Pampati V, Malla Y. Two-year follow-up results of fluoroscopic cervical epidural injections in chronic axial or discogenic neck pain: a randomized, double-blind, controlled trial. Int J Med Sci. 2014;11(4):309-20.
10. Horlocker TT. Regional anaesthesia in the patient receiving antithrombotic and antiplatelet therapy. Br J Anaesth. 2011;107(Suppl 1):i96-106.
11. Khan S, Pioro EP. Cervical epidural injection complicated by syrinx formation: a case report. Spine (Phila Pa 1976). 2010;35(13):E614-6.
12. Arora D, Mehta Y, Jain A, Trehan N. Headache and seizures after cervical epidural injection in a patient undergoing coronary artery bypass grafting. Ann Card Anaesth. 2012;15(3):244-6.
13. Mehta S, Khalil AA, Alshekhlee A. Air myelopathy following a cervical epidural injection. Pain Med. 2010;11: 1678 9.
14. Arguija AF. Cerebral venous thrombosis after cervical spine epidural injection. J Med Cases. 2013; 4:170-2.
15. Rustom DH, Gupta D, Chakrabortty S. Epidural Lipomatosis: a dilemma in interventional pain management for the use of epidural steroids. J Anaesthesiol Clin Pharmacol. 2013;29:410-1.
16. Collighan N, Gupta S. Epidural steroids. Contin Educ Anesth Crit Care Pain. 2010;10(1):1-5.
17. Stauber B, Ma L, Nazari R. Cardiopulmonary arrest following cervical epidural injection. Pain Physician. 2012;15(2):147-52.
18. Hodges SD, Castleberg RL, Miller T, Ward R, Thornburg C. Cervical epidural steroid injection with intrinsic spinal cord damage. Two case reports. Spine 1998;23(19):2137-42.
19. Lee SE, Joe HB, Park JH, Yi IK, Choi YH, Han KR, et al. Distribution range of cervical interlaminar epidural injections: a comparative study with 2.5 mL, 5 mL, and 10 mL of contrast. Pain Physician. 2013;16(2):155-64.

CHAPTER 30

Cervical Transforaminal Epidural Block

Shoji Ishigami, Steve M Aydin

ABSTRACT

Cervical epidurals are often done for the treatment of radiculopathy. The most common approach is the interlaminar approach and has been well described in the literature on its uses, treatment, and technique. Like the lumbar spine, in some cases, a transforaminal approach may be done. This technique is very specific and targeted to the nerve as it exits the neuroforamen. This approach has been documented as having risks. However, it may be helpful in a situation to treat one specific level, which is irritated in isolation, as well as help diagnose which nerve is specifically causing symptoms.

INTRODUCTION

The first cervical epidural injection was described by Dogliotti in the 1930s. However, for decades, cervical epidural injection was considered a high risk to be used as routine treatment for neck pain due to much narrower anatomical epidural space in the cervical spine (<2 mm at C7) compared to that of lumbar spine (<6 mm at L2). The risk was considerably minimized by advent of fluoroscopy and newer imaging technology, such as digital subtraction imaging.[1] Two main approaches, translaminar and transforaminal, are now commonly used to treat various types of pain that originate from the neck area used by interventional pain specialists.[2]

ANATOMY

As the name implies, epidural space is a space located outside the dura mater. Unlike the epidural space in the head, which is considered as a potential space, the epidural space in the spine is a true anatomical space that contains small arteries, intervertebral venous plexus, fatty tissues, lymphatics, and nerve roots.[2] The epidural space is contained anteriorly by the posterior longitudinal ligaments, posteriorly by the ligamentum flavum, and laterally by the pedicles and intervertebral foramina. It extends from the foramen magnum down to the sacrococcygeal junction.[3]

In cervical spine, the interspinous ligament is absent. The ligamentum flavum becomes thinner with higher cervical levels, and approximately half of individuals do not have fused ligament. Therefore, these structures provide less resistance to needle insertion and can mislead to dural or cord puncture when the loss-of-resistance technique is being used. The landmark for the cervical spine is C7 spinal process, which has the most prominent spinal process of the cervical spines and can be easily identified by palpation. The epidural space above C7 can be <2 mm and becomes much narrower at higher levels, making it more challenging to perform injection in the area. However, flexion of the head can increase the space to some extent.[2,4]

Another unique structure of the cervical spine is that the vertebral artery runs through the foramen transversarium of the transverse processes. The vertebral artery is in proximity to cervical nerve roots that traverse through their dura sleeves as they exit through intervertebral foramina. Intervertebral foramina are bordered above and below by the pedicles, anteriorly by vertebral artery and posteriorly by facet joint. The anterior and posterior tubercles on the pedicle create sleeve-like structure for the nerve root to sit on. The facet joint consists of the inferior articular process and the superior articular process of the vertebral body, above and below, respectively. In the cervical spine, the number of nerve root levels corresponds to the higher number of the two that create the intervertebral foramen (i.e., C3 nerve root comes out from C3-C4 intervertebral foramen).

It is also important to know that the epidural veins are located laterally within the epidural space with respect to spinal cord, making it more susceptible for venous puncture when a transforaminal approach is used.[3] Furthermore, the radiculomedullary artery, which feeds the anterior spinal artery, arises anywhere from C3 to C8. Occlusion of the radiculomedullary artery due to particulate injectate can cause anterior spinal cord syndrome.

INDICATIONS

The common indications for cervical epidural injections are:

- Cervical radiculopathy
- Cervical spondylosis
- Neck pain.[4]

Postherpetic neuralgia, complex regional pain syndrome resistant to sympathetic nerve block, postlaminectomy syndrome, and cervicogenic headache are also indicated; however, the supportive evidence is still lacking. Cervical epidural injection can also be utilized as a diagnostic tool when injected with short-acting anesthesia without steroid to identify the source neck pain.

According to a recent review of literatures, there is a good number of research evidence supporting the use of cervical epidural injection for cervical disk herniation or radiculitis.[5] The diagnostic cervical facet joint nerve block is also supposed by good evidence with a criterion standard of 75% or greater relief with controlled diagnostic blocks. However, a fair amount of evidence is present for axial or discogenic pain, spinal stenosis, and postcervical surgery syndrome. Also, there is a fair amount of evidence for conventional cervical radiofrequency neurotomy and cervical medial branch blocks. Lastly, evidence for use of cervical epidural steroid injection is limited for cervical intra-articular injections and cervical provocation discography.[6]

CONTRAINDICATIONS

Absolute Contraindications

Following are the absolute contraindications for cervical epidural injections:

- Patient refusal
- Infection at the injection site
- Coagulopathy
- Acute spinal cord compression
- Contrast allergy
- Bleeding disorders
- Pregnancy.

Relative Contraindications

Following are the relative contraindications for cervical epidural injections:

- Systemic infection
- Allergy to injectate
- Anatomic anomalies
- Severe cardiopulmonary conditions associated with decompensation triggered by postural changes required for injection procedure.

Careful medical screening should be provided to a patient's comorbidities, such as immune disorders, endocrine disorders, kidney diseases, and patients on anticoagulation or antiplatelet therapy.[5,6]

STEROID INJECTATES

Different steroid subtypes have different solubility properties in saline solution. Steroids such as methylprednisolone and triamcinolone tend to form large slugging aggregates of >100 μm.[7] Thus, methylprednisolone and triamcinolone sludge can block vasculature with diameter <100 μm—smaller arteries (20–50 μm), arterioles (10–15 μm), and capillaries (5–8 μm). Therefore, dexamethasone or betamethasone sodium phosphate, which has better solubility, is recommended for cervical epidural injection, especially for the transforaminal approach.[8]

EQUIPMENT IN THE PROCEDURE ROOM

A C-arm fluoroscopy should be used for proper visualization of the cervical spine anatomy from multiple angles. The procedure table should be able to accommodate prone and decubitus position of the patient and C-arm access. A motorized table with a prone headrest is recommended.[1,2]

Rescue protocols must be in place at any facilities at which cervical epidural injection is being performed. Transforaminal epidural steroid injections can result in potential life-threatening situations due to proximity to the vertebral arteries. The interlaminar epidural approach has a higher risk of hematoma, and subarachnoid or subdural injection can occur. Therefore, the procedure room must be equipped for advanced cardiopulmonary life support—suction, oxygen source, airway and intubation equipment, emergency antidotes and rescue drugs defibrillator, and cardiopulmonary monitoring equipment. All the patients should have intravenous access available prior to the procedure.[9]

Kit for Transforaminal Approach

- Sterile prep solution, either betadine or DuraPrep®
- Sterile clear fenestrated drape so that the patient's face can be visualized
- Three 3 mL syringes for local anesthetic, contrast, and steroid
- 25- or 27G needle, 5/8 to 1 inch for skin anesthesia
- Three extension tunings
- 25G, 2.5-inch short bevel needle
- 1% lidocaine for skin anesthesia
- Preservative-free 1% or 2% lidocaine
- Nonionic contrast—Omnipaque 240® or Isovue-M 200
- Betamethasone 6 mg/mL or dexamethasone 10 mg/mL.

Chlorhexidine can be used for patients with iodine allergy[10] for contrast, 1–2 mL of gadolinium (magnetized) can be used for patients who are allergic to nonionic contrast dye. However, gadolinium contrast shows up very faint under fluoroscopy and may not be suitable for transforaminal epidural injections.

PREPROCEDURE

As with any procedure, appropriate history should be obtained, and physical examination should be performed prior to the procedure. The risk for complications due to the procedure should be discussed with the patient, such as allergic reaction, bleeding, infection, nerve injury or damage, and postdural puncture headache (see complications below). After the risks and benefits are discussed, consent should always be signed by the patient and a witness prior to the procedure. Then, the patient is brought to the procedure room and the medical staff members in the procedure room should be introduced to the patient. A facial mask with a clear shield, lead apron, and radiation exposure badge should be always worn by the physician. All the instruments should be laid out on the sterile Mayo tray.[9]

The patient is secured in a prone position with a pillow under the chest with the neck flexed. The arms can be placed above the head or at the patient's sides if lateral X-ray is planned. The needle insertion area is prepped with skin prep using strict aseptic technique and left to dry. Sterile gloves should be worn, and sterile drapes should cover the patient's head and shoulders.[1,9]

If sedation is being administered, the patient should only receive minimal sedation so that the physician should be able to maintain verbal contact with the patient throughout the procedure.

The procedure should be paused or stopped if the patient becomes verbally unresponsive to lower the risk.

TRANSFORAMINAL EPIDURAL INJECTIONS

Technique

Although rare, transforaminal injection has a higher risk for arterial injection of particulate steroid resulting in thromboembolic ischemic infarct of spinal cord or cerebellum, resulting in death. Therefore, the physician who performs transforaminal epidural injection should be well trained in lumbar transforaminal epidural injection before attempting to perform cervical transforaminal epidural injection.[9]

The patient is placed in supine position (also oblique or lateral decubitus position can be done) and secured. Again, a minimal amount of sedation should be used on patient if sedation is required. As with cervical translaminar epidural injection, the patient should be able to feel painful stimuli and always maintain verbal communication with the physician.[7,8]

Patient's neck can be rotated slightly toward the contralateral side to maximize the surface area of the region of the neck to be injected.[11] The C-arm fluoroscopy is placed into an oblique plane and a 10–20° caudal tilt may be applied to best visualize the desired foramen in a straight line. The first intervertebral foramen visualized beneath the skull is comprised of C2-C3, and the C3 nerve root exits through this foramen **(Figs. 1A and B)**.[3]

The desired target site is the upper portion of the superior articular process at the tip of intervertebral foramen entrance. Thus, the needle should be aimed right above the nerve root of interest. After skin anesthesia with 1–2% local anesthetic is given, a 25 g, 2.5-inch short-bevel spinal needle is driven down to the upper portion of the superior articular process either under continuous fluoroscopic guidance or under small serial movements of the needle. The patient may complain about some pain in the neck or shoulder. However, if paresthesia is felt by the patient, then the needle needs to be withdrawn and redirected **(Figs. 2A and B)**.

Once the needle touches down on the superior articular process, the needle should be slightly withdrawn and redirected anteriorly or "walked off" the bone into the

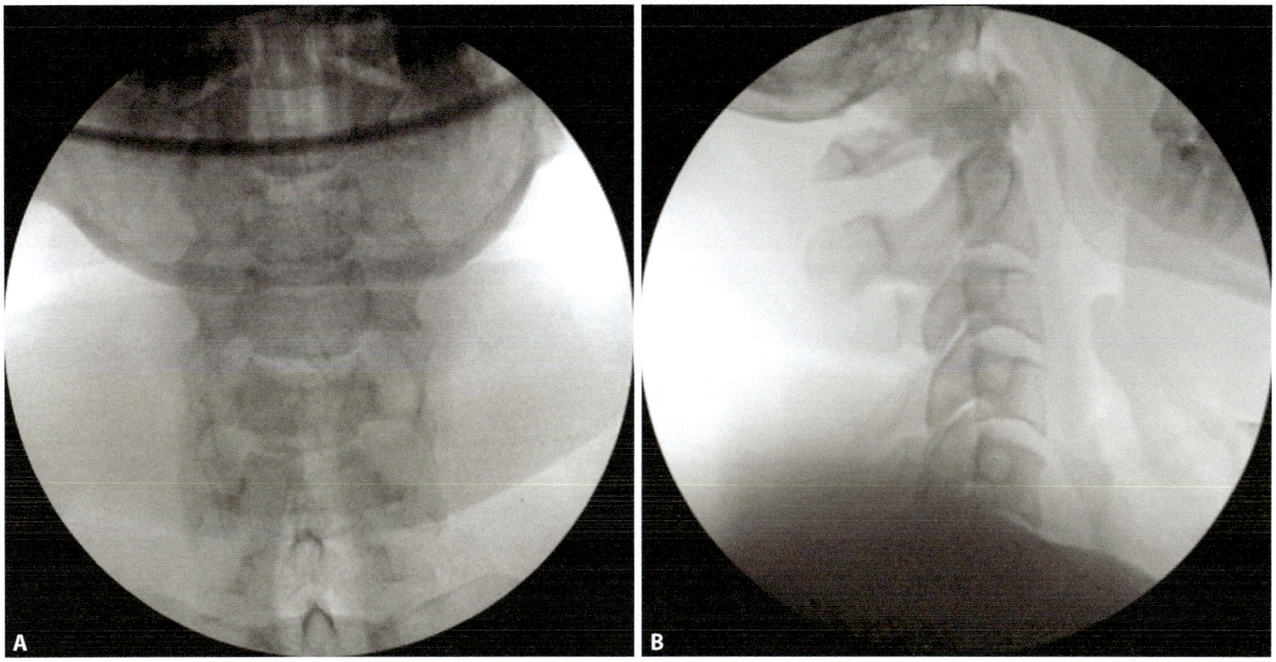

Figs. 1A and B: Anteroposterior and lateral cervical X-ray views of bony anatomy.

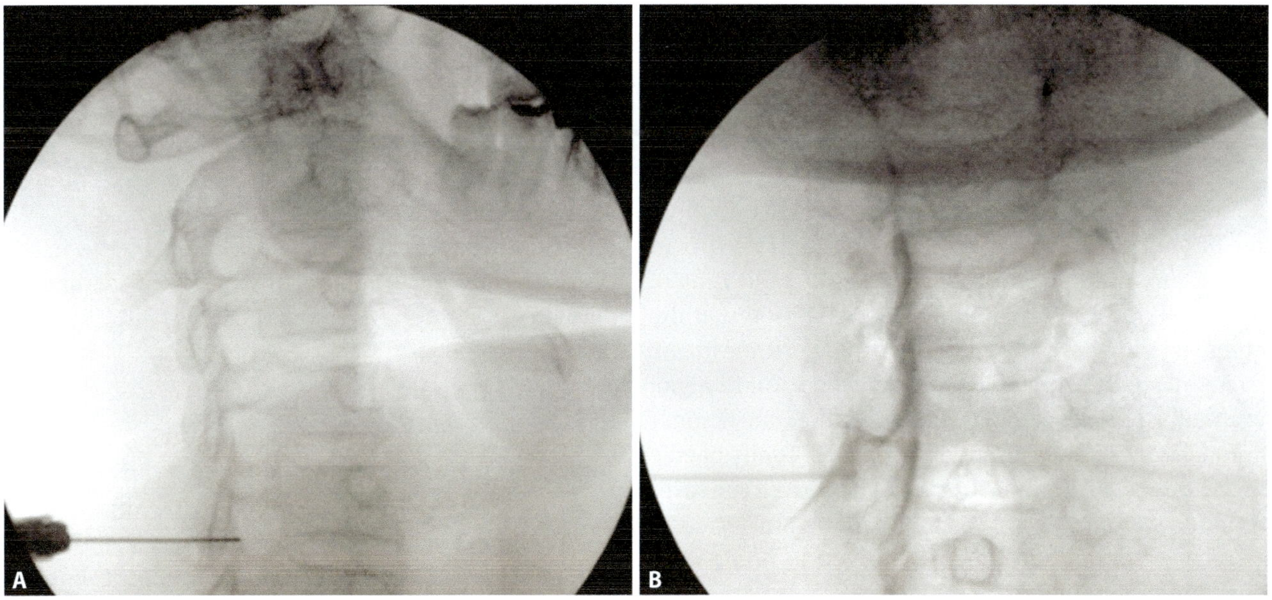

Figs. 2A and B: Oblique cervical view (A) with needle placement into the neuroforaminal, followed by anteroposterior view; (B) with contrast injection for epidural spread.

intervertebral foramen by only a few millimeters. Again, do not completely enter the foramen as the risk for arterial puncture becomes high. The needle position should be checked on anteroposterior (AP) image. Once the needle has been placed and no aspiration for cerebrospinal fluid and blood is confirmed, then 1 mL of nonionic contrast is injected. Again, contrast spread should be visualized by live fluoroscopy and the digital subtraction mode is very helpful to see the spread. If quick superior absorption of the contrast on live fluoroscopy is observed, this may

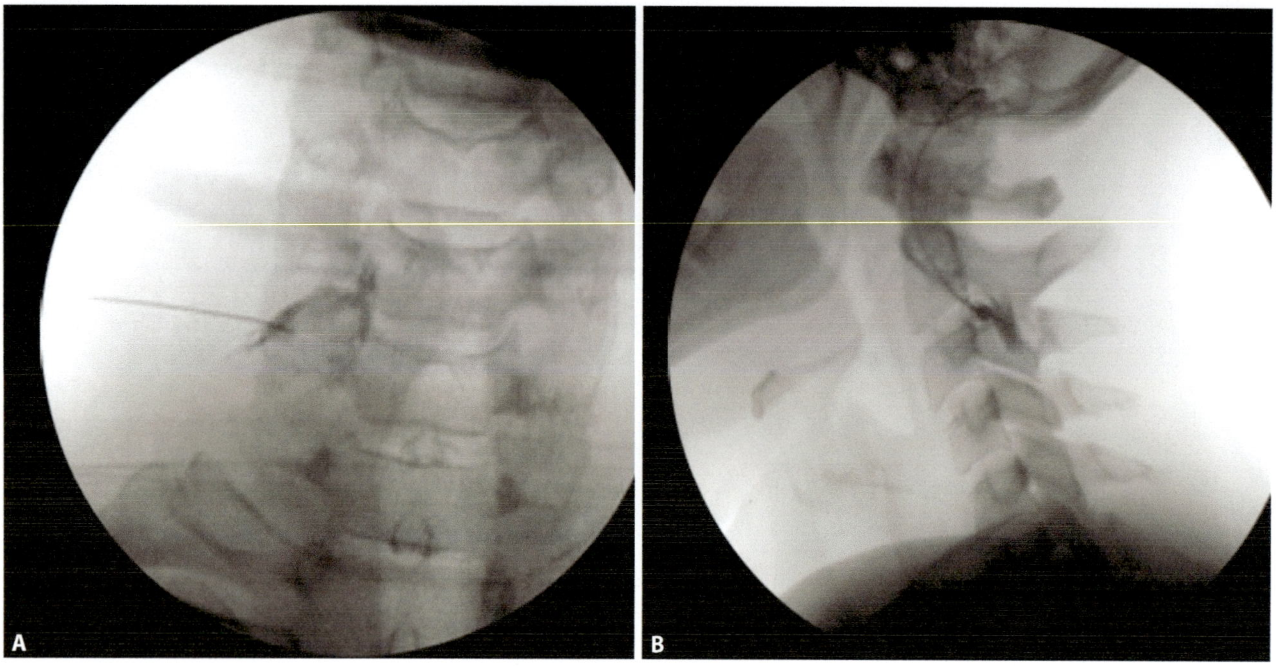

Figs. 3A and B: Anteroposterior (A) and lateral (B) views of needle placement and contrast for cervical transforaminal epidural steroid injections.

indicate a needle in the vertebral artery. Quick absorption with spread over the anterior surface of the vertebral body could signify flow into the radiculomedullary artery and anterior spinal artery. If either situation occurs, the needle is withdrawn and the procedure is aborted.[10] The needle should be repositioned if the subarachnoid flow of contrast is observed. If proper contrast spread tracking around the nerve root is observed, then 1 mL of 1% or 2% lidocaine can be injected. Make sure that the patient does not have any symptoms from local anesthetic toxicity. Then 6–12 mg of betamethasone or 10–12 mg of dexamethasone can be injected. As with the translaminar approach, the stylet is inserted back to the Tuohy needle before being withdrawn from the epidural space to minimize steroid tracking. The patient is transferred to the recovery room and then discharged to home after being found stable **(Figs. 3A and B)**.

Complications

The potential complications following transforaminal cervical epidural steroid injections are like those of translaminar epidural injections. However, there are additional complications, which should be noted. Notably, transient and increased radicular pain is one of the most common symptoms presented by the patient during the procedure and should go away with local anesthetic injection.

A severe complication is puncture into the radiculomedullary artery residing between C3 and C8, which can potentially cause anterior spinal cord syndrome by infracting anterior spinal artery.

Aside from direct spinal cord injury by the needle, thromboembolic ischemic infarct of the cerebellum through vertebral artery puncture can be fatal.[6]

CONCLUSION

Due to the nature of complex anatomy of the cervical spine, any attempt to perform epidural injections in this area should be approached with extreme caution. The physician who is performing the injection should have mastered lumbar epidural injections first. Advanced life support should be readily available when performing these procedures.

REFERENCES

1. Abbasi A, Malhotra G, Malanga G, Elovic EP, Kahn S. Complications of interlaminar cervical epidural steroid injections: a review of the literature. Spine (Phila Pa 1976). 2007;32(19):2144-51.
2. Braddom RL. Physical Medicine and Rehabilitation, 4th edition. Philadelphia, PA: Elsevier Inc; 2011. pp. 541-62.

3. Demondion X, Lefebvre G, Fisch O, Vandenbussche L, Cepparo J, Balbi V. Radiographic anatomy of the intervertebral cervical and lumbar foramina (vessels and variants). Diagn Interv Imaging. 2012;93(9):690-7.
4. Dogliotti AM. A new method of block anaesthesia: segmental peridural spinal anaesthesia. Am J Surg. 1933;20:107-18.
5. Han KR, Kim C, Park SK, Kim JS. Distance to the adult cervical epidural space. Reg Anesth Pain Med. 2003;28(2):95-7.
6. Huston CW. Cervical epidural steroid injections in the management of cervical radiculitis: interlaminar versus transforaminal. A review. Curr Rev Musculoskelet Med. 2009;2(1):30-42.
7. Tiso RL, Cutler T, Catania JA, Whalen K. Adverse central nervous system sequelae after selective transforaminal block: the role of corticosteroids. Spine J. 2004;4(4): 468-74.
8. Manchikanti L, Abdi S, Atluri S, Benyamin RM, Boswell MV, Buenaventura RM, et al. An update of comprehensive evidence-based guidelines for interventional techniques in chronic spinal pain. Part II: guidance and recommendations. Pain Physician. 2013;16(2)(Suppl 2):S49-283.
9. Safriel Y. Lumbar and cervical pain management procedures: when and how to do them. Appl Radiol. 2010;39(12):14-23.
10. Sviggum HP, Jacob AK, Arendt KW, Mauermann ML, Horlocker TT, Hebl JR. Neurologic complications after chlorhexidine antisepsis for spinal anesthesia. Reg Anesth Pain Med. 2012;37(2):139-44.
11. Windsor RE, Storm S, Sugar R, Nagula D. Cervical transforaminal injection: review of the literature, complications, and a suggested technique. Pain Physician. 2003;6:457-65.

31 CHAPTER

Cervical Medial Branch Block

Sanjeeva Gupta, Sanjay Varma, Risha Gupta

ABSTRACT

Cervical facet joints are the primary source of pain in 54% of patients complaining of neck pain postwhiplash injury after road traffic accident. In 54% of patients with cervicogenic headache, the source of pain is likely to be the C2/C3 facet joint. Of the lower cervical facet joints, the C5/C6 facet joint is most involved followed by C6/C7 and then C4/C5 and C7/T1 joints. Based on the pain referral maps shown in **Figure 1**, we can clinically identify the probable pathological joints to be blocked within ±one joint.

The cervical medial branch block (CMBB) and third occipital nerve block are diagnostic blocks to find out if the pain is originating from the facet joints blocked. In clinical practice, some patients get long-term pain relief (few weeks to few months) following these procedures. There are reported instances of local anesthetic and particulate steroids being injected into the blood vessels with catastrophic consequences. If steroids are used, a nonparticulate steroid such as a preservative-free dexamethasone is safer. Because of the high incidence of false-positive response following CMBB, it is recommended that patients get significant short-term pain relief following CMBB on two different occasions before radiofrequency denervation is considered. However, in clinical practice, significant short-term pain relief (on activities of daily living which produced pain before the injection) following the CMBB at the mid and lower cervical levels on one occasion is considered reasonable to proceed with radiofrequency denervation. It may also be reasonable to repeat the CMBB again if the block provided significant pain relief with improved quality of life for a prolonged duration.

INTRODUCTION

Cervical medial branch block (CMBB) and third occipital nerve block are diagnostic blocks to find out if the pain is originating from the facet joints blocked. Patients can have difficulty in understanding what a diagnostic procedure is and may expect the procedure to provide them with long-term pain relief and may get disappointed if their expectations are not met. In our experience it will be a good idea to explain the diagnostic nature of the procedure with the help of an Analogy/Metaphor "Electrical Light Switch (Facet Joint) > Electrical Wire (Nerve - Medial Branch) > Light Bulb (Brain)" and please refer to Chapter 7, page 56 in this book for more details. In clinical practice, some patients get long-term pain relief ranging between a few weeks to a few months following these procedures. This is difficult to explain but it is possible that the central sensitization that may have occurred due to poorly managed chronic pain that is blocked temporarily by the local anaesthesia used for medial branch block may contribute for the prolonged pain relief in addition the other factors. If CMBB provides significant pain relief for a short duration then radiofrequency denervation can be considered.

Cervical facet joints are the primary source of pain in 54% of patients complaining of neck pain postwhiplash injury after road traffic accident. Another common cause of facet joint pain is cervical spondylosis. The C3/C4 facet joint pathology can give rise to occipital headaches in addition to neck pain. In 54% of patients with cervicogenic headache, the source of pain is likely to be the C2/C3 facet joint. Of the lower cervical facet joints, the C5/C6 facet joint is most involved followed by C6/C7 and then C4/C5 and C7/T1 joints.

Dwyer et al.[1] studied the distribution of pain from cervical facet joints. Cervical facet joints from C2-C3 to C6-C7 were distended with contrast medium in volunteers. Each joint produced a clinically distinguishable, characteristic pattern of pain, which enabled the construction of pain maps **(Fig. 1)**. Other studies have also confirmed their findings.[2-4] There is some overlap between the distributions of pain produced by stimulating different joints.

Grubb and Kelly[5] studied 807 cervical discs over a period of 12 years and recorded the distribution of pain on stimulating the discs. Somatic referred pain originating from the cervical discs also follows a similar pattern of distribution as that produced by the facet joints. Diagnostic CMBB or provocation discography can inform us of the structure most likely responsible for pain. As CMBB is comparatively easier to perform it is prudent to investigate the facet joints first. Based on the pain referral maps shown in **Figure 1**, it may be possible to clinically identify the probable pathological joints to be blocked within ± one joint and decide which medial branches should be blocked.

There is a high incidence of false-positive response following CMBB. Barnsley et al.[6] studied 55 consecutive patients with neck pain for more than 3 months following a motor vehicle accident. Double blind controlled differential anesthetic blocks with 0.5% bupivacaine or 2% lignocaine were performed. The duration of pain relief was assessed in a double-blind fashion. Patients who had a longer duration of pain relief with bupivacaine were considered true positive. The incidence of false-positive rate with a single block was 27%. If patients have a positive response with the first block ideally it will be prudent to repeat the same block again to confirm the diagnosis before considering radiofrequency neurotomy. However, in clinical practice, significant short-term pain relief (on activities of daily living which produced pain before the injection) following the Cervical Medial Branch Blocks (CMBB) on one occasion at the mid and lower cervical levels is considered reasonable to proceed with radiofrequency denervation. It may also be reasonable to repeat the CMBB again if the previous block provided significant pain relief with improved quality of life for a prolonged duration. Please also consider going through to references 10 and 11 at the end of this chapter for additional information.

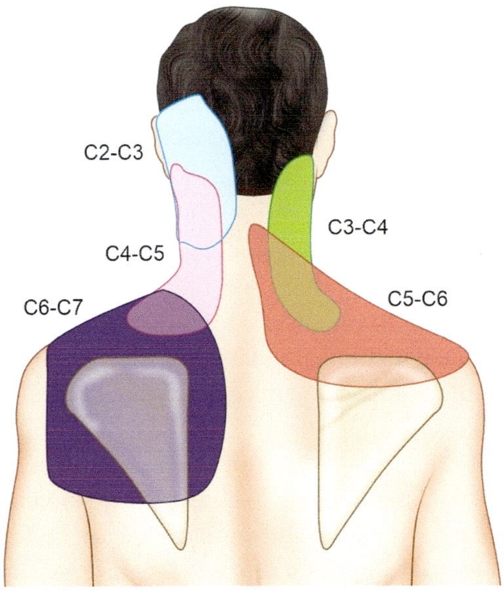

Fig. 1: Somatic referral pattern of pain originating from the cervical facet joints. It may be possible to localize the origin of pain within +one joint on the basis of this referral map.

GENERAL PRINCIPLES OF CERVICAL SPINE INTERVENTIONS

In the cervical spine, the structures are small and are close to each other. The spinal cord is vulnerable to overadvancement of the needle during interventions. The vascular structures such as the vertebral artery and epidural venous plexus are very close to the target point of injection **(Fig. 2)**. There are reported instances of local anesthetic and particulate steroid being injected into the

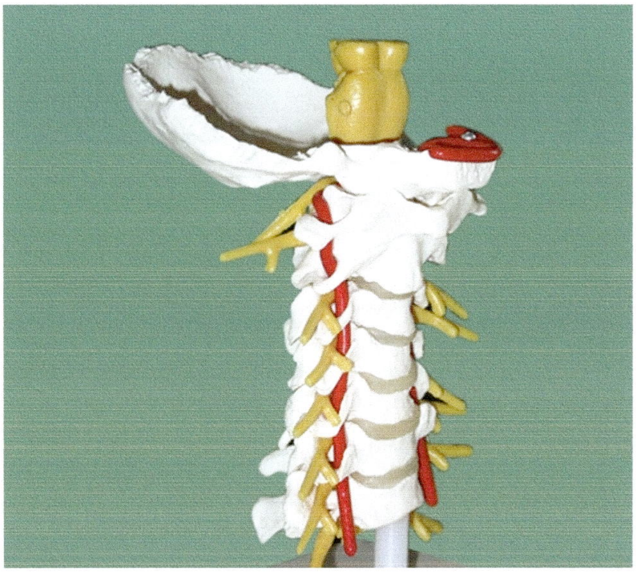

Fig. 2: Picture showing the structures around the cervical spine.

blood vessels with catastrophic consequences. The dome of the pleura can be injured causing pneumothorax when performing injections at or below C6 level, especially in patients with short neck. The esophagus and trachea can also be injured. The needle should be advanced very slowly and where necessary, fluoroscopic views should be obtained in multiple planes and proper interpretation of the contrast flow is important.

CERVICAL MEDIAL BRANCH BLOCKS

Anatomy: The cervical facet joint is formed by the inferior articular surface of the articular pillar above and the superior articular surface of the articular pillar below. The joint capsule is richly innervated. The articular branches from the C5 and C6 medial branches, which are the branches of the posterior primary rami, innervate the C5/C6 facet joint. The C6/C7 joint is innervated by the C6 and C7 medial branches and so on. Lord et al.[7] published a study in 1996 showing the variation in the location of the medial branches of the cervical dorsal rami which we think one should read before embarking on to cervical MBB/radiofrequency denervation.

The medial branches arise from the posterior primary rami and wrap around the waist of the respective articular pillar to give the rostral and caudal articular branches to supply the joints above and below as shown in **Figure 3**.

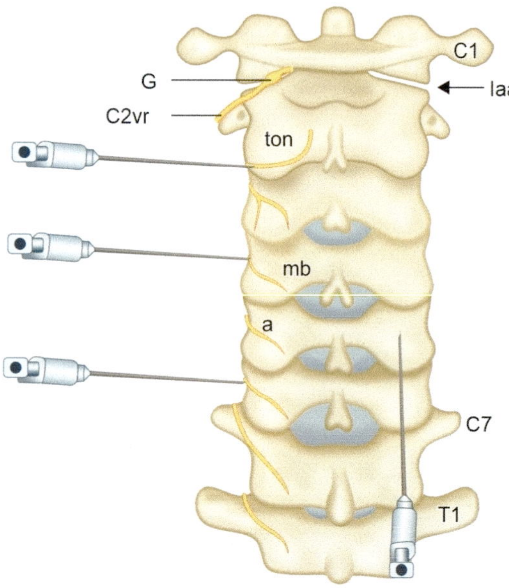

Fig. 3: Diagram showing the anteroposterior (AP) view of the cervical spine with medial branches (mb) and articular branches (a).

Indication

Neck pain not responding to conservative management.

Contraindications

- Patient unable to cooperate
- Patient allergic to medications used
- Operator unfamiliarity with the fluoroscopic image of the cervical spine or the landmarks for the CMBB not clearly visible on fluoroscopy.

Equipment

- Basic monitoring: *Noninvasive blood pressure* (NIBP) and SaO_2
- Resuscitation equipment
- Fluorescent table
- Image intensifier
- Cleaning agent and drapes
- 1% lignocaine for skin infiltration
- 22G intravenous (IV) cannula
- 5 cm (patient in lateral or supine position) or 10 cm (patient in prone position) curved tip 22G spinal needle
- 0.5% bupivacaine.

PATIENT POSITION, FLUOROSCOPIC ANATOMY AND PROCEDURE[8-11]

Cervical MBB can be done in prone, lateral, or supine position. We perform upper cervical MBB (up to C5 or C6 MBB) and the third occipital nerve block in lateral position and lower cervical MBB (C7 and sometimes C6 MBB) in prone position.

Cervical Medial Branch Block in Lateral Position

In the lateral fluoroscopic view of the cervical spine, the most prominent spinous process of C2 helps us to identify the levels of the cervical spine. Next, identify the vertebral body, the articular pillars and the spinous processes of each vertebra. To obtain appropriate fluoroscopic views appropriate patient positioning is critical. We ensure that appropriate fluoroscopic images have been obtained and target points identified before scrubbing for the procedure. If appropriate images are not obtained to facilitate the procedure it is reasonable to change the position, ask for help or cancel the procedure and come back another day. One of the authors (Dr Sanjeeva Gupta) has cancelled the procedure on at least one occasion as he could not identify the target points due to severe spondylosis of the cervical spine.

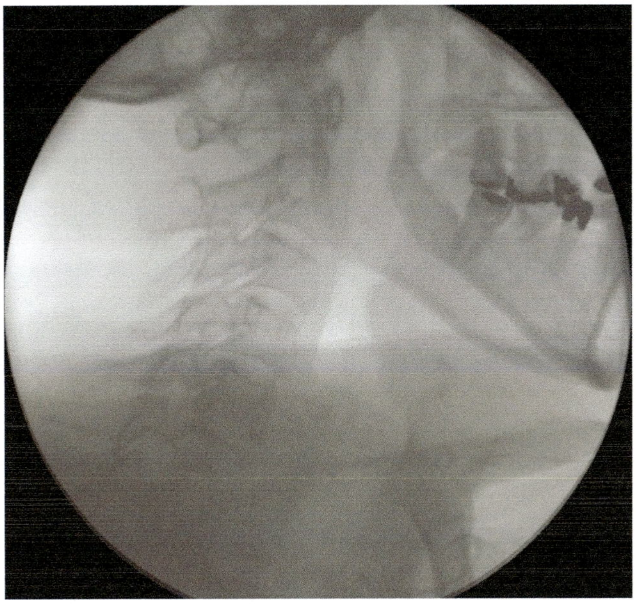

Fig. 4: Lateral image of cervical spine. The right and the left articular processes are not super-imposed. To get the correct image observe the movement of the vertical lateral margins of the articular process with right or left C-arm rotation under continuous fluoroscopy to super-impose the articular process in the vertical direction. Then tilt the C-arm in the cephalic or caudal direction to super-impose the facet joint lines in the horizontal direction to eliminate the parallax.

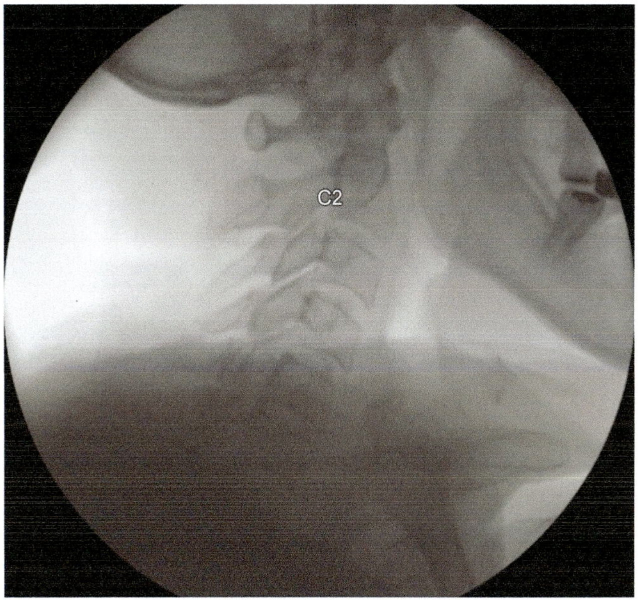

Fig. 5: After appropriate rotation of the C-arm to the right or left under continuous fluoroscopy and then tilting the C-arm in a cephalic or caudal direction, the right and the left articular pillars are superimposed. The facet joint lines appear crisp with the vertebral bodies and disk spaces outlined. This image is good to identify the target point for C3 medial branch block (MBB). The C-arm will need to be adjusted again if other MBBs are planned.

With the patient in the lateral position, either a pillow and/ or a folded sheet is kept under the head with the neck slightly flexed. The patient is asked to hold the flexed knee with their hands as this will retract the shoulders away from the neck/cervical spine and give a better fluoroscopic image. Fluoroscopic image is obtained to identify the landmarks for CMBB. The articular pillars of the right and left sides are superimposed by rotating the upper end of the image intensifier C-arm in the right or the left oblique direction under continuous fluoroscopy observing the direction of movement of the vertical sides of the articular pillars[8-12] **(Figs. 4 and 5)**. Once the articular pillars are superimposed we deliberately make it worse by rotating the C-arm to the right or left under continuous fluoroscopy to get the parallax image. This confirms that the initial image was appropriate as sometimes images obtained at the cervical level can be very deceptive and misguiding, which can lead to complications. The C-arm is then tilted toward the head (cephalad direction) or the feet (caudad direction) to superimpose the right and left facet joint line in the horizontal direction to obtain a crisp rhomboid image of the articular process at the level to be blocked **(Figs. 6 to 8)**. It may be necessary to follow the above process for each medial branch block.

Once an appropriate fluoroscopic image is obtained, the target point is identified, and local anesthetic injected to anesthetize the skin and subcutaneous tissue overlying the target area. A 22G 5 cm curved tip spinal needle is advanced in the direction of the X-ray beam using a gun barrel approach to contact the centroid of the articular pillar—the target area for the C4 to the C6 medial branch **(Figs. 9 and 10)**. Once the needle is in contact with the bone, it is withdrawn by about 1 mm and 0.5 mL of 0.5% bupivacaine is injected. This is repeated at each level to be blocked.

We use the prone position for C7 MBB, sometimes for C6 MBB and occasionally for C5 MBB if the patient has a short neck. When prone position is used a pillow is placed under the chest with the forehead resting on the bed with the head turned slightly to the opposite side to the proposed side of the intervention. The arm is tucked to the side and the shoulders are pulled toward the knees.

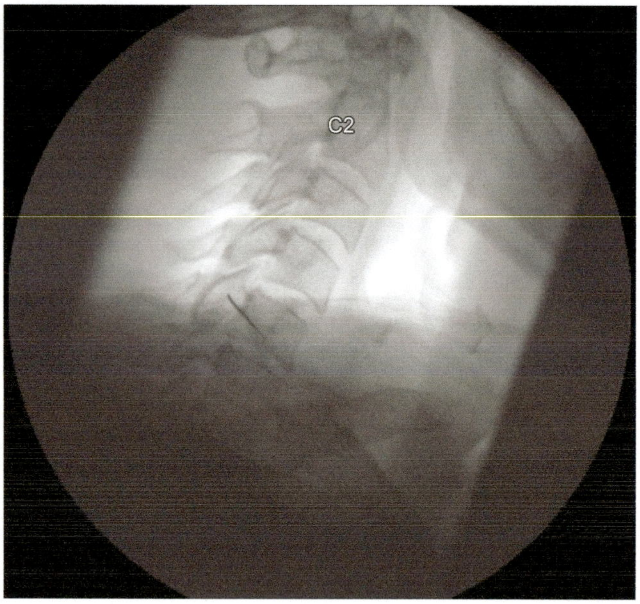

Fig. 6: Needle tip is at the target point to block the C5 medial branch block (MBB). Note that there is parallax at the C3 and C4 levels. The horizontal parallax along the facet joint line at the C4 level should be eliminated by cephalic or caudal tilt and the vertical parallax at the C3 level should be eliminated by right or left rotation before doing C4 and C3 MBB, respectively.

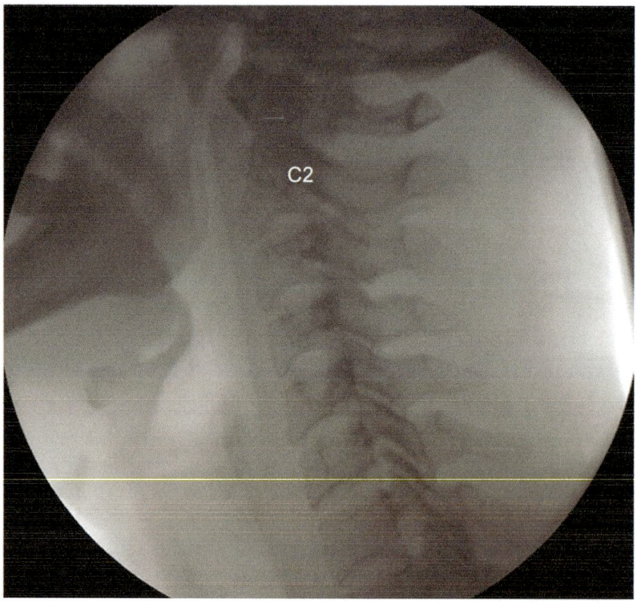

Fig. 7: In this image, there is parallax at the C5 and C6 levels. Tilting the C-arm in a cephalic or caudal direction will eliminate the parallax.

Prone position can be used for upper cervical MBB also and, in fact, may be safer for some interventionists provided they understand the fluoroscopic anatomy!

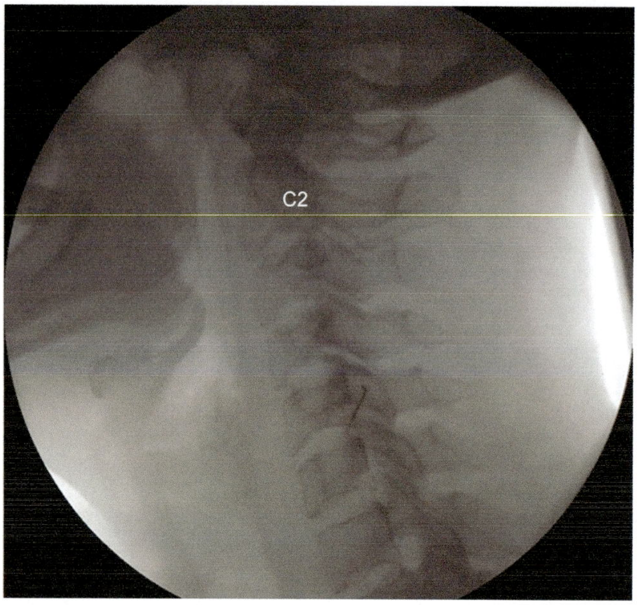

Fig. 8: Tilting the C-arm has eliminated the parallax at C5 level. The needle tip is at the target point for C5 medial branch block (MBB).

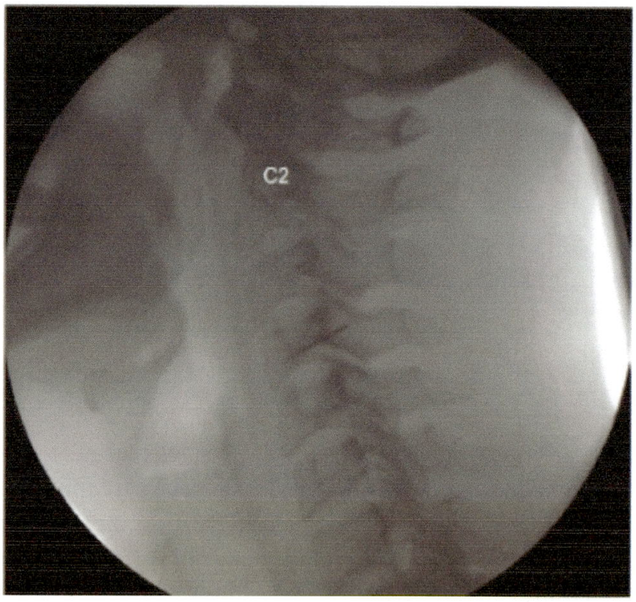

Fig. 9: Needle tip at target point for C4 medial branch block (MBB).

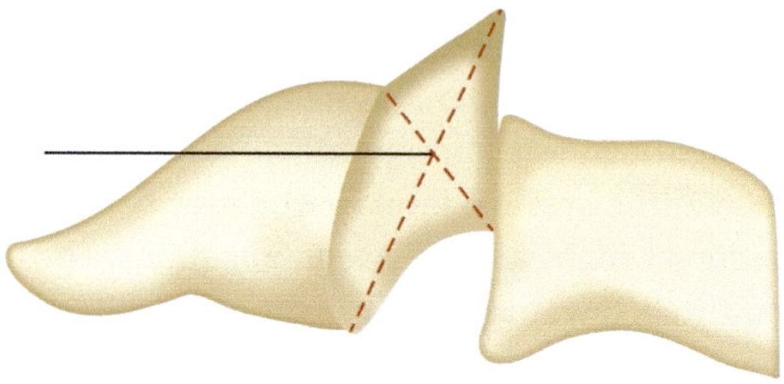

Fig. 10: Diagram showing the centroid of the articular pillar.

Cervical Medial Branch Block in Prone Position

A true anteroposterior (AP) view is obtained with the spinous processes in between the two pedicles. The C-arm is then tilted in the cephalad or caudad direction to display the facet joints which appear like transverse lines as can be seen in **Figures 11 and 12**. The skin and subcutaneous tissue over the target point which is in the lateral aspect of the mid-portion of the lamina as shown in **Figures 11 and 12** (most medial portion of the waist of the lamina) is infiltrated with 1% lignocaine. A 22G, 10 cm long spinal needle with a curved tip is aimed at the target point along the beam of the X-ray using the gun barrel technique. Once the needle is at the target point the position of the tip of the needle is adjusted in the lateral view to be in the center of the articular process/rhomboid and 0.5 mL of either 0.5% bupivacaine or 2% lignocaine is injected at each level. Sometimes it can be difficult to obtain a proper lateral view in prone position.

C7 MBB in prone position. The superior articular process (SAP) and the transverse process (TP) of C7 vertebra which will appear like the front of a "boot" is identified (Fig. 11—arrow pointing toward the junction of the SAP and TP; Fig. 13). The TP of the C7 points downwards and that of T1 points upwards. The location of the C7 medial branch can be variable. We use a 10 cm long 22G spinal needle when we perform cervical MBB in the prone position. The distal 5–7 mm of the needle is bent in

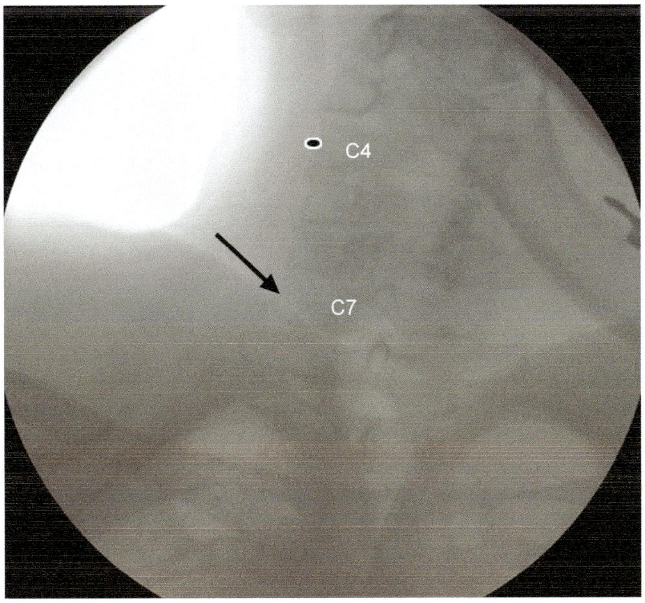

Fig. 11: Anteroposterior (AP) view of the cervical spine. The target point for the medial branch block (MBB) is the most medial aspect on the waist of the respective articular pillar. This image is appropriate for C4 MBB. The arrow points to the junction of the SAP and the TP of C7 which appears like the front of a "boot" (*see* text).

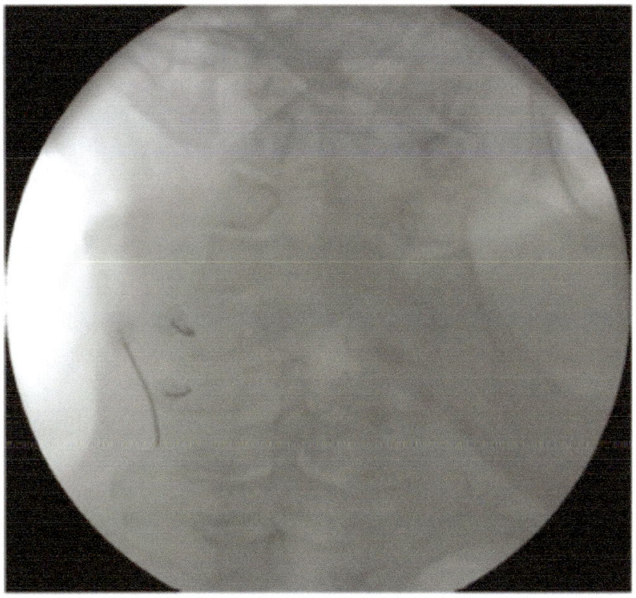

Fig. 12: Anteroposterior fluoroscopic image of cervical spine with needle tips in position for left C5, C6, and one of the target points for the C7 medial branch block (*see* text).

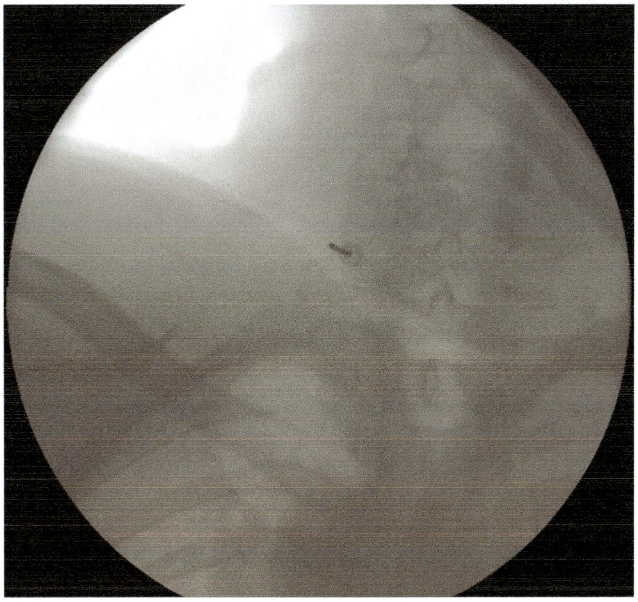

Fig. 13: Needle tip at the base of the superior articular process at its junction with the transverse process, one of the target points for C7 medial branch block (*see* text).

the direction of the bevel by about 5–7° to facilitate needle navigation to the target point. The needle is directed along the X-ray beam to the three target points:

1. The base of the SAP at its junction with the TP
2. The apex of the SAP of C7
3. The third point is collinear with the second point but lies 3 to 5 millimeters more superficially.

Bupivacaine 0.5%, 0.5 mL is injected at each of the three target points.

THIRD OCCIPITAL NERVE BLOCK

Anatomy

Two medial branches are formed from the C3 dorsal ramus. The deep medial branch is the same as the medial branches at the lower cervical levels and crosses the C3 articular pillar to innervate the C3/C4 facet joint along with the C4 medial branch.

The superficial medial branch of the C3 dorsal ramus is the third occipital nerve, which runs along or close to the C2/C3 facet joint and innervates the C2/C3 facet joint. It also innervates the skin over the suboccipital area.

Indications

- Cervicogenic headache
- Upper neck pain.

Contraindications

- Patient unable to cooperate
- Patient allergic to medications used
- Operator unfamiliarity with fluoroscopic image of the cervical spine or the land marks for the CMBB not clearly visible on fluoroscopy.

Patient Position, Fluoroscopy, and Procedure

We perform third occipital nerve block in lateral position. A true lateral view is obtained by right or left rotation and cephalad or caudal tilt as described for the CMBB. We particularly observe the upper border of C2 spinous process and eliminate double shadow to obtain a crisp single line of the upper border of the C2 spinous process. This maneuver invariably improves the visibility of the C2/C3 facet joint line. After obtaining the appropriate image as shown in **Figure 14**, we advance a 5 cm curved tip 22G spinal needle in the direction of the X-ray beam using a gun barrel approach to the three target points. The three target points are identified as under—an imaginary vertical line is drawn to bisect the C2/C3 facet joint line and the three target points are along this vertical bisector line as under **(Figs. 14 to 17)**:

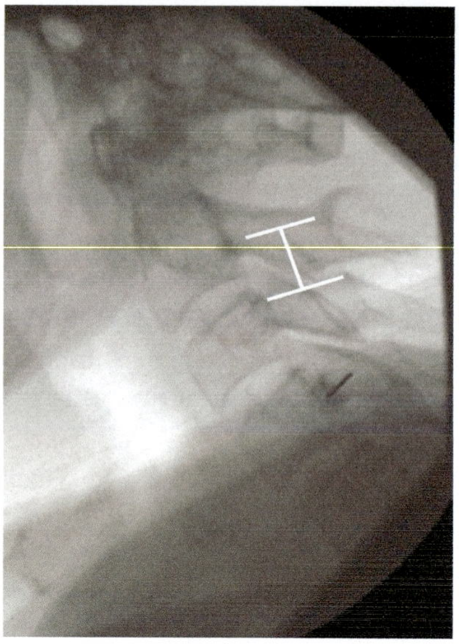

Fig. 14: Image shows the imaginary line bisecting the C2-C3 facet joint line and the upper and the lower target points along the bisecting line (*see* text).

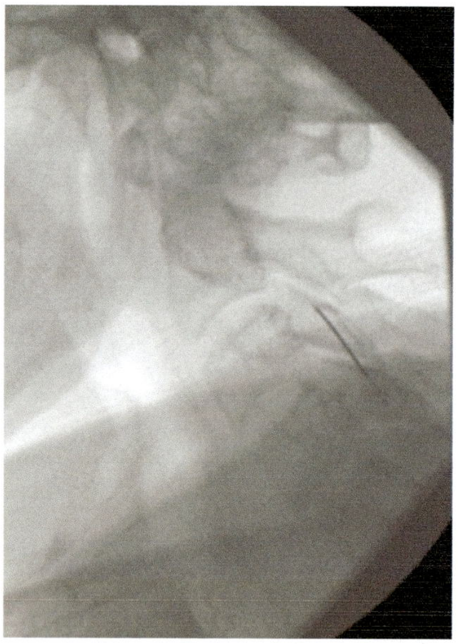

Fig. 15: Needle tip at the lower target area for third occipital nerve block (*see* text).

1. A point on the bisecting line at the level of the base of the C2-C3 intervertebral foramen, the target for the lowest location of the nerve
2. A point on the bisecting line opposite the apex of the SAP of C3, the target for the highest known location of the third occipital nerve

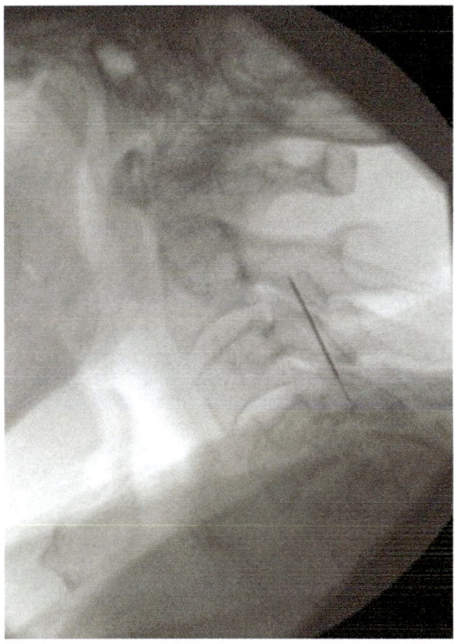

Fig. 16: Needle tip at the upper target area for third occipital nerve block (*see* text).

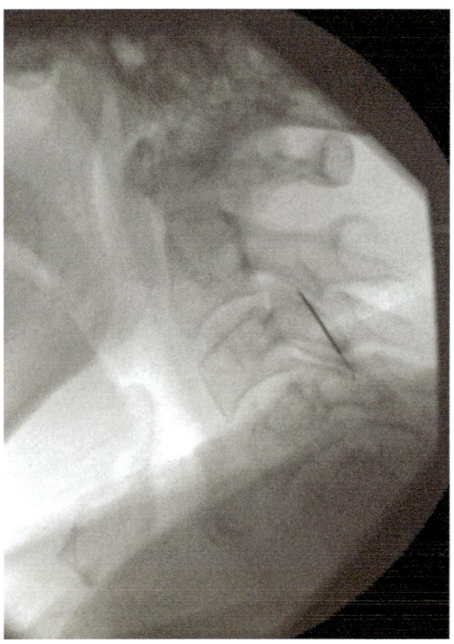

Fig. 17: Needle tip at the mid-target area for third occipital nerve. The needle tip should lie on the bone at the superior edge of the C3 articular process along the bisecting line (*see* text).

3. The third target point lies halfway between the first and the second points which is the most common location of the third occipital nerve. If this point is over the joint, there is a risk of entering the joint and hence it is recommended that the target point is chosen to lie over the most superior part of the C3 articular pillar along the bisecting line.

0.3 mL of 0.5% bupivacaine is injected at each of the three target points. For the third occipital nerve to be technically adequate, patient should develop an area of numbness in the corresponding occipital area. Images should be saved for medico-legal purposes and also to assist in planning for radiofrequency denervation procedures if this is necessary in the future. We normally block only one side at a time. As the upper cervical proprioceptors which are critical for tonic neck reflexes are anesthetized patients may report a sense of ataxia following the third occipital nerve block, especially if this is done bilaterally. If this occurs, to compensate, they should be advised to engage and rely on visual cues. Patients should be advised to always focus on horizontal objects such as window frames or door frames or the horizon itself. They should be warned that if they look downwards and if they look sideways to a companion they will incur the sense of unsteadiness and so must avoid these actions.[13] We do not do bilateral third occipital nerve block because of these reasons.

Assessment

As indicated earlier, CMBB and occipital nerve blocks are diagnostic procedures, and it is vital that the pain relief is assessed before the patient is discharged. We assess patients before the procedure and ask them to consider the pain they have at rest and on moving the neck in flexion, extension, and lateral bending as 100% of their pain. After the procedure, we assess the patients again before they are discharged (about 30–60 minutes after the procedure. Do not use sedation for diagnostic procedures). We assess the amount of pain relief they have had at rest and on moving the neck in different directions following the CMBB (compared to the pain they had before the procedure). We also ask the patient if the pain relief after the procedure is significant in their opinion. The percentage of pain relief after CMBB and if the pain relief is significant or not is recorded in the patient's notes. It is important to remember that there can be more than one pain generator in the neck and we may not be able to identify or treat each one of them.

Complications

Complications of CMBB include inadvertent spinal cord injury, dural puncture or injection into the dural sleeve. Obtaining appropriate fluoroscopic images can decrease the chances of such serious problems. Inadvertent injection of local anesthesia into the vertebral artery can cause serious problems. Injury to the dome of the pleura is a possibility if the block is done at or below the C6 level. We also advise patients to avoid an aeroplane journey up to 7 days post-procedure.

We recommend that physicians perform an adequate number of interventions (about 100 procedures) at the lumbar levels before performing interventions at the cervical and thoracic spine levels. We would also suggest that it may be a good practice to visit and observe your colleagues who are regularly performing procedures at the cervical spine levels and also consider having them with you when you start performing these procedures.

Clinical Pearls

To assist with assessing patients with neck pain and performing blocks subsequently, we have provided a flow diagram for the blocks to be considered when patients present with middle and lower neck pain **(Flowchart 1)** and upper neck pain **(Flowchart 2)**.

Assess the patient and find out if the pain is more in the upper or the lower part of the neck. We also put in some effort to find out if the patient has more pain on the right or the left side. We generally do the procedure on only one side at a time. In a good number of patients in our experience, the pain starts on one side and then spreads to the opposite side (referred pain) and in such cases,

Flowchart 1: Cervical facet joint pain algorithm in clinical practice (for middle and lower neck pain).

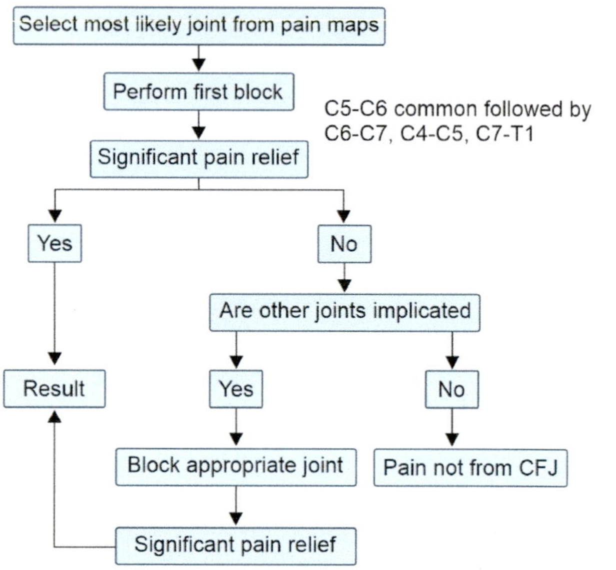

(CFJ: cervical facet joint)

Flowchart 2: Cervicogenic headache algorithm (for upper neck pain).

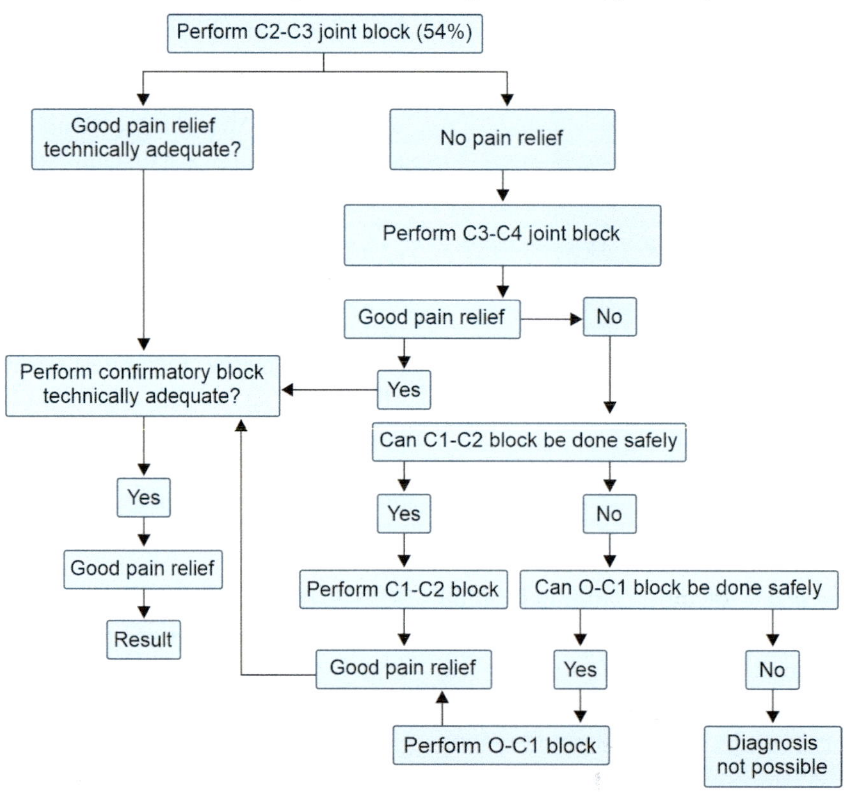

we do the CMBB on the side, where the pain originates and assess the pain relief on both sides after the procedure and document. This assists us to plan for the future.

If the pain is more in the upper part of the neck, look for referred pain in the occipital region and other parts of head. If the pain starts in the neck and then spreads to the occipital area and other parts of the head, suspect cervicogenic headache and consider performing the third occipital nerve block and assess the patient after the procedure.

If the pain starts in the lower part of the cervical spine and gets referred in between the scapula or the suprascapular area and/or the upper arm, then suspect lower cervical facet joint problem and block the C5, C6, +/-C4, +/-C7 MBB and assess the patient after the procedure.

CONCLUSION

Cervical MBB and third occipital nerve blocks are diagnostic blocks. If the patient derives good pain relief for a significant duration following the procedure they can be repeated.

Sound knowledge of the fluoroscopic anatomy of the cervical spine is essential when performing interventions in the cervical spine area. It is entirely appropriate to postpone or abandon the procedure if the target points are not identified on fluoroscopy. We would also suggest that it will be good practice to visit your colleagues who perform these procedures on a regular basis and also consider having them with you as a guide when you start performing procedures as the cervical spine level. Because of the high incidence of false-positive response following CMBB, some recommend that patients should get significant short-term pain relief following CMBB on two different occasions before radiofrequency denervation is considered. However, in clinical practice, significant short-term pain relief (on activities of daily living which produced pain before the injection) following the CMBB on one occasion at the mid and lower cervical levels is considered reasonable to proceed with radiofrequency denervation. It may also be reasonable to repeat the CMBB again if the procedure provided significant pain relief with improved quality of life for a prolonged duration.

REFERENCES

1. Dwyer A, Aprill C, Bogduk N. Cervical zygapophyseal joint pain patterns. I: A study in normal volunteers. Spine (Phila Pa 1976). 1990;15(6):453-7.
2. Barnsley L, Lord SM, Wallis BJ, Bogduk N. The prevalence of chronic cervical zygapophyseal joint pain after whiplash. Spine (Phila Pa 1976). 1995;20(1):20-6.
3. Aprill C, Dwyer A, Bogduk N. Cervical zygapophyseal joint pain patterns. II: A clinical evaluation. Spine (Phila Pa 1976). 1990;15(6):458-61.
4. Fukui S, Ohseto K, Shiotani M, Ohno K, Karasawa H, Naganuma Y, et al. Referred pain distribution of the cervical zygapophyseal joints and cervical dorsal rami. Pain. 1996;68(1):79-83.
5. Grubb SA, Kelly CK. Cervical diskography: clinical implications from 12 years of experience. Spine (Phila Pa 1976). 2000;25(11):1382-9.
6. Barnsley L, Lord S, Wallis B, Bogduk N. False-positive rates of cervical zygapophyseal joint blocks. Clin J Pain. 1993;9(2):124-30.
7. Lord SM, Barnsley L, Wallis BJ, McDonald GJ, Bogduk N. Percutaneous radio-frequency neurotomy for chronic zygapophyseal-joint pain. N Engl J Med. 1996;335(23):1721-6.
8. Gupta S, Dhandapani K. Applied anatomy and fluoroscopy for spinal interventions. In: Simpson K, Baranidharan G, Gupta S (Eds). Oxford Specialist Handbook in Pain Medicine: Spinal Interventions in Pain Management. Oxford: Oxford University Press; 2012. pp. 1-10.
9. The British Pain Society and Faculty of Pain Medicine of the Royal College of Anesthetists. Standards of Good Practice for Spinal Interventional Procedures in Pain Medicine. London: The British Pain Society; 2015.
10. Gupta S, Baranidharan G, Sharma M, Gupta H. Fluoroscopy for minimally invasive spinal and trigeminal procedures. In: Atlas of Interventional Pain Management Procedures - A Stepwise Approach. Eds: Baheti DK, Gupta S, Bakshi S, Gehdoo RP. Jaypee Brothers Medical Publishers, Ltd. India. 2023. pp 3-26.
11. Gupta S, Ghai B Cervical Medial Branch Block. In: Atlas of Interventional Pain Management Procedures—A Stepwise Approach. Eds: Baheti DK, Gupta S, Bakshi S, Gehdoo RP. Jaypee Brothers Medical Publishers, Ltd. India. 2023. pp 82-7
12. Cervical Medial Branch Blocks. In: Bogduk N (Ed). Practice guidelines for spinal diagnostic and treatment procedures, 2nd edition. San Francisco, California: International Spinal Intervention Society; 2013. pp. 101-39.
13. Third Occipital Nerve Blocks. In: Bogduk N (Ed). Practice guidelines for spinal diagnostic and treatment procedures, 2nd edition. San Francisco, California: International Spinal Intervention Society; 2013. pp. 141-63.

32 CHAPTER

Cervical Medial Branch Blocks and Radiofrequency Neurotomy

Shruti G Kapoor, Samir N Shah

ABSTRACT

Cervical spondylitis is a common and disturbing pain problem facing all age population. This chapter deals with a stepwise description of performing of cervical median branch neurotomy by using radiofrequency lesioning.

DEFINITION

It is estimated that the facet joint is a source of nociception in 36–67% of individuals with persistent neck pain.[1-3] Severe facet arthrosis can cause myelopathy[4] and degenerative spondylolisthesis of cervical spine.[5] Cervical medial branch block (CMBB) is a diagnostic procedure designed to assess if the patient's neck and/or shoulder pain is secondary to cervical facet arthropathy. To achieve this aim, the nerves innervating the zygapophysial or facet joints in the neck, medial branches of the cervical dorsal rami, are anesthetized using local anesthetic. If this leads to significant improvement in a patient's pain, the block can be followed by radiofrequency neurotomy of these nerves.

ANATOMY (FIG. 1)

Facet joints are "true joints"; that is, they are formed by two opposing cartilaginous surfaces and have a synovial lining. The facet joints are located posterolaterally, at the junction of the pedicle and transverse process. They are formed by the inferior articular pillar of the superior vertebral body and the superior articular pillar of the inferior vertebral body. In the cervical spine, the joints are oriented almost parallel to the axial plane. This allows for cervical flexion, extension, and rotation. The joints are innervated by the medial branch of the dorsal primary ramus.[6] This runs along the centroid of the articular pillar, where it can be easily targeted. Each joint is innervated by the nerve at that level and by a descending branch from the nerve above. Both these nerves are anesthetized to anesthetize the joint.

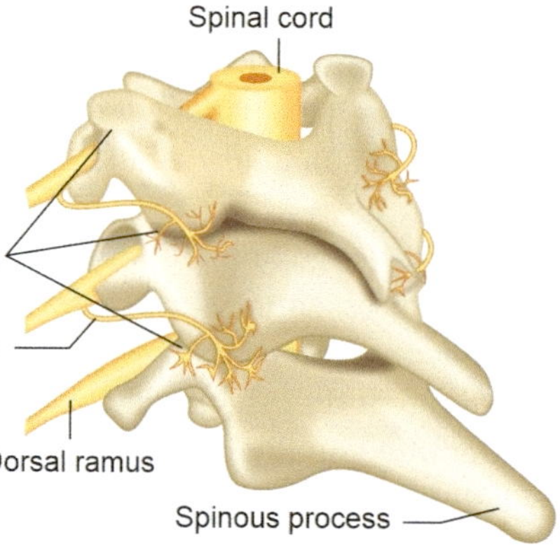

Fig. 1: Cervical facet joint anatomy.

CLINICAL PRESENTATION

Patients with facet arthropathy usually present with axial neck pain. They may report a gradual onset of pain years ago without any clear inciting events, followed by progressive worsening. Alternatively, pain may be of acute onset following a whiplash (sudden flexion–extension) injury, during a motor vehicle accident for instance. Patients describe the pain as a deep, dull ache that is worse with neck movement. Pain may refer to the shoulder. High cervical spine facet disease may also present with headaches, especially if the third occipital nerve is involved.

Physical examination typically reveals tenderness to palpation of paraspinal muscles. Range of motion is usually decreased in extension, and facet loading leads to pain. These physical examination findings, however, are not very sensitive or specific.[7]

These pain complaints, however, may also be explained by disk disease or muscle injury. Thus, to definitively diagnose facetogenic pain, diagnostic medial branch blocks are performed. These are diagnostic and in some ways predictive. Opinion varies as to how much relief should be achieved with diagnostic medial branch blocks before radiofrequency lesioning is performed.[8] It is agreed that significant relief following diagnostic medial branch blocks points to a facetogenic pain etiology and can be followed up by radiofrequency lesioning.

INDICATIONS

Cervical diagnostic medial branch blocks are performed in individuals complaining of axial neck pain that is thought to be facetogenic in nature. If diagnostic blocks lead to at least 50% pain relief, it may be followed by radiofrequency neurotomy.

CONTRAINDICATIONS

Contraindications to facet injections include a history of allergy to local anesthetics or steroids, coagulopathy (due to disease process or use of anticoagulants), localized or systemic infection, or patient refusal.

PREPROCEDURE PREPARATION

When the patient is seen in consultation, an informed consent may be obtained. This may be updated on the day of the procedure. If no coagulopathy is suspected, blood work is usually unnecessary. If the patient is on anticoagulants, multidisciplinary care will be needed to safely discontinue anticoagulants and resume after the procedure. If pain reports are axial only with no radicular pain in the arms, magnetic resonance imaging (MRI) of cervical spine is not absolutely necessary.

On the day of the procedure, informed consent is updated and any remaining patient questions are answered. An intravenous line is established for resuscitation in the rare case of complications. Resuscitation equipment including "code-cart" and ability to intubate the patient if needed should be available.

PROCEDURE

Positioning

After a time-out to confirm patient's name, date of birth, procedure being performed, and site/side of procedure, the patient lies prone on the procedure table. Vital signs are monitored throughout the procedure, and verbal contact is maintained with the patient. Cervical spine is positioned flexed for optimal visualization of cervical facets. This can be achieved by putting a pillow under the patient's forehead. The C-arm is rotated about 25° caudal to align it with the axis orientation of the facet joint. Oblique angulation of the C-arm is not required.

Block Technique

After sterile prep and drape, cervical facet levels are first demarcated by counting up from T1 (easily identified by the first rib) or counting down from C2 (easily identified by the odontoid process). The needle entry point is the skin overlying the middle ("waist") of the articular pillar of each medial nerve to be anesthetized. Using a 25G 1.5-inch needle, the skin overlying this entry point is anesthetized with 1% lidocaine. A 22- or 25G spinal needle (for diagnostic medial branch blocks) or 10 cm SMK cannula with a 5-mm active tip (for radiofrequency neurotomy) is then advanced in a co-axial fashion till it seats itself on the lateral border between the superior and the inferior articulating surfaces. It is important to make sure that bony contact is made at this point. Needle position is confirmed with anteroposterior (AP) and lateral views **(Figs. 2 and 3)**.

For diagnostic medial branch block, 0.5 mL of 2% lidocaine or 0.25–0.5% bupivacaine is then injected. For radiofrequency neurotomy, the needle tip is walked off the lateral edge of the vertebral body about 2–3 mm so

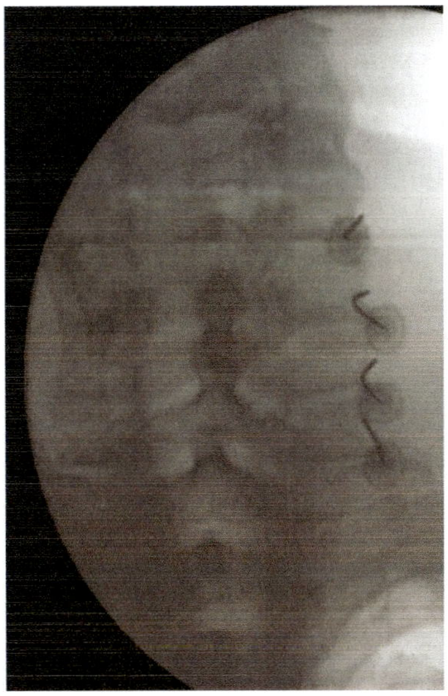

Fig. 2: Anteroposterior view needles at multiple facet joint.

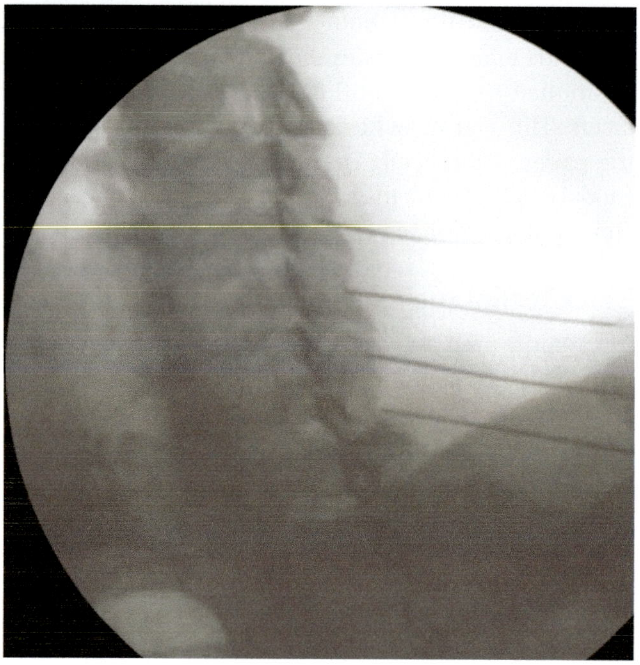

Fig. 3: Needles in lateral view.

that the active tip is now positioned parallel to the medial branch nerve. Sensory stimulation at 50 Hz, 0.3–0.5 V is desirable, followed by motor stimulation at 2 Hz up to 2 V to confirm that there is no motor nerve ablation. Each level is then anesthetized with 0.5 mL of 1% lidocaine for patient comfort. Radiofrequency neurotomy is then performed at a temperature of 60°C, for 60 seconds. The needles are then removed and the skin cleaned. A band-aid may be applied to the area if needed.

Of note, comparative medial branch blocks may be performed to increase the positive predictive value of the test.[9,10] For this approach, the block is performed on two occasions with two different anesthetics to reduce the false-positive rate associated with single block procedures.[11,12] This procedure involved the injection of 0.5 mL of either bupivacaine 0.5% or lidocaine 2% under fluoroscopic guidance onto the medial branch of the dorsal ramus of the target facet joint.

Postprocedure Care

The patient is assisted off the table and taken to the postprocedure area. Vital signs are monitored, and the patient is monitored for any complication. Postprocedure instructions, including ice to the region for 24 hours (if needed), using mild anti-inflammatory medications for postprocedure pain (if needed) and not driving are given to the patient. Care is transitioned over to the patient's caregiver.

Complications

- Postprocedure pain may be expected, and severity varies from patient to patient.
- Bleeding is usually minimal.
- If the needle is positioned close to the anterior primary ramus, injury may occur leading to weakness and loss of motor function. This can be avoided by careful motor stimulation.
- If the needle is positioned too anteromedially, it is fathomable that the needle tip enters the spinal canal. However, this catastrophic complication can be prevented by a careful, methodical approach to the procedure with good visualization using fluoroscopy.
- Other potential complications include spinal cord trauma, infection, intra-arterial or intravenous injection, spinal anesthesia, chemical meningitis, neural trauma, pneumothorax, radiation exposure, and facet capsule rupture.[13]

CONCLUSION

The use of radiofrequency to do cervical median branch neurotomy is an effective modality for cervical radicular pain. The steps suggested in the preceding text will be useful for upcoming and practicing pain physicians.

REFERENCES

1. Lord SM, Barnsley L, Wallis BJ, Bogduk N. Chronic cervical zygapophysial joint pain after whiplash. A placebo-controlled prevalence study. Spine (Phila Pa 1976). 1996;21:1737-44, discussion 1744-5.
2. Manchikanti L, Manchikanti KN, Pampati V, Brandon DE, Giordano J. The prevalence of facet-joint-related chronic neck pain in postsurgical and nonpostsurgical patients: a comparative evaluation. Pain Pract. 2008;8:5-10.
3. Manchikanti L, Singh V, Pampati V, Damron KS, Beyer CD, Barnhill RC. Is there correlation of facet joint pain in lumbar and cervical spine? An evaluation of prevalence in combined chronic low back and neck pain. Pain Physician. 2002;5:365-71.
4. Aizawa T, Ozawa H, Hoshikawa T, Kusakabe T, Itoi E. Severe facet joint arthrosis caused C7/t1 myelopathy: a case report. Case Rep Med. 2009;2009:481459.
5. Pellengahr C, Pfahler M, Kuhr M, Hohmann D. Influence of facet joint angles and asymmetric disk collapse on degenerative olisthesis of the cervical spine. Orthopedics. 2000;23(7):697-701.

6. Bogduk N. The clinical anatomy of the cervical dorsal rami. Spine (Phila Pa 1976). 1982;7(4):319-30.
7. King W, Lau P, Lees R, Bogduk N. The validity of manual examination in assessing patients with neck pain. Spine J. 2007;7(1):22-6.
8. Boswell MV, Colson JD, Sehgal N, Dunbar EE, Epter R. A systematic review of therapeutic facet joint interventions in chronic spinal pain. Pain Physician. 2007;10(1):229-53.
9. Bogduk N. International Spinal Injection Society guidelines for the performance of spinal injection procedures. Part 1: Zygapophysial joint blocks. Clin J Pain. 1997;13(4):285-302.
10. Lord SM, Barnsley L, Bogduk N. The utility of comparative local anesthetic blocks versus placebo-controlled blocks for the diagnosis of cervical zygapophysial joint pain. Clin J Pain. 1995;11(3):208-73.
11. Manchikanti L, Boswell MV, Singh V, Pampati V, Damron KS, Beyer CD. Prevalence of facet joint pain in chronic spinal pain of cervical, thoracic, and lumbar regions. BMC Musculoskelet Disord. 2004;5:15.
12. Barnsley L, Lord S, Wallis B, Bogduk N. False-positive rates of cervical zygapophyseal joint blocks. Clin J Pain. 1993;9(2):124-30.
13. Boswell MV, Colson JD, Spillane WF. Therapeutic facet joint interventions in chronic spinal pain: a systematic review of effectiveness and complications. Pain Physician. 2005;8(1):101-14.

33 CHAPTER

Thoracic Paravertebral Block

Lisa V Doan

ABSTRACT

Thoracic paravertebral blocks involve the injection of local anesthetic into the paravertebral space, an area lateral to the spinal column, resulting in somatic and sympathetic blockade. Several techniques have been described for placement of this block, including those based on landmarks, nerve stimulation, and ultrasound guidance.

INTRODUCTION

Thoracic paravertebral blocks involve injection of local anesthetic into the paravertebral space, ideally resulting in ipsilateral somatic and sympathetic nerve blockade. These are often used for unilateral acute and chronic pain. Bilateral blocks have also been described.

ANATOMY

The thoracic paravertebral space is a wedge-shaped space located lateral to the spinal column **(Fig. 1)**. Its posterior border is formed by the superior costotransverse ligament which runs from the inferior border of the transverse process to the superior border of the rib below. Anterolaterally, space is bordered by the parietal pleura. Medially, the space is bordered by the lateral aspect of the vertebral body and intervertebral foramen and contents. The paravertebral space contains the spinal nerve as well as the rami communicantes and the sympathetic chain. Paravertebral space communicates with the epidural space medially via the intervertebral foramen. Laterally, it is continuous with the intercostal space.[1]

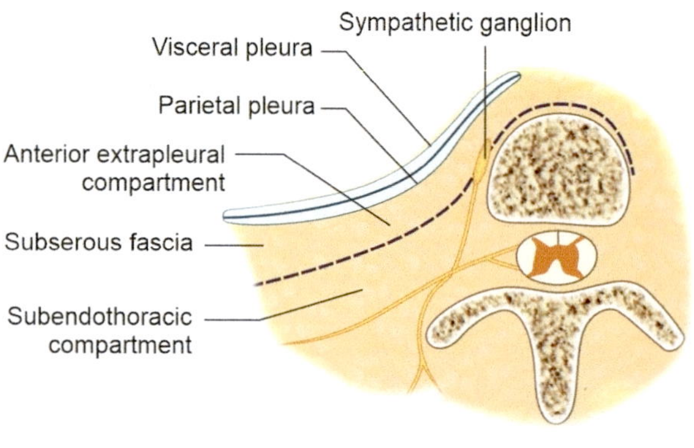

Fig. 1: Anatomy of the thoracic paravertebral space.

The thoracic paravertebral space is subdivided by the endothoracic fascia. The endothoracic fascia lines the inside of the thoracic cavity. It is continuous superiorly with Sibson's fascia. Dorsally, it merges with the prevertebral fascia. Inferiorly, it is continuous with the transversalis fascia that lines the abdomen. Between the endothoracic fascia and the parietal pleura is the subserous fascia which acts as a connective tissue investment.[2] The endothoracic fascia divides the thoracic paravertebral space into the anterior extrapleural paravertebral compartment and the posterior subendothoracic paravertebral compartment.[3]

The spread of local anesthetic solution after thoracic paravertebral injection can be variable. Some degree of epidural spread can be seen in 70% of injections.[4] Injection of 15 mL of local anesthetic at a single thoracic level caused on average sympathetic blockade over eight dermatomes. Somatic block occurred on average over five dermatomes, one cephalad and four caudad to the injection site.[5] Contralateral and lumbar spread occasionally associated with paravertebral block is likely related to the location of the injectate in relation to the endothoracic fascia.[3,5,6]

INDICATIONS

Thoracic paravertebral blocks are typically used for unilateral surgery though bilateral blocks have also been used. Surgical indications include thoracotomy, video-assisted thoracoscopic surgery, minimally invasive cardiac surgery, and breast surgery such as mastectomy. Other indications include analgesia for rib fractures, postherpetic neuralgia, and chronic post-thoracotomy or postmastectomy pain.

CONTRAINDICATIONS

Absolute Contraindications

Absolute contraindications include the following:

- Patient refusal
- Infection at the site of needle insertion
- Allergy to medications typically injected.

Relative Contraindications

Relative contraindications include the following:

- Lack of patient cooperation, including combativeness or agitation
- Coagulopathy
- Prior thoracotomy
- Altered chest or thoracic anatomy.

EQUIPMENT AND DRUGS

Equipment

- Antiseptic solution
- Sterile drape and sterile gauze
- Sterile gloves
- Marking pen
- 5 mL, 10 mL, and/or 20 mL syringes
- 25G needle for skin anesthesia
- 22G needle or 18G Tuohy needle for continuous paravertebral block with an epidural catheter
- Nerve stimulator, if applicable
- Ultrasound probe, if applicable, with sterile conductive gel and sterile probe cover.

Drugs

- 1% lidocaine for skin infiltration
- Bupivacaine or ropivacaine is often used for block.
    - 15–20 mL local anesthetic for a single-level injection
    - Up to 5-mL local anesthetic per level for multilevel injections
- For continuous infusion
    - 0.2% ropivacaine or 0.25% bupivacaine often used.
    - Infused at approximately 10 mL/hour.

PATIENT POSITION

The patient is placed in a sitting or lateral decubitus position. The area is sterilely prepared and draped.

PROCEDURE

Several techniques for thoracic paravertebral block have been described, including those based on landmarks, nerve stimulator guidance, and ultrasound guidance. For a continuous block, an 18G Tuohy needle is used. Approximately 5 mL of local anesthetic is injected, and the catheter is advanced 5 cm into the paravertebral space. Advancement of a catheter may be more challenging for the paravertebral space than for the epidural space. Typical levels to be blocked are listed in **Table 1**.

Landmark-based Technique

The spinous processes are palpated and marked. The insertion site is marked 2.5 cm from midline, corresponding to the transverse process of vertebra one level below that of the spinous process **(Fig. 2)**. After subcutaneous infiltration of local anesthetic, the needle is introduced 90° to all planes and advanced to touch the transverse process at a depth of 2.5–3.5 cm in the mid-thoracic area in an average-sized adult. The depth is noted. The needle is then redirected cephalad and advanced no more than 1 cm past the transverse process. The needle is aspirated to assess for blood, cerebrospinal fluid, or air. Local anesthetic is then slowly injected.

Loss-of-Resistance Technique

The first steps of this technique are as for the landmark-based technique, utilizing a Tuohy needle. After touching the transverse process, a syringe filled with air is attached to

TABLE 1: Level of paravertebral block placement.

Surgery	*Level of block*
Breast surgery	• Single level T1-T6 • Catheter T2-T3
Thoracotomy, thoracoscopy	• Single level T4-T9 • Catheter T4-T5
Cardiac surgery	• Single level T2-T9 • Catheter T4-T5

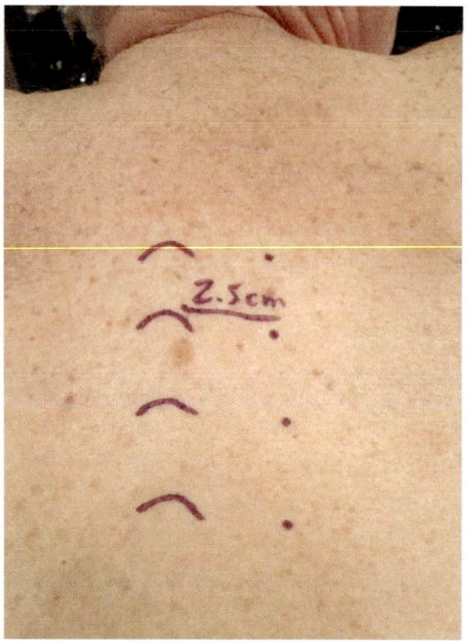

Fig. 2: Landmark-based technique of paravertebral block.

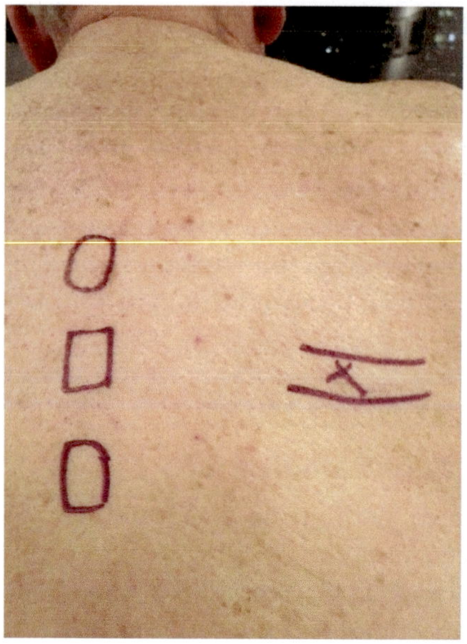

Fig. 3: Intercostal approach to continuous paravertebral block.

the needle. The needle is then redirected to the cephalad. Loss of resistance is felt when the needle traverses the superior costotransverse ligament. The loss is more subtle than that appreciated to locate the epidural space. The needle is aspirated to assess for blood, cerebrospinal fluid, or air. Local anesthetic is then slowly injected.[1]

Nerve Stimulator Technique

The insertion site is marked as for the landmark-based technique. A stimulating needle is connected to a nerve stimulator. A pulse width of 0.1 ms and a stimulating frequency of 2 Hz are used. An initial current of 2.5–5 mA is used. The needle is advanced watching for contraction of the intercostal or abdominal muscles. The needle position is considered optimal when muscle contractions are still present at 0.5–0.6 mA.[7]

Intercostal Approach

An intercostal approach for continuous paravertebral block has been described. The patient is placed in a sitting position. The rib at the level to be blocked is marked 8 cm lateral to the midline **(Fig. 3)**. The area is sterilely prepared and draped. The skin and subcutaneous tissue are anesthetized with local anesthetic. An 18G Tuohy needle is inserted and advanced to touch the rib. The needle is then oriented such that the tip is angled 45° cephalad and 60° medial to the sagittal plane. The needle is then walked off caudad and advanced 5–6 mm. 5 mL of local anesthetic is injected after negative aspiration, and a catheter is advanced through the needle at 8 cm beyond the needle depth. This technique was proposed as an alternative to the classical landmark-based approach to avoid risks such as inadvertent dural sleeve puncture and to overcome problems such as altered spinal anatomy or history of spine surgery.[8]

Ultrasound-guided Techniques

Several ultrasound-guided techniques have been proposed, including parasagittal and transverse approaches.

For a parasagittal approach, a linear array probe is placed longitudinally in the paravertebral area approximately 2.5 cm lateral to the spinous process. A view of the transverse processes, superior costotransverse ligament, and pleura is obtained **(Fig. 4)**. After local anesthetic infiltration of the skin and subcutaneous tissues, the needle is inserted at the inferior portion of the probe. The needle is advanced using an in-plane technique with cephalad orientation. The needle tip is advanced past the superior costotransverse ligament to lie in the paravertebral space. Injection of local anesthetic leads to anterior displacement of the parietal pleura.[9] An out-of-plane technique has also been described which is purported to cause less discomfort due to decreased needle traversal.

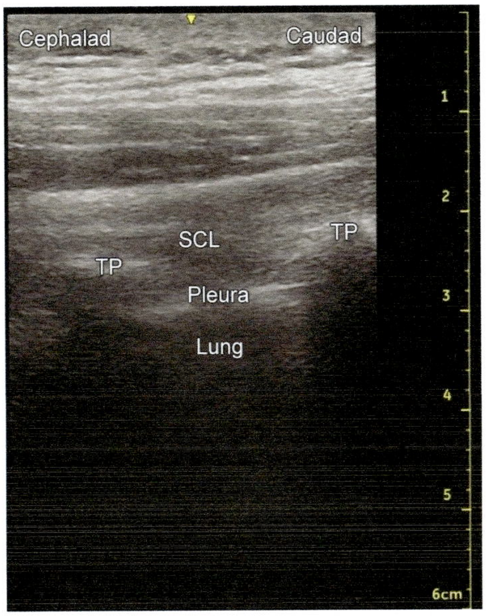

Fig. 4: Parasagittal approach to ultrasound-guided paravertebral block. (SCL: superior costotransverse ligament; TP: transverse process)

For a transverse approach, a linear array probe is placed in the horizontal plane. The spinous process is identified, and the ultrasound probe is moved laterally until the transverse process and pleura are identified. After the skin and subcutaneous tissues are anesthetized, the needle is inserted in an out-of-plane approach to be positioned between the internal intercostal muscle and the pleura. Anterior displacement of the parietal pleura is seen with injection of local anesthetic.[10]

An ultrasound-guided intercostal approach has been described for continuous paravertebral block. This technique also uses a transverse approach. A linear array probe is placed in the horizontal plane approximately 8 cm lateral to midline to identify the rib **(Fig. 5)**. The probe is then tilted to identify the muscles and pleura deep to the rib **(Fig. 6)**. After the skin and subcutaneous tissues are anesthetized, the needle is inserted in-plane at the lateral end of the probe. The tip is advanced to lie between the internal intercostal muscle and the pleura. Anterior displacement of the parietal pleura is seen with injection of local anesthetic, and the catheter is inserted 7 cm beyond the needle depth.[11]

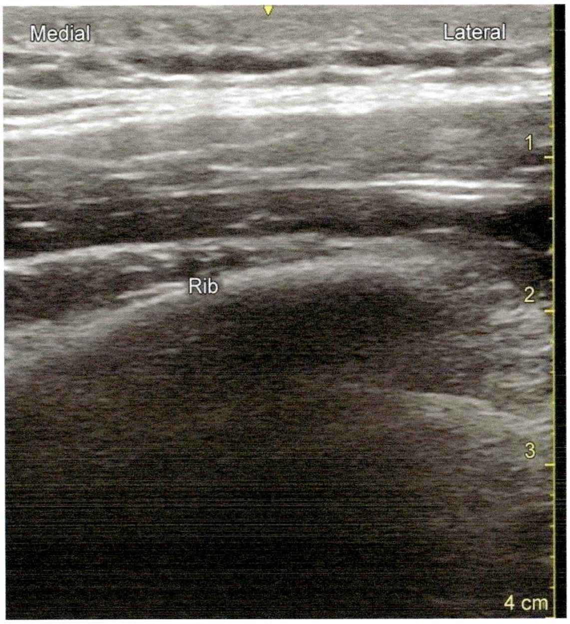

Fig. 5: Ultrasound-guided intercostal approach to continuous paravertebral block—view of rib.

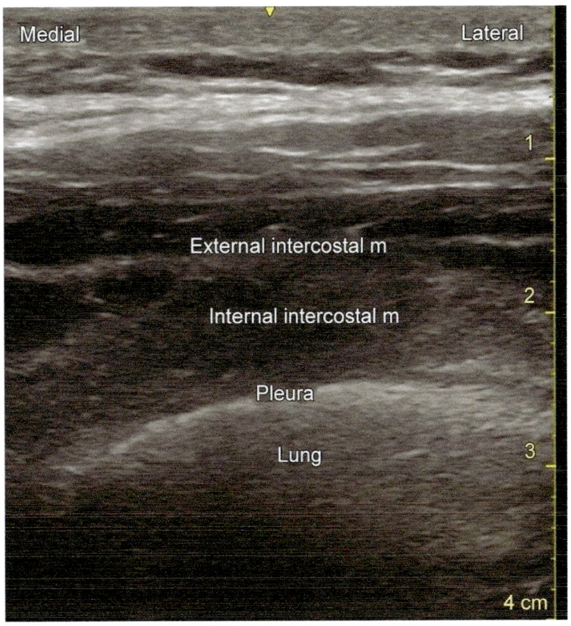

Fig. 6: Ultrasound-guided intercostal approach to continuous paravertebral block—view of muscles and pleura.

COMPLICATIONS

Complication rates vary based on experience, patient habitus and anatomy, and technique used. Possible complications are listed in **Box 1**.

The rate of failed blocks has been reported to be between 6.8% and 10% in studies using loss of resistance, nerve stimulator-guided, and ultrasound-guided techniques.[7,12,13] These rates are lower than that associated with thoracic epidural blockade.[14]

BOX 1: Complications of paravertebral blockade.

- Failed blocks
- Hypotension
- Vascular puncture/hematoma
- Pneumothorax
- Epidural or intrathecal spread
- Pain at site of injection
- Infection
- Nerve injury

Hypotension after paravertebral blockade has been reported to be approximately 4%.[7,12] This is lower than that reported with thoracic epidural blockade.[15] Hypotension is likely related to sympathetic blockade or epidural extension.

The rate of inadvertent vascular puncture, noted by blood on aspiration, has been reported to be between 3.8% and 6.8%. The incidence of hematoma formation at the site of injection is reported to be 2.4%.[7,12] Pulmonary hemorrhage has also been described in a patient planned for a repeat thoracotomy for repair of recurrent paraesophageal hernia. Paravertebral block was attempted using a loss-of-resistance technique. Blood was noted coming from the double-lumen tube. The procedure was aborted, and afterward a CT scan showed intrapulmonary hemorrhage. A subsequent procedure, in which paravertebral block was not attempted, revealed adhesions and obliteration of the paravertebral space. Thus, caution should be used in performing paravertebral block in patients who have already undergone a prior thoracotomy.[16]

The incidence of pneumothorax has been reported to be between 0.3% and 0.5% with loss-of-resistance or nerve stimulator techniques.[7,12] Pleural puncture has also been noted after ultrasound-guided techniques, primarily related to placement and advancement of catheters for continuous techniques.[17]

Significant epidural or intrathecal spread has been reported in approximately 1% of single-shot paravertebral blocks.[7] Postural headaches have been described after thoracic paravertebral blocks, likely due to inadvertent dural puncture. These headaches have been described after placement at sites 1 cm from midline as well as more lateral insertion sites 2.5 cm from midline. Dural sleeves may extend into the paravertebral space. Abnormalities such as dilated root sleeves or root cysts may also exist that could contribute to inadvertent dural puncture.[18,19]

Local pain at the site of injection has been reported in 1.3% of cases.[7] Rare complications, such as infection and nerve injury, may also occur.

NOVEL USES FOR CHRONIC PAIN

Thoracic paravertebral block is indicated for chronic pain conditions such as postherpetic neuralgia and other neuropathic pain syndromes including post-thoracotomy and postmastectomy pain. Novel techniques include radiofrequency and peripheral nerve stimulation of the nerve in the paravertebral space.[20,21] Further studies are needed to establish the efficacy of these techniques.

CONCLUSION

Thoracic paravertebral block offers an alternative to epidural block for acute pain. Its use in chronic pain continues to be investigated.

ACKNOWLEDGMENTS

The author thanks Herbert Mienert, Hersh Patel, and Daniel Kohut for assistance with images.

REFERENCES

1. Eason MJ, Wyatt R. Paravertebral thoracic block: a reappraisal. Anaesthesia. 1979;34:638-42.
2. Dugan DJ, Samson PC. Surgical significance of the endothoracic fascia. The anatomic basis for empyemectomy and other extrapleural technics. Am J Surg. 1975;130:151-8.
3. Karmakar MK, Chung DC. Variability of a thoracic paravertebral block. Are we ignoring the endothoracic fascia? Reg Anesth Pain Med. 2000;25:325-7.
4. Purcell-Jones G, Pither CE, Justins DM. Paravertebral somatic nerve block: a clinical, radiographic, and computed tomographic study in chronic pain patients. Anesth Analg. 1989:68:32-9.
5. Cheema SP, Ilsley D, Richardson J, Sabanathan S. A thermographic study of paravertebral analgesia. Anaesthesia.1995;50:118-21.
6. Karmakar MK, Kwok WH, Kew J. Thoracic paravertebral block: radiological evidence of contralateral spread anterior to the vertebral bodies. Br J Anaesth. 2000;84:263-5.
7. Naja Z, Lönnqvist PA. Somatic paravertebral nerve blockade. Incidence of failed block and complications. Anaesthesia. 2001;56:1184-8.
8. Burns DA, Ben-David B, Chelly JE, Greensmith JE. Intercostally placed paravertebral catheterization: an alternative approach to continuous paravertebral blockade. Anesth Analg. 2008;107:339-41.
9. Riain SC, Donnell BO, Cuffe T, Harmon DC, Fraher JP, Shorten G. Thoracic paravertebral block using real-time ultrasound guidance. Anesth Analg. 2010;110:248-51.
10. Marhofer P, Kettner SC, Hajbok L, Dubsky P, Fleischmann E. Lateral ultrasound-guided paravertebral blockade: an

anatomical-based description of a new technique. Br J Anaesth. 2010;105:526-32.
11. Ben-Ari A, Moreno M, Chelly JE, Bigeleisen PE. Ultrasound-guided paravertebral block using an intercostal approach. Anesth Analg. 2009;109:1691-4.
12. Lönnqvist PA, MacKenzie J, Soni AK, Conacher ID. Paravertebral blockade. Failure rate and complications. Anaesthesia. 1995;50:813-5.
13. Luyet C, Herrmann G, Ross S, Vogt A, Greif R, Moriggl B, et al. Ultrasound-guided thoracic paravertebral puncture and placement of catheters in human cadavers: where do catheters go? Br J Anaesth. 2011;106:246- 54.
14. Hermanides J, Hollmann MW, Stevens MF, Lirk P. Failed epidural: causes and management. Br J Anaesth. 2012;109:144-54.
15. Joshi GP, Bonnet F, Shah R, Wilkinson RC, Camu F, Fischer B, et al. A systematic review of randomized trials evaluating regional techniques for postthoracotomy analgesia. Anesth Analg. 2008;107:1026-40.
16. Thomas PW, Sanders DJ, Berrisford RG. Pulmonary haemorrhage after percutaneous paravertebral block. Br J Anaesth. 1999;83:668-9.
17. Kus A, Gurkan Y, Akgul AG, Solak M, Toker K. Pleural puncture and intrathoracic catheter placement during ultrasound guided paravertebral block. J Cardiothorac Vasc Anesth. 2013;27:e11-2.
18. Sharrock NE. Postural headache following thoracic somatic paravertebral nerve block. Anesthesiology. 1980;52:360-2.
19. Lin HM, Chelly JE. Post-dural headache associated with thoracic paravertebral blocks. J Clin Anesth. 2006;18:376-8.
20. Uchida K. Radiofrequency treatment of the thoracic paravertebral nerve combined with glucocorticoid for refractory neuropathic pain following breast cancer surgery. Pain Physician. 2009;12:E277-83.
21. Hegarty D, Goroszeniuk T. Peripheral nerve stimulation of the thoracic paravertebral plexus for chronic neuropathic pain. Pain Physician. 2011;14:295-300.

34 CHAPTER

Lumbar and Caudal Epidural Blocks

Sanjay Bakshi, Gerard W Abrahamsen

ABSTRACT

Epidural steroid injections are the placement of steroids into the epidural space. They were first described in 1953, and epidural steroids have been administered to millions of patients for the treatment of axial and radicular back pain. Traditionally, these injections were performed from a "blind approach" (without fluoroscopy) and lacked target specificity and contrast spread to confirm needle placement into the epidural space. With the advent and use of fluoroscopy, the transforaminal approach became widespread, with the thought that epidural steroids would be more effective if they were delivered more accurately to the site of pathology.[1-4]

The main clinical indications for epidural steroid injections include—disk degeneration or herniation, spinal nerve root compression, spinal nerve root inflammation, and spinal stenosis. Correlating the distribution of the patient's pain with their imaging study findings, the clinician can decide the epidural technique, level, and side of the spine at which the injection should be performed to achieve maximum benefit.

This chapter will discuss the indications to perform epidural steroid injections and the proper techniques used in performing interlaminar, transforaminal, and caudal epidural steroid injections. We will also review the recent national headlines in the United States, in regard to the widespread outbreak of fungal meningitis after epidural steroid administration, the Food and Drug Administration (FDA) statement on "Epidural Steroid Injection: Drug Safety Communication: Risk of Serious Neurological Problems" and review several journal articles pertaining to the efficacy of epidural steroid injections.

INTRODUCTION

Epidural steroid injections are the placement of steroids into the epidural space. They were first described in 1953 and epidural steroids have been administered to millions of patients for the treatment of axial and radicular back pain. Traditionally, these injections were performed with a "blind approach" (without fluoroscopy) and lacked target specificity and contrast spread to confirm needle placement into the epidural space. With the advent and use of fluoroscopy, the transforaminal approach became widespread, with the thought that epidural steroids would be more effective if they were delivered more accurately to the site of pathology.[1-4]

The basis behind the use of epidural steroid injections is that chemical mediators are released from a disk after injury to that disk. This results in the release of phospholipase A2 (PLA2) from the nucleus pulposus into the epidural space.[5] The PLA2 is an enzyme found in high concentrations in disk material. It is highly inflammatogenic and propagates an inflammatory cascade with the liberation of arachidonic acid with inflammatory responses via leukotrienes and prostaglandins.[6] Epidural steroids act by blocking PLA2 activity and can exert an anesthetic-like activity by blocking nociceptive C-fiber conduction.[7] This effect is reversed when the corticosteroid is removed, suggesting a direct membrane effect. Glucocorticoid receptor sites have also been located on norepinephrine and 5-hydroxytryptamine neurons within the dorsal horn substantia gelatinosa.[8,9]

Since our last publication, epidural steroid injections have been in the public eye for various reasons.

In 2012, epidural steroid injections made national headlines in the United States, when there was a widespread outbreak of fungal meningitis after epidural steroid injections. The Centers for Disease Control (CDC) determined that 751 patients across the country were affected with fungal meningitis after receiving epidural injections with preservative-free methylprednisolone acetate (MPA) manufactured at New England Compounding Center (NECC), located in Framingham, Massachusetts. The CDC reports that of the 751 patients, 64 died.

The NECC was a family-owned compounding pharmacy that was established in 1998. The pharmacy failed to comply with the standards of sterile compounding of medications that were ultimately used by multiple pain centers and administered during epidural injections. The NECC was investigated and later closed and has numerous lawsuits to date. This brought up discussions, concerns, and patient fear throughout the United States about the safety of epidural injections and the medications that are administered during the procedure.

The Food and Drug Administration (FDA) on April 23, 2014, released a statement, "Epidural Steroid Injection: Drug Safety Communication: Risk of Serious Neurological Problems". The focus was on corticosteroids, including methylprednisolone, hydrocortisone, triamcinolone, betamethasone, and dexamethasone. This statement outlined that the effectiveness and safety of epidural administration of corticosteroids have not been established and the FDA has not approved corticosteroids for this use. The FDA also required drug labels of corticosteroid injections into the epidural space to list the following rare but serious adverse events, including loss of vision, paralysis, stroke, or death.[10] This action by the FDA has been widely criticized as being without scientific analysis of the evidence or reliance on consensus.[11-13] The International Spinal Injection Society (ISIS) issued a response to the FDA steroid statement that the alert was misleading in its message regarding the safety of epidural steroid injections and contained inaccuracies regarding the effectiveness of this procedure.[14] The American Society of Interventional Pain Physicians (ASIPP) has also appealed the FDA statement with an official appeal letter, including the signatures of 1,040 practicing interventional pain physicians.[15]

The efficacy of epidural steroid injections has been criticized due to a lack of well-designed clinical trials demonstrating the safety and efficacy of these injections. However, recently in the interventional pain management community, there has been a push to perform literature reviews and design clinical studies to demonstrate the efficacy and preserve this procedure that has been used to safely treat millions of patients suffering from spinal pain throughout the world.[12,16,17]

Benyamin R, et al.[18] performed a systematic review of "the effectiveness of lumbar interlaminar epidural injections in managing chronic low back and lower extremity pain". 82 lumbar interlaminar trials were reviewed, and 15 randomized trials and 11 nonrandomized studies were included in the analysis to determine improvement in pain, functional status, psychological status, return to work, and reduction in opioid intake. The authors concluded that the evidence was good for lumbar epidural injections under fluoroscopy for radiculitis secondary to disk herniation with local anesthetics and steroids, fair with local anesthetic only, whereas it was fair for radiculitis secondary to spinal stenosis with local anesthetic and steroids and fair for axial pain without disk herniation with local anesthetic with or without steroids.[18]

The effectiveness of epidural steroid injections in a highly selective group of professional athletes, National Football League (NFL) players, has been investigated. Krych A, et al.[19] reviewed all NFL players who underwent an epidural steroid injection for acute lumbar disk herniation at their institution from 2003 to 2010. The purpose was to determine the success of the injections as defined as return to play. The study population included 17 players having a total of 37 injections for 27 distinct lumbar disk herniation episodes. The authors determined that the rate of success for returning an athlete to play for a given episode was 89%, four players required a repeat injection for the same episode, and three of these four players ultimately failed conservative management requiring surgery. Therefore, they concluded that in their selective group of professional athletes, epidural steroid injections are a safe and effective therapeutic option for the treatment of lumbar disk herniation.[19]

In January 2013, the North American Spine Society (NASS) released a reviewed and recommendation statement on lumbar transforaminal epidural steroid injections (TFESI). The intent of the statement was to present the current state of the evidence for the use of TFESI in treating lumbar radiculopathy/radiculitis resulting from herniated disk or spinal stenosis and provide evidence-based recommendations regarding their use in treating lumbar radicular pain.[20]

The NASS Statement Work Group looked at the efficacy of TFESI in the treatment of radicular pain from lumbar spinal stenosis and lumbar disk herniation. They determined that TFESI was found to be effective in providing pain relief for at least 1 month in >50% of patients. More than half of these patients continued to benefit for a year or more.[20-23]

The North American Spine Society also reported on complications associated with TFESI and reported that TFESI are safe procedures with minor transient side effects from medications.[24-26] It was also reported that catastrophic complications of lumbar TFESI, such as spinal cord injury or infarction, are rare but possible and can result from the vascular injection of particulate steroids.[27-29] Previous spine surgery is also a notable risk factor for the development of spinal cord injury following TFESI. Most patients who developed spinal cord infarction had prior lumbar surgery, possibly due to altered anatomy or changes to the vascular supply.[30,31] Digital subtraction fluoroscopy with real-time imaging has been demonstrated to reduce the incidence of intravascular injection.[32] However, at this time digital subtraction fluoroscopy remains investigational and is therefore not the current standard of care.

ANATOMY

The epidural space lies between the osseoligamentous structures lining the vertebral canal and the dural membrane surrounding the spinal cord and the nerve roots.[33] The anterior epidural space is bordered anteriorly by the vertebral body, intervertebral disk, and posterior longitudinal ligament and posteriorly by the thecal sac. The posterior epidural space is bordered anteriorly by the thecal sac and posteriorly by the ligamentum flavum and the laminae. Each spinal nerve exists within an intervertebral foramen, bordered anteriorly by the vertebral body and the disk, posteriorly by the facet joint, and superiorly and inferiorly by the pedicles of the adjacent vertebrae.

EVALUATION

Evaluation of a patient with back pain should begin with a detailed history and physical examination. Patients will often complain of lower back pain with radicular symptoms to the lower extremities, including pain, numbness, paresthesia, or weakness. Patients will often also describe symptoms consistent with neurogenic claudication. Physical examination may reveal paresthesia in a dermatomal distribution, weakness in a myotomal distribution, and a positive straight leg raise.

Imaging studies should be performed, including plain film radiographs and magnetic resonance imaging (MRI) or computed tomography (CT) scan, to confirm a diagnosis that will benefit from epidural steroid injections. Electrodiagnostic signs of radiculopathy may be helpful but are not an absolute prerequisite to epidural injections.

INDICATIONS

The main clinical indications for epidural steroid injections include disk degeneration or herniation, spinal nerve root compression, spinal nerve root inflammation, and spinal stenosis. Correlating the distribution of the patient's pain with the imaging study findings, the clinician can then decide the epidural technique, level, and side of spine at which the injection should be performed to achieve maximum benefit.

Epidural steroid injections should then be performed if the patient has a diagnosed cause of radiculopathy, has not responded to nonsurgical conservative measures, and whose pain is likely to have an inflammatory basis.

CONTRAINDICATIONS

Absolute contraindications to epidural steroid injections include patients who are unwilling to consent to the procedure, evidence of an untreated infection at the site of the injection, pregnancy, and bleeding diathesis. Relative contraindications are known allergy to the medications and dye administered, concurrent use of anticoagulant medication, known systemic infection, immunosuppression, severe respiratory or cardiovascular compromise, and anatomic, congenital, or surgical changes preventing safe administration of medication into the epidural space. If the patient has a known allergy to the medications used for the procedure, premedication may then be required depending on the severity of the allergic reaction.

EQUIPMENT/SUPPLIES

When performing epidural injections, a C-arm fluoroscope is required for precise needle placement and visualization of flow of contrast. The equipment and supplies needed include Tuohy epidural needles, 18- or 20G 3.5 inch (interlaminar) spinal needle, 22- or 25G 5-inch short bevel needle (transforaminal), 25G 1.5-inch needle for administration of local anesthetic, 5 mL syringe, or 10 mL glass or plastic syringe (for an interlaminar approach using "loss-of-resistance technique"), 10 mL plastic syringe, 3 mL syringe for injection of contrast, connection tubing, sterile gloves, drapes, gowns, and povidone-iodine or chlorhexidine prep. Typically, the supplies can be packaged in a custom epidural tray. Most patients also require intravenous (IV) access. In some cases, IV sedation is used. Physiological monitoring should also be used throughout the procedure.

MEDICATIONS

Medications used for epidural steroid injections vary but include preservative-free sterile saline, water-soluble, nonionic radiographic contrast medium (Isovue or Omnipaque), local anesthetic (lidocaine 1–2% or bupivacaine 0.125–0.5%), and a corticosteroid preparation (triamcinolone 20–80 mg, betamethasone 6–18 mg, depo-medrol 20–80 mg, or dexamethasone).[34,35]

Common volumes used for the injectate include: Interlaminar approach—a total volume of 6–8 mL, transforaminal approach—total volume of 2 mL, and caudal approach—total volume of 10–15 mL. The clinician will then combine 1–2 mL of corticosteroid with local anesthetic or normal saline to achieve the desired volume.

TECHNIQUES

The interlaminar approach, both midline and paramedian, involves insertion of an epidural needle midway between the laminae of the adjacent vertebrae, whereas the transforaminal approach involves insertion of a spinal needle into the superior portion of an intervertebral foramen just inferior to the pedicle.

PROCEDURE

Interlaminar Approach

After an informed consent is obtained, the patient is placed prone on the fluoroscopy table. It is advisable to place a small pillow under the lower abdomen to open up the interlaminar space. At this point, the skin is prepped and draped in a sterile fashion.

After carefully identifying the appropriate interlaminar space that you want to enter using fluoroscopy, make a skin mark over the lamina below the target interspace. The skin and subcutaneous tissues are now anesthetized using 1% lidocaine.

A 20G Tuohy needle is now advanced to the lamina. It is preferable to contact the superior border of the lower lamina so that you have a perception of the appropriate depth. The needle can now be walked off the lamina till it is felt to enter the ligamentum flavum. At this point, attach a "loss-of-resistance" syringe to the needle. Depending on the operator's preference, you can use either saline or air for the loss-of-resistance technique. Carefully advance the needle in small increments till you feel the loss of resistance on entering the epidural space. Once the epidural space is entered, 1–2 cc of radiocontrast dye is injected, and the dye spread is visualized under continuous fluoroscopy in the anteroposterior (AP) position. The C-arm is now rotated to the lateral position and appropriate dye spread is reconfirmed in the lateral position. The dye spread should be in the epidural space, and there should be no intravascular or intrathecal flow patterns. It is advisable to save the hard copy of the dye spread patterns in both AP and lateral views **(Figs. 1A to F)**.

Transforaminal Approach

The standard infrapedicular approach is described here. There have been various modifications to this technique that have been described, such as infraneural and dorsal,[36-38] with the hope of avoiding the radicular arteries and complications associated with that.[39-43] However, none of these different approaches has been proven to be safer.

After an informed consent is obtained, the patient is placed prone on the fluoroscopy table. Skin is prepped and draped in a sterile fashion.

After starting in the AP position, the C-arm is rotated slightly in an oblique fashion so that the typical Scotty dog picture can be visualized. The initial target is the 6 o'clock position of the pedicle. A skin mark is placed directly over this point. Skin and subcutaneous tissues are then anesthetized using 1% lidocaine. A 22- or 25G 5-inch short bevel needle is then advanced under fluoroscopic guidance toward the target point. The needle position is then checked initially in the AP position and subsequently in the lateral position to ensure that the tip of the needle is finally in the optimum position. At this point in the AP view, the tip of the needle should lie just below the midpoint of the pedicle and should not cross the facet joint line. In the lateral view, the needle tip should lie in the posterior–superior quadrant of the neural foramen. At this point, once the needle is felt to be in optimal position, 1 cc of radiocontrast dye is injected under continuous fluoroscopy. It is advisable to attach low-volume extension tubing to the needle and inject the dye

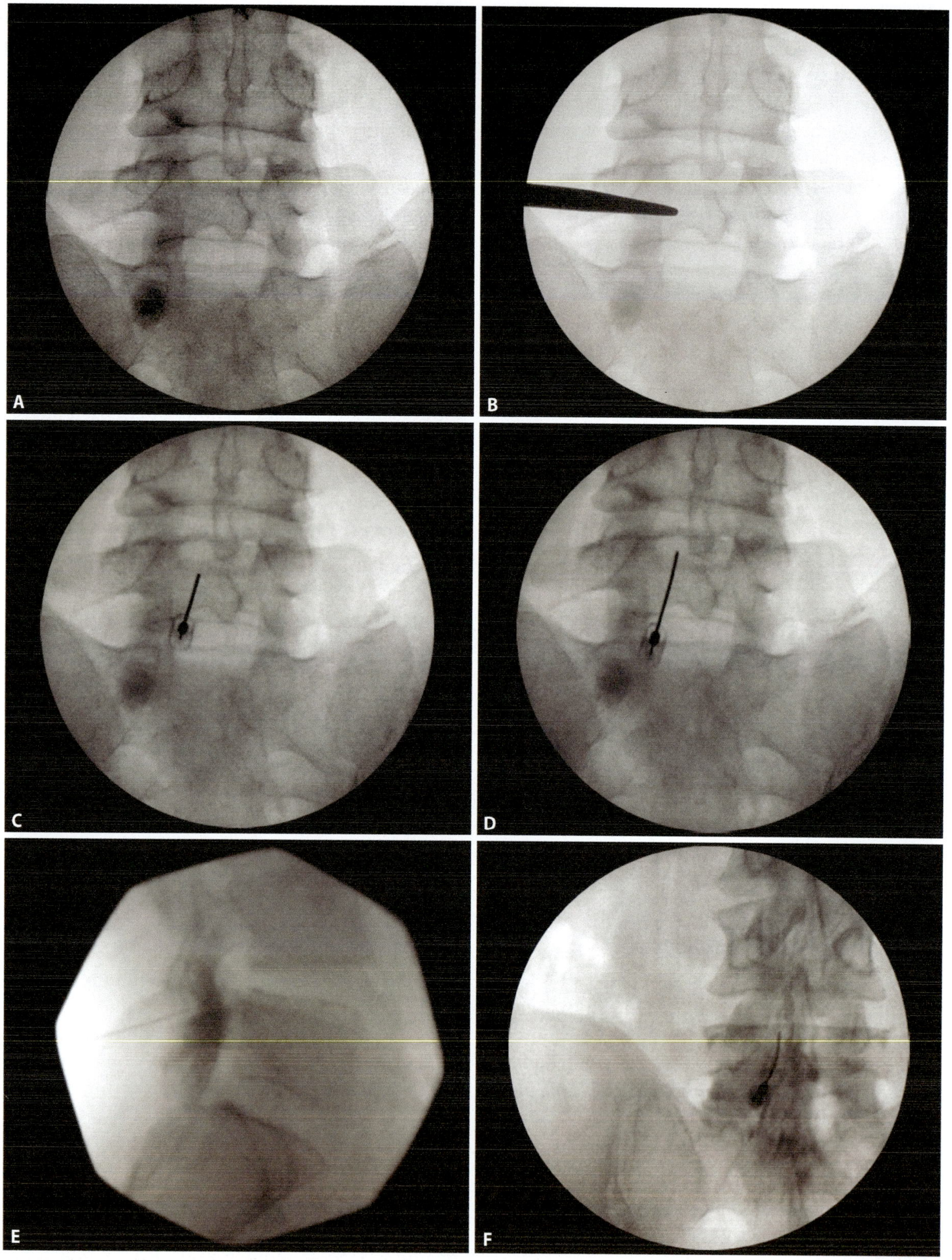

Figs. 1A to F: (A) Initial anteroposterior (AP) view; (B) Point of skin entry; (C) Needle headed to the lamina; (D) Needle walks off lamina; (E) Reconfirm position on the lateral view; (F) Anteroposterior view of dye spread.

and subsequent medications via the extension tubing under continuous fluoroscopy. Care is taken to see that there is an appropriate dye flow pattern, and it is critical to ensure that there is no intravascular dye spread. Continuous fluoroscopy is used because intravascular injection can be missed if intermittent fluoroscopy is used. In fact, some people recommend routine use of digital subtraction to rule out intravascular injection; however, this has not become a standard of care.

Once appropriate dye spread is confirmed, the steroid mixture can then be injected. The use of nonparticulate steroid preparation is preferable because then there is less chance of vascular thrombosis.

When using this approach for the L5-S1 interspace, it may require a caudal-cranial adjustment of the C-arm to get an appropriate visualization of the target by moving the superior articular process away.

The approach to the S1 foramen is different from the above. In this case, the needle is placed through the posterior S1 foramen onto the pedicle of S1. The C-arm needs to be adjusted slightly cephalocaudal and slightly ipsilateral oblique to superimpose the anterior and posterior S1 foramen. The needle enters the lateral margin of the posterior S1 foramen. The safe technique is to initially hit the bony surface of the sacrum first and then walk off into the foramen. At this point, depth is checked in the lateral position to make sure that the needle does not pass anteriorly into the pelvic cavity. Once the needle is felt to be in the appropriate position, radiocontrast dye is injected to ensure appropriate dye spread along the S1 nerve root sleeve. At this point, the mixture of cortisone is injected. Note that the dye and the subsequent medications should be injected under continuous fluoroscopy **(Figs. 2 and 3)**.

Caudal Approach

After informed consent, the patient is placed prone on the fluoroscopy table, with a pillow under the lower abdomen. Skin is prepped and draped in a sterile fashion. It is often helpful to have the patient rotate their feet inward.

This procedure is ideally started with the C-arm in the lateral position. It is helpful usually to manually feel for the indentation of the sacral cornua. At this point, skin and subcutaneous tissues are anesthetized.

Under the lateral view of the fluoroscope, the needle is advanced cephalad toward the sacral hiatus at a 45° angle. If you touch bone, readjust the needle angle and try to walk the needle into the caudal canal. You will initially feel the needle entering the sacrococcygeal ligament, followed by the loss of resistance. At this point, radiocontrast dye is injected and appropriate dye spread is reconfirmed in both lateral and AP positions. Careful negative aspiration is done before dye injection to ensure that no blood or cerebrospinal fluid (CSF) is aspirated.

Since the caudal canal is spacious, usually 10–15 cc of steroid mixture is injected **(Figs. 4A to E)**.

POSTPROCEDURAL CARE

Following the injection, the patient should be monitored with physiological monitoring for at least 30 minutes. If vital signs are stable and the patient is doing well, they may then be discharged. The patient should be advised of home care instructions, including possible bruising and increased pain at the incision site for the first few days following the procedure, in which ice packs may be beneficial, rest and abstinence from driving for 24 hours postprocedure, and increased activity as tolerated. The patient should notify the office of any skin rashes, hives, shortness of breath, wheezing, increase in pain level, persistent nausea or vomiting, persistent headache that worsens upon sitting, and fever >100°F.

COMPLICATIONS

Complications following epidural steroid injections are rare. However, possible risks and complications include pain at the injection site, nerve root injury, spinal cord injury, including spinal cord infract, epidural hematoma, epidural abscess, meningitis, osteomyelitis, and postdural puncture headache. Local anesthetic side effects include weakness in lower extremity secondary to motor block, cardiac arrhythmia, seizure, and hypotension. Patients should also be advised of potential steroid effects such as fluid retention, transient weight gain, hyperglycemia, hypertension, Cushing syndrome, facial flushing, and steroid myopathy.[24] Allergic reactions may also occur with any of the medications administered.

Added precaution should be used when performing TFESI. Case reports[44] warn of unexpected paraplegia following lumbar transforaminal injections. The mechanism of injury was not demonstrated but was referred to be inadvertent, intra-arterial injection of particulate steroids into a radicular artery that reinforced blood supply of the lower end of the spinal cord. This reinforces the need for careful attention when injecting the contrast medium to avoid possible intra-arterial injection of steroids.

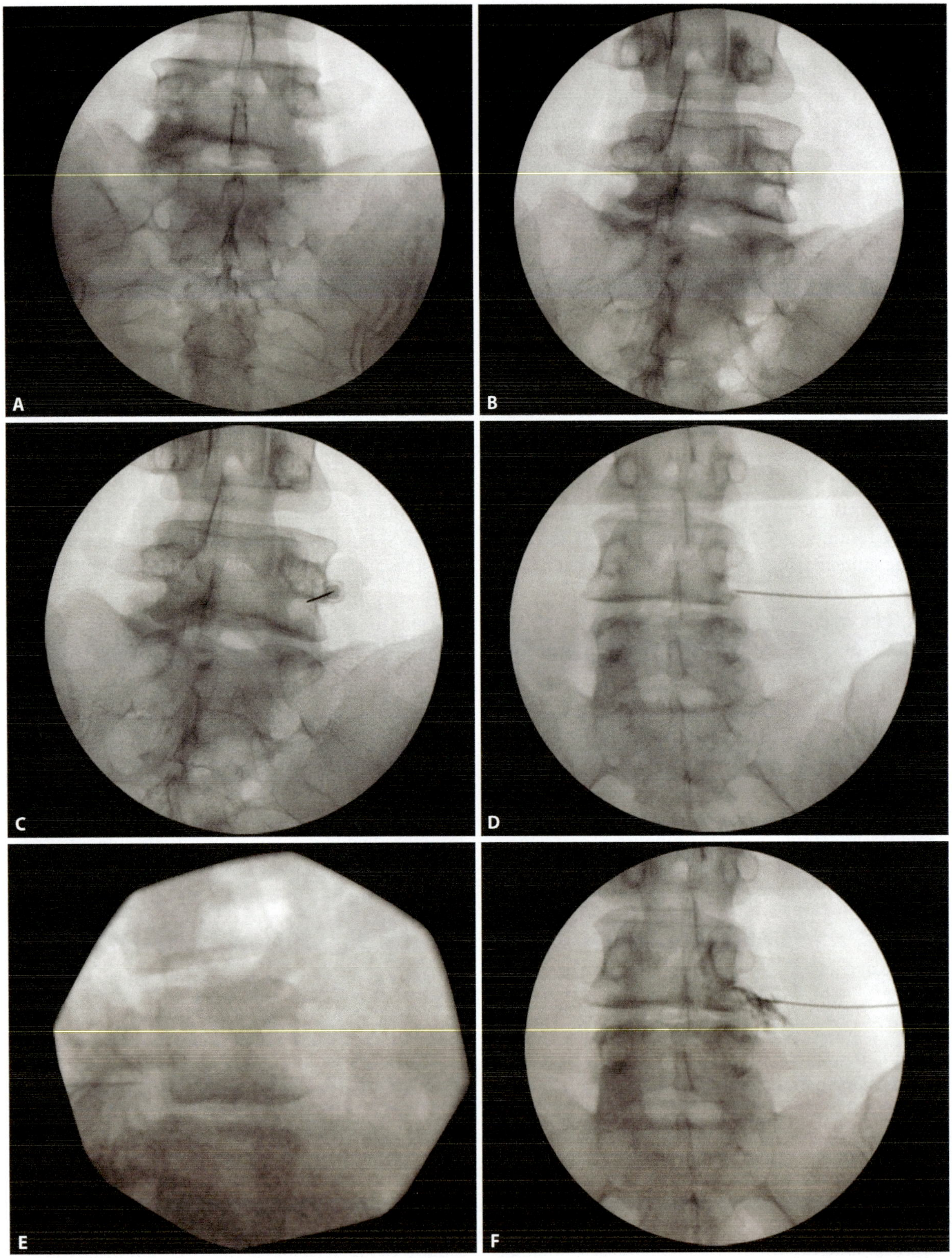

Figs. 2A to F: (A) Straight anteroposterior view; (B) Slight oblique angulation with a skin marker; (C) Needle entry—oblique view; (D) Reconfirm in anteroposterior view; (E) Lateral view of needle tip; (F) Final view of dye spread.

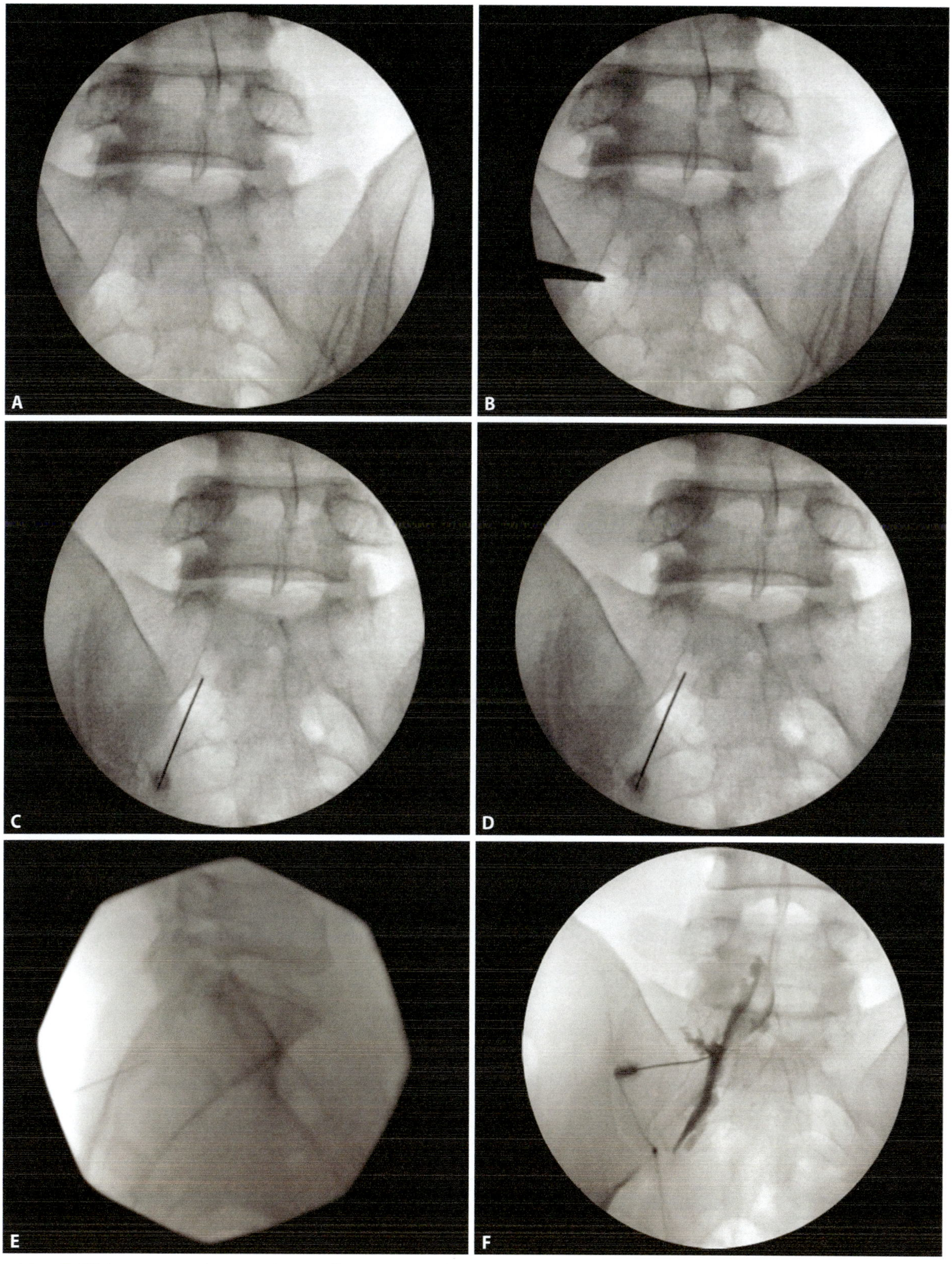

Figs. 3A to F: (A) Anteroposterior view; (B) Needle entry point for S1; (C) Needle headed toward S1 foramen; (D) Needle walks off the bone; (E) Reconfirm in lateral view; (F) Anteroposterior view of dye spread.

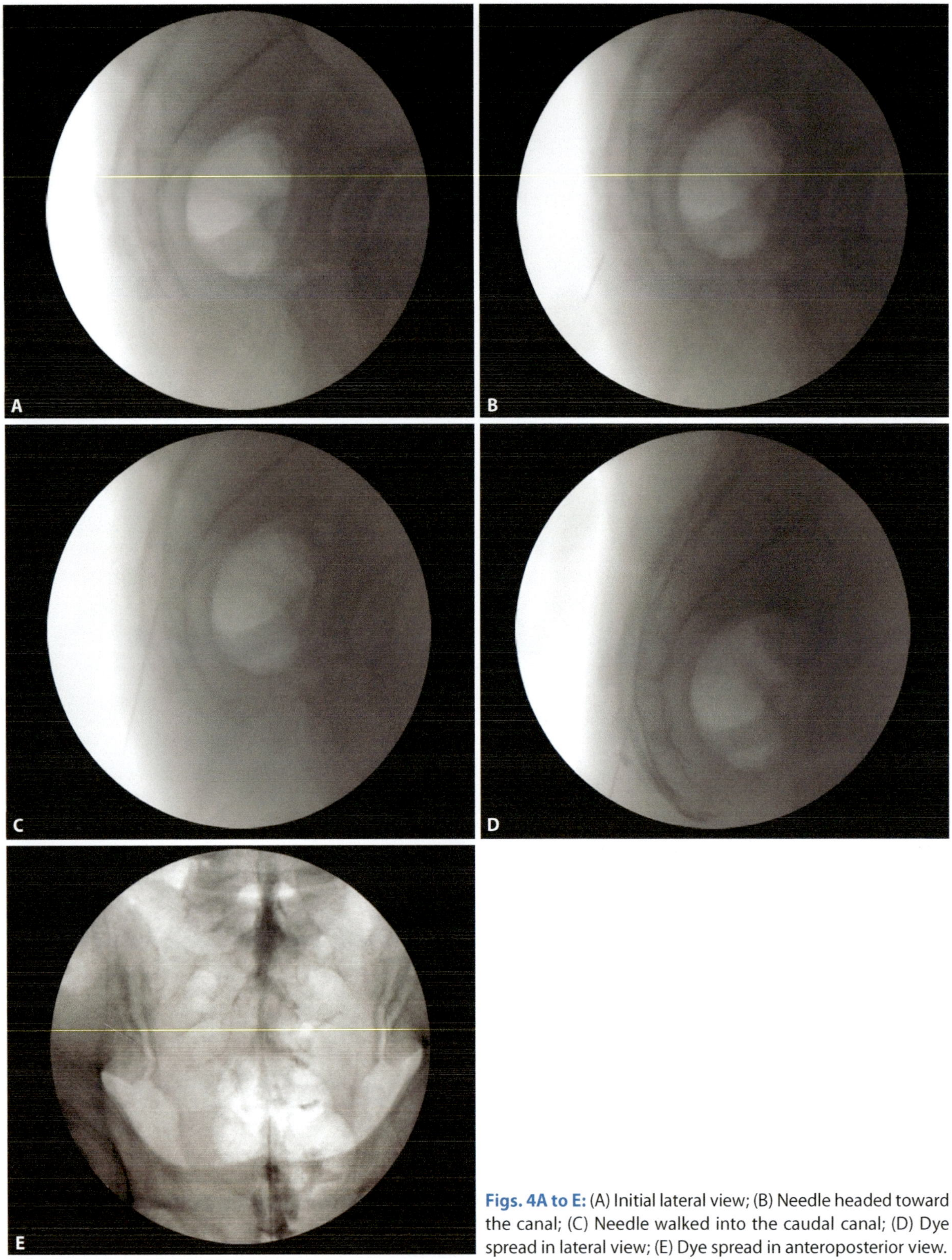

Figs. 4A to E: (A) Initial lateral view; (B) Needle headed toward the canal; (C) Needle walked into the caudal canal; (D) Dye spread in lateral view; (E) Dye spread in anteroposterior view.

Some of the techniques suggested are:

- Use of short bevel or blunt needles
- Using extension tubing and injecting under live fluoroscopy
- Use of nonparticulate steroids
- Digital subtraction angiography (DSA)
- Lidocaine test prior to injection of steroid.

CONCLUSION

Lumbar epidural steroid injections performed under fluoroscopic guidance are a safe and effective treatment modality for many conditions causing back pain and radicular symptoms. It should therefore be considered in the treatment plan in patients with a diagnosed, nonemergent cause of back pain who have failed more conservative treatment options.

REFERENCES

1. Derby R, Kine G, Saal J, Reynolds J, Goldthwaite N, White A, et al. Response to steroid and duration of radicular pain as predictors of surgical outcome. Spine (Phila Pa 1976). 1992;17(Suppl 6):S176-83.
2. Derby R, Bogduk N, Kine G. Precision percutaneous blocking procedures for localizing spinal pain: part 2. The lumbar neuraxial compartment. Pain Digest. 1993;3:175-88.
3. Bogduk N, Aprill C, Derby R. Epidural steroid injections. In: White AH (Ed). Spine Care: Diagnosis and Conservative Treatment St. Louis: Mosby; 1995. pp. 298-321.
4. Bogduk N. Epidural steroids. Spine (Phila Pa 1976). 1995;20(7):845-8.
5. Rydevik B, Brown MD, Lundborg G. Pathoanatomy and pathophysiology of nerve root compression. Spine (Phila Pa 1976). 1984;9(1):7-15.
6. Saal JS, Franson RC, Dobrow R, Saal JA, White AH, Goldthwaite N. High levels of inflammatory phospholipase A2 activity in lumbar disc herniations. Spine (Phila Pa 1976). 1990;15(7):674-8.
7. Snoek W, Weber H, Jørgensen B. Double-blind evaluation of extradural methyl prednisolone for herniated lumbar discs. Acta Orthop Scand. 1977;48(6):635-41.
8. Johansson A, Hao J, Sjölund B. Local corticosteroid application blocks transmission in normal nocioceptive C-fibers. Acta Anaesthesiol Scand. 1990;34(5):335-8.
9. Fuxe K, Härfstrand A, Agnati LF, Yu ZY, Cintra A, Wikström AC, et al. Immunocytochemical studies on the localization of glucocorticoid receptor immunoreactive nerve cells in the lower brain stem and spinal cord of the male rat using monoclonal antibody against rat liver glucocorticoid receptor. Neurosci Lett. 1985;60:1-6.
10. US Food and Drug Administration. (2014). Drug Safety Communications. FDA Drug Safety Communication: FDA requires label changes to warn of rare but serious neurological problems after epidural corticosteroid injections for pain. [online] Available from www.fda.gov/downloads/Drugs/Drug-Safety/ UCM394286.pdf. [Last accessed August, 2024].
11. Manchikanti L, Falco FJ, Benyamin RM, Gharibo CG, Candido KD, Hirsch JA. Epidural steroid injections safety recommendations by the Multi-Society Pain Workgroup (MPW): more regulations without evidence or clarification. Pain Physician. 2014;17(5):E575-88.
12. Manchikanti L, Candido KD, Singh V, Gharibo CG, Boswell MV, Benyamin RM, et al. Epidural steroid warning controversy still dogging FDA. Pain Physician. 2014;17(4):E451-74.
13. Candido KD, Knezevic NN, Chang-Chien GC, Deer TR. The Food and Drug Administration's recent action on April 23, 2014 failed to appropriately address safety concerns about epidural steroid use. Pain Physician. 2014;17(4):E549-52.
14. International Spinal Intervention Society. Update on ISIS Response to FDA Statement on ESIs. 2014;30:12.
15. Hamburg M, Lemtouni S. Office of the Center Director, Center for Drug Evaluation and Research, US Food and Drug Administration (FDA). Re: FDA Safe Use Initiative of Epidural Steroids Evaluation with Assignment of Responsibility to Multisociety Pain Workgroup (MPW) from American Society of Interventional Pain Physicians (ASIPP) and 1,040 Interventional Pain Physicians. 2014.
16. Manchikanti L, Falco FJ, Singh V, Pampati V, Parr AT, Benyamin RM, et al. Utilization of interventional techniques in managing chronic pain in the medicare population: analysis of growth patterns from 2000 to 2011. Pain Physician. 2012;15(6):E969-82.
17. Gupta S, Gupta M, Nath S, Hess GM. Survey of European pain medicine practice. Pain Physician. 2012;15(6):E983-94.
18. Benyamin RM, Manchikanti L, Parr AT, Diwan S, Singh V, Falco FJ, et al. The Effectiveness of lumbar interlaminar epidural injections in managing chronic low back and lower extremity pain. Pain Physician. 2012:15(4): E363-404.
19. Krych AJ, Richman D, Drakos M, Weiss L, Barnes R, Cammisa F, et al. Epidural steroid injections for lumbar disc herniation in NFL athletes. Med Sci Sports Exerc. 2012;44(2):193-8.
20. Akuthota V, Bogduk N, Easa JE, Patel AA, Prather H, Sharma A, et al. Lumbar Transforaminal Epidural Steroid Injections: Review and Recommendation Statement. North American Spine Society; 2013.
21. Ghahreman A, Ferch R, Bogduk N. The efficacy of transforaminal injection of steroids for the treatment of lumbar radicular pain. Pain Med. 2010;11(8):1149-68.
22. Ng L, Chaudhary N, Sell P. The efficacy of corticosteroids in periradicular infiltration for chronic radicular pain: a randomized, double-blind, control trial. Spine (Phila Pa 1976). 2005;30(8):857-62.

23. Ackerman WE 3rd, Ahmad M. The efficacy of lumbar epidural steroid injections in patients with lumbar disc herniations. Anesth Analg. 2007;104(5):1217- 22, tables of contents.
24. Botwin KP, Gruber RD, Bouchlas CG, Torres-Ramos FM, Freeman TL, Slaten WK. Complications of fluoroscopically guided tramsforaminal lumbar epidural injections. Arch Phys Med Rehabil. 2000;81(8):1045-50.
25. Gerszten PC, Smuck M, Rathmell JP, Simopoulos TT, Bhagia SM, Mocek CK, et al. Plasma disc decompression compared with fluoroscopy-guided transforaminal epidural steroid injections for symptomatic contained lumbar disc herniation: a prospective, randomized, controlled trial. J Neurosurg Spine. 2010;12(4);357-71.
26. Gonzalez P, Laker SR, Sullivan SW, Harwood JE, Akuthota V. The effects of epidural betamethasone on blood glucose in patients with diabetes mellitus. PM R. 2009;1(4):340-5.
27. Huntoon MA, Martin DP. Paralysis after transforaminal epidural injection and previous spine surgery. Reg Anesth Pain Med. 2004:29(5):494-5.
28. Kennedy DJ, Dreyfuss P, Aprill CN, Bogduk N. Paraplegia following image-guided transforaminal lumbar spine epidural steroid injection: two case reports. Pain Med. 2009;10(8):1389-94.
29. Somayaji HS, Saifuddin A, Casey AT, Briggs TW. Spinal cord infarction following therapeutic computed tomography-guided left L2 nerve root injection. Spine (Phila Pa 1976). 2005;30(4):E106-8.
30. Gharibo C, Koo C, Chung J, Moroz A. Epidural steroid injections: an update on mechanisms of injury and safety. Tech Reg Anesth Pain Manag. 2009;13(4):266-71.
31. Huntoon MA, Martin DP. Paralysis after transforaminal epidural injection and previous spinal surgery. Reg Anesth Pain Med. 2004;29(5):494-5
32. Siglar JD, Garvan C, McLean JP, Plastaras C, Rittenberg JD. Digital subtraction: does it matter? The rate of intravascular uptake in cervical epidural steroid injections with and without digital subtraction. Arch Phys Med Rehabil. 2008;89:E96.
33. Fenton DS, Czervionke LF. Image-guided spine intervention. Philadelphia: Saunders; 2003. pp. 99-126, 100.
34. Bogduk N, Aprill C, Derby R. Selective nerve root blocks. In: Wilson DJ (Ed). Interventional Radiology of the Musculoskeletal System. London: Edward Arnold; 1995. pp. 121-32.
35. Bogduk N, Aprill C, Derby R. Epidural steroid injections. In: White AH (Ed). Spine Care: Diagnosis and Conservative Treatment. St Louis: Mosby; 1995. pp. 322-43.
36. Glaser SE, Shah RV. Root cause analysis of paraplegia following transforaminal epidural steroid injections: the 'unsafe' triangle. Pain Physician. 2010;13(3): 237-44.
37. Helm S, Glase S, Falco F, Henry B. A medical-legal review regarding the standard of care for epidural injections, with particular reference to a closed case. Pain Physician. 2010;13(2):145-50.
38. Zhu J, Falco FJ, Formoso F, Onyewu O, Irwin FL. Alternative approach for lumbar transforaminal epidural steroid injections. Pain Physician. 2011;14(4):331-41.
39. Glaser SE, Falco F. Paraplegia following a thoracolumbar transforaminal epidural steroid injection. Pain Physician. 2005;8(3):309-14.
40. Jasper JF. Lumbar retrodiskal transforaminal injection. Pain Physician. 2007;10(3):501-10.
41. Helm S 2nd, Jasper JF, Racz GB. Complications of transforaminal epidural injections. Pain Physician. 2003;6(3):389-90.
42. Windsor RE, Falco FJ. Paraplegia following selective nerve root blocks. ISIS Scientific Newsletter. 2001;4:53-4.
43. Murthy NS, Maus TP, Behrns CL. Intraforaminal location of the great anterior radiculomedullary artery (artery of Adamkiewicz): a retrospective review. Pain Med. 2010;11(12):1756-64.
44. Houten JK, Errico TJ. Paraplegia after lumbosacral nerve root block: report of three cases. Spine J. 2002;2(1):70-5.

35 CHAPTER

Lumbar Facet Joint, Medial Branch, and Radiofrequency Procedures

Annu H Navani, Irina Melnik, Richard Derby, Jeong-Eun Lee

ABSTRACT

Effective treatment of chronic back pain requires accurate identification of the primary source of pain. It is known that spine has multiple potential pain generators, with lumbar facet joints being a frequent source of posterior elements disease, often contributing to chronic back pain and occasionally leg pain symptoms. Clinical presentation and imaging tests are not dependable in identification of the facet joint-mediated pain. Diagnostic facet joint blocks in the form of intra-articular injection of local anesthetics directly into the joints, or medial branch blocks (MBBs) when anesthetic is injected at the nerve that innervates the facet joint blocking the pain transmission, became the standard procedures of choice in identifying the source of the back pain. MBB became a "gold standard" diagnostic test, since it has a valid subsequent therapeutic procedure of choice, in the form of radiofrequency (RF) nerve ablation (RFA); MBB is easier and safer to perform, and it is associated with potentially higher prognostic value. Lumbar MBBs target each of the nerves that innervate a given joint (two branches per joint). The anatomy of these nerves is pivotal to the accurate conduct of diagnostic blocks and subsequently to the accurate conduct of medial branch (MB) RFA treatment.[1] As with any diagnostic test, the downside of the MBB is a potential presence of false-positive and false-negative rates. One of the most important goals of MBB is in its prognostic value. When used as a prognostic tool, the false-negative and false-positive rates of MBB depend on the eventual outcome of RFA, with its confirmed rate of success.[2] The positive-predictive value of MBB greatly improved by using additional confirmatory block and by optimizing the "cutoff value" of the pain relief following the MBB test at above 70%.[3] RFA treatment has gained popularity as a minimally invasive percutaneous procedure of choice in patients with refractory back pain due to facet joint disease, using thermal heating of the MBs innervating affected joint. The success of procedure and the duration of pain relief have been shown to correlate with RF electrode size and proper anatomic positioning of the electrode close to the MB in a parallel manner.[4] RFA is considered a safe, palliative procedure that can be safely and easily repeated with few associated complications when performed by a well-trained practitioner.

INTRODUCTION

The lumbar facet joint has long been a significant source of low-back pain. The facet joint is a true synovium-lined joint located in the posterior compartment of the spine that allows the spine to flex, extend, and rotate.[5] The most common cause of facet joint-mediated pain is due to degenerative changes including osteoarthritis.

For this reason, facet-mediated pain is most common in the elderly population. The prevalence by some sources of facet joint-mediated pain contributing to low-back pain is 15% in younger-aged, injured workers with chronic back pain to 40% in older, noninjured patients with degenerative or rheumatic problems.[6]

By convention, lumbar medial branch blocks (MBBs) are used to test a patient's pain originating from the given lumbar zygapophyseal joint (facet joint). For that purpose, the nerves that innervate the joint are anesthetized. This is based on the argument that of all the structures innervated by medial branches (MBs) of the lumbar dorsal rami, the zygapophyseal joints are the only structure that might harbor a discrete focal source of chronic pain.[7]

HISTORICAL BACKGROUND

The development of lumbar MBBs was prompted in as early as 1971 when Rees claimed that the pain arising from the lumbar zygapophyseal joint could be treated by severing the nerves and Shealy claimed that these could be coagulated with the radiofrequency (RF) electrode.[8-13] Subsequently, studies describing intra-articular injections dominated the literature on zygapophyseal joint pain during the 1980s.[7] However, once it was established that intra-articular injections of steroids did not provide lasting relief from lumbar zygapophyseal joint pain, lumbar MB neurotomy remained the only means of providing relief from this pain and MBBs as their precursor diagnostic blocks. In 1997–1998, Dreyfuss and colleagues performed studies demonstrating that lumbar MBBs were target-specific provided that precise target points were accurately identified and needles placed in a particular direction.[14] Kaplan and colleagues further showed that normal volunteers were protected from experimentally induced facet-mediated pain if the appropriate MBs were anesthetized.[15] Once the diagnosis of facet-mediated pain via lumbar MBBs was established, numerous studies followed showing dramatic and long-lasting relief of pain following lumbar MB neurotomy. van Kleef and colleagues demonstrated that the lumbar MB neurotomy was not a placebo.[16]

CLINICAL PRESENTATION

The diagnosis of facet-mediated pain is established with detailed history, comprehensive physical examination, review of diagnostic studies, and lastly corroboration of facts obtained from these sources. First of all, it is important to make sure that all serious possible causes of back pain, such as infection, tumors, and vascular or metabolic diseases, have been excluded by careful and thorough history and examination, laboratory tests, and medical imaging if necessary.

Although there are no clinical features that allow a physician to predict with confidence that the patient with back pain will respond positively to lumbar MBBs, there are certain features that increase the likelihood of zygapophyseal joint pain, such as age >65 years, pain relieved by recumbency and absence of aggravation of pain by coughing, forward flexion or rising from flexion. Typically, the lumbar facet pain presents as low back pain that is aggravated by hyperextension or extension-rotation.[17] If five or more of these criteria are satisfied, the likelihood ratio for positive response to block is 3.[18]

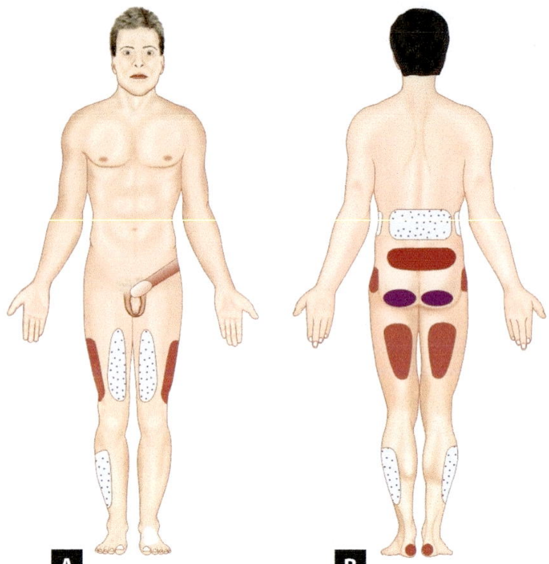

Figs. 1A and B: Pain referral patterns from the lumbar facet joints. In descending order, the most common referral patterns extend from the darkest (low back) to the lightest (flank and foot) regions.[21]

Consequently, the presence of these features triples the likelihood of zygapophyseal joint blocks being positive. Somatic referred pain in the lower limb is not a contraindication for lumbar MBBs **(Figs. 1A and B)**. Although those symptoms are more commonly representative of radiculitis or radiculopathy, they have been reported to be relieved by anesthetizing lumbar zygapophyseal joints are the past.[19,20]

ANATOMICAL CONSIDERATION

The lumbar spine can be divided into two to three compartments—anterior, middle, and posterior. The anterior compartment consists of vertebral bodies and disk spaces, the middle compartment consists of epidural space and neural foramina, and the posterior compartment consists of facet joints. The vertebrae articulate anteriorly through the disks and posteriorly through the two facet joints, one on each side. The facet joints are paired diarthrodial synovial joints formed by the inferior articular process of one vertebra and the superior articular process (SAP) of the subjacent vertebrae below. Biomechanically, this produces a complex tripod structure that has evolved into distinctive patterns at each spinal level. The facet joints share the same general characteristics of the synovial joint. The articular surface is covered by cartilage and the synovial membrane bridges the margins of the cartilage of two facets in each joint. Covering the synovial membrane superiorly, posteriorly, and inferiorly is a thick fibrous joint capsule, however, anteriorly the synovial membrane lacks of true fibrous capsule and instead is in direct contact with the ligamentum flavum. Superiorly and inferiorly, the fibrous joint capsule forms a pocket connected to the lumbar facet joint between the capsule pocket and synovium are two structures. The first has been referred to a meniscoid. There are several descriptions of these meniscoids, but probably they are best understood as a fold of synovium that contains adipose tissue, collagen, and some blood vessels. The normal function of these meniscoids is not clear although in the diseased facet joints, they have been implicated as a source of damage to the articular cartilage causing the facet joints to lock. The second structure is simply adipose tissue, which occupies any leftover space beneath the capsule. The superior and inferior parts of the capsule each have a hole. The superior hole connects the intracapsular fat to the epidural space. The capsule is attached to the margins of the articular process of the adjacent vertebra, accessory ligaments unite the lamina, transverse process (TP), and spinous process is to help stabilize the joint.[5]

The zygapophyseal joints are innervated by articular branches that arrive from the MBs of the dorsal primary rami of the spinal nerves as these nerves pass posteriorly and inferiorly and lie in grooves on the posterior surfaces of medial parts of the TP. Each articular branch supplies two adjacent joints; therefore, each joint is supplied by two nerves, the nerve at the same level and the level above; for example, L4-L5 joint is innervated by L3 and L4 MBs. A list of the appropriate MBs innervating specific facet joints is as follows:

- L2-L3 joint innervated by L1-L2 MBs
- L3-L4 by L2 and L3 MBs
- L4-L5 with L3 and L4 MBs
- L5-S1 with L4 and L5 MBs

For the L1-L4 MBs, the target point is at the junction of SAP and TP at which the target nerve crosses midway between the superior border of the TP and the location of mamillo-accessory notch. The numbering of the MBs differs as per the location; thus, L4 MB crosses over the L5 TP and L3 MB over the L4 TP. At the L5 level, the target nerve is not the MB, but the L5 dorsal ramus proper. The nerve crosses the ala of the sacrum in a manner analogous to the passage of upper MBs and crosses the TP.

Although a posterior approach is possible, the easiest and most convenient approach is an oblique approach. On the oblique view, the target can be identified in either of the two ways. Figuratively, the target point lies above and behind the eye of the "Scotty dog". The term "Scotty dog" is often referred to the appearance of vertebral silhouette in oblique view **(Fig. 2)**.

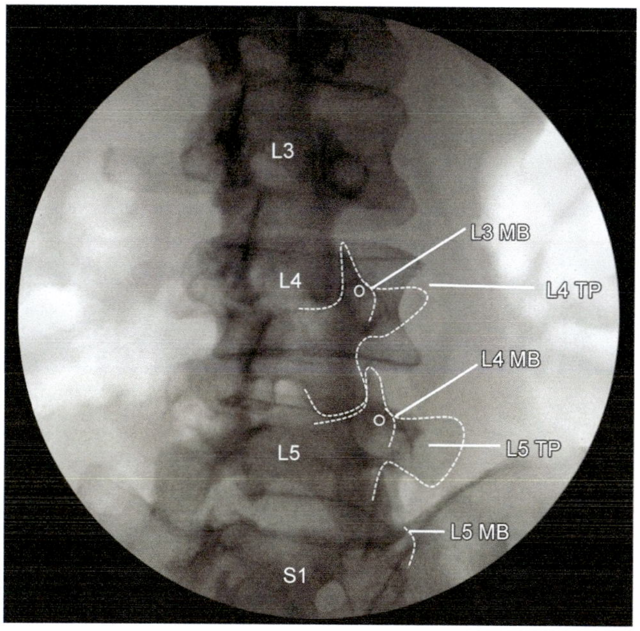

Fig. 2: Scotty dog appearance in oblique view. (MB: medial branch; TP: transverse process)

The MBs anteroposterior (AP) compartments of the back by curving around the concavity of the ventral edge of the neck of the SAP and subsequently turning medially under the mamillo-accessory ligament (MAL) through the mamillo-accessory notch. A line can be visualized between these two points (ventral edge of the neck of the SAP and the mamillo-accessory notch). The target point for blocks lies on this line, above its midpoint.

For any given zygapophyseal joint, both the nerves that innervate the joint will need to be anesthetized. Correct placement is confirmed by obtaining a posteroanterior (PA) view. In this view, the tip of the needle should be at least opposite the lateral margin of the silhouette of SAP and preferably slightly medial to its margin. This is because SAP often bulges laterally overlapping the target point dorsally. If the tip lies lateral to this margin, it has struck the base of the thick TP and SAP. Once the needle is in correct position, the bevel should be directed medially so as to avoid spread of injections to the intervertebral foramina. Oblique view provides the easiest and safest approach, with the needle tip target positioned at the

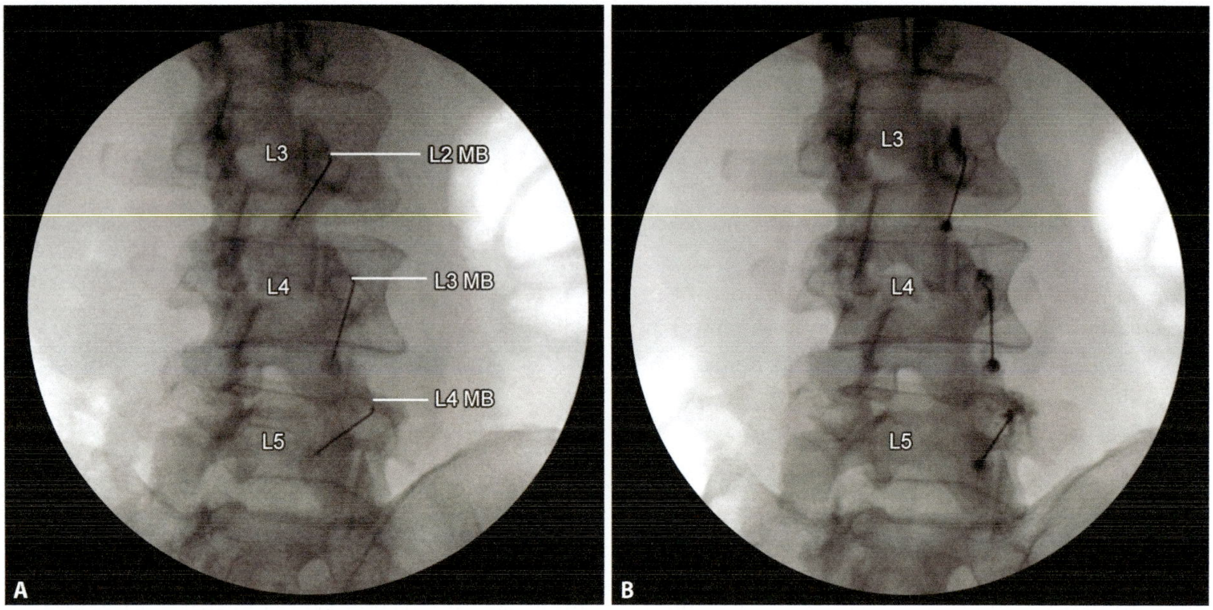

Figs. 3A and B: Medial branch needle placement for L2, L3, L4 medial branch blocks, over the transverse processes (TP) of L3, L4, L5, respectively. (A) Without contrast; (B) With contrast. (MB: medial branch)

"eye of the Scotty dog" **(Fig. 3A)**. Once this has been done, 0.1–0.3 mL of contrast medium is injected to test the correct positioning of the needle as well as to exclude venous uptake. If it does, the needle must be readjusted by 1 or 2 mm and the contrast injection repeated. If there is no venous uptake, 0.5 mL of local anesthetic is injected at the target nerve. Both nerves that innervate the target joint are anesthetized in the same way **(Fig. 3B)**.

For L5 dorsal ramus block, the protocol is the same as the higher levels **(Fig. 4A)**. The difference is that the target nerve is not MB but the dorsal ramus itself and that the target point is the junction of the ala of sacrum and the SAP of the sacrum. This target point is recognized in PA views as a notch between the two bones. The target point lies opposite to the middle of the base of the SAP and hence likely below the silhouette of the top of the ala of the sacrum. A higher placement is associated with the spread of injected into the L5-S1 epidural space and lower placement is associated with the spread to the S1 posterior sacral foramen.[14] Insertion is monitored to ensure that the needle is not straight over the top of the sacrum. Insertion is terminated once the needle strikes the bone at the target point. The AP view should show the tip of the needle tucked against the SAP of the sacrum and under its lateral margin **(Fig. 4B)**. If bone is reached, but not precisely at the target point, the needle is readjusted and a well correct position is obtained. Once the needle is in correct position, the bevel is directed to face medially. This reduces the risk of inadvertent spread of injected to either L5-S1 intervertebral foramina or S1 posterior foramen. Contrast medium should be injected both to confirm the accurate placement of the needle and to exclude venous uptake.

PRINCIPLES AND TECHNIQUES

The International Spine Intervention Society recommends lumbar MBB to replace or should replace intra-articular injections for diagnosis of lumbar zygapophyseal joints for the reasons mentioned above. If the MBBs' diagnostic test is positive, the patient can be considered for radiofrequency ablation (RFA)/MB neurotomy described later in this chapter.

As noted earlier, the lumbar MBBs have replaced the intra-articular injections and diagnosis of lumbar zygapophyseal joint pain for the most part.[7] The main advantages of approaching the joint via MB nerves rather than intra-articularly are as follows:

- MBBs are relatively easier to perform.
- MBBs are safer and more expedient.
- MBBs are more easily subjected to control.
- Intra-articular blocks therapeutic utility; that is, if they are positive, they lack valid subsequent treatment.

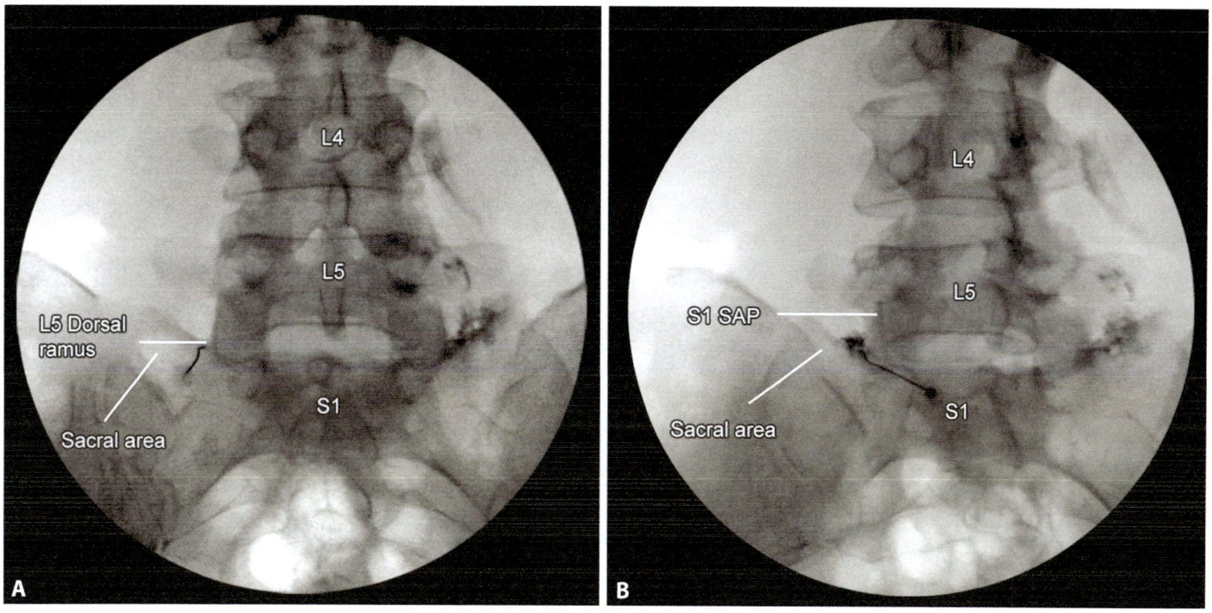

Figs. 4A and B: Medial branch (MB) needle placement for L5 dorsal ramus over the sacral ala. (A) Anteroposterior (AP) view without contrast; (B) Oblique view with contrast. (SAP: superior articular process)

- MBBs do have therapeutic utility for, if positive, the pain can be treated with RF neurotomy.

The purpose of performing MBBs is to conclude diagnostically if the patient's back pain is emanating from the facet joints if by anesthetizing the innervations to the facet joints by blocking the MBs. Typically, 70% or more reduction of a patient's typical preprocedure pain is considered as a positive response. The clinician interpreting the results of the block must also consider the placebo effect, and MBBs are often repeated with the short-acting local anesthetic. The patient with two positive MBBs concordant with the duration of action of local anesthetics should be considered for MB rhizotomy.

The intra-articular facet block can also be considered for suspected facetogenic pain. This injection involves injecting a combination of short- or long-acting local anesthetic with a steroidal agent. The technique is thought to have a twofold effect of diagnosing suspected facetogenic pain with added benefit of reducing inflammation from within the joint providing long-lasting resolution of symptoms; however, since the benefits of the RF neurotomy after diagnosis with MBs are longer lasting, this pathway is noted to be more beneficial than intra-articular injection with steroidal agents. The volume that the facet joint accommodates is only 0.5–0.8 cc thereby limiting the dose of steroid and thereby long-term effects. These blocks are performed in oblique view as described below.

INDICATIONS

The fundamental indication of lumbar MBB is to desire or need to know if the patient's pain is mediated by MBs of the lumbar dorsal rami. The only validated treatment for pain mediated by lumbar MBs is percutaneous RF neurotomy. If this treatment is not available, the conduct of MBBs can be justified only on grounds of the diagnostic utility. However, if RF neurotomy is available, MBBs are an essential prerequisite before entertaining the long-acting procedure, RF neurotomy.

Medial branch blocks are not indicated for acute back pain. There is a high chance of acute back pain recovering regardless of or even despite conservative treatment, and RF neurotomy is not indicated for acute pain. Therefore, it is not necessary and becomes a waste of resources to perform diagnostic block in patients with acute back pain. In principle, therefore, MBBs are indicated only for patients with chronic pain; however, these can be considered for investigating back pain in patients of sub-acute duration when the pain is not improving or responding to conservative management. This is justified based on the fact that pinpointing the source of pain and promptly treating it in these patients could avoid the onset of chronic pain behavior.

CONTRAINDICATIONS

Absolute contraindications for lumbar MBBs are conditions in which needle interventions under X-ray may jeopardize a patient's health. These include but are not necessarily limited to bacterial infections, systemic or localized, in the region of the blocks to be performed. The other absolute contraindication is the patient's refusal of the procedure, bleeding diathesis due to hematological disease or anticoagulants, and possible pregnancy.

Relative contraindications that do not preclude lumbar MBBs but will require special consideration are, for example, allergy to contrast medium, which may require coverage with corticosteroid, H1 and H2 antagonists, allergy to local anesthetic which may require identification, and use of a class of anesthetic to which the patient is not allergic and concurrent treatment with nonsteroidal anti-inflammatory medication including aspirin, which may compromise coagulation in which case medication may need to be suspended for an appropriate period prior to conduct of the blocks.

EQUIPMENT AND FACILITY REQUIREMENTS

These interventions should be performed in fluoroscopy suite under sterile technique using C-arm fluoroscope. Fluoroscopy is mandatory for conducting lumbar MBBs. The preferred equipment is C-arm fluoroscope that allows for X-ray beam to be directed at any angle. This will help document accurate placement of needle and spread of contrast medium. The device must be available to obtain either hardcopy film or images specialized paper or permanent digital image.

Additional equipment needed would be solutions for skin preparation, such as iodine-based solutions or alcohol-based antiseptic solutions, sterile gloves, local anesthetic agents with syringes, needles, and extension tubing. Please note that intravenous solutions, sedation, or antibiotics are not mandatory and not required. Sterile gowns and drapes are necessary to create a sterile surgical environment. Agents most commonly used to anesthetize the MBs are bupivacaine 0.5% and lidocaine 2%. Other concentrations that can be used are bupivacaine 0.75% and 0.25% and lidocaine 1% and 4%. Because small volumes are used, it is generally considered that high concentration of the local anesthetics be used in order to obtain the most effective anesthetic effect. For MBBs, not more than 0.5 mL is required to block the nerve adequately. Contrast medium is required to test for intravascular placement of the block needle.

Intra-articular Facet Joint Block

After discussion of risks and benefits and completion of the informed consent, the patient is asked to lie supine on the fluoroscopy table with a pillow under the lower abdomen to straighten the lumbar lordosis. Skin is prepped and draped in a sterile fashion. The initial AP view of the spine is visualized once the exact level is confirmed **(Fig. 5A)**. The fluoroscopic beam is rotated obliquely 10–40° lateral from the midline on the site of the facet joint to be blocked **(Fig. 5B)**. The upper lumbar joints have a different orientation than the lower lumbar facet joints. The posterior joints space may start to open as the obliquity of the fluoroscope increases. The best fluoroscopic image of the joint may be obtained at angle 5–10° more oblique than the best angle for the needle to enter the joint. The ideal point of skin entry is just lateral to the inferior edge of the inferior articular process. Usually, this is the widest part of the joint and is easiest to enter. The point is marked on the skin and 1% lidocaine is used to anesthetize the skin and subcutaneous tissue using a 27G 1.5-inch needle. After the local anesthetizing, a 22- or 25G spinal needle is used to enter the joint space using a tunnel approach directly under the beam of the fluoroscope. Often a pop is felt as one enters the joint; this may or may not reproduce the patient's typical concordant pain. Injecting about 0.25 cc of radiocontrast dye into the joint reconfirms the appropriate position of the needle in the joint **(Fig. 5C)**. Once appropriate placement of the needle in the joint has been confirmed, a mixture of local anesthetic and corticosteroid is injected in the joint as noted in **Figures 5A to C**. Typically, the joint is demonstrated as an S-shaped joint; the contrast dye is identified in a dumbbell shape in the oblique view and a discoid shape in the AP view.

Lumbar Medial Branch Block

After informed consent is obtained, the patient is placed on the fluoroscopy table in a prone position with a pillow under the lower abdomen. Skin is prepped and draped in a sterile fashion.

The procedure is started in straight AP position of the C-arm and vertebral levels are identified, numerically counting from either the last rib or the sacrum up. The C-arm is then rotated in the oblique fashion till the "Scotty dog" configuration is visualized.

For MBs L1 to L4, the largest position of the needle lies in the junction of the base of the TP and SAP. Under fluoroscopic guidance, the needle is introduced

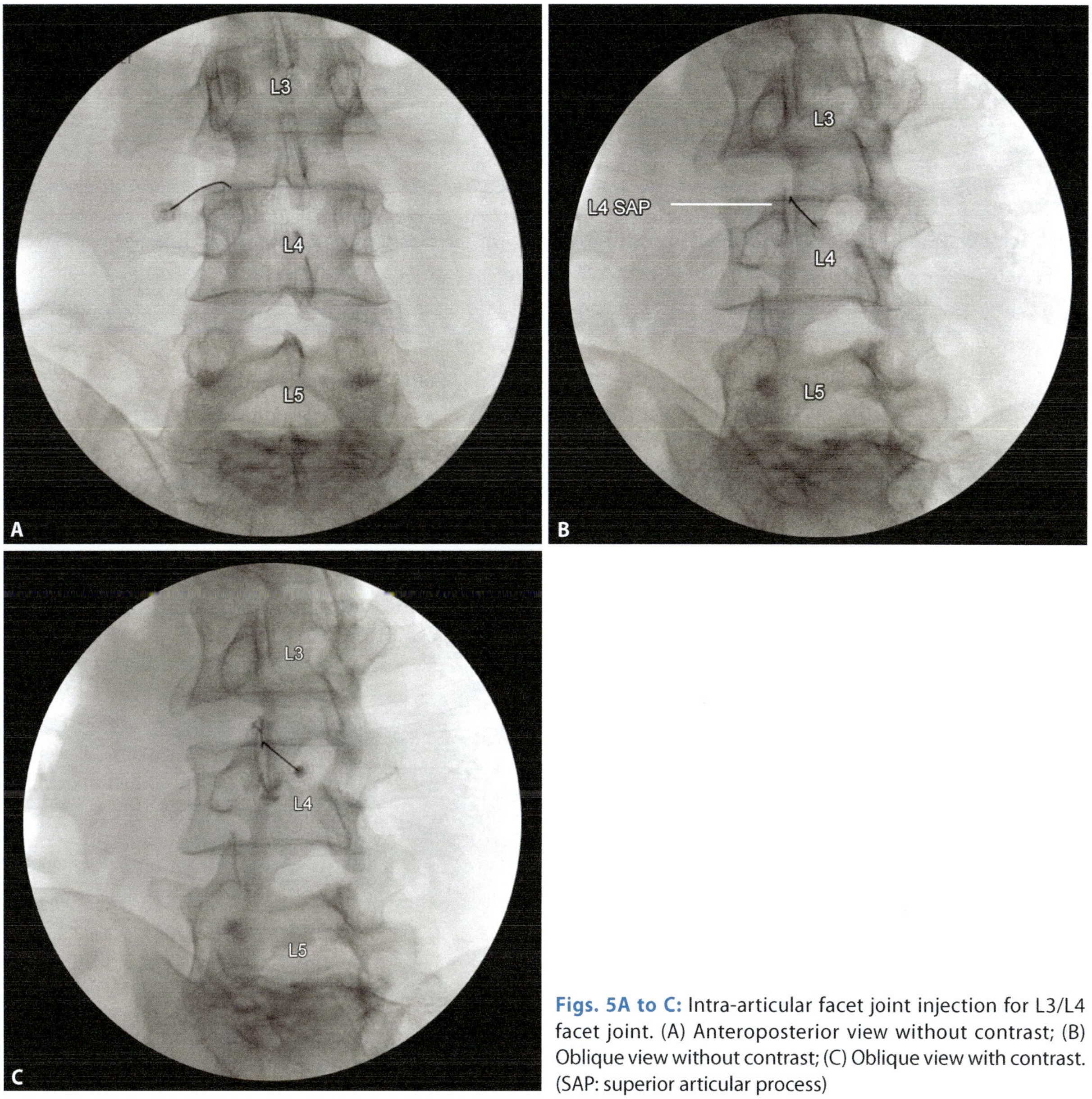

Figs. 5A to C: Intra-articular facet joint injection for L3/L4 facet joint. (A) Anteroposterior view without contrast; (B) Oblique view without contrast; (C) Oblique view with contrast. (SAP: superior articular process)

approximately 5 cm lateral from the midline and directed obliquely to avoid the overhanging articular process. For L1 to L4, the MBs are blocked where it lies in the gutter on the dorsal surface of the TP just caudal to the most medial end of the superior edge of the TP. At the lumbosacral junction, the posterior primary ramus of L5 is blocked, as it runs into the groove between the ala of the sacrum and the superior articulate process of the sacrum. For the injection to be reliably diagnostic, the needle location needs to be precisely placed and preferably with the bevel facing medially and inferiorly for L1 through L4 and medially at L5. The ideal target point is midway between the upper border of TP and the MAL. Blocking a single joint requires two medial nerves to be injected from the same level and the level above. To minimize unwarranted spread of injection, the injection is precisely targeted and only a small volume of local anesthetic is used. Once the needle has contacted the bone, the final needle position is checked in the oblique and lateral views. It is critical to ensure that appropriate nerves are selected depending upon which joint is being investigated; for example, if one wants to block L4-L5 joint, the MBs to be blocked will be L3 and L4 and L4 and L5 for L5-S1 blocks. Once that has been done, 0.5 cc of contrast dye is injected followed by 0.5 cc of local anesthetic.

DISCHARGE INSTRUCTIONS

The patient is instructed to call the interventionist back if there is fever, tenderness, any unusual symptoms, or pain following the procedure such as fever, tenderness greater than what may be expected from the needle track, any signs of infection, or any new neurological symptoms. The patient should also be instructed to carefully document movements and activities of daily living that are customarily restricted by pain in order to determine the efficacy of the block. The patient is typically asked to maintain a pain journal and document their pain, axial pain score with movements, especially extension and lateral rotation every hour for the next 5 hours.

The patient can resume normal activities the following day and should refrain from driving and operating heavy machinery on the day of the procedure. If steroids are used, it may take up to 3–5 days for the full effect of the medications to take place.

Although experienced operators may be more efficient and faster than beginners, there are a few parameters that have been recommended by the International Spine Interventional Society[7] to define the minimal level of competence and proficiency for performance of lumbar MBBs. It is recommended to not have more than eight adjustments or corrections of the course of needle from insertion to reaching the target point and not >1.5 minutes of total radiation exposure time to block the given nerve which includes exposure time to identify the target point, puncture point and prior to reinsertion of the needle. This will help the interventionalists self-guide their performance.

POTENTIAL COMPLICATIONS

The MBBs and intra-articular injections are relatively safe procedures. Potential complications may include as with any spine injection, such as bleeding, infection, postprocedure radicular back pain, thecal sac puncture, spinal headache, allergic reaction to medications, and possible vasovagal reaction.

RADIOFREQUENCY NEUROTOMY

Percutaneous RF neurotomy is a therapeutic procedure in which a Teflon-coated electrode with an exposed tip is inserted close to the peripheral nerve in such a manner that when higher frequency electric current is applied to the electrode, it concentrates around the exposed tip, heats the immediately surrounding tissues, and coagulates them including the target nerve. Percutaneous RF of the lumbar MB is a specific application of this procedure when the target nerve is the MB of the lumbar dorsal ramus.

Historical Background

Since the pioneering work of White and Sweet in 1969,[22] RF neurotomy has been used successfully in the treatment of trigeminal neuralgia. That success inspired its application for the treatment of spinal pain. Its use for lumbar spinal pain was first promoted by Shealy,[12,13,23] between 1974 and 1976; others soon adopted the procedure and reported good results. Other neurodestructive procedures such as cryolesioning, chemical neurolysis, and lasers have been used over the years; however, RFA stands as unrelenting efficacious treatment for long-term relief of pain from the lumbar facets.

Clinical Relevance

Radiofrequency lesioning is generated by RF generator, which is connected to the electrode placed on the body. The current flows between the tissues the active electrode is positioned on where the heat lesion has to be made and the other electrode which is a large grounding pad, not intended to produce heat lesioning. The mechanism of the tissue heating is primary ionic. The RF voltage on the tip of the needle sets up an electric field in the space around the needle and the heat is generated. It is important to understand that the tip of the needle does not actually heat up. The tip of the needle has a sensor, which gives a temperature reading. The equilibrium is usually reached about in 60 seconds. The size of the lesion depends on the electrode tip length as well as diameter and temperature of the tip.

Principles

Radiofrequency denervation is performed by alternating high-frequency electric current between the large surface area of the grounding pad and a small surface area, which is an uninsulated tip of the needle. The current approaches the electric tip, the electric field becomes denser and stronger, and the current alternates causing the charged molecules to oscillate. Oscillation heats the tissue sufficiently to coagulate it. The volume of the coagulated tissue assumes the shape of a long spheroid whose long axis is formed by the uninsulated tip of the needle. Coagulation occurs principally along the long axis of the needle. A small amount of coagulation occurs distal to the tip of the needle. The size of the lesion and dimensions are proportional to the size of the electrode, the length of the electrode, and the diameter of the electrode.

The concept of the lesion size and diameter is important as placing the electrode perpendicular to the nerve will create a very small lesion which may miss it. Consequently, a full optimal coagulation electrode should be placed parallel to the nerve. In case of perpendicular needle placement or use of a small-sized electrode, multiple lesions have to be made to get the most optimal response. For the optimal lesioning, the RF needle trajectory (at L1-L4 MB levels) needs to be oblique to the sagittal plane, placed parallel from below the target nerve at 15–20° **(Fig. 6A)**. This will help to avoid the needle deflection by the MAL and improve the nerve exposure to the active electrode tip at the most accessible part of the MB, laying at the anterolateral aspects of the curved neck of the SAP, providing the most optimal lesioning **(Fig. 6B)**. This does not apply to the neurotomy of the L5 dorsal ramus, for a MAL does not obstruct the course of an electrode at the S1 level, allowing more sagittal placement **(Figs. 7A and B)**.

The size of the lesion also depends on the duration of coagulation. As the temperature of the electrode reaches 65°C, the coagulation starts on the surface. The volume of coagulation tissue expands as the temperature increases to 80°C. At 30 seconds, the lesion increases to 85% of its maximum size. Once the temperature reaches 80°C, the lesion size is 60% of its maximum size. After 60 seconds, it reaches 94% of the size which is attained by maintaining 80°C for 90 seconds. Thereafter, increasing the time further does not increase the size of the lesion, so the optimal duration of coagulation is between 60 and 90 seconds.

The electrode of choice for lumbar RF is 100 mm 18- or 20G long straight probe with a 10-mm active tip. Most common coagulation parameters are 80°C for 90 seconds. At lesser duration than 60–90 seconds, the lesions made may be too small to coagulate the target nerve accurately. Raising the temperature too fast risks cavitation occurring in the lesion and production of a lesion that is irregular in shape and size.[24] Impedance is an important parameter

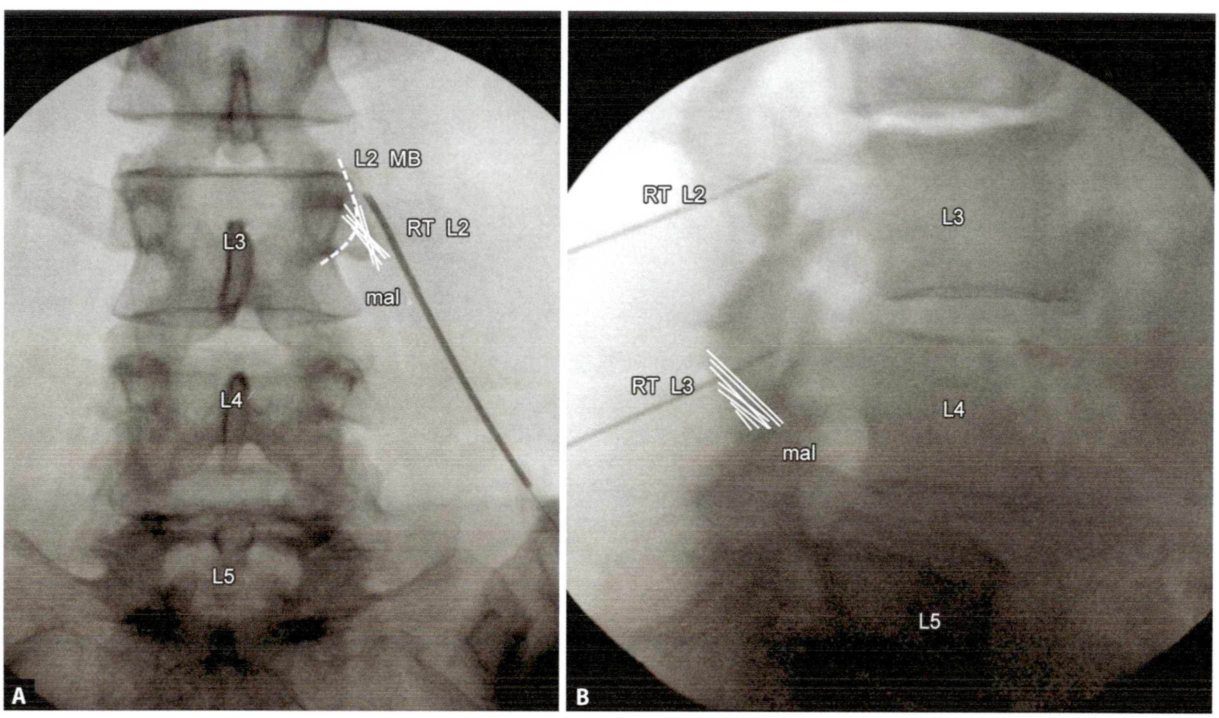

Figs. 6A and B: Views of radiofrequency needle placement with optimal trajectory to medial branches of L2, L3, avoiding mamilloaccessory ligaments. (A) Anteroposterior view; (B) Lateral view.

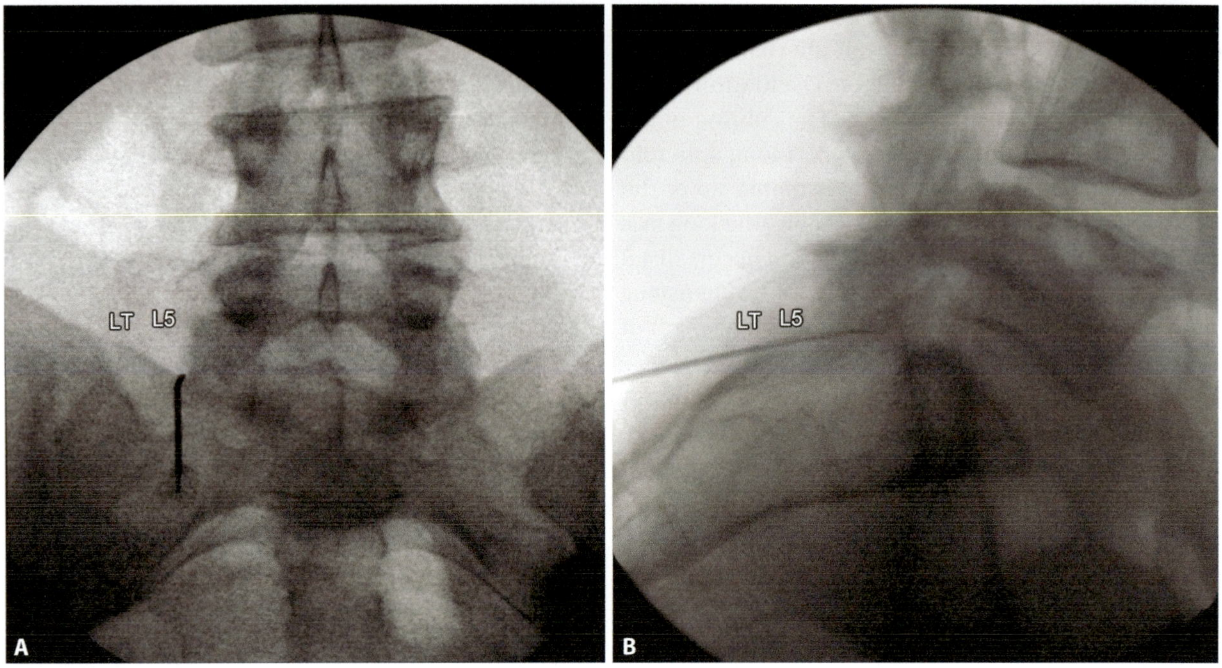

Figs. 7A and B: An example of correct radiofrequency electrode position for L5 dorsal ramus neurotomy over the sacral ala. (A) Anteroposterior (AP) view; (B) Lateral view.

that needs to be maintained as the power and temperature are increased. Erratic behavior of the impedance and fluctuations in the temperature indicate faulty equipment or connections or presence of blood or other fluid in the area of lesion.

Radiofrequency coagulation lesions the entire nerve; electrodiagnostic studies have shown that even alpha motor neurons are coagulated.[24] RF neurotomy, therefore, is a nonselective method of coagulating peripheral nerves.

Patient's Selection

The optimal patient for lumbar RF denervation is a patient with pain for at least 3 months with no indications of resolving by natural history and who has not responded to conservative treatments. The pain is focal, axial in nature, appears to be coming from facet etiology, and has undergone controlled diagnostic blocks of the target MBs with different local anesthetics, each time getting significant pain relief greater than at least 50% pain relief corresponding to the duration of the local anesthetic. Previous surgery or presence of radicular symptoms does not exclude the candidacy for RF denervation if the patient meets the above-listed criteria.

Procedural Considerations

After informed consent is obtained, the patient is placed on the fluoroscopy table in a prone position with a pillow under the lower abdomen. Skin is prepped and draped in a sterile fashion.

The needles are placed under fluoroscopy guidance in a manner similar to the MBB. Once the depth is known, the needle is withdrawn and slightly readjusted to pass along the neck of the SAP no more than a few millimeters. At this view, the AP view of the placement is done, and lateral view shows the target area **(Figs. 8A to D)**. Once that is accomplished, the probe is inserted and sensory testing of MBs is performed at 50 Hz. The current is advanced in 0.1 mA increments and the patient is asked for reproduction of his back pain, pressure, or buzzing sensation in the back. Patients are also instructed to inform if the pain starts radiating in a radicular pattern down the leg. Usually with good placement, sensory stimulation is noted to be <0.5 V. Once sensory testing is over, motor stimulation is carried out at 2 Hz, which should be done up to three times of the sensory threshold. At this time stimulation of paravertebral or multifidus muscle is usually noted, but there should be no motor stimulation of the lower extremities. Once these parameters are noted at each level, 0.5 mL of 2%

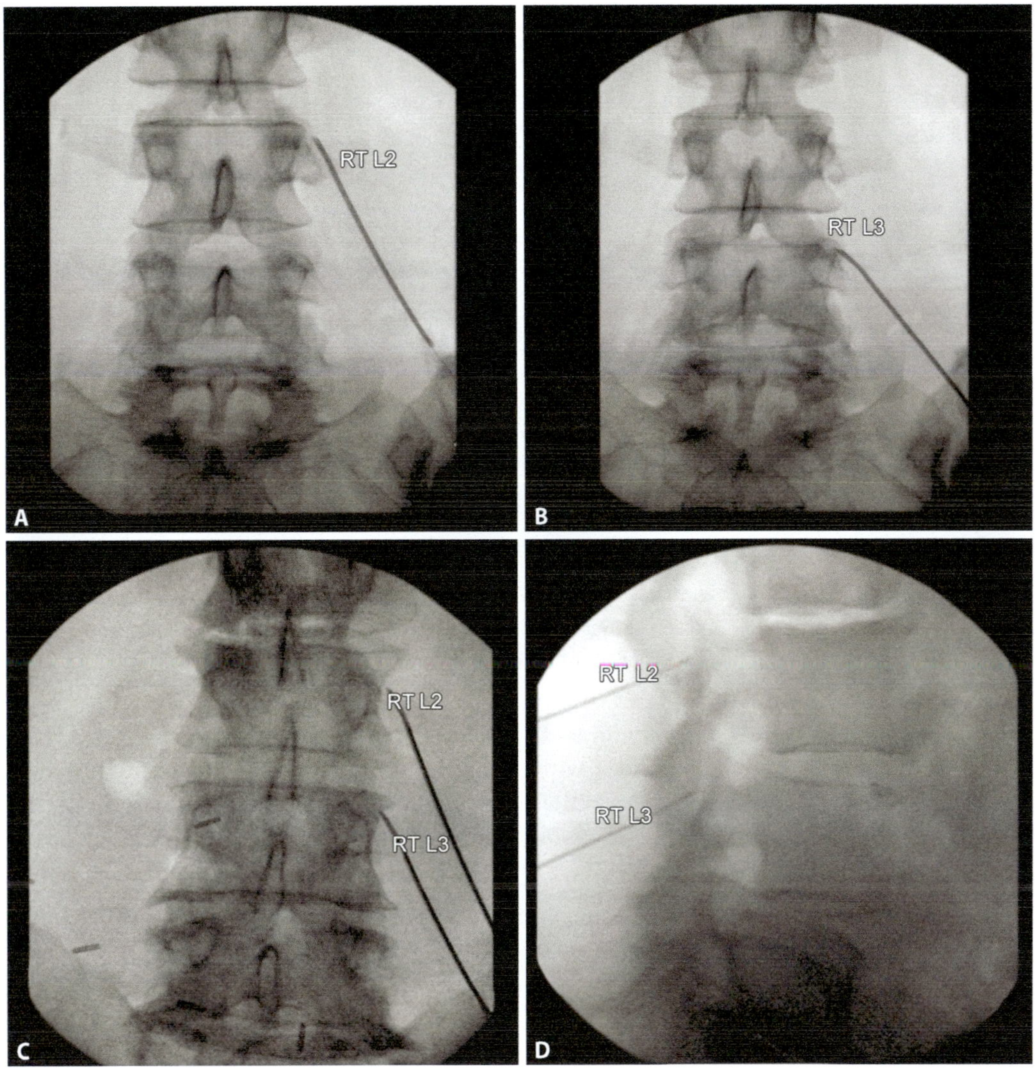

Figs. 8A to D: An example of correct radiofrequency electrode position for L2 and L3 medial branch (MB) neurotomy over the L3 and L4 transverse processes, respectively. (A to C) Anteroposterior view; (D) Lateral view.

lidocaine is given through each needle to anesthetize the MB, and RF coagulation is carried out usually at 80° for 90 seconds at each level. Prior to coagulating and in some cases after the procedure is done, a small amount of corticosteroid and local anesthetic is injected to decrease the incident of postprocedure pain and neuritis. The electrodes and needles are removed. The areas are clean. Small bandages are applied and similar precautions as with MBBs are carried out.

Contraindications

Absolute contraindications of lumbar RF denervation are like the ones for MBBs. The specific ones that apply to RF denervation are the patient being medically or psychologically unstable and pregnancy. Relative contraindications are patients with pacemaker, anatomical derangement that would compromise safe placement of the electrode, coexisting medical illness, immunosuppression, unrealistic patient, or family expectation.

Also, other absolute contraindications are indeterminate results of diagnostic nerve blocks and other relative contraindications are patients using anticoagulants whose treatment can be suspended temporarily, coexisting diseases producing significant respiratory or cardiovascular compromise that may affect the safe and comfortable conduct of the procedure, immunosuppression, unrealistic

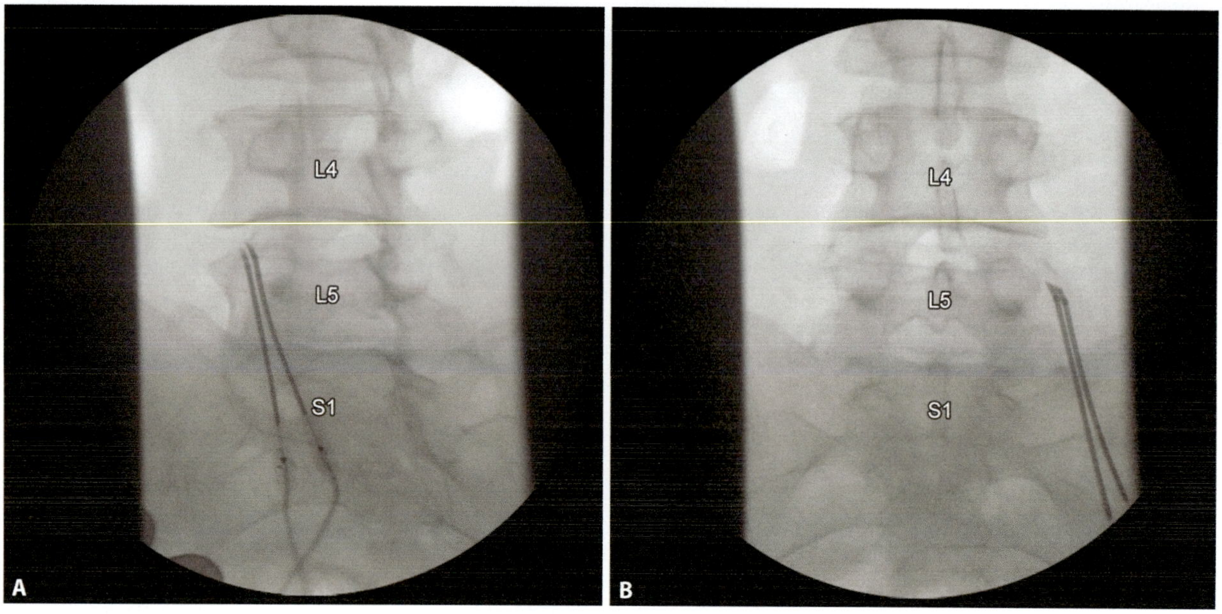

Figs. 9A and B: Bipolar radiofrequency (RF) needle positioning for the bilateral L4 medial branch (MB) neurotomy. (A) Oblique view; (B) Anteroposterior (AP) view.

family or patient expectation, uncooperative patient who is unlikely to tolerate the procedure or compliant with postoperative care instructions, inadequate pain relief, or relief less than 3 months' duration following previous neurotomy.

Technical Variations

Radiofrequency ablation can be conducted in a variety of ways. It can be carried out with different temperature settings, by creating multiple lesions along the course of the nerve, by using larger versus smaller gauge electrodes, and by using hollow versus solid needles. Pulsed RF can be used for MBs but is kept reserved for the peripheral nerves that cannot tolerate complete coagulation resulting in tissue and function loss.[25] The coagulation commences when the temperature at the electrode tip reaches 65°C. As noted earlier, the most optimal temperature and duration are noted to be 80°C and 90 seconds, respectively, for the best ablation outcome. The decision regarding multiple lesions should be made based on the size of the active electrode tip and the size of the target zone. If the length of the active electrode tip covers the length of the target zone, only one lesion will be required. If, however, the target zone is larger than the active tip, creating a second lesion along the target nerve, which overlaps with the first lesion slightly, increases the length of the nerve coagulated. The larger gauge electrodes are more likely to thoroughly coagulate the target nerve. A newer RFA bipolar technique **(Figs. 9A and B)** has been gaining popularity, using two 18G needles with a 1 cm exposed tip placed in a parallel fashion at a target MB tangentially, within one needle width of each other.[4,26] This approach has been shown to produce larger size of the nerve ablation,[27] contributing to the improvement of some postprocedure outcome measures, including duration of pain relief and activities of daily leaving.[28]

Radiofrequency of MBs can also be repeated. It does not permanently destroy the nerve. The cell body of the nerve remains intact and thus the nerve regenerates and the pain occasionally recurs. On average, the patient can be expected to get approximately 350–400 days of complete pain relief. Frequently, when the pain recurs, it is usually not as severe. Repeat RFs can be performed but repeating within 6 months to 1 year is not recommended.

POSTPROCEDURE CARE

Upon removal of the needle, the skin is cleaned to remove the antiseptic or any blood. A small adhesive patch can be applied to the puncture site but is unnecessary. If the patient complains of any untoward side effects following the procedure, appropriate neurological examination and imaging study should be conducted. Blood pressure and pulse observation are done in resting supine position. Rarely any further investigation is needed. Otherwise, the procedure is usually well tolerated. The patient may be allowed to dress and wait in the recovery room for 20–30 minutes and then the patient is discharged from a stable condition.

CONCLUSION

Percutaneous procedures designed for facet joint-mediated pain are the second most common type of interventions performed in pain management centers throughout the United States. MBBs and intra-articular facet injections are appropriate diagnostic and treatment options for a patient's axial low-back pain coming from the posterior elements of the lumbar spine including facet joints. These procedures need to be done carefully under fluoroscopic guidance following appropriate guidelines. RF lesioning of nerves supplying painful tissues can provide an effective treatment after the pain source is established. Used appropriately, such procedures have the potential to offer relief of chronic pain when less invasive treatments and natural history have failed, and when the patient is not interested in perusing surgical interventions. RFA is a palliative procedure, designed to relieve pain from a facet joint by coagulation of its afferent nerve supply. Its outcome highly depends on rigorous patient selection, use of controlled comparative anesthetic MBB protocol with cutoff pain relief values recommended to exceed 70%, on proper electrode position, and on the size of a cannula. When performed correctly, by a well-trained practitioner, using well-established protocols, RFA is a safe and effective procedure with few associated complications and side effects and can offer a long-term solution of relief from facet joint-mediated pain.

Most of these procedures are well tolerated, minimally invasive, requiring minimal recovery time, and are typically performed on the outpatient type of basis, which increases a patient's convenience and satisfaction.

REFERENCES

1. Bogduk N. Evidence-informed management of chronic low back pain with facet injections and radiofrequency neurotomy. Spine J. 2008;8(1):56-64.
2. Derby R, Melnik I, Choi J, Lee JE. Indications for repeat diagnostic medial branch nerve blocks following a failed first medial branch nerve block. Pain Physician. 2013;16(5):479-88.
3. Derby R, Melnik I, Lee JE, Lee SH. Correlation of lumbar medial branch neurotomy results with diagnostic medial branch block cutoff values to optimize therapeutic outcome. Pain Med. 2012;13(12):1533-46.
4. Lau P, Mercer S, Govind J, Bogduk N. The surgical anatomy of lumbar medial branch neurotomy (facet denervation). Pain Med. 2004;5(3):289-98.
5. Gray DP, Bajwa ZH, Warfield CA. Facet block and neurolysis. In: Waldman SD (Ed). Interventional Pain Management, 2nd edition. Philadelphia, PA: Saunders; 2001. pp. 446-83.
6. Schwarzer AC, Aprill CN, Derby R, Fortin J, Kine G, Bogduk N. Clinical features of patients with pain stemming from the lumbar zygapophysial joints. Is the lumbar facet syndrome a clinical entity? Spine (Phila Pa 1976). 1994;19(10):1132-7.
7. Bogduk N. Practice Guidelines for Spinal Diagnostic and Treatment Procedures, 2nd edition. San Francisco, USA: International Spine Intervention Society; 2004.
8. Rees WE. Multiple bilateral subcutaneous rhizolysis of segmental nerves in the treatment of the intervertebral disc syndrome. Ann Gen Pract. 1971;16:126-7.
9. Rees WS. Multiple bilateral percutaneous rhizolysis. Med J Aust. 1975;1(17):536-7.
10. Shealy CN. Facets in back and sciatic pain. A new approach to major pain syndrome. Minn Med. 1974;57(3):199-203.
11. Shealy CN. The role of the spinal facets in back and sciatic pain. Headache. 1974;14(2):101-4.
12. Shealy CN. Percutaneous radiofrequency denervation of spinal facets. Treatment for chronic back pain and sciatica. J Neurosurg. 1975;43(4):448-51.
13. Shealy CN. Facet denervation in the management of back and sciatic pain. Clin Orthop Relat Res. 1976;(115):157-64.
14. Dreyfuss P, Schwarzer AC, Lau P, Bogduk N. Specificity of lumbar medial branch and L5 dorsal ramus blocks. A computed tomography study. Spine (Phila Pa 1976). 1997;22(8):895-902.
15. Kaplan M, Dreyfuss P, Halbrook B, Bogduk N. The ability of lumbar medial branch blocks to anesthetize the zygapophysial joint. A physiologic challenge. Spine (Phila Pa 1976). 1998;23(17):1847-52.
16. van Kleef M, Barendse GA, Kessels A, Voets HM, Weber WE, de Lange S. Randomized trial of radiofrequency lumbar facet denervation for chronic low back pain. Spine (Phila Pa 1976). 1999;24(18):1937-42.
17. Revel M, Poiraudeau S, Auleley GR, Payan C, Denke A, Nguyen M, et al. Capacity of the clinical picture to characterize low back pain relieved by facet joint anesthesia. Proposed criteria to identify patients with painful facet joints. Spine (Phila Pa 1976). 1998;23(18):1972-6.
18. Bogduk N. Commentary on the capacity of the clinical picture to characterize low back pain relieved by facet joint anesthesia. Pain Med J Club. 1998;4:221-2.
19. McCall IW, Park WM, O'Brien JP. Induced pain referral from posterior lumbar elements in normal subjects. Spine (Phila Pa 1976). 1979;4(5):441-6.
20. Mooney V, Robertson J. The facet syndrome. Clin Orthop Relat Res. 1976;(115):149-56.
21. Cohen SP, Raja SN. Pathogenesis, diagnosis, and treatment of lumbar zygapophyseal (facet) joint pain. Anesthesiology. 2007;106(3):591-614.

22. Taha JM. Percutaneous radiofrequency trigeminal ganglionolysis. In: Burchiel K (Ed). Surgical Management of Pain, 2nd edition. New York, USA: Thieme Medical Publishers; 2002. pp. 841-8.
23. Shealy CN. The role of the spinal facets in back and sciatic pain. Headache. 1974;14(2):101-4.
24. Dreyfuss P, Halbrook B, Pauza K, Joshi A, McLarty J, Bogduk N. Efficacy and validity of radiofrequency neurotomy for chronic lumbar zygapophysial joint pain. Spine (Phila Pa 1976). 2000;25(10):1270-7.
25. Navani A, Mahajan G, Kreis P, Fishman SM. A case of pulsed radiofrequency lesioning for occipital neuralgia. Pain Med. 2006;7(5):453-6.
26. Bogduk N, Macintosh J, Marsland A. Technical limitations to the efficacy of radiofrequency neurotomy for spinal pain. Neurosurgery. 1987;20(4):529-35.
27. Derby R, Lee CH. The efficacy of a two needle electrode technique in percutaneous radiofrequency rhizotomy: an investigational laboratory study in an animal model. Pain Physician. 2006;9(3):207-13.
28. Derby R, Melnik I, Lee JE, Fernandez R. Outcome results of medial branch neurotomy using a bipolar technique. International Spine Intervention Society (ISIS) - 2013, 21st Annual Scientific Meeting Research Abstracts. Pain Med. 2013;14(8):1269-76.

36 CHAPTER

Lumbar Plexus Block

Mohammed Piracha, Kingsuk Ganguly, Neel Mehta

ABSTRACT

The lumbar plexus block is an advanced lower extremity block useful in surgical anesthesia for the lower extremity, with potential application for chronic pain syndromes. While traditional approaches have been under landmark and nerve stimulation, ultrasound guidance is providing for a safe alternative approach. Although it is not a neuraxial block, similar precautions should be taken, and awareness of complications should be paramount.

INTRODUCTION

The lumbar plexus is a lower extremity plexus involving the anterior primary rami of the L1-L4 nerve roots with occasional contributions from T12 and L5. Some of the eventual regional nerves of the lumbar plexus include the femoral nerve, lateral femoral cutaneous nerve, obturator nerve, iliohypogastric nerve, ilioinguinal nerve, and genitofemoral nerve. Thus, along with a sciatic nerve block, a lumbar plexus block can achieve complete surgical anesthesia of the lower extremity.[1]

INDICATIONS

- Lower extremity surgeries such as hip, femoral fractures, anterior thigh, knee, and above knee amputations. Postoperative opioid consumption has been shown to be reduced when it is used as part of a multimodal analgesic approach in total knee and hip arthroplasties.[1]
- Acute herpes zoster infection of the lower extremity. One case study showed successful management of acute pain secondary to herpes zoster infection with a lumbar plexus block in an elderly patient with multiple medical comorbidities.[2] The patient also developed a sympathetic block, with signs of skin flushing, increased temperature, and loss of pinprick and temperature discrimination.
  - As diagnostic measure for complex regional pain syndrome (CRPS) it will help pain physician while evaluating such patients, as sympathetic block is unilateral and postganglionic.

CONTRAINDICATIONS

- Patient refusal
- Patients reporting allergies to local anesthetics
- An active infection close to the needle site, such as a psoas abscess
- An elevated international normalized ratio (INR), the potentially devastating complications of a retroperitoneal hematoma.

TECHNIQUE

The most recent American Society of Regional Anesthesia and Pain Medicine (ASRA) guidelines should be followed, which recommend applying the neuraxial guidelines to lumbar plexus blocks. Although it is not a neuraxial block, the lumbar plexus block is considered to be an advanced procedure. Given the plexus location relatively deep within the psoas muscle, which is why the procedure is also referred to as a psoas compartment block with the nerve roots in proximity to the epidural space.[3] Both of these factors can contribute to a potential systemic toxicity. Patient discomfort is not uncommon given the deep location that the needle must traverse through. Standard monitors should be placed along with an intravenous line for sedation and patient safety.

Traditionally, landmark techniques have been used to achieve this block. First, the patient is placed in the lateral decubitus position with the operative side up and the nonoperative side in the dependent position. A slight forward tilt of the pelvis will often help facilitate palpation of the anatomical landmarks.[3] The anatomical landmarks include the iliac crest, the spinous processes, and a point that is 3–4 cm lateral to the intersection of these two landmarks. After palpation and identification of the iliac crest, a vertical line can be drawn across the patient's back beginning at the lateral edge of the pelvic bone and across the spinous processes. Upon palpation and identification of the midline spinous processes, a horizontal line can be drawn across the midline that intersects with the lateral line. This point of intersection may often be the spinous process of L4 and should be noted as it is from here that a 3–4 cm measurement is made laterally. The lateral point to this intersection will be the needle entry site.[3]

A similar approach involves using the posterior superior iliac spine as a landmark and drawing a horizontal line parallel to the spinous processes, which eventually intersects with the vertical line of the iliac crest. This intersection, which can be about 5 cm lateral to the spinous process of L4 in most patients, is then determined to be the needle point of entry **(Fig. 1)**.[1,4-7]

The procedure must be performed in a sterile manner. The back is cleaned with antiseptic solution and a drape should be placed over the field. The skin and subcutaneous tissue of the needle entry site can be infiltrated with local anesthesia. The palpating hand should be close to the entry site and can be pushed in to facilitate the distance between the site of the plexus and the needle. A peripheral nerve stimulator will be necessary and a 10 cm, 21 gauge insulated needle should suffice for most patients. The needle should enter perpendicular to the skin. Using nerve stimulation, the current can be set at 1.5 mA. The initial twitches seen upon advancement will be the paravertebral muscles. The needle should be advanced until the twitches of the ipsilateral quadriceps muscle are seen. This usually happens at a depth between 6 and 8 cm.[3] Upon seeing these twitches, the current should be reduced to 0.5–1.0 mA with preservation of twitches. Twitches should not be observed below 0.5 mA as this may indicate intradural placement.[3] If twitches are still seen between 0.5 and 1.0 mA, about 30–40 mL of local anesthetic can then be slowly delivered to this area. Ideally, the local anesthetic will spread within the psoas fascial plane with an onset of action within 20–30 minutes.[3]

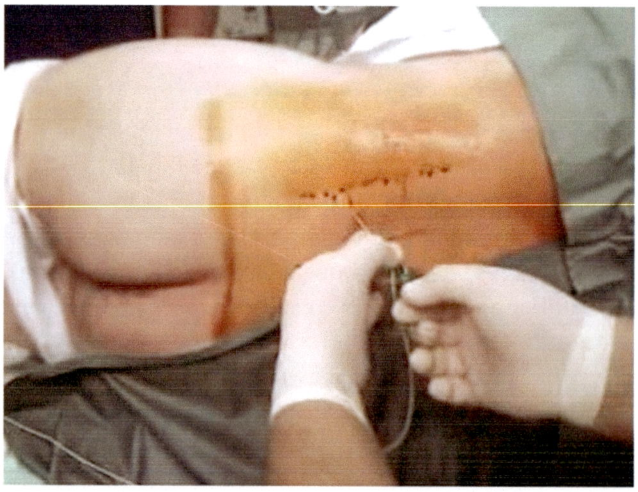

Fig. 1: A needle is inserted perpendicular to the skin plane, 4 cm lateral to the midline at the level of L3-L5.

Others advocate intentionally contacting the L4 transverse process with the needle.[4-7] Variations exist as to the actual depth of the lumbar plexus depending on the patient's body habitus, but multiple sources indicate that once the transverse process is contacted, the lumbar plexus is no more than 2 cm distal.[1] The plexus can be reached by walking off the transverse process caudally and then advanced until stimulation of the quadriceps is seen, which can range from 20 mm to 2 cm. Further advancement increases the risk of retroperitoneal injury.

Ultrasound Technique

The advent of ultrasound has dramatically shifted the approach to most regional anesthetic techniques. Its use in lumbar plexus blocks is more limited, however, as the visualization of this deep structure is challenging. Bony landmarks, such as the L4 transverse process, can be confirmed and identified, which can assist the operator during needle guidance. A low-frequency (4–5 MHz) curved transducer will provide a more optimal image of the deep structures. Beginning with a paramedian scan with the probe oriented in the longitudinal paravertebral plane, one can begin to identify the lumbar interspinous processes. It is best to start caudally at the sacrum and move the probe cranially. Under ultrasound, the sacrum should be seen as a hyperechoic line. As the probe moves cranially, the discontinuation of this hyperechoic line should denote the L5/S1 interspace. As one continues to move the probe cranially, identifying the interspaces as they go, the kidney may be visualized around the L3/L4 area.[1] This is important to note to prevent renal injury during placement of the block. The longitudinal paravertebral plane views will help identify the transverse process and the peritoneum. Measuring the distance of these two landmarks from the skin is important as the operator can remain aware of these depths during needle advancement. The probe can then be moved to the midline of the spinous processes and rotated 90° in a transverse orientation, usually at the L3/L4 interspace, where the paravertebral muscles, quadratus lumborum, and psoas muscle may be identified **(Fig. 2)**.[1] The roots of the lumbar plexus usually lie in the posterior to middle one-third of the psoas muscle, which is the planned destination for the needle tip.[1] The needle tip can be advanced in-plane or out-of-plane to the posterior one-third of the psoas muscle, where the local anesthetic can be deposited.

An alternative approach involves maintaining the probe in the longitudinal paravertebral plane about 3–4 cm lateral to the spinous processes and identifying the transverse processes of L2-L4 and their respective acoustic shadows. These shadows form a "trident" through which the psoas muscle runs.[8] The needle can then be entered in-plane from a caudal to cranial direction into the space between the L3 and L4 transverse processes and eventually into the posterior part of the psoas muscle. Both techniques require steep angulation, and visualization of the entire shaft may not be possible. Methods such as hydrodissection with saline or nerve stimulation may need to be concomitantly used to confirm appropriate placement.

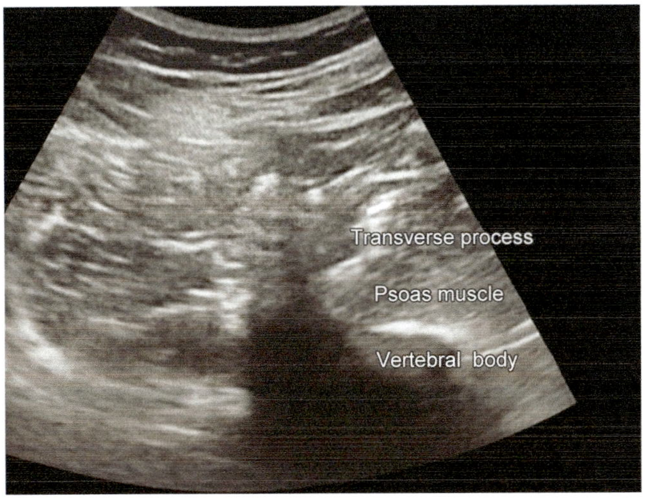

Fig. 2: In-plane view at L4 vertebral body.

The lumbar plexus block is essentially a compartment block within the fascial plane of a large muscle such as the psoas, therefore, a higher volume of local anesthetic is required to achieve the desired effect.[3] Up to 25–40 mL of local anesthetic is recommended for this procedure. Given the vascularity of the psoas muscle and the large volume of local anesthetic required, total dose should be kept in mind to reduce the risk of local anesthetic toxicity. Multiple sources indicate that up to 40 mL of bupivacaine (0.25%), ropivacaine (0.25–0.5%), or mepivacaine (1%) can be safely delivered.[9-11] The choice and dose of local anesthetic can depend on whether a dense surgical block is needed or if it is for pain management. Other factors include desired time of onset, which would be faster for mepivacaine (10–15 minutes vs. 20–30 minutes for bupivacaine) or duration (4–5 hours for bupivacaine vs. 2.5–3 hours for mepivacaine).[3] The duration of postoperative analgesia after a single injection can range anywhere from 6 to 24 hours depending on the choice of local anesthetic.[3]

A catheter can also be placed in these blocks for postoperative pain management. The technique and approach are similar to a single injection, other than the fact that a Tuohy needle will need to be used to thread the catheter caudally and laterally, following the trajectory of the lumbar plexus.[3] It is often helpful to inject 5–10 mL of local anesthetic prior to threading the catheter to help create a space for the catheter to migrate to. Threading the catheter of about 5 cm distal to the tip of the Tuohy is usually appropriate.[3] If the plan is to begin the infusion immediately, the initial bolus dose can be reduced to 15–20 mL. It would be more prudent to use a long-acting agent such as 0.2% ropivacaine for the infusion, which can be set at a basal rate of 5 mL/hour with an optional bolus dose of 5 mL/hour. If a patient is experiencing breakthrough pain, a bolus should always be delivered as simply increasing the rate is insufficient.[3] The catheter can be tested for efficiency by injecting a bolus dose of a local anesthetic with a faster onset time, such as lidocaine or mepivacaine. This can then help determine the appropriate course of action.

PITFALLS

Given the deep location of the lumbar plexus, many common pitfalls arise. Upon insertion and advancement of the needle, if no quadriceps stimulation is seen, a stepwise approach to troubleshooting should be taken. The needle should be pulled back to the skin, followed by a minimum change of angulation. The needle can then be advanced cranially, caudally, medially, or laterally. The needle should be pulled back to skin prior to each directional angulation change to minimize trauma and bending of the needle. If there is still no quadriceps stimulation noted, the needle should be pulled out and reinserted in a new position 2 cm cranially or caudally.[3]

If flexion of the thigh is seen during stimulation, the needle is too deep and is stimulating the psoas muscle. The needle should be withdrawn and repositioned. Stimulation of the hamstring muscles may be seen indicating that the needle tip is too caudal and medial from the lumbar plexus and is instead stimulating the sciatic nerve. The needle should be withdrawn and then advanced more cephalad and lateral.[3]

When using the L4 transverse process to walk off caudally to the plexus, bone may continue to be encountered despite a steep caudal angulation. This may mean that the tip is too medial, contacting lamina, and should be pulled back and advanced laterally.[4-7]

COMPLICATIONS

The deep location of the lumbar plexus with its proximity to the epidural space and muscles makes the lumbar plexus block a regional anesthetic technique that carries a higher risk of local anesthetic toxicity. The risk can be pronounced in continuous infusions if the maximum dose recommendations are exceeded, especially if the patient has a concomitant sciatic nerve catheter. Epidural diffusion, rather than injection, has been considered one of the more common complications.[12] The risk of local anesthetic toxicity can be minimized by mixing a short-acting anesthetic with a long-acting anesthetic to decrease the overall dose and toxicity.[3] A slow injection can reduce the risk of epidural diffusion. Infection is a complication with any invasive procedure and can be prevented following sterile aseptic technique.

Intrathecal and intravascular injections are also possible complications. When using nerve stimulation, if quadriceps contractions are still seen below 0.5 mA, there is an elevated risk that the needle tip is in the dural sleeve, and the tip should be retracted.[3] Intravascular injection should be monitored with intermittent aspiration upon injection of the local anesthetic.

Nerve injury is a rare but possible complication. The way to reduce this is to assess how the patient is doing during the injection. One should immediately stop if the patient complains of pain on injection. Excessive resistance during injection may also be a sign of intraneural injection. Minute changes in the position of the tip can be made before reinjection. Femoral nerve injury secondary to hematoma has been reported in the literature.[13,14] A hematoma into the retroperitoneal space is troublesome as its deep location does not allow the area to be compressible. Renal injury is a possibility when the needle is in the retroperitoneal space. Keeping needle insertions at a minimum is important to prevent this.

Hemodynamics should always be monitored in these patients. The vicinity of the epidural and intrathecal space along with the ipsilateral lumbar sympathectomy can cause hemodynamic variability. The intricacies of this block are not minute and mandate close monitoring.

CONCLUSION

While lumbar plexus blocks may not be the primary analgesic modality for the hip and lower extremity, it is an important block to know for the pain physician. Its ability to treat and diagnose pain syndromes affecting a specific area of the lower extremity makes it a useful skill set to have.

REFERENCES

1. Benzon H, Raja SN, Fishman SM, Liu S, Cohen SP. Essentials of Pain Medicine, 3rd edition. Philadelphia: Elsevier/Saunders; 2011.
2. Hadzić A, Vloka JD, Saff GN, Hertz R, Thys DM. The "three-in-one block" for treatment of pain in a patient with acute herpes zoster infection. Reg Anesth. 1997;22:575-8.
3. Hadzic A. Hadzic's peripheral nerve blocks and anatomy for ultrasound-guided regional anesthesia, 2nd edition. New York: McGraw Hill Medical; 2012.
4. Awad IT, Duggan EM. Posterior lumbar plexus block: anatomy, approaches, and techniques. Reg Anesth Pain Med. 2005;30:143-9.
5. Capdevila X, Coimbra C, Choquet O. Approaches to the lumbar plexus: success, risks, and outcome. Reg Anesth Pain Med. 2005;30:150-62.
6. Farny J, Drolet P, Girard M. Anatomy of the posterior approach to the lumbar plexus block. Can J Anaesth. 1994;41:480-5.
7. Kirchmair L, Entner T, Kapral S, Mitterschiffthaler G. Ultrasound guidance for the psoas compartment block: an imaging study. Anesth Analg. 2002;94:706-10.

8. Karmaker MK, Ho AM, Li X, Kwok WH, Tsang K, Kee WD. Ultrasound-guided lumbar plexus block through the acoustic window of the lumbar ultrasound trident. Br J Anaesth. 2008;100:533-7.
9. Seeberger M, Urwyler A. Paravascular lumbar plexus block: block extension after femoral nerve stimulation and injection of 20 vs. 40 mL mepivacaine 10 mg/mL. Acta Anaesthesiol Scand. 1995;39:769-73.
10. Ng HP, Cheong KF, Lim A, Lim J, Puhaindran ME. Intraoperative single-shot "3-in-1" femoral nerve block with ropivacaine 0.25%, ropivacaine 0.5% or bupivacaine 0.25% provides comparable 48-hr analgesia after unilateral total knee replacement. Can J Anaesth. 2001;48:1102-8.
11. Weber A, Fournier R, Van Gessel E, Riand N, Gamulin Z. Epinephrine does not prolong the analgesia of 20 mL ropivacaine 0.5% or 0.2% in a femoral three-in-one block. Anesth Analg. 2001;93:1327-31.
12. De Leeuw MA, Zuurmond WW, Perez RS. The psoas compartment block for hip surgery: the past, present, and future. Anesthesiol Res Pract. 2011;2011:159541.
13. Uhrbrand A, Jensen TT. Iatrogenic femoral nerve neuropathy after blockade of lumbar plexus (3-in-1 block). Ugeskr Laeger. 1988;150:428-9.
14. Jöhr M. A complication of continuous blockade of the femoral nerve. Reg Anaesth. 1987;10:37-8.

37 CHAPTER

Sacroiliac Joint Radiofrequency Denervation

Sanjeeva Gupta

ABSTRACT

Sacroiliac joint (SIJ) pain is the source of pain in between 15% and 25% of patients presenting with low back pain. SIJ was found to be a source of pain in 32% of patients who presented with low back pain after lumbar fusion surgery. Low back pain which is maximum below L5 vertebral body level in a multiparous woman with tenderness over the SIJ is a good predictor of SIJ pain. If diagnostic SIJ injection provides significant short-term pain relief then SIJ radiofrequency denervation (SIJ-RFD) can be considered. SIJ-RFD should be performed under strict aseptic conditions and the different available techniques are described in this chapter. Please also consider referring to the chapters on SIJ block[1] and SIJ-RFD[2] in the book, *Atlas of Interventions Pain Management Procedures—A Stepwise Approach,* published by the same publisher as this book in 2023.

INTRODUCTION

In my clinical practice, if the sacroiliac joint (SIJ) injection with local anesthesia and steroid provides patients with good pain relief for 3–6 months or more, I repeat the same injection again up to twice a year if appropriate and encourage patients to do regular physiotherapy exercises and lifestyle modification among other methods of managing persistent pain. However, if the duration of pain relief is not significant, then I offer patients the choice of SIJ radiofrequency denervation (SIJ-RFD). However, the decision to go ahead with SIJ-RFD should be individualized based on the pain specialist's experience and patient's preference. Simplicity III probe and the SInergy-cooled radiofrequency techniques for SIJ-RFD are described in this chapter. After SIJ-RFD, I encourage patients to do regular physiotherapy exercises and consider lifestyle modification among other methods of managing persistent pain. Please also consider referring to the chapters on SIJ block[1] and SIJ-RFD[2] in the book, *Atlas of Interventions Pain Management Procedures—A Stepwise Approach*, published by the same publisher as this book in 2023.

In some situations, due to the variations in anatomy or difficulty in getting the required equipment, or the excessive costs involved to perform the SIJ-RFD with Simplicity probe or the SInergy-cooled RF technique it may be reasonable to consider alternative techniques such as using a radiofrequency needle to lesion the lateral branches of S1, S2, S3 and dorsal rami of L5 which supply the SIJ. Understanding the nerve supply of the SIJ and the direction in which the nerves travel from the nerve root or dorsal rami to supply the SIJ is important when modifying techniques in certain circumstances.

INDICATION

Significant short-term pain relief with SIJ injection with local anesthesia ± steroid.[1]

CONTRAINDICATIONS

- *Absolute contraindications:* Systemic or localized bacterial infection in the region of the block to be performed, and pregnancy.
- *Relative contraindications:* If a patient has a pacemaker or spinal cord stimulator, the company manufacturing these devices should be contacted for advice.

EQUIPMENT

- All the equipment needed for SIJ injection
- Simplicity III probe and a compatible radiofrequency generator or a SInergy-cooled radiofrequency system with appropriate probe. An 18G or 16G 100 mm long radiofrequency needle with at least 10 mm active tip
- Appropriate monitoring is essential if sedation/analgesia is used. In addition to local anesthesia, I use alfentanil analgesia in some patients to help the procedure. The patient should be verbally communicable throughout the procedure.

RADIOFREQUENCY DENERVATION OF SACROILIAC JOINT WITH SIMPLICITY III PROBE

The procedure is carried out under aseptic conditions. Patient is in prone position with a pillow(s) under the lower abdomen and/or pelvis. The anteroposterior (AP) view of the SIJ to be denervated is obtained. The C-arm is rotated to the right or the left side to move the overhanging iliac crest laterally to help advancement of the Simplicity probe. The C-arm may need to be tilted in the cephalic direction to identify the sacral foramen as this will facilitate placement of the Simplicity probe a few millimeters lateral to the sacral foramen.

Once proper images are obtained, a skin entry point is chosen in an area which is medial to and in the upper one-third of the ipsilateral hip joint image on fluoroscopy **(Fig. 1)**. The skin entry point suggested is only a guide as each patient may require a different skin/needle entry point and one learns this with experience. The skin entry point can vary depending on several factors including patient position, weight of the patient, and the curvature of the sacrum.

Once the skin entry point is identified, 0.25% bupivacaine is infiltrated into the skin and subcutaneous tissue with a 25G hypodermic needle, and then a 22G 10 cm long spinal needle can be used to infiltrate 0.25% bupivacaine into the deeper subcutaneous tissue and over the projected path of insertion of the simplicity probe. Try to contact the posterior plate of the sacrum with the spinal needle at around the ipsilateral S4 foramen level and then advance the spinal needle a few millimeters lateral to the sacral foramen. Also obtain a lateral view to look at the spinal needle trajectory, to assess the curvature of the sacrum, and to confirm that the spinal needle stays posterior to the posterior sacral plate and then inject 0.25% bupivacaine along the tract of the needle. Another skin entry point with the spinal needle proximal to the first

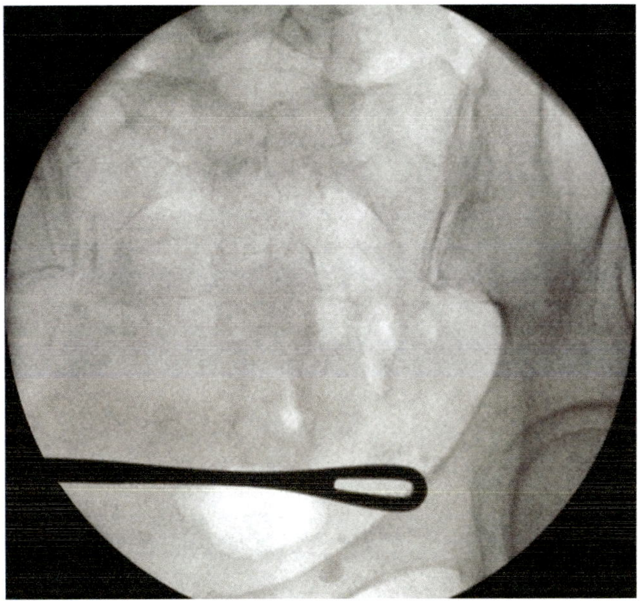

Fig. 1: Approximate skin puncture point is chosen for sacroiliac joint (SIJ) radiofrequency denervation using Simplicity III probe. A skin entry point is chosen in an area which is medial to and in the upper one-third of the ipsilateral hip joint image on fluoroscopy (See text for more details).

one may be necessary to anesthetize the entire length of the area of the projected probe insertion path. 20–25 mL of 0.25% bupivacaine may be necessary.

Alternatively, the L5 dorsal rami and the S1 to S3 lateral branches supplying the ipsilateral SIJ can each be blocked with 0.25% bupivacaine separately by placing 22G 10 cm long spinal needles in the area of the L5 dorsal rami and the lateral branches (in an area lateral to the respective sacral foramens).[2] Obtain a lateral view with all the block needles in place to assess the depth on the posterior sacral plate from the skin and assess the curvature of the sacrum to plan the Simplicity probe insertion/trajectory. It may be reasonable to leave the spinal needles in place until the simplicity probe is appropriately placed. However, the spinal needles should be removed before the radiofrequency lesioning is started.

Once the skin, subcutaneous tissue, and the projected tract of the Simplicity probe is anesthetized, the Simplicity III probe is inserted via the skin puncture site identified before and advanced toward the posterior sacral plate to make bone contact at around the S4 foramen level. A lateral view is obtained to confirm that the probe is posterior to the sacral plate.

The Simplicity probe is then gradually advanced toward the junction of the S1 superior articular process and the ala of the sacrum. Repeated AP and lateral fluoroscopic imaging

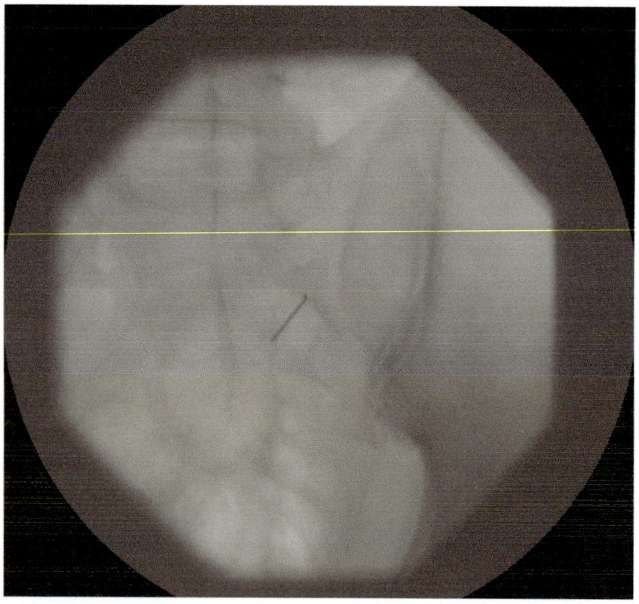

Fig. 2: Anteroposterior (AP) view of the right hemipelvis. Needle tip lateral to right S2 foramen for injecting local anesthetic.

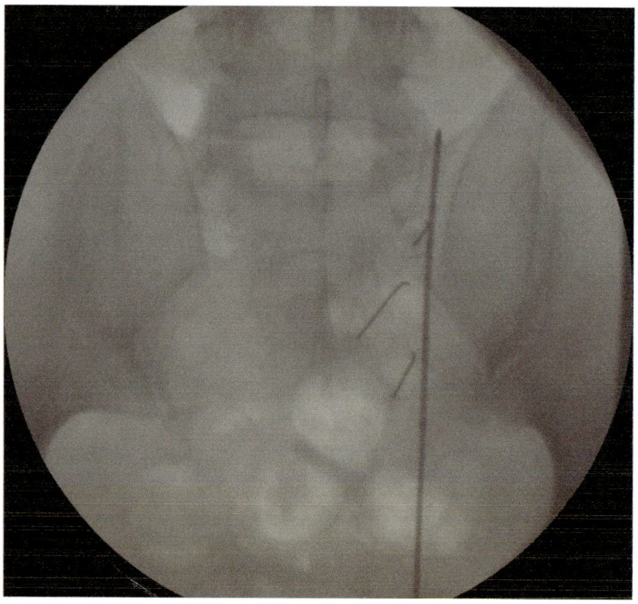

Fig. 3: Anterioposterior (AP) view. The Simplicity III probe is in place. The three spinal needles that were used to inject local anesthetic can also be seen.

Source: With permission from Jani SR et al.[2]

is used to confirm that the Simplicity III probe is advancing in the correct direction and depth. Once the Simplicity probe is correctly placed, it is connected to the compatible radiofrequency generator and the lesion performed for 7.5 minutes at 80°C as per the protocol **(Figs. 2 to 5)**.

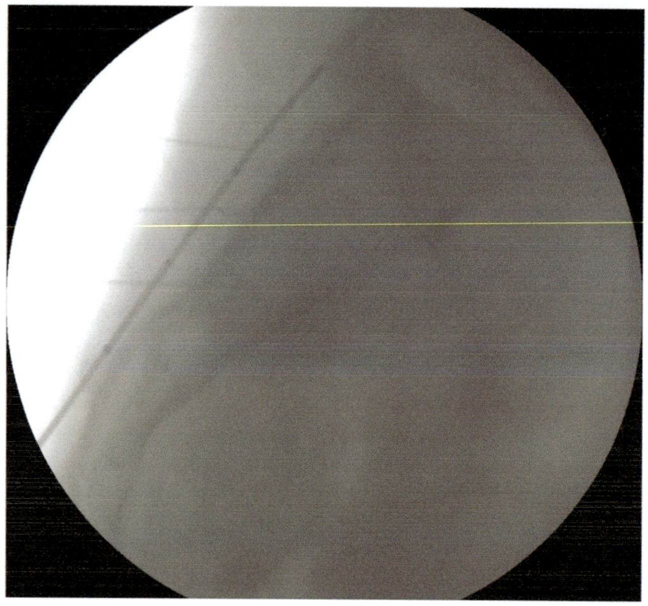

Fig. 4: Lateral view shows the Simplicity III probe in place. A lateral view before inserting the Simplicity III probe can help decide the skin entry point of the probe taking into consideration the curvature/anatomy of the sacral plate.

Source: With permission from Jani SR et al.[2]

The patient should be monitored for any unexpected symptoms (e.g., radicular pain in the lower limb, symptoms in the genital or anal or perineum area, etc.)

The RFD of the L5 dorsal rami is done as described in the chapter on *Lumbar Radiofrequency* in this book. Please also refer to Reference 2 for more details.

RADIOFREQUENCY DENERVATION OF SACROILIAC JOINT WITH SINERGY-COOLED RADIOFREQUENCY TECHNIQUE

SInergy-cooled radiofrequency technique generates a much larger lesion than a standard radiofrequency and since the lesions are concentric it is more reliable over the sacrum which has an uneven surface. The course that the lateral branches of S1, S2, and S3 take to innervate the SIJ can vary, and it is recommended that lesions are performed such that it covers the areas as shown in **Figure 5**. After the probe is placed in the correct area, the radiofrequency energy is applied for 150 seconds at a set temperature of 60°C using pain management radiofrequency generator (Kimberly-Clark Health Care, USA). The 60°C radiofrequency setting adjusts the probe surface to this temperature accordingly, while the lesioned tissue may reach temperatures between 75°C and 80°C as a result. One lesion is performed at L5 dorsal rami level and three lesions are performed at S1 and S2 levels and two lesions at S3 level as shown in **Figures 5 and 6**.

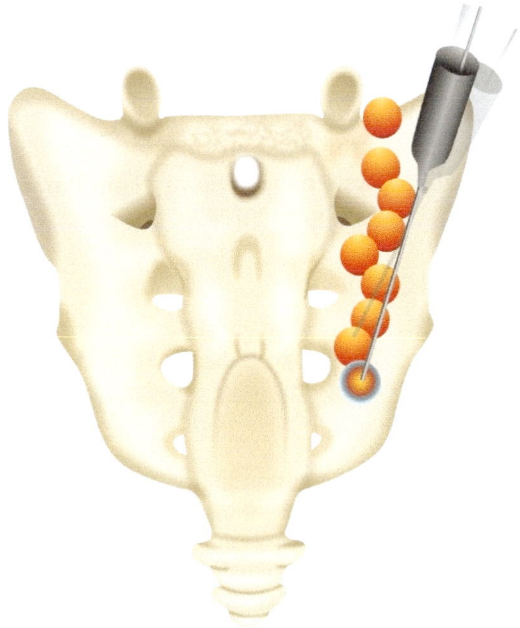

Fig. 5: *SInergy-cooled radiofrequency (RF) technique:* Figure showing the lesions to be performed. One lesion is performed at L5 dorsal rami level, and three lesions are performed at S1 and S2 levels, and two lesions at S3 level.
Source: Figure provided by Halyard Health Inc.

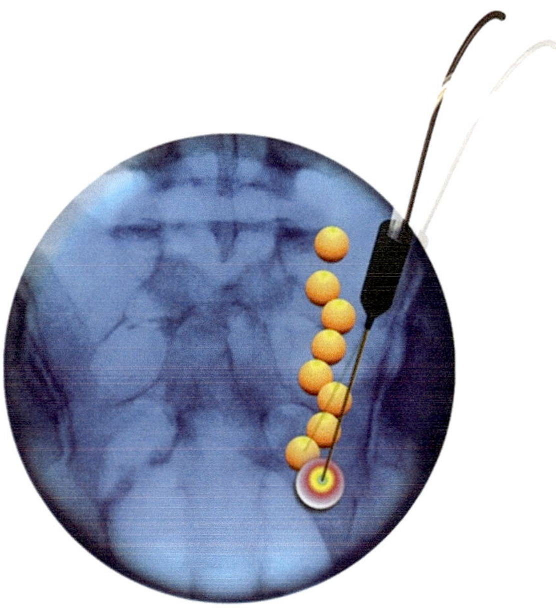

Fig. 6: *SInergy-cooled radiofrequency (RF) technique:* The lesions superimposed on an X-ray image.
Source: Figure provided by Halyard Health Inc.

Most of the published studies on the outcome of SIJ denervation have used the SInergy-cooled radiofrequency technique.[3,4]

RADIOFREQUENCY DENERVATION OF SACROILIAC JOINT WITH AN 18G OR A 16G RADIOFREQUENCY NEEDLE WITH AT LEAST 10 MM ACTIVE TIP

The SIJ-RFD may also be performed by placing the radiofrequency needles lateral to the S1, S2, and S3 foramen and at the L5 dorsal rami area and performing multiple lesions at each level. Sensory stimulation-guided SIJ denervation has been described by Yin et al.[5]

In some situations, due to the variations in anatomy or difficulty in getting the required equipment, or the excessive costs involved to perform the SIJ-RFD with Simplicity probe or the SInergy-cooled RF technique it may be reasonable to consider alternative techniques such as using a radiofrequency needle to lesion the lateral branches of S1, S2, S3 and dorsal rami of L5 which supply the SIJ. Understanding the nerve supply of the SIJ and the direction in which the nerves travel from the nerve root or dorsal rami to supply the SIJ is important when changing techniques that suit certain circumstances.

An 18G or 16G, 10 cm long radiofrequency needle with at least 10 mm active tip is used for the procedure. The radiofrequency needle is placed in such a way that the active tip is about 5–7 mm away from the sacral foramen. Multiple lesions are performed lateral to the respective sacral foramen at each level to cover the areas between *1 o'clock* and *5 o'clock* position (in relation to the respective sacral foramen) on the right side and from *11 o'clock* to *7 o'clock* position on the left side. These lesions are likely to denervate the lateral branches supplying the ipsilateral SIJ at the respective levels. The L5 dorsal rami is denervated as described in the chapter on lumbar radiofrequency. **Figure 7** is a diagrammatic representation of the approximate area to be covered during denervation lateral to the S1, S2 and the S3 foramen. The author is not aware of any published studies using this technique and the physician performing this technique takes the full responsibility of any risks associated with this technique.

It is recommended that before performing SIJ denervation with any of the above-mentioned techniques, it is very important to visit some of your colleagues who perform these techniques on a regular basis

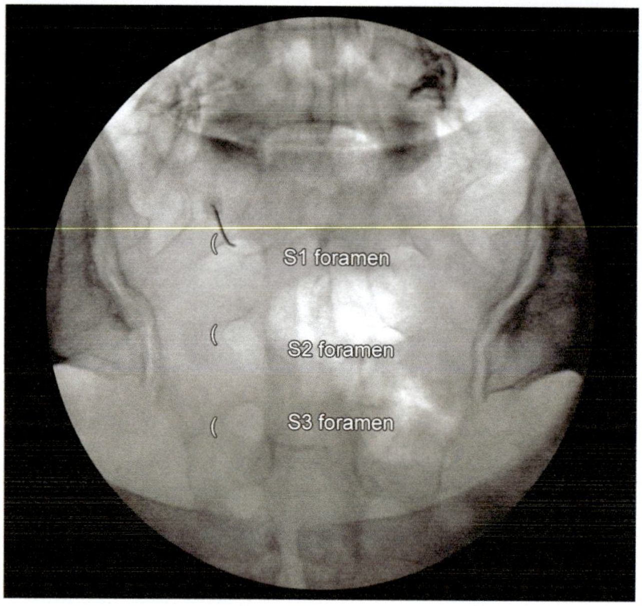

Fig. 7: An 18G or 16G radiofrequency (RF) needle with at least 10 mm active tip is used to perform multiple lesions at S1, S2, and S3 foramen area at least 5–7 mm lateral to the lateral foraminal opening to cover the areas between 1 o'clock and 5 o'clock position (in relation to the respective sacral foramen) on the right side and from 11 o'clock to 7 o'clock position on the left side.

and observe the technique. It may also be a good idea to initially have a colleague who performs these procedures regularly to be present when you start doing these procedures.

CONCLUSION

Sacroiliac joint pain is underdiagnosed and is also difficult to treat. *The combination of pain which is maximum below L5 level in a multiparous woman with tenderness over the SIJ is a good predictor of SIJ pain.* If the local anesthesia +/– steroid injection provides good pain relief and if the pain relief does not last long enough, then SIJ-RFD should be considered. However, the decision to proceed with SIJ-RFD should be individualized based on the pain specialist's experience and patient's preference. After SIJ-RFD, I encourage patients to do regular physiotherapy exercises and consider lifestyle modification among other methods of managing persistent pain. Please also consider referring to the chapters on SIJ block[1] and SIJ-RFD[2] in the book, *Atlas of Interventions Pain Management Procedures—A Stepwise Approach*, published by the same publisher as this book in 2023.[1,2] The evidence is summarized in a systematic review in Pain Physician in 2015[6] and in the randomized trial by Dr Patel.[3]

REFERENCES

1. Gupta S. Sacroiliac joint block. In: Baheti DK, Gupta S, Bakshi S, Gehdoo RP (Eds). Atlas of Interventional Pain Management Procedures: A Stepwise Approach. India: Jaypee Brothers Medical Publishers; 2023. pp. 153-5.
2. Jani SR, Gupta S, Baranidharan G. Sacroiliac joint radiofrequency denervation. In: Baheti DK, Gupta S, Bakshi S, Gehdoo RP (Eds). Atlas of Interventional Pain Management Procedures: A Stepwise Approach. India: Jaypee Brothers Medical Publishers, Ltd.; 2023. pp. 156-69.
3. Patel N. Twelve-month follow-up of a randomized trial assessing cooled radiofrequency denervation as a treatment for sacroiliac region pain. Pain Pract. 2016;16:154-67.
4. Cohen SP, Hurley RW, Buckenmaier CC 3rd, Kurihara C, Morlando B, Dragovich A. Randomized placebo-controlled study evaluating lateral branch radiofrequency denervation for sacroiliac joint pain. Anesthesiology. 2008;109:279-88.
5. Yin W, Willard F, Carreiro J, Dreyfuss P. Sensory stimulation-guided sacroiliac joint radiofrequency neurotomy: technique based on neuroanatomy of the dorsal sacral plexus. Spine (Phila Pa 1976). 2003;28:2419-25.
6. Simopoulos TT, Manchikanti L, Gupta S, Aydin SM, Kim CH, Solanki D, et al. Systematic review of the diagnostic accuracy and therapeutic effectiveness of sacroiliac joint interventions. Pain Physician. 2015;18:E713-56.

38

CHAPTER

Sciatic Nerve Block (Subgluteal)

Yashwant L Nankar

ABSTRACT

The sciatic nerve supplies most of the motor and sensory function to the lower limb. The sciatic nerve block is a useful procedure for patients with lower limb pain. It can give patients a very good relief from chronic neuropathic pain conditions, such as chronic sciatic radiculopathy, herpetic neuralgia, and diabetic neuropathy. It is also useful to manage severe ischemic pain in lower extremities, such as rest pain due to critical limb ischemia and during endovascular treatment. In emergency departments, it is also helpful for controlling acute pain emergencies such as acute sciatic radiculopathy, distal lower limb fractures, and for postoperative pain control. Apart from the use of local anesthetics for short-term, long-term relief can be obtained with steroids, neurolytics, or use of continuous catheter technique. In this chapter, we will focus mainly on the technical aspect of ultrasound-guided nerve block from a pain physician's point of view.

INTRODUCTION

Sciatic nerve block (SNB) is useful in the management of distal lower extremity pain sustained by the sciatic nerve. The sciatic nerve is the important nerve of the lower extremity, supplying the vast majority of the motor and sensory function to the lower limb. It supplies motor function to the posterior thigh and all muscles below the knee. Sensory function is provided to the posterior thigh, posterior knee joint, and everything below the knee except a narrow band on the medial lower leg. This area is supplied by the saphenous nerve, which is derived from the lumbar plexus. The sciatic nerve can be approached from multiple locations. This procedure can be performed under peripheral nerve stimulator guidance with imagining techniques such as ultrasound guidance, C-arm, computed tomography (CT) guidance, or even blind. Subgluteal sciatic block under ultrasound guidance has become the standard of practice. In this chapter, we describe a single-injection method for SNB using an ultrasound-guided infragluteal approach where the nerve is located along the lateral border of the biceps femoris muscle.

ANATOMY

Sciatic nerve arises from anterior divisions of L4-S3 nerve roots and exits pelvis through greater sciatic foramen. Then it descends between the greater trochanter of the femur and the ischial tuberosity between the piriformis and gluteus maximus, and then it lies posterior to the quadratus femoris muscle just lateral to the ischial tuberosity at which position it is accessible to nerve block. Distally in the posterior thigh it lies in the plane anterior to the biceps femoris muscle before entering the popliteal triangle. The nerve may be approached at any of these locations however, a common site is in the proximal infragluteal location.[1]

INDICATIONS

- *Neuropathic pain in lower extremities:*[2]
    - Chronic sciatic radiculopathy[3]
    - Herpetic neuralgia[4]
    - Diabetic neuropathy[5]
- *Ischemic pain in lower extremities:*
    - Chronic ischemic leg pain[6]
    - Rest pain due to critical limb ischemia, during endovascular treatment[7]

- *In emergency department for controlling acute pain emergencies such as:*[8]
  - Acute sciatic radiculopathy
  - Distal lower limb fractures
  - Postoperative pain control.

CONTRAINDICATIONS

- Local infection
- Refusal of a competent patient to undergo the procedure.

EQUIPMENT AND DRUGS

Needles:
- 25G ¾-inch needle, for local infiltration
- Insulated needle 50–100 mm 22G
- 22G spinal needle
- 18G Tuohy

Syringes: 5 mL, 10 mL, and 2 mL, each 2

Equipment:
- Peripheral nerve stimulator
- Syringe pump or elastomeric pump

Imaging modalities:
- Ultrasonography
- Computed tomography

Drugs:
- Lignocaine 2%
- Bupivacaine 0.5%
- Normal saline
- Depot steroids triamcinolone or alpha-methylprednisolone 40 mg
- Phenol 3% for neurolysis.

PREPARATION

History and physical examination of the local area before the procedure.

Laboratory investigation: Preoperative blood investigation and coagulation profile.

Preoperative patient explanation and consent:
- Risks and benefits, expected outcome, written informed consent, and large bore intravenous access
- Patient monitoring—blood pressure, heart rate, and pulse oximetry to observe any potential cardiac effects

Sedation: Usually not necessary for block with local anesthetics

POSITION

- The lateral decubitus position **(Fig. 1)**, with the side to be blocked up, rolled forward, and the knee flexed to 90°.
- The foot positioned so that twitches of the foot are easily seen in response to nerve stimulation.

PROCEDURE

- Preoperative antibiotic might be given depending on institutional practice.
- Bony landmarks are identified, and surface marking is done **(Fig. 2)**.
- First skin disinfection with chlorhexidine 2%.

Probe Position (Fig. 3)

- Low frequency convex probe, 2–5 MHz
- Initial probe position—over the subgluteal region in a transverse plane, between the greater trochanter and the ischial tuberosities.

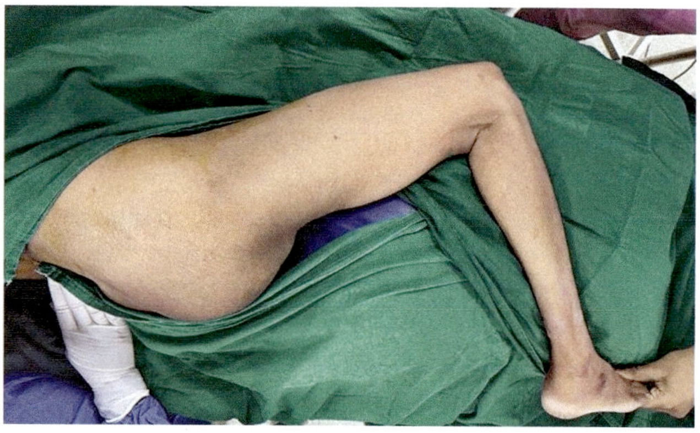

Fig. 1: Patient in lateral decubitus position with the block limb uppermost.

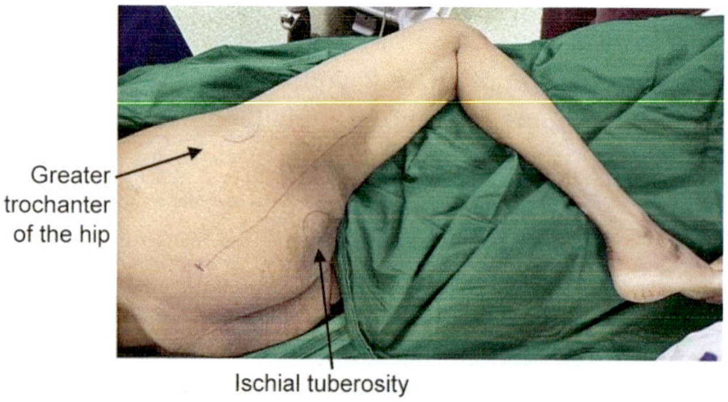

Fig. 2: Surface marking for bony landmarks—greater trochanter, ischial tuberosity.

Identify structures from superficial to deep and medial to lateral **(Fig. 4)**:
- Gluteus maximus muscle
- Quadratus femoris muscles
- Greater trochanter laterally
- Ischial tuberosity medially
- Sciatic nerve as a hyperechoic and lip-shaped oval structure inside a space lined by a hyperechoic margin formed by the surrounding muscles.

Needle Entry

It can be approached with either an in-plane approach **(Fig. 4)** or an out-of-plane approach.

In-Plane Approach

The curvilinear convex ultrasound probe is placed initially over the greater trochanter of the femur, and its bony shadow is identified.

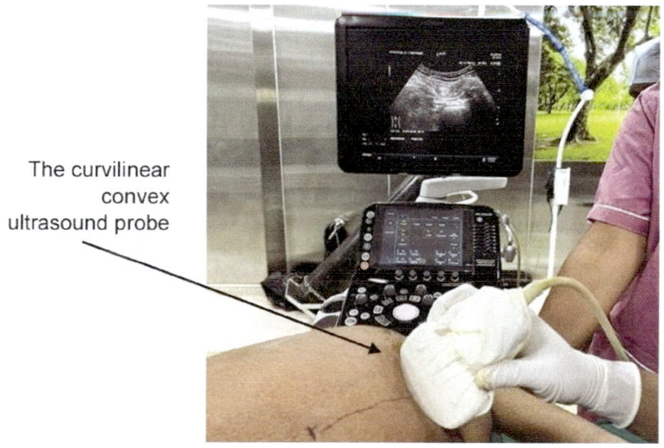

Fig. 3: The curvilinear convex ultrasound probe position to visualize transverse scan of sciatic nerve.

The probe is moved medially to identify the curvilinear bony shadow of the ischial tuberosity.

The sciatic nerve is visible in a sling between these two hyperechoic bony shadows **(Fig. 4)**. It usually appears as a wedge-shaped hyperechoic structure that is easier to identify more proximally, and then followed down to the infragluteal region.

The skin is infiltrated with lidocaine at the point of insertion of the block needle.

Entry point is from the lateral side to the medial part of the thigh, pushing the needle tip reaching the perineural space close to the sciatic nerve **(Fig. 5)**.

The needle tip is tracked at all times.

Needle-tip position is often confirmed from the movement of the tissues around it, and by injections of small volumes of distilled water, local anesthetic, or air.

Electrical stimulation can be used to help confirm needle-to-nerve contact.[9]

The stimulation frequency is set at 2 Hz, pulse width at 100 seconds, and the intensity of the stimulating current is set to deliver 1.0–1.2 mA.

Observation: Plantar flexion or inversion of the ipsilateral foot or a dorsiflexion of the foot at 0.4 mA.

It is useful to use ultrasound to observe the pattern of local anesthetic spread around the sciatic nerve in perineural space in real time. The aim is to obtain circumferential spread of injectate around the nerve.

For Continuous Block

- Needle used—18G Tuohy
- After confirming needle tip position:

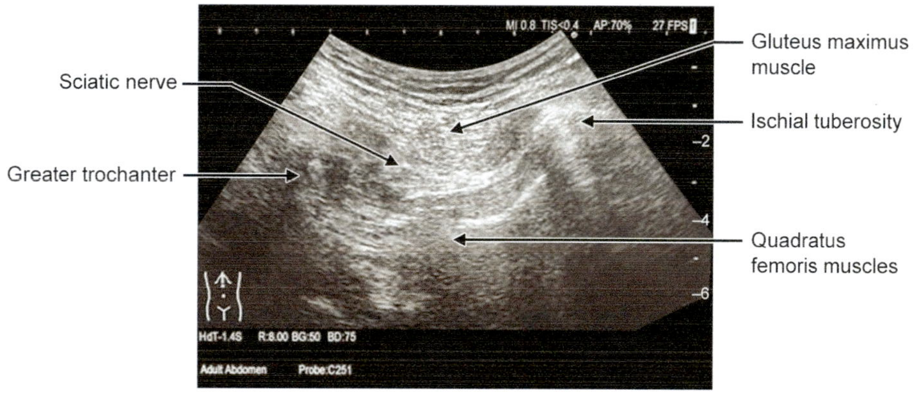

Fig. 4: USG transverse scan of sciatic nerve.

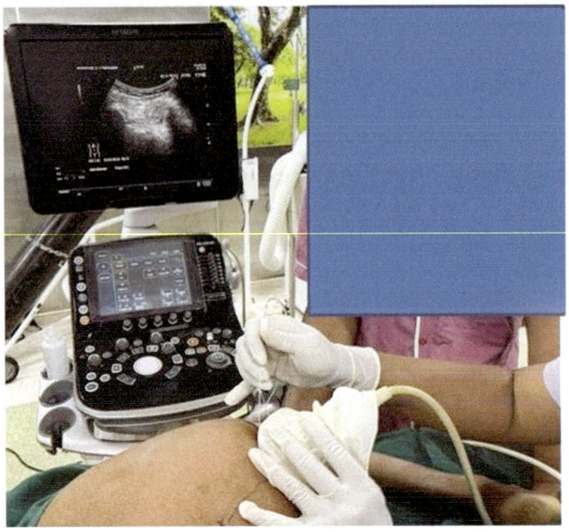

Fig. 5: Needle entry point: In-plane approach.

- Epidural catheter inserted under real-time ultrasound guidance and advanced 3 cm over the needle tip into the perineural space.
- The needle is then withdrawn.
- Confirm optimal catheter positioning with real-time assessment of saline solution spread.
- Secure catheter with Tegaderm transparent dressing.

Drugs Used

For sciatic radiculopathy in emergency department: 10 mL of 0.5% bupivacaine mixed with 8 mg of dexamethasone.

For continuous technique: Local anesthetic, 10 mL bolus, followed by 6 mL 2 hourly depending on pain score response from patient.

The recommended duration for infusion of local anesthetic in continuous peripheral nerve blockade is not well defined in literature, must not exceed 48–72 hours, depending on the patient's comorbidities, extreme age, renal failure, hepatic failure, increased risk of local anesthetic toxicity due to alteration of absorption and elimination and therefore the concentration of local anesthetic can remain high in the circulation for longer periods.

NEUROLYSIS

Popliteal-SNB with a subneurolytic dose of phenol (3%) produced significant reduction in the rest pain scores in an ischemic leg. Phenol is reported to have a differential effect disrupting predominantly the pain fibers, retaining the other sensory functions and motor power. This provides sufficient analgesia for 3–6 months.[6]

COMPLICATIONS

Potential complications related to SNBs include infection at the injection site, bleeding, nerve injury, and local anesthetic toxicity.

CONCLUSION

Infragluteal SNB is reliable, efficient, safe, and well tolerated by patients. Technically simple, use easily identifiable landmarks, produce minimal patient discomfort, and provide prompt onset of analgesia. Neuropathic pain in lower extremities can be managed by repeated SNBs, which provide effective pain relief, reduce or discontinue analgesics, and improve quality-of-life. In diabetic patients with refractory neuropathic pain, this technique appears to be an effective lifesaving tool providing long-term relief and improving the quality-of-life of patients. It should be commonly used by pain physicians for helping patients suffering from acute, neuralgic, chronic, and cancer pain in lower extremity.

REFERENCES

1. Enneking FK, Chan V, Greger J, Hadzić A, Lang SA, Horlocker TT. Lower-extremity peripheral nerve blockade: essentials of our current understanding. Reg Anesth Pain Med. 2005;30:4-35.
2. Kouroukti I, Asimakopoulos T, Botou P, Hristodoulou A, Gika A, Tomara H, et al. (Greece) Sciatic Nerve Block for Neuropathic Pain Management: A Case Report, 13th Congress of the European Pain Federation. Budapest, Hungary: EFIC; 2023.
3. Vrsajkov V, Lukić-Šarkanović M, Ilić N. ESRA19-0024 Interventional treatment with peripheral nerve blocks can positively influence chronic sciatic pain resistant to standard analgesic treatment. Abstracts of the European Society of Regional Anesthesia. Regional Anesth Pain Med. 2019;44(Suppl 1).
4. Bagaphou TC, Santonastaso D, Gargaglia E, Norgiolini L, Tiburzi C, Cristallini S, et al. Ultrasound guided continuous sciatic nerve block for acute herpetic neuralgia. Case Rep Anesthesiol. 2019;2019:7948282.
5. Schaeffer E, Le Saché F. Sciatic catheters: an analgesic alternative in diabetic patients. Can J Anesth. 2016;63:468-74.

6. Vergheese DC, Valiaveedan S, Thomas MK, Aftab S, Thomas T. Sub-neurolytic dose of phenol for popliteal-sciatic nerve block under ultrasound guidance for the relief of ischemic leg pain. Int J Med Res Health Sci. 2016;5:66-72.
7. Gedikoglu M, Eker HE. Ultrasound-guided popliteal sciatic nerve block: an effective alternative technique to control ischaemic severe rest pain during endovascular treatment of critical limb ischaemia. Pol J Radiol. 2019;84: e537-41.
8. Herrala J, Nagdev A, Gullikson J, Sobrero M, Schwimmer H, Duggan N, et al. 248, Ultrasound-guided transgluteal sciatic nerve block in emergency department patients with sciatic radiculopathy: a multicenter rospective study. Ann Emerg Med. 80(4):S108-9.
9. Sukhani R, Candido KD, Doty R Jr, Yaghmour E, McCarthy RJ. Infragluteal-parabiceps sciatic nerve block: an evaluation of a novel approach using a single-injection technique. Anesth Analg. 2003;96:868-73.

39 CHAPTER

Coccygeal Nerve Block

Yashwant L Nankar

ABSTRACT

Coccygeal nerve block is a useful procedure for diagnosis and treatment of chronic pain patients with pain in coccygeal and perineal region, specifically in the rectum and the coccyx. It can give patients very good relief from chronic pain conditions such as coccygodynia, pain following surgery for rectal cancer, or pain due to anococcygeal nerve (ACN) injury due to falls, exercise, and complication from surgery. The advantage of this nerve block is that both bowel and bladder functions are not affected. This procedure can be performed under image guidance with C-arm or computed tomography (CT) guidance. Long-term relief can be obtained with radiofrequency ablation or use of neurolytics.

INTRODUCTION

The coccygeal plexus is a small nerve plexus formed by the fifth sacral nerve (S5) with a contribution from S4 and the coccygeal nerve. The coccygeal plexus gives rise to the anococcygeal nerve (ACN). The ACN is a nerve in the pelvis, which supplies the skin in the coccygeal region as well as the sacrococcygeal joint and the area near the coccyx bone. Coccygeal nerve block is useful for the diagnosis and treatment of intractable perineal pain in this region.[1] Chronic pain in this region can develop as an occupational hazard seen in persons with habit of sitting for long time, using poor posture while sitting, prolonged bicycle riding, parturition, or a serious accident, such as a fall. In cancer patients, the intractable perineal pain often appears in the anal region following abdominoperineal resection, with osseous metastasis or the local recurrence of cancer.[2] Different studies[2-4] have demonstrated that coccygeal nerve blocks have the ability to provide almost immediate relief from these conditions. This chapter describes a paracoccygeal approach alongside the coccyx under fluoroscopy using the lateral view and ability to easily use the shorter, thinner spinal needle.

ANATOMY

The coccyx is a large triangular bone located directly beneath the sacrum **(Fig. 1)**.

The coccyx consists of three to five spinal bones that are fused into one narrow, curved structure. The main purpose of the coccyx is to bear the weight of the body, but it is also the main point of attachment for muscles, ligaments, and tendons.

The coccygeal plexus is formed by ventral branches of S4 and S5 sacral nerves and coccygeal spinal nerve. The coccygeal plexus gives rise to the ACN, which is the 31st pair of spinal nerves **(Fig. 2)**.

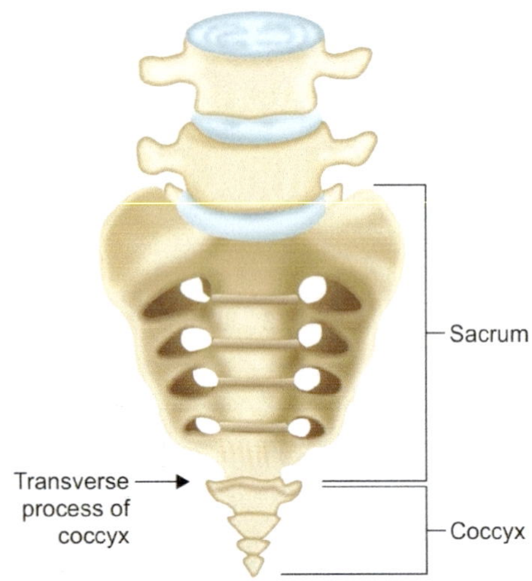

Fig. 1: Anatomy of sacrum, coccyx, and transverse process of coccyx.

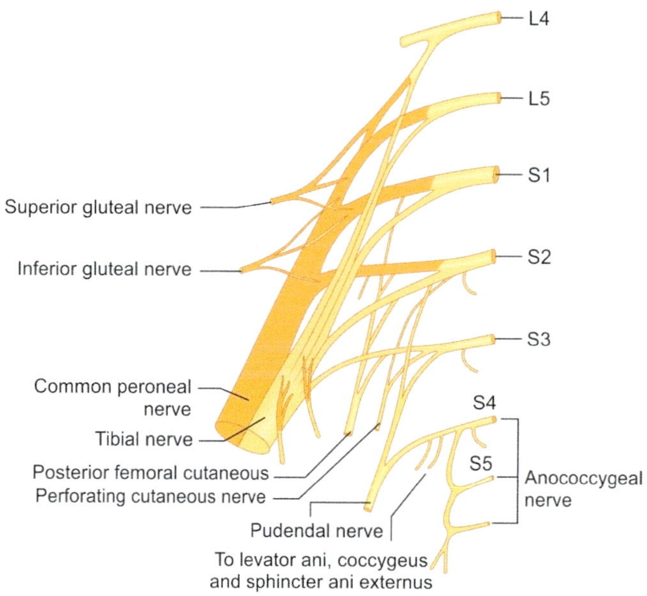

Fig. 2: Coccygeal nerve plexus.

Coccygeal nerve passes through the sacral hiatus running along the dorsal surface of the coccygeal bone, turning around the base of coccygeal angle, and passing between the coccygeal vertebrae, enters the adipose tissue surrounding sacrotuberous ligament where it unites with the fifth sacral nerve. ACN supplies the skin in the coccygeal region as well as the sacrococcygeal joint and the area near the coccyx bone. There are no named motor branches.

INDICATIONS

Coccygeal nerve block is indicated for the following:

Chronic pain conditions such as:

- Coccygodynia due to childbirth
- Injury or partial dislocation of the sacrococcygeal joint
- Levator ani myofascial pain syndrome
- Meningeal cyst
- Obesity (due to excess pressure on the coccyx when sitting)
- Pudendal nerve injury or neuropathic pain (e.g., in bike riders)
- Tarlov pilonidal cysts
- Sacrococcygeal synchondrosis
- Sacrospinal ligaments dysfunction
- Sacrotuberous ligament dysfunction
- Chronic pain after anus, rectum, and perineal surgery.

EQUIPMENT AND DRUGS

Needles:

- 25G ¾-inch needle, for local infiltration
- 22G spinal needle

Syringes: 1 mL, 2 mL, and 5 mL, each 2

Equipment:

- Marker pen
- Metal marker
- Radiation safety devices for all

Imaging modalities:

- C-arm
- Computed tomography (CT)

Drugs:

- Lignocaine 2%
- Bupivacaine 0.5%
- Normal saline
- Depot steroids triamcinolone or alpha methylpred nisolone 40 mg
- Alcohol 99%; phenol 6% for neurolysis
- Radiopaque contrast media.

FLUOROANATOMY

In anteroposterior (AP) view, identify the sacrococcygeal junction and the transverse process of coccyx which is a small bony projection lateral to the upper end of the bone immediately below the sacral hiatus. The site of drug entry is just AP to transverse process of coccyx **(Figs. 3A and B)**.

POSITION

Place the patient in prone position with pillow under abdomen to correct lordosis **(Fig. 4)**.

PROCEDURE

Step 1:

- After identifying the site, preparing and draping the area, direct C-arm toward the sacrococcygeal junction and take AP image to view the transverse process of coccyx.
- Put metal marker on the most inferior aspect of the sacral hiatus **(Fig. 5)**.
- The needle entry point is about 1 cm lateral to the lateral border of coccyx.

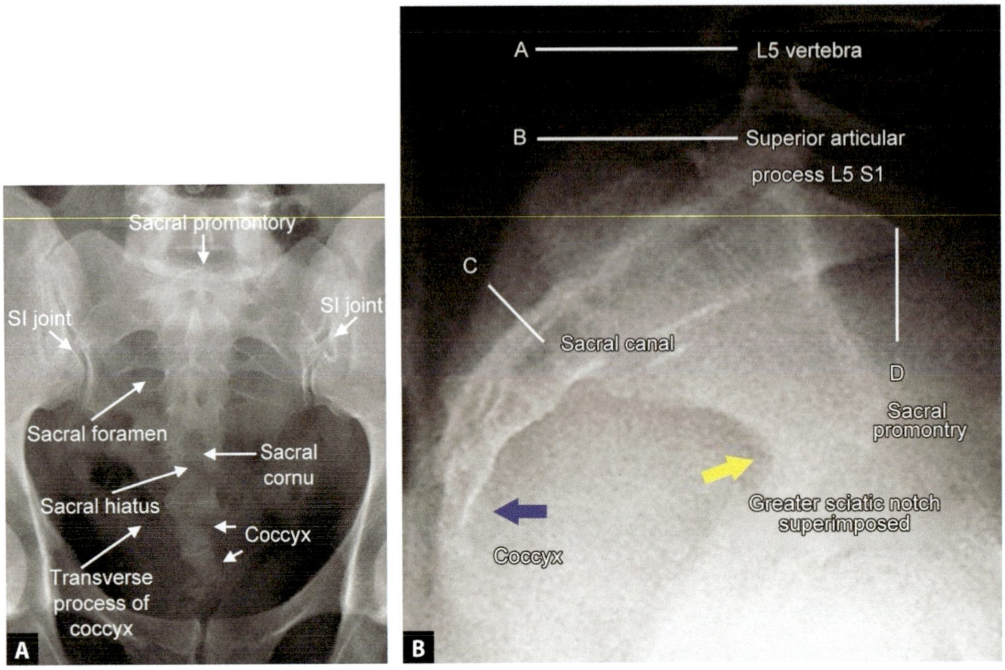

Figs. 3A and B: (A) Fluroanatomy of anteroposterior (AP) view of sacrum, coccyx. (SI: sacroiliac); (B) Fluroanatomy lateral view sacrum, coccyx (SI: sacroiliac).

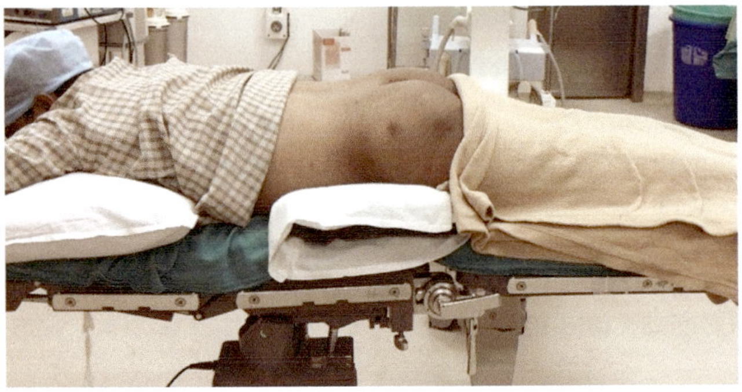

Fig. 4: Prone position with pillow under abdomen.

Step 2:

- After infiltration with 1% lignocaine, take a 22 or 25G spinal needle with slightly bending the tip (20–30°) **(Fig. 6)** and advance under fluoroscopic guidance.
- The needle trajectory is angled to directly contact lateral aspect of coccyx, thus, giving tactile sensation **(Fig. 7A)**.
- The needle is then carefully advanced in lateral view with tip just anterior to anterior margin of coccyx **(Fig. 7B)**.
- Inject 1 mL of omnipaque and confirm in AP and lateral view **(Figs. 8A and B)**.

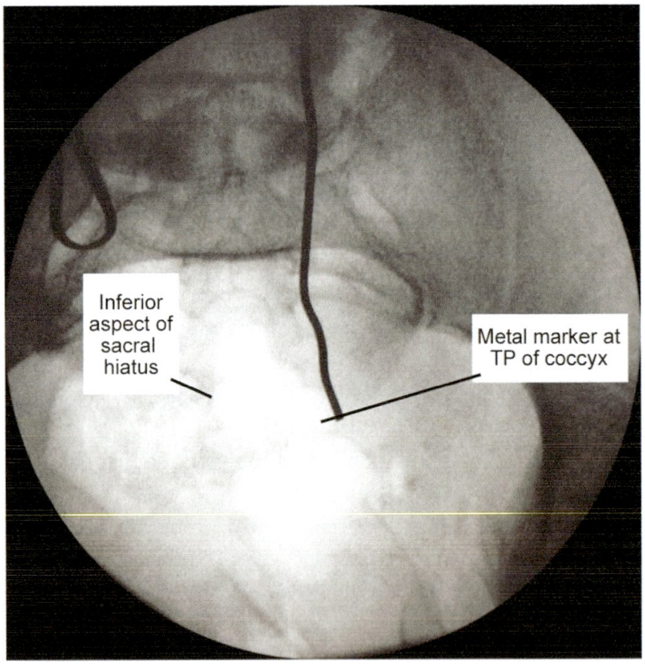

Fig. 5: Metal marker tip on the most inferior aspect of the sacral hiatus at transverse process of coccyx.

- After negative aspiration, inject 0.25% bupivacaine with or without steroid about 2 cc.
- Patient is shifted to recovery room.

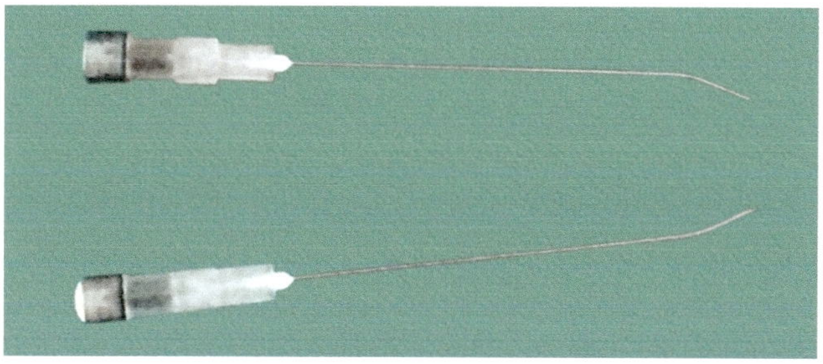

Fig. 6: Needles with bent tip.

POSSIBLE COMPLICATIONS

Coccygeal nerve block is a minimally invasive technique but may cause the following:

- Bleeding
- Infection
- Nerve damage that may occur due to a needle puncture
- Tingling or numbness in the extremities
- Side effects with relation to local anesthetic, alcohol, or phenol.

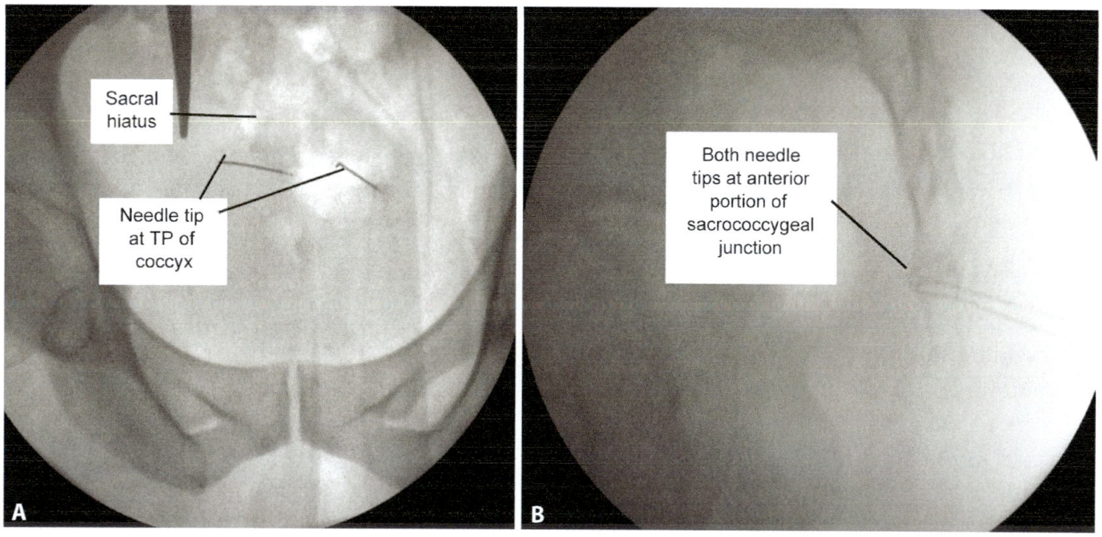

Figs. 7A and B: (A) Anteroposterior (AP) view with needles tip at tip of coccygeal transverse process; (B) Lateral view with needles tip at anterior portion of sacrococcygeal junction.

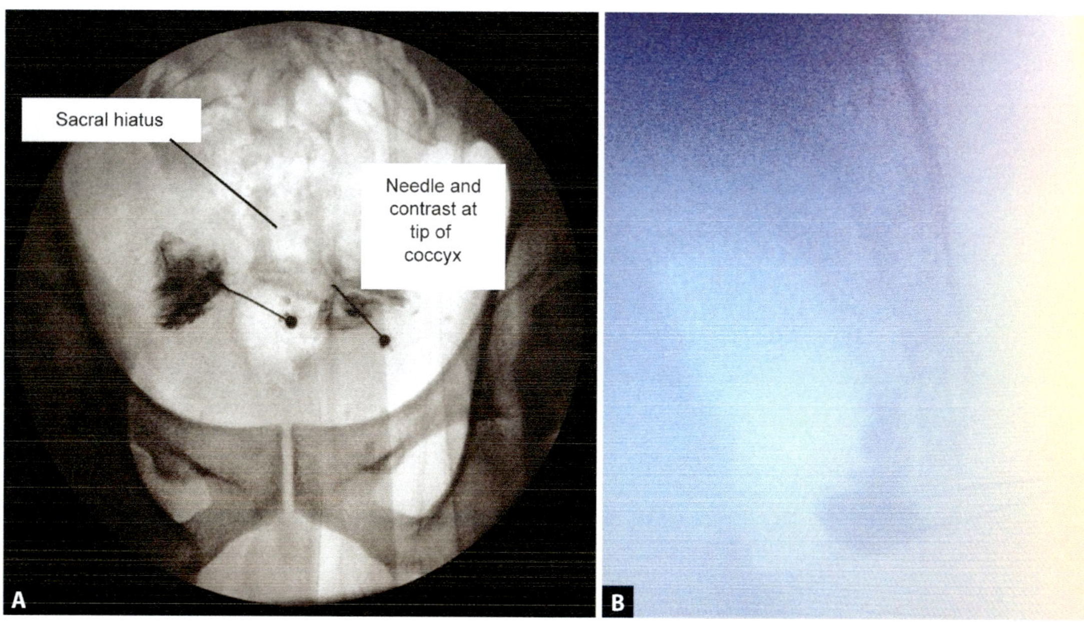

Figs. 8A and B: (A) Anteroposterior (AP) view with contrast; (B) Lateral view with contrast.

NEUROLYTIC

Neurolytics such as alcohol and phenol can be used for long-term relief.

Absolute alcohol when used as the neurolytic agent its effect is both profound and long-lasting. The effect of phenol is both less pronounced and shorter-acting. The disadvantage of using alcohol as a neurolytic agent is that patients sometimes experience burning pain after an alcohol injection, even though they have been pretreated with a local anesthetic. This may be due to either the diffusion of alcohol to surrounding tissues, because the 2 mL injection (1 mL bupivacaine and 1 mL alcohol) exceeds the capacity of the space, or if the tip of the needle is dislocated while alcohol is being injected. It is advisable to pretreat patients with an extradural sacral block for the pain caused by the alcohol injection.

Intractable perineal pain often appears in the anal region following abdominoperineal resection in the treatment of rectal cancer. The occurrence of such pain is often associated with osseous metastasis or the local recurrence of cancer, but many patients can continue their normal routines of daily life, if the pain is adequately controlled.

The coccygeal nerve block using alcohol is a useful method to provide adequate relief of localized intractable perineal pain.[2] The analgesic effect lasted for about 3-11 months without complications, such as sensory paralysis of the pudendum, dysuria, or weakness in the lower limbs.

De Vésian[5] in 1907 reported the use of 60% alcohol in an obstinate case of reflex coccygodynia, getting the idea from the treatment of facial neuralgia by the injection of alcohol. The patient was pain-free for 4 months. Ralph Duffy[6] reported similar result in his case. He recommended this procedure for patients who resist excision.

CONCLUSION

Coccygeal nerve block is a very useful procedure. This procedure is extremely useful, because site-specific perineal pain can be selectively blocked. The technique is simple; there is no danger of infection in the intrathecal or extradural space, and there is no need to keep the patient immobilized for a long time after the procedure as against intrathecal neurolytics. The procedure can be repeated, if required. It should be commonly used by pain physicians for helping patients suffering from acute, neuralgic, chronic, and cancer-related pain in coccygeal region.

REFERENCES

1. Alimehmeti RH, Schuenke MD, Dellon AL. Anococcygeal nerve and sitting pain: differential diagnosis and treatment results. Ann Plast Surg. 2022;88:79-83.
2. Yamada K, Ishihara Y, Saito T. Relief of intractable perineal pain by coccygeal nerve block in anterior sacrococcygeal ligament after surgery for rectal cancer. J Anesth. 1994; 8(1):52-4.
3. Wray CC, Easom S, Hoskinson J. Coccydynia. Aetiology and Treatment. J Bone Joint Surg Br. 1991;73(2):335-8.
4. Mitra R, Cheung L, Perry P. Efficacy of fluoroscopically guided steroid injections in the management of coccydynia. Pain Physician. 2007;10(6):775-8.
5. De Vésian. Revue Pratique de Gynocologie. d' Obstétrique, et de Pédiatrie. 1907.
6. Duffy R. Coccygodynia: causes and treatment. Boston Med Surg J. 1914;171(27):1011-2.

40 CHAPTER

Obturator Nerve Block

Beatriz Nistal-Nuño, Arthur Atchabahian

ABSTRACT

The obturator nerve block can be used for postoperative analgesia after knee surgery as well as for the management and diagnosis of chronic hip pain to reduce adductor spasticity and as an adjunct for transvesical tumor resection. Some residual adductor power will be preserved even after a successful block because of cross-innervation by the femoral and sciatic nerves. In some cases, the accessory obturator nerve might have to be blocked as well. Techniques of obturator nerve blockade using neurostimulation, ultrasound guidance, and fluoroscopy have been described. Complications are rare but can involve needle entry into the pelvis or hemorrhage.

INTRODUCTION

The obturator nerve (ON) arises from the lumbar plexus and innervates most of the adductors in the medial compartment of the thigh as well as part of the medial femur. It is used to supplement femoral and sciatic nerve blocks for analgesia after knee surgery, diagnosis and management of painful conditions of the hip, treatment of adductor spasticity, and as an adjunct for endoscopic urological transurethral resections of inferolateral bladder wall tumors, to prevent ipsilateral obturator stimulation and thigh adductor muscle contraction during the procedure.

INDICATIONS

There are morphine-sparing effects of obturator nerve block (ONB) after major surgical procedures on the knee or the medial thigh. In blocks in which multiple nerves of the lower extremity are targeted (e.g., the posterior lumbar plexus block or the anterior "3 in 1" block), the ON has a relatively low block success rate.[1] A recent study showed that the ON is almost never blocked following a fascia iliaca compartment block, even when a suprainguinal approach is used.[2] Therefore, the ONB can be a valuable adjunct to femoral and lateral femoral cutaneous nerve blocks for surgeries of the knee or for analgesia for surgical tourniquets placed on the thigh. In a group of 60 patients, ONB provided superior analgesia when combined with femoral and sciatic nerve blocks for total knee replacement versus those cases unaccompanied by ONB.[3,4]

Other indications for ONB include diagnosis and management of painful conditions of the hip (radiofrequency lesioning of sensory branches of the nerve has been successfully used to treat hip joint pain in 14 patients),[3,5] treatment of adductor spasticity,[1] and as an adjuvant to femoral nerve blockade in pain therapy.[6]

While the ON and AON (if present) contribute to the innervation of the anterior capsule of the hip,[7] the interadductor ONB used in clinical practice might be too distal to provide effective hip analgesia, and another technique such as the PENG block[8] is needed to reliably block those branches.

The nerve may also be blocked as an adjunct for endoscopic urological transurethral resections of inferolateral bladder wall tumors, to prevent ipsilateral obturator stimulation and thigh adductor muscle contraction during the procedure,[6] since subarachnoid block or general anesthesia without the aid of muscle relaxants does not routinely prevent adductor muscle contractions that could contribute to bladder perforation, bleeding or incomplete resection.[3,9-12] However, it is difficult to predict whether the block is necessary in urological surgery only on the basis of the tumor site.[6,13]

ANATOMY

The ON is a mixed nerve and contains both motor and sensory nerve fibers. The large number of motor fibers makes the ON a frequent choice for the electromyographic (EMG) recording of compound motor action potentials (CMAPs).[1]

It originates from the L2-L4 branches of the lumbar plexus, although the contribution from L2 is frequently small or even nonexistent.[3,14] The nerve emerges at the upper level of the medial border of the psoas major muscle at the approximate level of the sacroiliac joint, passing over the psoas major muscle[3,15] and passes behind the iliac vessels from which it is separated by the fascia iliaca.[3] It continues its downward course, descending into the pelvis with the iliac vessels and obturator artery and vein along the obturator groove and passes through the obturator foramen into the thigh.[3] In the lesser pelvis, it is adjacent to the obturator fascia, which covers the outer part of the internal obturator muscle.[16] It runs close to the prostatic urethra, bladder neck, and inferolateral bladder wall within the pelvic cavity.[17-19] At the level of the obturator foramen, which lies beneath the superior pubic ramus, the nerve bifurcates into two terminal branches (anterior and posterior).[3] The position of the obturator arteries with respect to the obturator divisions is variable.[1] The anterior branch (superficial nerve) supplies sensation through an articular branch to the anterior hip joint and innervates the anterior adductor muscles (pectineus, adductor longus, and adductor brevis).[3,20] In some patients, branches entering the adductor brevis can be visualized giving the appearance of three divisions to the ON.[1] It makes, to a varying extent, a small cutaneous sensory contribution to the medial and inferior aspects of the thigh.[3] The posterior branch innervates the deep adductor muscles (adductor brevis and magnus, obturator externus) and frequently sends a variable contribution to the medial portions of the knee joint.[3,20,21] This small contribution may be important for analgesia following knee surgery.[3,22]

The decrease in adductor power is the best method for assessing ONB. However, even with complete ONB, there is some residual adductor strength because of the pectineus (femoral nerve innervation) and part of the adductor magnus (sciatic nerve innervation) muscles.[1]

Up to 30% of individuals may have a small accessory obturator nerve (AON). The AON can be derived from the ventral rami of L3 and L4[3] or branch off the ON as this nerve (ON) runs along the lateral wall of the small pelvis. It runs along the posterior aspect of the external iliac artery.[23] Unlike the ON, it branches off by extending downward over the superior pubic ramus on the remainder of its route.[23] This accessory nerve partially contributes to motor innervation of the pectineus muscle and hip joint.[3,24] It was observed that the AON innervates the hip joint and pectineus muscle (100%) and supplies branches to the trunk of the ON (6.1%), the anterior branch of the ON (14.3%), the posterior branch of the ON (4.65%), and the anastomosing branch to the femoral nerve (2.3%).[23] The AON follows a different path from that of the ON and may limit the efficacy of an ONB block if it is not blocked.[23] The AON may contribute to continued adductor spasm despite ON blockade.[25] It is, thus, important to ensure that this branch is also blocked. If there is insufficient ON blockade, adding a block of the AON should be considered, particularly in surgeries of the hip. For ideal analgesia, all these branches should be blocked. The blockade of all branches innervating the hip joint is essential for complete hip anesthesia and analgesia.[23]

CONTRAINDICATIONS

There are few specific contraindications for this block in addition to contraindications to nerve blocks in general, such as patient refusal and skin lesions or infection in the inguinal area, and relative contraindications, such as pre-existing neuropathy or significant clotting disorders. Limited mobility at the joints does not affect the eligibility for the block unless it prevents positioning the patient in the lithotomy position.[16]

TECHNIQUE USING NEUROSTIMULATION

Different approaches to ON[26,27] have been proposed since 1928.[16] Because of a lack of clear anatomic landmarks, significant patient discomfort and inconsistent results, the classic method (Labat's technique) remained forgotten until 1967, when this method was simplified.[28] Currently, this classical pubic approach is still commonly used for ONB using a nerve stimulator, although the success rate varies (60.5-91.7%).[29,30] In 1993, the interadductor approach was described, in which a needle is inserted behind the upper end of the adductor longus muscle.[27] Recently, a simple and reliable new method (the inguinal approach), in which the needle is inserted at the midpoint between the femoral arterial pulse and the inner side of the adductor longus muscle on the inguinal crease, was described by Choquet et al.[31]

Classic Pubic Approach (of Labat)

The patient is placed in the supine position with the legs slightly abducted and externally rotated.[17] After identification of the pubic tubercle, a 21- or 22G, 10 cm needle is inserted aiming posteriorly and 20° laterally through a skin wheal 2 cm lateral and 2 cm inferior to the tubercle **(Fig. 1)**.[31,32] The needle is advanced until it makes contact with the inferior border of the superior pubic ramus bone at a depth of 2–4 cm.[33] As the needle is advanced medially toward the superior pubic ramus, small amounts of local anesthetic are injected to decrease patient discomfort.[32] The needle is then withdrawn by 3 cm and redirected caudad and laterally at an angle of 45° to enter the obturator foramen until contraction of the thigh adductor muscles is observed.[33] Stimulation is begun using a current of 1.2 mA with a twitch duration of 0.1 ms and a frequency of 2 Hz. The current is gradually decreased, and the needle is redirected as needed to maintain the muscle twitch below 0.5 mA. At that time, 10–20 mL of local anesthetic is injected after confirmation that no blood is seen during aspiration.[17,31,33,34]

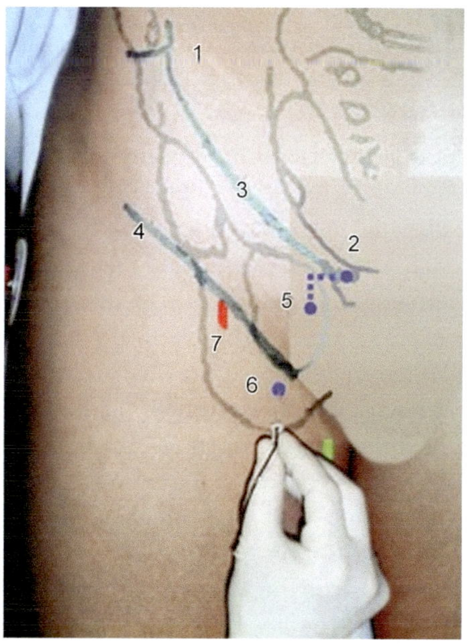

Fig. 1: Illustration of the traditional pubic and the inguinal approach for obturator nerve block. In the pubic approach, the insertion point of the needle is 2 cm lateral and 2 cm inferior to the pubic tubercle. In the inguinal approach, the insertion point of the needle is at the midpoint of the line drawn between the femoral arterial pulse and the inner border of the adductor longus tendon. 1, Superior anterior iliac spine; 2, pubic tubercle; 3, inguinal ligament; 4, inguinal crease; 5, insertion point of needle in the pubic approach; 6, insertion point of the needle in the inguinal approach; 7, femoral pulse; 8, inner border of the adductor longus tendon

Source: Used with permission from Choquet O, Capdevila X, Bennourine K, Feugeas JL, Bringuier-Branchereau S, Manelli JC. A new inguinal approach for the obturator nerve block: anatomical and randomized clinical studies. Anesthesiology. 2005;103(6):1238-45.

The block is technically difficult as the nerve is deep. It is classified as a block with an intermediate level of difficulty.[33] The success rate of ONB with this method varies from 60.5 to 91.7% using a nerve stimulator.[29,30] Even in the most experienced hands, this block can be unsuccessful.[17] Wassef[27] studied the degree of patient discomfort with the pubic approach and found that 90% of patients reported moderate-to-severe discomfort.[31] For the pubic approach, the pubic tubercle is the most definitive landmark. Sometimes, the identification of the pubic tubercle is difficult in obese patients or patients with a blunt pubic bone. If the tubercle is not correctly identified, the needle could pass above the pubic ramus and cause damage to the surrounding structures (bladder, rectum, spermatic cord).[31,35,36] Furthermore, this approach is performed in a highly vascularized region.[17,37] The ON crosses the obturator canal close to the obturator vessels.[31] The incidence of vascular injury is also frequent due to proximity to the obturator vessels.[33] The circumflex arteries and veins are in close proximity to the obturator foramen. Intravascular injection and hematoma may occur.[18,38] The vascular connections between the obturator and external iliac systems behind the pubic ramus (i.e., the corona mortis) can be life-threatening in case of injury.[19] Careful approach is mandatory with this technique to avoid damaging surrounding structures and vessels.[17] A safer and less complicated approach is, therefore, desirable for a wider applicability of ONB.[33]

Accessory Obturator Nerve Blockade

In addition to inducing ON blockade using a classic approach, the technique described below can be used to block the accessory branch **(Fig. 2)**. It is to be noted, however, that this technique was only studied in cadavers and never applied to live patients.[23] The needle is inserted at about 2 cm lateral and caudal to the pubic tubercle, just as described for the ONB. However, the needle is directed laterally and slightly cranially to contact the lateral bony edge of the obturator canal. The blockade needle is then withdrawn to subcutaneous tissue and redirected about 30° lateral from its initial position, targeting the

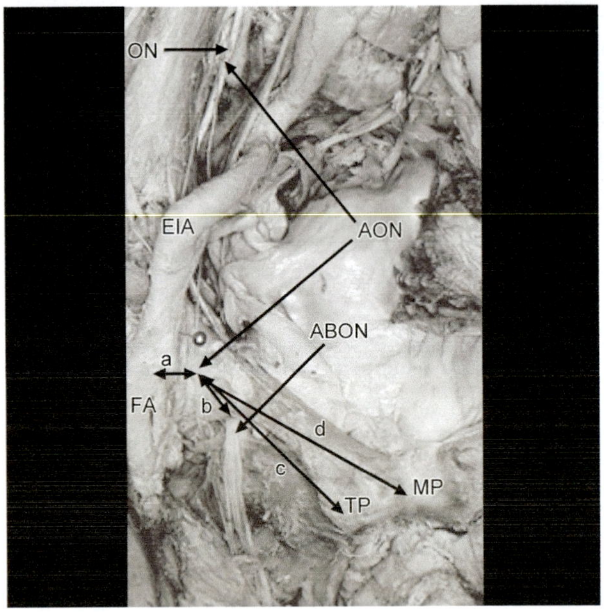

Fig. 2: Accessory branch and measured distances. a, Distance of the AON to the FA; b, upper wall of external opening of obturator canal; c, pubic tubercle; d, median plane. (AON: accessory obturator nerve; ABON: anterior branch of obturator nerve; EIA: external iliac artery; FA: femoral artery; MP: median plane; ON: obturator nerve; TP: pubic tubercle)

Source: Used with permission from Akkaya T, Comert A, Kendir S, Acar HI, Gumus H, Tekdemir I, Elhan A. Detailed anatomy of accessory obturator nerve blockade. Minerva Anestesiol. 2008;74(4):119-22.

superior edge of the superior pubic ramus. The needle is then advanced toward the superior pubic ramus until it contacts the anterior wall of the bone and walks off cephalad about 1 cm further on the superior (cephalad) surface of the bone. This location is the final position of the needle, and 5-10 mL of local anesthetic is injected after aspiration. Attention must be paid not to position the needle too laterally to avoid any injury to the femoral artery (FA). To aid in doing this, a trace of FA should be drawn on the skin prior to beginning the blockade procedure. During the procedure, the FA should be pushed laterally by using the other hand to avoid a puncture. The tip of the needle should not be positioned too far laterally.[23]

Interadductor Approach

Kakinohana et al.[30] proposed an interadductor approach. This method involves the insertion of a needle behind the adductor longus tendon combined with nerve stimulation to identify the ON. In their study, it proved to be faster and more successful than the traditional approach in terms of shortening the time from needle insertion to adductor motor response.[15]

The modification of the interadductor approach (described by Wassef) does not necessitate changing the patient's position[16] to locate the long adductor tendon **(Figs. 3A to C)**. A stimulating needle is inserted approximately 2 cm lateral to the tendon's attachment to the pubic bone in the palpable crevice below the muscle. The needle is directed toward the patient's head at a slight angle so that after inserting the needle 2–4 cm deep, its tip lies below the long adductor muscle **(Figs. 3A to C)**.[16,39] The current is initially set at 1.5 mA; once an adductor response is elicited, the current is reduced down to 0.5 mA, and 10 mL of local anesthetic is administered after an aspiration test.[16] This interadductor approach for ONB is easy, which is further confirmed by the lack of a statistically significant correlation between the anesthesiologist's experience and the success rate. Patient's sex, age, and body mass index (BMI) do not seem to affect the efficacy, which makes it possible to use this block in every patient group.[16]

Inguinal Approach

Choquet et al.[31] described the inguinal approach, which involves blockade of the anterior and posterior branches of ON at the inguinal level. Complications are less likely with this approach as the nerve is located superficially at that level, with no major vessels in its proximity.[33] The inguinal approach is also more acceptable to the patient because palpation and penetration of the pubic area are avoided.[31]

The patient, placed in a supine position and with the legs slightly abducted, is first asked to slightly flex his or her hip, and a line is drawn using a skin marker to locate the inguinal crease. After identification of the adductor longus tendon at the pubic tubercle, as the most superficial palpable tendon in the medial part of the thigh, a mark on the skin is made in the inguinal crease at the midpoint of the line drawn between the femoral arterial pulse and the inner border of the adductor longus tendon **(Fig. 1)**. This point corresponds to an easily palpable groove between the vascular bundle and the adductor longus muscle.[31] This approach is performed in two stages. First, a 21G, 5 cm stimulating needle is inserted 0.5 cm below the skin mark in a cephalad direction with a 30° angle to the skin until adductor muscle (adductor longus or gracilis) contractions are elicited.[17] The adductor longus response of the ON (anterior branch) is observed at the anterior part of the inner thigh. Weak contraction of the gracilis, which frequently accompanies the former, forms a narrow muscular band down to the medial part of the knee.[31]

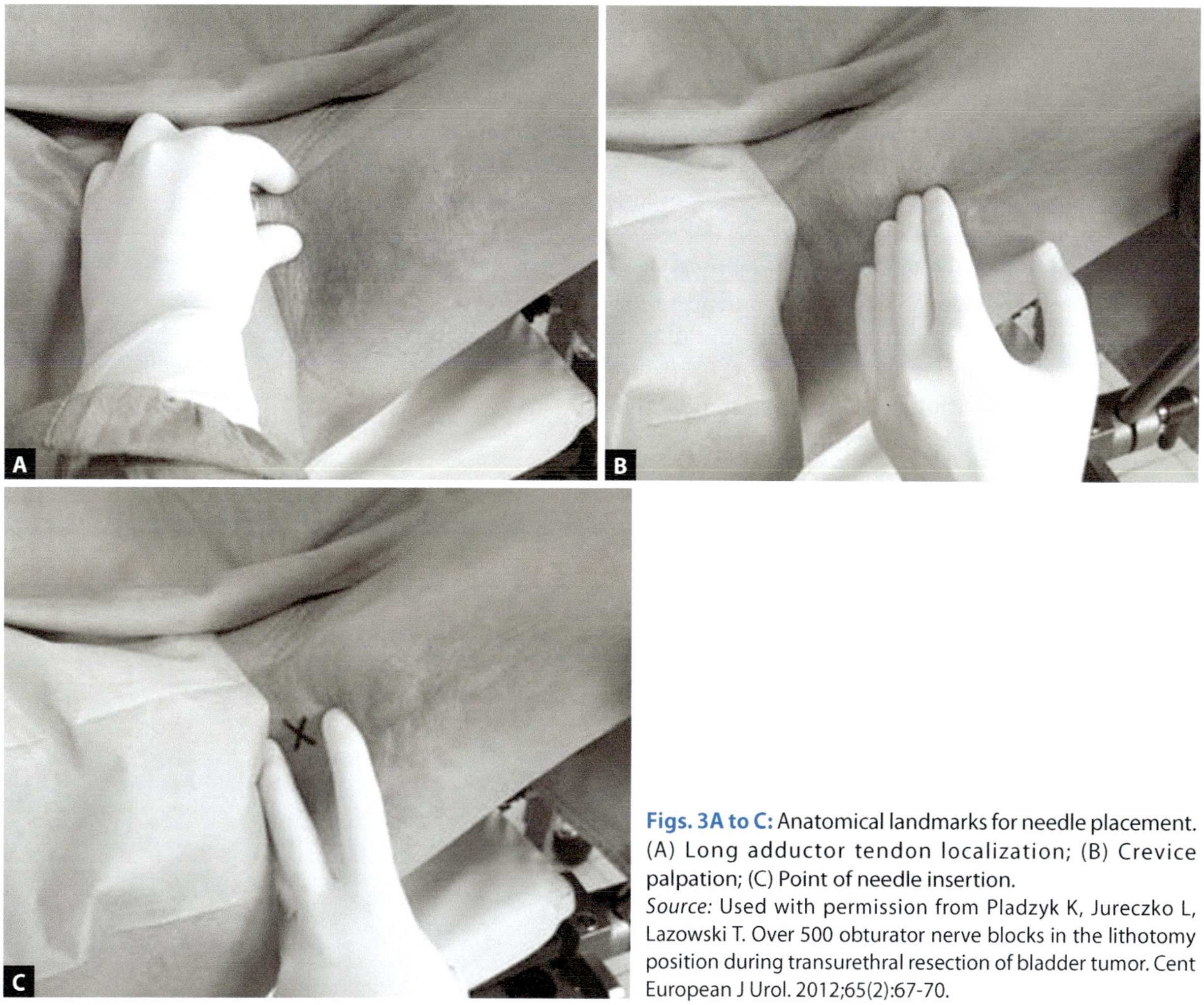

Figs. 3A to C: Anatomical landmarks for needle placement. (A) Long adductor tendon localization; (B) Crevice palpation; (C) Point of needle insertion.
Source: Used with permission from Pladzyk K, Jureczko L, Lazowski T. Over 500 obturator nerve blocks in the lithotomy position during transurethral resection of bladder tumor. Cent European J Urol. 2012;65(2):67-70.

When a muscle response is maintained at a current below 0.5 mA, 5 mL of local anesthetic is injected to block the anterior branch of the ON. The needle is then advanced about 0.5–1 cm while reorienting it about 5° laterally.[17,31] The adductor magnus response is felt in the posterior aspect of the inner thigh and produces a noticeable hip adduction.[31] Similarly, 5 mL of local anesthetic is then injected to block the posterior branch block.[17] At the inguinal level, the anterior and posterior branches are only separated by the adductor brevis muscle. An injection near a single branch could thus potentially achieve a complete block of both branches.[31] Fesenthal,[40] however, asserts that both anterior and posterior divisions must be blocked to accomplish an effective ONB to reduce spasticity.[31]

This approach significantly decreases discomfort and pain during performance of the block and the time taken to achieve a similar quality of sensory and motor blockade compared with the classic pubic tubercle approach. The risk of penetrating the pelvic cavity is present but lower than with the classic approach.[31] The puncture at a distance from the pelvis and large vessels in the inguinal approach minimizes the risk of complications and allows compression in the event of a hematoma.[31] The main limitation is the failure to reach branches contributing to hip joint innervation, which frequently arise before passage of the nerve into the thigh.[31] With bilateral ONB, the total dose of local anesthetic[12] must be taken into consideration.[31]

Transvesical Block

Khorrami also describes a transvesical ONB in 30 patients, but in 20% of them, the lidocaine was applied blindly because the nerve could not be detected with stimulation. In one case, the adductor contraction was sustained despite the ONB.[16,41]

TECHNIQUE USING ULTRASOUND

The anterior and posterior divisions of the ON converge proximally along the lateral border of the adductor brevis muscle. The ON divisions are thin and flat as the fascicles disperse to the muscle groups. The ON divisions have a "white bands" appearance on sonography.[42] It is important that the flat surfaces of the ON divisions be perpendicular to the sound beam to enhance their echo brightness. It is important to note that, although the anterior and posterior divisions converge along the lateral border of the adductor brevis, they do not actually merge there in most (75–80%) subjects because the divisions remain separated by the obturator externus muscle.[31] Therefore, the ONB is best performed as a multiple-injection technique targeting each of the two divisions separately.[1]

Different approaches have been proposed for ultrasound-guided ONB, both in plane and out of plane, either before or after the bifurcation of the ON into its anterior and posterior branches.[6] Helayel et al.[43] used an out-of-plane approach for the anterior branch of the ON, which appears as a flat, hyperechoic structure between the pectineus, adductor longus, and adductor brevis muscles. Simeoforidou et al.[44] proposed an out-of-plane approach for both ON branches with dual guidance. After placing the patient in the supine position with the leg slightly abducted, a linear high-frequency ultrasound probe is positioned to bisect the angle formed by the inguinal crease and adductor longus, perpendicular to the skin to visualize the pectineus muscle, as well as the adductor longus, adductor brevis, and part of the adductor magnus muscles **(Fig. 4)**. The anterior division of the ON is identified between the adductor longus and brevis muscles, whereas the posterior division lies below the adductor brevis **(Fig. 5)**. A more proximal approach to the ON, before its bifurcation, has also been proposed by Akkaya et al.[6,45]

Gray[1] proposed to visualize the obturator divisions and the adductor brevis muscle in short-axis view in the medial thigh. This is best accomplished by sliding the transducer back and forth between proximal and distal locations to observe the convergence of the divisions along the lateral border of the adductor brevis. An out-of-plane approach is often used because of the proximity of the femoral vessels with a lateral-to-medial in-plane approach. The block is usually performed at the level where the anterior and posterior divisions are just separated by the adductor brevis muscle, with the deeper posterior division targeted first.

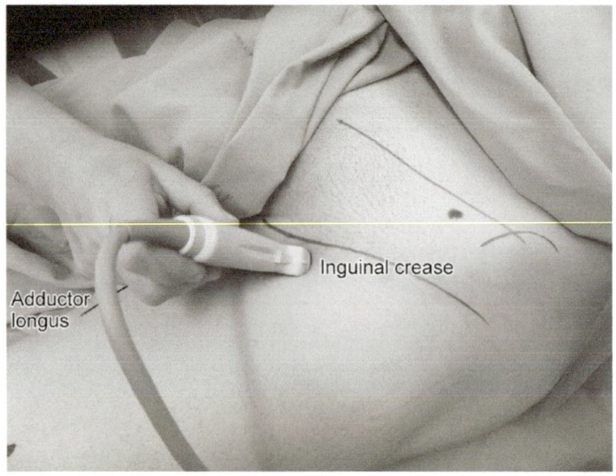

Fig. 4: Position of the ultrasound probe: Opposite the angle that is formed by the inguinal crease and adductor longus, with its short diameter in the course of the dichotomous of the angle.
Source: Used with permission from Simeoforidou M, Bareka M, Basdekis G, Tsiaka K, Chantzi E, Vretzakis G. Peripheral nerve blockade as an exclusive approach to obturator nerve block in anterior cruciate ligament reconstructive surgery. Korean J Anesthesiol. 2013;65(5):410-7.

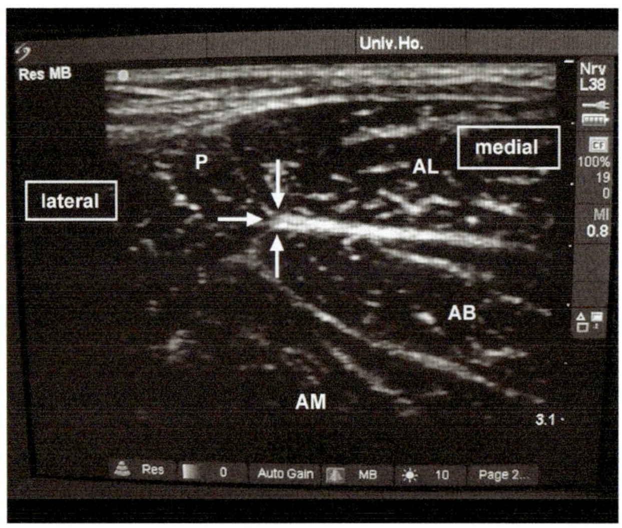

Fig. 5: Ultrasound image where next to pectineus and below adductor longus, a "spider net" image is visualized. Arrows indicate the position of the nerve in the short-axis view. (AB: adductor brevis; AL: adductor longus; AM: adductor magnus; P: pectineus)
Source: Used with permission from Simeoforidou M, Bareka M, Basdekis G, Tsiaka K, Chantzi E, Vretzakis G. Peripheral nerve blockade as an exclusive approach to obturator nerve block in anterior cruciate ligament reconstructive surgery. Korean J Anesthesiol. 2013;65(5):410-7.

The local anesthetic distribution should be within the fascia that invests the adductor brevis and the obturator divisions. If the ON divisions cannot be visualized, a transadductor brevis injection can be performed. Care is taken to avoid puncture of the adjacent obturator arteries.[1,38]

Sinha et al.[46] demonstrated that the injection of half of the local anesthetic solution between the pectineus and adductor brevis muscles, and half between the adductor brevis and adductor magnus muscles, without attempting to visualize the nerves, under ultrasound guidance leads to a mean muscle strength reduction of 82% in 93% of their population (30 patients scheduled for knee surgery),[6] and thus a fairly complete ONB.

Almeida described in one patient a novel, posterior approach that might also block the pudendal nerve, but it remains to be tested in a larger series.[47]

FLUOROSCOPIC RADIOFREQUENCY ABLATION

The patient is placed supine under the image intensifier. A local anesthetic skin wheal is performed at the site of injection (same as for the classic Labat approach). A 22G 10 cm electrode with a 4-mm exposed tip and a radiofrequency generator are used. Under fluoroscopy, the needle is advanced perpendicular to the skin until it reaches the superior-lateral corner of the obturator foramen and contacts the superior ramus of the pubic bone. It is then redirected to pass underneath it. The needle is advanced slightly obliquely to enter the obturator canal to position the needle parallel to the nerve.[13] Needle placement is checked using the C-arm in anteroposterior (AP), oblique, and lateral views and confirmed by electrical stimulation of the target nerve.[11] With sensory stimulation at 50 Hz, paresthesias should be elicited in the groin and hip areas at 0.6 V. After negative aspiration, 1 mL of 2% lidocaine is injected, and then a radiofrequency ablation of the articular branch of ON is carried out at 80°C for 90 seconds twice.[48]

CONCLUSION

The ONB can be used for postoperative analgesia as well as for the management and diagnosis of chronic pain and spasticity. Some residual adductor power will be preserved even after a successful block because of cross-innervation by the femoral and sciatic nerves. In some cases, the AON might have to be blocked as well. Techniques of ON blockade using neurostimulation, ultrasound guidance, and fluoroscopy have been described. Complications are rare but can involve needle entry into the pelvis or hemorrhage.

REFERENCES

1. Gray AT. Obturator Nerve Block. In: Gray AT (Ed). Atlas of Ultrasound-Guided Regional Anesthesia. Philadelphia: Saunders Elsevier; 2010.
2. Hoope WT, Smulders PS, Baumann HM, Hermanides J, Beenen LF, Oostra RJ, et al. A radiological cadaveric study of obturator nerve involvement and cranial injectate spread after different approaches to the fascia iliaca compartment block. Sci Rep. 2023;13(1):12070.
3. Benzon HT, Raja SN, Liu SS, Fishman SM, Cohen SP. Obturator nerve block. In: Narouze H, Candido M (Eds). Essentials of Pain Medicine, 3rd edition. Philadelphia: Elsevier; 2011.
4. McNamee DA, Parks L, Milligan KR. Post-operative analgesia following total knee replacement: an evaluation of the addition of an obturator nerve block to combined femoral and sciatic nerve block. Acta Anaesthesiol Scand. 2002;46:95-9.
5. Kawaguchi M, Hashizume K, Iwata T, Furuya H. Percutaneous radiofrequency lesioning of sensory branches of the obturator and femoral nerves for the treatment of hip joint pain. Reg Anesth Pain Med. 2001;26:576-81.
6. Ghisi D, Delaunay L, Fanelli A. Use of ultrasound for lower extremity. Curr Opin Anaesthesiol. 2014;27:528-37.
7. Short AJ, Barnett JJG, Gofeld M, Baig E, Lam K, Agur AMR, et al. Anatomic study of innervation of the anterior hip capsule: implication for image-Guided Intervention. Reg Anesth Pain Med. 2018;43(2):186-92.
8. Girón-Arango L, Peng PWH, Chin KJ, Brull R, Perlas A. Pericapsular nerve group (PENG) block for hip fracture. Reg Anesth Pain Med. 2018;43(8):859-63.
9. Atanassoff P, Weiss B, Horst A, Kulling D, Stein R, Theiler I. Electroneurographic study on the obturator nerve. Anesthesiology. 1994;81:A1043.
10. Atanassoff PG, Weiss BM, Brull SJ, Horst A, Külling D, Stein R, et al. Compound motor action potential recording distinguishes different onset of motor block of the obturator nerve in response to etidocaine or bupivacaine. Anesth Analg. 1996;82:317-20.
11. Atanassoff PG, Weiss BM, Brull SJ, Horst A, Külling D, Stein R, et al. Electromyographic comparison of obturator nerve block to three-in-one block. Anesth Analg. 1995;81:529-33.
12. Atanassoff PG, Weiss BM, Brull SJ. Lidocaine plasma levels following two techniques of obturator nerve block. J Clin Anesth. 1996;8:535-9.
13. Mihara T, Itoh H, Hashimoto K, Goto T. Trans-resectoscope stimulation predicts the need to block adductor response during bladder tumor resection. Anesth Analg. 2013;117:740-4.
14. Bridenbaugh P, Wedel D. The lower extremity. Somatic blockade. In: Cousins MJ, Bridenbaugh DL (Eds). Neural Blockade in Clinical Anesthesia and Management of Pain, 3rd edition. Philadelphia: Lippincott-Raven; 1998. pp. 373-94.
15. Thallaj A, Rabah D. Efficacy of ultrasound-guided obturator nerve block in transurethral surgery. Saudi J Anaesth. 2011;5:42-4.
16. Pladzyk K, Jureczko L, Lazowski T. Over 500 obturator nerve blocks in the lithotomy position during transurethral

resection of bladder tumor. Central European J Urol. 2012;65(2):67-70.
17. Jo YY, Choi E, Kil HK. Comparison of the success rate of inguinal approach with classical pubic approach for obturator nerve block in patients undergoing TURB. Korean J Anesthesiol. 2011;61(2):143-7.
18. Brown DL. Atlas of Regional Anesthesia. Philadelphia, PA: WB Saunders; 1992. pp. 103-8.
19. Berberoğlu M, Uz A, Ozmen MM, Bozkurt MC, Erkuran C, Taner S, et al. Corona mortis: an anatomic study in seven cadavers and an endoscopic study in 28 patients. Surg Endosc. 2001;15:72-5.
20. Iwanaga J, Reina F, Ishak B, Reina MA, Dumont AS, Tubbs RS. Revisiting the muscular innervation of the obturator nerve: application to neurotization procedures. Kurume Med J. 2023;68(2):75-80.
21. Meier G, Buttner J. Obturator nerve block. Pocket Compendium of Peripheral Nerve Blocks, 4th edition. Germany: Arcis Publishing Company; 2006.
22. Tran J, Peng PWH, Chan VWS, Agur AMR. Overview of innervation of knee joint. Phys Med Rehabil Clin N Am. 2021;32(4):767-78.
23. Akkaya T, Comert A, Kendir S, Acar HI, Gumus H, Tekdemir I, et al. Detailed anatomy of accessory obturator nerve blockade. Minerva Anestesiol. 2008;74:119-22.
24. Sunderland S. Obturator Nerve. Nerves and Nerve Injuries. Edinburgh: Harcourt Brace/Churchill Livingstone;1968. pp. 1096-109.
25. Vloka JD, Hadić A. Obturator and genitofemoral nerve blocks. Techn Reg Anesth Pain Manage. 1999;3:28-32.
26. Labat G. Regional Anesthesia: Its Technic and Clinical Application. Philadelphia: W.B Saunders; 1928. pp. 286-7.
27. Wassef MR. Interadductor approach to obturator nerve blockade for spastic conditions of adductor thigh muscles. Reg Anesth. 1993;18:13-7.
28. Parks CR, Kennedy WF Jr. Obturator nerve block: a simplified approach. Anesthesiology. 1967;28:775-8.
29. Macalou D, Trueck S, Meuret P, Heck M, Vial F, Ouologuem S, et al. Postoperative analgesia after total knee replacement: the effect of an obturator nerve block added to the femoral 3-in-1 nerve block. Anesth Analg. 2004;99:251-4.
30. Kakinohana M, Taira Y, Saitoh T, Hasegawa A, Gakiya M, Sugahara K. Interadductor approach to obturator nerve block for transurethral resection procedure: comparison with traditional approach. J Anesth. 2002;16:123-6.
31. Choquet O, Capdevila X, Bennourine K, Feugeas JL, Bringuier-Branchereau S, Manelli JC. A new inguinal approach for the obturator nerve block: anatomical and randomized clinical studies. Anesthesiology. 2005;103:1238-45.
32. Morgan GE, Mikhail MS, Murray MJ. Peripheral Nerve Blocks. Clinical Anesthesiology, 3rd edition. New York: McGraw-Hill Medical Lange; 2002.
33. Moningi S, Durga P, Ramachandran G, Murthy PV, Chilumala RR. Comparison of inguinal versus classic approach for obturator nerve block in patients undergoing transurethral resection of bladder tumors under spinal anesthesia. J Anaesthesiol Clin Pharmacol. 2014;30:41-5.
34. Tekgül ZT, Divrik RT, Turan M, Konyalioğlu E, Şimşek E, Gönüllü M. Impact of obturator nerve block on the short-term recurrence of superficial bladder tumors on the lateral wall. Urol J. 2014;11(1):1248-52.
35. Hong Y, O'Grady T, Lopresti D, Carlsson C. Diagnostic obturator nerve block for inguinal and back pain: a recovered opinion. Pain. 1996;67:507-9.
36. Shulman MS, Vellayappan U, Monaghan TG, Coukos WJ, Krenis LJ. Simultaneous bilateral obturator nerve stimulation during transurethral electrovaporization of the prostate. J Clin Anesth. 1998;10:518-21.
37. Miller RD. Miller's Anesthesia, 6th edition. Philadelphia: Churchill Livingstone; 2005. pp. 1695-704.
38. Akata T, Murakami J, Yoshinaga A. Life-threatening haemorrhage following obturator artery injury during transurethral bladder surgery: a sequel of an unsuccessful obturator nerve block. Acta Anaesthesiol Scand. 1999;43:784-8.
39. Ciechomski M. Obturator nerve blockade during resection of bladder tumor. Urol Pol. 2004;57(4):58-61.
40. Fesenthal G. Nerve blocks in the lower extremities: anatomic considerations. Arch Phys Med Rehabil. 1974;55:504-7.
41. Khorrami MH, Javid A, Saryazdi H, Javid M. Transvesical blockade of the obturator nerve to prevent contraction in transurethral bladder surgery. J Endourol. 2010; 24(10):1651-4.
42. Soong J, Schafhalter-Zoppoth I, Gray AT. Sonographic imaging of the obturator nerve for regional block. Reg Anesth Pain Med. 2007;32:146-51.
43. Helayel PE, da Conceição DB, Pavei P, Knaesel JA, de Oliveira Filho GR. Ultrasound-guided obturator nerve block: a preliminary report of a case series. Reg Anesth Pain Med. 2007;32:221-6.
44. Simeoforidou M, Bareka M, Basdekis G, Tsiaka K, Chantzi E, Vretzakis G. Peripheral nerve blockade as an exclusive approach to obturator nerve block in anterior cruciate ligament reconstructive surgery. Korean J Anesthesiol. 2013;65:410-7.
45. Akkaya T, Ozturk E, Comert A, Ates Y, Gumus H, Ozturk H, et al. Ultrasound-guided obturator nerve block: a sonoanatomic study of a new methodologic approach. Anesth Analg. 2009;108:1037-41.
46. Sinha SK, Abrams JH, Houle TT, Weller RS. Ultrasound-guided obturator nerve block: an interfascial injection approach without nerve stimulation. Reg Anesth Pain Med. 2009;34:261-4.
47. Almeida CR. The novel obturator fascia compartment block: a technical report. Korean J Anesthesiol. 2022;75(6):541-3.
48. Kasliwal P, Iyer V, Kasliwal S. Percutaneous radiofrequency ablation for relief of pain in a patient of hip joint avascular necrosis. Indian J Pain. 2014;28:121-3.

41 CHAPTER

Piriformis Muscle Injection

Yashwant L Nankar

ABSTRACT

The injection of piriformis muscle is the procedure for diagnosis and management of chronic pain syndromes known as piriformis muscle syndrome (PMS) or piriformis syndrome. The diagnosis of piriformis syndrome has been difficult due to lack of means to identify and selectively inject into this muscle as it lies deep to the buttock, adipose tissue, and gluteus maximums muscle. This chapter describes a simple, safe, and reproducible technique to inject the piriformis muscle under fluoroscopic guidance with a nerve stimulator.

INTRODUCTION

Piriformis muscle syndrome is a less common cause of lower extremity radicular pain which may result from sciatic nerve irritation or compression by the piriformis muscle.[1,2] This syndrome must be differentiated from other causes of low back pain, typically related to lumbar disk disease or spinal stenosis. The treating physician must have a high index of suspicion for the problem, lest it be overlooked. If left untreated, a patient may undergo unsuccessful back surgery for a disk herniation; however, a coexisting occult piriformis syndrome can result in a failed back syndrome.[3] Diagrammatic representation of the piriformis muscle in relation to sciatic nerve is provided in **Figure 1**.

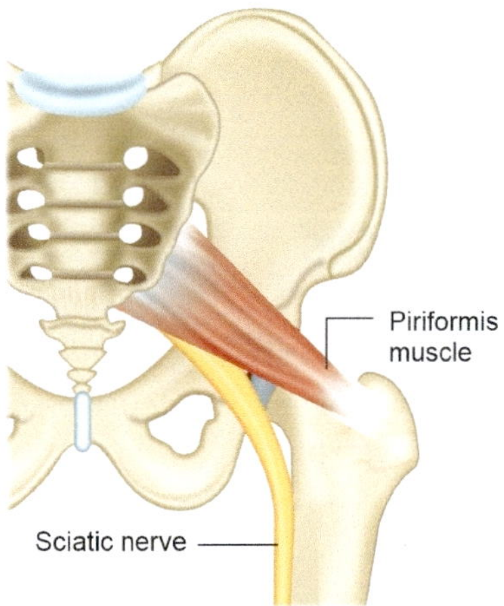

Fig. 1: Piriformis muscle and sciatic nerve post-view.

SYMPTOMS

Piriformis muscle syndrome has a variety of symptoms including pain, tingling, and numbness in the buttocks descending down the lower thigh, leg, and all toes (multiple dermatomes). The pain can be severe while walking, climbing stairs, sitting for long periods of time, getting up from bed, during bowel movement, scrotal region or labia majora, and in female patients there may be dyspareunia.

Fifty percent of patients with piriformis syndrome have a history of trauma, with either a direct buttock contusion or a hip or lower back torsion injury; the remaining 50% of cases are of spontaneous onset.[4]

DIAGNOSTIC CRITERIA

Physical Examination

- The patient may have difficulty sitting due to an intolerance of weight bearing on the buttock
- Piriformis muscle spasm often is detected by careful, deep palpation.
- Tenderness in buttock from the sacrum to the greater trochanter
- The reproduction of sciatica-type pain with weakness results from resisted abduction or external rotation **(Pace test-Refer to Video No. 9)**.

- The Freiberg's test is another diagnostic sign that elicits pain upon forced internal rotation of the extended thigh **(Refer to Video No. 9)**.
- A digital rectal or per vaginal examination may reveal a tenderness on the lateral pelvic wall that reproduces symptoms.

Imaging Studies

- Diagnostic imaging of the lumbar spine is mandatory to exclude associated discogenic and/or osteoarthritic contributing pathology.
- Diagnostic ultrasonographic imaging of the piriformis muscle has demonstrated a significant correlation of piriformis muscle morphology abnormality.

INDICATIONS

- Patient with lower extremity radicular pain in whom the PMS is suspected.
- Patient refractory to conservative regimen.

CONTRAINDICATIONS

- Unwilling patient
- Local infection
- Bleeding disorders.

INVESTIGATIONS

- Hemogram
- *X-ray:* Hip, sacroiliac (SI) joint, lumbosacral (LS) spine
- Magnetic resonance imaging (MRI) LS spine
- Computed tomography
- Ultrasonography (USG) pelvis
- Electromyograph.

EQUIPMENT

- C-arm compatible surgical table
- C-arm with radiation safety devices
- Stimuplex set
- Nerve stimulator with needle 22G 4 inch or longer
- Marker pen, metal marker
- 26G, ½ inch and 18G, 1½ inch needle
- 2 mL, 5 mL, and 10 mL syringes.

DRUGS

- Inj. iohexol (Omnipaque)
- Inj. normal saline (0.9%)
- Inj. lidocaine (2%)
- Inj. bupivacaine or ropivacaine (0.5%), preservative-free
- Inj. Aurocort (preservative-free triamcinolone acetonide), methylprednisolone
- Inj. botulinum toxin.

PREPROCEDURE PREPARATION

- Rule out red flags such as infection, trauma, tumor, and significant neurological deficit
- Informed written consent
- Basic investigations such as bleeding time (BT), clotting time (CT), blood sugar level (BSL)
- Intravenous (IV) line with 20G cannula
- Anesthetist standby with monitoring of pulse, blood pressure (BP), oxygen saturation (SaO_2), electrocardiogram (ECG)
- Antibiotics as per institutional protocol.

PROCEDURE

Step 1

- After position of patient **(Fig. 2)**, rotate the fluoroscope to identify the corresponding hemipelvis and acetabular region. Now place a metal marker on the most inferior aspect of the SI joint and on the most superior-lateral aspect of the acetabulum. On this line, about one-third of the way medial from the acetabular landmark is the needle entry point **(Fig. 3)**.
- After painting and draping, inject 1% lignocaine; care must be taken to avoid the deeper structures to prevent loss of stimulating ability of the nerve stimulator by the local anesthetic.

Step 2 (Needle Placement)

A 4-inch Stimuplex insulated needle **(Fig. 4)** is inserted and advanced under fluoroscopic guidance. Now, stimulation output is obtained at 1.5–2.0 mA and 2 Hz frequency to

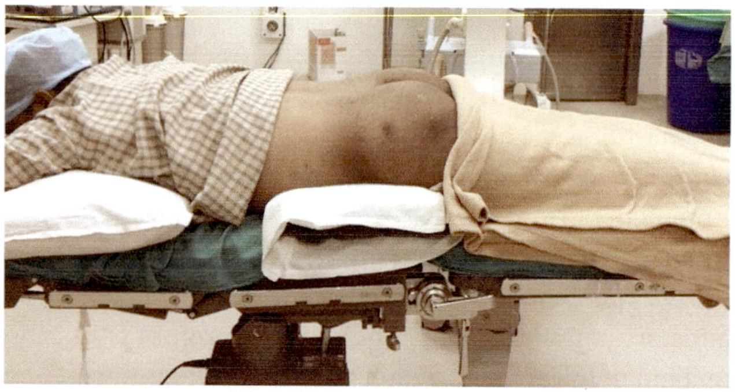

Fig. 2: Prone position with pillow under pelvis.

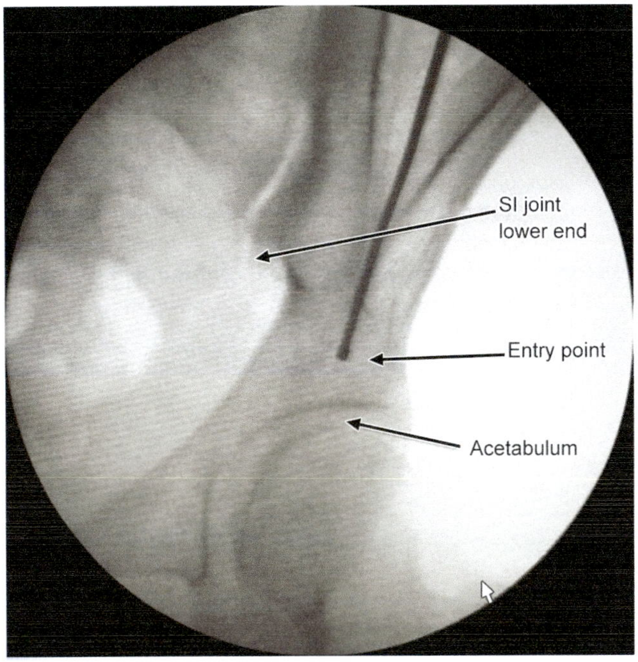

Fig. 3: Fluoroscopic anteroposterior view with landmark around piriformis muscle. (SI: sacroiliac)

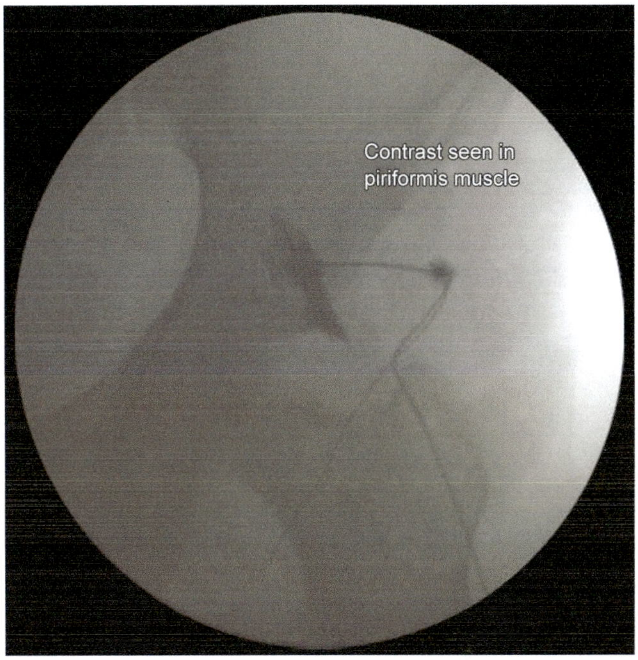

Fig. 5: Myogram of piriformis muscle.

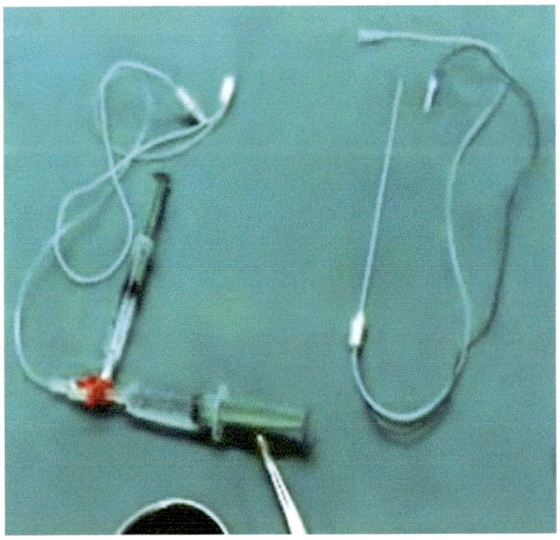

Fig. 4: 4-inch stimuplex needle.

obtain contraction of the gluteus maximus muscle. Then, the stimulator output is reduced until only a moderate gluteal twitch is observed.

Step 3

Now, advance the needle until contraction of the gluteus is markedly diminished. The output is reduced to <0.6 mA and the needle tip adjusted until there is just a discernable twitch noted at the needle hub and at the hip, which identifies the piriformis muscle **(Refer to Video No. 9)**.

Precautionary Tips

- In case the dorsal aspect of the ileum is encountered, the needle should be pulled back 1–2 mm. The output is then adjusted until a slight twitch is obtained.
- In case paresthesias or contractions of the calf or foot muscles are seen, it indicates close proximity to the sciatic nerve.
- Never inject if the patient is feeling sharp pain shooting down their leg as the needle tip may be inside the sciatic nerve. Move the needle and retry.

Step 4

Inject 1 mL of radiopaque contrast to obtain myogram of piriformis muscle **(Fig. 5)**. Contrast should flow in a diagonal pattern from cephalad to caudad as it goes toward the femoral attachment site of the piriformis muscle.

Step 5

- Now, inject 3 cc mixture of 0.25% bupivacaine with or without steroid into the piriformis muscle after negative aspiration for blood.
- In patients who are refractory to local and/or steroid medication, injection botulinum toxin 100 IU is beneficial.

COMPLICATIONS

Inadvertent direct injection of the sciatic nerve, which usually results in a nondisabling and temporary sciatic mononeuropathy.

CONCLUSION

A less common but important cause of lower extremity radicular pain may result from nerve irritation by the piriformis muscle, known as PMS. The multimodal approach includes medication and piriformis muscle injection followed by rehabilitation with physical therapy. The role of the piriformis muscle in radicular pain may be more effectively addressed with accurate diagnosis and precision injection of medication.

REFERENCES

1. Fishman LM, Dombi GW, Michaelsen C, Ringel S, Rozbruch J, Rosner B, et al. Piriformis syndrome: diagnosis, treatment, and outcome—a 10-year study. Arch Phys Med Rehabil. 2002;83(3):295-301.
2. Fishman LM, Anderson C, Rosner B. BOTOX and physical therapy in the treatment of piriformis syndrome. Am J Phys Med Rehabil. 2002;81(12):936-42.
3. Wyant GM. Chronic pain syndromes and their treatment. III. The piriformis syndrome. Cand Anaesth Soc J. 1979; 26(4):305-8.
4. Benson ER, Schutzer SF. Posttraumatic piriformis syndrome: diagnosis and results of operative treatment. J Bone Joint Surg Am. 1999;81(7):941-9.

42 CHAPTER

Popliteal Nerve Block of Sciatic Nerve

Yashwant L Nankar

ABSTRACT

The popliteal block of the sciatic nerve is a proven and safe technique used extensively to provide pain relief for distal lower extremity. This chapter describes a simple and reproducible technique for safely performing this block with the help of peripheral nerve stimulator and putting catheter for prolonged analgesia.

INTRODUCTION

The introduction of peripheral nerve stimulators,[1,2] along with ultrasound-guided,[3,4] approaches has allowed continuous block with better safety profile. Better nerve identification reduces patient discomfort and improves the blockade efficacy with a high success rate.

In comparison to proximal approaches to the sciatic nerve, the nerve block into the popliteal fossa preserves hamstring function, allowing easier ambulation of the patient.

Popliteal nerve block is mainly used for postoperative analgesia and also in treatment for a patient with severe acute or long-term pain in the lower limb.

ANATOMY

The sciatic nerve is the largest nerve supplying the lower extremity. It is formed by the union of the first three sacral spinal nerves and the fourth and fifth lumbar nerves. It leaves the pelvis through the greater sciatic foramen and runs toward the posterior aspect of the thigh between the greater trochanter and the ischial tuberosity. It separates into its terminal branches about 6 cm proximal to the popliteal crease into the tibial nerve and the common peroneal nerve. These nerves innervate the entire leg below the knee, except the anteromedial leg and foot which are innervated by the saphenous nerve (L2-L4). The tibial nerve supplies the heel and the sole of the foot. The common peroneal, also known as the common fibular nerve, innervates the lateral aspect of the leg and dorsum of the foot.

INDICATIONS

- Acute pain management in emergency department[5]
- Postoperative pain therapy at home for ambulatory surgery setting[6]
- Treatment of complex regional pain syndrome (CRPS I) patients to alleviate pain and allow intense physiotherapy[7]
- To increase blood flow after vascular accidents[8]
- Trauma patients to provide analgesia during transport to distal treatment center, especially from battlefield wounds[9]
- Cancer-related pain in lower limbs.[10]

CONTRAINDICATIONS

Absolute

- Unwilling patient
- Local infection
- Bleeding disorders
- Allergy to local anesthetics.

Relative

- Nonavailability of needle insertion site because of a splint/cast/dressing
- Systemic infection.

INVESTIGATIONS

- Hemogram

EQUIPMENT

- An insulated stimulating needle (which can be connected to a nerve stimulator)
- Nerve stimulator
- Marker pen, metal marker
- 26G, ½ inch for local infiltration
- 18G, 1½ inch needle
- 2 mL, 5 mL, and 10 mL syringes.

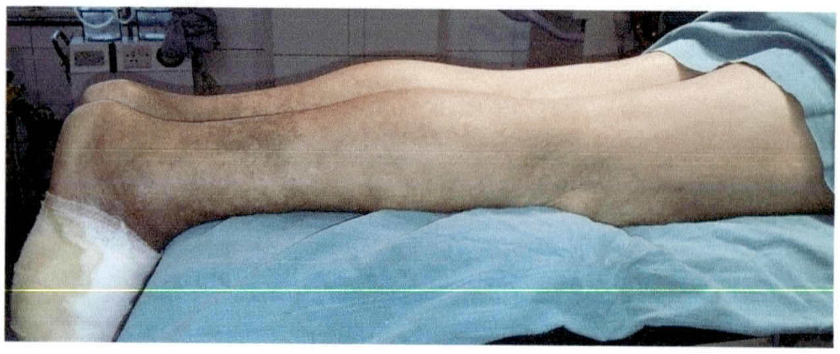

Fig. 1: Position for popliteal nerve block.

DRUGS

- Inj. lidocaine 2% (maximum dosage 300 mg plain, 500 mg with epinephrine. Duration is 1–1.5 hours plain, and 2–3 hours with epinephrine)
- Inj. bupivacaine or ropivacaine, 0.5%, preservative-free (maximum dosage 250 mg. Duration is 2–8 hours)
- Inj. normal saline (0.9%).

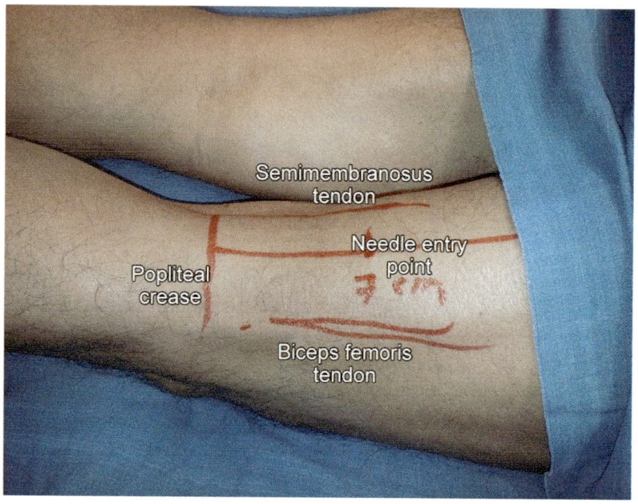

Fig. 2: Surface marking with labeling for popliteal crease.

PREPROCEDURE PREPARATION

- Rule out red flags like infection, trauma, tumor, and significant neurological deficit.
- Obtain written informed consent.
- Blood investigations such as bleeding time (BT), clotting time (CT), triple H and blood sugar.
- Secure intravenous line.
- Anesthesiologist standby with monitoring of pulse, blood pressure, oxygen saturation (SaO_2), and electrocardiogram (ECG)
- Antibiotics as per institutional protocol.

PROCEDURE (Refer to Video No. 13)

Step 1

After position **(Fig. 1)**, the three landmarks **(Fig. 2)** are identified and marked with a pen: (1) Popliteal crease, (2) tendons of biceps femoris (lateral), and (3) semitendinosus (medial).

After local anesthesia, a Stimuplex needle is inserted at an entry point that is about 7 cm superior to the popliteal crease at the midpoint between each identified tendon, which is approximately 1 cm lateral to the apex of the popliteal triangle.

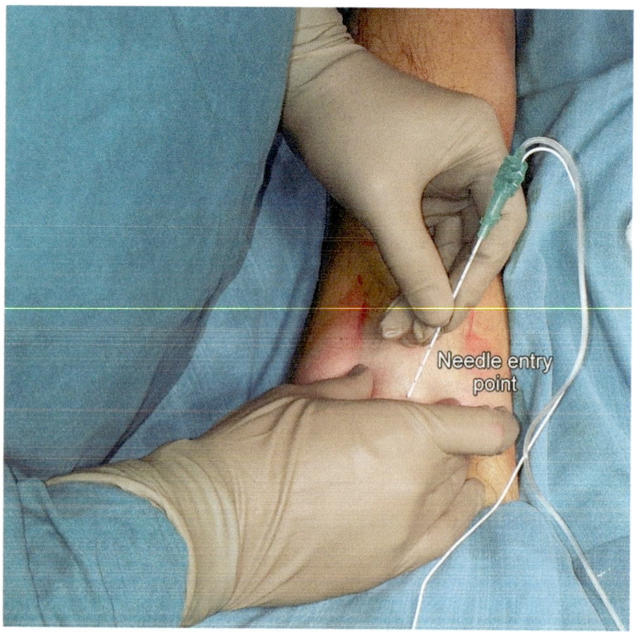

Fig. 3: Needle entry point.

Step 2: Needle Placement

- Needle is advanced at a 45°–60° angle to the skin in a cephalad direction **(Fig. 3)** for about an inch.
- Set the nerve stimulator initially between 1.0 and 1.2 mA.
- Advance anteriorly until the desired nerve is stimulated.

Step 3: Stimulation Response (Refer to Video No. 13)

- Inversion of the foot indicates stimulation of the tibial and deep peroneal nerves.
- Eversion of the foot indicates stimulation of the superficial peroneal nerve.
- Plantar flexion indicates stimulation of the posterior tibial nerve.
- Dorsiflexion indicates stimulation of the deep peroneal nerve.

When stimulation response is localized, the output current of the nerve stimulator is gradually adjusted to the lowest current at which these responses are still obtained (goal is <0.4 mA).

If stimulation is obtained at <0.2 mA, the needle should be slightly withdrawn as stimulation at such a small current intensity may indicate an intraneural placement of the needle.

Step 4: Drug Injection

After appropriate stimulation at the desired current level and aspiration of the needle to ensure nonintravascular placement, injection of 30–40 cc of local anesthetic may be injected for block.

CONTINUOUS TECHNIQUE (Refer to Video No. 13)

With the patient in the prone position, landmarks are marked. The site of puncture is between the upper muscular borders of the popliteal fossa, in the midline, at least 7 cm above the popliteal skin crease. A Contiplex needle connected to a peripheral nerve stimulator is introduced at an angle of 45° to the skin and advanced in an anterior and cephalad direction. Its position is judged adequate when output <1 mA elicits a slight motor response of the foot. The stylet of the needle is then removed and a catheter is introduced. After an aspiration test, the drug is injected, needle removed, and dressing applied to fix the catheter. Drug is injected intermittently as bolus or a continuous infusion with pump.

Few Tips

- Studies have shown that inversion of the foot leads to the best sensory and motor block and dorsiflexion of the foot is the second best.
- Occasionally, a local twitch of the biceps femoris muscle is elicited after needle insertion, indicating that needle placement is too lateral and must be redirected slightly medial.
- Conversely, if local twitching of the semitendinosus and semimembranosus muscles occurs, needle placement is too medial and must be redirected slightly more lateral.
- If no motor response is obtained with initial stimulation, subsequent attempts should be made more lateral (rather than more medial, which causes a risk of inadvertent vascular penetration).
- Vascular puncture and intravascular injection are rare with this block because the nerve is superficial to the popliteal artery and vein at this location.
- Stimulation should be attempted as cephalad as possible in the popliteal fossa, making it less likely that the sciatic nerve has divided at that point and improving block success.

COMPLICATIONS

- Increased pain in area of injection
- Infection[11]
- Hematoma.

CONCLUSION

Popliteal sciatic block is a good primary analgesic modality for the lower two-thirds of lower extremity; it is an important block to know for the pain physician. Its ability to treat and diagnose pain syndromes affecting a distal area of the lower extremity makes it a useful skill set to have.

REFERENCES

1. Singelyn FJ, Gouverneur JM, Gribomont BF. Popliteal sciatic nerve block aided by a nerve stimulator: a reliable technique for foot and ankle surgery. Reg Anesth. 1991;16(5):278-81.
2. Vloka JD, Hadzic A, Koorn R, Thys DM. Supine approach to the sciatic nerve in the popliteal fossa. Can J Anaesth. 1996;43(9):964-7.
3. McCartney CJL, Brauner I, Chan VWS. Ultrasound guidance for a lateral approach to the sciatic nerve in the popliteal fossa. Anaesthesia. 2004;59(10):1023-5.
4. Buys MJ, Arndt CD, Vagh F, Hoard A, Gerstein N. Ultrasound-guided sciatic nerve block in the popliteal fossa using a lateral approach: onset time comparing separate tibial and common peroneal nerve injections versus injecting proximal to the bifurcation. Anesth Analg. 2010;110(2):635-7.
5. Phillips WJ, Troutman G, Lerant A. Nerve stimulator-assisted sciatic nerve block for painful procedures in the ED. Am J Emerg Med. 2011;29(9):1130-5.

6. Ilfeld BM, Morey TE, Wang RD, Enneking FK. Continuous popliteal sciatic nerve block for postoperative pain control at home: a randomized, double-blinded, placebo-controlled study. Anesthesiology. 2002;97(4): 959-65.
7. Everett A, Mclean B, Plunkett A, Buckenmaier C. A unique presentation of complex regional pain syndrome type I treated with a continuous sciatic peripheral nerve block and parenteral ketamine infusion: a case report. Pain Med. 2009;10(6):1136-9.
8. Hashimoto A, Ito H, Sato Y, Fujiwara Y. Automated intermittent bolus infusion for continuous sciatic nerve block: a case report. Masui. 2011;60(7):873-5.
9. Buckenmaier CC, Rupprecht C, McKnight G, McMillan B, White RL, Gallagher RM, et al. Pain following battlefield injury and evacuation: a survey of 110 casualties from the wars in Iraq and Afghanistan. Pain Med. 2009;10(8): 1487-96.
10. Fischer HB, Peters TM, Fleming IM, Else TA. Peripheral nerve catheterization in the management of terminal cancer pain. Reg Anesth. 1996;21:482-5.
11. Maheshwari A, George JE, Esa WA, Turan A, Mounir-Soliman L. Images in anesthesiology: severe posterior thigh abscess as a complication of popliteal sciatic nerve catheter. Anesthesiology. 2013;118(4):955.

43 CHAPTER

Ilioinguinal Nerve Block

Beamy S Sharma, Arthur Atchabahian

ABSTRACT

The ilioinguinal/iliohypogastric nerve block has been used for intraoperative and postoperative pain control as well as treatment for chronic pain secondary to ilioinguinal neuralgia. This can be achieved with small volumes of an intermediate to long-acting, low-concentration local anesthetic. Steroids can be added for inflammatory pain. There are two approaches to this block—landmark technique and ultrasound guidance; however, ultrasound has demonstrated greater precision and efficacy. The block is associated with minimal side effects, but peritoneal entry and bowel perforation can be a rare, yet serious complication.

INTRODUCTION

The ilioinguinal nerve block, along with the iliohypogastric nerve block, was first described in the 1980s for postoperative pain relief for children undergoing procedures in the inguinal region. It was later applied to the adult population as well.[1] The ilioinguinal nerve block can be a supplemental peripheral nerve block for surgeries affecting the inguinal region, as well as a treatment for patients suffering from ilioinguinal neuralgia.

INDICATIONS

The ilioinguinal block is used most commonly to provide analgesia following surgery in the inguinal region, such as inguinal herniorrhaphy or orchiopexy, and even bilaterally for cesarean sections. The transversus abdominis plane block often spares the L1 distribution; therefore, the ilioinguinal nerve block is preferred for procedures in the inguinal area.[2-5] It is also preferred over the caudal block in children, because it provides the same amount of analgesia while requiring a smaller dose of local anesthetic.[6] Furthermore, it causes less urinary retention and no motor block.[7] It is usually combined with the iliohypogastric nerve block, as both nerves have an almost parallel course and cannot be selectively blocked.[8] However, it cannot be used as a sole anesthetic for hernia surgeries because of the visceral pain from surgical traction and manipulation of the spermatic cord. Spinal or general anesthesia, or infiltration by the surgeon, is needed.[9,10] The addition of this nerve block has been associated with decreased postoperative pain with less analgesic consumption, less postoperative nausea, and shorter discharge times from the postanesthesia care unit.[11-17] The addition of steroids to the injected solution also improved abdominal pain after discharge.[18]

For patients suffering from chronic groin pain, usually from nerve injury or entrapment after surgery, this block serves both a therapeutic and diagnostic purpose.[19] 10% of patients who have undergone inguinal hernia repair end up suffering from neuralgia, although this number is probably underestimated. A study looking at 49 patients who suffered from neuralgia after inguinal hernia repair showed that 81% suffered from ilioinguinal nerve damage and 23% from iliohypogastric nerve damage.[20] Local anesthetic can be injected to block the ilioinguinal nerve, and if the pain subsides, it is evidence of neuralgia of that nerve. At this point, the options for pain control are frequent nerve blocks or ablation of the nerve (neurectomy). A small study of 20 patients demonstrated 70% of patients with either refractory genitofemoral or ilioinguinal neuralgia improved with a nerve block.[21] If the pain does not subside, this indicates there is another source for the abdominal pain, either from another nerve or a different etiology altogether, such as hip disease or L1 root injury.

CONTRAINDICATIONS

The contraindications for this block are similar to other peripheral nerve blocks. They include patient refusal, infection in the area, known local anesthetic allergy, and severe coagulation abnormalities.[22] There are no specific contraindications.

ANATOMY

The ilioinguinal nerve **(Fig. 1)** provides sensation to the upper portion of the medial thigh, the root of the penis, and upper scrotum in men and the mons pubis and lateral part of labia majora in women.[22] It arises from the lumbar plexus, specifically L1 and occasionally T12, and emerges between the psoas major and quadratus lumborum, then spans around to the abdominal wall. It initially travels between the transverse abdominis and internal oblique muscles, and some variable distance after crossing the anterior-superior iliac spine (ASIS), it crosses the internal oblique to then travel between the internal and external oblique muscles **(Fig. 2)**. The longest course of the nerve is between the internal oblique and transversus abdominis muscles,[2] as it usually becomes superficial closer to the inguinal ring.

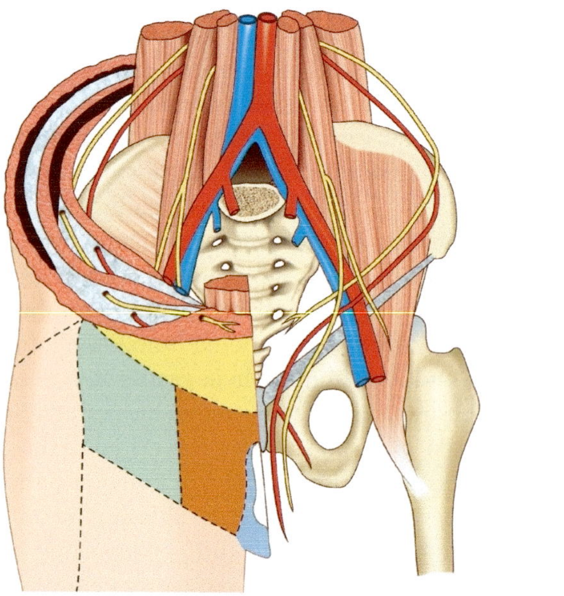

Fig. 1: Innervation of the ventral abdominal wall by iliohypogastric (yellow), ilioinguinal (orange), and genitofemoral nerves (green).[23]

The iliohypogastric nerve runs adjacent to the ilioinguinal nerve, both medial and superior.[2] It also arises from the lumbar plexus, originating from T12 and L1. The nerve divides into lateral and anterior branches after penetrating the transversus abdominis muscle. The lateral branch provides sensation to the posterior lateral

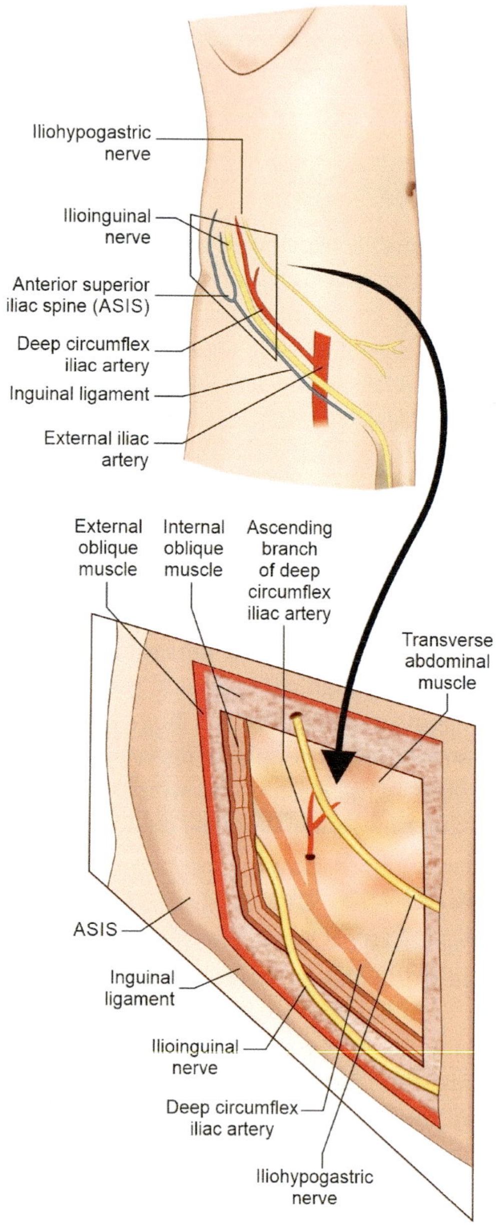

Fig. 2: Applied anatomy. The superficial muscular layer contains ilioinguinal and iliohypogastric nerves that lie between the internal and external oblique muscles. In the deep fascial layer (inset), ilioinguinal and iliohypogastric nerves lie between the internal oblique and transverse muscles at the same plane as the branch of the deep circumflex iliac artery.[24]

gluteal region and the anterior branch provides sensation to the suprapubic region.[19,22] After passing the ASIS, the iliohypogastric nerve courses between the internal oblique and external oblique muscle layers.[19] Branches of the deep circumflex iliac artery also accompany the nerves. Eventually, the nerve becomes superficial near the inguinal canal.

MEDICATIONS

The local anesthetic of choice is ideally intermediate- to long-acting with a low concentration. Frequent choices are 1% lidocaine, 1% mepivacaine, 0.25% bupivacaine, or 0.2% ropivacaine.[9] This is a low-volume block and 5–15 mL of local anesthetic solution is usually adequate. Furthermore, the surgeon will often inject additional local anesthetic near the spermatic cord for inguinal hernia repair, and this needs to be considered when deciding the amount of local anesthetic to be injected for the ilioinguinal block.[9]

Methylprednisolone can be injected with the local anesthetic for patients with an inflammatory component to their chronic groin pain. Generally, 80 mg is given as the initial dose, followed by daily doses of 40 mg.[22] The addition of steroids has also been shown to prolong the analgesic effects of the block.[18,25] There are also reports of adding clonidine to the solution in both surgical and chronic pain patients, but while some studies have shown that it can significantly prolong the blockade, others failed to show a significant difference in block duration.[26-29]

PREPARATION

The patient is placed in the supine position. The ASIS and umbilicus should be identified and marked. The area is prepped in a sterile manner. The local anesthetic of choice is drawn up and a 20–22 g, 5 cm short-bevel needle is available.

LANDMARK TECHNIQUE

There are two possible approaches for the landmark technique:[19]

1. In one approach, the needle is inserted at 2–3 cm medial and 2–3 cm inferior to the ASIS, pointing in medial and inferior directions, toward the pubic symphysis. The needle is entered perpendicular to the skin, resistance is felt as the needle crosses the external oblique muscle, followed by a popping sensation as it pierces the underlying fascia. 2 mL of local anesthetic solution is injected. The needle is further advanced so that it then pierces the internal oblique and an additional 2 mL of solution is injected. The needle is retracted to the skin and angled 45° medial. Again, the needle should pass the external oblique and fascia where 2 mL of solution is injected, and then pass the internal oblique and fascia where another 2 mL is injected. This is repeated once more after the needle is retracted to the skin, but this time it is angled 45° lateral. The planes between both the external and internal obliques and internal oblique and transversus abdominis are infiltrated, because the level at which the ilioinguinal nerve crosses the internal oblique muscle and becomes more superficial is variable.[10,30]
2. In the other method, a line is drawn between the ASIS and the umbilicus **(Fig. 3)**. The needle is inserted 3 cm from the ASIS along that line (~2 cm medial and 2 cm superior) from ASIS. The injection of local anesthetic is the same as described above with the double plane injections. No difference has been shown between the two different landmark approaches.[31,32]

ULTRASOUND GUIDANCE

Studies comparing the landmark technique and the ultrasound technique showed greater satisfaction with pain control and earlier ambulation and discharge in patients receiving the block using ultrasound guidance.[33,34] Using

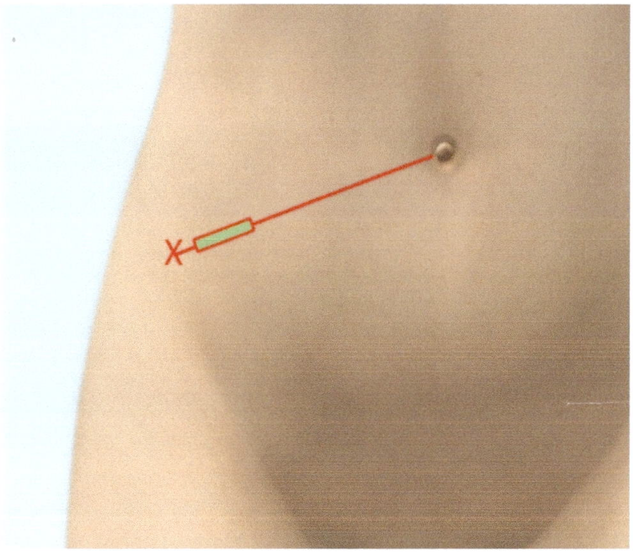

Fig. 3: Landmark for block performance. X marks the anterior-superior iliac spine (ASIS). A line is drawn from the ASIS to the umbilicus. The green rectangle marks the typical position of the ultrasound probe.

ultrasound imaging, Weintraud et al. also demonstrated in pediatric patients that with the landmark approach, only 14% of the injections delivered local anesthetic in the intended location.[35] The variable anatomy limits the efficacy of the landmark approach.[30,36] Furthermore, this approach allows for smaller volumes of local anesthetic to be injected.[34,37,38] Additionally, a study focusing on the pharmacokinetics indicated that the use of ultrasound led to a higher maximum plasma concentration of local anesthetic and faster absorption; therefore, a lower volume of local anesthetic should be used with the ultrasound technique.[39]

With this approach, the patient is again in the supine position. The ASIS is identified. The ultrasound probe is placed 2 cm medial and 2 cm superior to the ASIS, along the line running between ASIS and umbilicus **(Fig. 3)**. The three muscle's layers should be identified: (1) External oblique, (2) internal oblique, and (3) transversus abdominis **(Fig. 4)**. Of the three layers, the internal oblique tends to be the thickest and the transversus abdominis is usually very thin.[40] The muscles are hypoechoic, contrasting with the hyperechoic fascial layers.[41] Care should be taken to locate the muscles starting from the peritoneum toward the surface, as especially in obese patients, the subcutaneous fat can be interspersed with linear images that could be mistaken for fascial planes between muscles. A needle is inserted entering from the lateral or medial side, using an in-plane approach, although an out-of-plane approach is possible as well. The nerves are hypoechoic compared to the surrounding hyperechoic subcutaneous tissue and can be located between either of muscle layers. They are small and sometimes difficult to identify. The location of the nerves may also be identified using the deep circumflex artery that runs alongside them, using color Doppler.[2] If the nerves are not seen, both fascial planes (between external and internal oblique, and between internal oblique and transversus abdominis) should be infiltrated. Typically, 5 mL of local anesthetic is injected to surround the nerves **(Fig. 5)**, taking care not to injure the artery. For chronic pain treatment, steroids can also be injected, as discussed earlier.

COMPLICATIONS

There are few complications associated with this peripheral nerve block. Hematoma formation is the most significant complication. This is more likely to occur if the area is injected more than once. While this is unlikely to put the patient in increased harm, it can make the surgical procedure more difficult.[9] Other complications include local infection, intravascular injection, and inadvertent nerve block, usually the femoral nerve or lateral cutaneous femoral nerve.[19]

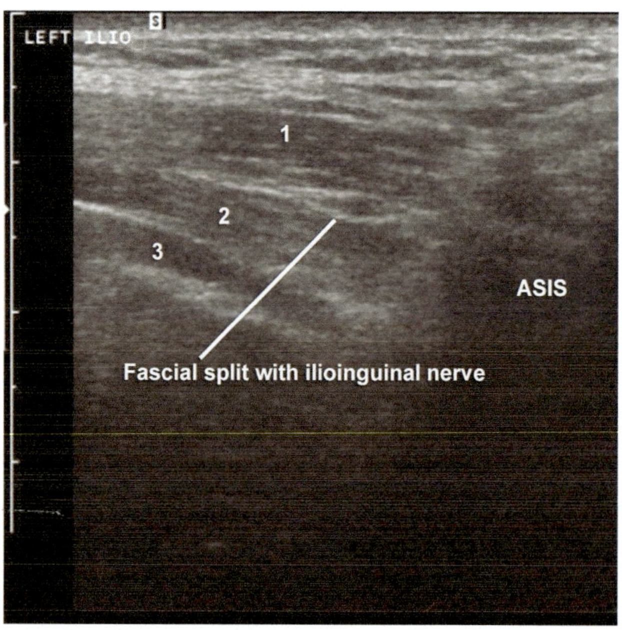

Fig. 4: Ultrasound view of the area of block performance, with the probe straddling the anterior-superior iliac spine (ASIS). Fascial split containing the ilioinguinal nerve indicates: (1) Exterior oblique muscle, (2) interior oblique muscle, and (3) transverse muscle.[24]

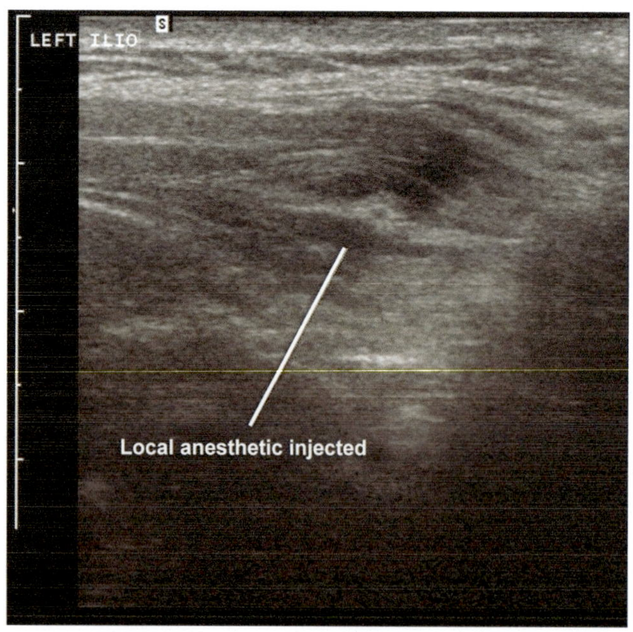

Fig. 5: Site of injection of local anesthetic. The anesthetic solution encircles the ilioinguinal nerve, which is clearly visualized as a hypoechoic structure.[24]

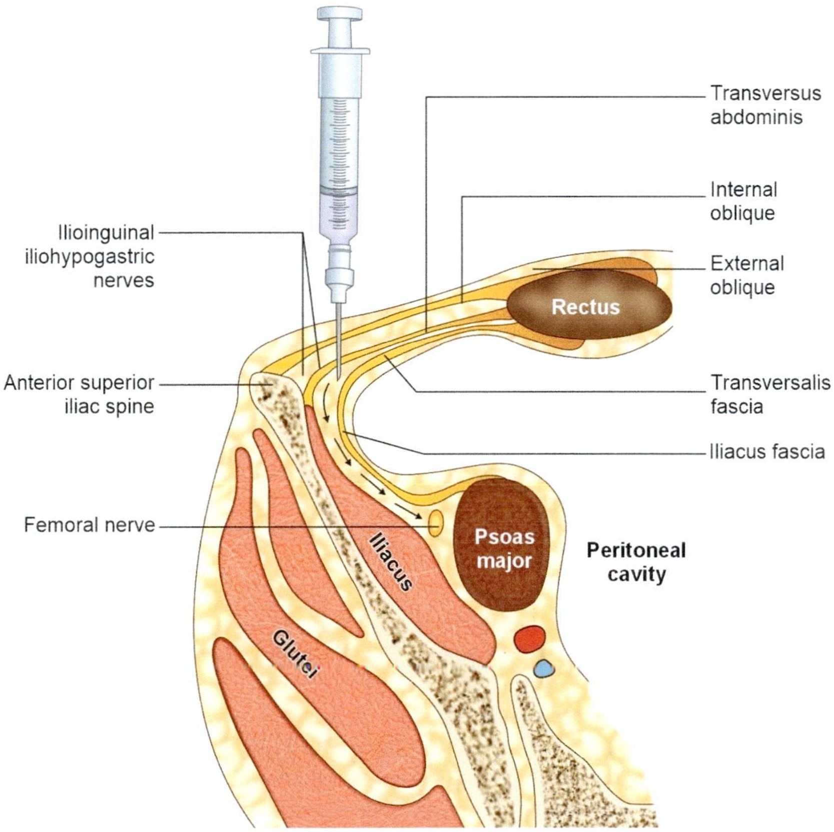

Fig. 6: Cross-sectional diagram of the pelvis at the level of the anterior superior iliac spine (ASIS) demonstrating reflection of the transversalis fascia as the iliacus fascia and the femoral nerve lying in the natural gutter lateral to the psoas.[43]

The femoral nerve can be affected by diffusion of local anesthetic medially under the fascia iliaca, which is continuous to the transversalis fascia and where the femoral nerve lies **(Fig. 6)**. This is more likely to occur if local anesthetic is injected deep to the internal oblique muscles.[42,43] Patients should be assessed for quadriceps weakness before being allowed to ambulate to prevent falls.

A rarer yet serious complication is peritoneal entry and perforation of the colon or small intestine, as the transversus abdominis is a thin muscle.[2] There are few case reports of bowel injury, either hematoma or perforation, all involving children, suggesting that the pediatric population is at increased risk for this complication.[44-46]

CONCLUSION

The ilioinguinal and iliohypogastric nerve blocks provide effective analgesia, both in the perioperative setting and for chronic pain patients. The use of ultrasound has led to greater block success and should be the standard of care.

REFERENCES

1. Bhalla T, Sawardekar A, Dewhirst E, Jagannathan N, Tobias JD. Ultrasound-guided trunk and core blocks in infants and children. J Anesth. 2013;27(1):109-23.
2. Gray A (Ed). Atlas of Ultrasound-Guided Regional Anesthesia, 1st edition. Philadelphia, PA, USA: Elsevier-Saunders; 2013.
3. Børglum J, Jensen K, Christensen AF, Hoegberg LC, Johansen SS, Lönnqvist PA, et al. Distribution patterns, dermatomal anesthesia, and ropivacaine serum concentrations after bilateral dual transversus abdominis plane block. Reg Anesth Pain Med. 2012;37(3):294-301.
4. Tran TM, Ivanusic JJ, Hebbard P, Barrington MJ. Determination of spread of injectate after ultrasound-guided transversus abdominis plane block: a cadaveric study. Br J Anaesth. 2009;102(1):123-7.
5. Fredrickson MJ, Paine C, Hamill J. Improved analgesia with the ilioinguinal block compared to the transversus abdominis plane block after pediatric inguinal surgery: a prospective randomized trial. Paediatr Anaesth. 2010;20(11):1022-7.
6. Abdellatif AA. Ultrasound-guided ilioinguinal/iliohypogastric nerve blocks versus caudal block for postoperative analgesia in children undergoing unilateral groin surgery. Saudi J Anaesth. 2012;6(4):367-72.

7. Caetano AM, Falbo GH, Lima LC. Comparison among three techniques of postoperative regional analgesia with ropivacaine in children. Rev Bras Anestesiol. 2006;56(6):561-70.
8. Schmutz M, Schumacher PM, Luyet C, Curatolo M, Eichenberger U. Ilioinguinal and iliohypogastric nerves cannot be selectively blocked by using ultrasound guidance: a volunteer study. Br J Anaesth. 2013;111(2):264-70.
9. Brown D. Atlas of Regional Anesthesia, 1st edition. Philadelphia, PA, USA: Saunders-Elsevier; 2010.
10. Kaye AU, Vadivelu N. Essentials of Regional Anesthesia, 1st edition. New York, NY, USA: Springer; 2012.
11. Gürkan I, Utebey G, Özlü O. Comparison of ilioinguinal-iliohypogastric nerve block versus spinal anesthesia techniques for single sided inguinal herniorrhaphy. Agri. 2013;25(3):108-14.
12. Bærentzen F, Maschmann C, Jensen K, Belhage B, Hensler M, Børglum J. Ultrasound-guided nerve block for inguinal hernia repair: a randomized, controlled, double-blind study. Reg Anesth Pain Med. 2012;37(5):502-7.
13. Wolfson A, Lee AJ, Wong RP, Arheart KL, Penning DH. Bilateral multi-injection iliohypogastric-ilioinguinal nerve block in conjunction with neuraxial morphine is superior to neuraxial morphine alone for postcesarean analgesia. J Clin Anesth. 2012;24(4):298-303.
14. de Castro Santos G, Braga GM, Queiroz FL, Navarro TP, Gomez RS. Assessment of postoperative pain and hospital discharge after inguinal and iliohypogastric nerve block for inguinal hernia repair under spinal anesthesia: a prospective study. Rev Assoc Med Bras (1992). 2011;57(5):545-9.
15. Shoeibi G, Babakhani B, Mohammadi SS. The efficacy of ilioinguinal-iliohypogastric and intercostal nerve co-blockade for postoperative pain relief in kidney recipients. Anesth Analg. 2009;108(1):330-3.
16. Oriola F, Toque Y, Mary A, Gagneur O, Beloucif S, Dupont H. Bilateral ilioinguinal nerve block decreases morphine consumption in female patients undergoing nonlaparoscopic gynecologic surgery. Anesth Analg. 2007;104(3):731-4.
17. Yazigi A, Jabbour K, Jebara SM, Haddad F, Antakly MC. Bilateral ilioinguinal nerve block for ambulatory varicocele surgery. Ann Fr Anesth Reanim. 2002;21(9):710-2.
18. Feng LJ. Painless abdominoplasty: the efficacy of combined intercostal and pararectus blocks in reducing postoperative pain and recovery time. Plast Reconstr Surg. 2010;126(5):1723-32.
19. Benzon H. Essentials of Pain Medicine, 1st edition. St Louis, Mo, USA: Elsevier-Saunders; 2011.
20. Vuilleumier H, Hübner M, Demartines N. Neuropathy after herniorrhaphy: indication for surgical treatment and outcome. World J Surg. 2009;33(4):841-5.
21. Acar F, Ozdemir M, Bayrakli F, Cirak B, Coskun E, Burchiel K. Management of medically intractable genitofemoral and ilioingunal neuralgia. Turk Neurosurg. 2013;23(6):753-7.
22. Waldman S. Atlas of Interventional Pain Management, 1st edition. Philadelphia, PA, USA: Saunders-Elsevier; 2009.
23. van Ramshorst GH, Kleinrensink GJ, Hermans JJ, Terkivatan T, Lange JF. Abdominal wall paresis as a complication of laparoscopic surgery. Hernia. 2009;13(5):539-43.
24. Gofeld M, Christakis M. Sonographically guided ilioinguinal nerve block. J Ultrasound Med. 2006;25(12):1571-5.
25. Movafegh A, Razazian M, Hajimaohamadi F, Meysamie A. Dexamethasone added to lidocaine prolongs axillary brachial plexus blockade. Anesth Analg. 2006;102(1):263-7.
26. Maaliki H, Naja Z, Zeidan A. Repeated ilioinguinal block using a catheter technique for pain relief in inguinal neuralgia. Pain Pract. 2008;8(2):144-6.
27. Pöpping DM, Elia N, Marret E, Wenk M, Tramer MR. Clonidine as an adjuvant to local anesthetics for peripheral nerve and plexus blocks: a meta-analysis of randomized trials. Anesthesiology. 2009;111(2):406-15.
28. Kaabachi O, Zerelli Z, Methamem M, Abdelaziz AB, Moncer K, Toumi M. Clonidine administered as adjuvant for bupivacaine in ilioinguinal-iliohypogastric nerve block does not prolong postoperative analgesia. Paediatr Anaesth. 2005;15(7):586-90.
29. Beaussier M, Weickmans H, Abdelhalim Z, Lienhart A. Inguinal herniorrhaphy under monitored anesthesia care with ilioinguinal-iliohypogastric block: the impact of adding clonidine to ropivacaine. Anesth Analg. 2005;101(6):1659-62.
30. Klaassen Z, Marshall E, Tubbs RS, Louis RG Jr, Wartmann CT, Loukas M. Anatomy of the ilioinguinal and iliohypogastric nerves with observations of their spinal nerve contributions. Clin Anat. 2011;24(4):454-61.
31. Seyedhejazi M, Daemi OR, Taheri R, Ghojazadeh M. Success rate of two different methods of ilioinguinal-iliohypogastric nerve block in children inguinal surgery. Afr J Paediatr Surg. 2013;10(3):255-8.
32. Kundra P, Sivashanmugam T, Ravishankar M. Effect of needle insertion site on ilioinguinal-iliohypogastric nerve block in children. Acta Anaesthesiol Scand. 2006;50(5):622-6.
33. Demirci A, Efe EM, Türker G, Gurbet A, Kaya FN, Anil A, et al. Iliohypogastric/ilioinguinal nerve block in inguinal hernia repair for postoperative pain management: comparison of the anatomical landmark and ultrasound guided techniques. Rev Bras Anestesiol. 2014;64(5):350-6.
34. Willschke H, Marhofer P, Bösenberg A, Johnston S, Wanzel O, Cox SG, et al. Ultrasonography for ilioinguinal/iliohypogastric nerve blocks in children. Br J Anaesth. 2005;95(2):226-30.
35. Weintraud M, Marhofer P, Bösenberg A, Kapral S, Willschke H, Felfernig M, et al. Ilioinguinal/iliohypogastric blocks in children: where do we administer the local anesthetic without direct visualization? Anesth Analg. 2008;106(1):89-93.
36. Hong JY, Kim WO, Koo BN, Kim YA, Jo YY, Kil HK. The relative position of ilioinguinal and iliohypogastric nerves in different age groups of pediatric patients. Acta Anaesthesiol Scand. 2010;54(5):566-70.

37. Willschke H, Bösenberg A, Marhofer P, Johnston S, Kettner S, Eichenberger U, et al. Ultrasonographic-guided ilioinguinal/iliohypogastric nerve block in pediatric anesthesia: what is the optimal volume? Anesth Analg. 2006;102(6):1680-4.
38. Nan Y, Zhou J, Ma Q, Li T, Lian QQ, Li J. Application of ultrasound guidance for ilioinguinal or iliohypogastric nerve block in pediatric inguinal surgery. Zhonghua Yi Xue Za Zhi. 2012;92(13):873-7.
39. Weintraud M, Lundblad M, Kettner SC, Willschke H, Kapral S, Lönnqvist PA, et al. Ultrasound versus landmark-based technique for ilioinguinal-iliohypogastric nerve blockade in children: the implications on plasma levels of ropivacaine. Anesth Analg. 2009;108(5):1488-92.
40. Rankin G, Stokes M, Newham DJ. Abdominal muscle size and symmetry in normal subjects. Muscle Nerve. 2006;34(3):320-6.
41. Sviggum HP, Niesen AD, Sites BD, Dilger JA. Trunk blocks 101: transversus abdominis plane, ilioinguinal-iliohypogastric, and rectus sheath blocks. Int Anesthesiol Clin. 2012;50(1):74-92.
42. Rosario DJ, Skinner PP, Raftery AT. Transient femoral nerve palsy complicating preoperative ilioinguinal nerve blockade for inguinal herniorrhaphy. Br J Surg. 1994; 81(6):897.
43. Rosario DJ, Jacob S, Luntley J, Skinner PP, Raftery AT. Mechanism of femoral nerve palsy complicating percutaneous ilioinguinal field block. Br J Anaesth. 1997;78(3):314-6.
44. Amory C, Mariscal A, Guyot E, Chauvet P, Leon A, Poli-Merol ML. Is ilioinguinal/iliohypogastric nerve block always totally safe in children? Paediatr Anaesth. 2003;13(2): 164-6.
45. Frigon C, Mai R, Valois-Gomez T, Desparmet J. Bowel hematoma following an iliohypogastric-ilioinguinal nerve block. Paediatr Anaesth. 2006;16(9):993-6.
46. Jöhr M, Sossai R. Colonic puncture during ilioinguinal nerve block in a child. Anesth Analg. 1999;88(5):1051-2.

44 CHAPTER

Genicular Nerve Block and Motor-Sparing Neural Ablation Techniques for Persistent Knee Pain

Annie Wong, Prit Anand Singh

ABSTRACT

Symptomatic osteoarthritis of the knee is present in 20–30% of the elderly population aged >65 years, and its prevalence is increasing. In some cases when conservative treatment with medications/physiotherapy is not helpful and knee replacement is not considered appropriate, diagnostic genicular nerve block followed by radiofrequency (RF) procedure or chemical neurolysis to the nerve supply of the knee joint can be considered. Four key target sites are identified—superolateral, superomedial, inferomedial, and inferolateral genicular nerves. If the diagnostic genicular nerve block provides good short-term pain relief of >50%, RF procedure, chemical neurolysis, or cryoablation can be considered in appropriately selected patients.

INTRODUCTION

Osteoarthritis (OA) of the knee joint is a very common disease of advanced age, with an overall global prevalence ranging from 14% to 18%. In addition to pain, OA of knee can reduce mobility and cause psychosocial problems. Symptomatic OA of the knee is present in 20–30% of the elderly population aged >65 years and its prevalence is increasing. Excess body weight, injury to the knee joint, metabolic bone disease, and occupation involving excessive lifting are some of the factors that can contribute to OA of the knee.[1]

Failure of chondrocytes to maintain homeostasis between the synthesis and degradation of the extracellular matrix is believed to be the cause of OA knee.

Chronic knee pain can develop because of disuse/overuse, injuries of the knee joint, due to neurological conditions (e.g., multiple sclerosis), patients who have had total knee surgeries (TKR), etc. Pain and disabilities are the major consequences of OA knees, with 25% of patients suffering from severe arthralgia.

Patients with knee pain are initially treated with conservative measures such as analgesics following the World Health Organization (WHO) analgesic ladder [paracetamol, nonsteroidal anti-inflammatory drugs (NSAIDs), COX-2 inhibitors, opioids], adjuvant drugs, physiotherapy, rehabilitation, transcutaneous electrical nerve stimulation (TENS) machine, and even local application of capsaicin/NSAIDs cream among other modalities. Other integrative pain therapies including acupuncture/acupressure/ultrasound/laser therapies may also be used for the management of pain, with low or no evidence of benefit from literature. Intra-articular local anesthetic with steroid and hyaluronic acid/platelet-rich plasma injections into the knee joint have been used as well with some benefits.

In some cases when conservative treatment is not helpful and knee replacement is not considered appropriate, diagnostic genicular nerve block followed by motor-sparing radiofrequency (RF) ablation, chemical neurolysis can be considered.

NEUROANATOMY

The knee joint is innervated by the articular branches of various nerves, including the femoral, common peroneal, saphenous, tibial, and obturator nerves. The cutaneous and articular sensory innervation of the knee region is complex and displays considerable variation.[2]

To elucidate knee innervation, it is convenient to divide it into anterior and posterior compartments, further subdividing the anterior compartment into four quadrants. The genicular nerves—superolateral genicular nerves (SLGN), superomedial genicular nerves (SMGN), inferolateral genicular nerve (ILGN), and inferomedial genicular nerves (IMGN)—are primarily responsible for innervating each respective quadrant anteriorly. Additionally, various cadaveric studies suggest contributions from supplementary branches including the recurrent peroneal nerve, nerves to the vastus medialis, intermediate, lateralis, and the infrapatellar branch.[2]

- *SLGN:* Courses around the femur shaft amid the vastus lateralis and the lateral epicondyle, aligned with the accompanying genicular artery.
- *SMGN:* Follows the trajectory of the superomedial genicular artery around the femur shaft, passing between the adductor magnus tendon and the medial epicondyle subjacent to the vastus medialis.
- *ILGN:* Tracks around the tibial lateral epicondyle beneath the lateral collateral ligament, in concordance with the accompanying genicular artery just superior to the fibular head.
- *IMGN:* Travels horizontally beneath the medial collateral ligament amid the tibial medial epicondyle and the collateral ligament insertion, accompanying the genicular artery.

Recurrent peroneal nerve: Originates from the common peroneal nerve in the inferior popliteal region, circumferentially navigates around the fibula before passing just inferior to the fibula head and ascending superiorly to the anterolateral tibial epicondyle, alongside the recurrent tibial artery.

The nerves do not follow a fixed vascular supply to the anterior knee joint although a very small artery and vein are intimately associated with each nerve.

The posterior compartment is supplied by branches of sciatic nerve and not usually ablated for knee pain; however, some practitioners have used pulsed RF denervation.

DIAGNOSTIC GENICULAR NERVE BLOCK

Indications

The following are the conditions where diagnostic genicular nerve block is indicated:

- Chronic knee pain due to arthritis
- Postoperative knee pain, uncontrolled by systemic analgesia/supplemental analgesic trial
- Patients for conservative management of knee pain.

Contraindications

The following are the contraindications for diagnostic genicular nerve block:

- Active infection—local or systemic
- Full anticoagulation
- Patient refusal
- Allergy to local anesthetics.

Equipment

- *Ultrasound machine:* Linear high-frequency transducer (may need curvilinear probe)
- 22G, short-bevel needle or hypodermic needle
- Local anesthetic/steroid (if used as a single shot diagnostic/therapeutic injection to prolong analgesia)
- X-ray C-arm (operator dependent)
- Facility with monitoring/resuscitation equipment.

Procedure

The procedure can be performed in clinic/operating theater area. Patient can be either in a supine or sitting-up position with ipsilateral knee flexed slightly. Procedure is performed under strict aseptic technique with an intravenous (IV) access and ASA-stipulated minimum monitoring for patient safety.

Up to four target sites are identified; however, the procedure should only be done on the site of pain after history and thorough clinical examination.

- Superolateral genicular nerve, where the lateral femoral shaft meets the epicondyle
- Superomedial genicular nerve, where the medial femoral shaft meets the epicondyle
- Inferomedial genicular nerve, where the medial tibial shaft meets the epicondyle
- Inferolateral geniculate nerve, above the fibular head, under the lateral collateral ligament.

This procedure is commonly performed using ultrasonography, either a cart-based or a portable machine. The skin and soft tissues can be anesthetized with 1% lidocaine. At each target, needle is advanced next to the vessel (if seen) or till bony contact is felt using either an in-plane or out-of-plane approach. After confirming the correct position, 2–4 mL of local anesthetic is injected. The ILGN is usually target for single-shot block, but RF ablation is not carried out, as it may be too superficial/issues with involvement of the superficial peroneal nerve.

SLGN: Position the transducer in a coronal plane over the lateral epicondyle of the femur, then move it proximally to

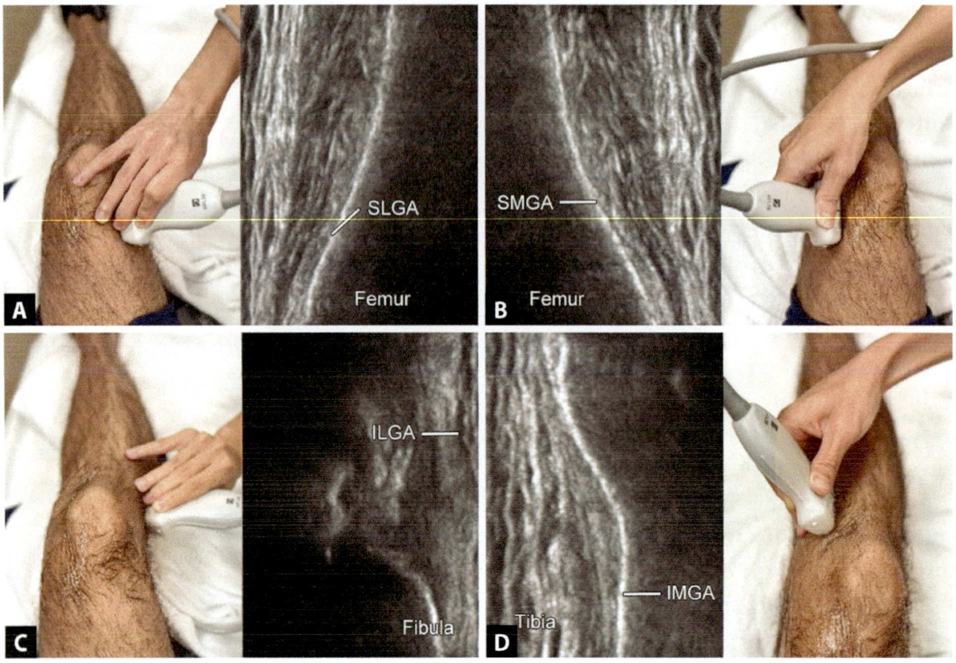

Figs. 1A to D: Sonoanatomy of the genicular nerves in a coronal plane. (A) Superolateral genicular artery (SLGA) with transducer position and sonoanatomy of the superomedial genicular nerve; (B) Superomedial genicular artery (SMGA) with transducer position and sonoanatomy of the inferomedial genicular nerve; (C) Inferolateral genicular artery (ILGA) with transducer position and sonoanatomy of the superolateral genicular nerve; (D) Inferomedial genicular artery (IMGA) with transducer position and sonoanatomy of the inferolateral genicular nerve.

visualize the metaphysis. The superolateral genicular artery can be discerned in most cases between the deep fascia of the vastus lateralis and the femur at this level **(Fig. 1A)**.

SMGN: Position the transducer in a coronal plane over the medial epicondyle of the femur, and slightly proximally to visualize the metaphysis anterior to the adductor tubercle. Here, identify the artery between the deep fascia of the vastus medialis and the femur **(Fig. 1B)**.

ILGN: Place the transducer coronally over the lateral aspect of the knee's distal end. After identifying the lateral epicondyle of the tibia, move the transducer distally to visualize the fibular head. The inferolateral genicular artery is situated between the collateral ligament and the lateral condyle of the tibia **(Fig. 1C)**.

IMGN: Place the transducer in a coronal plane over the medial condyle of the tibia and move it distally to visualize the metaphysis. At this level, observe the inferomedial genicular artery, which is seen beneath the medial collateral ligament in most cases **(Fig. 1D)**.

If ultrasound guidance is not available, it may be reasonable to do a diagnostic block using fluoroscopy imaging.

DENERVATION OF THE GENICULAR NERVE

Indications

It is indicated in case of good short-term pain relief following diagnostic genicular nerve blocks. As a rough rule, >50–75% improvement in pain scores after the diagnostic block is an indication for denervation, otherwise it is suggested to review the history and clinical examination to rule out other causes of knee pain.

Contraindications

Contraindications are similar, as for a diagnostic block.

GENICULAR NERVE RADIOFREQUENCY DENERVATION

Equipment

Cooled RF or conventional RF system with machine and needles.

Procedure

The patient should be in a comfortable supine position. The procedure is performed under strict aseptic conditions in an operating theater area. IV access, sedation/analgesia, American Society of Anesthesiologists (ASA)-stipulated minimum monitoring is needed as the denervation is a painful procedure and aim should be to avoid any nocebo response from the procedure. Operative knee is elevated slightly with the use of a foam bolster, pillow, or sandbag to obtain better lateral X-ray images. A true anteroposterior (AP) image is initially taken to identify true landmarks. A combined ultrasound and fluoroscopy (CUF) technique can be used to identify landmarks and blood vessels for the procedure, with in-plane use of ultrasound (US) for initial insertion of the RF cannula. The sites remain the same as diagnostic procedure.

The skin and soft tissues are anesthetized with 1% lidocaine. At each target, cannula is advanced using "tunnel technique" until bony contact is made, and a lateral image is obtained to confirm in two planes. At each target, fine adjustments may be needed to confirm needle tip is positioned appropriately (halfway to two-thirds across the thickness of the femur and tibia in lateral view) **(Figs. 2 to 4)**. The stylet is removed and the RF probe is inserted, to stimulate each genicular nerve branch to get sensory response at around 0.3–0.5 V (patient may report tingling, warmth, pressure-type sensation around the needle or in the area of "usual" pain) and no motor response at 2 Hz up to 1 V to make sure that there is no motor nerve in the way of the lesion. The inferior lateral genicular branch is deliberately omitted to avoid lesioning of the common peroneal/fibular nerve.

If no motor response is observed at 2 Hz, then 2 mL of local anesthetic is utilized before ablation. For cooled RF lesioning, the machine is programed at 60°C for 2.5 minutes at each site.

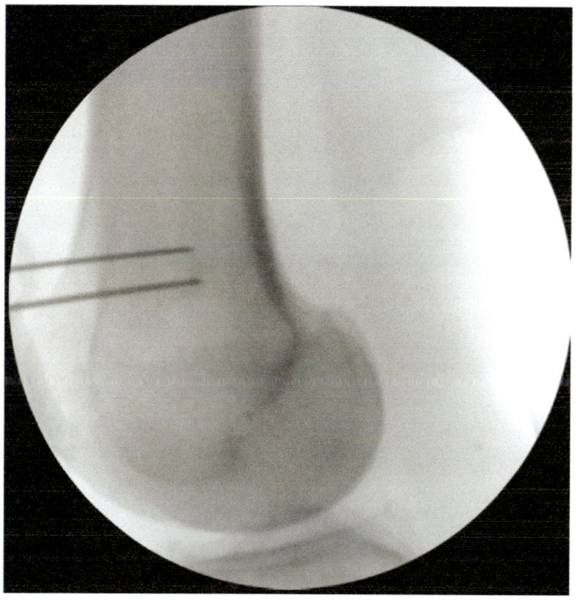

Fig. 3: Probe positioning for superior genicular radiofrequency neurotomy (superolateral and superomedial)—lateral view.

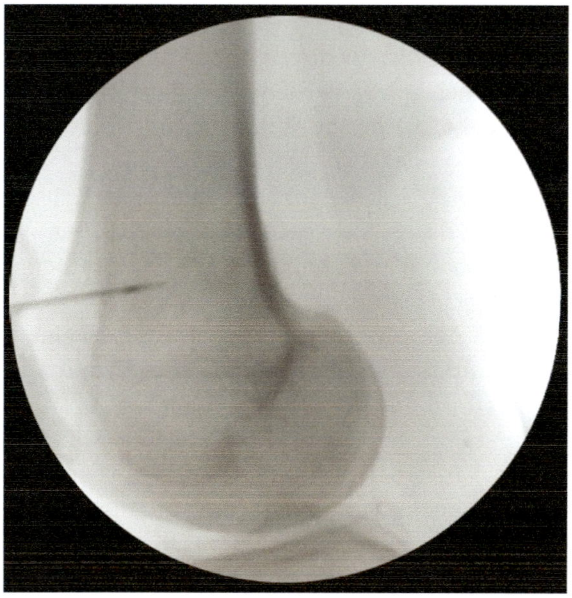

Fig. 2: Probe positioning for superior genicular radiofrequency neurotomy—lateral view.

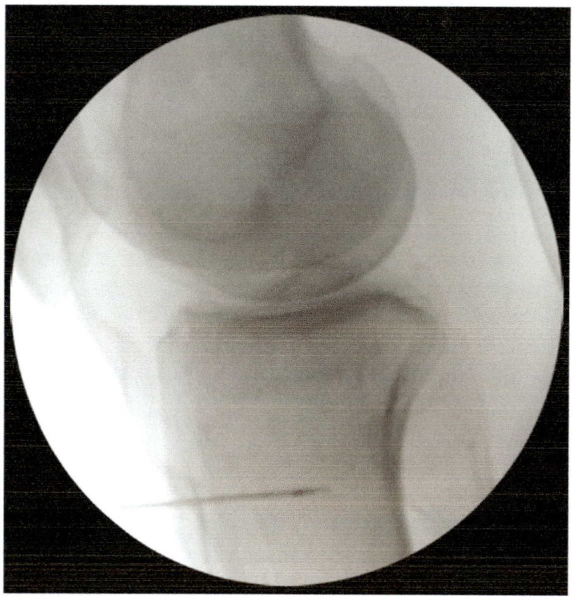

Fig. 4: Probe positioning for inferomedial genicular radiofrequency neurotomy—lateral view.

The needles are manipulated and two lesions at each site should be done, taking into account anatomical variations and the spread of small sensory nerves **(Figs. 5 and 6)**. Some operators use steroid after the procedure; however, the evidence is currently lacking to suggest the routine use to prevent neuritis.

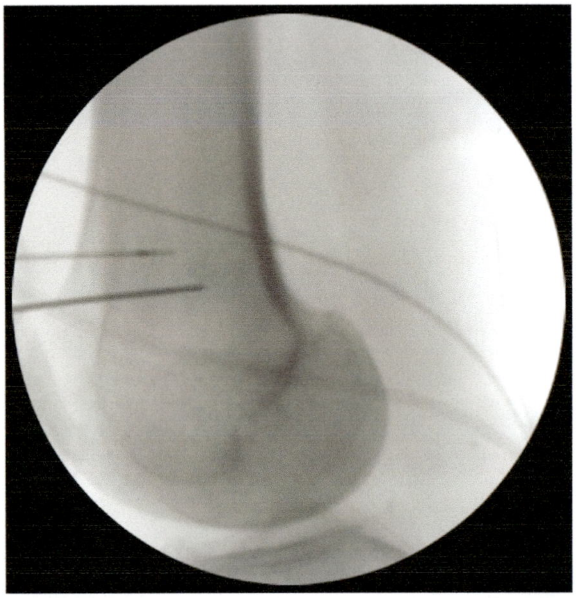

Fig. 5: One of the radiofrequency probes in Figure 3 has been withdrawn by 1 cm for another lesión.

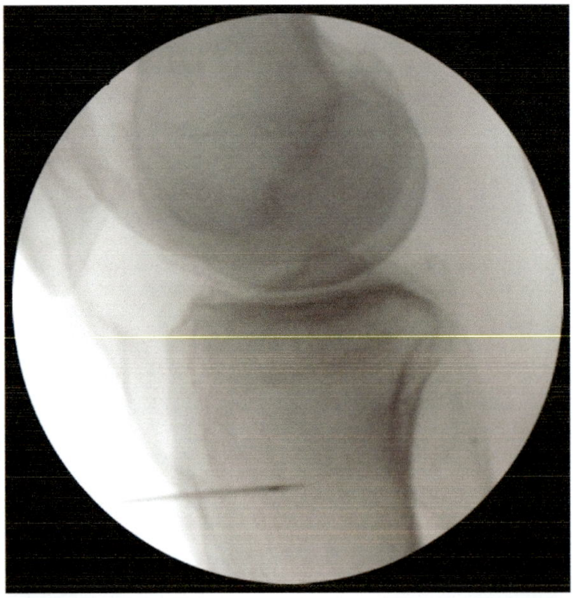

Fig. 6: Probe withdrawn by about 1 cm compared to Figure 4 to continue inferomedial genicular radiofrequency neurotomy—lateral view.

The procedure can be performed using conventional RF needle. 18G or 16G, 10/15 cm long curved tip RF needle with 10 mm active tip is used for the knees. It has to be kept in mind that the lesions with conventional RF needles with smaller gauge will have a smaller diameter c.f. Cooled RF needle of same gauge. Secondly, in extremely thin patients, the minimal tibial bone distance from skin should be 20 mm to avoid skin burns during/after the procedure.

ULTRASOUND-GUIDED CHEMICAL NEUROLYSIS (CHEMOABLATION) OF GENICULAR NERVES

The targets are SMGN, SLGN, and IMGN. This procedure is performed under real-time ultrasound guidance. A CUF-guided approach can be used as well.

Diagnostic block of the genicular nerve is preferred to confirm the source of pain. However, for patients with significant medical, social, biological, and other issues, both diagnostic block and chemical neurolysis can be performed at the same sitting.

Technique

- Patient should be in supine position with the knee slightly flexed by placing a pillow in the popliteal fossa.
- Skin prepped with antiseptic solution
- 0.5–1.0 mL of 1% lidocaine to skin as local anesthesia
- A linear ultrasound probe is usually used.
- 22G echogenic needle or a hypodermic needle is utilized depending on chemoablation agent.
- The target site for SLGN, SMGN, and IMGN remains the same as diagnostic blocks above.
- 3–5 mL of 66% alcohol or any concentration above 5% phenol is deposited to each target site.
- Patient should be monitored closely postprocedure for any adverse reactions.

Alcohol neurolysis is usually followed by chemical neuritis, and patient may complain of pain for a few days afterward and should be counseled accordingly. Some operators do use steroids alongside the solution. Some local anesthetics at the site (1–2 mL) can be used before alcohol injection to dull the pain. The relief lasts for 6–24 weeks in most patients. Repeat injections can be done in appropriate patients; however, no long-term studies for follow-ups have been noted in the literature.

ASSESSMENT

For all the procedures described above, appropriate assessment of patient's pain and function is carried out before and after the procedure to find out how much pain relief and improved function the procedure has provided to guide further management. This is documented in the patient's record. After the procedure, a repeat clinical examination is performed to reassess the range of movement, muscle strength, pain score, and presence of side effects. Patient may report numbness in area of injection covering "usual" pain. If the patient reports significant short-term reduction of pain score and improved quality of life following diagnostic procedure, consider RF in appropriately selected patients.

The WOMAC (Western Ontario McMaster Universities Osteoarthritis) score is a common tool used to assess patients with OA knee. It has three domains, namely pain, stiffness, and function, and contains a total of 24 questions. Each question is rated between 0 and 4, depending on the severity.

If the patient gets good pain relief, it is extremely important that the window of opportunity should be utilized appropriately. Patients should have already been referred to a skilled physiotherapist, so that appropriate physiotherapy can be commenced in a paced manner. This principle applies to all the procedures described in this chapter.

DISCUSSION

Chronic OA of the knee joint is one of the most common diseases of advanced age, and it is also extremely disabling. Motor-sparing ablation techniques of genicular nerves are a safe, effective, and minimally invasive therapeutic procedure for chronic knee OA patients who respond with short-term excellent pain relief following diagnostic blocks. Pericapsular denervation techniques for the major joints have opened a new chapter for pain interventions involved in management of OA knee. While regenerative injection therapy is proven to be useful in reducing and improving function in patients with OA knee, its value remains questionable with conflicting literature results.

However, one should note that recent cadaver studies demonstrated that articular innervation is far more complex than what is known. Apart from the techniques discussed earlier, there is also some evidence for the use of intra-articular pulsed RF for knee pain. The aim is to deliver an electrical field effect to the C fibers, hence modulate the pain via needle electrode positioned intra-articular in the knee joint. This is thought to have the anti-inflammatory protective effects and regenerative properties of intra-articular cartilage.

In a case series on motor-sparing neural ablation for knee pain by Ng et al.,[3] they reported drop in WOMAC score by 34–53.7% in the patients who underwent thermal RF ablation and chemical neurolysis. This group demonstrated that overall benefit of alcohol neurolysis appeared to be noninferior to the traditional denervation by the thermal RF ablation. No transient neuritis or an initial pain flare-up was detected in any of these patients.

Choi[4] compared genicular nerve RF with Sham procedure. Thirty-eight patients between 61 and 75 years of age were included in the study. Among them, 19 had RF of genicular nerve and 19 had sham treatment. Visual analog scales (VAS) and Oxford knee score (OKS) were measured at 1, 4, and 12 weeks. In the RF group, 10/17 (59%), 11/17 (65%), and 10/17 (59%) achieved at least 50% knee pain relief at 1, 4, and 12 weeks, respectively. VAS scores showed that the RF group had less knee joint pain at 4 (p <0, 0.01) and 12 (p <0,0.01) weeks compared with the control group; OKS showed similar findings (p <0.001). No adverse events occurred. Hence, it was concluded that RF neurotomy of genicular nerves led to significant pain reduction and functional improvement.

Ikeuchi[5] studied 35 patients aged between 69 and 85 years. 18 had RF and 17 had local anesthetic block. VAS and WOMAC scores were measured at 4, 8, and 12 weeks. Statistically significant pain relief (according to VAS scores) was noted for the RF group at 4, 8, and 12 weeks. No adverse events were identified.

Risso et al.[6] studied 43 patients with chronic knee pain secondary to OA. Ultrasound-guided diagnostic blocks of genicular nerves (superomedial, inferomedial, and superolateral) with 1.5 mL of 0.25% bupivacaine at each site were performed on them and those who reported >50% reduction in Numeric Rating Scale (NRS) went on to undergo chemical neurolysis, using 1.5 mL 7% glycerated phenol in each genicular nerve. NRS and WOMAC scores improved at all points up to 6 months postintervention. Rushin[7] reported two cases of patient post-chemical neurolysis who showed significant improvement in pain intensity and quality-of-life in both patients with chronic knee pain for 6 weeks. Walgea et al.[8] suggested option of image-guided injection of neurolytic agents tagged with contrast dye to achieve a more optimal target site injection under live fluoroscopy. This method accounts for the anatomic variability of genicular nerve location.

CONCLUSION

Thermal or cooled RF ablation and chemical neurolysis of genicular nerves are effective, minimally invasive techniques for management of knee pain due to various etiologies. Patients with moderate-to-severe pain and comorbidities with significant risk of perioperative management can be offered this treatment as a viable method of management. Although it remains debatable whether partial denervation would be sufficient to provide adequate pain relief, many randomized control trials and case series have shown significant improvement in disability in patients. These are safe (small risk of complications) and easy to learn and perform (following simple steps) nonsurgical techniques that should be taken into thoughtful consideration while managing patients with chronic knee pain.

REFERENCES

1. Cui A, Li H, Wang D, Zhong J, Chen Y, Lu H. Global, regional prevalence, incidence and risk factors of knee osteoarthritis in population-based studies. EClinicalMedicine. 2020; 29-30:100587.
2. Tran K, Peng PWH, Lam K, Baig E, Agur AMR, Gofeld M. Anatomical study of the innervation of anterior knee joint capsule: implication for image-guided intervention. Reg Anesth Pain Med. 2018;43:407-14.
3. Ng TKT, Lam KHS, Allam AES. Motor-sparing neural ablation with modified techniques for knee pain: case series on knee osteoarthritis and updated review of the underlying anatomy and available techniques. Hindawi, Biomed Res Int. 2022;2022:2685898.
4. Choi WJ, Hwang SJ, Song JG, Leem JG, Kang YU, Park PH, et al. Radiofrequency treatment relieves chronic knee osteoarthritis pain: a double-blind randomized controlled trial. Pain. 2011;152(3):481-7.
5. Ikeuchi M, Ushida T, Izumi M, Tani T. Percutaneous radiofrequency treatment for refractory anteromedial pain of osteoarthritic knees. Pain Med. 2011;12(4):546-51.
6. Risso RC, Ferraro LHC, Frederico TN, Peng PWH, Luzo MV, Debieux P, et al. Chemical ablation of genicular nerve with phenol for pain relief in patients with knee osteoarthritis: a prospective study. Pain Pract. 2021; 21(4):438-44.
7. Dass RM, Kim E, Kim HK, Lee JY, Lee HJ, Rhee SJ. Alcohol neurolysis of genicular nerve for chronic knee pain. Korean J Pain. 2019;32(3):223-7.
8. Walega DR, McCormick ZL. Chemical neurolysis of the genicular nerves for chronic knee pain: reviving an old dog and an old trick. Pain Med. 2018;19:1882-4.

7

SECTION

Advanced Pain Management

45 CHAPTER

Percutaneous Adhesiolysis in Chronic Low Back Pain

Laxmaiah Manchikanti, Mahendra Sanapati, Gabor B Racz

ABSTRACT

Percutaneous adhesiolysis is an interventional modality for managing chronic low back and lower extremity pain, specifically pain that is secondary to postlumbar surgery syndrome, spinal stenosis, and severe degenerative disk disease. Pain and disability in the low back and lower extremities following lumbar spine surgery have been hypothesized to be secondary to multiple causes, including epidural fibrosis. The purpose of percutaneous epidural adhesiolysis is to minimize the deleterious effects of epidural scarring. This scarring may prevent the direct application of drugs to the nerve and other spinal tissues for treating chronic low back and lower extremity pain. Percutaneous adhesiolysis was first reported by Racz et al. utilizing mechanical lysis of adhesions, epidural hypertonic saline injection, and hyaluronidase. The mechanical aspect of the lysis follows the compartmental filling idea of Angelo Rocco where the fluid from the strategically placed ventral lateral epidural catheter tip by following the path of least resistance fills up one compartment after the other. The procedure has evolved into a commonly utilized low back pain treatment in patients with chronic, intractable, recalcitrant pain after the failure of conservative modalities and epidural injections.

Over the years, significant evidence has accumulated. Based on high-quality relevant randomized controlled trials, there is level II evidence for adhesiolysis for managing postsurgery syndrome, lumbar central spinal stenosis, and chronic pain from disk herniation.

INTRODUCTION

Chronic low back pain is the most common of all chronic spinal problems, resulting in significant healthcare expenditures and disability.[1-6] Pain and disability in the low back and lower extremities following lumbar spine surgery have been hypothesized to be secondary to multiple causes, including epidural fibrosis, disk herniation, diskogenic pain, spinal stenosis, arachnoiditis, facet joint pain, and inappropriate surgery. Debate continues whether epidural fibrosis is the major cause of pain after lumbar spine surgery, with some authors arguing there is no association and others arguing there is a significant association. Postsurgery syndrome and spinal stenosis are multifactorial disorders, with variable clinical presentations.

Treating low back pain with an epidural injection was first reported soon after the turn of the 20th century[7] with epidurography first reported two decades later.[8] Intrathecal cold hypertonic saline was first used for pain in 1967.[9] Intrathecal cold saline was afterward used as a cancer pain treatment.[10] The solution's hypertonicity rather than its thermal quality accounts for its therapeutic value.[11]

Racz and colleagues[12-16] first used hypertonic saline in the epidural space for facilitating lysis of adhesions. They also tested in vitro canine dura permeability and found hypertonic saline to have slow transdural equilibration. To accelerate the onset and extent, intensity, and duration of caudal anesthesia, hyaluronidase was added.[17-19]

Over the years, multiple investigators[5,12-14,20-42] have studied the effectiveness of adhesiolysis and hypertonic saline neurolysis with or without hyaluronidase in postsurgery syndrome, spinal stenosis, and disk herniation.

APPLIED ANATOMY

- The spine comprises three compartments. They are the anterior, neuraxial, and posterior.[43]
  - The anterior compartment contains the vertebral body and the intervertebral disk **(Fig. 1)**.
  - The epidural space structures and neural pathways make up the neuraxial compartment; the posterior lamina, zygapophysial joints, and bony vertebral arch structures make up the posterior compartment **(Fig. 1)**.
- There is variation in the vertebral spinous processes' orientations along the spinal axis.
  - In the lumbar spine, the spinous processes are directly above the widest portion of the inter-laminar space. This facilitates midline and paramedian approaches **(Figs. 2A to C)**.
- The structures within the osseous and ligamentous boundaries of the spinal canal comprise the neuraxial compartment **(Fig. 1)**.
  - The epidural space is in the neuraxial compartment.
  - Fat, epidural veins, epidural arteries, and lymphatics are present in the epidural space.[44,45]
- The spinal canal extends from the foramen magnum to the sacrum. Structures surrounding the spinal canal include the ligamentum flavum and periosteum, posteriorly; the posterior longitudinal ligament that lies over the dorsal aspects of the vertebral bodies and disks, anteriorly and by pedicles and intervertebral foramen, laterally **(Fig. 3)**.[46]
  - The spinal cord ends at L1 or L2 in adults. The dural sac extends to the spinal cord and conus to the level of S2 **(Figs. 1 and 3)**.[46]
- The dural sac sits on the floor of the vertebral canal **(Fig. 3)**.
- The anterior relations of the dural sac are the backs of the vertebral bodies and the intervertebral disks. The posterior longitudinal ligament covers them.
  - The anterior spinal arteries and sinuvertebral nerves run across the base of the vertebral canal. They are located anterior to the dural sac.

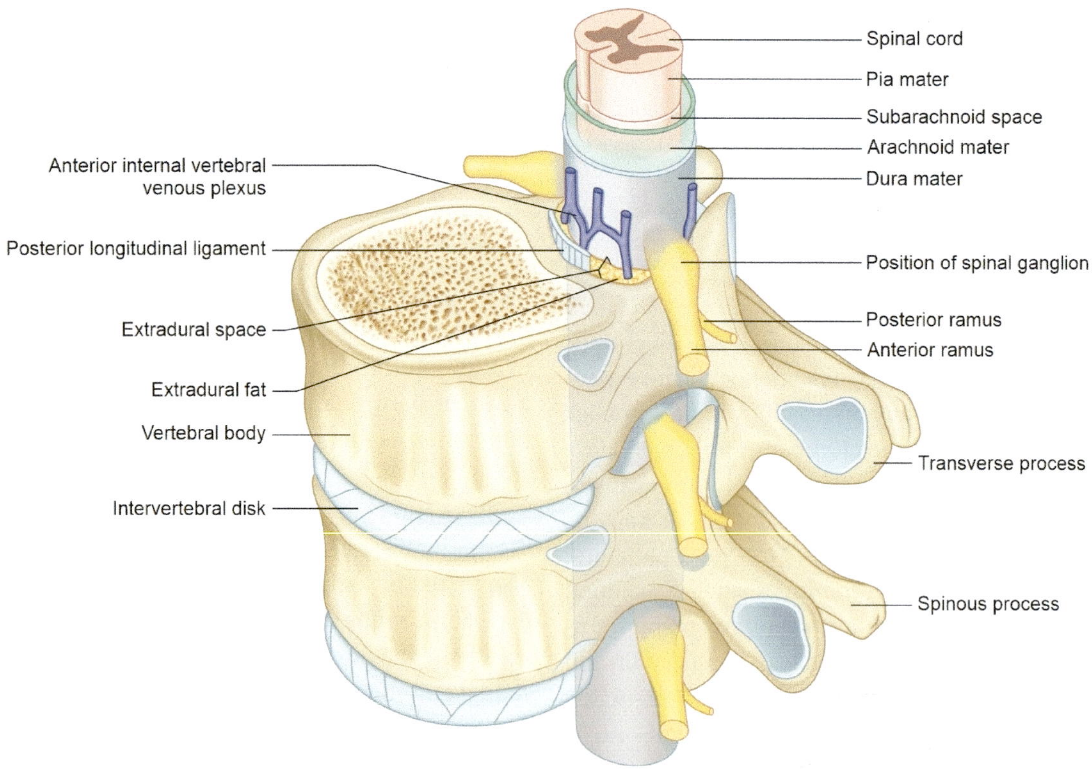

Fig. 1: Lumbar vertebral canal and its contents, showing anterior, neuraxial, and posterior compartments.
Source: Reproduced from Gray's Anatomy for Students, Drake, ©2004, with permission from Elsevier.
This is Fig. 11.6 from Manchikanti L, Schultz DM, Atluri S, Glaser SE, Falco FJE. Lumbar Epidural Injections. In: Manchikanti L, Kaye AD, Falco FJE, Hirsch JA (Eds). Essentials of Interventional Techniques in Managing Chronic Spinal Pain. New York, NY: Springer; 2018. pp. 141-86..

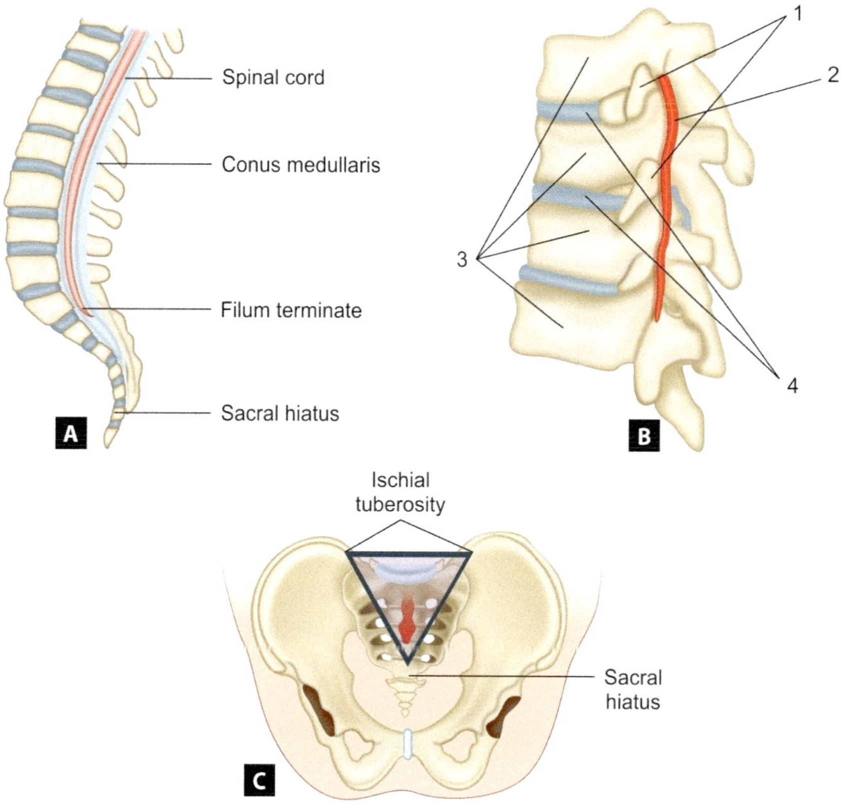

Figs. 2A to C: Anatomy of lumbosacral epidural space. (A) Median sagittal section of the lumbosacral part of the vertebral column; (B) The ligamentum flavum: (1) intervertebral foramen, (2) ligamentum flavum, (3) vertebral body, (4) intervertebral disk; (C) Identification of the sacral hiatus anatomical landmarks.

  - The dural sac posteriorly is related to the roof of the vertebral canal, the laminae, and ligamentum flava.
- The epidural space is a potential space between the dural sac and the osseoligamentous boundaries of the vertebral canal **(Fig. 3)**.
  - The epidural membrane is a thin layer of areolar connective tissue. Its structure varies from diaphanous to pseudomembranous.[46]
  - The epidural membrane surrounds the dural sac and lines the deep surface of the laminae and pedicles.
  - The epidural membrane lines the back of the vertebral body and then passes medially deep to the posterior longitudinal ligament, where it detaches to the anterior surface of the deep portion of the ligament, ventrally, opposite the vertebral bodies.
  - The posterior longitudinal ligament laterally covers the disk's back, thus preventing the epidural membrane from covering the back of the annulus fibrosus.
  - The epidural space extends from the foramen magnum to the end of the dural sac at S2. The actual size of the posterior epidural space varies greatly. It expands to 4–6 mm at its greatest width in the mid-lumbar spine and gradually decreases to about 3 mm at S1.
- The epidural space surrounds the dural sac.
  - It is bordered posteriorly by the ligamentum flavum and periosteum, and anteriorly by the posterior longitudinal ligament and vertebral bodies.
  - Laterally, it is bordered by the pedicles and intervertebral foramina.
  - The epidural space is widest in the midline underneath the junction of the lamina and narrows laterally beneath the zygapophysial joint.
  - Laterally, the ligamentum flavum joins the joint capsule of the adjacent zygapophysial joint.
  - The actual size and shape of the epidural space depends on the way the dural sac is attached to the walls of the spinal canal, as well as the spinal canal's shape at different levels.

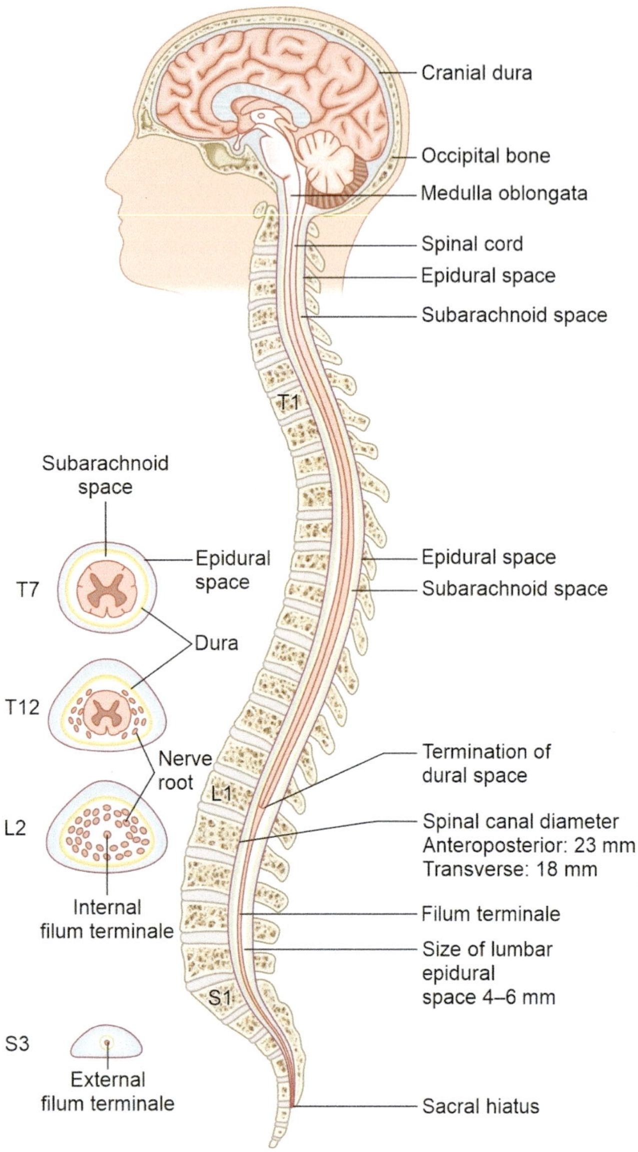

Fig. 3: Illustration of contents of the vertebral canal and epidural space.

Source: Reproduced from Gray's Anatomy, 39th ed, Standring. ©2005, with permission from Elsevier

This is Fig. 11.7 from Manchikanti L, Schultz DM, Atluri S, Glaser SE, Falco FJE. Lumbar Epidural Injections. In: Manchikanti L, Kaye AD, Falco FJE, Hirsch JA (Eds). Essentials of Interventional Techniques in Managing Chronic Spinal Pain. New York, NY: Springer; 2018. pp. 141-86.

- The lumbar epidural space has a dorsomedian connective tissue band. This dorsomedian connective tissue band (plica median dorsalis) and additional transverse connective tissue bands divide the posterior epidural space.
- However, controversy exists about whether the dorsomedian connective tissue is continuous, fenestrated, or interrupted.
- The epidural space may be compartmentalized, which can account for the limitation of injected substances.

▪ The ligamentum flavum has been proposed to be joined in the midline. There appears to be a paired nature to the ligament having both a right and left portion.
  - Cryomicrotome sectioning performed on the epidural space has shown that there is a variable degree of fusion of the ligamentum flavum in the midline.
  - The ligamentum flavum in the lumbar spine is thicker than in the cervical and thoracic spine.

▪ The sacrum is a triangular bone, dorsally convex, that consists of five fused sacral vertebrae **(Figs. 2A to C)**. It articulates cephalad with the fifth lumbar vertebra and caudad with the coccyx.[47]
  - The concave anterior surface features four parts of large anterior sacral foramina that provide passage from the midline sacral canal for the anterior rami of the upper four sacral nerves.
  - The anterior foramina are unsealed and provide a ready escape passage for solutions injected into the sacral canal.
  - The dorsal surface of the sacrum is variably convex and irregular, with important prominences representing the fused elements of the sacral vertebrae.
  - In the midline, there is a median crest with three or more, but commonly four, prominent tubercles which are variable, representing the sacral spinous processes.[43] Lateral to the crest and medial to the four posterior sacral foramina is the intermediate sacral crest, with a row of four tubercles, which represents the upper four sacral articular processes **(Figs. 2A to C)**.
  - The remnants of the S5 inferior articular processes are prominent and palpable through the skin and constitute the sacral cornua and, together with adjacent coccygeal cornua which they abut, are key landmarks for identification of the sacral hiatus and successful caudal blockade.

▪ The coccyx is a small triangular bone consisting of three to five fused rudimentary vertebrae **(Figs. 2 and 3)**.
  - The coccyx attaches to the lower part of the sacrum. The tip of the coccyx is an important landmark.

BOX 1: Indications for lysis of epidural adhesions.

- Duration of pain of 3–6 months
- Average pain levels of >5 on a scale of 0–10
- Intermittent or continuous pain causing functional disability
- Chronic low back and/or lower extremity pain which has failed to respond or poorly responded to noninterventional and nonsurgical conservative management and fluoroscopically directed epidural injections
- Chronic low back and/or lower extremity pain resulting from:
  - Postsurgery syndrome
  - Epidural fibrosis
  - Spinal stenosis
  - Radiculopathy
  - Herniated disk

- The sacral hiatus is a defect in the lower part of the posterior wall of the sacrum, formed by the failure of laminae of S5, and usually part of S4, to meet and fuse in the median plane.
  - A variable space is left which is described as an inverted *U* or *V*, covered by the thick fibrous posterior sacral coccygeal ligament.[47]
  - Direct access to the caudal canal is obtained by penetration of the sacrococcygeal ligament.
  - There is significant variation in the normal anatomy in this area, with a widely and highly variable (in sizes and shapes) the sacral hiatus. The hiatus lies higher than the lower one-third of the S4 in about 50% of specimens.[47]
  - The distance between the tip of the dural sac and the apex of the hiatus is highly variable from 20 to 45 mm.
  - Absent hiatus has been described in approximately 7% of specimens, and very small (<2 mm) anteroposterior (AP) diameter of the canal at the apex of the hiatus in 5% of specimens. However, in practice, absent hiatus is probably seen in <1% of patients.

INDICATIONS AND CONTRAINDICATIONS

Percutaneous adhesiolysis is performed to eliminate the deleterious effects of scar formation. Such scars can obstruct drugs from making their way to nerves or other tissues for treating chronic back pain with or without radiculopathy.

Indications are listed in **Box 1**. Contraindications are listed in **Box 2**.

Dural tug is an indication not only of back pain but for example thoracic pain with severe mid-thoracic on provocation. Dural tug occurs when flexion and movement of the head and neck pulls on the dura where it is adhered to the posterior longitudinal ligament. Posterior longitudinal ligament is the most richly innervated structure that will respond with pinpoint accuracy for pain upon movement of the dura **(Figs. 4 to 8)**.

BOX 2: Potential contraindications for lysis of epidural adhesions.

- Large contained or sequestered herniation
- Cauda equina syndrome
- Compressive radiculopathy
- Uncontrolled major depression or psychiatric disorders
- Arachnoiditis
- Syrinx formation
- Uncontrolled or acute medical illnesses
- Chronic severe conditions that could interfere with the interpretations of the outcome assessments for pain and bodily function
- Pregnancy and lactation
- History of adverse reaction to local anesthetic, steroids, hypertonic saline, or contrast
- Patients unable to understand the informed consent and protocol
- Patients unable to be positioned in prone position to perform the procedure
- Infection
- Anticoagulant therapy
- Non-aspirin antiplatelet therapy

The lateral recess stenosis cannot only constrict or compress nerve roots but can obstruct venous runoff, and fluid foraminotomy from ventral lateral catheter placement can open high pressure veins by allowing runoff **(Fig. 9)**.

Racz and others[15-17,20,25] described adhesiolysis of epidural scar tissue as follows: On day 1, epidurography, adhesiolysis, and injection of hyaluronidase, bupivacaine, triamcinolone diacetate, and 10% sodium chloride solution; on days 2 and 3, injections of bupivacaine and hypertonic sodium chloride solution. This 3-day protocol was modified by Manchikanti et al.[5,14-16] to a 1-day protocol.

CLINICAL EFFECTIVENESS

- Evidence is determined based on a best evidence synthesis,[48] ranging from level I to V.
  - Level I evidence is the highest level of evidence. It is obtained from multiple, relevant, high-quality randomized controlled trials (RCTs).
  - Level II evidence is obtained from at least one relevant high-quality RCT, or multiple relevant moderate or low-quality RCTs.

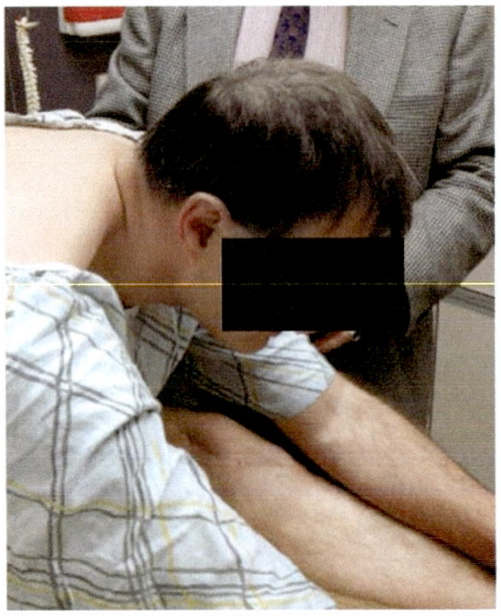

Fig. 4: The "dural tug" maneuver being performed prior to percutaneous neuroplasty.

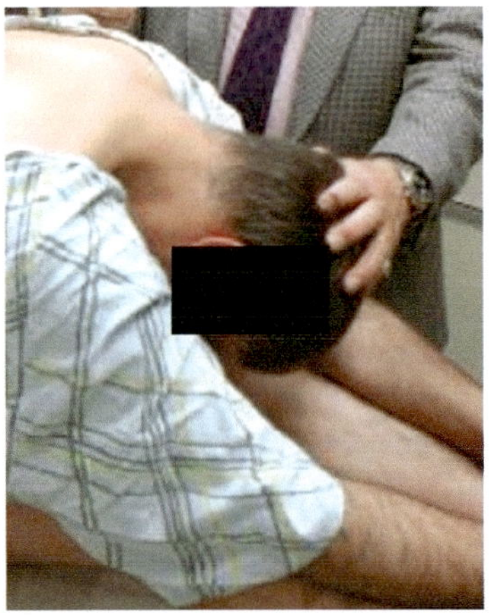

Fig. 5: Note pain reproduction prior to full neck flexion secondary to dural adhesions.

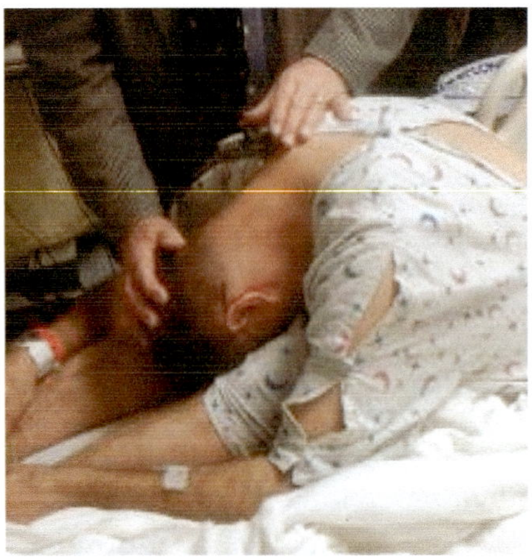

Fig. 6: Patient after percutaneous neuroplasty with pain-free neck and back flexion due to treatment of dural adhesions.

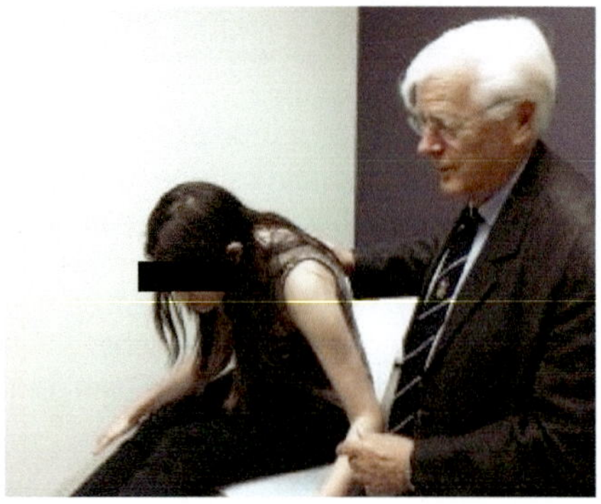

Fig. 7: There is decreased spine flexion prior to treatment secondary to dural adhesions. The pain generator was subsequently documented to be T9-T10 dural adhesion from an annular tear.

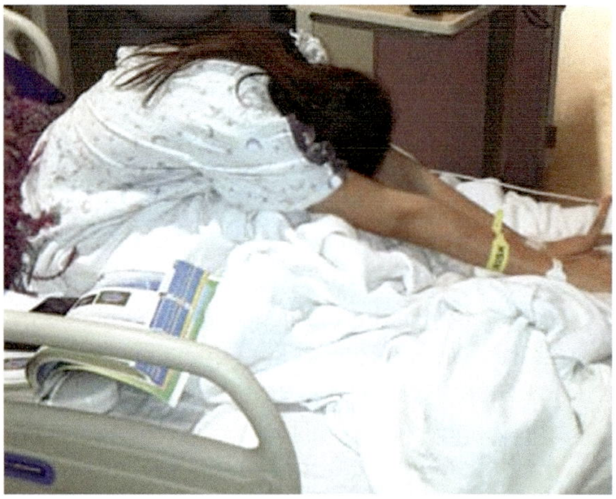

Fig. 8: After treatment, the same patient demonstrates increased painless flexion of the spine.

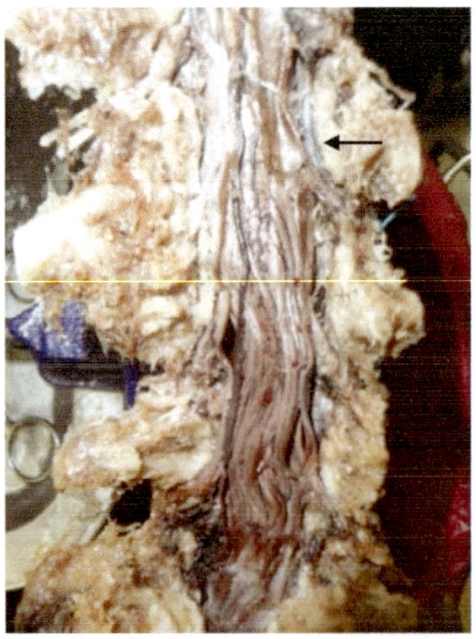

Fig. 9: Engorged blood vessels in the epidural cavity in cadaver. See vein on right side next to the nerve root target site for fluid foraminotomy and opening venous runoff and decompression.

TABLE 1: Evidence of therapeutic effectiveness of percutaneous adhesiolysis in the lumbar spine.

	Evidence	*Systematic reviews/ guidelines*	*Therapeutic studies*
Postsurgery syndrome	Level II	Manchikanti et al.[4,32,34] Helm et al.[20]	Heavner et al.[22] Manchikanti et al.[23,25] Veihelmann et al.[24] Lee and Lee[30] Chun-jing et al.[35] Akbas et al.[36]
Central spinal stenosis	Level II	Manchikanti et al.[4,33] Helm et al.[20]	Manchikanti et al.[26] Karm et al.[37] Choi et al.[38] Choi et al.[39]
Disk herniation/ radiculitis	Level II	Manchikanti et al.[4,31] Helm et al.[20]	Gerdesmeyer et al.[27,28]

  - Level III evidence incorporates not only evidence from randomized trials but also from nonrandomized trials.
  - Levels IV and V evidence is based on observational studies and consensus.
- Evidence for percutaneous adhesiolysis for postsurgery syndrome, central spinal stenosis, chronic disk herniation, or radiculitis in the lumbar spine is level II for both short-term and long-term improvement as shown in **Table 1**.
  - Evidence for percutaneous adhesiolysis for degenerative disk disease in the lumbar spine is not available.
- A cost-utility analysis performed by Manchikanti et al.[29] of 1-day percutaneous adhesiolysis for postsurgery syndrome, as well as for spinal stenosis in patients who have failed conservative management, including fluoroscopically directed epidural injections, was $3,710 per 1-year quality-adjusted life-year (QALY). First prospective, randomized, double-blind study by Heavener et al.[22] showed reduction of additional procedures.

TECHNICAL CONSIDERATIONS

The technique of lumbar adhesiolysis involves accessing the lumbar epidural space through a caudal, interlaminar, or transforaminal approach. Entry is obtained with a 16G RK needle.

Racz Technique

The technique employed by Racz and colleagues[12,22] is described as percutaneous epidural neuroplasty. It is compared to the modified technique by Manchikanti et al.[23] in **Table 2**.

Safety is determined through demonstration of lateral runoff which converts high-pressure veins through low-pressure veins. If loculation occurs, especially in the cervical spine, it is demonstrated by the development of perivenous counter spread (PVCS). Flexion and rotation of the head and neck can open up lateral runoff and release the pressure through the enlarged neural foramina **(Fig. 10)**.

General Principles

- All possible complications related to the procedure should be listed in the consent form.
- Intravenous (IV) access is strongly recommended.
  - It may be necessary to sedate the patient with midazolam and fentanyl. Although sedation is given, it is important that the patient be awake and responsive during the procedure to ensure that the spinal cord is not compressed during the injection.
- Fluoroscopy is mandatory.
- A water-soluble, nonionic contrast medium is used because of the possibility of unintended subarachnoid injection.

Caudal Approach

- The patient is placed prone with firm padding under the pelvis or abdomen in order to straighten the lumbar spine, with toes pointing inward.
- Electrocardiography sensors, a pulse oximeter, and a blood pressure cuff are applied.
- The sacral area is prepared with sterile technique and draped from the top of the iliac crest to the bottom of the buttocks.
  - The sacral cornua and the sacral hiatus are palpated with the index finger of the operator's nondominant hand.
  - The entry point through the skin, approximately 1–2 cm lateral and 2 cm inferior to the sacral hiatus, is in the gluteal fold opposite the affected side.
  - The entry point is infiltrated with a local anesthetic such as lidocaine.
  - A 16G RK needle is passed through the described entry point or 15–16G RX-2™ Coudé® needle for the caudal, lumbar, thoracic, and transforaminal is

TABLE 2: Percutaneous adhesiolysis techniques as described by Racz and colleagues and Manchikanti et al.

3-day technique (Racz and colleagues)	***1-day technique (Manchikanti et al.)***
In the operating room: • Place epidural needle • Inject iohexol (Omnipaque 240) and visualize spread of contrast medium (epidurogram) • If filling defect corresponding to area of pain is present, thread Racz Tun-L-Kath (Epimed) catheter into filling defect (scar), while injecting normal saline through the catheter; observe fluoroscopically to visualize washout of contrast medium and opening of scar • Inject additional iohexol to ascertain opening of scar and spread of injectate within the epidural space • Inject preservative-free saline (2–20 mL) with or without hyaluronidase (Hylenex) • Inject 0.25% bupivacaine or 0.2% ropivacaine plus corticosteroid (4 mg dexamethasone or 10–40 mg methylprednisolone or triamcinolone) • Tape catheter in place	*In the operating room:* • Place epidural needle • Inject Omnipaque 240 and visualize spread of contrast medium with caudal or lumbar epidurogram • After identification of the filling defect corresponding to the area of the pain, thread a Racz catheter into the filling defect • Inject additional Omnipaque 240 to ascertain opening of the scar and spread of injectate within the epidural space and nerve roots • May inject preservative-free saline, 2–20 mL • Inject 2% Xylocaine, 5 mL • Tape the catheter in place in a sterile fashion
In the postoperative care unit: • After ascertaining absence of motor blockade, inject 0.9% or 10% saline 30 minutes after steroid/local anesthetic injection	*In the recovery room:* • After ascertaining for lack of motor blockade, inject 6 mL of 10% saline in two divided doses of 3 mL each, 15–30 minutes after injection of local anesthetic
In clinic area: • Once on each of the following 2 days, inject 0.25% bupivacaine or 0.2% ropivacaine; 30 minutes later, inject 0.9% or 10% saline* • After the last treatment, remove the epidural catheter	• Inject 6 mg of Celestone Soluspan or nonparticulate Celestone, or alcohol-free 40 mg of triamcinolone • Inject 0.5–1 mL of normal saline and remove the catheter

Note: *The above daily injection has been modified to two additional local anesthetic and hypertonic saline injections 6–8 hours apart during an "observational admit" in order to reduce costs.

The injection of hypertonic saline should not be painful. If pain occurs during infusion, it should be stopped and additional 2–3 mL of local anesthetic injected. Complete the infusion in a few minutes.

Source: Adapted and updated from Heavner JE et al.[22] and Manchikanti L et al.[23] with permission from the authors and the American Society of Interventional Pain Physicians.

preferred by Racz as movement of the needle tip is less likely to cause injury and is more directional. Also, 18G RX-2® Coudé™ needle for cervical site-specific delivery of medications with a 22G VERSA- KATH®.

- The needle is advanced to a point below the S3 foramen to prevent S3 nerve root damage.

- Placement is confirmed by lateral and anteroposterior fluoroscopic views.
  - After aspiration is negative for blood and cerebrospinal fluid (CSF), 10 mL of iohexol (Omnipaque®-240) or metrizamide (Amipaque®) is injected under fluoroscopy.
- Next, insert a catheter into the scarred area.
  - The ideal epidural catheter is a stainless steel, fluoropolymer-coated, spiral-tipped Racz Tun-L-Kath-XL0 (Epimed International Inc.) as illustrated in **Figures 11A to D**.
  - The bevel of the needle should face the ventrolateral aspect of the caudal canal on the affected side.
  - Multiple passes may be necessary to place the catheter into the scarred area.
  - Catheter tip placement should be lateral of the dural boundary and target specific ventral lateral. Avoid midline catheter placement to reduce likelihood of subdural or subarachnoid.
  - To facilitate steering of the catheter into the desired location, a 15° bend is placed at its distal end.
- After final placement of the catheter and negative aspiration, another 5–10 mL of contrast medium is injected through the catheter.
  - This additional contrast should spread into the area of previous filling defect and outline the targeted nerve root **(Figs. 12A to E)**. 1,500 units of hyaluronidase (Wydase®) in 10 mL of preservative-free saline are injected rapidly.

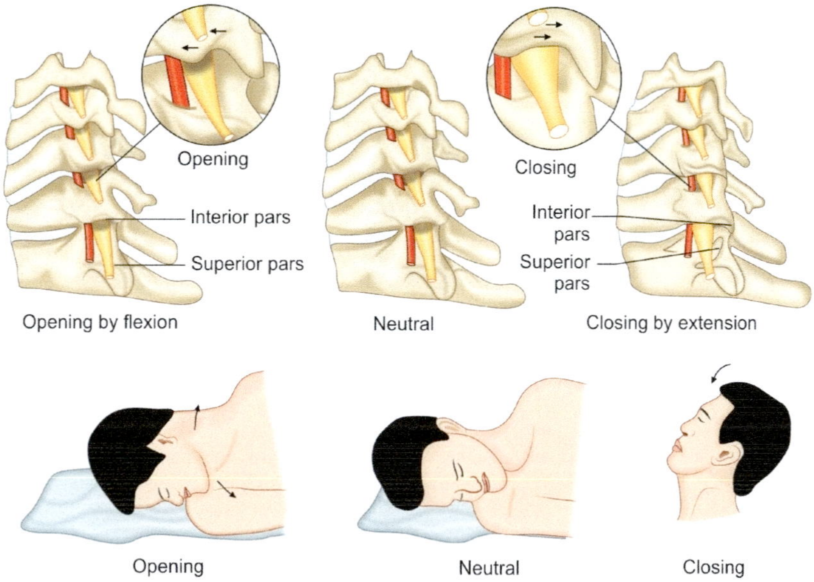

Fig. 10: Flexion rotation, left to right regardless patient position. The neural foramen enlarges on flexion rotation and gets smaller with extension. The inferior pars slides forward over the superior pars to enlarge the foramen. This allows lateral runoff and pressure release with perivenous counter spread.

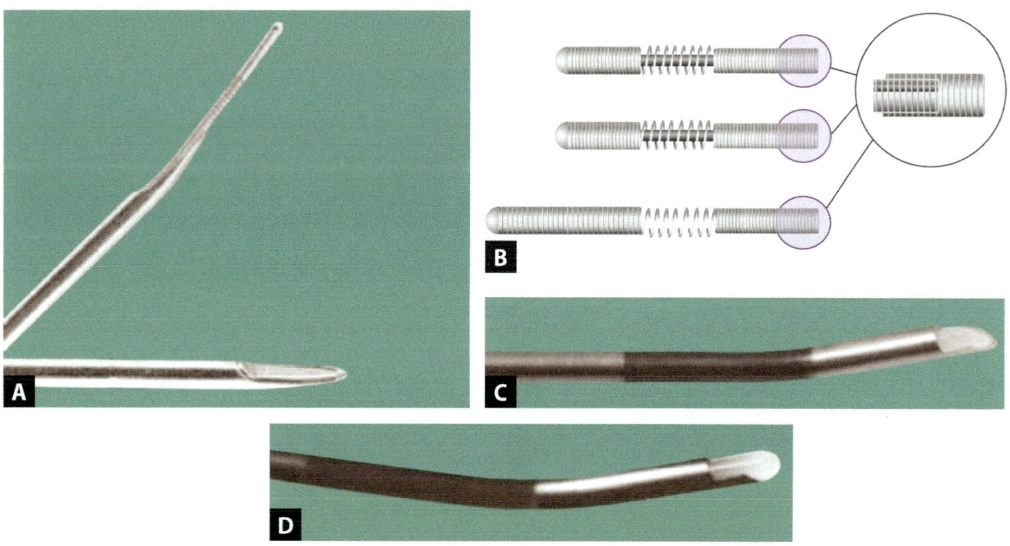

Figs. 11A to D: Special needle and catheter for adhesiolysis. (A) RK epidural needle (close up); (B) Tun-L-Kath and Tun-L-XL/24 epidural catheters; (C) RX Coudé® epidural needle; (D) RX-2™ Coudé® epidural needle.
Courtesy: Epimed International, Gloversville, NY, with permission.

- Afterward, 10 mL of 0.2% ropivacaine or 0.25% bupivacaine and 40 mg of triamcinolone or methylprednisolone are injected through the catheter in divided doses. Other corticosteroids may also be used.
- When the procedure is completed, the catheter should be secured to the skin with 2–0 nylon on a cutting needle, with application of antibiotic ointment and gauze.
- The catheter is connected to an adapter and to a bacteriostatic filter that is not removed until three daily injections have been completed. The filter is capped, and the catheter is taped to the flank of the patient.
- During the procedure, the patient is given IV broad-spectrum antibiotics, 1 g/day, to prevent bacterial colonization that is especially hazardous because of the epidurally administered steroid.

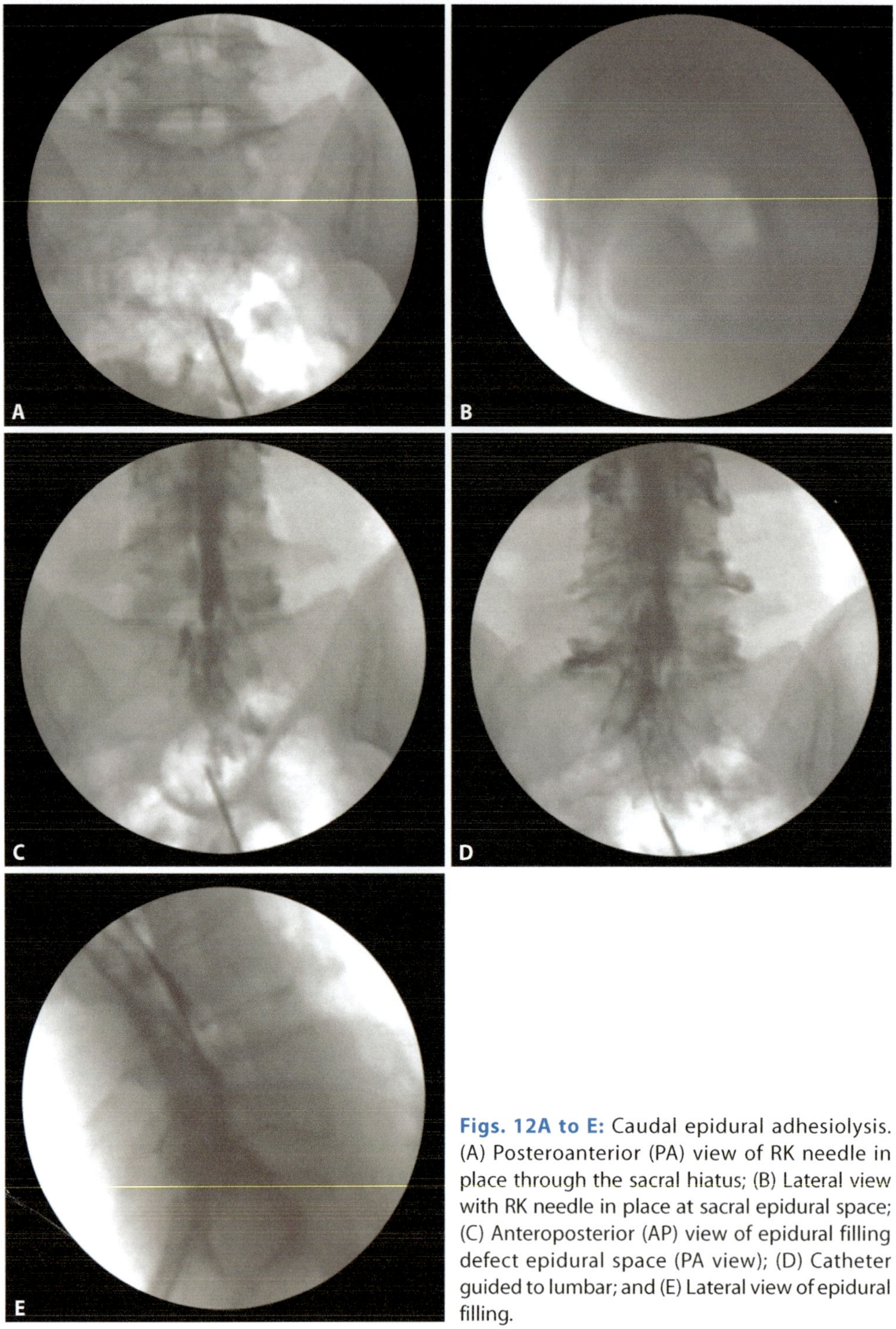

Figs. 12A to E: Caudal epidural adhesiolysis. (A) Posteroanterior (PA) view of RK needle in place through the sacral hiatus; (B) Lateral view with RK needle in place at sacral epidural space; (C) Anteroposterior (AP) view of epidural filling defect epidural space (PA view); (D) Catheter guided to lumbar; and (E) Lateral view of epidural filling.

- Once the patient is taken to the recovery room (placed with the affected side down) and vital signs are checked, 9 mL of 10% hypertonic saline is infused over 20–30 minutes.
- Occasionally, the patient may complain of severe burning pain during the infusion. The cause is usually the introduction of hypertonic saline into nonanesthetized epidural tissue.

   - Should the patient complain of pain, the infusion must be stopped and another 3–5 mL bolus of local anesthetic is given. After 5 minutes, the hypertonic saline infusion can be restarted without incident.
   - After completion of the hypertonic saline infusion, 1.5 mL of preservative-free normal saline is used to flush the catheter. Once this task is completed, the cap is replaced on the filter.
- The catheter is left in place for 3 days.
   - On the second and third days, it is injected once a day with 10 mL of 0.2% ropivacaine after negative aspiration from the catheter. 15 minutes later, 10 mL of 10% saline is infused over 20 minutes for patient comfort.
   - As in any hypertonic saline infusion series, the catheter must be flushed with 1.5 mL of preservative-free normal saline.
   - On the third day, the catheter is removed 10 minutes after the last injection.
   - A triple antibiotic ointment is placed on the wound, which is covered with a bandage or other appropriate dressing.

Interlaminar Lumbar Approach

The technique for lysis of epidural adhesions in these areas of the spinal cord must be modified to ensure that initially the needle is positioned in the epidural space and that spinal cord compression by subsequent injections is avoided.

- The patient is placed in the lateral or prone position on the fluoroscopy table.
   - Sterile preparation and draping is carried out.
   - Skin entry should be 1.5–2 levels below the desired epidural entry to facilitate catheter placement.
- After local anesthetic is used on the skin, an 18G needle is inserted through the same puncture site to form an entry wound.
   - Through the puncture site, a 16G RK needle is first advanced under fluoroscopic guidance (AP view) to determine the direction of the needle.
   - Next, in the lateral view, the needle is advanced to the point just before the "straight line" formed by the fluoroscopic image of the anterior border of the spinous process in the lateral view (the insertion site of the ligamentum flavum).
   - The lateral view under fluoroscopy demonstrates the depth of needle placement.
   - Lastly, an AP view is checked again to confirm the direction of the needle.
   - When the direction is satisfactory, the loss of resistance technique is used to advance the needle into the epidural space.
- Inject contrast to outline the filling defect.
- A Racz Tun-L-Kath or Racz Tun-L-Kath-XL epidural catheter is passed in an anterocephalad direction toward the filling defect outlined by the contrast until the catheter tip enters the scarred area.
   - After negative aspiration, 1–3 mL of nonionic contrast is injected while observing the fluoroscope screen for spread within the adhesions and runoff of contrast is observed.
   - Once an outflow or runoff tract is seen (i.e., either opening of the neuroforamina or caudal spread), 3–5 mL of 0.9% preservative-free saline with 1,500 units hyaluronidase is injected.
   - Lastly, 0.2% ropivacaine (4 mL) and 40 mg (1 mL) triamcinolone diacetate are injected after negative aspiration, while attention is directed to watch for displacement of the contrast.
   - For safety purposes, the local anesthetic is given in divided doses to first rule out intrathecal subdural (1–2 mL) or intravascular injection. 5 minutes later, the rest of the volume of the local anesthetic and steroid is injected.

Modified Manchikanti Technique

The technique utilized by Manchikanti et al.[23,25,26] is outlined in **Table 2** and illustrated in **Figures 13 and 14**.

Facilities

The procedure is performed in a sterile operating room under appropriate sterile precautions utilizing fluoroscopy, RK needle, and a spring-wire catheter.

Preparation

After the initial evaluation, the patient is transferred to the holding area, where appropriate preparation is carried out, including preoperative evaluation, with IV access, and administration of antibiotic, based on protocol and patient condition.

Consent

An appropriate detailed consent is obtained from all patients.

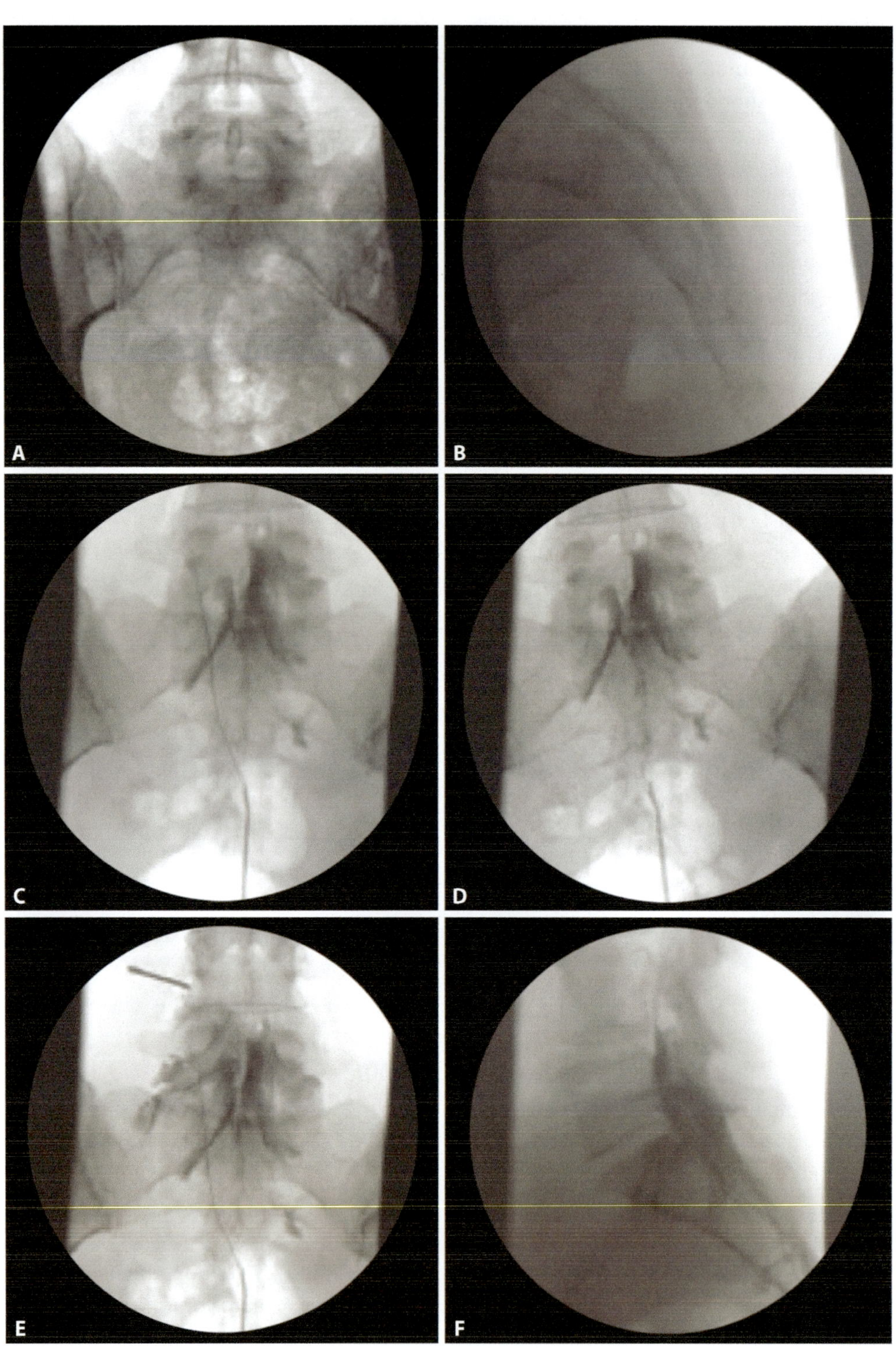

Figs. 13A to F: Percutaneous adhesiolysis with caudal approach—positioning, preparation, and fluoroscopy. (A) Fluoroscopic view in anteroposterior (AP) position; (B) Fluoroscopic view in lateral position; (C) AP fluoroscopic view after injection of 5 mL of contrast medium showing lack of filling on the left side in L5 distribution; (D) Placement of Racz catheter and adhesiolysis and positioning of the catheter over the L5 body to the left laterally; (E) Contrast medium injection after placement of the catheter following adhesiolysis showing excellent filling of the L5 nerve root; (F) Lateral fluoroscopic view showing nerve root filling along with ventral and dorsal filling of the epidural space.

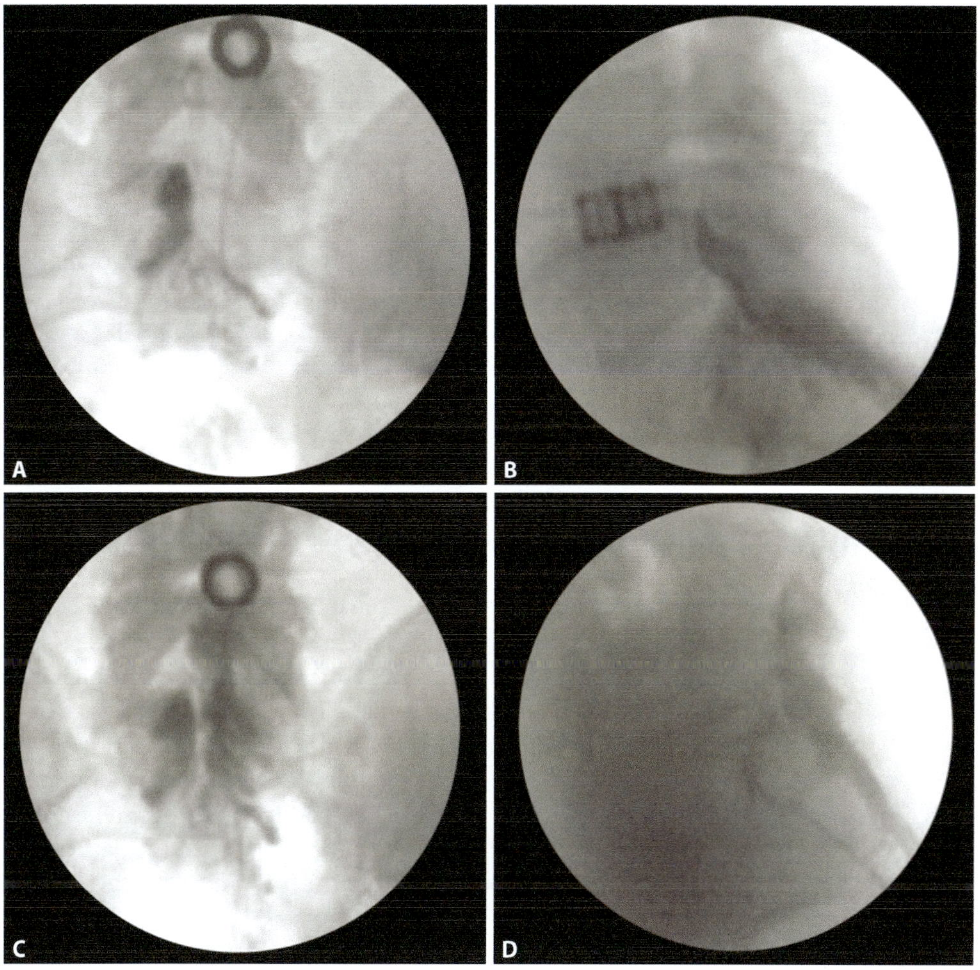

Figs. 14A to D: Example of caudal epidural adhesiolysis. (A) Posteroanterior (PA) view showing defect on right with Racz catheter in place; (B) Lateral view prior to adhesiolysis with catheter in place; (C) PA view following appropriate adhesiolysis illustrating nerve root filling; (D) Lateral view with filling defect on right side after adhesiolysis.

Operating Room

- Procedural steps are illustrated in **Table 2** and **Figures 13A to F**.
  - Patient is positioned in prone position with firm padding under pelvis.
  - Sterile preparation is carried out with povidone-iodine (betadine) preparation.
  - Draping is carried out to cover the patient, extending into the mid-thoracic or cervical region.
  - Appropriate monitoring of blood pressure, pulse, and pulse oximetry is carried out.
  - Sedation is slowly administered.
  - The fluoroscope is adjusted over the lumbosacral region for AP and lateral views.
  - A physician, scrubbed and in sterile gown and gloves, infiltrates the area for needle insertion with local anesthetic.
  - An RK needle is introduced into the epidural space under fluoroscopic utilization.
  - Once the needle placement is confirmed to be in the epidural space, a lumbar epidurogram is carried out utilizing approximately 2–5 mL of contrast. Finding the filling defects by examining the contrast flow into the nerve roots is the purpose of the epidurogram.
- After appropriate determination of epidurography, a Racz catheter, which is a spring-guided, reinforced catheter, is slowly passed through the RK needle to the area of the filling defect or the site of pathology

determined by magnetic resonance imaging (MRI), computed tomography (CT), or patient symptoms.
  - Following the positioning of the catheter into the appropriate area by mechanical means, adhesiolysis is carried out.
  - After completion of the adhesiolysis, a repeat epidurogram is carried out by additional injection of contrast.
  - If appropriate adhesiolysis is completed, nerve root filling as well as epidural filling will be noted. **Figures 14A to D** illustrate an example of the procedure.
  - **Figures 15A to C** illustrate subarachnoid injection of contrast.
- At this time, variable doses of local anesthetic are injected. Commonly injected is 5–10 mL of 2% lidocaine hydrochloride or 5–10 mL of 0.25% bupivacaine.
- Following completion of the injection, the catheter is taped utilizing bio-occlusive dressing, and the patient is turned to the supine position and transferred to the recovery room.

Recovery Room

- The patient is very closely monitored for any potential complications or side effects. If no complications are observed and the patient reports good pain relief without any motor weakness, hypertonic saline neurolysis is carried out at this time by injection of variable doses of 10% sodium chloride solution.
  - Hypertonic neurolysis may be carried out by an infusion pump or repeat injections in doses of 2–3 mL, ranging from 6 to 10 mL total, followed by injection of steroid (Celestone 6–12 mg or Depo-Medrol 40–80 mg).
- The catheter is flushed with normal saline, removed, and checked for intactness.
  - The wound is also checked at this time.
- The patient is ambulated if all parameters are satisfactory. IV access is removed and the patient is discharged home with appropriate instructions.

Transforaminal Approach

- A transforaminal approach may be used when the lesion cannot be reached caudally.
  - This is indicated for most lesions cephalad to L4. Most lesions above L4 should be approached transforaminally.
  - Fluoroscopic views of 15–20° oblique and 25–30° caudocephalad should be obtained to visualize the advancement of a 16G RX Coudé epidural needle. The needle is directed toward a point just lateral to the superior pars interarticularis of the vertebrae that comprise the caudal aspect of the neural foramen **(Figs. 16A to D)**.
  - If the needle tip is rotated in the neural foramen or the spinal canal, the RX-2™ Coudé® needle is preferred. The RX-2™ Coudé® comes with a second stylet that can be inserted and interlocked with the needle to convert the needle tip to a blunt needle shape to reduce the likelihood of cutting dura or other structures.
  - The advancing needle should contact bone. When it does, it should be rotated 180°. After advancing 2–3 mm past the bone, the needle should be rotated back. Then get a lateral fluoroscopic image.
  - The needle's tip should be in the posterior neural foramen, about 2–3 mm. Inject 1–2 mm of Omnipaque 240. Confirm the epidural spread in the following views: lateral, anteroposterior, and oblique.
- The catheter—A Tun-L-Kath or Tun-L-XL/24 **(Figs. 16A to D)** is then inserted.
  - The catheter should advance easily, but do not advance it past the midline. The needle may be removed once the catheter is in the epidural space.
  - If the catheter meets resistance, remove it and then check and/or adjust the needle's placement. Never force the catheter.
  - The needle may need to be advanced or withdrawn 1–2 mm.
- The medication guideline is the same as for caudal or interlaminar approaches, but the injectate volume is reduced by 25–50%
- L2 transforaminal needle placement as described by Racz is shown in **Figures 16A to D**.
  - The fluoroscopic C-arm is rotated laterally until the superior pars interarticularis of L2 is visible. Caudal rotation is initiated until the superior pars interarticularis obscures the disk space, resulting in the end plates being squared.

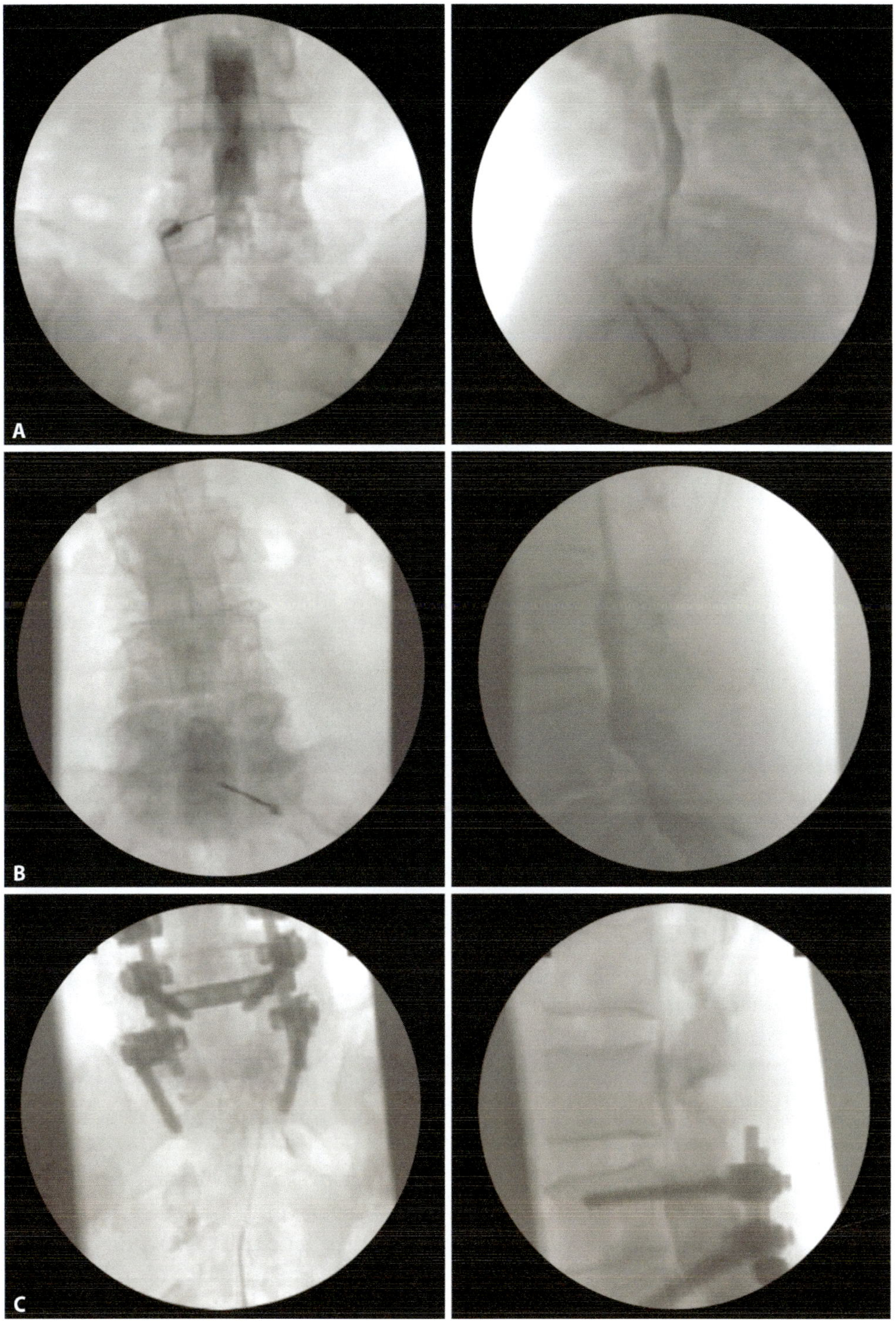

Figs. 15A to C: Subarachnoid pattern of contrast injection. (A) Lumbar interlaminar epidural with subarachnoid filling patterns—anteroposterior (AP) and lateral views; (B) Lumbar interlaminar epidural with subarachnoid filling patterns—AP and lateral views; (C) Caudal epidural adhesiolysis—subarachnoid distribution of contrast—AP and lateral views.

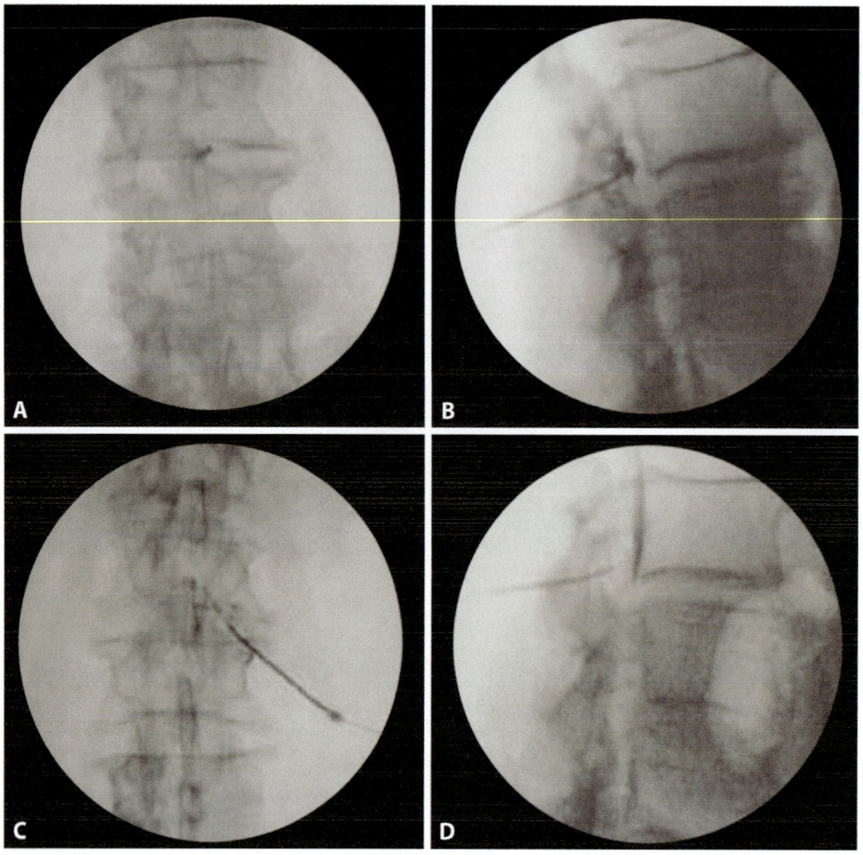

Figs. 16A to D: Transforaminal epidural adhesiolysis in a postfusion patient with left L5 radiculitis. (A) C-arm positioning; (B) Lateral view with contrast injection; (C) Anteroposterior (AP) view with catheter placement; (D) Lateral view with ventral spread.

- This technique's goal is not to square the end plates, it is to visualize the superior parts.
- Use a lateral view to aim the needle at the pars interarticularis and then rotate around **(Fig. 16A)**.
- The needle tip will be seen to pass through the interior transverse ligament. To confirm correct foraminal placement, inject ¼ mL of Omnipaque 240.
  - Place a small bend near a Brevi-XL catheter's tip and thread it into the needle. The needle should pull the catheter into the ventral epidural space **(Fig. 16B)**.
- Anteroposterior view of the transforaminal catheter shows the position in the ipsilateral side of the ventral lateral epidural space.
  - 5 mL of Omnipaque 240 contrast medium is injected and spreads cephalad and caudad just below the catheter. The shadow of spinal stenosis is visible secondary to the hypertrophic ligamentum flavum and the bulging L2 disk **(Fig. 16C)**.

SIDE EFFECTS AND COMPLICATIONS

- Lumbar adhesiolysis is generally a safe procedure, but complications can occur. The most troubling and common are dural puncture, spinal cord compression, catheter shearing, infection, and a reaction to steroids, hypertonic saline, or hyaluronidase.[20,23,49-64]
  - Complications are listed in **Table 3**. Unintended subarachnoid or subdural puncture from injection of local anesthetic or hypertonic saline is one of the major complications of the procedure.
  - Cardiac arrhythmias, myelopathy, paralysis, and loss of sphincter control have all been reported due to injection of hypertonic saline in the subarachnoid space.[51]
  - Subarachnoid leakage of hypertonic saline has rarely been blamed for arachnoiditis incidents.[52]
  - Catheter placement targeting should not be midline, but ventral and lateral to the painful area.

TABLE 3: Potential complications of percutaneous adhesiolysis.

Pain	• Pain at the site of the needle insertion • Exacerbation of existing pain • Pain in the low back
Infection	• Soft tissue abscess • Epidural abscess • Meningitis • Encephalitis
Bleeding	• Soft tissue hematoma • Epidural hematoma • Spinal cord hematoma • Nerve root sheath hematoma
Trauma	• Soft tissue • Nerve root • Spinal cord
Inadvertent	• Dural puncture
Injection	• Subdural injection • Intrathecal injection • Intravascular injection
Miscellaneous	• Spinal cord compression • Cauda equina syndrome • Arachnoiditis • Paraplegia • Increased intrathecal pressure • Increased intraocular pressure • Retinal hemorrhage • Torn catheter • Retained catheter

- The second specific complication of percutaneous epidural adhesiolysis is related to catheter shearing and its retention in the epidural space.[49,56,59]
  - Over 20 Racz catheter shearing reports are listed on the Food and Drug Administration (FDA) website.
    - The catheter remnant was surgically removed in seven patients.
    - It is likely that Racz catheter shearing and breakage occur more often since the MedWatch System uses voluntary reporting of adverse events.
    - Generally, it is believed that only 5% of adverse events are reported to the FDA.[60]
    - Patients who have retained Racz catheter fragments should not undergo MRI studies. There have been no reported complications.
  - Controversy surrounds whether to surgically remove broken neuraxial catheters or manage the patient conservatively.
  - Current practice, based on ease of retrieval, is to observe the patient if a standard removal technique fails to retrieve it.
    - However, there is also a potential for neurologic and/or infectious complications with any foreign body.
- Spinal cord compression following rapid injections into the epidural space, epidural infection, direct trauma to the spinal cord, neural trauma, and occasional sensitivity (3%) to hyaluronidase are the potential complications.[65]
  - Other side effects are related to the administration of steroids and are generally attributed to the chemistry or pharmacology of the steroids.[50,55]
    - However, appropriate therapeutic doses of epidural steroids were done without complications.[64]
- The list of potential complications is long, but the actual incidence is extremely low considering there have been over 2.5–3 million catheters used for various spinal and peripheral nerve block indications.

PRECAUTIONS

- Iatrogenic subdural or subarachnoid spread of any injectate is possible, no matter which approach is used. Physicians should exercise caution and pay attention to proper technique.
  - Injecting a local anesthetic before adhesiolysis is performed is not advised, even though it was done in the past.
    - Do not inject hypertonic saline through the needle into the epidural space; the catheter should be used. Hypertonic saline should be injected incrementally 15 minutes after the administration of short-acting local anesthetics and 30 minutes after the administration of long-acting local anesthetics.
  - Motor block can occur if local anesthetic spreads subdurally; this can occur 15–18 minutes after administration. The patient should be observed this long before injecting the hypertonic saline.
  - If hypertonic saline spreads to the subdural space, vascular structures within the space can become compressed due to osmotic fluid expansion.
    - Resulting symptoms include pain, weakness, numbness, paralysis, and bowel and bladder

denervation. Avoid injecting patients who have arachnoiditis. If delayed onset paralysis occurs, aspirate the loculation.[66,67]

- Alternate approaches are:
    - Injection of steroid at the end after the injection of hypertonic saline; however, the deviation should never occur with regards to injection of local anesthetic (specifically a long-acting local anesthetic) prior to the lysing and confirmation of the position of the catheter and lack of subarachnoid spread.
    - Injection of hypertonic saline through the needle is not recommended under any circumstances.
    - Injection of hypertonic saline, without appropriate waiting time, through the catheter is not recommended under any circumstances.
- The injection procedures with such deviations as described above may result in serious complications, including arachnoiditis, which may be attributed to the injection, even though there is no substantial proof at the present time to indicate that 10% sodium chloride solution in fact causes arachnoiditis.

- Relative contraindications to interventional techniques have been described for patients being treated with antithrombotics and anticoagulants.
    - American Society of Interventional Pain Physician (ASIPP) guidelines[4,68] and American Society of Regional Anesthesia and Pain Medicine (ASRA) guidelines[69] have provided guidance for epidural procedures for patients receiving antithrombotic therapy. Guidelines on anticoagulants and antithrombotics are described on the ASIPP website (http://www.asipp.org/), which is regularly updated.[70]
- Prior to the percutaneous adhesiolysis procedure, patients on warfarin therapy should have their prothrombin time checked and documented to be at acceptable levels.
    - In stopping anticoagulant therapy, one should take into consideration the risk or benefit ratio of the procedure.
    - In addition, the pain physician may also wish to consult with the physician in charge of the patient's anticoagulant therapy.
    - It is prudent to advise the patient to contact the physician in charge of the anticoagulant therapy and let him/her make the decision regarding the appropriateness of discontinuing anticoagulant therapy.
    - Other anticoagulants including rivaroxaban (Xarelto) and apixaban (Eliquis) should be stopped for 24 hours for Xarelto and 48 hours for Eliquis for caudal approach. However, for other approaches including cervical, thoracic, lumbar interlaminar entries, these must be stopped earlier with 3 days for Eliquis and 2 days for Xarelto. A patient's renal function must also be taken into consideration, and the dosage must be adjusted based on renal function.
- Multiple antiplatelet agents, including phosphodiesterase inhibitors, have been recommended to be continued prior to these procedures.
    - Platelet aggregation inhibitors including clopidogrel (Plavix), prasugrel (Effient), and ticlopidine (Ticlid) may be continued or may be stopped for 7 days for clopidogrel and prasugrel, and for 14 days for ticlopidine.
    - Other antithrombotics include dabigatran (Pradaxa) may be stopped for 5 days.
        - Aspirin and nonsteroidal anti-inflammatory drugs (NSAIDs) alone are considered safe.[4,68,69]
    - The combination of multiple drugs with aspirin and NSAIDs or other antiplatelet therapy with clopidogrel or ticlopidine may increase the risk of spinal hematoma.
    - The risk and potential discontinuation may be considered by the physician in charge of the antiplatelet therapy.

CONCLUSION

The effectiveness of the procedures gets better with experience. The safety of the procedures also improves by incorporating principles such as making sure there is no loculation, evidenced by pain covering a bigger area of the body than just the nerve root and resolving loculation-related pain by facilitating lateral runoff. Flexion rotation has led to better dispersal of injected medication and enhanced lateral runoff.

Postprocedure neural flossing exercises increase effectiveness of the lysis procedure by increasing nerve root mobility. Recognition that any sharp needle movement within the spinal canal can increase the risk of injury to the dura and other structures whereas using the second stylet in the RX-2™ Coudé® needle converts the needle tip to a blunt which reduces the chance of such injuries. The increasing list of recent reference publications without any negative information places the lysis procedure significantly ahead of spine surgical interventions. Additionally, reducing pain enhances effectiveness of neuromodulation and instances where neuromodulation is failing to relieve pain, the lysis procedures may be indicated.

ACKNOWLEDGMENT

The authors would like to thank Angela Pranivong and transcriptionists Tonie M Hatton and Diane E Neihoff, for their assistance with the preparation of this manuscript.

REFERENCES

1. US Burden of Disease Collaborators. The State of US Health, 1999-2010: burden of diseases, injuries, and risk factors. JAMA. 2013;310:591-606.
2. Martin BI, Turner JA, Mirza SK, Lee MJ, Comstock BA, Deyo RA. Trends in health care expenditures, utilization, and health status among US adults with spine problems, 1997-2006. Spine (Phila Pa 1976). 2009;34:2077-84.
3. Gaskin DJ, Richard P. The economic costs of pain in the United States. J Pain. 2012;13:715-24.
4. Manchikanti L, Knezevic NN, Navani A, Christo PJ, Limerick G, Calodney AK, et al. Epidural interventions in the management of chronic spinal pain: American Society of Interventional Pain Physicians (ASIPP) comprehensive evidence-based guidelines. Pain Physician. 2021;24:S27-208.
5. Manchikanti L, Kaye AM, Knezevic NN, Giordano J, Applewhite MK, Bautista A, et al. Comprehensive, evidence-based, consensus guidelines for prescription of opioids for chronic non-cancer pain from the American Society of Interventional Pain Physicians (ASIPP). Pain Physician. 2023;26:S7-126.
6. Dieleman JL, Cao J, Chapin A, Chen C, Li Z, Liu A, et al. US health care spending by payer and health condition, 1996-2016. JAMA. 2020;323:863-84.
7. Sicard MA. Extradural drug injections by saracoccygiane route. C R Seances Soc Biol Fil. 1901;53:396-8.
8. Sicard JA, Forestier J. Methode radiographique d'exploration de la cavite epidurale par le Lipiodol. Rev Neurol. 1921;2:1264.
9. Hitchcock E. Hypothermic subarachnoid irrigation for intractable pain. Lancet. 1967;1:1133-5.
10. Ventrafridda V, Spreafico R. Subarachnoid saline perfusion. In: Bonica II (Ed). Advances in Neurology. Volume 4. New York: Raven Press; 1974. pp. 477-84.
11. Hitchcock E. Osmolytic neurolysis for intractable facial pain. Lancet. 1969;1:434-6.
12. Racz GB, Holubec JT. Lysis of adhesions in the epidural space. In: Racz GB (Ed). Techniques of Neurolysis. Boston, MA: Kluwer Academic Publishers; 1989. pp. 57-72.
13. Racz GB, Racz GJ, Racz TA. Interventional pain procedures. In: Carl Noe (Ed). Pain Management for Clinicians: A Guide to Assessment and Treatment. Berlin, Germany: Springer; 2020. pp. 523-654.
14. Manchikanti L, Heavner JE, Racz GB. Lumbar percutaneous adhesiolysis. In: Manchikanti L, Singh V, Falco FJE, Kaye AD, Soin A, Hirsch JA (Eds). Manchikanti's Essentials of Interventional Techniques in Managing Chronic Pain, 2nd edition. New York, NY: Springer; 2023, in press.
15. Manchikanti L, Bakhit CE. Percutaneous lysis of epidural adhesions. Pain Physician. 2000;3:46-64.
16. Manchikanti L, Racz GB. Percutaneous adhesiolysis for failed back surgery syndrome and other applications. In: Baheti DK, Bakshi S, Gupta S, Gehdoo RS (Eds). Interventional Pain Management: A Practical Approach, 2nd edition. New Delhi, India: Jaypee Brothers Medical Publishers (P) Ltd.; 2016. pp. 311-29.
17. Racz GB, Heavner JE, Smith JP, Noe CE, Al-Kaisy A, Matsumoto T, et al. Epidural lysis of adhesions and percutaneous neuroplasty. In: Racz GB, Noe CE (Eds). Pain and Treatment. InTech; 2014.
18. Payne JN, Rupp NH. The use of hyaluronidase in caudal block anesthesia. Anesthesiology. 1951;12:164-72.
19. Moore DC. The use of hyaluronidase in local and nerve block analgesia other than spinal block. 1520 cases. Anesthesiology. 1951;12:611-26.
20. Helm S 2nd, Racz GB, Gerdesmeyer L, Justiz R, Hayek SM, Kaplan ED, et al. Percutaneous and endoscopic adhesiolysis in managing low back and lower extremity pain: a systematic review and meta-analysis. Pain Physician. 2016;19:E245-82.
21. Manchikanti L, Heavner JE, Racz GB. Percutaneous adhesiolysis. In: Manchikanti L, Kaye AD, Falco FJE, Hirsch JA (Eds). Essentials of Interventional Techniques in Managing Chronic Spinal Pain. New York, NY: Springer; 2018. pp. 241-72.
22. Heavner JE, Racz GB, Raj PP. Percutaneous epidural neuroplasty: prospective evaluation of 0.9% NaCl versus 10% NaCl with or without hyaluronidase. Reg Anesth Pain Med. 1999;24:202-7.
23. Manchikanti L, Rivera JJ, Pampati V, Damron KS, McManus CD, Brandon DE, et al. One day lumbar epidural adhesiolysis and hypertonic saline neurolysis in treatment of chronic low back pain: a randomized, double-blind trial. Pain Physician. 2004;7:177-86.
24. Veihelmann A, Devens C, Trouillier H, Birkenmaier C, Gerdesmeyer L, Refior HJ. Epidural neuroplasty versus physiotherapy to relieve pain in patients with sciatica: a prospective randomized blinded clinical trial. J Orthop Sci. 2006;11:365-9.
25. Manchikanti L, Singh V, Cash KA, Pampati V. Assessment of effectiveness of percutaneous adhesiolysis and caudal

epidural injections in managing lumbar post surgery syndrome: 2-year follow-up of randomized, controlled trial. J Pain Res. 2012;5:597-608.

26. Manchikanti L, Cash KA, McManus CD, Pampati V. Assessment of effectiveness of percutaneous adhesiolysis in managing chronic low back pain secondary to lumbar central spinal canal stenosis. Int J Med Sci. 2013;10:50-9.
27. Gerdesmeyer L, Wagenpfeil S, Birkenmaier C, Veihelmann A, Hauschild M, Wagner K, et al. Percutaneous epidural lysis of adhesions in chronic lumbar radicular pain: a randomized double-blind, placebo- controlled trial. Pain Physician. 2013;16:185-96.
28. Gerdesmeyer L, Noe C, Prehn-Kristensen A, Harrasser N, Al Muderis M, Weuster M, et al. Long-term efficacy of percutaneous epidural neurolysis of adhesions in chronic lumbar radicular pain: 10 year follow-up of a randomized controlled trial. Pain Physician. 2021;24:359-67.
29. Manchikanti L, Helm S 2nd, Pampati V, Racz GB. Cost utility analysis of percutaneous adhesiolysis in managing pain of post-lumbar surgery syndrome and lumbar central spinal stenosis. Pain Pract. 2015;15:414-22.
30. Lee JH, Lee SH. Clinical effectiveness of percutaneous adhesiolysis versus transforaminal epidural steroid injection in patients with postlumbar surgery syndrome. Reg Anesth Pain Med. 2014;39:214-8.
31. Manchikanti L, Knezevic E, Knezevic NN, Sanapati MR, Kaye AD, Thota S, et al. The role of percutaneous neurolysis in lumbar disc herniation: systematic review and meta-analysis. Korean J Pain. 2021;34:346-68.
32. Manchikanti L, Knezevic NN, Sanapati SP, Sanapati MR, Kaye AD, Hirsch JA. Is percutaneous adhesiolysis effective in managing chronic low back and lower extremity pain in post-surgery syndrome: a systematic review and meta-analysis. Curr Pain Headache Rep. 2020;24:30.
33. Manchikanti L, Knezevic NN, Sanapati MR, Boswell MV, Kaye AD, Hirsch JA. Effectiveness of percutaneous adhesiolysis in managing chronic central lumbar spinal stenosis: a systematic review and meta-analysis. Pain Physician. 2019;22:E523-50.
34. Manchikanti L, Soin A, Boswell MV, Kaye AD, Sanapati M, Hirsch JA. Effectiveness of percutaneous adhesiolysis in post lumbar surgery syndrome: a systematic analysis of findings of systematic reviews. Pain Physician. 2019;22:307-22.
35. Chun-jing H, Hao-xiong N, Jia-xiang N. The application of percutaneous lysis of epidural adhesions in patients with failed back surgery syndrome. Acta Cir Bras. 2012;27: 357-62.
36. Akbas M, Elawamy AR, Salem HH, Fouad AZ, Abbas NA, Dagistan G. Comparison of 3 approaches to percutaneous epidural adhesiolysis and neuroplasty in post lumbar surgery syndrome. Pain Physician. 2018;21:E501-8.
37. Karm MH, Choi SS, Kim DH, Park JY, Lee S, Park JK, et al. Percutaneous epidural adhesiolysis using inflatable balloon catheter and balloon-less catheter in central lumbar spinal stenosis with neurogenic claudication: a randomized controlled trial. Pain Physician. 2018;21:593-606.
38. Choi SS, Lee JH, Kim D, Kim HK, Lee S, Song KJ, et al. Effectiveness and factors associated with epidural decompression and adhesiolysis using a balloon-inflatable catheter in chronic lumbar spinal stenosis: 1-year follow-up. Pain Med. 2016;17:476-87.
39. Choi E, Nahm FS, Lee PB. Evaluation of prognostic predictors of percutaneous adhesiolysis using a Racz catheter for post lumbar surgery syndrome or spinal stenosis. Pain Physician. 2013;16:E531-6.
40. Cho PG, Ji GY, Yoon YS, Shin DA. Clinical effectiveness of percutaneous epidural neuroplasty according to the type of single-level lumbar disc herniation: a 12-month follow-up study. J Korean Neurosurg Soc. 2019;62:681-90.
41. Funao H, Yokosuka K, Ukai J, Nakanishi K, Paku M, Tomita T, et al. Efficacy of minimally invasive trans-sacral canal plasty between patients with and without failed back surgery syndrome. Medicina (Kaunas). 2022;58:251.
42. Cho JH, Lee JH, Song KS, Hong JY, Joo YS, Lee DH, et al. Treatment outcomes for patients with failed back surgery. Pain Physician. 2017;20:E29-43.
43. Bogduk N. The innervation of the lumbar spine. Spine (Phila Pa 1976). 1983;8:286-93.
44. Standring S. Macroscopic anatomy of the spinal cord and spinal nerves. In: Standring S (Ed). Gray's Anatomy: The Anatomical Basis of Clinical Practice. London: Churchill Livingstone; 2005. pp. 775-88.
45. Bowsher D. A comparative study of the azygous venous system in man, monkey, dog, cat, rat and rabbit. J Anat. 1954;88:400-6.
46. Woollam DH, Millen JW. The arterial supply of the spinal cord and its significance. J Neurol Neurosurg Psychiatry. 1955;18:97-102.
47. Willis RJ. Caudal epidural blockade. In: Cousins MJ, Bridenbaugh PO (Eds). Neural Blockade in Clinical Anesthesia and Management of Pain. New York: Lippincott-Raven Press; 1998. pp. 323-42.
48. Manchikanti L, Falco FJE, Benyamin RM, Kaye AD, Boswell MV, Hirsch JA. A modified approach to grading of evidence. Pain Physician. 2014;17:E319-25.
49. Viesca CO, Racz GB, Day MR. Special techniques in pain management: lysis of adhesions. Anesthesiol Clin North Am. 2003;21:745-66, vi.
50. Manchikanti L. Role of neuraxial steroids in interventional pain management. Pain Physician. 2002;5:182-99.
51. Lewandowski EM. The efficacy of solutions used in caudal neuroplasty. Pain Digest. 1997;7:323-30.
52. Aldrete JA, Zapata JC, Ghaly R. Arachnoiditis following epidural adhesiolysis with hypertonic saline. Report of two cases. Pain Digest. 1996;6:368-70.
53. Kim RC, Porter RW, Choi BH, Kim SW. Myelopathy after intrathecal administration of hypertonic saline. Neurosurgery. 1988;22:942-5.

54. Nelson DA. Intraspinal therapy using methylprednisolone acetate. Twenty-three years of clinical controversy. Spine (Phila Pa 1976). 1993;18:278-86.
55. Lucas JS, Ducker TB, Perot PL Jr. Adverse reactions to intrathecal saline injections for control of pain. J Neurosurg. 1975;42:557-61.
56. Manchikanti L, Bakhit CE. Removal of a torn Racz catheter from lumbar epidural space. Reg Anesth. 1997;22:579-81.
57. Perkins WJ, Davis DH, Huntoon MA, Horlocker TT. A retained Racz catheter fragment after epidural neurolysis: implications during magnetic resonance imaging. Anesth Analg. 2003;96:1717-9.
58. Lingenfelter RW. Hazard of a new epidural catheter. Anesthesiology. 1983;58:292-4.
59. Ellis JS Jr, Ramamurthy S. More problems with the Arrow-Racz epidural catheter. Anesthesiology. 1986;65:124-6.
60. Landow L. Monitoring adverse drug events: the Food and Drug Administration MedWatch reporting system. Reg Anesth Pain Med. 1998;23:190-3.
61. Kushner FH, Olson JC. Retinal hemorrhage as a consequence of epidural steroid injection. Arch Ophthalmol. 1995;113:309-13.
62. Bromage PR, Benumof JL. Paraplegia following intracord injection during attempted epidural anesthesia under general anesthesia. Reg Anesth Pain Med. 1998;23:104-7.
63. Rathmell JP, Garahan MB, Alsofrom GF. Epidural abscess following epidural analgesia. Reg Anesth Pain Med. 2000; 25:79-82.
64. Manchikanti L, Pampati V, Beyer C, Damron K, Cash K, Moss T. The effect of neuraxial steroids on weight and bone mass density: a prospective evaluation. Pain Physician. 2000;3:357-66.
65. Horlocker TT, Wedel DJ, Benzon H, Brown DL, Enneking FK, Heit JA, et al. Regional anesthesia in the anticoagulated patient: defining the risks (the second ASRA Consensus Conference on Neuraxial Anesthesia and Anticoagulation). Reg Anesth Pain Med. 2003;28:172-97.
66. Racz GB, Day MR, Heavner JE, Smith JP. The Racz procedure: lysis of epidural adhesions (percutaneous neuroplasty). In: Deer TR, Leong MS, Buvanendran A, Gordin V, Kim PS, Panchal SJ, Ray AL (Eds). Comprehensive Treatment of Chronic Pain by Medical, Interventional and Integrative Approaches. New York: Springer; 2013. pp. 521-34.
67. Racz GB, Heavner JE. Complications associated with lysis of epidural adhesions and epiduroscopy. In: Rathmell JP, Neal J (Eds). Complications in Regional Anesthesia and Pain Medicine, 2nd edition. Philadelphia: Lippincott Williams and Wilkins; 2013. pp. 373-84.
68. Manchikanti L, Falco FJE, Benyamin RM, Caraway DL, Kaye AD, Helm S 2nd, et al. Assessment of bleeding risk of interventional techniques: a best evidence synthesis of practice patterns and perioperative management of anticoagulant and antithrombotic therapy. Pain Physician. 2013;16(2 Suppl):SE261-318.
69. Narouze S, Benzon HT, Provenzano D, Buvanendran A, De Andres J, Deer T, et al. Interventional spine and pain procedures in patients on antiplatelet and anticoagulant medications (Second Edition): Guidelines from the American Society of Regional Anesthesia and Pain Medicine, the European Society of Regional Anaesthesia and Pain Therapy, the American Academy of Pain Medicine, the International Neuromodulation Society, the North American Neuromodulation Society, and the World Institute of Pain. Reg Anesth Pain Med. 2018;43:225-62.
70. Manchikanti L, Sanapati M, Kaye AD, Kaye AM. Antiplatelet and anticoagulant therapy in interventional pain management. In: Manchikanti L, Singh V, Falco FJE, Kaye AD, Soin A, Hirsch JA (Eds). Manchikanti's Essentials of Interventional Techniques in Managing Chronic Pain, 2nd edition. New York, NY: Springer; 2023, in press.

46 CHAPTER

Epiduroscopy for Patients with Lumbosacral Radicular Pain

Jan Willem Kallewaard, Sanjeeva Gupta, Jonathan Richardson

ABSTRACT

The development of miniature endoscopic instruments has given us a better insight into the contents of the epidural space and has helped in targeted therapy in the spinal canal. It also allows us to diagnose and treat patients while awake and without the need for an open surgical incision. This results in reduced risk, less trauma, shorter recovery time, and reduced cost. Patients who have lower limb radicular pain following spinal surgery with no surgically correctable pathology on imaging and who have failed to respond to conservative management and transforaminal epidural steroid injections (TFESI) are reasonable candidates for epiduroscopy (spinal endoscopy). The pathophysiology of radicular pain, proposed treatment algorithm for radicular pain management, indications and contraindications, technique of performing epiduroscopy, the proposed mechanism by which epiduroscopy helps, and the evidence are presented in this chapter.

INTRODUCTION

Endoscopic surgical procedures are one of the most significant advances in modern medicine. The development of miniature endoscopic instruments has given us a better insight into the contents of the epidural space and has helped in targeted therapy in the spinal canal. It also allows us to diagnose and treat patients while awake and without the need for an open surgical incision. This results in reduced risk, less trauma, shorter recovery time, and reduced cost. We propose a treatment algorithm for lumbosacral radicular pain **(Flowchart 1)**.

TECHNICAL REQUIREMENTS

New outpatient-based endoscopy procedures are made possible by miniaturized specialized instruments. Advantage of these technical developments is that procedures can be performed with patients awake or under light sedation.

For spinal endoscopy (epiduroscopy), we need high-quality optics, a cold light source, flexibility, steerability, and a system for constant administration of a distending medium of saline. All this has to be made with as small an outside diameter as possible, and it is really in the two decades that these requirements have been met.

How does epiduroscopy differ from gadolinium-enhanced magnetic resonance imaging, which is the best available method of imaging to identify fibrous tissue in the spinal canal?

Epiduroscopy is better than magnetic resonance imaging scan in identifying nerve root vascularity, nerve root inflammation, nerve root sensitivity, identification of fibrous tissue, diagnostic localization of pain, and therapeutic aspect of pain management.[1,2]

Magnetic resonance imaging scan is better than epiduroscopy in delineating nerve root anatomy, identifying disk prolapse, assessment of spinal canal size, and exclusion of serious pathology.

PATHOPHYSIOLOGY OF RADICULAR PAIN

For generation of radicular pain, ischemia and/or inflammation is necessary. The nucleus pulposus which contains phospholipase A2 and other irritant chemicals can leak from damaged intervertebral disks and can initiate an inflammatory reaction in the nerve root or dorsal root ganglion and can also subsequently promote fibrosis. Studies have shown that application of nucleus pulposus material to the nerve roots slows down nerve conduction and impairs nerve function.[3-5] Cytokines present in the

Flowchart 1: Proposed treatment algorithm for lumbosacral radicular pain.

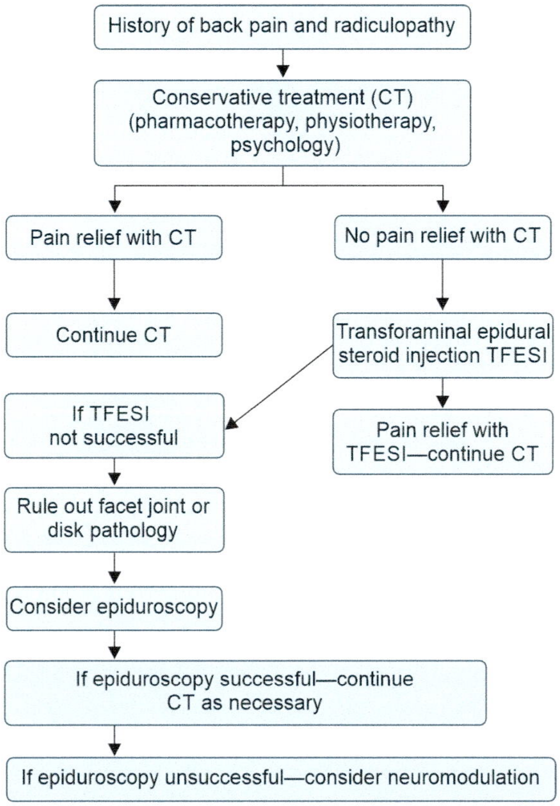

(TFESI: transforaminal epidural steroid injection)

synovial fluid of the facet joints can leak due to rupture of the joint capsule and cause nerve root irritation. Trauma, ischemia, inflammation of the nerve root, and surgery can promote fibrosis, which can alter blood and cerebrospinal fluid (CSF) flow and compromise nutrition of the nerve root.

INDICATIONS (PATIENT SELECTION)

Patients who have lower limb radicular pain with no surgically correctable pathology on imaging (almost all of these patients will have already had spinal surgery in the past) and who have failed to respond to conservative management and transforaminal epidural steroid injections are suitable for epiduroscopy. Before embarking on epiduroscopy, one should be convinced that the pain is not arising from the facet joints or the intervertebral disks.

Persistent spinal pain syndrome (PSPS) refers to chronic axial pain and/or extremity pain. Two subtypes have been defined: PSPS-type 1 is chronic pain without previous spinal surgery and PSPS-type 2 is chronic pain, persisting after spine surgery, and was formerly known as failed back surgery syndrome (FBSS) or postlaminectomy syndrome.[6] Patients with PSPS-type 2 can have a combination of severe nociceptive and neuropathic symptoms and possible nociplastic symptoms with superadded psychological component as treatment fails and time goes on. Between 5 and 50% of surgical interventions on the lumbar spine result in chronic pain. Approximately 37,500 patients with this syndrome are generated annually each year in the USA. As epiduroscopy can mobilize adhesions by mechanical and hydrostatic neuroplasty, it may have a specific role to play for these patients without causing any further major trauma.

CONTRAINDICATIONS

Contraindications for epiduroscopy include lack of consent, local infection at the sacral entry site, use of anticoagulants or a bleeding diathesis, hypersensitivity to amide local anesthetics or contrast media, pregnancy, marked obesity, and uncontrolled hypertension. The patient needs to be able to lie prone for at least an hour.

HOW DOES SPINAL ENDOSCOPY RELIEVE BACK PAIN?

The proposed mechanisms are that the saline flush helps in diluting and "washing out" phospholipase A2 and other irritant materials leaked from the intervertebral disks and the facet joints. Nerve roots with their inherent structural weakness, poor blood supply, and nutritional reliance on CSF are easily engulfed by adhesions, compromising their nutrition. Epiduroscopy may improve nerve root nutrition and vascularity by breaking down adhesions. This is done by the saline flush used, which helps in hydrostatic adhesiolysis (neuroplasty) and by mechanical adhesiolysis by the tip of the epiduroscope. Stereotactic placement of medications, such as local anesthetic, steroid, clonidine, and hyaluronidase provides targeted therapy. Studies have shown that up to 50% of epidural drug delivery may not be in the right place. Adhesions in the epidural space can prevent solutions from reaching their target.[6]

EPIDUROSCOPY: INSTRUMENTATION AND PROCEDURE

Epiduroscopy is a diagnostic and therapeutic procedure. It is commonly performed via the caudal approach, but the epidural space can also be visualized by carefully passing the spinal endoscope through a Tuohy needle at any level of the spine.

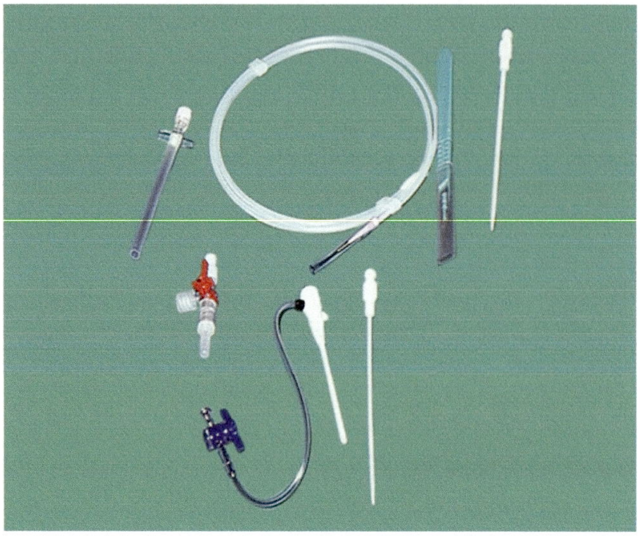

Fig. 1: Epidural access kit.

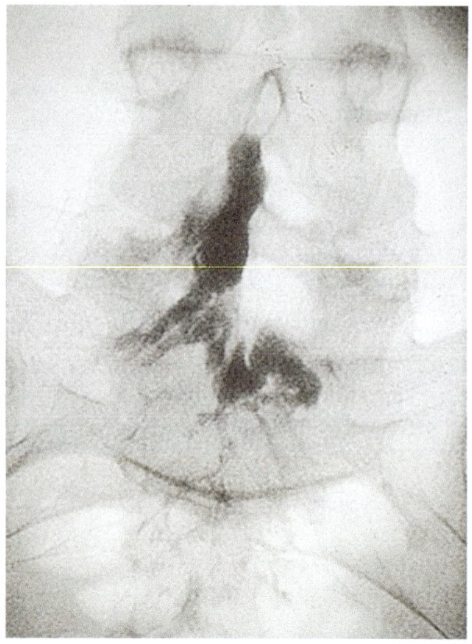

Fig. 2: Preprocedure epidurogram showing filling defect in the symptomatic right S1 nerve root area. There is also a filling defect around the right L4 and L5 area, but this patient did not have any symptoms in the area supplied by right L4 and L5 and the filling defect was ignored.

For epiduroscopy, patients are awake OR have conscious sedation and in prone position with their feet inverted, as this improves access to the caudal epidural space. Soft pillows are placed under the patient as the procedure takes approximately 1 hour. The lumbar, sacral, and caudal areas are cleaned with betadine and draped as in any other surgical procedure.

In patients who are not allergic to penicillin, cefuroxime 1.5 g is given intravenously as antibiotic prophylaxis preoperatively.

Epidural Access Kit (Fig. 1)

Epidural access kit includes needles and syringes to inject local anesthetic into the skin, 18G Tuohy needle, guidewire, dilator, and epidural sheath (similar to pulmonary artery catheter sheath).

The procedure is carried out under conscious sedation. A sensible verbal contact must be maintained with the patient during the entire procedure. Lignocaine 1% is injected into the skin over the sacrococcygeal area and the caudal epidural space is entered with an 18G Tuohy needle under lateral fluoroscopic guidance. Once the caudal epidural space is identified, radio-contrast dye is injected to obtain a baseline epidurogram. This may identify areas of filling defect that may correspond to the patient's symptom **(Fig. 2)**. A guidewire is then advanced into the epidural space through the Tuohy needle under fluoroscopy **(Fig. 3)**. The Tuohy needle is removed and a bold incision made at the entry point of the guidewire to facilitate smooth entry of the dilator along with the epidural sheath into the caudal epidural space. Adequate care is taken to prevent the guidewire from becoming kinked.

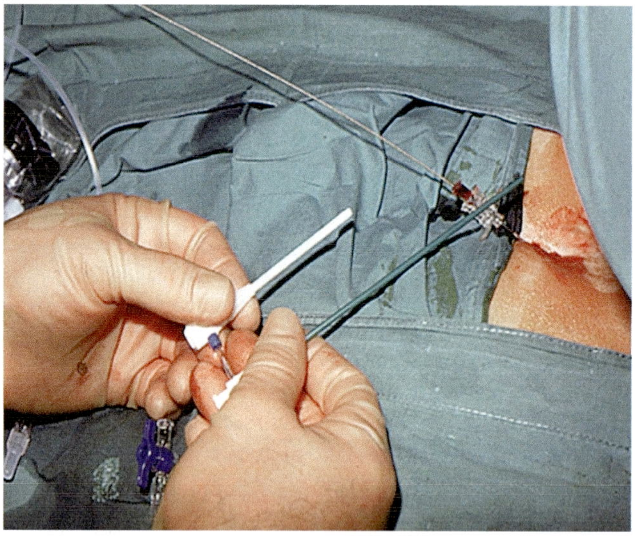

Fig. 3: Epidural needle with guidewire in place. The epidural sheath and the dilator are being assembled to pass over the guidewire into the caudal epidural space.

Video-guided Catheter or Steering Device (Fig. 4)

Video-guided catheter (VGC) is radiopaque and guides the flexible fiberoptic endoscope in the epidural space.

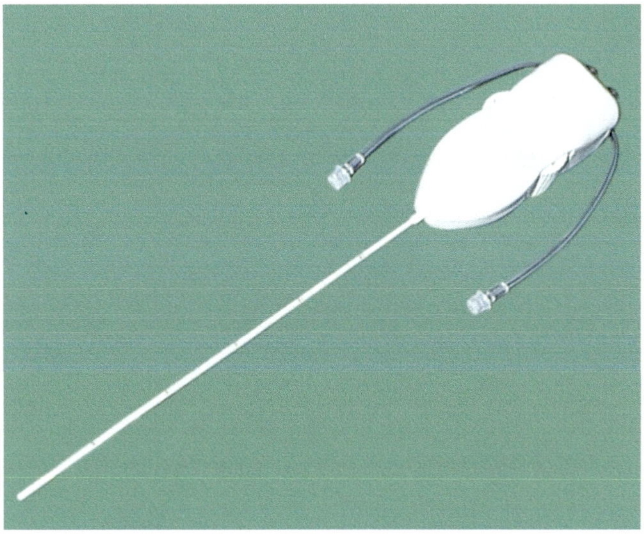

Fig. 4: The video-guided catheter or the steering device with the handle which contains the steering device.

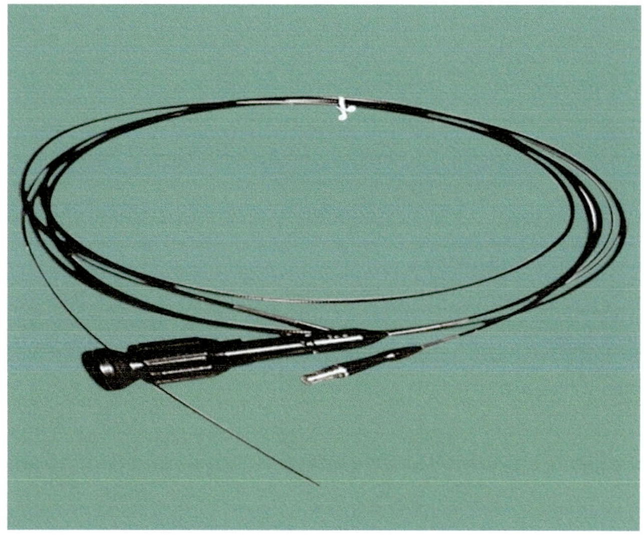

Fig. 5: The fiberoptic scope.

The VGC we use is 2.7–3, 0 mm in external diameter. It has two 1.3 mm working channels with a four-way steering mechanism and a radiopaque tip. The two working channels can be used—one for the fiberscope and the other for saline flush or instrumentation.

- *Side port:* There are two side ports that terminate with standard female luer locks. One side port is used for saline infusion and to monitor the epidural space pressure and the other port is left open to air to act as a vent for excess saline, thus preventing excessive rise in epidural pressure.
- *Accessory port:* This port contains a Tuohy Borst adapter, duckbill valve, and side port channel. These ports are used to pass accessories through the working lumina of the catheter, i.e., fiberoptic scope and instruments.
- *Handle assembly:* Houses the steering mechanism and is used to hold and direct the VGC.
- *Steering dial:* Controls the steering mechanism that manipulates the tip of the VGC and thus the fiberscope can be directed in two different directions. This is exactly like using a fiberoptic bronchoscope.
- *VGC shaft:* Flexible shaft with steerable tip
- *VGC distal tip:* Radiopaque tip of VGC can be viewed under fluoroscopy.

Flexible Fiberoptic Endoscope (Figs. 5 to 7)

The flexible fiberoptic endoscope works in conjunction with the VGC to provide direct visualization of the targeted

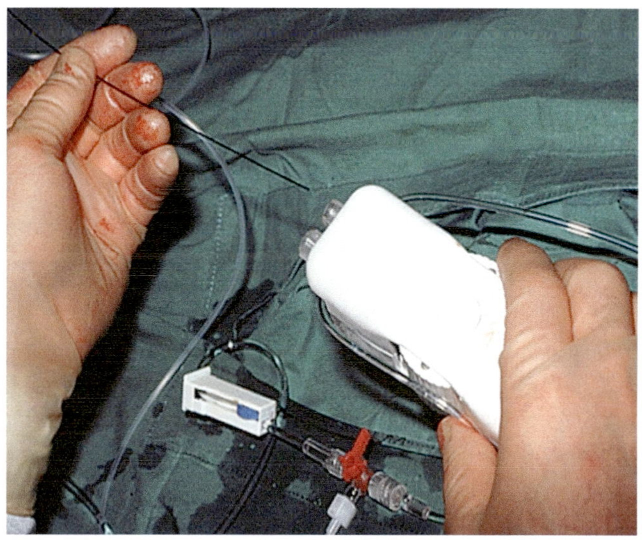

Fig. 6: The fiberoptic scope is being passed through the accessory port of the video-guided catheter.

pathology. The fiberoptic scope we use is 0.9 mm in external diameter and 125 cm long. Magnification is 40× and has a resolution of 10,000 pixels. It has a standard 32 mm eyepiece that couples to the video coupler. The distal tip incorporates the microlens assembly.

The scope is connected to a cold light source and further connected to a video staking system to obtain images on the screen. The flexible fiberoptic scope is passed through one of the lumina of the VGC and threaded to project about 1 mm beyond the tip of the VGC. The side port of the VGC is connected to saline flush, which

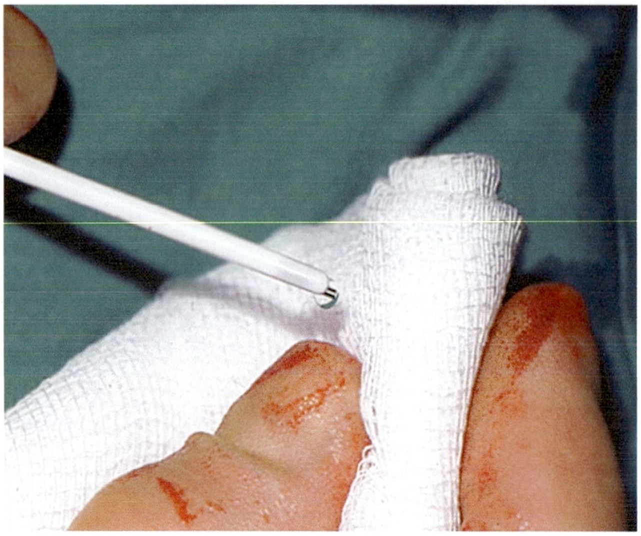

Fig. 7: The fiberoptic scope projects about 1 mm beyond the tip of the video-guided catheter and is being focused.

is hung about 1 meter above the level of the patient. A pressure-monitoring device may also be connected via a three-way tap to monitor epidural space pressure. It is important to keep the epidural pressure as low as possible and at least below the mean arterial pressure. Side effects, such as headache, paresthesia and back pain, are directly proportional to the epidural space pressure.

The VGC along with the microendoscope is introduced into the epidural space through the epidural sheath. Saline is necessary for visibility and helps in hydrostatic adhesiolysis (neuroplasty). The tip of the VGC is guided toward the suspected sites of nerve root pathology under fluoroscopy **(Fig. 8)**. Hydrostatic pressure and movement of the tip of the VGC help in releasing epidural adhesions and improve visibility and further spread of saline. With time, the epidural space clears and it will be possible to identify structures such as nerve roots **(Figs. 9 to 11)**. When the nerve root(s) responsible for the patient's symptom is touched, it produces exactly the same type and pattern of the patient's pain. After achieving satisfactory adhesiolysis and identifying the pathological nerve root, an epidurogram is performed and can be compared with the preprocedure image. Generally, a better spread of dye is noted **(Fig. 12)**. A steroid-containing solution is injected at this site through one of the side ports of the VGC.

The VGC along with the fiberoptic endoscope and the epidural sheath is removed. The wound is covered with steristrips. The patient is kept supine for the next 1 hour and then discharged home.[7]

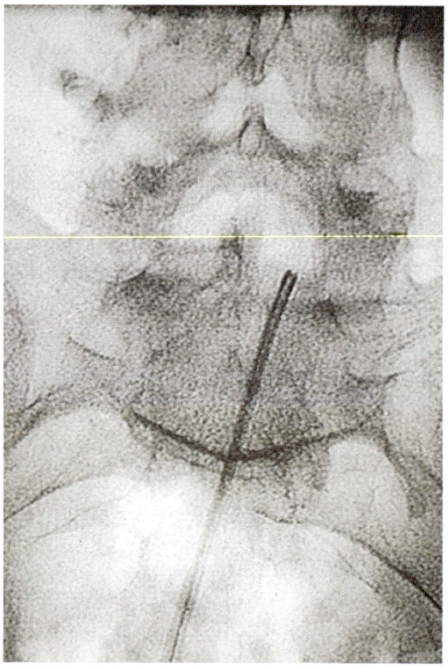

Fig. 8: The video-guided catheter which houses the fiberoptic scope is guided to the suspected site of pathology under fluoroscopic and video guidance.

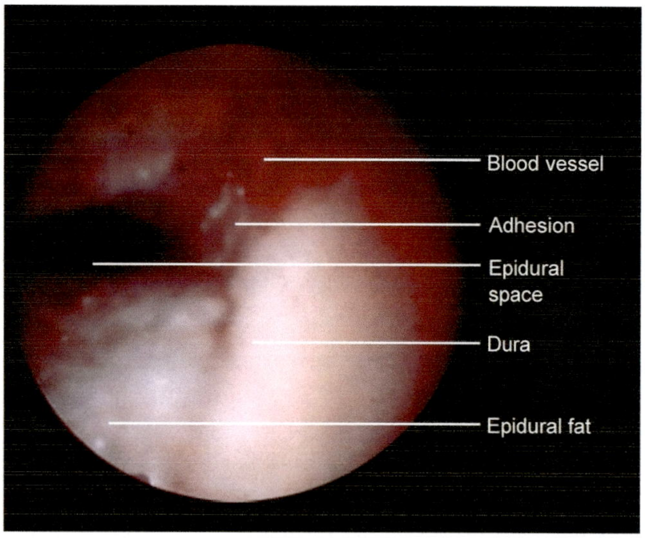

Fig. 9: Epiduroscopic picture showing adhesion which appears white, epidural fat which appears glistening, blood vessel, epidural space, and dura.

Sterilization Procedure for Fiberoptic Scope

- *NU-CIDEX:* It contains 3,500 ppm peracetic acid. If the equipment is immersed in NU-CIDEX for 5 minutes, it acts as a disinfectant and if immersed for 10 minutes it sterilizes the equipment.
- Ethylene oxide gas sterilization can also be used.

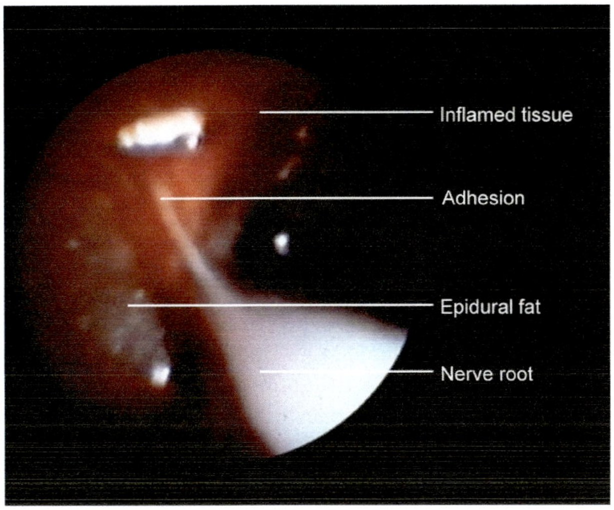

Fig. 10: Epiduroscopic picture showing inflamed tissue, adhesions, epidural fat, and nerve root.

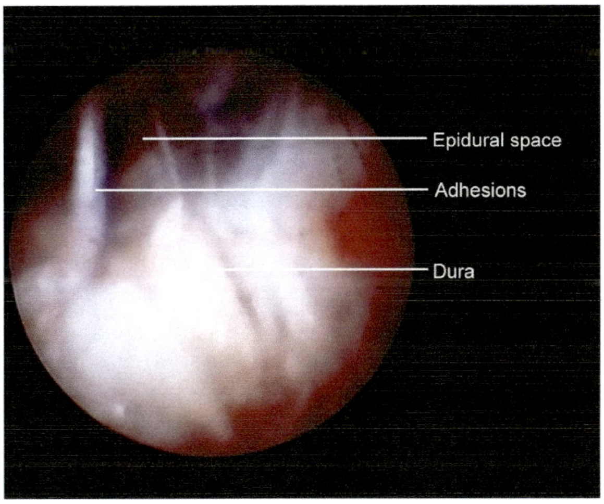

Fig. 11: Epiduroscopic picture showing adhesions.

Safety Considerations

Patient must be awake as they serve as their own monitor. Epidural space pressure due to saline infusion should not exceed mean arterial pressure.

The procedure should be stopped if patient reports pressure, paresthesia, or complains of headache, ear pressure, neck or shoulder pain as these symptoms indicate a rise in epidural space pressure. If these symptoms do not decrease, the procedure may have to be abandoned.

Side Effects

- Pain at the insertion site
- Headache during or after the procedure

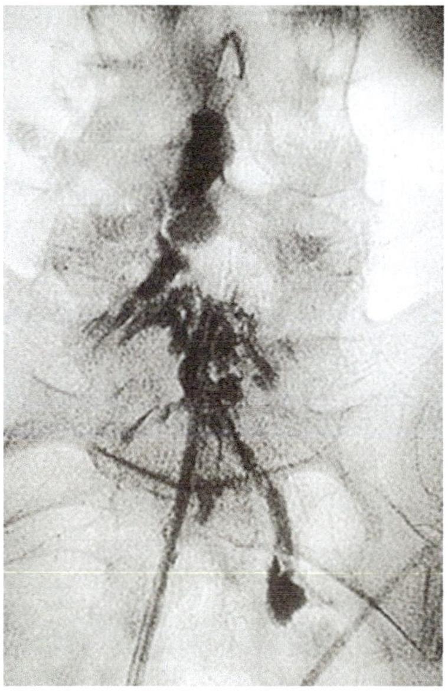

Fig. 12: Postprocedure epidurogram showing good dye spread along the right S1 nerve root, which was the pathological site in this patient.

- Small amounts of drainage from the epidural sheath insertion site
- Paresthesia during the procedure.

Complications

- Macular hemorrhage due to the transmission of epidural space pressure due to the hydraulics of CSF
- Dural puncture headache
- Epidural infection and/or abscess
- Numbness
- Tingling
- Paresthesia
- Nerve root avulsion
- Meningitis
- Arachnoiditis.

To our knowledge there are no reported incidences of paralysis, although this can be a potential complication.

OUTCOME STUDIES FOLLOWING EPIDUROSCOPY

A recent review article by Kallewaard et al. summarizes the available evidence and outcome with favorable treatment outcomes in 30–50% of patients. Other published studies indicate that about one-third of patients derive significant pain relief and improved function after epiduroscopy and another third derive no benefit from the procedure.[8-14]

Geurts et al.[10] concluded that 45% of their patients have more than 50% pain relief at 12 months following the procedure. There are several case reports suggesting favorable outcome following epiduroscopy. Application of holmium: Yttrium garnet laser and radiofrequency technique to promote adhesiolysis has also been described.[15,16] However, Raffaeli et al.[17] had three potentially lethal complications out of 10 patients' examinations. These involved serious medullar irritation resulting in seizures, bradycardia, and respiratory depression requiring emergency drug treatment and assisted ventilation. These events probably resulted from the large volume of epidural fluid that was used during the procedure (up to 1,200 mL), as well as heavy sedation. Excess epidural space pressure is transmitted throughout the neuroaxis via the hydraulics of the CSF. The resulting intracranial pressures would have been very high. With our own examinations, lasting approximately 1 hour, we use approximately 100 mL of saline.

CONCLUSION

Back pain is a major problem in the society. No satisfactory treatment is yet available in all cases. The number of patients with FBSS is rising. If conservative measures or epidural steroid injections fail, epiduroscopy is a safe and effective daycare treatment option in carefully selected patients who have low back pain and radiculopathy. Outcome results are encouraging, although further studies are urgently needed. The use of laser[15] or radiofrequency co-ablation technique[15] to facilitate adhesiolysis in the epidural space appears promising.

REFERENCES

1. Igarashi T, Hirabayashi Y, Shimizu R, Saitoh K, Fukuda H. Thoracic and lumbar extradural structure examined by extraduroscope. Br J Anaesth. 1998;81:121-5.
2. Igarashi T, Hirabayashi Y, Shimizu R, Mitsuhata H, Saitoh K, Fukuda H, et al. Inflammatory changes after extradural anaesthesia may affect the spread of local anaesthetic within the extradural space. Br J Anaesth. 1996;77: 347-51.
3. Otani K, Arai I, Mao GP, Konno S, Olmarker K, Kikuchi S. Nucleus pulposus-induced nerve root injury: relationship between blood flow and motor nerve conduction velocity. Neurosurgery. 1999;45(3):614-20.
4. Olmarker K, Myers RR. Pathogenesis of sciatic pain: role of herniated nucleus pulposus and deformation of spinal nerve root and dorsal root ganglion. Pain. 1998; 78:99-105.
5. Byröd G, Rydvik B, Nordborg C, Olmarker K. Early effects of nucleus pulposus application on spinal nerve root morphology and function. Eur Spine J. 1998;7:445-9.
6. van de Minkelis J, Peene L, Cohen SP, Staats P, Al-Kaisy A, Boxem KV, et al. Persistent spinal pain syndrome type 2. Pain Pract. 2024.
7. Gupta S, Richardson J. Epiduroscopy for chronic low-back pain and radiculopathy. In: DK Baheti, S Bakshi, S Gupta, RP Gehdoo (Eds). Interventional Pain Management—A Practical Approach, 1st edition. New Delhi: Jaypee Brothers Medical Publishers; 2009. pp. 233-43.
8. Kallewaard JW, Vanelderen P, Richardson J, Van Zundert J, Heavner J, Groen GJ. Epiduroscopy for patients with lumbosacral radicular pain. Pain Pract. 2014;14(4):365-77.
9. Richardson J, McGurgan P, Cheema S, Prasad R, Gupta S. Spinal endoscopy in chronic low back pain with radiculopathy. A prospective case series. Anaesthesia. 2001; 56(5):454-60.
10. Geurts JW, Kallewaard JW, Richardson J, Groen GJ. Targeted methylprednisolone acetate/hyaluronidase/clonidine injection after diagnostic epiduroscopy for chronic sciatica: A prospective, 1-year follow-up study. Reg Anesth Pain Med. 2002;27(4):343-52.
11. Igarashi T, Hirabayashi Y, Seo N, Saitoh K, Fukuda H, Suzuki H. Lysis of adhesions and epidural injection of steroid/local anaesthetic during epiduroscopy potentially alleviate low back and leg pain in elderly patients with lumbar spinal stenosis. Br J Anaesth. 2004;93:181-7.
12. Manchikanti L, Pampati V, Bakhit CE, Pakanati RR. Non-endoscopic and endoscopic adhesiolysis in post-lumbar laminectomy syndrome: a one-year outcome study and cost effectiveness analysis. Pain Physician. 1999;2:52-8.
13. Manchikanti L, Rivera JJ, Pampati V, Damron KS, Beyer CD, Brandon DE, et al. Spinal endoscopic adhesiolysis in the management of chronic low back pain: a preliminary report of a randomized, double-blind trail. Pain Physician. 2003;6:259-67.
14. Dashfield AK, Taylor MB, Cleaver JS, Farrow D. Comparison of caudal steroid epidural with targeted steroid placement during spinal endoscopy for chronic sciatica: a prospective, randomized, double-blind trial. Br J Anaesth. 2005;94:514-9.
15. Ruetten S, Meyer O, Godolias G. Application of holmium: YAG laser in epiduroscopy: extended practicabilities in the treatment of chronic back pain syndrome. J Clin Laser Med Surg. 2002;20(4):203-6.
16. Raffaeli W, Righetti D. Surgical radio-frequency epi-duroscopy technique (R-ResAblator) and FBBS treatment: preliminary evaluations. Acta Neurochir Suppl. 2005; 92:121-5.
17. Raffaeli W, Pari G, Visani L, Balestri M. Periduroscopy: preliminary reports—technical notes. The Pain Clinic. 1999;11(3):209-12.

47 CHAPTER

Spinal Cord Stimulation

Sanjay Bakshi, Gerard W Abrahamsen

ABSTRACT

Spinal cord stimulation (SCS) can be successfully used for many intractable pain conditions including angina, peripheral vascular disease, and chronic pain syndromes, such as failed back syndrome, complex regional pain syndrome (CRPS), phantom limb pain, and arachnoiditis. However, in the United States, the primary indications for SCS are failed back syndrome and CRPS. In contrast, in Europe, SCS is commonly used as treatment for chronic intractable angina and peripheral vascular disease. SCS is also being used for pelvic pain, urologic disorders, occipital neuralgia, and various other neuropathic pain conditions.

When considering SCS therapy, the patient should have exhausted all conservative treatment modalities. The patient should also not be a candidate for corrective surgery, which may alleviate the patient's symptoms. At this point, an SCS trial may be considered using a multidisciplinary approach including neuropsychological screening to ensure appropriate patient selection. Possible candidates for SCS therapy should also be reasonably intelligent to use the device, interpret the reduction of symptoms, and have good home support.

This chapter will discuss the indications, contraindications, and proper technique used in the placement of a spinal cord stimulator. We will also discuss new products available for SCS and provide updates on the new approaches of stimulation, including dorsal root ganglion stimulation, high-frequency stimulation, and burst stimulation.

INTRODUCTION

Chronic pain is often a difficult and costly condition to treat. In many cases, a patient's symptomatology will fail to improve with traditional treatment modalities, such as pharmacotherapy [non-steroidal anti-inflammatory drugs (NSAIDs) and neuropathic pain medications], physical therapy, chiropractic treatment, interventional spinal injections (epidural steroid injections, facet joint injections, sacroiliac joint blocks, stellate ganglion blocks, sympathetic blocks, etc.), and surgery. In these cases, treatment can be very frustrating for the clinician and patient and will often result in escalating doses of opioid pain medications. At this point in a patient's treatment plan, a clinician may consider modalities, such as spinal cord stimulation (SCS). SCS has shown to be very effective and has been used worldwide for the treatment of angina, peripheral vascular disease, epilepsy, and chronic pain syndromes, such as failed back syndrome, complex regional pain syndrome (CRPS), phantom limb pain, and arachnoiditis.[1-3]

Spinal cord stimulation therapy blocks neuropathic pain by applying electrical stimulation over the spinal cord. This modality is most successful at alleviating neuropathic appendicular pain, but studies have also shown resolution of neuropathic axial pain.[4] SCS was first introduced in 1967 by Norman Shealy and colleagues.[5] Rosenthal et al. reported on the clinical outcomes of SCS for axial back pain and radicular pain in a large sample of patients. 79 patients implanted with Boston Scientific Precision® at a single pain management clinic were contacted. 50 patients responded to the survey, 62% with primarily axial back pain and 38% with primarily radicular pain. It was determined that 61% with radicular pain reported pain relief in their limbs, 54% with axial back pain reported relief in their backs, and all patients reported reduced pain from baseline by 56%.[6]

MECHANISM OF ACTION

The mechanism of action of SCS still remains controversial. The most accepted mechanism is based on the gate control theory of pain published by Melzack and Wall in 1965.[7] This theory first proposed that painful "electrochemical" nociceptive information in the periphery is transmitted to the spinal cord in small diameter, unmyelinated C fibers and lightly myelinated A-δ fibers. These fibers terminate at the substantia gelatinosa of the dorsal horn, the gate of the spinal cord. Sensation, such as touch and vibration, is carried in large myelinated A-β fibers and also terminates at this gate in the spinal cord. Therefore, the basis of this theory is that reception of large fiber information, such as touch or vibration, would turn off or close the gate to reception of small fiber information, resulting in analgesia.[8] It has also been proposed that electrical stimulation may release putative neurotransmitters or neuromodulators, which affect prolonged pain relief.[9,10]

Stimulation is now being studied with a variety of new approaches and for new indications. This includes dorsal root ganglion (DRG) stimulation, high-frequency stimulation, and burst stimulation. DRG stimulation is being tested for its effectiveness in chronic pain. This approach can be considered when traditional SCS cannot achieve the desired distribution of stimulation or if the traditional SCS approach is providing unwanted stimulation. The DRG contains cell bodies of sensory neurons that bring information from the periphery to the spinal cord. This makes the DRG a prime target to achieve stimulation in the regions of the body that are often difficult to achieve with traditional SCS, such as axial back pain, groin pain, foot pain, CRPS of an extremity, foot pain, and chest wall pain. Schu et al. performed a retrospective review of SCS of the DRG for groin pain and concluded that neuromodulation of the DRG may be an effective treatment for chronic neuropathic pain conditions in the groin region. DRG stimulation also provided excellent cross-dermatomal paresthesia coverage in patients with discrete pain areas.[11] Deer et al. also performed a prospective study of DRG stimulation for the relief of chronic pain. They looked at 10 patients with chronic uncontrolled trunk and/or limb pain and also concluded that DRG stimulation can reduce uncontrolled chronic pain and may provide additional benefits over traditional SCS including better coverage in difficult-to-reach areas of stimulation, such as the back and feet.[12]

The mechanism of action of traditional SCS is mentioned earlier and uses a low-frequency state that produces paresthesia that is often mapped in the distribution of a patient's pain. Recent advances have led to the development of high-frequency stimulation to provide pain relief without the need for paresthesia. High-frequency SCS can be used to treat failed back surgery syndrome and patients with axial back pain. Clinical evidence obtained in a multicenter prospective fashion was positive and only supports the frequency at 10,000 kHz. Attempts at 5,000 kHz were no better than placebo.[13] Burst stimulation is also being studied as a new approach to provide closely spaced, high-frequency stimuli to the spinal cord to also produce pain relief without generating paresthesia. De Ridder et al. performed a randomized placebo-controlled trial looking at burst stimulation for limb and back pain. The authors concluded improvement in back, limb, and general pain over tonic stimulation.[14]

INDICATIONS

As mentioned earlier, SCS can be successfully used for many intractable pain conditions including:

- Angina
- Peripheral vascular disease
- Chronic pain syndromes, such as failed back syndrome, arachnoiditis, CRPS, phantom limb pain
- Vagus nerve stimulation for epilepsy
- Sacral nerve stimulation for overactive bladder
- Urinary retention not caused by obstruction
- Chronic bowel incontinence
- Nausea and vomiting associated with gastroparesis
- Deep brain stimulation for Parkinson's disease, essential tremor, dystonia, and obsessive-compulsive disorder.

However, in the United States, the primary indications for SCS are failed back syndrome[15] and CRPS.[16-20] In contrast, in Europe, SCS is commonly used as treatment for chronic intractable angina[21-23] and peripheral vascular disease. SCS is also being used for pelvic pain, urologic disorders, occipital neuralgia, and various other neuropathic pain conditions. When considering SCS therapy, the patient should have exhausted all conservative treatment modalities. The patient should also not be a candidate for corrective surgery which may alleviate the patients' symptoms. At this point, an SCS trial may be considered using a multidisciplinary approach including neuropsychological screening to ensure appropriate patient selection.[24] Possible candidates for SCS therapy should also be reasonably intelligent to use the device, interpret their reduction of symptoms, and have good home support.

CONTRAINDICATIONS

Neuropsychological clearance should rule out any underlying personality disorders, substance abuse, secondary gain issues, or unrealistic expectations from treatment that may alter the results from the trial. Other contraindications to SCS treatment include:

- Systemic infection
- Women who are pregnant or lactating
- Patients with a demand-type cardiac pacemaker
- Coagulopathy
- Patients who experience discomfort from the sensation of transcutaneous electrical nerve stimulation
- Individuals who fail to achieve <50% reduction of pain during trial stimulation.

After SCS has been implanted, magnetic resonance imaging (MRI) and diathermy are also contraindicated. However, Medtronic has a compatible device with MRI.

TRIAL STIMULATION

Prior to permanent implantation of SCS, all patients should undergo a trial. The most common trial method is a percutaneous trial, where leads are inserted into the epidural space percutaneously and left in for a period of a few days to a week. At the end of the trial period, the leads are removed in the office by pulling them out of the skin. Some people prefer to do the trial by securing the leads in place surgically and connecting them to a temporary extension that is externalized.

Some people also do an "on the table" trial. This trial addresses only the distribution of the stimulation pattern. It does not address the reduction of the patient's symptoms prior to permanent implantation of the device.

For this reason, this method is infrequently used and may result in a higher rate of implantation of the stimulator device. The patient should be assessed for a 50–70% reduction of the patient's typical pain, increase in the ability to perform activities of daily living, and possible reduction in patient's narcotic medication usage. Although SCS may reduce pain, it does not eliminate pain.[25-28] The benefit of an SCS trial is that the patient can experience the sensation of stimulation and assess the percentage of pain relief prior to surgical implantation.

SURGICAL IMPLANTATION

Following a successful trial, planning for surgical implantation of the leads and generator should begin. As with any surgical procedure, preoperative clearance and informed consent should be obtained. Prior to the procedure, the clinician should discuss with the patient a suitable implantation site for the pulse generator. It should be in a location that the patient would be able to reach with a remote to activate the device. Depending on operator and patient preference, the pulse generator or battery can be implanted in the flank, lower abdominal wall, or buttocks. Poorly placed pulse generators can lead to discomfort at the internal pulse generator (IPG) site which may require surgical revision.

The clinician will also need to decide whether to use a laminotomy or percutaneous lead. The other decision to be made is whether to have a standard or rechargeable battery.

EQUIPMENT

Currently, the three major manufacturers of SCS devices in the United States are Medtronics Inc., Advanced Neuromodulation Systems (ANS), and Boston Scientific. The actual device should be decided on a case-by-case basis to suit an individual patient's needs. The basic components of the system are the lead and the battery. The leads are percutaneous and laminotomy leads **(Figs. 1 and 2)**.

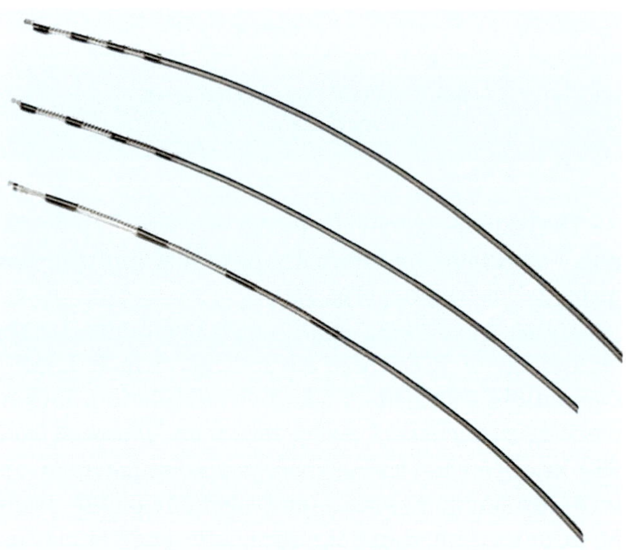

Fig. 1: Different types of percutaneous leads.
Source: Medtronic, USA.

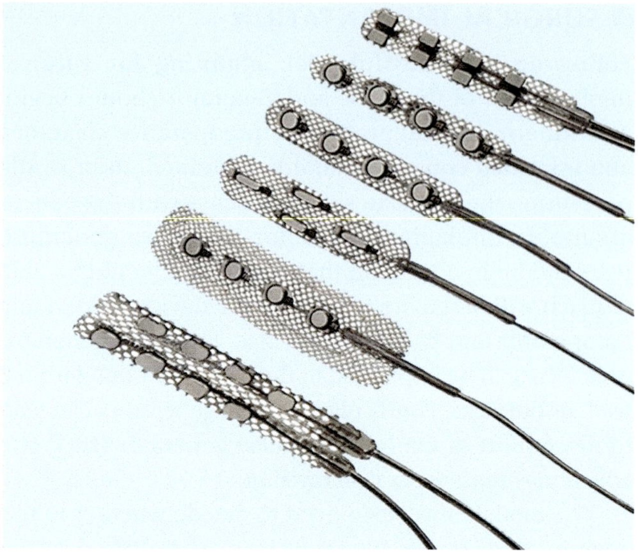

Fig. 2: Different types of laminotomy leads.
Source: Medtronic, USA.

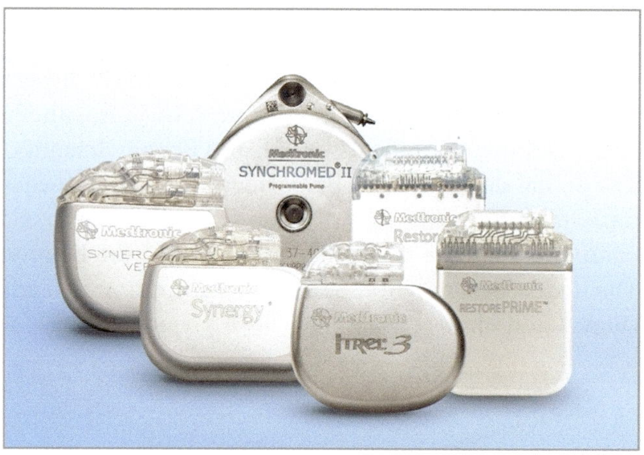

Fig. 3: Different types of batteries.
Source: Medtronic, USA.

The batteries are radiofrequency or externally powered, pulse generator or internally powered, and the new rechargeable batteries **(Fig. 3)**.

There have been many advancements in the technology of SCS. These advancements include MRI-compatible stimulators, adaptive stimulation, locking mechanical anchors to reduce migration, improved leads with more contacts for better programming, percutaneous lead introduction sheaths, and steerable paddle leads. Medtronics Sure Scan neurostimulator and Vectris Sure Scan leads allow patients to safely undergo an MRI without worrying about the previous complications of lead heating, device damage, unintentional stimulation, and magnetic pulling.[29,30] Accelerometer additions, such as Medtronic.

Adaptive Stim, reduce stimulation changes with changes in the patient's body positions. Using technology similar to that used in smartphones, the device can now detect if you are standing or lying down and can automatically change the stimulation settings to your last comfortable setting by either sitting, lying, standing, or being active.[31]

The Epiducer lead introduction system by St. Jude Medical (SJM) allows for the introduction of multiple lead arrays as well as steerable paddle leads through a single percutaneous entry point. The SJM steerable percutaneous paddle leads are placed through the Epiducer and permits the placement of a paddle lead without a laminotomy. The benefits of a paddle lead include unidirectional stimulation, delivery of focused energy resulting in better battery longevity, decreased longitudinal and lateral migration, and avoidance of uncomfortable stimulation of the ligamentum flavum.[32] The device by Boston Scientific has electrode with 16 contacts.

PROCEDURE

Step 1: Trial Stimulation

Most often, the trial is done percutaneously and this technique will be discussed here. The procedure described here is for placement of leads in the thoracic epidural space for treatment of back and leg pain. The patient lies on the table in the prone position with a pillow placed under the abdomen. Mild sedation is used for the procedure. The procedure may be performed in a fluoroscopy suite or an operating room setting. Strict aseptic techniques are used. Antibiotics are given prophylactically before the procedure. Initially, fluoroscopy is used to count the levels. The author usually places a spinal needle across T10, so it serves as a landmark and you do not need to recount which level you are at. You can also make markings on the skin with a marking pen. The entire procedure is done using fluoroscopy. Needle entry is usually at the T12-L1 level or L1-L2 level. Note that the angle of entry is much more shallow than a regular epidural. This makes it easier to thread the lead in the epidural space. It is preferable to first hit the lamina below to get an idea of depth. The needle is then walked off the lamina into the interlaminar space. Epidural space is identified using the loss-of-resistance technique. Once the epidural space is identified, the lead is inserted and threaded up to the T8 level. At this point, you should check a lateral view to make sure that the lead is in the posterior epidural space. Sequential trialing is then done to check at which level the patient gets appropriate coverage of the painful area. Depending on the patient's pain distribution, either one or two leads may be used. It is critical that the patient should not be too sedated, otherwise he/she will not be able to give you adequate feedback about his/her stimulation pattern if it is appropriately covering their area of pain. Once you are satisfied that there is good overlap between the patient's painful area and stimulation pattern, the needle is removed, with the lead left in place. After removal of the needle, make sure that the lead has not moved. This is done by comparing it with the previous fluoroscopy picture. The lead is then fixed to the skin and sterile dressing is applied. Hard copies of the fluoroscopy films are saved for later reference during permanent implantation.

At this stage, the patient can be discharged home for an extended trial or admitted for an inpatient trial depending on the operator's preference and the patient's medical condition. If the patient is being discharged home, it is advisable to observe the patient for a few hours after the procedure to make sure that they do not develop any neurological deficits. Antibiotics are prescribed for the entire period that the leads remain in the patient during the trial. After the trial, the leads can be removed right in the doctor's office. If the patient reports >50% relief of pain and has improved activities of daily living during the trial period, then they are considered appropriate candidates for a permanent implantation. Ideally, they should use less pain medications during the trial period but that is not an absolute requirement for the trial to be considered successful **(Figs. 4 to 9)**.

Postprocedure Care following Surgical Implantation

Following surgical implantation, routine incision management and suture removal should be followed. Typically, the SCS is activated following removal of sutures. The patient should also refrain from any strenuous activity or reaching above the head until approximately 6 weeks. At this time, the system is said to have matured, forming a fibrous capsule around the implant. The patient should also have a thorough explanation on how to use the device. In some cases, the patient will have multiple programs and will require different degrees of stimulation throughout the day to achieve pain reduction.

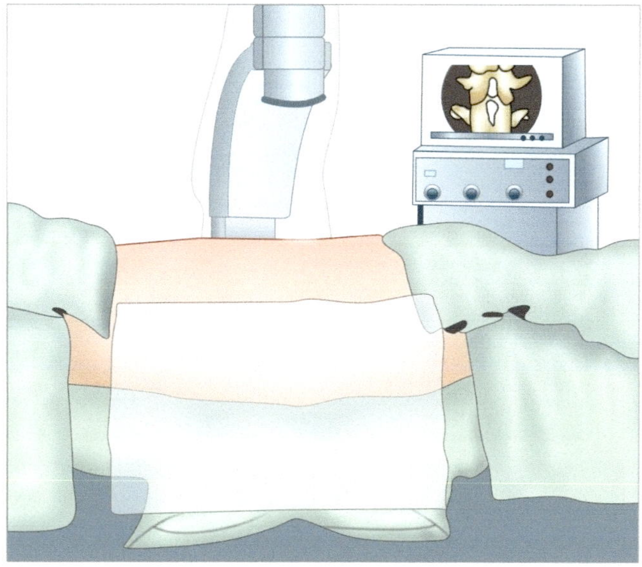

Fig. 4: Initial position of patient.
Source: Medtronic, USA.

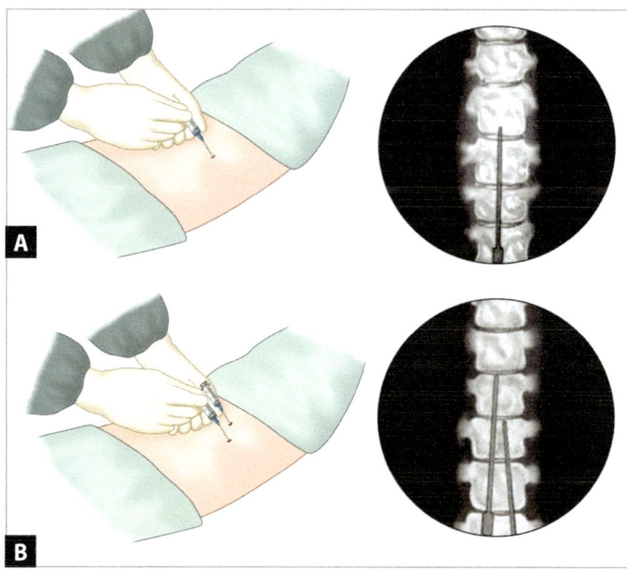

Figs. 5A and B: Needle entry percutaneous approach.

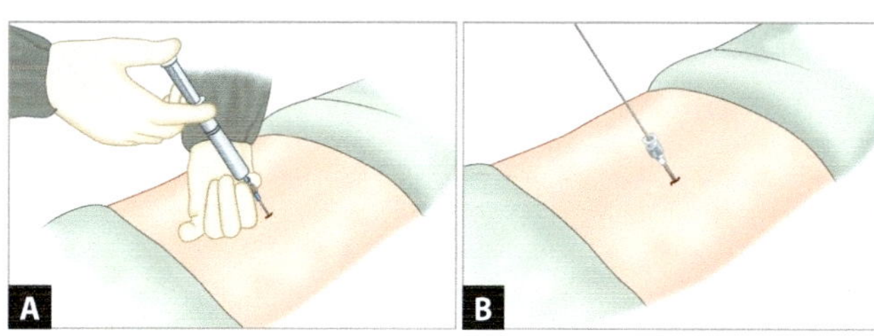

Figs. 6A and B: Loss-of-resistance technique.
Source: Medtronic, USA.

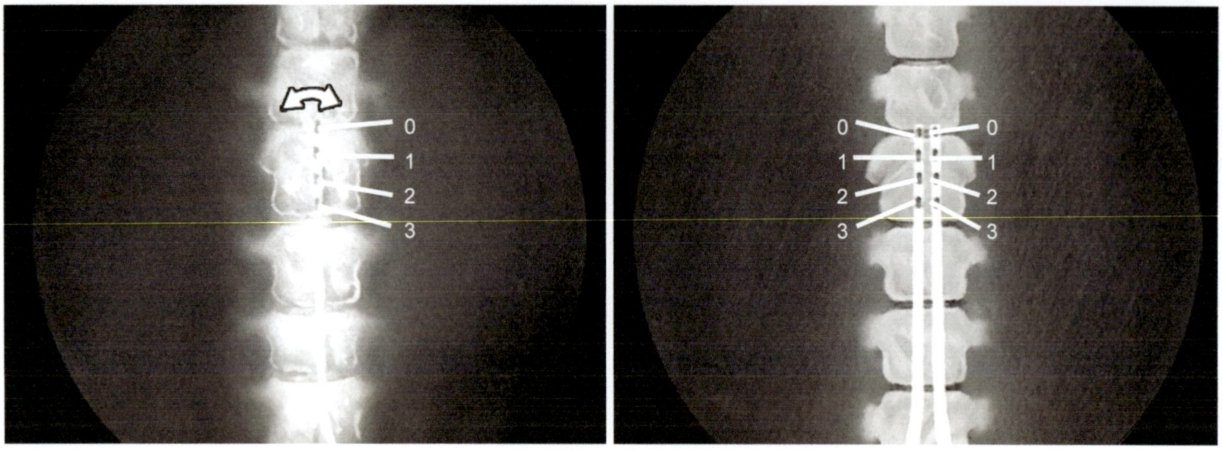

Fig. 7: Fluoroscopic view of lead position.
Source: Medtronic, USA.

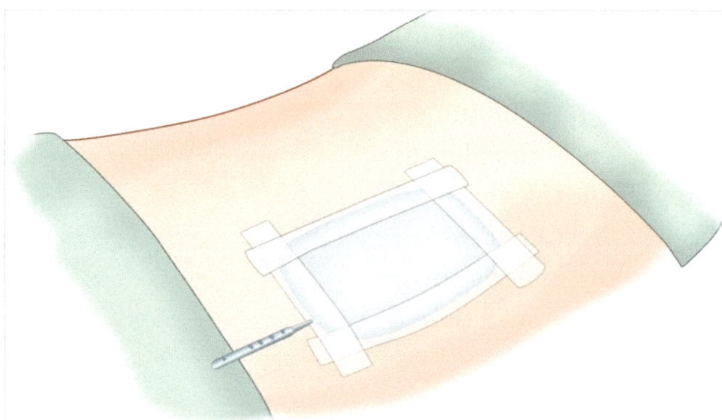

Fig. 8: Sterile dressing applied at the end of the procedure.
Source: Medtronic, USA.

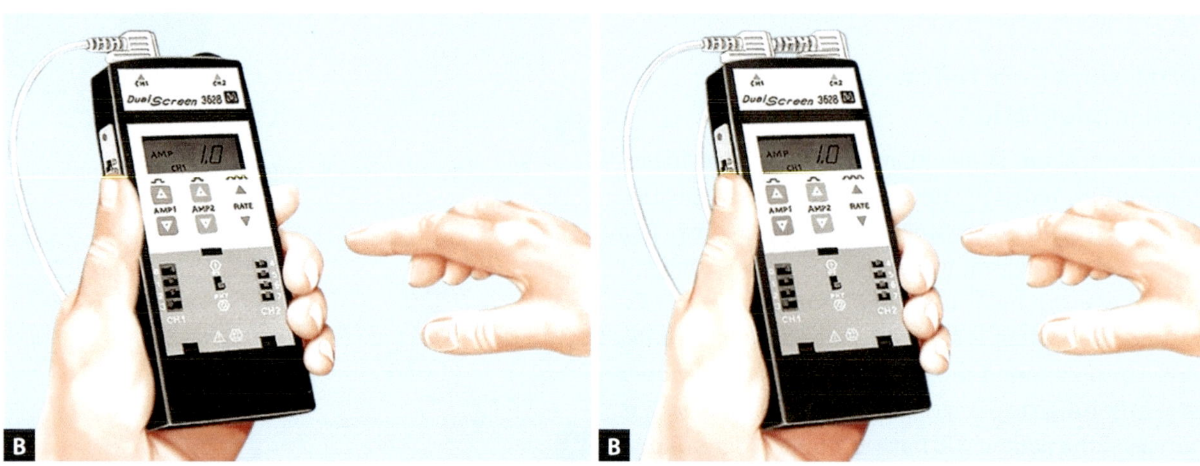

Figs. 9A and B: Programmer to check stimulation pattern.
Source: Medtronic, USA.

STEP 2: PERMANENT IMPLANTATION

Once the patient is felt to be a successful candidate depending on the trial, the permanent implantation is performed. Prior to the procedure, the implanting physician needs to have a detailed discussion with the patient about which type of battery would be appropriate and the preferred site of implantation of the battery. The battery can be inserted in the flank, upper abdominal wall, or the buttocks. On the day of the procedure, the battery site should be marked out in the holding area prior to the procedure. On the operating table, the patient is positioned in the prone position. Initial steps are exactly the same as for the trial. Once the leads are in place, and the patient has appropriate coverage similar to or better than the trial, an incision is made around the lead and dissected down to the supraspinous ligament. The lead is now anchored to the supraspinous ligament. This is probably the most important part of the procedure since the most common complication is movement of the leads. Therefore, the leads need to be carefully secured to the supraspinous ligament. The next step is the preparation of the pocket for the battery. The pocket is created so that there is adequate space for the battery as well as any excess lead or extension which needs to be tucked behind the battery. A radiofrequency generator should be generated no deeper than 1 cm below the skin, whereas a pulse generator is placed deeper, but no deeper than 1 inch below skin. Once the pocket is created, tunneling is done between the pocket and the lead site, and the system is connected between the lead and the battery, either via an extension or directly to the battery itself. The entire system is checked at this point. If appropriate coverage is still present, the incisions are both closed in layers. The patient is usually discharged home the same day or the next day **(Figs. 10 to 18)**.

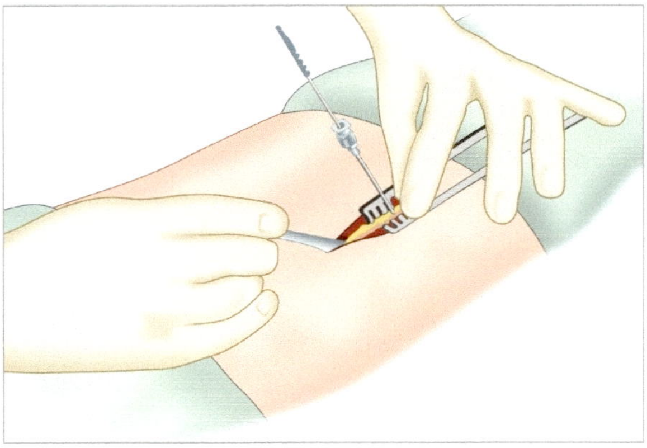

Fig. 10: Incision around needle.
Source: Medtronic, USA.

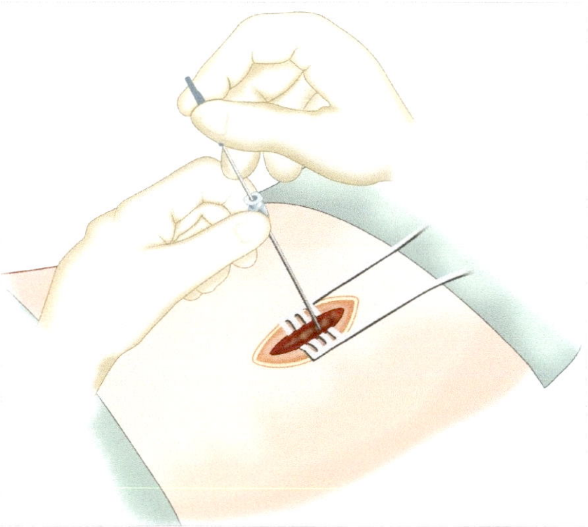

Fig. 11: Needle removed—lead left in place.
Source: Medtronic, USA.

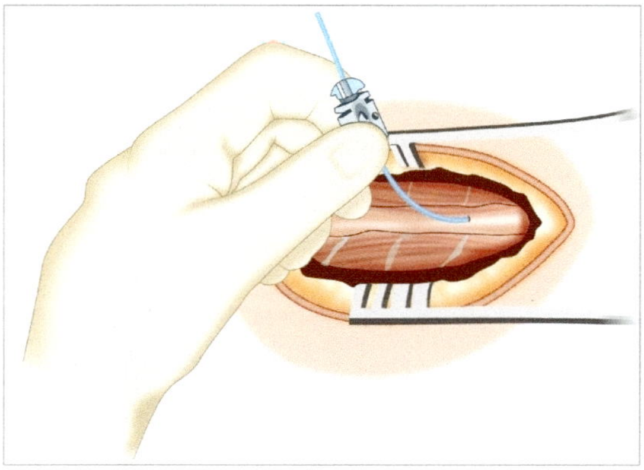

Fig. 12: Anchor being threaded in.
Source: Medtronic, USA.

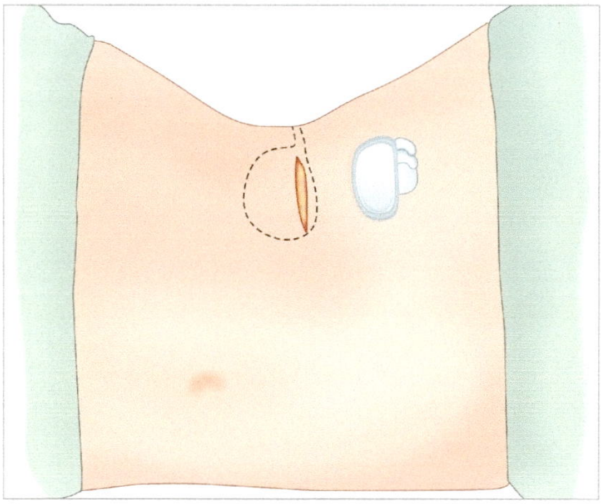

Fig. 13: Pocket created for battery.
Source: Medtronic, USA.

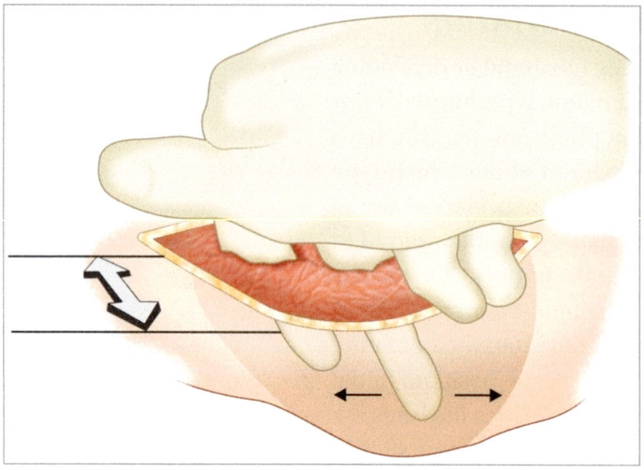

Fig. 14: Pocket being prepared for battery.
Source: Medtronic, USA.

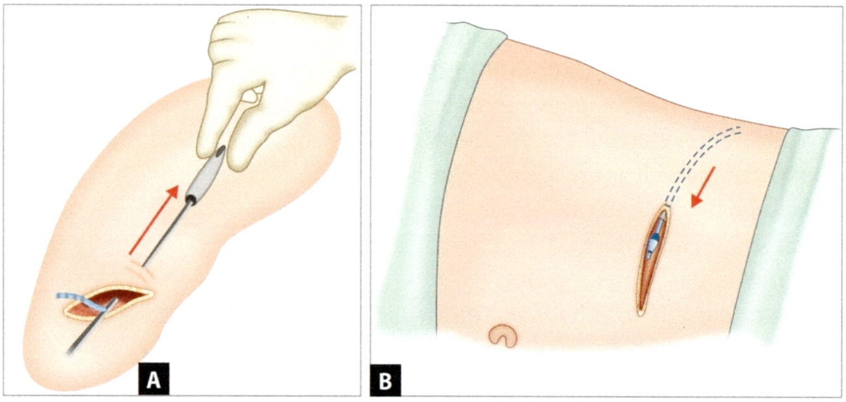

Figs. 15A and B: Tunneling between lead and battery site.

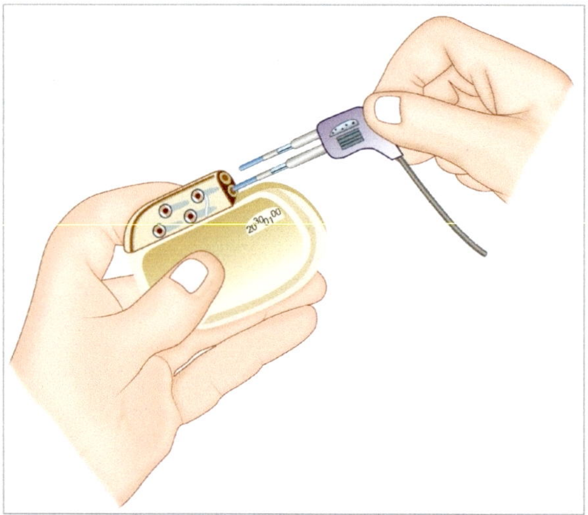

Fig. 16: Battery being connected.
Source: Medtronic, USA.

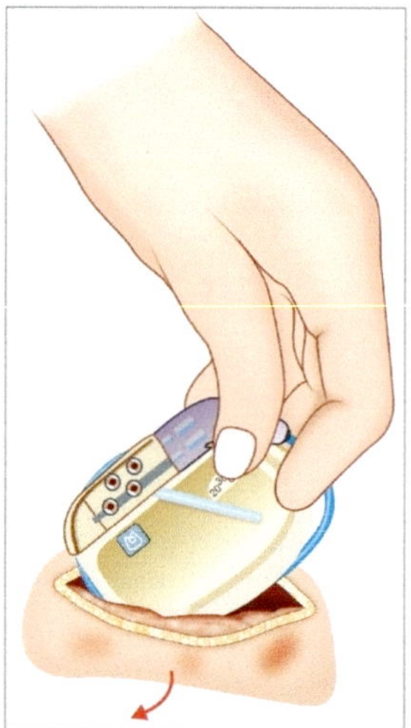

Fig. 17: Battery being placed into pocket.
Source: Medtronic, USA.

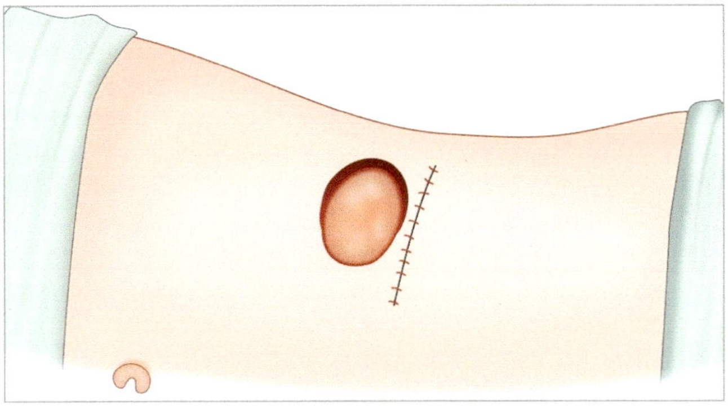

Fig. 18: Incision closed in layers.

COMPLICATIONS

Potential complications following SCS implantation include:

- Epidural hematoma
- Dural puncture headache
- Infection (including meningitis, epidural abscess)
- Lead migration
- Pocket seroma
- Stitch abscess
- Equipment failure.

The most serious complications are epidural hematoma and epidural abscess. Clinically, they are very rare and can be minimized by meticulous surgical technique and ensuring that the patients are not on any anticoagulation medication.

Dural puncture headache will typically resolve on its own; however, some patients may require an epidural blood patch for symptomatic relief.

If a dural puncture headache occurs during an SCS trial, it is recommended to abort the trial until resolution of the symptoms because the results of the trial may not be as accurate. Pocket seroma is an unlikely complication. This may require drainage if the seroma is severe or infected. Lead migration is the most common complication following SCS implantation. When a lead migrates, the patient will experience a change or complete loss of stimulation. Patients should be informed of the complication and the possibility of further surgical exploration to correct lead positioning.

Any part of the SCS system can fail at any point. Battery life is the most frequent issue. Numerous variables will affect the duration of battery life. These variables include the hours of use per day, the number of active electrodes, and program settings including amplitude, pulse width, and frequency. Newer pulse generators now have a rechargeable battery option, which may be considered in patients whose settings require more demand on the battery. However, patients should be informed that the rechargeable battery will also require replacement at some point.

CONCLUSION

Spinal cord stimulation can be a very valuable tool in the management of a wide variety of intractable chronic pain syndromes. It should be considered only when conservative measures have been exhausted and surgery is not a viable option. The success rate of this treatment modality can be high if performed with a multidisciplinary approach, in an appropriate candidate, using meticulous surgical technique, and with long-term follow-up.

REFERENCES

1. Vulink NC, Overgaauw DM, Jessurun GA, Tenvaarwerk IA, Kropmans TJ, van der Schans CP, et al. The effects of spinal cord stimulation on quality of life in patients with therapeutically chronic refractory angina pectoris. Neuromodulation. 1999;2(1):33-40.
2. Claeys LG. Spinal cord stimulation and chronic critical limb ischemia. Neuromodulation. 1999;2:1-3.
3. Kumar K, Toth C, Nath RK, Laing P. Epidural spinal cord stimulation for treatment of chronic pain--some predictors of success. A 15-year experience. Surg Neurol. 1998; 50(2): 110-21.
4. Law JD. Spinal stimulation: statistical superiority of monophasic stimulation of narrowly separated, longitudinal bipoles having rostral cathodes. Appl Neurophysiol. 1983; 46(1-4):129-37.
5. Shealy CN, Mortimer JT, Reswick JB. Electrical inhibition of pain by stimulation of the dorsal columns: preliminary clinical report. Anesth Analg. 1967;46:489-91.
6. Rosenthal RM, Foster A. Axial Back Pain Relief and Patient Satisfaction Profiles with Spinal Cord Stimulation (SCS): 50-Patient Series. Presented at the 2008 Annual Meeting of the American Academy of Pain Medicine (AAPM).
7. Melzack R, Wall PD. Pain mechanisms: a new theory. Science. 1965;150(3699):971-9.
8. Krames ES. Neuroaugmentation. Mechanisms of action of spinal cord stimulation. Intervention Pain Management, 2nd edition. 2001;53;561-5.
9. Levin BE, Hubschmann OR. Dorsal column stimulation: effect of human cerebrospinal fluid and plasma catecholamines. Neurology. 1980;30:65-71.
10. Meyerson BA, Brodin E, Linderoth B. Possible neuro-humoral mechanisms in CNS stimulation for pain suppression. Appl Neurophysiol. 1985;48:175-80.

11. Schu S, Gulve A, ElDabe S, Baranidharan G, Wolf K, Demmel W, et al. Spinal cord stimulation of the dorsal root ganglion for groin pain - a retrospective review. Pain Pract. 2015;15(4):293-9.
12. Deer TR, Grigsby E, Weiner RL, Wilcosky B, Kramer JM. A prospective study of dorsal root ganglion stimulation in the relief of chronic pain. Neuromodulation. 2013;16(1): 67-72.
13. Van Buyten JP, Al-Kaisy A, Smet I, Palmisani S, Smith T. High-frequency spinal cord stimulation for the treatment of chronic back pain patients: results of a prospective multicenter European clinical study. Neuromodulation. 2013;16(1):59-66.
14. De Ridder D, Plazier M, Kamerling N, Menovsky T, Vanneste S. Burst spinal cord stimulation for limb and back pain. World Neurosurg. 2013;80(5):642-9.e1.
15. North RB, Ewend MG, Lawton MT, Piantadosi S. Spinal cord stimulation for chronic, intractable pain: superiority of "multi-channel" devices. Pain. 1991;44(2):119-30.
16. Oakley JC, Weiner RL. Spinal cord stimulation for complex regional pain syndrome: a prospective study of 19 patients at two centers. Neuromodulation. 1999;2(1):47-50.
17. Bennett DS, Aló KM, Oakley J, Feler CA. Spinal cord stimulation for complex regional pain syndrome I [RSD]: a retrospective multicenter experience from 1995 to 1998 of 101 patients. Neuromodulation. 1999;2(3):202-10.
18. Broseta J, Roldan P, Gonzalez-Darder J, Bordes V, Barcia-Salorio JL. Chronic epidural dorsal column stimulation in the treatment of causalgic pain. Appl Neurophysiol. 1982;45(1-2):190-4.
19. Barolat G, Schwartzman R, Woo R. Epidural spinal cord stimulation in the management of reflex sympathetic dystrophy. Stereotact Funct Neurosurg. 1989;53(1): 29-39.
20. Stanton-Hicks M. Spinal cord stimulation for the management of complex regional pain syndromes. Neuromodulation. 1999;2(3):193-201.
21. Mannheimer C, Augustinsson LE, Carlsson CA, Manhem K, Wilhelmsson C. Epidural spinal electrical stimulation in severe angina pectoris. Br Heart J. 1998;59(1):56-61.
22. Augustinsson LE. Spinal cord electrical stimulation in severe angina pectoris: surgical technique, intraoperative physiology, complications, and side effects. Pacing Clin Electrophysiol. 1989;12(4 Pt 2):693-4.
23. Murphy DF, Giles KE. Dorsal column stimulation for pain relief from intractable angina pectoris. Pain. 1987; 28(3):365-8.
24. Olson KO, Bedder MD, Anderson VC, Burchiel KJ, Villanueva MR. Psychological variables associated with outcome of spinal cord stimulation trails. Neuromodulation. 1998;1(1):6-13.
25. North RB, Ewend MG, Lawton MT, Kidd DH, Piantadosi S. Failed back syndrome: 5-year follow-up after spinal cord stimulator implantation. Neurosurgery. 1991;28(5):692-9.
26. Kumar K, Nath R, Wyant GM. Treatment of chronic pain by epidural spinal cord stimulation: a 10-year experience. J Neurosurg. 1991;75(3):402-7.
27. Racz GB, McCarron RF, Talboys P. Percutaneous dorsal column stimulator for chronic pain control. Spine (Phila Pa 1976). 1989;14(1):1-4.
28. North RB, Kidd DH, Zahurak M, James CS, Long DM. Spinal cord stimulation for chronic, intractable pain: experience over two decades. Neurosurgery. 1993;32(3):384-95.
29. Risk Management Report for Sure Scan (MRI compatible) Implantable Neurostimulation System and 1×8 Vectris Percutaneous Leads. NDHF1173— 126742.
30. MRI Standard Letter. Spinal Cord Stimulation Systems. 2011.
31. Medtronic advanced pain therapy using neurostimulation for chronic pain. Clinical Summary. 2011;M221494A006.
32. North RB, Kidd DH, Olin JC, Sieracki JM. Spinal cord stimulation electrode design: prospective, randomized, controlled trial comparing percutaneous and laminectomy electrodes-part I: technical outcomes. Neurosurgery. 2002;51(2):381-90.

48 CHAPTER

Diskography

Eric Lee, Corey Hunter, Sudhir Diwan

ABSTRACT

This chapter identifies possible benefits of diskogram as a tool to diagnose pain generators. The diskogram highlights indications and contraindications in order to perform disk procedure and to know the source of pain and perform the diskectomy. It further gives recommendations in how to perform the procedure at various levels in the spinal column, including cervical, thoracic, and lumbar levels, and also reviews possible side effects and complications that may occur when performing the procedure to make practitioners aware of the importance of evaluating the risk benefit of any intervention.

INTRODUCTION

The challenge in identifying the extent to which structures contribute to low back pain has always been one of great importance to the pain physician.[1] One structure that may play an integral role in low back pain is the intervertebral disk. In addition to history, physical examination, and imaging studies, interventional physicians have been trying to utilize tests that further evaluate both anatomical and functional information about a disk.[2]

Provocative diskography is the term applied for the procedure to reproduce diskogenic pain by injecting contrast into the nucleus pulposus of the disk. The pain is reproduced by two ways—first, by chemical irritation of sensitive tissue and second, by increasing the intradiskal pressure due to volume and stretching the annular fibers of the disk.

Diskography helps to evaluate disk morphology and confirms the diagnosis for consideration of various surgical treatments.[3] It also helps to confirm normal disks.

WHY DO INTERVERTEBRAL DISKS CAUSE PAIN?

In the cervical region, disk pain is transmitted through sensory nerves that innervate the disk.[4] In the lumbar spine, it is believed that only the outer third of the annulus fibrosus has sensory nerve supply; however, in damaged or degenerated disks, the innervation fibers spread into the nucleus pulposus.[5,6] This leads to growth of sensory fibers into the inner third with neovascularization and neural expression inflammatory factors, such as substance P, interleukin (IL)-6, IL-8,[7] and C-reactive protein.[8] These changes in nerve fibers play an important role in the pathogenesis of diskogenic low back pain.

At least one-third of patients with chronic low back pain have internal disk derangement (IDD). Disk degeneration is a progressive condition that gradually involves the entire nucleus and spreads radially to the annulus. IDD can happen with an intact annulus. Imaging, such as computed tomography (CT) and magnetic resonance imaging (MRI), may help identify IDD; however, it cannot identify if one of these disks is painful.[9] Therefore, diskography is the gold standard to determine IDD and if that disk is painful.

- To confirm the source of pain in patients with a documented disk bulge.
- As a preoperative procedure to confirm the vertebral level for spinal fusion and if adjacent disks can support a fusion.[10]
- Diskography may help to distinguish the source of pain either from the disk or from the scar tissue in postsurgical patients.
- In patients, who are status postsurgery, who continue to have persistent pain, diskography can be used to see whether or not the disks adjacent to the fusion are the source of the patient's symptoms.

- Assessment of candidates for minimally invasive surgery who have confirmed disk herniation. To determine if other treatment modalities, e.g., intradiskal electrothermal therapy, nucleoplasty, and chemonucleolysis, would be of benefit for the patient's pain.
- Persistent pain where other diagnostic tests have failed to confirm disk as a source of pain.

CONTRAINDICATIONS

- Patients unable to understand the procedure and unwilling to provide informed consent including psychiatric condition that contributes to this
- Systemic infection or localized infection at the site of procedure to be performed
- Patients with known bleeding disorder or on anticoagulation therapy
- Allergy to contrast medium
- Significant myelopathic changes due to risk of aggravation of myelopathy
- Pregnancy
- Solid bone fusion preventing access to disk
- Severe spinal canal compromise at disk level of interest.

CERVICAL DISKOGRAPHY

Anatomy of Cervical Spine (Figs. 1A and B)

- Cervical disks have certain characteristics distinct from other parts of the spine.
- Radicular pain originating exclusively from cervical disk herniation is much less common than in the lumbar region.
- The posterior longitudinal ligament in the cervical region is thicker, with a double layer, enclosing the posterior and lateral parts of the disk, while it is a much thinner, single layer, with weaker lateral protection in the lumbar area.
- The facet joints **(Fig. 2)** protect the cervical nerve roots from impingement by interposing a bony wall between the disk and the nerve root.
- The nuclear material of the cervical disk lies more anterior than it does in the lumbar spine; therefore, posterior displacement is less likely to occur unless great forces are applied on the disk.
- The outer annulus is substantially thicker in the posterior portion of the cervical disk, which reduces the disk's ability to bulge posteriorly.
- Treatment of cervical diskogenic pain has been difficult because the disk receives sensory input from various different sources,[11] and there is no clear consensus which among them is responsible for pain, although there are several studies attempting to elucidate this further.[12]
- The anterior aspect of the disk receives sensory innervation from the sympathetic chain and the posterior aspect receives innervation from the sinuvertebral nerves. It is thought that these nerves provide innervation to the facet joints as well.[13]

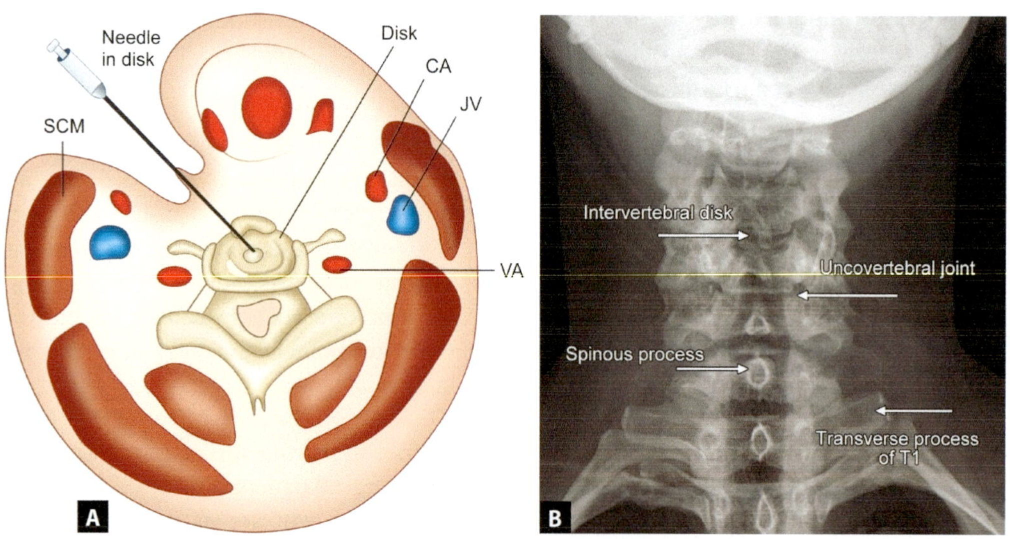

Figs. 1A and B: (A) Diagrammatic representation of the technique for the anterior approach to the cervical disk; (B) Fluoroscopic anatomy of cervical spine.
(CA: carotid artery; JV: jugular vein; SCM: sternocleidomastoid muscle; VA: vertebral artery)

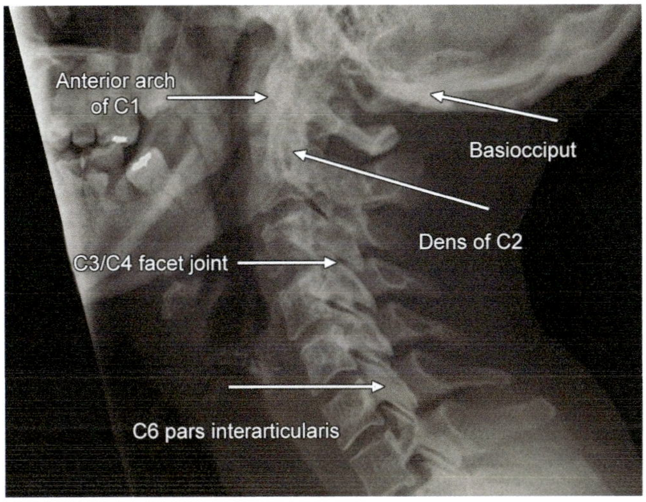

Fig. 2: Cervical facet joints anatomy.

Indications of Cervical Diskography

There are several indications for performing cervical diskography. The primary goal of this procedure is to identify a painful cervical disk as well as display internal derangements.[14]

- In surgical naïve patients, cervical diskography is used to determine the source of pain in patients with documented evidence of a disk bulge on modern imaging studies, such as MRI or CT scan.[15]
- Diskography may be used to reproduce pain in patients with persistent radicular pain where imaging studies may not show any significant anatomical abnormalities.
- Cervical diskography can also be used as part of the preoperative workup for patients who are candidates for cervical fusion. It helps to determine the level of fusion by finding the disk that is most symptomatic.
- Cervical diskography can also be used to distinguish whether the etiology of a patient's pain is from a disk herniation or a scar tissue.

Technique for Cervical Diskography

Fluoroscopic suite or operating room with C-arm fluoroscope is mandatory to perform the diskogram at any level.[16] The C-arm is rotated to 20–25° obliquely and angled either cephalad or caudad to align the vertebral endplates of the intervertebral disk space.

- Prophylactic antibiotics should be considered, such as cefazolin 1 g intravenously within 1 hour before the procedure or clindamycin 600 mg intravenously 1 hour before the procedure (if allergic to cephalosporin or penicillin).[17]
- The patient is placed in the supine position with the neck in the neutral position.
- The right side of the neck is preferred due to the leftward orientation of the esophagus at this level. The neck is prepped and draped in the normal sterile fashion.
- Important structures must be noted at this level including the trachea, carotid artery, jugular vein, and esophagus.
- The medial border of the sternocleidomastoid muscle is palpated and local anesthetic is injected subcutaneously at the chosen level of cervical disk.
- A 25G, 3.5-inch styletted needle is placed through the skin and advanced to the middle of the disk in question **(Figs. 3A and B)**.
- The needle is advanced incrementally with imaging. If a paresthesia is elicited, the needle should be withdrawn and then readvanced cephalad toward the middle of the disk.
- Once the disk is contacted, the needle is advanced incrementally under lateral view of the C-arm until the middle of the disk is penetrated. Imaging is performed in order to avoid exiting the back of the disk into either the spinal canal or the pleura.
- 0.3 mL of contrast is injected with careful attention being paid to resistance to injection, patient's response, and whether or not pressure is maintained or dissipated in the disk via manometry.[16]
- The diskogram in anteroposterior and lateral views **(Figs. 4A and B)** should be evaluated for the integrity of the disk, and a decision should be made whether the adjacent disk needs to be studied or whether local anesthetic should be injected in the disk of question.
- The decision to inject local anesthetic into the disk space can give erroneous information if adjacent disks are to be evaluated. The local anesthetic can possibly track in the epidural space or can anesthetize some of the nerves that provide sensory input to the adjacent disks.

Imaging Details with X-ray

- The images of the injected disk should be evaluated to see whether or not the disk and its components are intact.
- The condition of the disk will determine where the contrast will collect.
- A normal disk will appear as a lobulated mass with some posterolateral clefts due to the normal aging process of the disk.

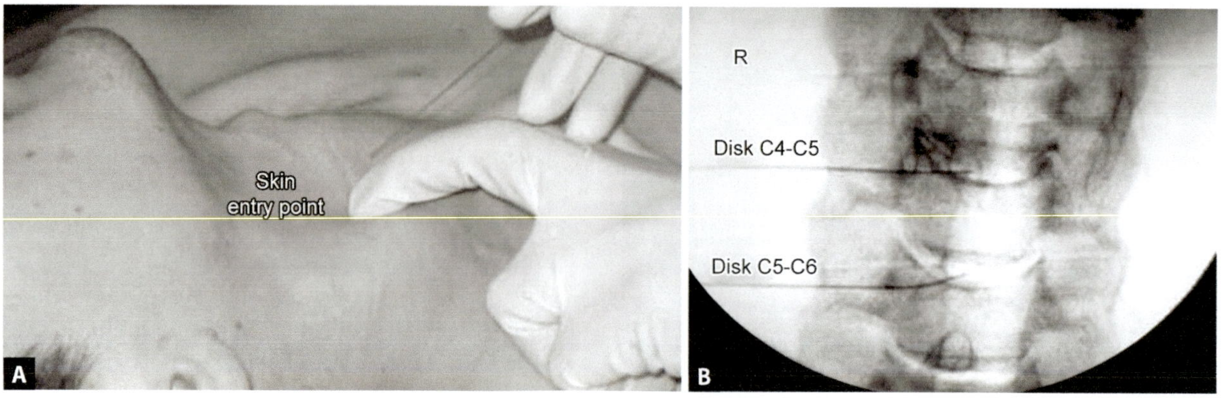

Figs. 3A and B: (A) Skin entry point cervical disk; (B) Needle entry in cervical disk.

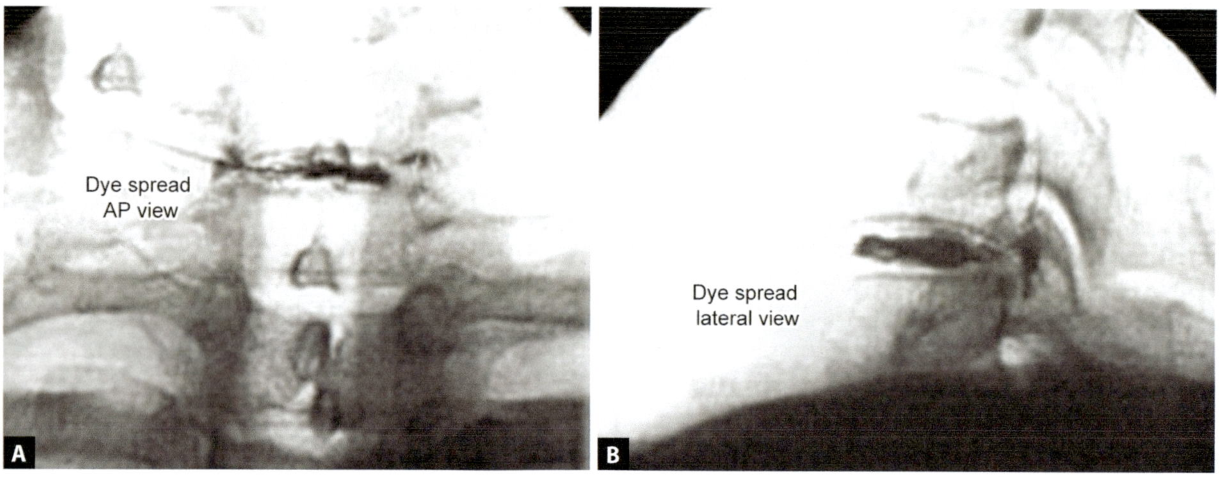

Figs. 4A and B: Cervical diskogram dye spread: anteroposterior (AP) and lateral views.

- If the inner annulus is torn, a transverse pattern of contrast will show on the nucleogram or if the tears of the annulus extend to the outer layer, a radial pattern will be noted.
- It is also possible for the contrast to flow into the epidural space or the endplate of the vertebra if the annulus is completely disrupted.
- In certain situations, the injected contrast may flow between the layers of the annulus.

THORACIC DISKOGRAM

Anatomy of Thoracic Spine (Fig. 5)

- Thoracic disks are located between the cartilaginous end plates of the vertebrae above and below it.
- The disk of the thoracic spine is characterized by a thick fibroelastic annulus that surrounds a gelatinous nucleus pulposus.

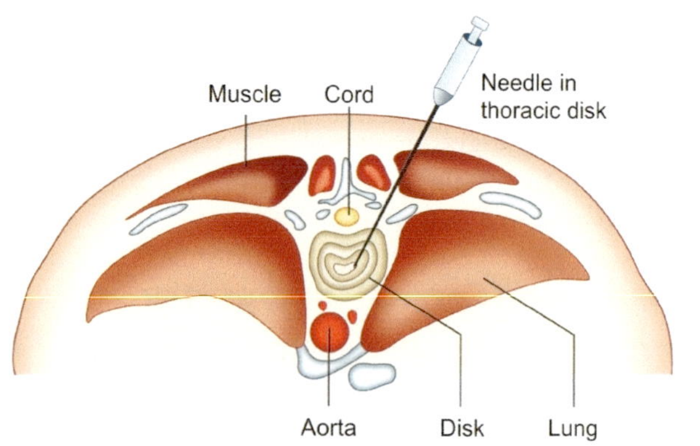

Fig. 5: Diagrammatic anatomy of thoracic disk with needle in disk.

- These annular fibers run in an oblique direction from adjacent vertebrae.
- These annular fibers receive sensory input from various sources including sinuvertebral nerves (posteriorly) and the sympathetic chain (anteriorly).

- Nerve roots leave laterally through the intervertebral foramina.
- The disk can impinge the nerve roots if herniated laterally.
- The disk can impinge the spinal cord if herniated posterolaterally.

Indications for Thoracic Diskography

- Often most useful in determining the source of pain but performed the least due to least likelihood of a thoracic disk to herniate.
- Patients with pain in whom testing has been normal or unrevealing.
- In postsurgical patients with persistent pain, one may want to differentiate scar tissue from disk tissue or evaluate the disks adjacent to a fusion.
- In presurgical candidates, diskography may be used to further evaluate the levels to be fused.

Technique for Thoracic Diskography

Prophylactic antibiotics should be considered, such as cefazolin 1 g intravenously within 1 hour before the procedure or clindamycin 600 mg intravenously 1 hour before the procedure (if allergic to cephalosporin or penicillin).[15]

- Patient is placed in prone position with a pillow under the lower chest in order to flex the spine.
- If CT is being used, make careful note of pleura, lung, ribs, nerve roots, and spinal cord.
- The spinous process above the disk of question is located and the skin 1.5 inches laterally on either side is prepped, draped, and anesthetized.
- A 22G, 3.5-inch styletted needle is placed through the skin and advanced to the middle of the disk of question.
- The needle is advanced incrementally with imaging. If a paresthesia is elicited, the needle should be withdrawn and then redirected and advanced more cephalad toward the middle of the disk.
- Once the disk is contacted, the needle is advanced incrementally until the middle of the disk is penetrated. Imaging is performed in order to avoid penetration of the back of the disk either into the spinal canal or into the pleura.
- Similar to the cervical diskogram, 0.3 mL of contrast suitable for intrathecal use is injected with careful attention being paid to resistance to injection, patient's response, and whether or not a pressure is maintained or dissipated in the disk via manometry.
- Take note also of the amount of contrast injected, volume at which the patient experienced pain, pressure at which the patient experienced pressure or pain, and pain response (location, character, distribution, intensity, and concordance with chronic pain)
- The diskogram needs to be evaluated to check the integrity of the disk, and a decision needs to be made if there is a need to evaluate the adjacent disk spaces or to inject local anesthetic in the disk of question.
- The decision to inject local anesthetic into this disk space can give erroneous information if the adjacent disks are to be evaluated. The local anesthetic can possibly track epidurally or can anesthetize some of the nerves that provide sensory input to the adjacent disks.

Imaging Details with X-ray

- The images of the injected disk need to be evaluated to see whether or not the disk and its components are intact.
- The spread of the contrast will determine the condition of the disk.
- A normal disk will appear as a lobulated mass with some posterolateral clefts due to the normal aging process of the disk.
- If the inner annulus is torn, a transverse pattern of contrast will show on the nucleogram or if the tears of the annulus extend to the outer layer, a radial pattern will be noted.
- It is also possible for the contrast to flow into the epidural space or the end plate of the vertebra if the annulus is completely disrupted.
- In certain situations, the injected contrast may flow between the layers of the annulus.

LUMBAR DISKOGRAPHY

Anatomy of Lumbar Spine

- Radicular pain of diskogenic origin is much more common in the lumbar region than any other region.
- Unlike the cervical region, the bony facets do not protect the nerve roots.
- The posterior longitudinal ligament of the lumbar spine is thinner and less protective. This is especially true in the lateral aspects of the spine.
- The nuclear material in the lumbar spine is located more posterior than that of the cervical or thoracic spine.

- The nerve roots leave the spinal cord laterally and the laterally herniated disk can easily cause classic radicular symptoms.
- The innervation of the lumbar disks is very similar to that of the disks of the cervical and thoracic spine. The outer third of the annulus fibrosis of the disk is supplied by multiple sensory nerves.

Indications for Lumbar Diskography

- To determine the source of pain in patients with documented disk bulge from previous studies
- Patients with pain in whom testing has been normal or equivocal
- In presurgical candidates, diskography may be used to further evaluate the levels needed to be fused.
- If low back pain is not responding to conservative treatment measures and pain persists for an extended period of time, no evidence of contraindications occurs, such as severe spinal stenosis, resulting in intraspinal obstruction, infection, or predominately psychogenic pain.[18]
- Persistent pain where other diagnostic tests have failed to confirm disk as the source of pain

Technique for Lumbar Diskography (Fig. 6): Fluoroscopy of Lumbar Spine

- Patient is placed in the prone position with a pillow under the abdomen to slightly flex the lumbar spine.
- Imaging can be obtained to locate vital organs such as lungs, ribs, aorta, vena cava, kidneys, nerve roots, and spinal cord.
- The spinous process below the disk of question is palpated and the skin 1.5 inches laterally is sterilely prepped, draped, and anesthetized with 1% lidocaine.
- A 22G, 5-inch styletted needle is placed through the skin and advanced to the middle of the disk of question.
- The needle is advanced incrementally with imaging. If a paresthesia is elicited, the needle should be withdrawn and then redirected cephalad toward the middle of the disk.
- Once the disk is contacted, the needle is advanced incrementally until the middle of the disk is penetrated. Inject 0.3 mL of contrast **(Fig. 7)**. Imaging is performed in order to avoid penetration through the back of the disk or too laterally either into the spinal canal or the pleura (in L1 diskography).
- Take note also of amount of contrast injected, volume at which the patient experienced pain, pressure at which the patient experienced pressure or pain, and pain response (location, character, distribution, intensity, and concordance with chronic pain).
- The diskogram needs to be evaluated to check the integrity of the disk, and a decision needs to be made if there is a need to evaluate the adjacent disk spaces or to inject local anesthetic in the disk of question.

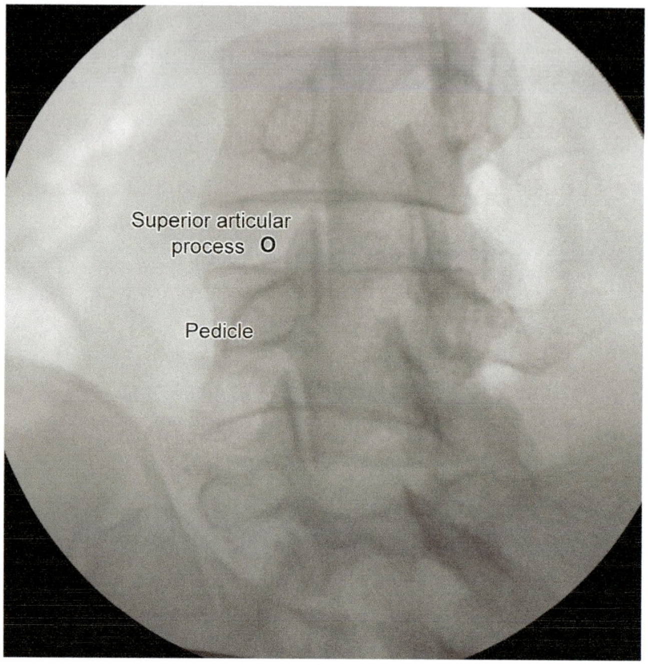

Fig. 6: Lumbar spine anatomy.

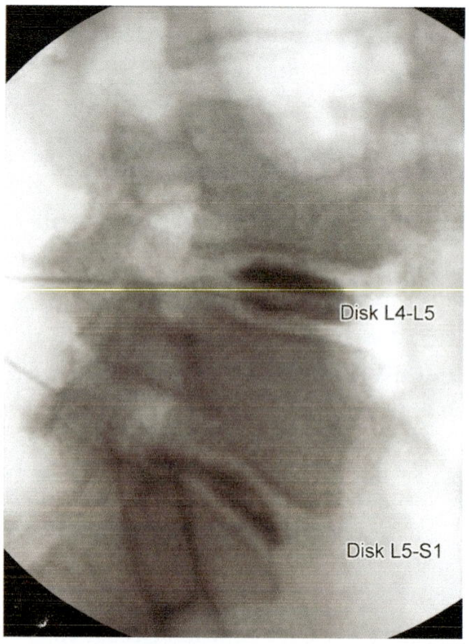

Fig. 7: Lumbar diskogram dye spread.

9. The decision to inject local anesthetic into this disk space can give erroneous information if the adjacent disks are to be evaluated. The local anesthetic can possibly track into the epidural space or it can anesthetize some of the nerves that provide sensory input to the adjacent disks.

Imaging Details of X-Ray

- The images of the injected disk need to be evaluated to see whether or not the disk and its components are intact.
- The condition of the disk will determine where the contrast will collect.
- A normal disk will appear as a lobulated mass with some posterolateral clefts due to the normal aging process of the disk.
- If the inner annulus is torn, a transverse pattern of contrast will show on the nucleogram or if the tears of the annulus extend to the outer layer, a radial pattern will be noted.
- It is also possible for the contrast to flow into the epidural space or the end plate of the vertebra if the annulus is completely disrupted.
- In certain situations, the injected contrast may flow between the layers of the annulus.

SIDE EFFECTS AND COMPLICATIONS OF DISKOGRAPHY

- Increased pain
- Headache
- Seizures
- Nausea
- Diskitis 1%[19,20]
- Sympathetic block
- Diarrhea
- Urticaria
- Spinal headache
- Meningitis
- Intrathecal hemorrhage
- Arachnoiditis
- Epidural abscess or hematoma
- Trauma to nerve roots or spinal cord or cauda equina
- Allergic reaction to contrast
- Severe reaction to accidental intradural injection
- Damage to the disk
- Diskography does not result in herniation of nucleus material or annular deterioration. Long-term follow-up studies have not demonstrated damage to normal disks after diskography.
- Some suggest that incidence of diskitis may be reduced when a double-needle technique is used.
- The incidence of diskitis might decrease further when prophylactic antibiotics are used.[18]
- The patients are instructed to ice the injection sites and to call if they have any fever or any systemic signs of infection such as rigors, chills, or shaking.
- Pneumothorax (upper lumbar, thoracic, and lower cervical)
- Hemothorax (upper lumbar, thoracic, and lower cervical)
- Retroperitoneal hematoma (lumbar)

CONCLUSION

Diskography can be a useful tool in the interventional pain physicians' skill set. It is a diagnostic test that attempts to help delineate pain generators in patients with back pain. A diskogram can help identify pathology that will dictate treatment options for patients and help in assessing the risk versus benefit for future procedures. As with any interventional procedure, there are potential side effects and complications. Therefore, it is important for the practicing physician to understand what those are and use good clinical judgment to minimize those risks. In the future, continued large-scale clinical research and studies would help to further elucidate the risk versus benefits of the diskogram procedure itself.

REFERENCES

1. Manchikanti L, Singh V, Pampati V, Damron KS, Barnhill RC, Beyer C, et al. Evaluation of the relative contributions of various structures in chronic low back pain. Pain Physician. 2001;4:308-16.
2. WCG Peh. Provocative discography: current status. Biomed Imaging Interv J. 2005;1(1):e2.
3. Menkowitz M, Stieber JR, Wenokor C, Cohen JD, Donald GD, Cresanti-Dakinis C. Intradiscal pressure monitoring in the cervical spine. Pain Physician. 2005;8:163-6.
4. Onyewu O, Manchikanti L, Falco FJ, Singh V, Geffert S, Helm S 2nd, et al. An update of the appraisal of the accuracy and utility of cervical discography in chronic neck pain. Pain Physician. 2012;15:E777-806.
5. Peng B, Hao J, Hou S, Wu W, Jiang D, Fu X, et al. Possible pathogenesis of painful intervertebral disc degeneration. Spine. 2006;31:560-6.
6. Freemont AJ. The cellular pathobiology of degenerate intervertebral disc and discogenic back pain. Rheumatology (Oxford). 2009;48:5-10.

7. Burke JG, Watson RW, McCormack D, Dowling FE, Walsh MG, Fitzpatrick JM. Intervertebral discs which cause low back pain secrete high levels of proinflammatory mediators. J Bone Joint Surgery. 2002;84-B:196-201.
8. Le Gars L, Borderie D, Kaplan G, Berenbaum F. Systemic inflammatory response with plasma C-reactive protein elevation in disk related lumbosciatic syndrome. Joint Bone Spine. 2000;67:452-5.
9. Manchikanti L, Dunbar EE, Wargo BW, Shah RV, Derby R, Cohen SP. Systematic review of cervical discography as a diagnostic test for chronic spinal pain. Pain Physician. 2009;12:305-21.
10. Kapural L, Boutwell K, Sakic K. Provocative discography and minimally invasive procedures for the treatment of discogenic pain. Periodicium Biologorum. 2009; 111(2):197-202.
11. Fujimoto K, Miyagi M, Ishikawa T, Inoue G, Eguchi Y, Kamoda H, et al. Sensory and autonomic innervation of the cervical intervertebral disks in rats: the pathomechanics of chronic discogenic neck pain. Spine (Phila Pa 1976). 2012;37:1357-62.
12. Sugiura A, Ohtori S, Yamashita M, Yamauchi K, Inoue G, Suzuki M, et al. Effect of applying p75 NTR saporin to a punctured intervertebral disc on calcitonin gene-related peptide expression in a rat dorsal root ganglion neurons. J Orthop Sci. 2010;15:407-13.
13. Ohtori S, Takahashi K, Chiba T, Yamagata M, Sameda H, Moriya H. Sensory innervation of the cervical facet joints in rats. Spine. 2001;26:147-50.
14. Falco FJ, et al. Cervical discography. In: Machika L, Singh V (Eds). Interventional Techniques in Chronic Spinal Pain. Paducah: ASIPP Publishing; 2007. pp. 567-80.
15. Motimaya A, Arici M, George D, Ramsby G. Diagnostic value of cervical discography in the management of cervical discogenic pain. Conn Med. 2000;64:395-8.
16. Schellhas KP, Garveya TA, Johnsona BA, Rothbarta PJ, Polleia SR. Cervical discography: analysis of provoked responses at C2-C3, C3-C4 and C4-C5. Am J Neuroradiol. 2000;21:269-75.
17. Fenton DS, Czervionke LF. Image-Guided Spine Intervention, 1st edition. Philadelphia: Saunders; 2002. p. 229.
18. Walker III J, Abd OE, Isaac Z, Muzin S. Discography in practice: a clinical and historical review. Curr Rev Musculoskeletal Med. 2008;1:69-83.
19. Williams PC, Jacobs WCH, Duinkerke ES, de Kleuver M. Lumbar discography: should we use prophylactic antibiotics? A study of 435 consecutive discograms and a systemic review of the literature. J Spinal Disord Tech. 2004; 17:243-7.
20. Kapoor SG, Huff J, Cohen SP. Systematic review of the incidence of discitis after cervical discography. Spine J. 2010;10(8):739-45.

49 CHAPTER

Intradiskal Electrothermal Therapy

Anil K Sharma

ABSTRACT

Intradiskal electrothermal therapy is a minimally invasive technique used to treat highly selective patients with chronic low back pain because of internal disk disruption (diskogenic) or annular tear. It is used in the lumbar spine only. Initially, the reports suggested effective therapy; however, new studies suggest much lower effectiveness. Its use has been on a decline because of lack of efficacy.

INTRODUCTION

Since the last chapter was written in 2008, the popularity of these procedures had been declining because of the lack of efficacy. The effectiveness of intradiskal electrothermal therapy (IDET) is <50% in recent studies even after using minimal clinical improvement standard, which is greater than 2-point change in visual analog scale (VAS). This procedure continues to be on the decline. In general, treatment of diskogenic low back pain is difficult and so far, no treatment has proven to be effective. Promising development in biology is going on which hopefully will be the treatment of future.

Intradiskal electrothermal therapy was developed by Saal and Saal in the 1990s as a treatment for chronic low back pain. Chronic low back pain can be caused by intervertebral disk derangement. It has also been postulated that annular disruption can be the source of back pain. In a normal disk, nociceptive nerve fibers innervate only the outer third of the disk, but as a result of degenerative changes and internal disk disruption (IDD), the nerves and the blood vessels can grow into the deeper layers of the annulus and can cause clinically severe diskogenic low back pain.[1,2]

About 30–50% of cases of low back pain are due to IDD.[3] IDD is a biochemical, biophysical, and morphological disruption of the nucleus pulposus and annulus fibrosis of the disk, which is categorized by radial or circumferential fissures extending from the nucleus pulposus to the outer third of the annulus. The presence of fissures or tears within the annulus can cause chronic inflammatory and mechanical stress on the intervertebral disk, which can result in nerve growth and new vascularization causing sensitization and pain.

Diskogenic back pain can be treated with conservative treatment including activity modification, pain medications, anti-inflammatories, physical therapy, steroid injections, chiropractic care, acupuncture, and other modalities. Surgical fusion is also an accepted treatment for diskogenic low back pain, which has not responded to conservative treatment. There has been significant variation in the outcome following surgical fusion, which is also associated with surgical risks including infection, adjacent segmental instability, and pseudoarthrosis.

Intradiskal electrothermal therapy is a minimally invasive technique used to treat highly selective patients with chronic low back pain as a result of IDD or annular tear. It is used in the lumbar spine only.

Internal disk disruption is diagnosed based on diskography where there is reproduction of back pain, which is concordant at low pressures <50 psi. The pain intensity should be >6/10 on a VAS and the CT scan after diskography shows grade 3 or greater annular tear, which extends to the outer third of the annulus, and controlled disk stimulation at the adjacent level is normal without any pain.

The possible mechanisms of action of IDET are still debatable, the most likely causes are alteration in spinal segment mechanics via collagen modification, thermal nociceptive fiber destruction in the annulus, biochemical mediation of inflammation, and decrease in vascular in-growth as well as possible healing of the annular tear.[4]

Intradiskal electrothermal therapy uses radiofrequency energy, which is converted to thermal energy. Initially, the technique was used by Slutter for radiofrequency lesioning of the nociceptive fibers on the disk annulus, where the radiofrequency heat was delivered to the annulus through a needle.[5] The technique produced a relatively small lesion because of the needle. Subsequent to that, Hayashi showed contraction of collagen fibers when exposed to temperature >65°C during surgery of the shoulder joint capsules using radiofrequency heat energy. Intradiskal electrothermal therapy uses a thermal-resistive catheter placed intradiskally at the side of the radial or circumferential annular tear where radiofrequency energy is delivered to the posterior or posterolateral annulus which gets converted into heat and causes thermal lesioning of the disk annulus. Temperatures above 55°C result in shrinkage of collagen fibers. Heat-labile hydrogen bonds can form triple helix of the collagen molecules to unwind and transition into a less organized, random, and contracted state. Subsequent to thermal treatment, fibroblast activity increases and new more stable, stiffer collagen is formed, and the nerve endings are destroyed.[6-8]

INDICATIONS

This procedure is indicated for patients suffering from chronic low back pain for >3 months, who had adequate conservative and nonoperative treatment with no improvement. They have no neurologic deficits and have normal neurological examinations with normal straight leg raising test. MRI reveals intact disk height or at least 80% of disk height maintenance with no significant herniation which might show annular tears or degenerative changes. There is no evidence of spondylolisthesis or segmental instability. Also, psychological factors and serious medical conditions are evaluated. After that, the patient undergoes diagnostic provocative diskography and satisfies the criteria for IDD.

TECHNIQUE

Intradiskal electrothermal therapy procedure is performed similar to a standard diskography approach to the disk, which is posterolateral. Informed consent is obtained from the patient. The procedure is explained in detail, including the physical limitations as well as explanation that pain relief might not be obtained for 3–6 months. Subsequent to that, prophylactic antibiotics are given. Cephazolin 1 g is given intravenously. If allergic to penicillin, clindamycin 600 mg intravenous is given. Antibiotics are given 30 minutes prior to the procedure.

The procedure is performed in a sterile environment with very mild sedation. Most of the patients require only 1–2 mg of midazolam and 100 mg of fentanyl. Occasionally, the patient might also need propofol. It is important to keep the patient awake during the insertion of the introducer needle as well as during the heating procedure to look for any radicular pain. The procedure is performed under fluoroscopy guidance on a radiolucent table.

The patient is placed in a prone position with one to two pillows under his stomach to obliterate the lumbar lordosis, and it also makes it easier to access the L5-S1 disk. A lap sheet with Ioban is used for draping. Subsequent to that, under fluoroscopy guidance, an appropriate level is identified. Under anteroposterior (AP) fluoroscopy guidance, the end plates are lined up and then an oblique fluoroscopy view is obtained to place the superior articular process (SAP) roughly into the center of the disk space **(Fig. 1)**. Entering from the opposite side of the patient's pain or from the opposite side of the annular tear is suggested. For example, if the annular tear is on the left side, enter the disk from the right side. A skin mark is placed just lateral to the SAP and is infiltrated with 1% lidocaine. A spinal needle is used to infiltrate the local anesthetic up to the SAP **(Fig. 2)**. Again, it is very important not to use too much local anesthetic in the deep tissue plane so as to avoid infiltrating the nerve root. A 17G, 6-inch long introducer needle is then introduced through the skin. A small incision is made with a #11 blade to make the entry of the needle easier. The needle is entered under fluoroscopy guidance. The tip of the needle is kept in the medial direction toward the SAP **(Fig. 3)**. The needle should be curved slightly for access to the L5-S1 disk if there is a high iliac crest. Once the SAP process is passed, advance the needle very slowly making sure that the nerve root is not irritated. It is important to keep the patient awake at this point. Once the nerve root is passed, the annulus is entered, and the cannula is placed into the posterior central aspect of the corresponding disk **(Fig. 4)**. AP and lateral views are obtained **(Fig. 5)**. The trocar is removed and the IDET catheter is introduced. The catheter

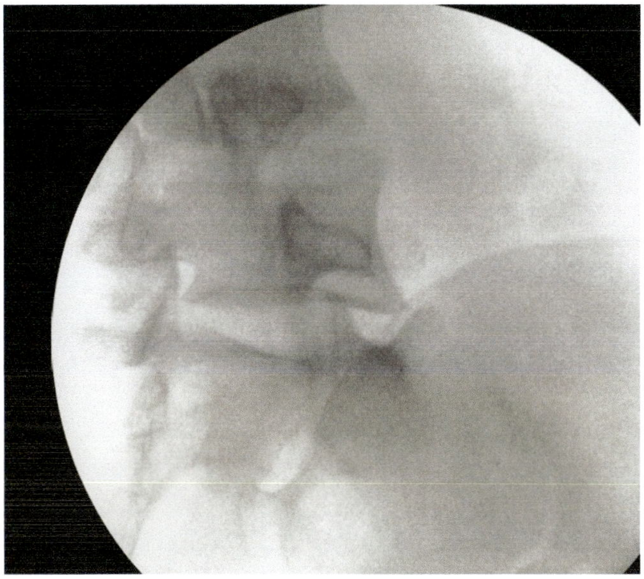

Fig. 1: An oblique fluoroscopy view of the patient undergoing an L5-S1 intradiskal electrothermal therapy procedure. The patient is placed in a prone position with two pillows under the stomach to move the iliac crest away. Approach to L5-S1 disk is identified in this patient, which is a triangle, formed by the superior articular process of S1, the iliac crest, and the L5 vertebral body on the top. L5-S1 disk is usually the most difficult disk to approach through the posterolateral approach for any percutaneous procedures, especially in males because of high iliac crest.

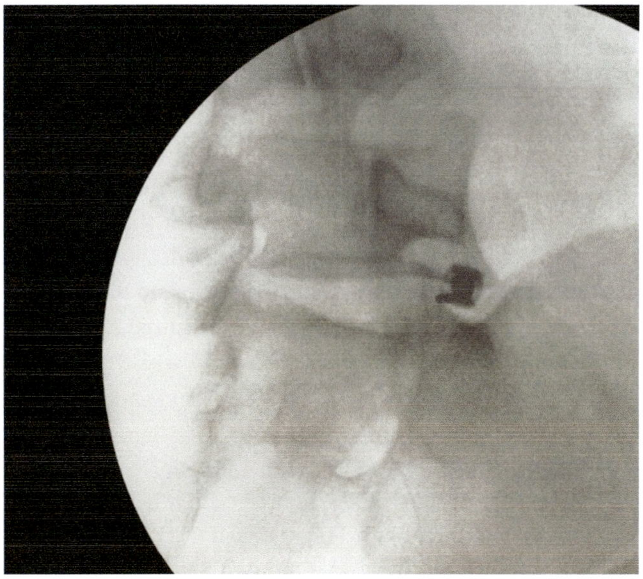

Fig. 2: *Oblique fluoroscopy view:* A needle is introduced, and bony contact is made with the lateral aspect of the superior articular process to note the depth of insertion as well as to keep the needle as close to the superior articular process so as to avoid injuring the nerve root. Again, note that this procedure is being performed under end-on view.

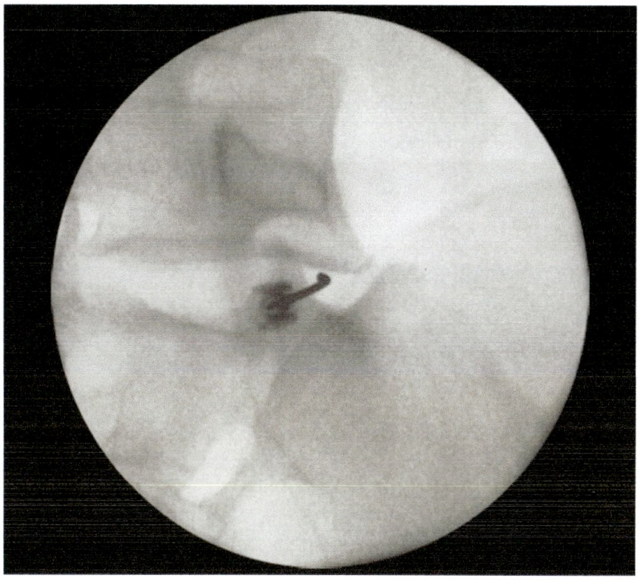

Fig. 3: The needle is slightly withdrawn and redirected just lateral to the superior articular process. At this point, it is important to ask the patient if he notices any pain down the leg as the needle is advanced further. The resistance of the annulus is usually felt as the tip goes through the annulus and then the resistance goes away.

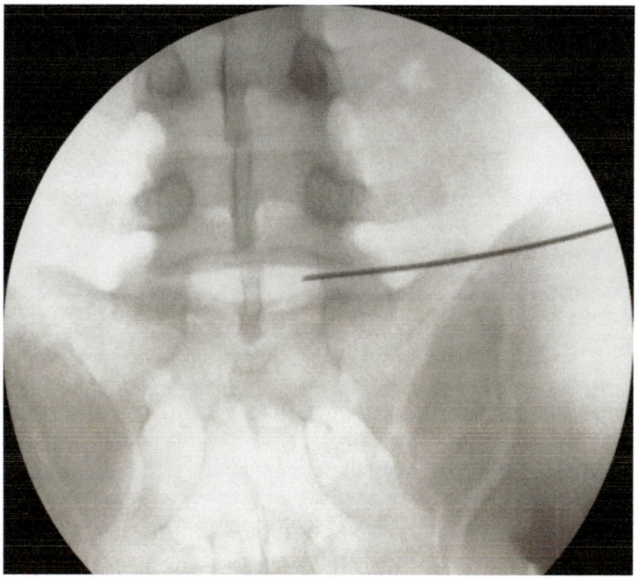

Fig. 4: *Anteroposterior fluoroscopy view:* The needle tip is beyond the annulus into the nucleus; again, endplates are lined up so as to make sure that the needle is placed in the center of the disk space.

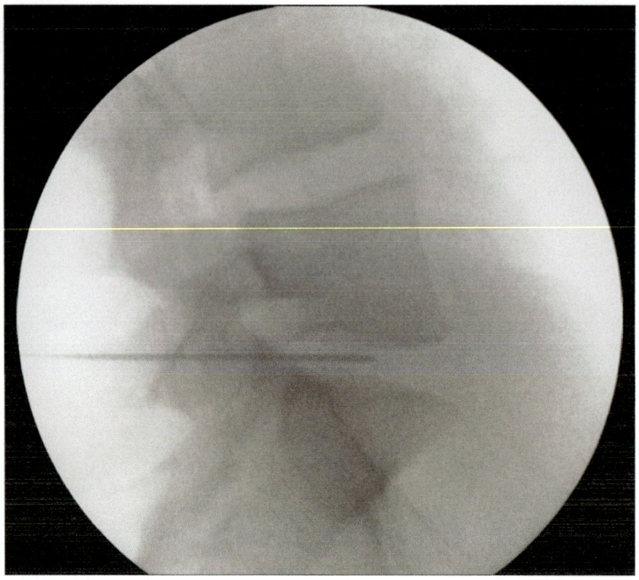

Fig. 5: *Lateral fluoroscopy view:* Again, note the needle to be in the center of the disk space.

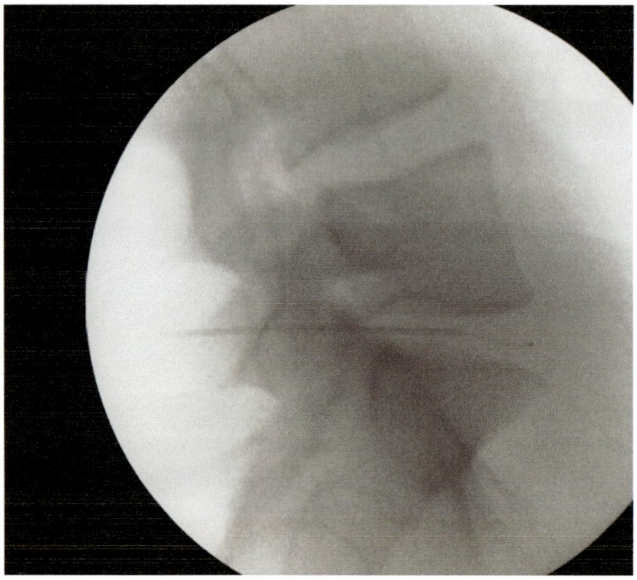

Fig. 6: Intradiskal electrothermal therapy catheter is advanced under lateral fluoroscopy view. The two proximal and distal markers can be seen. The catheter is advanced and has started to curve back after contacting the inner annulus.

is then slowly advanced under lateral fluoroscopy view as it starts to come around the posterior annulus **(Fig. 6)**. The catheter should not enter the spinal canal through an annulus tear. Once the catheter has successfully navigated the posterolateral aspect of the annulus, the view is changed to AP view and then the catheter is advanced from one pedicle to the other **(Fig. 7)**. Sometimes, resistance is

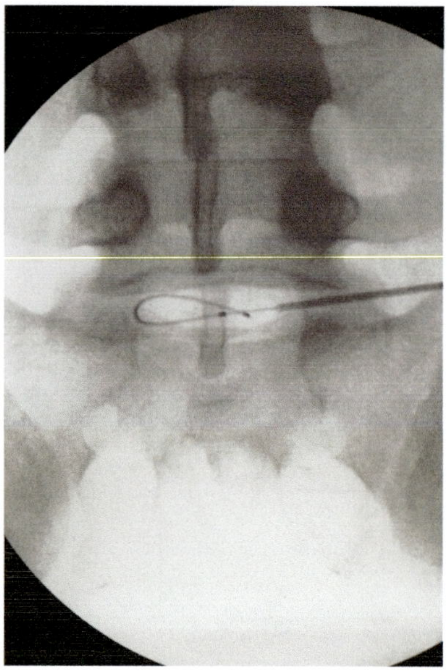

Fig. 7: Anteroposterior fluoroscopy of intradiskal electrothermal therapy catheter is advanced further and can be seen wrapping around the posterior annulus. Both proximal and distal markers are out of the needle. At this point, the distal marker needs to be advanced slightly more so as to cover most of the posterior annulus.

encountered because of the catheter tip lodging into the annular tear. At this point, watch for kinking of the catheter even with slight resistance. If kinking is noted, the catheter is withdrawn, redirected, and again attempts to navigate through the posterior annulus. If after a few attempts it is unable to do so, move the introducer needle in a more central or more posterior location and then reintroduce the catheter. On occasion, it is possible not to be able to cover the whole posterior annulus. In that case, the technique can be performed from both sides with another needle introduced from the opposite side and the catheter navigated to the opposite posterior annulus. Again, it is important not to use too much pressure while navigating the catheter as kinking can occur. If there is a kink in the catheter, a new catheter has to be used.

After appropriate positioning of the catheter, final AP and lateral fluoroscopy views are obtained to confirm the placement of the catheter **(Figs. 8 and 9)**. Following that, a P90 protocol developed by Saal and Saal is used, which involves heating the catheter up to a total of 16.5 minutes with a maximum temperature of 90°C. There are also other protocols available. Sometimes, the patients are not able to tolerate this maximum temperature because of the significant back pain, which starts as the catheter starts to

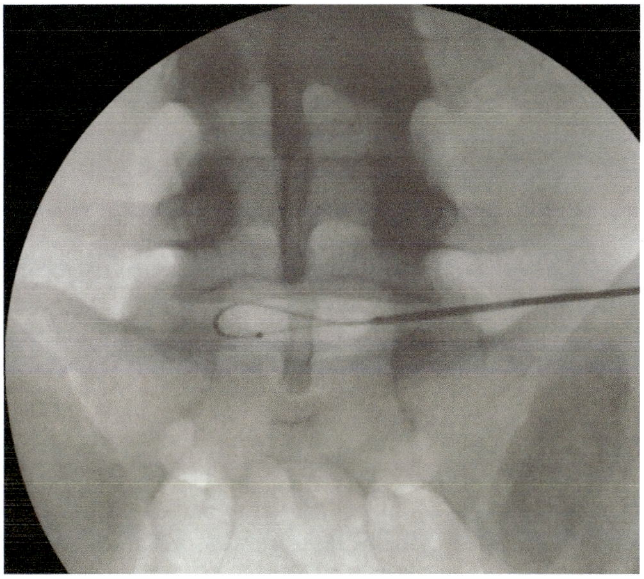

Fig. 8: The catheter is advanced further, and both proximal and distal markers are lying along the posterior annulus from pedicle to pedicle. The distal marker is being shadowed by the introducer needle.

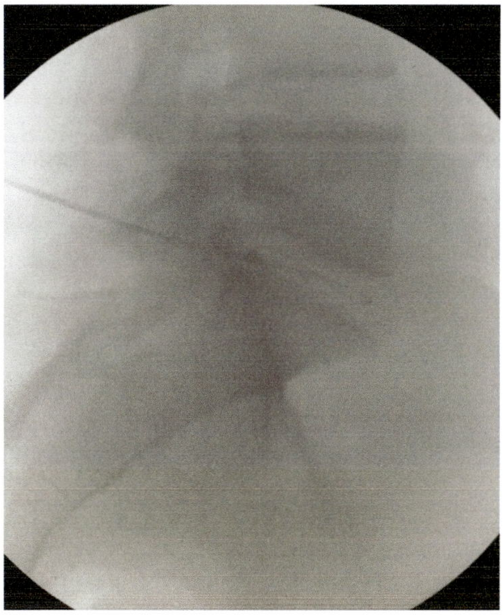

Fig. 9: Lateral view to confirm the catheter is not in the spinal canal.

heat up to 85°C. During the process of heating, the patient is asked to let us know if he starts to notice any pain going down his legs. Back pain is common during the heating part as the pain radiates into the buttocks and thighs.

Once the heating is done, the catheter is removed slowly making sure that there is no resistance. If there is resistance, then the catheter and needle are removed together. The catheter is removed and verified that the tip of the catheter is intact. Subsequent to that, 0.75% Marcaine mixed with 3 mg of clindamycin 1.5 mL is used for the disk as a prophylactic intradiskal antibiotic to prevent diskitis. The needle is subsequently removed. A bandage is usually applied and then the patient is taken to the recovery room.

POSTOPERATIVE INSTRUCTIONS

The patient has to wear a brace for 6 weeks after the IDET procedure. A lumbar-sacral orthosis (LSO) brace is usually prescribed. The patient is instructed to limit their sitting from 30 to 40 minutes at a time for the first 4 weeks. He can perform sedentary activity 1–3 weeks after the procedure but should avoid excessive sitting. Again, the patient can drive after the first few days, but should limit driving time to 30 minutes. The patient is instructed not to lift >10 pounds for the first 4 weeks. He can walk 20 minutes daily and advance to 20 minutes twice daily after 2 weeks.

The patient is usually seen in our office 2 weeks after the procedure. Subsequent to that, his activity increased slightly. At 6–8 weeks, he is sent for physical therapy and resumes daily activity with attention to back care and subsequent strengthening program.

COMPLICATIONS

Complications from this procedure can be related to needle injury of the nerve root, possibility of infection or diskitis, and catheter tip breakage or dislodgement. Postoperatively, the patient can develop herniation if physical activity is not limited because of the weakness of collagen fibers.[9]

There have also been cases reporting spinal cord injury and nerve root injury secondary to catheter misplacement which was not diagnosed prior to the heating process.[10,11]

STUDIES RELATED TO INTRADISKAL ELECTROTHERMAL THERAPY

In 1998, Saal and Saal presented 25 IDET patients. These patients underwent 6 months of conservative treatment followed by diskography. The patients reported functional improvement and reduction of pain medicine. The initial study was not successful as it lacked control. Also, the researchers were the inventors of the IDET.

Saal and Saal published a 2-year follow-up data of 62 IDET patients.[12] Out of 62 patients, 4 did not follow up in

1 year. The patients had the same inclusion and exclusion criteria. They were also excluded if they had any prior back surgery. At 24 months, the reported mean VAS was 3.4 as compared to 6.5 preprocedurally; 50% of the patients experienced a 4-point reduction in the VAS and 71% patients experienced a 2-point reduction in the VAS. They also showed an improvement in the quality of life. They did not report any complications in their study. This study was criticized for lack of randomization and lack of control group as well as the investigators who were the developers of this technology.

Bogduk and Karasek published a 2-year follow-up study on IDET patients with chronic low back pain.[13] VAS for pain, work status, and opioid use were used as outcome measures at 3 months. At 3 months, the pretreatment median VAS dropped from 8.0 to 3.4. At 24 months, 50% of the IDET patient group had at least 50% relief of pain and 20% were completely pain free. The authors also concluded that the results are related to the catheter placement as close as possible to the annular tear and the fissures.

Lee et al. conducted a prospective nonrandomized study in 62 patients with chronic low back pain.[14] They also included patients who had prior diskectomy. There was a statistically significant improvement in low back pain. The study was also nonrandomized and had no placebo control.

Pauza performed a randomized placebo control IDET study.[15] Uncompensated volunteers were selected. A total of 264 people were eligible. Patients were excluded from the study if they had any prior spine surgery, radicular pain, herniated disk, spinal stenosis, scoliosis, or narcotic usage >100 mg of morphine. Also, the patients were excluded if they had workman compensation issues or personal injuries. A total of 64 patients were candidates for randomization. These patients underwent psychological testing, diskography, and clinical examination.

The patients were randomized for IDET procedure or sham procedure. All the patients had the introducer needle introduced into the annulus. Randomized decision took place at the time of insertion of the introducer needle. The IDET group underwent standard heating of the IDET probe to 90°C. The sham group experienced the same visual and auditory environment as the treatment group. Following that, both groups were subjected to graded physical rehabilitation and follow-up was maintained for 12 months. Results showed that 40% of patients treated with IDET experienced 50% or more pain relief, but 50% of patients experienced no notable improvement, 6% of patients showed worsening of pain, and 21% of patients showed >80% reduction of pain.

CONCLUSION

In general, IDET is a minimally invasive technique that shows significant promise for treatment of low back pain coming from IDD or diskogenic etiology after receiving failed conservative treatments. It is a procedure which carries minimal risk if performed appropriately and promises that half of the patients will notice significant improvement of back pain. The results are not as encouraging as they were with the initial studies, but this procedure is suggested to be performed on carefully selected patients who have primarily back pain and have undergone testing, including diskography, and have not lost >80% of the disk height.

REFERENCES

1. Freemont A, Peacock T, Goupille P, Hoyland J, O'Brien J, Jayson M. Nerve ingrowth into diseased intervertebral disc in chronic back pain. Lancet. 1997;350:178-81.
2. Coppes M, Marani E, Thomeer RT, Groen GJ. Innervation of "painful" lumbar discs. Spine. 1997;22:2342-9.
3. Karasek M, Bogduk N. Intradiscal electrothermal annuloplasty: percutaneous treatment of chronic discogenic low back pain. Tech Reg Anesth Pain Manage. 2001;5:130-5.
4. Saal JA, Saal JS. Intadiscal electrothermal therapy for the treatment of chronic discogenic low back pain. Clin Sports Med. 2002;21(1):167-87.
5. Sluijter ME. The use of radiofrequency lesions for pain relief in failed back patients. Int Disabil Stud. 1988;10:37-43.
6. Saal JA, Saal JS. Intradiscal electrothermal treatment for chronic discogenic low back pain: prospective outcome study with a minimum 2-year follow-up. Spine. 2000;27:966-74.
7. Heary R. Intradiscal electrothermal annuloplasty: the IDET procedure. J Spinal Disord. 2001;14:353-60.
8. Narvani A, Tsiridis E, Wilson L. High intensity zone, intradiscal electrothermal therapy, and magnetic resonance imaging. J Spinal Disord Tech. 2003;16:130-6.
9. Cohen S, Larkin T, Polly D. A giant herniated disc following intradiscal electrothermal therapy. J Spinal Disord Tech. 2002;15:537-41.
10. Hsia A, Isaac K, Katz J. Cauda equina syndrome from intradiscal electrothermal therapy. Neurology. 2002;55:320-8.
11. Djurasovic M, Glassman S, Dimar J, Johnson J. Vertebral osteonecrosis associated with the use of intradiscal electrothermal therapy: a case report. Spine. 2002;27:325-8.

12. Saal JA, Saal JS. Thermal characteristics of lumbar disc: evaluation of a novel approach to targeted intradiscal thermal therapy. Presented at the 13th Annual Meeting of the North American Spine Society; October 28-31, 1998, San Francisco, California.
13. Bogduk N, Karasek M. Two-year follow up of a controlled trial of intradiscal electrothermal anuloplasty for chronic low back pain resulting from internal disc disruption. Spine. 2002;2:343-50.
14. Lee M, Cooper G, Lutz C, Hong H. Intradiscal electrothermal therapy (IDET) for treatment of chronic lumbar discogenic pain: a minimum 2-year clinical outcome study. Pain Physician. 2003;6:443-8.
15. Pauza KJ, Howell S, Dreyfuss P, Peloza JH, Dawson K, Bogduk N. A randomized placebo-controlled trial of intradiscal electrothermal therapy (IDET) for the treatment of discogenic low back pain. Spine. 2004;4:27-35.

50 CHAPTER

Vertebroplasty and Kyphoplasty

Kevin H Trinh, Steve M Aydin

ABSTRACT

Vertebroplasty and kyphoplasty are two minimally invasive percutaneous vertebral augmentation procedures developed to treat painful osteoporotic compression fractures. Performed under fluoroscopy, these procedures involve the transpedicular introduction of polymethylmethacrylate (PMMA) cement through the use of a bone biopsy needle. The purpose of the aforementioned procedures is to decrease pain via the reconstruction and stabilization of the endplates and vertebral body segment. There is class I evidence that supports the superiority of vertebral augmentation procedures over nonsurgical management. In addition, vertebral augmentation of osteoporotic compression fractures has been shown to be far superior to nonsurgical management in terms of reducing pain and subsequent fractures.

INTRODUCTION

Vertebral compression fractures are the most common type of fractures in patients with osteoporosis, affecting an estimated 1.5 million Americans every year.[1] Approximately 25% of all postmenopausal women will have a compression fracture during their lifetime, and the prevalence of this condition has been known to increase with age, reaching approximately 40% by the age of 80 years.[2,3] Vertebral compression fractures can cause progressive kyphosis of the thoracic spine leading to decreased pulmonary function, poor nutrition, chronic pain, clinical depression, and increased morbidity and mortality.[4] Traditional treatment strategies for osteoporotic vertebral compression fractures consist of bed rest, analgesic medications, and bracing. However, in the elderly, this conservative approach can lead to an increased rate of demineralization due to decreased mobility.[5] Surgical treatment may be considered in patients with vertebral compression fractures if there is spinal instability and neurologic compromise, although the success rate of surgery is limited by the patients' bone quality and general medical condition. As for minimally invasive techniques to treat painful vertebral compression fractures, there are currently two percutaneous vertebral augmentation methods for cement application into the vertebral body: Vertebroplasty and kyphoplasty.

Percutaneous vertebroplasty was introduced in 1984 in France by an interventional neuroradiologist, Herve Deramond. This process involves the injection of cement into the vertebral body under image guidance. He found this procedure to be useful in treating vertebral fractures secondary to benign and malignant tumors as well as osteoporotic compression fractures.[6] Neuroradiologists in the United States (US) adopted this technique in 1993, with the first case series in 1997.[7]

Kyphoplasty was developed by Dr Mark Reiley, an orthopedic surgeon, in the early 1990s. This procedure utilizes an inflatable balloon device (balloon tamp), which is placed percutaneously into the vertebral body to restore vertebral body height and minimize the associated kyphotic deformity before cement injection **(Fig. 1)**.

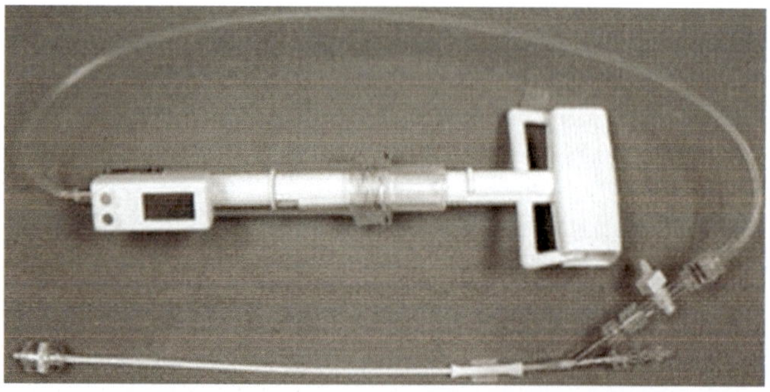

Fig. 1: Inflatable balloon and pressure gauge.[5]

INDICATIONS

According to the Guidelines of National Societies,[8] the main indications of vertebroplasty and kyphoplasty are:

- Intractable pain from osteoporotic vertebral compression fractures
- Painful vertebrae from aggressive primary tumors
- Painful vertebrae with osteolysis after malignant infiltration
- Painful fracture with osteonecrosis
- Chronic nonunion of fracture fragments after trauma.

CONTRAINDICATIONS

According to Interventional Radiology Quality assurance guidelines for percutaneous vertebroplasty,[8] contraindications for vertebroplasty and kyphoplasty are as follows:

- Retropulsion of bone into the spinal canal
- Unmanageable bleeding disorder
- Improvement of symptoms with conservative management
- Asymptomatic vertebral body fracture
- Local or generalized infection
- Allergy to bone cement
- Tumor mass with involvement of the spinal canal.

MECHANISM OF ACTION

There has been debate on the mechanism of analgesic effect from vertebral augmentation. Pain reduction has been attributed to the mechanical effects of reconstruction and stabilization of the endplates and vertebral body segment. Also, it is believed that there is a therapeutic effect from the exothermic reaction of the cement, assuming that the pain originates from intraosseous nerve endings.[9] Vertebroplasty provides stabilization and pain relief, without improvement in deformity. In comparison, kyphoplasty helps realign fractured vertebrae and restore vertebral height with the use of a balloon tamp to create a void for introduction of polymethylmethacrylate (PMMA). Although both procedures depend on mechanical stabilization by injection of PMMA cement, there is controversy on whether height restoration is clinically significant.

PROCEDURE

Both kyphoplasty and vertebroplasty are performed in a fully operational radiology suite or an operating room. Fluoroscopy is used during the procedure to define the anatomy for optimal needle placement. The chosen procedure can be performed under local anesthesia with conscious sedation in most patients. However, for uncooperative or very agitated patients, general anesthesia may be required. Intravenous (IV) access is mandatory and IV antibiotics should be used prophylactically. The skin should always be prepared and draped in a sterile fashion.

Vertebroplasty

Vertebroplasty is the percutaneous injection of PMMA into a vertebral body fracture using bone biopsy needles. The most important factor that influences the result of vertebroplasty is the visualization of needle placement and cement application.

The steps for vertebroplasty are as follows:[10]

1. Align the fluoroscope such that the spinous process is midline and the vertebra endplates are sharp for a true anteroposterior (AP) projection **(Fig. 2)**.
2. Center the pedicle within the vertebral bodies; the goal is to have the needle traverse within the central portion of the vertebral body.
3. Rotate the image intensifier 5° laterally for a lateral oblique view **(Fig. 3)**. A 13G bevel tipped bone biopsy needle (Jamshidi) is then selected. The goal is to target the lateral margin of the pedicle with the needle. For a left-sided approach, aim for the 9 o'clock position of the pedicle. Advance the needle along the axis of the image

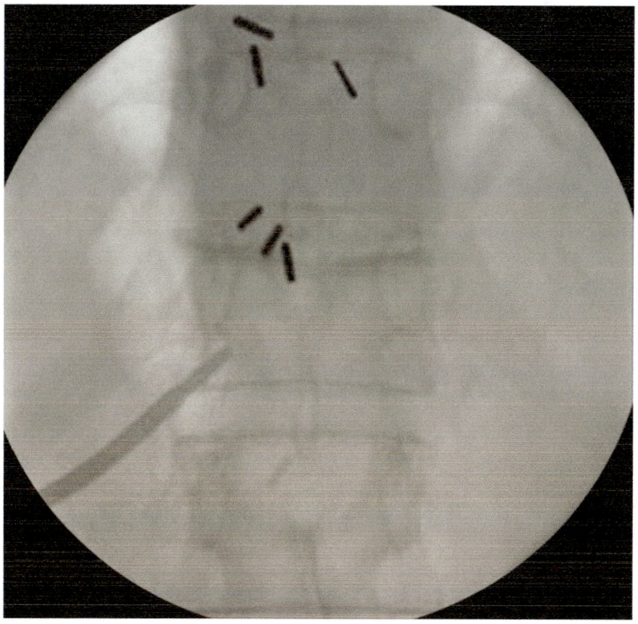

Fig. 2: Alignment of the image intensifier.

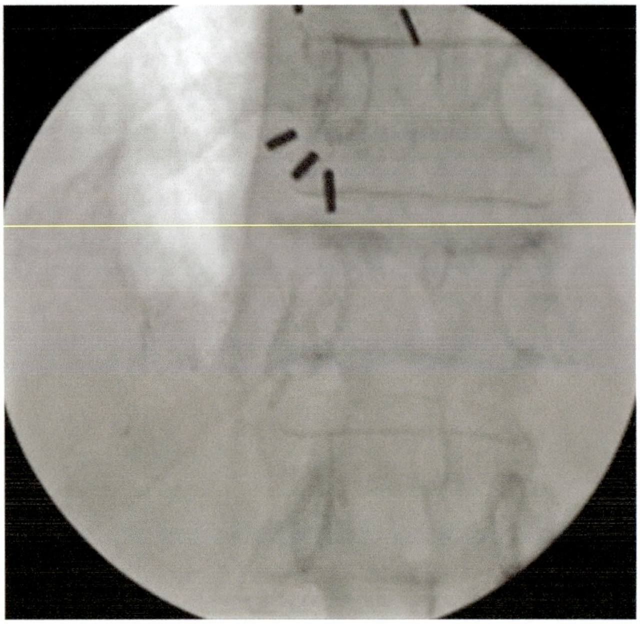

Fig. 3: 5° lateral oblique view.

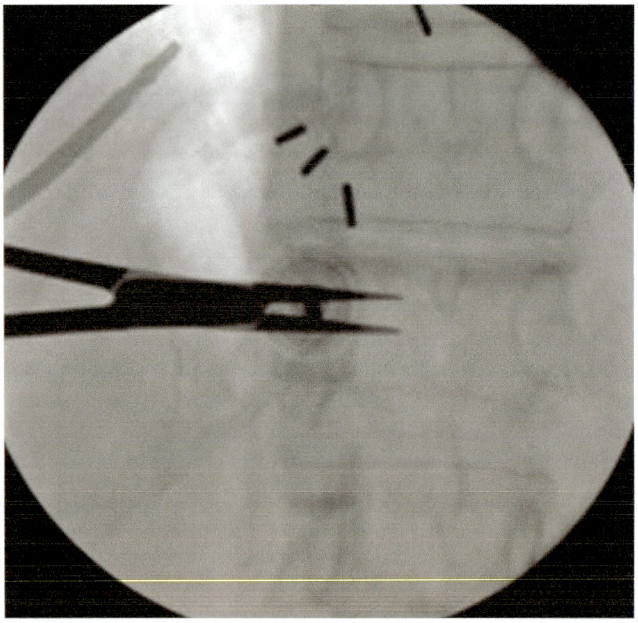

Fig. 4: Lateral margin of the pedicle is targeted and needle advanced along the axis of the fluoroscope in "bull's eye" view.

intensifier (bull's eye). Gentle hammering may be required in addition to hand-screwing motion during advancement of the needle into the bone **(Fig. 4)**. The purpose of obliquity is to offset the needle hub from the needle tip in AP view.

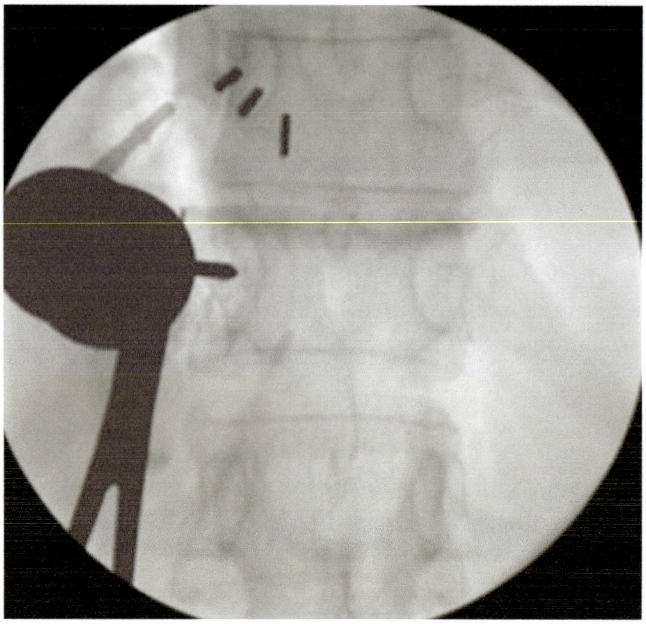

Fig. 5: Anteroposterior (AP) projection, needle tip visualized, needle advanced to the midline of the pedicle.

4. Return to the AP projection to view the tip of the needle. While utilizing the lateral and AP views, advance the needle to the midline of the pedicle **(Fig. 5)**.
5. Check the lateral projection during advancement of the needle; if the needle is anterior to the posterior margin of the vertebral body, the spinal canal has been cleared **(Fig. 6)**. Continue to advance the needle in the lateral projection until about 1 cm short of the anterior cortex of the vertebral body.
6. While in the lateral projection, inject the cement with continuous fluoroscopic monitoring **(Fig. 7)**. There should be no shine to the cement's appearance and the consistency should be like toothpaste. Pay attention to the posterior margin of the vertebral body at the epidural space. Halt cement injection if the cement reaches beyond 5 mm anterior to the posterior margin of the vertebral body. The cement volume should be no more than 1 cc on each side for a high thoracic, 2 cc on each side for a lower thoracic, and no more than 3 cc on each side for the lumbar. Watch for cement leaks into the surrounding tissue or vessels with continuous fluoroscopy.

Kyphoplasty

Kyphoplasty is a variation of vertebroplasty that involves the introduction of a cannula into the vertebral body, followed by the insertion of an inflatable balloon tamp. The

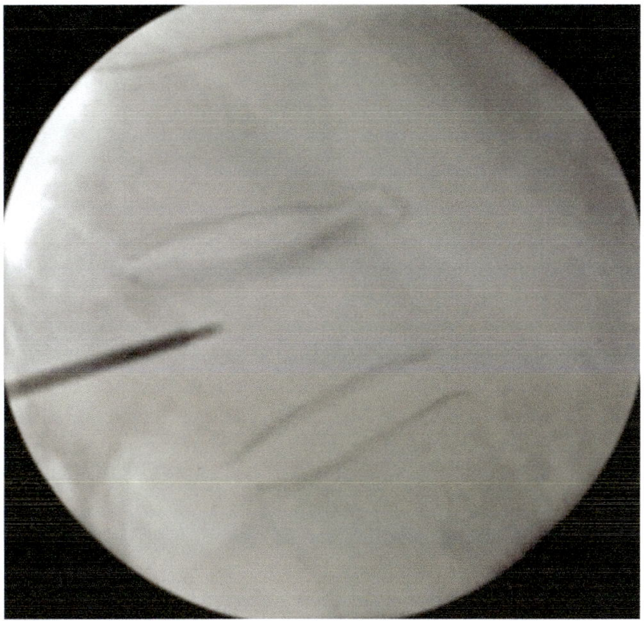

Fig. 6: Lateral projection where the needle is anterior to the posterior margin of the vertebral body and therefore the spinal canal has been cleared.

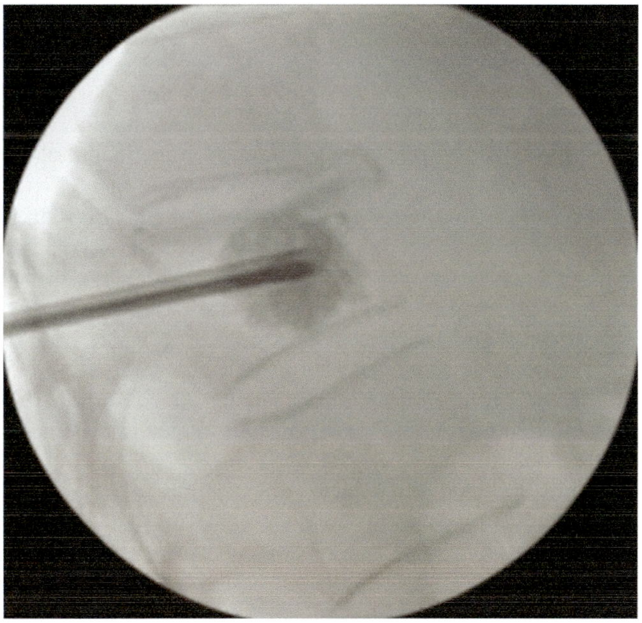

Fig. 7: Cement is injected in the lateral projection.

balloon tamponade is designed to reduce the vertebral body back to its original height while creating a cavity to be filled with bone cement.[5]

- Similar to the percutaneous route of vertebroplasty, a guidepin is inserted via a transpedicular entry point into the vertebral body.
- Place a cannulated obturator over the guidewire.
- A working cannula is placed over the obturator and advanced until the tip of the cannula is at the desired position in the posterior portion of the vertebral body.
- A hand-mounted drill is used to ream a corridor for the balloon tamponade to be placed through.
- Inflation is slowly performed under fluoroscopy. Inflation is continued until the maximum size-dependent balloon volume is reached or up to a maximum pressure of 220 psi.
- When a cavity is produced, PMMA cement is then injected.
- Filling is performed under fluoroscopic guidance and cement filling is stopped when the cement mantle reaches two-thirds of the way back to the posterior vertebral body cortex (viewed in the lateral fluoroscopic image).

POSTOPERATIVE PROTOCOL

If the patient reports increased pain immediately after vertebroplasty:

- Hold pressure after removal of the needle from the puncture site for approximately 10 minutes
- Sit the patient upright
- Consider narcotic therapy
- If pain persists after 2 hours, consider computed tomography (CT) imaging to exclude a complication[10]
- Any patient experiencing lower extremity weakness or bladder/bowel incontinence should be immediately imaged and referred to a spine surgeon.

COMPLICATIONS

Reported complications that are significant are low (<10%) and include increased pain, spinal cord compression, radiculopathies, pulmonary embolism, infection, and rib fractures.[11] In patients with metastasis or myeloma with a pathologic fracture, cement leakage leading to radiculopathy or spinal cord injury can be more common when compared to osteoporotic fractures. Uncommonly reported complications are anaphylaxis and increased pain due to thermal necrosis.

RESULTS

There is class I evidence to support the superiority of vertebral augmentation procedures over nonsurgical management.[12] A recent study by Papanastassiou et al.[13] found that vertebral augmentation was superior to nonsurgical management in the treatment of osteoporotic vertebral compression fractures in terms of reducing pain and subsequent fractures. They also noted that balloon kyphoplasty was superior to vertebroplasty and nonsurgical management in terms of quality of life. Even though research has shown positive results from vertebroplasty and kyphoplasty in the short-term, long-term effects of the cement have not been extensively studied. In addition, regardless of which procedure is chosen, outcomes often depend on the imaging equipment, adequate cement opacification, and operator experience. Therefore, careful use of either procedure is important in the safe treatment of pain associated with vertebral compression fractures.

CONCLUSION

Kyphoplasty and vertebroplasty can offer significant and immediate relief for patients suffering from back pain due to compression fractures. They are relatively safe and rewarding. Functional return and gains for the patient are paramount and can have added effects of reducing chronic pain medications, alterations in gait, and further increase of fall or fractures. Both kyphoplasty and vertebroplasty procedures have similar outcomes in regard to relief and functional improvement. Given the addition of the balloon component, kyphoplasty does have increased procedure time, whereas vertebroplasty has shown to have a slightly higher increase in cement migration relative to kyphoplasty. Both procedures have shown long-term improvements in pain; however, kyphoplasty has demonstrated slightly longer fracture-free survival when compared.[14] Procedure choice is up to treating physician and may depend on the patient, the fracture, and the ability to perform one or the other.

REFERENCES

1. Alexandru D, So W. Evaluation and management of vertebral compression fractures. Perm J. 2012;16(4):46-51.
2. Greenberg M. Handbook of Neurosurgery, 6th edition. New York: Thieme Publishing Group; 2005.
3. Black DM, Cummings SR, Karpf DB, Cauley JA, Thompson DE, Nevitt MC, et al. Randomised trial of effect of alendronate on risk of fracture in women with existing vertebral fractures. Lancet. 1996;348(9041):1535-41.
4. Kado DM, Browner WS, Palermo L, Nevitt MC, Genant HK, Cummings SR. Vertebral fractures and mortality in older women: a prospective study. Arch Intern Med. 1999;159(11):1215-20.
5. Lieberman I, Dudeney S, Reinhardt RN, Bell G. Initial outcome and efficacy of "kyphoplasty" in the treatment of painful osteoporotic vertebral compression fractures. Spine (Phila Pa 1976). 2001;26(14):1631-8.
6. Galibert P, Dermond H, Rosat P, Le Gars D. Preliminary note on the treatment of vertebral angioma by percutaneous acrylic vertebroplasty. Neurochirurgie. 1987;33(2):166-8.
7. Jensen ME, Evans AJ, Mathis JM, Kallmes DF, Cloft HJ, Dion JE. Percutaneous polymethylmethacrylate vertebroplasty in the treatment of osteoporotic vertebral compression fractures: technical aspects. Am J Neuroradiol. 1997; 18(10):1897-904.
8. Gangi A, Sabharwal T, Irani FG, Buy X, Morales JP, Adam A. Quality assurance guidelines for percutaneous vertebroplasty. Cardiovasc Intervent Radiol. 2006;29(2): 173-8.
9. Siemionow K, Lieberman IH. Vertebral augmentation in osteoporosis and bone metastasis. Curr Opin Support Palliat Care. 2007;1(4):323-7.
10. Syed MI, Shaikh A. Vertebroplasty: a systematic approach. Pain Physician. 2007;10(2):367-80.
11. Weill A, Chiras J, Simon JM, Rose M, Sola-Martinez T, Enkaoua E. Spinal metastases: indications for and results of percutaneous injection of surgical cement. Radiology. 1996;199(1):241-7.
12. Wardlaw D, Cummings SR, Van Meirhaeghe J, Bastian L, Tillman JB, Ranstam J, et al. Efficacy and safety of balloon kyphoplasty compared with non-surgical care for vertebral compression fracture (FREE): a randomized controlled trial. Lancet. 2009;373(9668):1016-24.
13. Papanastassiou ID, Phillips FM, Van Meirhaeghe J, Berenson JR, Andersson GB, Chung G, et al. Comparing effects of kyphoplasty, vertebroplasty, and non-surgical management in a systematic review of randomized and non-randomized controlled studies. Eur Spine J. 2012;21(9):1826-43.
14. Dohm M, Black CM, Darce A, Tillman JB, Fueredi G, KAVIAR investigators. A randomized trial comparing balloon kyphoplasty and vertebroplasty for vertebral compression fractures due to osteoporosis. Am J Neuroradiol. 2014; 35(12):2227-36.

51 CHAPTER

Nucleoplasty

Kyriacos Kyriakides

ABSTRACT

Chronic low back pain is a common condition affecting a considerable proportion of the population. Increasingly, this pain is being attributed to early degeneration of the intervertebral disk manifesting as disk bulging (and/or annular tears) on magnetic resonance imaging scanning and is referred to as diskogenic back pain. Nucleoplasty is a minimally invasive pain interventional procedure which appears as a promising new therapy for this select group of patients.

INTRODUCTION

Chronic back pain is a common condition that affects a considerable proportion of the population. In most individuals, pain resolves spontaneously within several weeks. However, for some people, pain persists despite specific causes of back pain, such as herniated disks, facet joint pathology, and fractures, being excluded. Increasingly, this pain is being attributed to early degeneration of the intervertebral disk manifesting as disk bulging (and/or annular tears) on magnetic resonance imaging scanning and referred to as diskogenic back pain.[1] Small disk protrusions and broad-based disk bulges can also cause persistent spinal nerve irritation and ongoing leg pain in some individuals.

Surgical diskectomy is a poor treatment option for these patients as there is no disk herniation that can be removed without causing further disruption of the normal disk architecture, which potentially can increase the risk of full disk herniation. This small, but important, group of patients has often gone untreated. Percutaneous disk decompression or nucleoplasty appears as a promising new therapy for this select group of patients. In May 2006, the National Institute for Health and Clinical Excellence (NICE) in the United Kingdom approved nucleoplasty and produced guidance in its use.[1]

WHAT IS NUCLEOPLASTY?

Nucleoplasty is a minimally invasive procedure performed on an outpatient basis. It makes use of a variant of radiofrequency technology (coblation technology), which delivers a focused field of energy between closely spaced electrodes at the tip of a rigid treatment probe **(Figs. 1A and B)**.

Energized particles within the created focused plasma possess sufficient energy to break down molecular bonds, thus excising/dissolving soft nucleus pulposus tissue at temperatures between 40 and 70°C with minimal damage to adjacent tissue and structures. Once within the nucleus pulposus, and according to a standardized protocol, the probe creates a series of channels within the disk **(Figs. 2A and B)**, thereby reducing intradiskal pressure and the size of the contained disk protrusion.

INDICATIONS

Radicular and axial back pain caused by contained disk protrusions that have failed to respond to conservative management including rest, physical therapy, medical treatment, and transforaminal/interlaminar steroid epidural injections and/or multidisciplinary program are given below:

- *Radicular symptoms:*
    - Small (<6 mm) contained disk protrusion
    - Disk height >50%
    - Diskography concordant (if indicated)
- *Axial symptoms (little supporting evidence):*
    - Small (<6 mm) contained disk protrusion
    - Disk height >75%
    - Diskography concordant (if indicated).

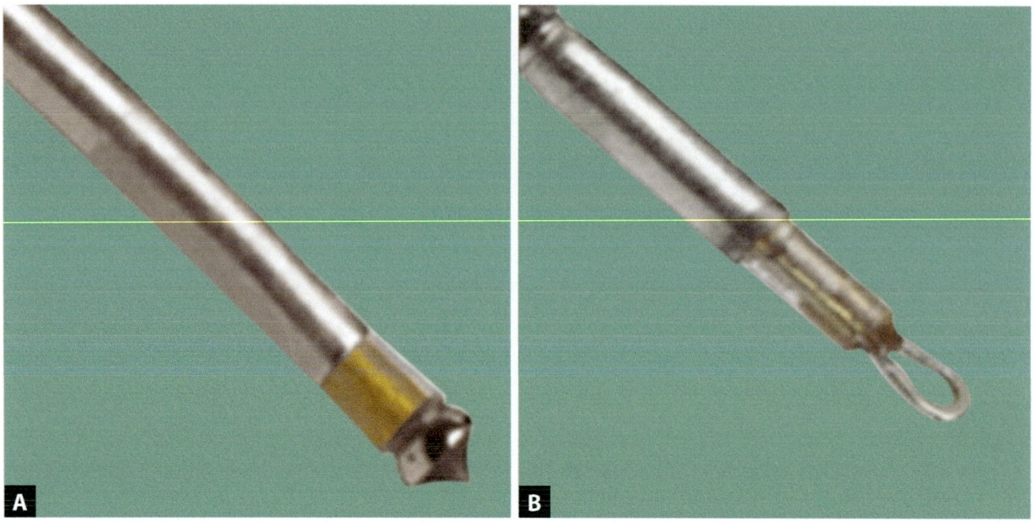

Figs. 1A and B: Treatment probes for nucleoplasty. (A) DLG SpineWand; (B) DC SpineWand.

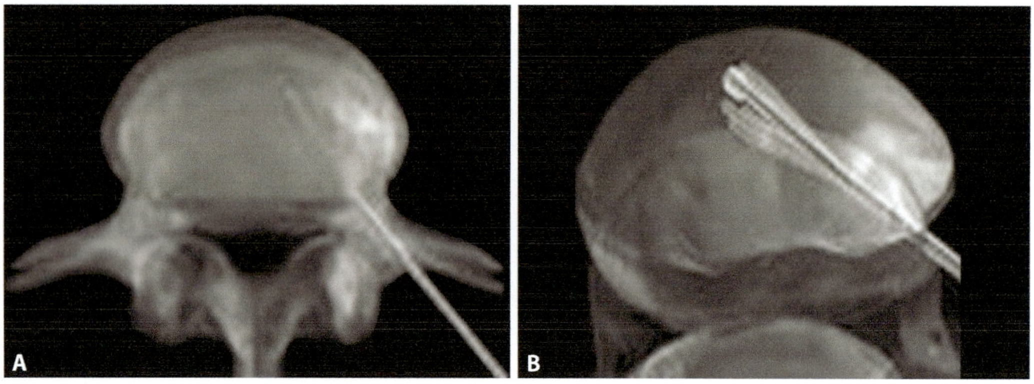

Figs. 2A and B: Schematic axial diagram of the (A) introducer needle and treatment device and (B) used to perform nucleoplasty.

CONTRAINDICATIONS

- Local or systemic sepsis
- Coagulopathy
- Complete annular disruption/extruded disk
- Severe disk degeneration (>50% loss in disk height)
- Moderate-to-severe spinal stenosis
- Spinal fracture/tumor.

TECHNIQUE

Preprocedure Preparation

The procedure is usually performed on an outpatient basis with local anesthesia and mild sedation (with appropriate monitoring as per local and national guidelines). It is important that the level of sedation should allow ongoing communication with the patient so as to be able to report any paresthesia or excess discomfort before neural injury occurs. Appropriate full sterile technique is observed. Use of antibiotics is not usually required. However, many pain physicians will administer antibiotics anytime the annulus is penetrated due to the theoretical risk of infection leading to diskitis. Treating one disk typically takes 30 minutes and two disks about 60 minutes.

Patient Positioning

Under fluoroscopic guidance, placement of the introducer needle for nucleoplasty is identical to that for needle placement during diskography. The patient lies prone with a pillow placed under the abdomen, above the iliac crest, in order to reduce the lumbar lordosis. The C-arm is first rotated 25–35° obliquely and then in a cephalad/caudal angulation (to align the vertebral plates) so that the X-ray beam is centered on the disk space to be treated **(Figs. 3A and B)**. Proper alignment of the C-arm is critical to the safety and success of the procedure.

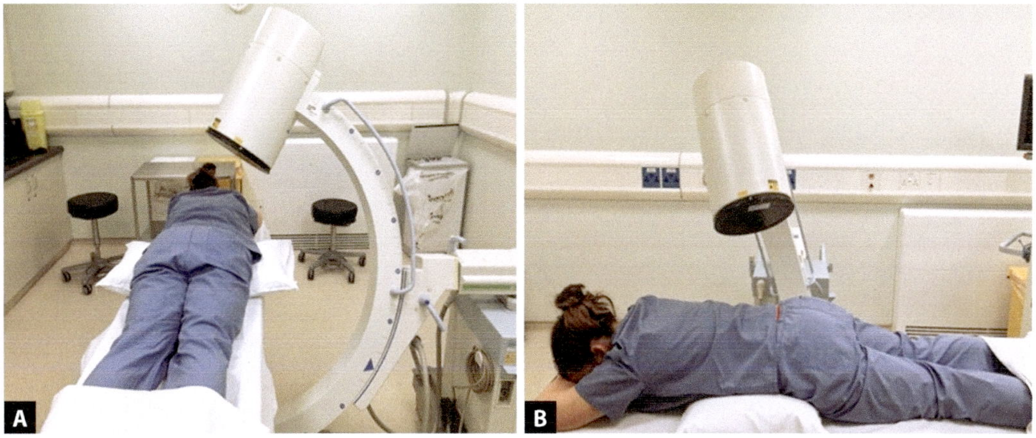

Figs. 3A and B: The patient is placed prone. The C-arm is rotated 25–35° obliquely and centered on the disk space to be studied. The C-arm is then angled in a cephalad direction that will vary from patient to patient, depending on the disk level to be studied and the patient's degree of lordosis.

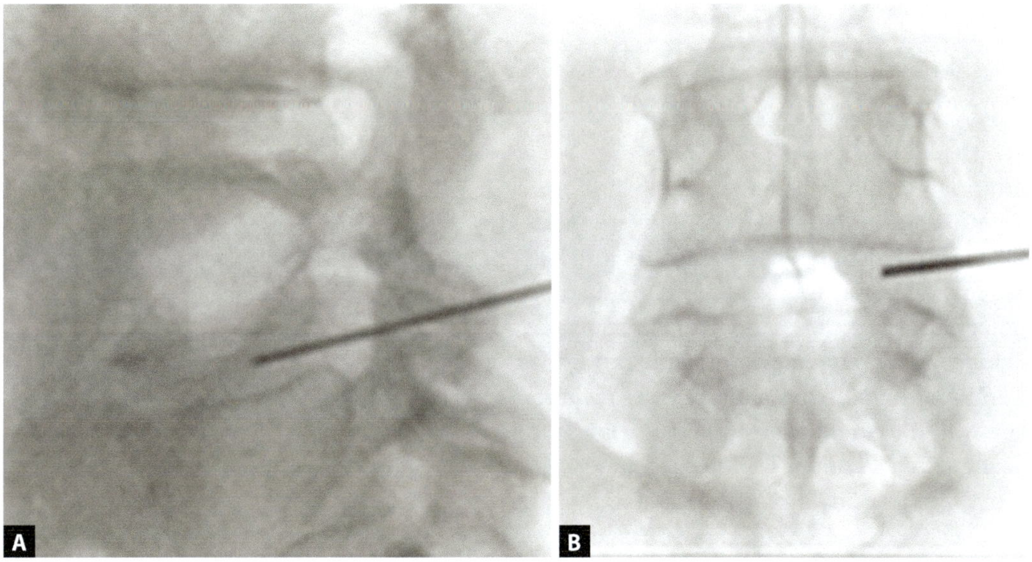

Figs. 4A and B: (A) Lateral and (B) anteroposterior radiographs of lumbar spine demonstrating placement of introducer needle for nucleoplasty at the L4/L5 disk level.

Introducer–Needle Placement

The 17G introducer needle supplied by the manufacturer is guided through the skin/tissues in a plane which is coaxial with the axis of the X-ray beam. The direction of the introducer needle is checked after every 1–1.5 cm of needle advancement and adjusted appropriately to stay coaxial. Once the needle comes in contact with the annulus fibrosus, there will be a notable increase in resistance. At this stage, the C-arm should be rotated to a lateral position and the introducer needle advanced one-third of the posterior to the anterior margin distance of the disk. The final placement is then checked in the anteroposterior (AP) plane **(Figs. 4A and B)**, ensuring that the tip of the introducer needle is again one-third from the ipsilateral to contralateral lateral disk margin. This allows for the creation of channels within the nucleus pulposus, which extend across the greatest distance from the posterolateral aspect of the nucleus on one side of the disk to the anterolateral aspect on the opposite side.

Disk Decompression

Once the introducer needle is placed optimally, a specialized probe (wand) is passed through the needle into the target disk. The probe is advanced through the

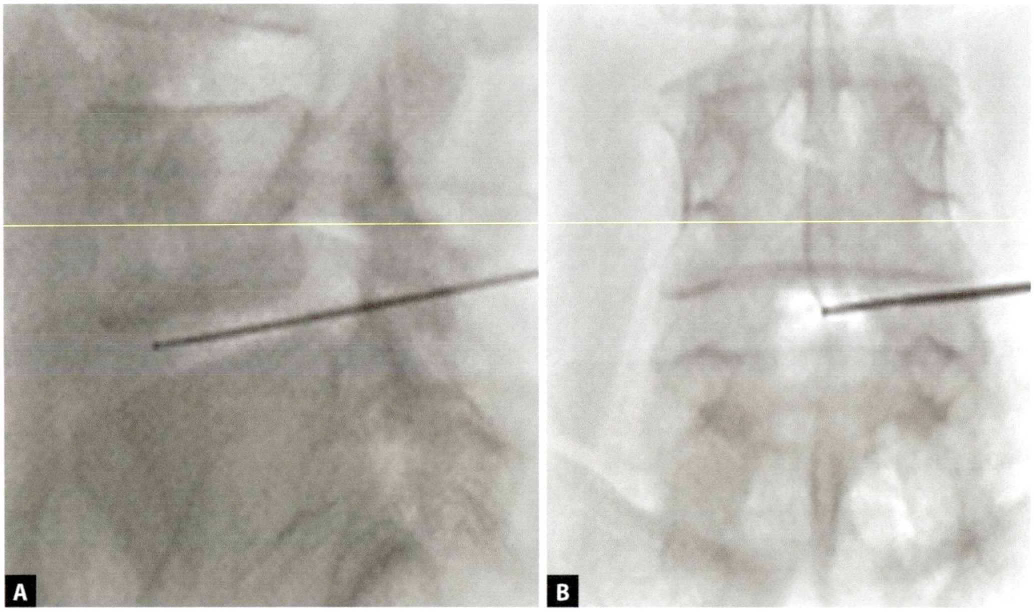

Figs. 5A and B: (A) Lateral and (B) anteroposterior radiographs of lumbar spine showing deployment of the nucleoplasty probe at the L4/ L5 disk level.

introducer until increase in resistance is felt when the probe tip meets the anterior inner margin of the annulus confirmed on lateral and AP radiographs **(Figs. 5A and B)**. A spring-loaded marker device is moved down the shaft of the introducer needle to mark this anterior-most extension and used as a guide for subsequent passes of the probe.

The distal end of the probe has a discrete area where the energy is delivered to the nucleus pulposus tissue. It is also slightly angulated so that a series of channels can be created by rotating and advancing the heated device (at 2, 4, 6, 8, 10, and 12 hours on a clock face). The device is heated up to 40–70°C, ablating the tissue. In this way, a discrete volume of nucleus pulposus is removed (the low-molecular-weight gases produced by ablation pass out of the disk via the introducer needle), lowering the pressure within the disk and reducing the size of the bulging disk/contained disk herniation.

Postprocedure Rehabilitation

A rehabilitation protocol is recommended, but not necessarily required for nucleoplasty. Most centers have utilized the same rehabilitation guidelines as they utilize for other interventional spine procedures. An appropriate rehabilitation procedure should incorporate progressive use of stretching and strengthening exercises, followed by staged return to more normal activities.

COMPLICATIONS

As with any procedure, there are some inherent risks. However, adverse events are uncommon and there are no cases in the reported literature of serious complications. Potential risks include but are not limited to:

- Bleeding/bruising/pain at the needle insertion point
- Increased severity of preprocedural back pain
- Infection (superficial or deep) including theoretical risk of diskitis (exact incidence unknown; diskitis following diskography reported to be <1:1,000)
- Transient neurological symptoms (e.g., numbness/tingling/weakness) due to irritation/injury of a nerve root.

EFFICACY OF NUCLEOPLASTY

Nucleoplasty has been substantiated by scientific and clinical evidence highlighted in a number of peer-reviewed published articles. The methodological quality of this evidence[2-7] consists of randomized controlled trials with important limitations (inconsistent results, methodological faults, indirect, or imprecise) and strong evidence from observational studies. These studies have clearly demonstrated a reduction in intradiskal pressure, positive intradiskal biochemistry changes because of coblation, and positive improvements in a number of clinical standardized outcome measures.

CONCLUSION

Nucleoplasty is a minimally invasive pain interventional procedure which appears as a promising new therapy for patients with chronic low back pain of diskogenic origin. Nucleoplasty has been substantiated by scientific and clinical evidence highlighted in a number of peer-reviewed published articles.

REFERENCES

1. NICE. (2006). Percutaneous disc decompression using coablation for lower back pain. [online] Available from https://www.nice.org.uk/guidance/ipg173 [Last accessed October, 2015].
2. Alexandre A, Coro L, Azuelos A, Pellone M. Lumbar nucleoplasty for discoradicular conflict. Acta Neurochir Suppl. 2005;92:83-6.
3. Gerszten PC, Smuck M, Rathmell JP, Simopoulos TT, Bhagia SM, Mocek CK, et al. Plasma disc decompression compared with fluoroscopy-guided transforaminal epidural steroid injections for symptomatic contained lumbar disc herniation: a prospective, randomized, controlled trial. J Neurosurg Spine. 2010;12(4):357-71.
4. Bokov A, Skorodumov A, Isrelov A, Stupak Y, Kukarin A. Differential treatment of nerve root compression pain caused by lumbar disc herniation applying nucleoplasty. Pain Physician. 2010;13(5):469-80.
5. Sinan T, Sheikh M, Buric J, Dashti K, Al-Mukhaimi A. Percutaneous coblation nucleoplasty in patients with contained lumbar disc prolapse: 1 year follow-up in a prospective case series. Acta Neurochir Suppl. 2011;108:107-12.
6. Kallás JL, Godoy BL, Andraus CF, Carvalho FG, Andraus ME. Nucleoplasty as a therapeutic option for lumbar disc degeneration related pain: a retrospective study of 396 cases. Arq Neuropsiquiatr. 2013;71(1):46-50.
7. Manchikanti L, Abdi S, Atluri S, Benyamin RM, Boswell MV, Buenaventura RM, et al. An update of comprehensive evidence-based guidelines for interventional techniques in chronic spinal pain. Part II: guidance and recommendations. Pain Physician. 2013;16(2 Suppl.):S49-283.

52 CHAPTER

Ozone Nucleolysis

Gautam Das

ABSTRACT

Low back pain, with or without radiation to leg, is very common. Disk prolapse with compression and/or inflammation of nerve root is one of the common reasons for this condition. When conservative management fails, surgery is one of the important treatment modalities for this condition. But complications of conventional surgery are very high, and thus, scientists were in search of some safer treatment modalities.

Ozone is a highly reactive unstable molecule which was found to denature disk glycoprotein molecule. Thus, osmolality of nucleus pulposus is reduced and it gets dehydrated. Thus, disk is reduced in size and decompresses nerve root. Ozone also has anti-inflammatory effect and thus reduces nerve root inflammation too. Ozone nucleolysis is a process of injecting an ozone–oxygen mixture inside the disk and around nerve root at neural foramen after injection of local anesthetics under radiological guidance.

Ozone nucleolysis is safe, low cost, and effective alternative treatment of prolapsed intervertebral disk.

INTRODUCTION

Low back pain, with or without sciatic nerve involvement, affects roughly 80% of the population at least once in their lifetime. In addition, low back pain is the leading cause of lost working days, which has a major effect on national healthcare spending.[1] Since disk prolapse was first diagnosed by Dandy and subsequently by Mixter and Barr, it has been implicated as one of the important causes of low back pain radiating to limbs.[2] Multiple modes of treatment had been prescribed with lot of debate involving each mode. Apart from conservative therapy, all other forms of treatment aim at decompressing the nerve roots. These can be done by either removing disk by conventional surgical method or by decompressing the foramen and disk by minimally invasive interventions. The various treatment options have confused clinicians due to significant failure rate associated with different kind of surgeries as well as with different interventions.[3]

Outcome studies of lumbar disk surgeries document a success rate between 49 and 95% and reoperation after lumbar disk surgeries ranging from 4 to 15%. Reasons for this failure include:

- Dural fibrosis
- Arachnoidal adhesions
- Muscle and fascial fibrosis
- Mechanical instability resulting from the partial removal of bony and ligamentous structures required for surgical exposure and decompression
- Presence of neuropathy.[4-11]

There has been surge of interest in search of safer alternative method of decompressing the nerve roots while maintaining the structural stability even on surgical approach such as microdiskectomy and by the same time, there was lot of nonsurgical approaches such as interventional injections, percutaneous diskectomy, and radiofrequency techniques. Epidural steroid injection and transforaminal epidural procedure, which are very frequently done, have a high success rate (up to 85%). But, chances of recurrences are there, especially if these interventions are done at a later stage. Chemonucleolysis using chymopapain also has high success rate (approximately 80%) with low recurrences, but was not popular owing to the chances of anaphylaxis following intradiskal chymopapain injection.[12] Injection of ozone for diskogenic radiculopathy (low back pain with radiation to legs) has developed as an alternative to chemonucleolysis and disk surgery owing to its high success rate, less invasiveness, fewer chances of recurrences, and remarkably fewer side effects.[10,13]

OZONE IN SPINE-RELATED PAIN

Ozone has been known since ancient times. It was the smell we can feel on early morning seashores. In fact in Greek, "ozein" means "smelling gas". Ozone was discovered in 1785 by Dutch physicist Martinus Van Marum while conducting experiment with electrostatic machines generating electric shocks, which gave off a distinctive, unique, and pungent odor. But, it was not until May 1840 that the German chemist Christian Friedrich Schönbein synthesized it.[14] In 1900, medical ozone was used in the United States by Nikola Tesla by using high voltage, high frequency, low amperage alternating current system. Since then, medical ozone had been used in multiple diseases. Initially, high dose was suspected to cause lot of tissue damage, then low dose concept was introduced to prevent tissue damage and it was found to be safer by inducing redox reaction. By then, different modes of ozone therapy for low back pain were introduced including breathing through oil, oils saturated with ozone, ozonated water, rectal insufflation, subcutaneous injection, and intramuscular injection[15] with lot of debates. It was Muto who suggested intradiskal injection of ozone for disk hernia in 1998 under computed tomography (CT) guidance.[10] Leonardi popularized fluoroscopy-guided ozone injection into the intervertebral disk. After that, successful outcomes have been reported from various European centers. It is very important to note from those reports that complications are remarkably few. Not even a single serious life-threatening complication was found even after 30,000 cases of ozone nucleolysis, which stresses the safety of these procedures.[16]

Ozone is an unstable, colorless, irritant gas with a pungent odor, which has a strong oxidizing power as well as good antiseptic, disinfectant, and antiviral properties. It is chemically the triatomic, allotropic form of oxygen, having the chemical symbol O_3, and a molecular weight of 48 kDa. Ozone, under standard atmospheric temperature and pressure, is an unstable gas with a half-life of 20 minutes that decomposes readily into molecular oxygen. For injection, it is always freshly prepared before administration, wherein only ozone-resistant syringes should be used.

PREPARATION OF OZONE

Ozone for medical practice is obtained from specialized generators. The ozone generators commonly used today employ the corona discharge principle. This technique utilizes a high-tension electrode and a ground electrode mounted in a spaced relation with a vitreous dielectric membrane covering one of the electrodes. The electrodes are connected to an electric power source to set up an electrostatic field.

The electrode must be constructed from a material that:

- Can withstand constant exposure to high-voltage electric fields
- Does not succumb to structural damage due to heat
- Discharges in a smooth energy field without creation of any "sparking" or "arcing" when energy is delivered.

Quartz glass is an ideal material to create electrodes as:

- It has no occlusions and impurities.
- It is impervious to the effects of a high-energy field.
- It is 100% resistant to the oxidative effects of ozone. Other materials used are Kynar and Teflon.

The ozone generator is fed with oxygen from an oxygen cylinder or an oxygen concentrator. Oxygen is the main raw material from which ozone is generated. Air contains 78% nitrogen and 21% oxygen. In the ozone generator, the free oxygen molecule combines with nitrogen to form nitric oxide, which is highly toxic. Inside the generator, oxygen passes between a high-quality double-walled quartz glass and the electrode. The electrical energy is converted into heat and ozone is produced. This heat should be removed as it will cause rapid decomposition of ozone into oxygen.

Parts of a Basic Ozone Generator

The following are the parts of a basic ozone generator **(Fig. 1)**:

- Power switch
- Flow meter
- Ozone ratio controller
- Ozone indicator
- Oxygen/air inlet port with replaceable tube
- Built-in syringe port with replaceable filter.

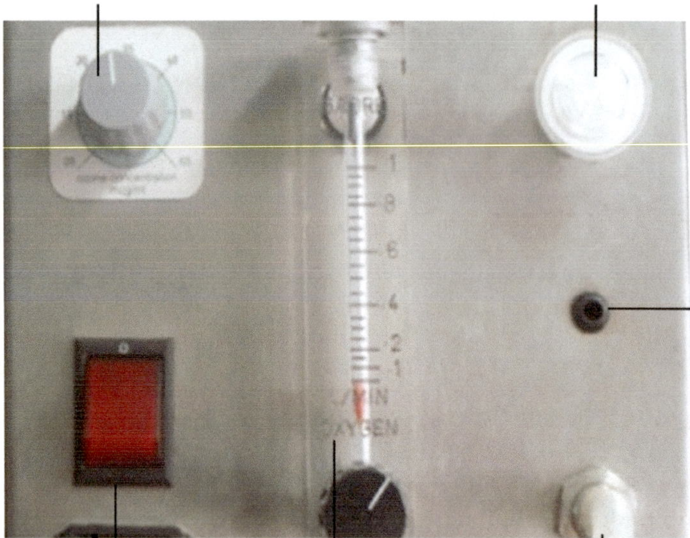

Fig. 1: Front view of ozone generator.

Steps to Generate Ozone

The following are the steps to generate ozone:

- The oxygen source is connected to the generator through the gas-feeding tube.
- The oxygen flow is set at 0.5–1 L/min.
- The desired ozone concentration is set on the ozone ratio controller.
- The machine is turned on.
- Ozone generation is usually indicated through the detection of a pungent smell or by an indicator in some machines.
- The initial volume of the ozone is discarded, and the rest is filled in ozone-resistant syringes.

The following precautions must be taken during ozone generation:

- It is essential that high concentrations of ozone are prevented from entering the air. This is only possible if an external or internal catalytic ozone destruct is provided with the ozone equipment. The best destruct units are those that use iron crystals and avoid carbon, as it can cause explosions.
- Proper ventilation in the form of vents and exhaust fans should be present to dissipate the heat.
- Do not breathe directly as it can cause bronchospasm.
- Ozone should not be applied directly to the skin and eyes as it produces dryness.
- Do not allow water to enter into the machine.
- Use filters to prevent bacteria or any metal impurities to enter into the syringe.

Other methods of preparation of ozone involve ultraviolet light, electrolysis, and the radiochemical method.[17] Cold plasma generators are nowadays available, which is long-lasting than other generators. Ozone is administered in the form of an oxygen–ozone gas mixture, medical ozone, at nontoxic concentrations varying from 1 to 40 µg of ozone per milliliter of oxygen.[18] Empirical studies performed in vivo on rabbits and in vitro on resected human disk specimens have demonstrated that for intradiskal administration, the optimal concentration of ozone per milliliter of oxygen is 27 µg.

Mechanisms of Action

The following are the mechanisms by which ozone provides relief in low back pain and radiculopathy:

- It had been postulated that in addition to mechanical compression, inflammatory mediators also play important role in low back pain and radiculopathy. Ozone has

an effect on the inflammatory cascade by altering the breakdown of arachidonic acid to inflammatory prostaglandins. As a result, inflammatory mediators are reduced, thereby subsequent decrease in pain.
- Herniation can impinge on the venous and arterial flow and cause phlebostasis and arteriostenosis, which leads to a serious hypoxemia of the area, thereby inducing inflammation. By applying the ozone to the herniated site, hyperoxygenation of the area occurs, which reduces the pain by direct and indirect mechanisms.
- Ozone is a rapid and strong oxidizing agent. When ozone is injected into the disk, the active oxygen atom called the singlet oxygen or the free radical attaches with the proteoglycan bridges in the jelly-like material or nucleus pulposus. They are broken down and no longer capable of holding water. As a result, disk shrinks and mummifies, and there is decompression of nerve roots. It is almost equivalent to surgical diskectomy and so the procedure is called ozone diskectomy or ozonucleolysis.
- The stimulation of fibroblastic activity by ozone will result in the initiation of the repair process by stimulating collagen deposition.[19,20]

All these lead to decompression of nerve roots, decreased inflammation of nerve roots, and increased oxygenation to the diseased tissue for repair work.

Methods of Injection

Ozone gas free of metallic and organic impurities is usually used in low back pain patients. These are prepared freshly from machine using sterile bacterial filters. Minimally invasive methods include intradiskal, paravertebral, and juxtaforaminal injection techniques. Although all of these methods have been shown to be effective, it seems that not all of the mechanisms of action mentioned above exist for all of them. In fact, the direct method, namely intradiskal injection in ozone therapy, seems to have an effect on all the mechanisms of action; however, the paravertebral muscle probably uses only the first mechanism listed above, which is the anti-inflammatory effect, and the juxtaforaminal method lacks the third one.

INDICATIONS

Ozone nucleolysis may be done in most kinds of disk-related pain disorders provided the disk has signs of hydration and inflammatory edema in magnetic resonance imaging, for example,
- Internal disk disruption with diskogenic pain
- Contained, hydrated disk prolapse or bulge with root irritation
- Noncontained, hydrated, extruded, and sequestrated disk with root irritation.

It can be also tried in other low back pain conditions including:
- Canal stenosis
- Postsurgical fibrosis (Failed back surgery syndrome)
- Facet joint arthropathy
- Calcified herniation
- Intervertebral osteochondrosis
- Pseudoanterolisthesis.

CONTRAINDICATIONS

There are few conditions where this procedure should not be performed, which include the following described here.

Absolute Contraindications

- Local or systemic infection
- Coagulopathy and patient on anticoagulants without adequate recommended drug-free period
- Lack of consent
- Active hypothyroidism
- Glucose-6-phosphate dehydrogenase (G6PD) deficiency.

Relative Contraindications

- Pregnancy
- Patient not able to lie prone
- Noncooperative patient
- Patient with severe cognitive dysfunction
- Allergy to any of the drugs used for procedure
- Unstable vital parameters
- Previous surgery
- Anatomical variation.

STEPS IN LUMBAR OZONE NUCLEOLYSIS (C-ARM GUIDED)

Ozone nucleolysis can be done either by CT or C-arm guidance depending on the availability of facilities.

Preparation

- Rule out red flags
- Informed and written consent is foremost important step.

- Patient should be explained about the procedure:
  - Why is it done?
  - How is it done?
  - What to expect from procedure?
  - Side effects and complications
  - Further plan of management depending on results
  - Alternative methods, if available
  - Basic cost involved in procedure
- Assess patient general and cardiorespiratory status with appropriate consultation and investigation before procedure.
- Whenever we are planning for procedure, we do certain basic investigations, which include bleeding, coagulation profile, and blood sugar.
- Get conventional lumbar X-ray to rule out anatomical difficulty in procedure.
- Get financial clearance from insurance bodies or other governing bodies before admission, if possible.
- Advise for standard preprocedural fasting.
- Advise to come with accompanying person on day of procedure.

Preprocedure Protocol

- Confirm identity, diagnosis, consent, and clearance for procedure.
- Check for availability of laboratory reports and radiological studies, which may be required during procedure.
- Start intravenous 20 g cannula in nondominant hand.
- Administer prophylactic antibiotic such as ceftriaxone 1 g intravenous (IV) or cefazolin 900 mg 20 minutes before procedure or as per institutional protocol. For patients allergic to cefazolin, clindamycin 600 mg, ciprofloxacin 400 mg, or vancomycin 900 mg may be preferred.
- Patient can be sedated with titrating dose of midazolam or propofol or sometimes with opioids so that patient will be comfortable during procedure.

Requirements

- C-arm with radiation safety devices
- C-arm compatible surgical table
- Metal locator
- Sterile gauze pieces
- Gloves according to performer
- Betadine/chlorhexidine solution
- Sterile drapes
- 26G, 1.5 inches, needle for skin infiltration
- 2 mL syringe for local anesthetic injection
- 5 mL syringe for contrast injection
- 10 mL syringe for ozone injection
- 1% lidocaine for skin infiltration
- Contrast solution such as iohexol or iopamidol
- 18G, 3.5 inches introducer needle
- 22G, 12 cm Quincke needle or diskography needle for intradiskal procedures
- 22G, 9 cm Quincke needle for periganglionic injection
- Adhesive tapes
- Sterile gown.

Position and Monitoring

- Place the patient in prone position.
- Keep pillow of appropriate size under abdomen to correct lordosis.
- Keep the patient comfortable with adequate head and leg rest and keep both arms by the side of head.
- Attach standard basic monitoring as recommended by the American Society of Anesthesiologists.
- Prepare the skin with betadine/chlorhexidine and drape the site with sterile materials.
- Instruct the patient to inform any paresthesia along any nerve root so that needle can be introduced in different path.

Procedure Steps

- Start with C-arm in anteroposterior (AP) position with X-ray tube below patient.
- Keep optimal working space between patient and image intensifier.
- Use automatic brightness mode, if available.
- Identify the side and level of intervertebral disk. Cross-check the level of vertebral body with X-ray.
- Take AP image with spinous process exactly in midline **(Fig. 2)**.
- Align end plate of target vertebral body by craniocaudal tilt **(Fig. 3)**. For upper lumbar disk, move image intensifier caudally and for lower lumbar, move image intensifier cranially
- Then, move the image intensifier in ipsilateral oblique direction until the superior articular pillar lies in the middle one-third of the disk **(Fig. 4)**.
- Needle entry is marked to a point in front of superior articular process targeted toward the center of disk **(Fig. 5)**.

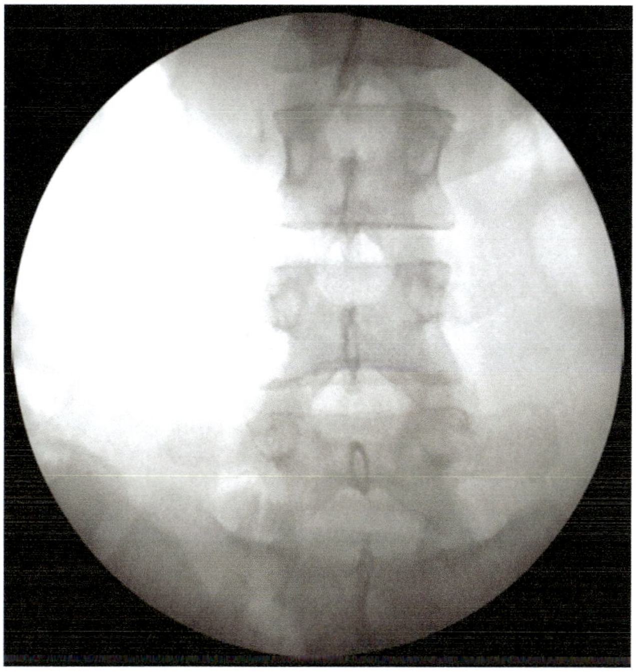

Fig. 2: Anteroposterior image of lumbar spine showing spinous process in midline.

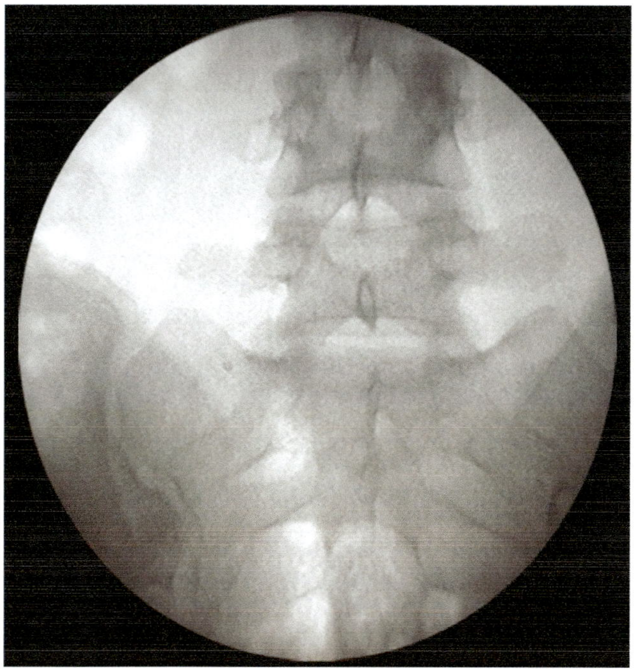

Fig. 3: Squaring of vertebral bodies.

- Infiltrate the entry point with 1% lignocaine and wait for 1 minute.
- It is advised to follow two needle techniques.

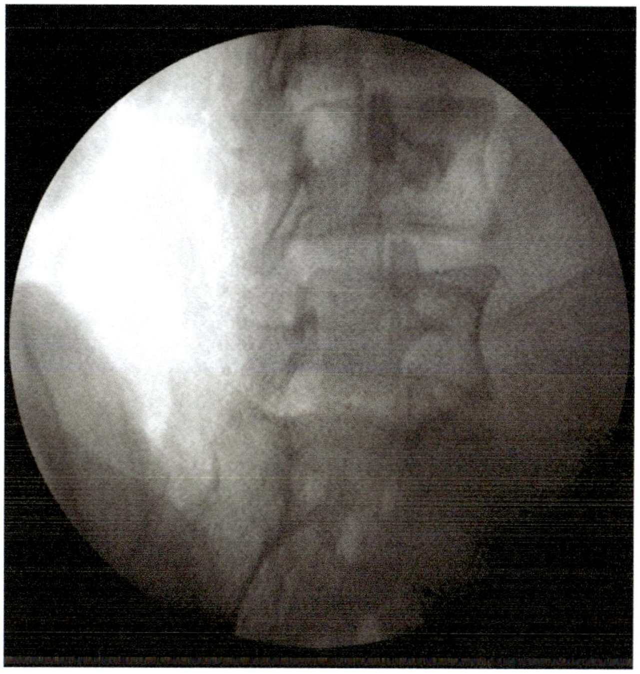

Fig. 4: Oblique view showing superior articular process of L5 at middle of lower endplate of L4.

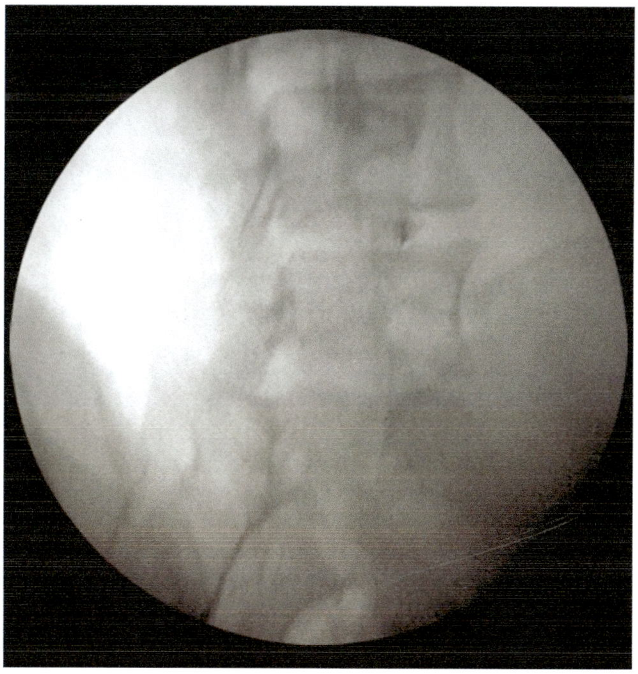

Fig. 5: Image showing needle in front of L5 superior articular pillar.

- 18G, 3.5 inches needle is inserted on end on view until annulus fibrosus **(Fig. 6)**.
- 22G, 12 cm needle is inserted through introducer needle and entered into annulus fibrosus.

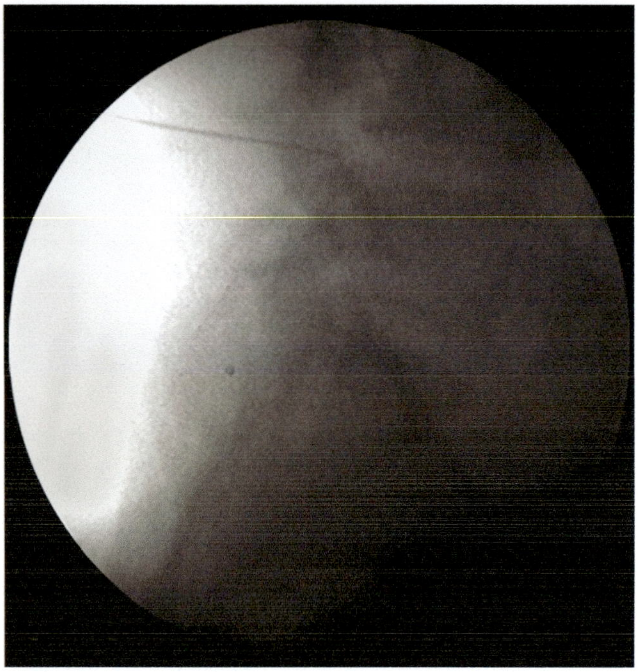

Fig. 6: Image showing needle about to enter annulus fibrosus.

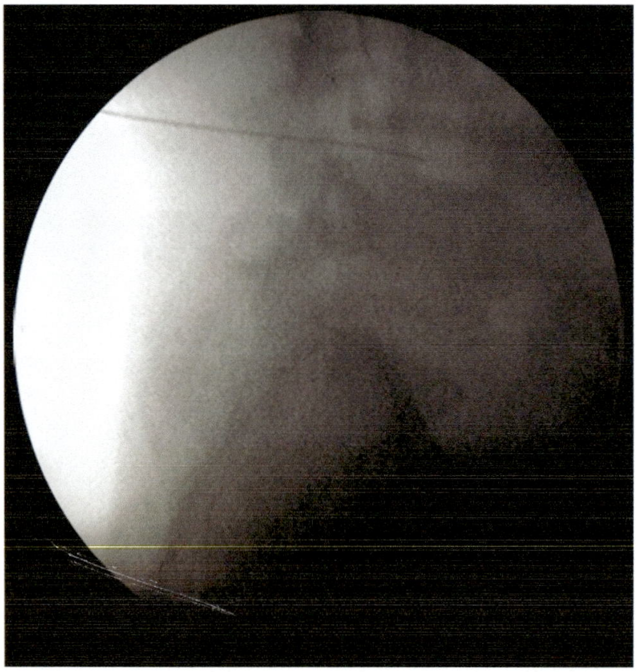

Fig. 7: Lateral view showing needle tip in the center of intervertebral disk.

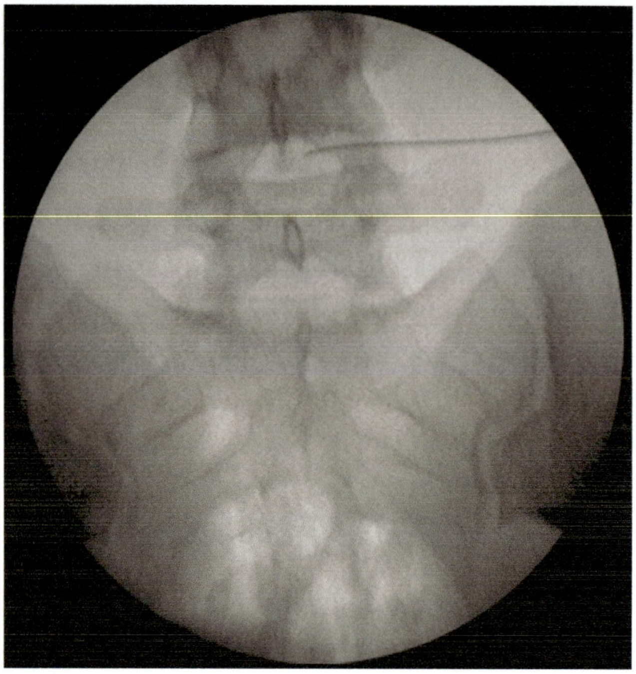

Fig. 8: Anteroposterior image showing needle in near center of intervertebral disk.

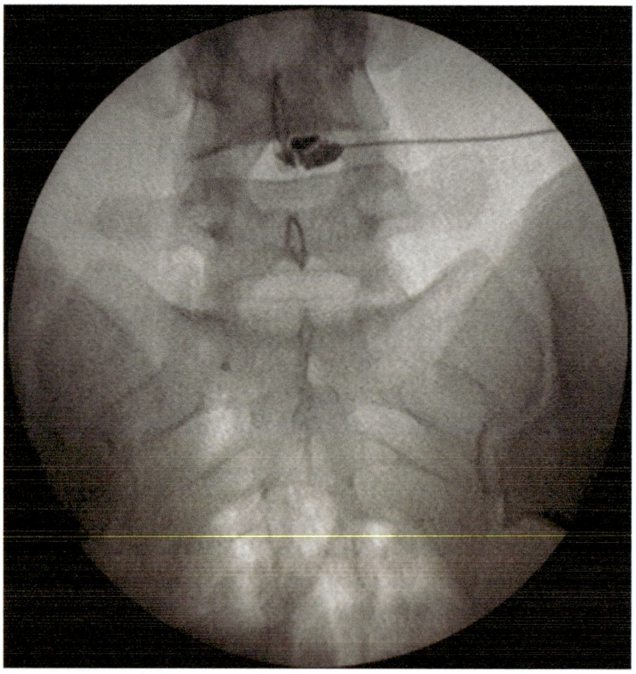

Fig. 9: Anteroposterior image showing dye spread in intervertebral disk.

- Now, C-arm is changed to lateral position and the needle is advanced until the needle lies between the endplates of the vertebra and to the center of the disk **(Fig. 7)**.
- Final needle position is confirmed by AP image **(Fig. 8)**.
- Some small amount of radiopaque dye (omnipaque) may be injected for diskogram, which is optional **(Figs. 9 and 10)**.

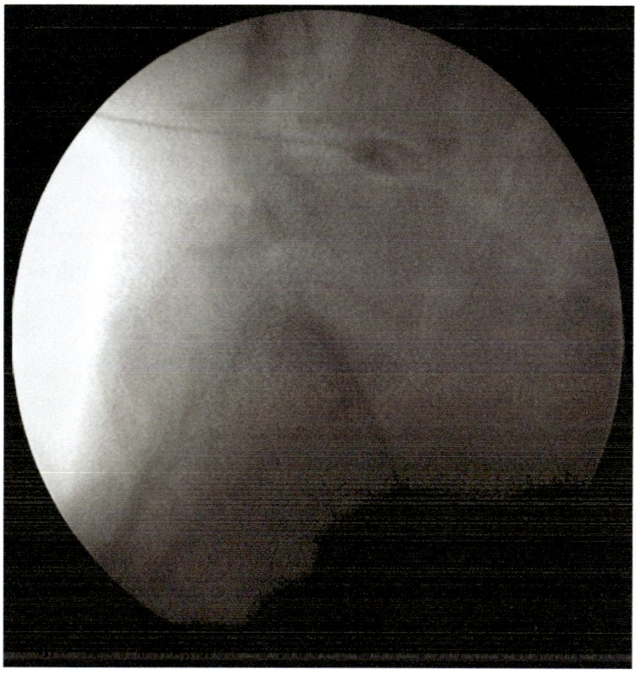

Fig. 10: Lateral image showing dye spread in intervertebral disk.

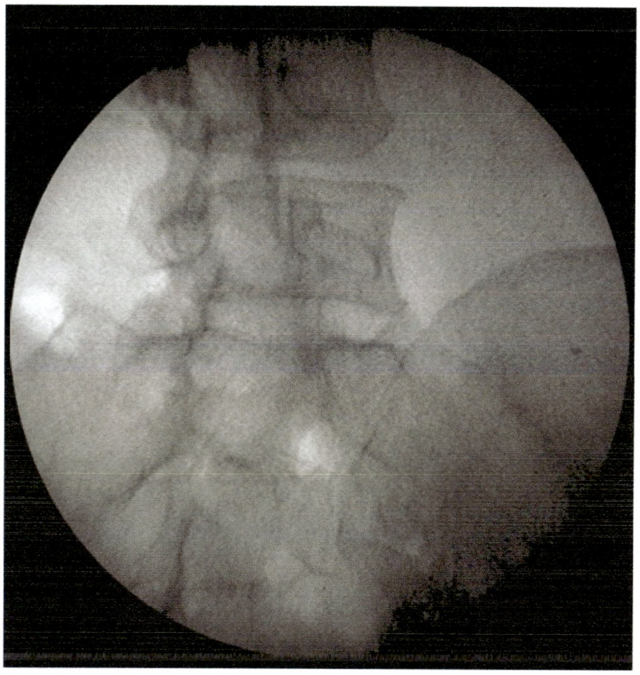

Fig. 11: Oblique view showing superior articular process of lower vertebra at 6 o'clock position of pedicle or upper vertebra.

- Then, 3–10 mL of oxygen-ozone mixture (at a concentration of 27–40 mg/mL) is injected into the disk. Ozone at this concentration is not all harmful for the surrounding tissues. Even when ozone spreads to the surrounding tissues including spinal cord, there is no harm. While needle with the syringe is taken out, some amount of oxygen-ozone mixture is also injected into the paraspinal muscle and pararadicular soft tissue to reduce nerve root inflammation and increase oxygenation of the paraspinal muscles.

Periganglionic Ozone Injection Steps

- Steps are the same as above up to squaring of vertebral body
- C-arm is moved to ipsilateral oblique direction until superior articular pillar of lower vertebral body lies at 6 o'clock position of upper vertebra. Needle entry is targeted at space between the two structures **(Fig. 11)**.
- 22G, 9 cm Quincke needle is inserted with bevel end targeting the pedicle so as to hit the 6 o'clock position of pedicle **(Fig. 12)**.
- Once it hit the pedicle, bevel end is turned inferior so as to slip off from pedicle
- Now, C-arm is moved to lateral position and needle tip should be in upper posterior quadrant

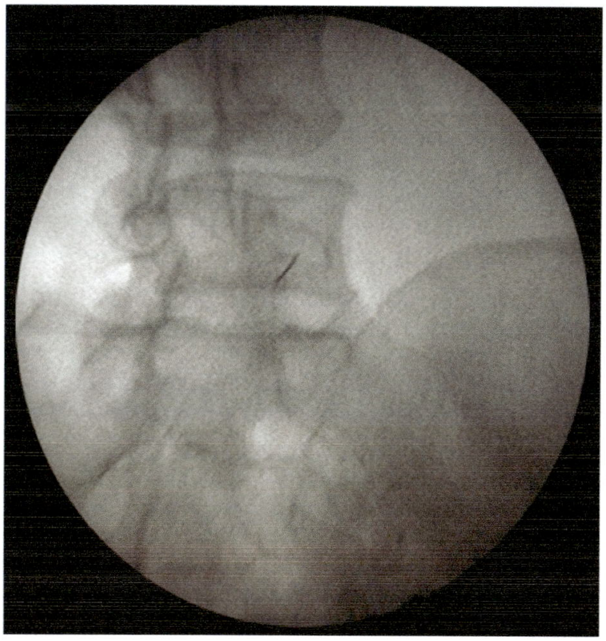

Fig. 12: Needle tip hitting at 6 o'clock position of pedicle.

- Needle tip position is confirmed in AP view **(Fig. 13)**
- Contrast is injected which spreads along the nerve root **(Fig. 14)**
- Once confirmed, 8–10 mL of oxygen-ozone mixture (at a concentration of 27–40 μg/mL) is injected.

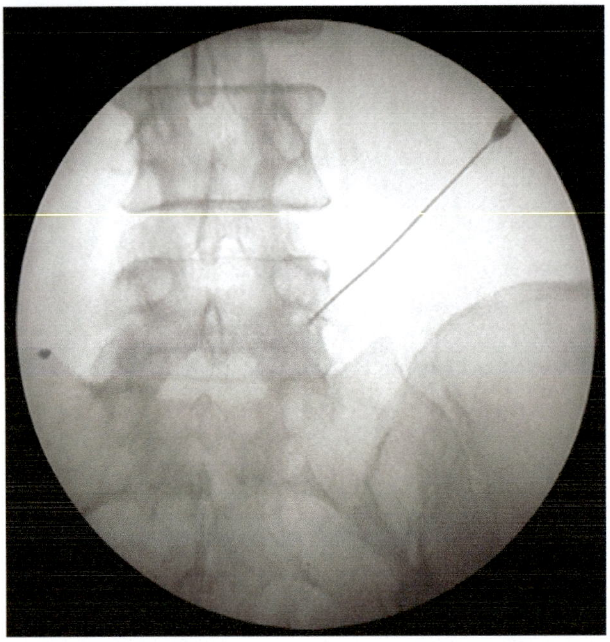

Fig. 13: Image showing needle in root of L5 nerve.

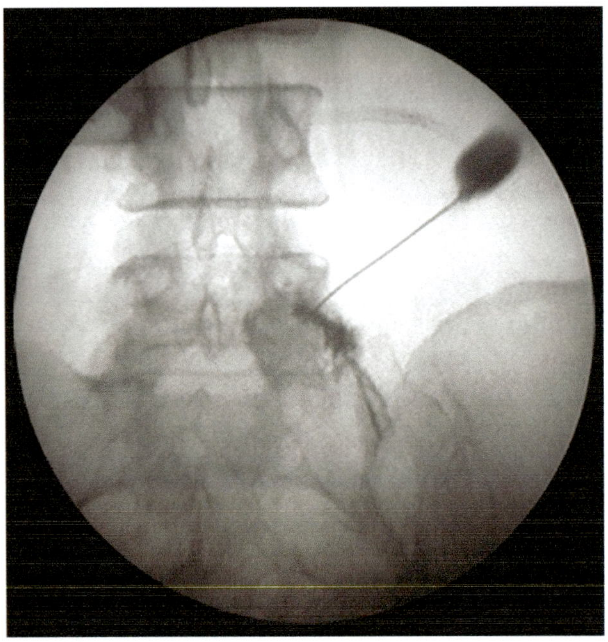

Fig. 14: Contrast spreads along L5 nerve and also spreads into epidural space.

Paravertebral Injection Steps

- Start with C-arm in AP view.
- 22G, 9 cm needle is targeted to hit lamina or articular pillar.
- Withdraw slightly from periosteum and inject 1–2 mL of 1% lignocaine and wait for 2 minutes.
- Inject 5–20 mL of oxygen-ozone mixture at a concentration of 10–20 µg/mL.
- Patients may feel some heaviness on back.

CERVICAL OZONE NUCLEOLYSIS

- Patient is placed in supine position with head slightly turned to opposite side.
- The neck may be extended by placing small pillow in between shoulder girdle.
- Arms are placed by the side of the body.
- For lower cervical disk, Swimmer's view can be used, or arms can be pulled down.
- Patient is instructed neither to move nor to talk in between and can raise their hands on any problem.
- C-arm is started in lateral view and level of vertebral body confirmed.
- Craniocaudal tilt can be done so as to square the vertebral body.
- Then, rotate the C-arm 20–30° until the anterior margin of the uncinate process is moved approximately one-quarter of the distance between the anterior and posterior lateral vertebral margins.
- Needle entry point is in between sternocleidomastoid and trachea on right side so as to avoid esophagus on left side.
- Constant retraction force is applied with index finger on sternocleidomastoid so as to retract carotid vessels laterally.
- The needle entry point is just 3 mm anterior to uncinate process.
- 23G, 9 cm Quincke needle is inserted anterior to uncinate process and once needle enters annulus fibrosus, C-arm is moved to AP view.
- The needle is advanced to the center of intervertebral disk.
- Contrast can be injected (optional) to confirm the needle position.
- Once confirmed, 3–4 mL of oxygen-ozone mixture at a concentration of 27–40 µg/mL is injected.

COMPLICATIONS

Complications are very rare. They include postprocedural muscle spasm and burning pain (these are transient) and diskitis (very rare due to the bactericidal effect of ozone). Other complications are similar to diskographic procedure. Some rare reports of vitreoretinal hemorrhage, thunderclap headache, and stroke had been documented, but it was usually owing to technical errors than by ozone itself.

ADVANTAGES

Ozone nucleolysis has a success rate of about 80%. On the other hand, surgical diskectomy has much higher side effects compared to remarkably fewer side effects of ozone diskectomy. Ozone diskectomy is usually a day care procedure and general anesthesia is not usually required. It is gaining popularity in different countries including India owing to low cost, less hospital stay, fewer post-procedural discomforts and morbidity, and very few side effects.

CONCLUSION

Ozone nucleolysis is a safer alternative treatment when conservative management fails. It is effective, low cost, and reasonably safe. Ozone nucleolysis works better when disk is adequately hydrated as it works by dehydration and reduction of the disk nucleus pulposus size. Though it is safe, complications such as diskitis have been reported. Thus, strict asepsis is mandatory while doing this procedure.

REFERENCES

1. Czervionke LF. Lumbar intervertebral disc disease. Neuroimag Clin North Am. 1993;3:465-85.
2. Mixter WJ, Barr JS. Rupture of the intervertebral disc with involvement of the spinal canal. N Eng J Med. 1934;211:210-5.
3. Das G, Ray S, Ishwarari S, Roy M, Ghosh P. Ozone nucleolysis for management of pain and disability in prolapsed lumbar intervertebral disc. Interv Neuroradiol. 2009;15:330-4.
4. Crock HV. Observation on the management of failed spinal operations. J Bone Joint Surg Br. 1976;58:193-9.
5. Greenwood J, McGuire TH, Kimbell F. A study of the causes of failure in the herniated intervertebral disc operation: an analysis of 67 reoperated cases. J Neurosurg. 1952;9:15-20.
6. Law JD, Lehman RW, Kirsch WM. Reoperation after lumbar intervertebral disc surgery. J Neurosurg. 1978;48:259-63.
7. Matsui H, Terahata N, Tsuji H. Hirano N, Naruse Y. Familial predisposition and clustering for juvenile lumbar disc herniation. Spine. 1992;17:1323-8.
8. Pheasant H. Sources of failure in laminectomies. Orthop Clin North Am. 1975;6:319-29.
9. Spaziante R. La terapia chirurgica nel conflitto disco-radicolare. Riv Neuroradiol. 1997;10:545-50.
10. Muto M, Avella F. Percutaneous treatment of herniated lumbar disc by intradiscal oxygen-ozone injection. Intervent Neuroradiol. 1998;4(4):279-86.
11. Iliakis E. Ozone treatment in low back pain. Orthopaedics. 1995;1:29-33.
12. Nordby EJ, Fraser RD, David MJ. Chemonucleolysis. Spine. 1996;21:1102- 5.
13. Muto M, Adreula C, Leonardi M. Treatment of herniated lumbar disc by intradiscal and intraforaminal oxygen-ozone (O2-O3) injection. J Neuroradiol. 2004;31(3):183-9.
14. Masennikov OV, Kontorshchikova CN, Gribkova IA. (2008). Ozone Therapy in Practice-Health Manual. State Medical Academy of Nizhny Novgorod: Nizhny Novgorod (Russia). [online] Available from http://www.absoluteozone.com/assets/ozone_therapy_in_practice.pdf [Last accessed July, 2024].
15. Torri G. Della GA, Casadei C. Clinical experience in the treatment of lumbar disc disease, with a cycle of lumbar muscle injection of an oxygen + ozone mixture. Int J Med Biol Environ. 1999;27:177-83.
16. Steppan J, Meaders T, Muto M, Murphy KJ. A metaanalysis of the effectiveness and safety of ozone treatments for herniated lumbar discs. J Vasc Interv Radiol. 2010;21:534-48.
17. Smith W. Principles of Ozone Generation. Australia: Watertec Engineering Pty. Ltd.; 2002.
18. Bocci VA. Scientific and medical aspects of ozone therapy. State of the art. Arch Med Res. 2006;37:425-35.
19. Sagai M, Bocci V. Mechanisms of action involved in ozone therapy: is healing induced via a mild oxidative stress? Med Gas Res. 2011;1:29.
20. Borrelli E. Mechanism of action of oxygen ozone therapy in the treatment of disc herniation and low back pain. Acta Neurochir Suppl. 2011;108:123-5.

53 CHAPTER

Percutaneous Transforaminal Endoscopic Lumbar Diskectomy

Girish Datar

ABSTRACT

The most common treatment for lumbar radicular pain due to disk herniation is diskectomy.[1] Since 1938, open diskectomy has been used to relieve pain caused by herniated disks. The success rate for this operation has been satisfactory, but complications may occur, including bleeding, prolonged pain, and scar formation. Furthermore, the soft tissue dissection and bony resection required to gain access to the disk herniation may lead to segmental instability and pain.

Minimally invasive techniques, such as endoscopic diskectomy, have been developed over the past 20 years and provide an opportunity to avoid the potential morbidity of traditional open surgery.[2] The early techniques were lacking in standardization and training, and the lack of instrumentation also made the procedure technically demanding. Over the past 15 years, major improvements in instrumentation and technique have been made, and their use is gradually increasing in acceptance.[3] The main advantages of the endoscopic approach are less skin and muscle trauma, maintenance of bony integrity, and minimization of nerve root trauma due to local anesthesia, which may translate into quicker recovery. Many papers report outcomes equivalent to those of open diskectomy, but with less surgical morbidity.

INTRODUCTION

Conventional diskectomy is one of the most common treatments for herniated nucleus pulposus with radicular pain. Though this procedure produces a successful outcome, it exposes the patient to potential complications such as infections, neurological injury, bleeding, scar formation, and epidural fibrosis. Stripping of paraspinal musculature, removal of bone, and retraction of neurological structures are necessary just to gain access to the site of the pathology, which may decompensate the degenerating spine, leading to secondary instability.[2]

To overcome some of the potential complications of conventional diskectomy, percutaneous transforaminal endoscopic lumbar diskectomy (PTELD) was developed. The advantages of this newly developed procedure are given in **Table 1**. PTELD causes pain relief by:

- Diskectomy and osteophytectomy under endoscopic and fluoroscopic guidance
- Washing out of inflammatory mediators with continuous irrigation
- Denervation of ingrown chronic nerve fibers by radiofrequency and laser.

INDICATIONS

Percutaneous transforaminal endoscopic lumbar diskectomy is indicated in:

- Protrusion, prolapse, extrusion, sequestration, and migrated herniations
- Decompression of lateral recess stenosis and foraminal stenosis
- Patients with disk herniation with failed conservative and/or interventional management
- Central, paracentral, foraminal, and extraforaminal herniations (far lateral type) **(Fig. 1)**
- Internal disk disruption
- Excision of synovial cysts
- Debridement of disk in diskitis and in preparation for interbody device
- Recurrent herniation and in patients with epidural fibrosis.

TABLE 1: Comparison between conventional diskectomy and percutaneous transforaminal endoscopic lumbar diskectomy (PTELD).

	Conventional diskectomy	*PTELD*
Approach	Posterior through the interlaminar window with or without laminotomy	Posterolateral through the intervertebral foramen
Anesthesia	General, spinal, or epidural anesthesia	Local anesthesia (procedure is performed in awake and aware state)
Size of skin incision	7.5 cm or more	<1 cm
Paraspinal musculature	Affected due to stripping (may lead to instability)	Not affected
Lamina or bone	Affected due to laminotomy (may cause instability)	Not affected
Ligamentum flavum	Affected due to opening (leads to instability and epidural fibrosis)	Not affected
Bleeding	Possible	Minimal
Retraction of neurological structures	Is must to access the site of pathology (This can cause neurological injury in an anesthetized patient)	Not necessary (Neurological injury is not possible as the patient is in an awake and aware state during the entire procedure and can report pain on handling neurological structures)
Epidural fibrosis	Possible due to invasion of dorsal epidural space	Minimal
Postoperative	Longer rehabilitation	Shorter rehabilitation

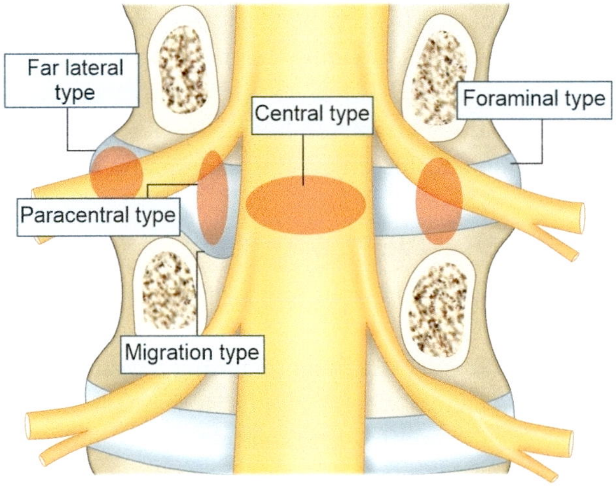

Fig. 1: Types of herniation.

CONTRAINDICATIONS

Percutaneous transforaminal endoscopic lumbar diskectomy is contraindicated in:

- Patients with red flag signs and cauda equina syndrome
- Patients with severe neurological deficits
- Patients with central spinal stenosis
- Pregnancy and bleeding disorders
- Relative contraindications may include sequestrated and migrated fragments that are out of reach of the endoscope through the foraminal approach and that are better approached with traditional techniques.[2] The relative contraindications are dependent on the skill and experience of the surgeon and their ability to perform additional procedures such as foraminoplasty and partial pediculectomy to approach the sequestrated and migrated fragment.

COMPLICATIONS

The following complications, though rare, should be discussed with the patient:

- *Diskitis (0.01%):* Usually presents weeks after the procedure with persistent back pain, difficulty in changing position, elevated C-reactive protein, and erythrocyte sedimentation rate. Repeat magnetic resonance imaging (MRI) may show marrow edema of the vertebral bodies and rarely a collection. Diskitis can be effectively treated with endoscopic debridement, rest, and intravenous (IV) antibiotics. Some patients may show erosion of vertebral bodies, which may need open decompression and stabilization. Adhering to strict aseptic principles and patient screening will reduce the incidence of this complication.
- Dysesthesia (Sunburn syndrome), which occurs in 15% of cases, usually lasts 3-6 weeks and causes Sunburn effect in the lower limbs after PTELD.

The exact cause of this is not known, but thermal, mechanical, and vascular factors may be responsible for this effect. Patients with mild symptoms respond to gabapentin and pregabalin, and those with severe symptoms need repeated transforaminal steroid blocks.[4]

- Lumbar plexopathy, a rare peripheral nerve problem due to injury to the nerve plexus, lymphatics, or vasculature, can be caused by approaching the neural foramina too close to the midline (within 8 cm). This is characterized by pain, numbness, spasms, tingling, weakness, or hypersensitivity in L1-L4 segments in lumbar plexopathy and L5-S3 segments in sacral plexopathy. This complication can be prevented by keeping at least 10 cm from the midline. Lumbar plexopathy is confirmed by electromyography and nerve conduction velocity and is treated with transforaminal epidural steroid, gabapentin, and muscle relaxants when necessary.
- Superficial or deep hematoma can occur in the subcutaneous tissue or between the psoas major and psoas minor muscles, respectively. Treatment with compression is necessary for superficial hematoma and observation by MRI for absorption of blood is required for deep layer hematoma. Rarely if the hematoma is causing neural compression with symptoms, it may call for surgical drainage.
- In conditions with high iliac crest, especially when accessing L5-S1 foramen, reduced intervertebral space, very narrow foramen, and the presence of abnormal neural tissue in the foramen (furcal nerve or conjoint nerve), the surgeon may not be able to access the site of the pathology and hence abandon the procedure and plan an alternative procedure. Careful preoperative planning will help choose the right patient for PTELD.
- In the case of compensated spine or in spine with existing instability, further increase in instability can occur after PTELD, which will need open or percutaneous instrumentation for stabilization. To reduce the chances of instability after PTELD, limiting annulotomy during the procedure may be helpful.
- Recurrent herniation is common in young patients with chronic symptoms and large herniations. Primary disk herniation causes permanent weakness in the annulus and makes it prone for recurrent herniation. Changing the lifestyle is critical to avoid repetitive stress on the spinal segment. As a surgeon, there is little that can be done to avoid this complication except for limiting annulotomy and removing all loose and degenerated fragments from the disk. The key to management of this problem is early detection and prompt treatment.[3]
- Chronic low back pain can be a complaint in some patients with advanced degeneration. Rehabilitation with core strengthening exercises and interventional procedures, such as facet or sacroiliac joint block and medial branch rhizotomy, can relieve back pain in majority of patients.[1] Those patients unresponsive to these treatments may need to undergo instrumented spinal fusion.
- Missed disk fragments are usually met in sequestrated, fragmented, and migrated disk herniations. Occasionally, if they are missed during the procedure and are causing symptoms, a second reoperation may be necessary to retrieve the missed fragment.[4]
- PTELD does not provide satisfactory pain relief of leg/buttock pain. This can be because of damage to the nerve due to long-standing chemical-mediated inflammation and mechanical compression. Occasionally, it can be due to a missed fragment, coexisting lateral canal stenosis, and preexisting neuropathy.

PREOPERATIVE PROTOCOL

The following steps must be followed before planning for PTELD:

- Detailed history obtained including aggravating and relieving factors, history of other diseases in the past, drug history, clinical and neurological examination, and exclude all red flag signs
- MRI of the lumbar spine with screening of thoracic and cervical spine. X-rays of the lumbar spine to rule out instability, pars defect, spondylolisthesis, and to study bony anatomy, especially iliac crest in L5-S1 disk herniation. Computed tomography (CT) scan may be useful to detect the bony boundaries of the foramen, detect pars defect, and identify the composition of the disk herniation—soft, hard, calcification, and osteophytes **(Table 2)**.
- Hematological, serological, and biochemical investigations
- Preoperative medical and anesthetic fitness

Preoperative Planning (Figs. 2A to C)

The success of PTELD is dependent on the best trajectory to the site of the pathology. Planning is done based on the MRI images and X-rays.

Step 1: Identify the site of the pathology on the axial and sagittal cut of the MRI.

Step 2: On the axial cut, draw the line "A" dividing the disk in right and left halves. Draw the second and third line "B" at the medial pedicular border on either side. Draw fourth and fifth line "C" midway between the central and medial pedicular line on either side.

Step 3: On the sagittal cut, draw the first line "1" at the inferior pedicular border of the superior vertebra and line "2" at the superior pedicular border of the inferior vertebra. Draw the line "3" in the center of the disk.

TABLE 2: Comparison of imaging modalities for evaluation of disk-related pathologies.

	X-ray	*CT scan*	*MRI*
Disk herniation		##	###
Neural structure			###
Bony anatomy	#	###	##
Spondylolysis	#	###	##
Calcification	#	###	#
Osteophytes	#	###	#
Instability	###		
Modic changes (1 and 2)			###
Modic changes (3)	#	##	###

#: Low sensitivity; ##: Moderate sensitivity; ###: High sensitivity (CT: computed tomography; MRI: magnetic resonance imaging)

Step 4: Identify the location of the herniation from these two images, plot it on the X-ray images which will serve as a guide during the procedure.

PATIENT POSITIONING AND ANESTHETIC TECHNIQUE

The patient is positioned on a radiolucent, height adjustable operating table in a prone position with soft bolsters under the chest and pelvis. We need to ensure that the abdomen is free, and patient is comfortable in this position. No attempts are made to correct the kyphosis and lordosis in the lumbar spine. The image intensifier comes in from the opposite side of the surgeon and the operating area. The height of the operating table is adjusted in the lateral imaging position of the image intensifier at its lowest position.

The anesthesiologist secures an IV line, and oxygen is delivered through a mask or nasal prongs. 1% preservative-free lignocaine is used by the surgeon for skin and subcutaneous infiltration. No local anesthetic is used in the foramen except for annular infiltration, so as not to block the exiting and traversing root, and that the patient can confirm pain during needle, dilator, and cannula insertion. To supplement it, the anesthesiologist uses a combination of fentanyl 50–100 µg, diclofenac sodium injection 100 mg or paracetamol 1 g IV, and midazolam 2–3 mg. The doses are titrated in such a way that the patient is awake, aware, and communicable during the entire procedure and does not perceive pain. Mild discomfort during the procedure is expected and is normal.

INSTRUMENTATION

Instruments used are shown in **Figures 3 to 9**.

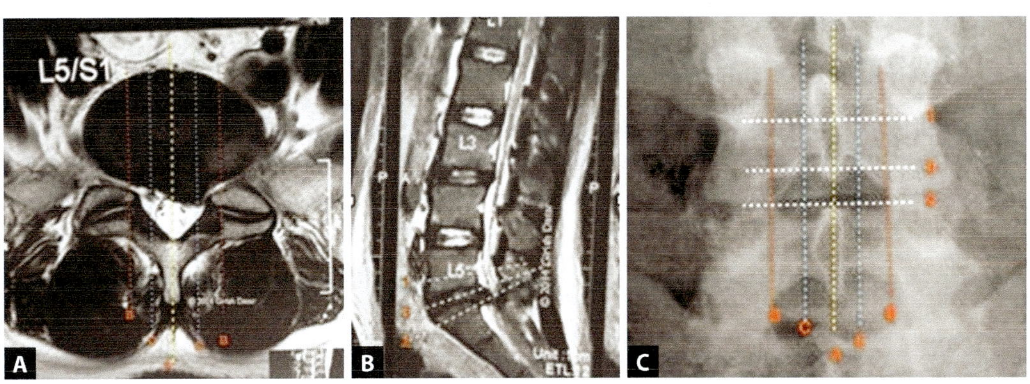

Figs. 2A to C: Preoperative planning using the magnetic resonance imaging (MRI) and X-rays.

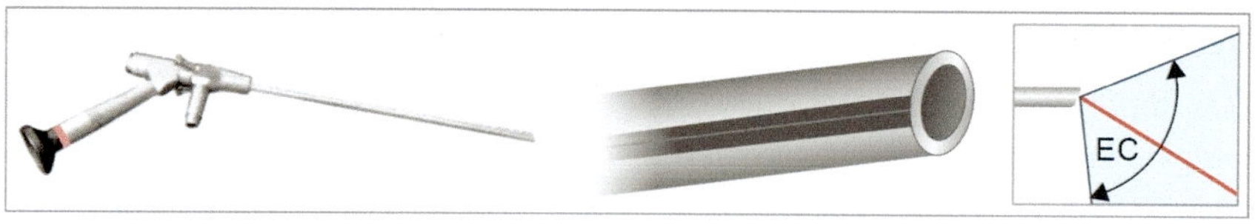

Fig. 3: 30° endoscope with integrated working channel, fiber-optics, camera, and irrigation port.

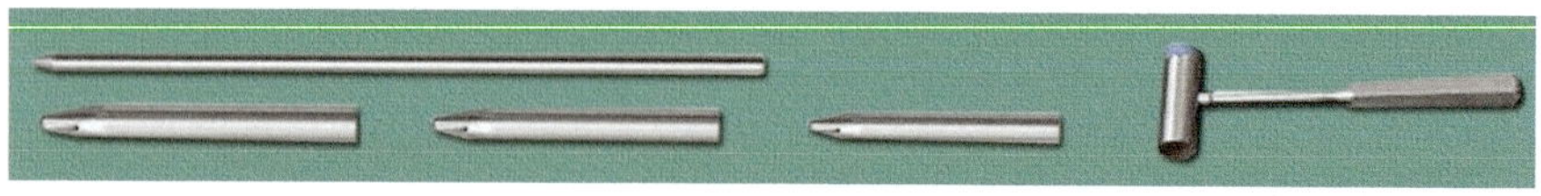

Fig. 4: Two-channel dilator with mallet.

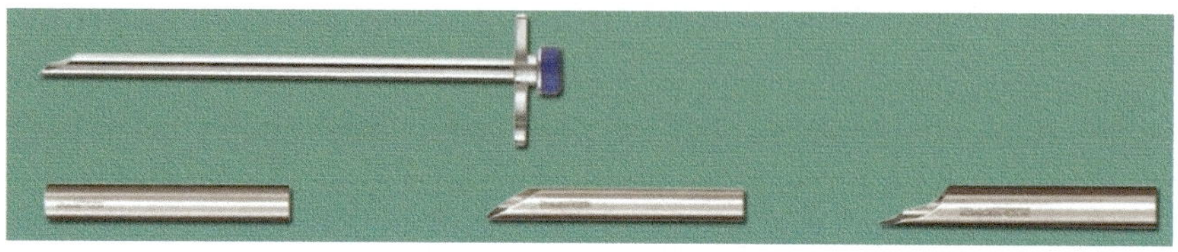

Fig. 5: Working cannula.

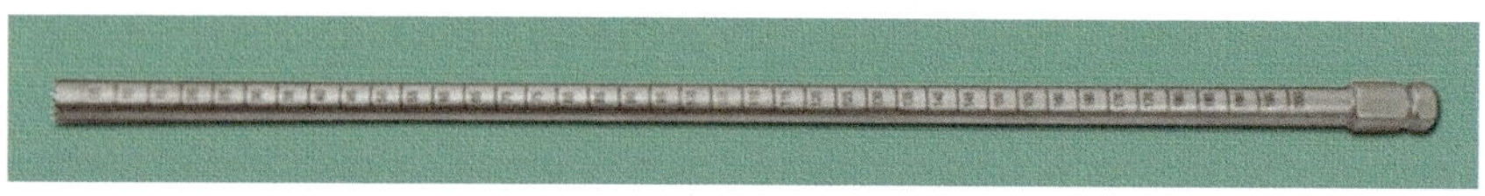

Fig. 6: Trephine.

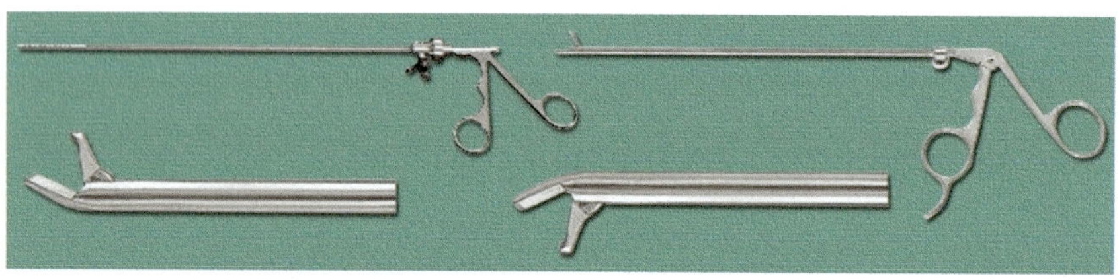

Fig. 7: Rongeurs and punch.

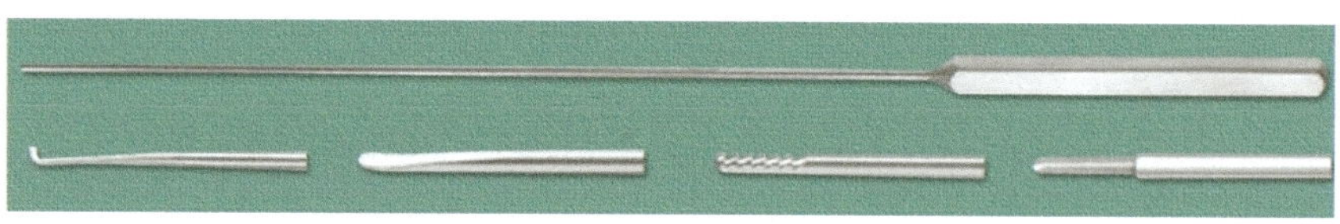

Fig. 8: Handheld instruments: Probes, annulotome, and rasp.

Identifying the Needle Entry Point on the Skin

With the patient lying prone on the radiolucent, height adjustable operating table, the image intensifier (II) is brought from the opposite side and oriented in a posterior-anterior (PA) position. The height of the operating table is adjusted in the lateral imaging position of the image intensifier at its lowest position. The following steps need to be followed for the identification of skin entry point:

- With the II oriented in PA position, ensure that the lumbar spine is well centered on the II screen.

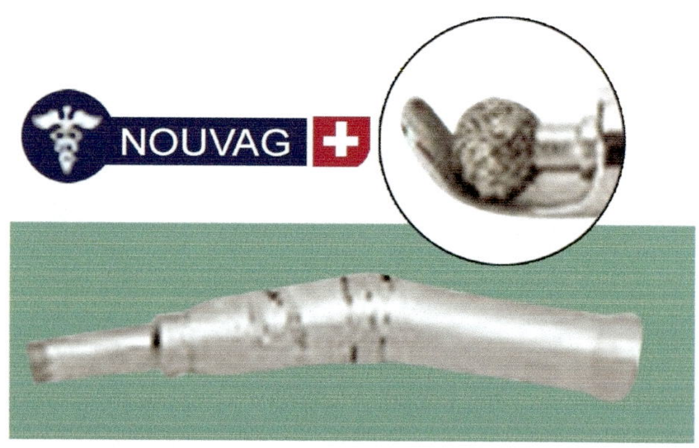

Fig. 9: Burr.

Confirm that spinous process is well centered between both the pedicles and there is no rotational component due to paraspinal spasm, which usually occurs due to spinal pathology. If any rotation is detected, it is corrected by repositioning the patient.

- Mark line "1" connecting tip of the spinous processes under II guidance using a radiolucent rod and a skin marking pen.
- Draw line "2" at the level of disk, where proposed surgery is planned. The point of intersection of line "1" and line "2" is the anatomic center of the disk **(Fig. 10)**.
- Draw the line "3" (In case of L5-S1) from the anatomic center of the disk to the highest point on the iliac crest **(Fig. 10)**.
- Now orient the II in lateral and mark the disk by placing the radio opaque marker on the side of the patient by adjusting the disk inclination either kyphotic, neutral, or lordotic as seen in the patient. Draw this line "4" from the anterior border of the disk to the back **(Fig. 11)**.
- Record the distance "x" from the anterior border of the disk to the posterior surface of the skin over the back. Transfer this distance "x" on the line "2" from the anatomic center of the disk **(Fig. 12)**.
- The point of intersection of the line "2" and line "4" is the needle entry point for that level **(Fig. 12)**.
- In some situations where the disk inclination is too high or too low, the line "2" and line "4" may not intersect as seen in **Figure 13**, in that situation the distance "y" which is calculated from the anterior border of the disk to the posterior surface of the skin over the back is plotted over the line "2" and a perpendicular drawn from this point will intersect the line "4" either above the line "2" or below the line "2" depending upon the lordosis or kyphosis, respectively. This intersection point is the needle entry point **(Fig. 13)**.
- In case of access to L5-S1 disk with high iliac crest, minor adjustments with respect to the iliac crest must be made. The coordinates are marked as explained and

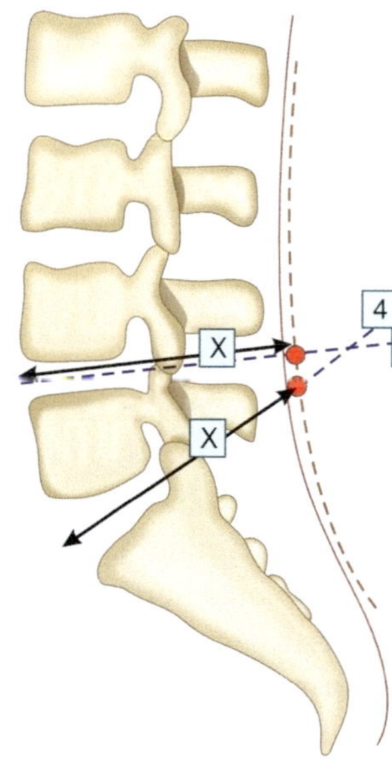

Fig. 11: Surface line marking to identify needle entry point.

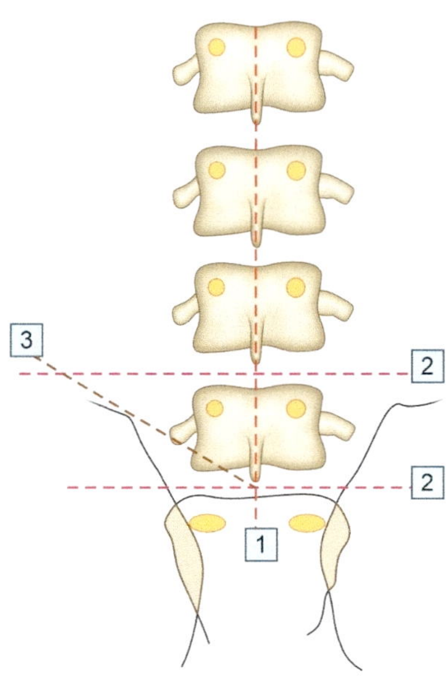

Fig. 10: Surface line marking to identify needle entry point.

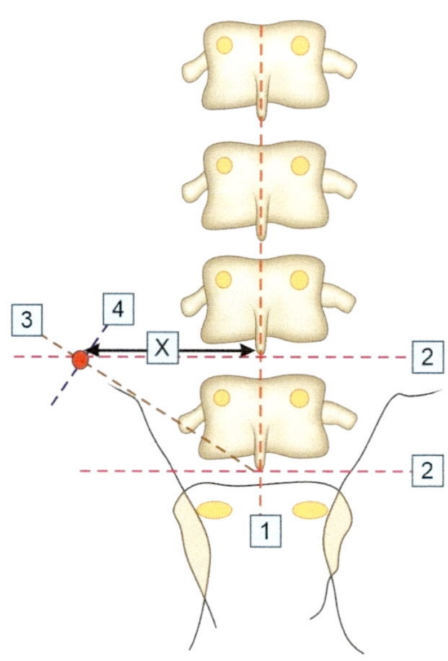

Fig. 12: Surface line marking to identify needle entry point.

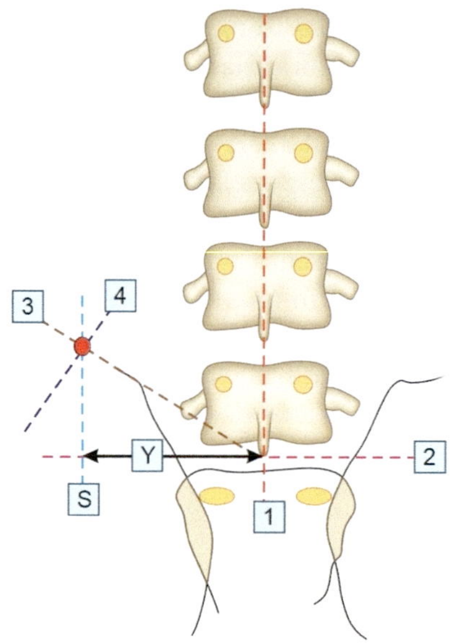

Fig. 13: Surface line marking to identify needle entry point.

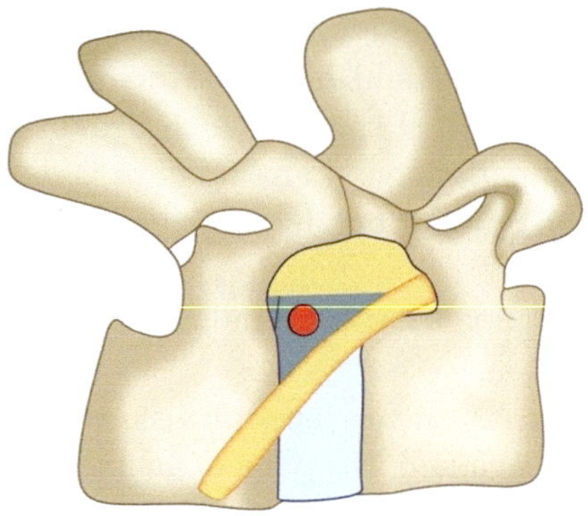

Fig. 14: Kambin's triangle.

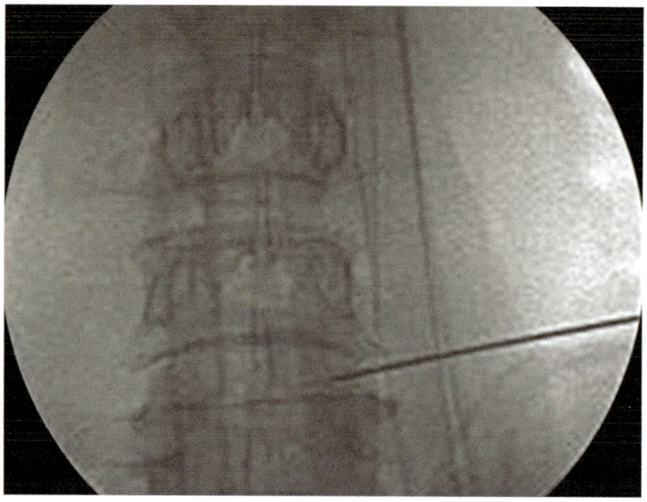

Fig. 15: Needle entry on the posterior–anterior image intensifier view.

with reference to the line "3", i.e., the iliac crest line, the needle entry point is selected superiorly and medially. Additional procedures such as medialization of annulotomy and/or foraminoplasty may be necessary to access centrally located herniations at L5-S1.

- In cases with hypertrophied superior articular process, one should be prepared to use the trephine or burr on the superior articular process to create more room in the foramen to gain access to the disk through the foramen.

Needle Insertion

Preoperative scrubbing, painting, and draping are done with large drapes and a lateral drape to protect the surgical site from contamination during intraoperative lateral imaging of the spine.

An 18G, 20 cm styletted needle is used for accessing the disk. The skin and subcutaneous tissue is infiltrated with 8-cc preservative-free 1% lignocaine. A stab incision is created at the point of entry. Creating a stab incision for the needle entry prevents inoculation of the disk with skin contaminants if any, thus preventing diskitis. The needle is progressed ahead with the bevel of the needle facing ventrally, so that the needle tends to travel dorsally and prevent inadvertent ventral entry. 2 cc of 1% preservative-free lignocaine is infiltrated all along the track till the needle reaches the first bony landmark, i.e., the superior articular process also called the lateral facet. 1/2 cc of local anesthetic is infiltrated at this site and stylet introduced, so as to clear the local anesthetic from the lumen of the needle. At this point, the spine is imaged in lateral, and position of the needle confirmed. At this point, the bevel of the needle is turned dorsally, and the lateral facet escaped, thereby entering the Kambin's triangle in the foramen.

Kambin's triangle is a triangular space bounded medially by the traversing root laterally by the exiting root and inferiorly by the superior endplate of the inferior vertebra. This is a three-dimensional potential space which can be used to enter the disk safely **(Fig. 14)**.[1]

Once the needle reaches the medial pedicular line on PA and posterior vertebral border on the lateral, the position of the needle is in the Kambin's triangle **(Figs. 15 and 16)**.

Chromatodiskography (Figs. 17 to 21)

Once the position of the needle is confirmed, the needle is advanced through the full thickness of the annulus. At this stage, chromatodiskography is performed. Selective staining of the degenerated nucleus is done with a mixture of nonionic radiopaque dye (omnipaque) and indigo carmine. Indigo carmine stains the acidic degenerated nucleus, making it visible during endoscopy for removal. The radiopaque dye aids in the radiographic control of the procedure and also confirms the status of the disk, location of the herniation, and the annular tear. The radiopaque dye and indigo carmine are mixed in a proportion of 9:1, respectively for selective staining **(Figs. 19A to C)**.

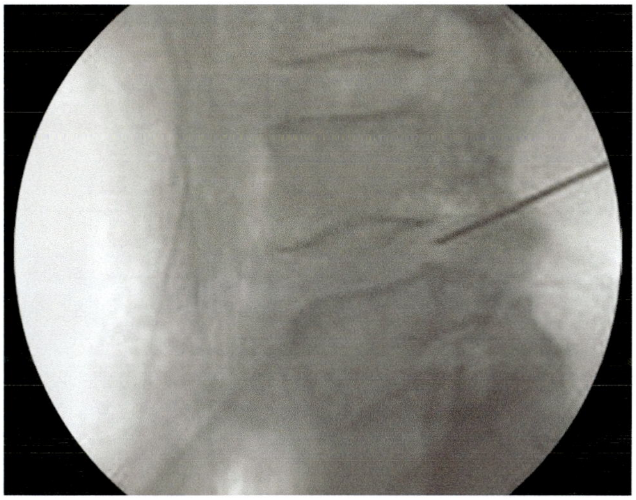

Fig. 16: Needle entry on the lateral image intensifier view.

Placement of the Guidewire, Dilator, and the Cannula

Once chromatodiskography has been performed, a long guidewire is introduced through the needle and anchored well in the disk, so that it does not come out during removal of the needle. The needle is gradually removed by rotatory action holding the guidewire in place. The skin incision is enlarged to about 0.8 mm to 1.0 cm to accommodate the dilator and the cannula. A blunt, conical, and two-channel dilator is introduced over the guidewire with gentle rotatory movement taking care that the guidewire does not bend during introduction of the dilator. Once the dilator reaches the superior articular process, the patient experiences mild back pain, which can be tackled with 1/2 cc of local anesthetic. With firm pressure on the dilator, the conical tip of the dilator is introduced in the foramen till the tip of the dilator reaches the surface of the annulus at the mid- or medial pedicular border, every time confirming that the patient does not have leg pain and he is able to move his ankle and toes. This is the last chance in case you need to change the trajectory and direction in PA and lateral. Once the dilator engages in the annular layers, it will be impossible to change direction. At this point, the dilator is held firmly over the annulus and the guidewire removed. Using the accessory channel in the dilator, four quadrant annular infiltration with 0.5 cc of 1% preservative-free lignocaine with a 20G needle, the dilator is gently tapped bluntly fenestrating the annulus. This is the painful part of the procedure and anesthesiologist needs to be informed to supplement

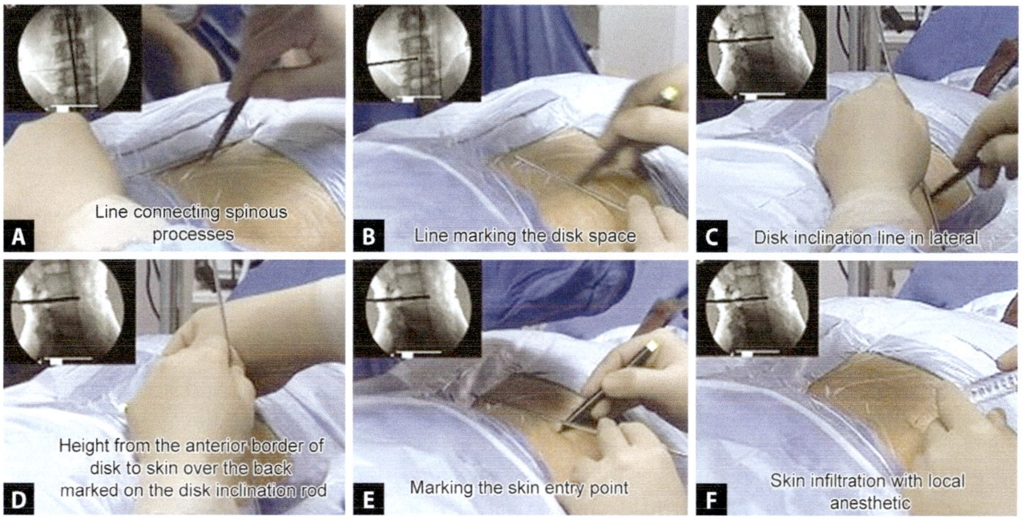

Figs. 17A to F: *Procedure:* Line marking and skin infiltration.

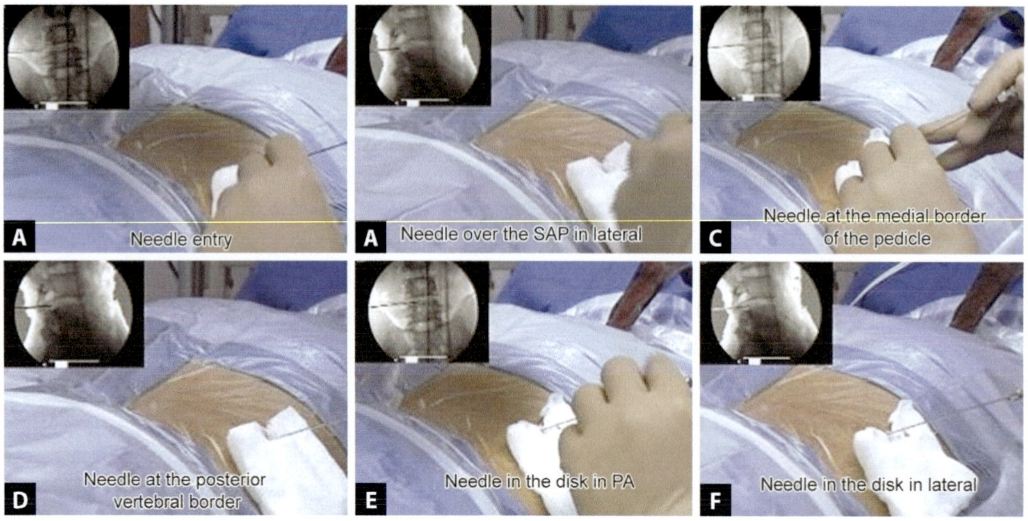

Figs. 18A to F: *Procedure:* Needle entry.

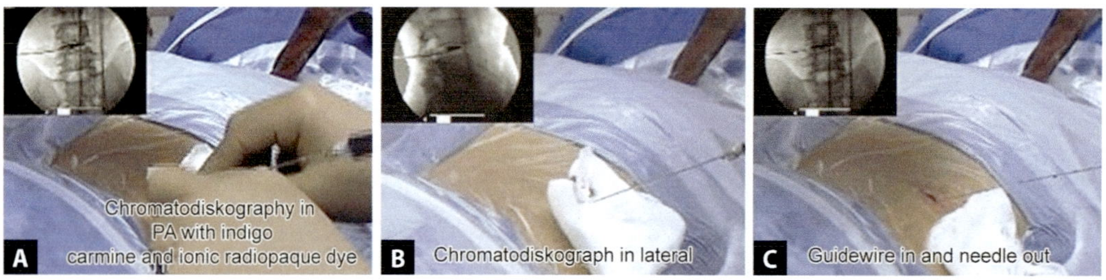

Figs. 19A to C: *Procedure:* Chromatodiskography.

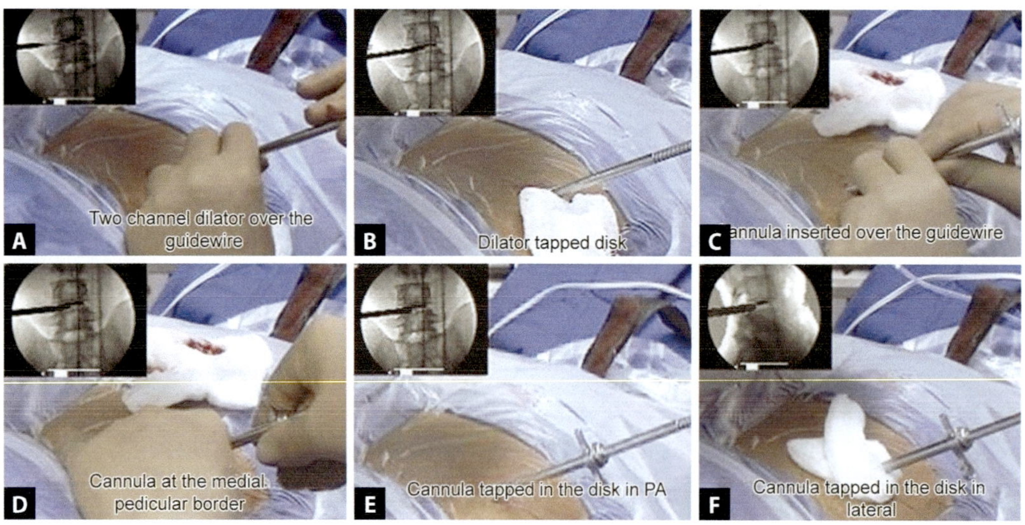

Figs. 20A to F: *Procedure:* Introduction of dilator and working sleeve.

the patient with extra doses of fentanyl, taking care that the patient should be able to report pain in the leg at all the time if any. Leg pain reported by the patient at any point of time should not be ignored and the dilator is adjusted till the time patient has no leg pain. Sometimes situation demands introduction of the cannula and scope to inspect the foramen and the surface of the annulus to work safely. Dilator is continued to be tapped till the

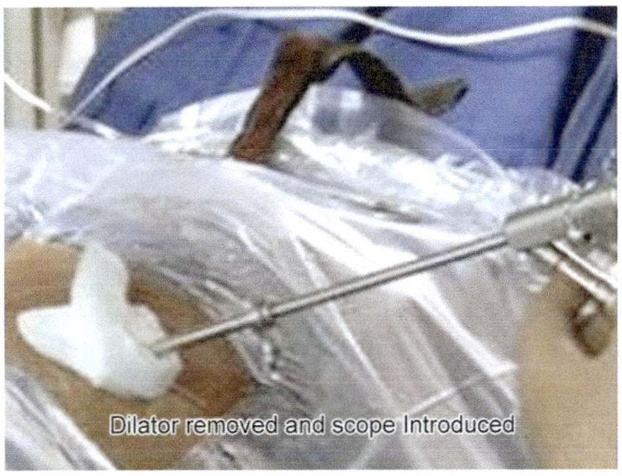

Fig. 21: *Procedure:* Introduction of endoscope.

tip reaches the center of the disk. A beveled cannula is introduced over the dilator and tapped in to reach the base of the herniation. The dilator is removed and scope introduced through the working cannula.

Diskectomy

The working channel of the endoscope accommodates various instruments for diskectomy and epidural clearance. Diskectomy is progressed with creating a space underneath the apex of the herniation. This technique is also called as inside out technique. Once this working cavity is created beneath the apex of the herniation as confirmed endoscopically and by the image intensifier, we start with cutting the annular collar so that the herniation is released from the annular rent wall and can be easily pulled out from within the disk through the pathological rent created by the herniation itself. This is achieved using Ho-YAG laser and the punch. Care should be exercised not to get too deep in the epidural space to jeopardize the integrity of thecal sac and the traversing nerve. The herniated nucleus many times along with flakes of cartilage from the end plate is loose and moves with Valsalva maneuver. Epidural bleeding encountered during this stage is controlled with 4.1 MHz radiofrequency. Once loosened, this herniated fragment can gently be teased and removed out either as a single fragment or piecemeal depending upon the consistency of the herniation. The herniation is initially teased out in the working cavity and then pulled out. If the fragment is large and cannot accommodate the working channel of the endoscope, it is removed along with the endoscope. Once the herniation is cleared, it is mandatory to check the epidural space for any missed fragment and if any removed. Turning the cannula and the scope 90° cranially will allow visualization of the exiting root. Confirmation of decompression of the traversing and exiting root is confirmed by:

- Visual confirmation of removal of the entire herniation
- Epidural oozing
- Free fluttering of the annular flaps and the epidural fat
- Relief of pain as confirmed by the patient
- Visualization of decompressed, traversing, and exiting root
- Free fluttering of the epidural tissue on cough impulse
- Free pulsations of the neurological structures.

Bony entrapment of the nerve is met many a times along with disk herniation. An experienced surgeon performs foraminotomy and/or foraminoplasty to decompress the neurological structures from bone, osteophytes, ligamentum flavum, superior foraminal ligament, fibrosis, and mobilize the exiting and traversing root. The floor, i.e., the annulus is removed by performing partial annulectomy. In addition, the ventral surface of the facet is laser ablated, thereby releasing hypertrophic ligamentum flavum attached to the anterior edge of the superior articular process. A trephine can be used to more aggressively decompress the undersurface of the superior articular process as well as the tip of the facet to expose the undersurface of the inferior facet. High-speed burrs can remove bone and smooth out the bony surface. The Ho-YAG laser is an effective tool that can be used to remove bone and ligamentous tissue. The end point is the identification of fat in the foramen or the visualization of a pulsating traversing and exiting nerve.

CLINICAL OUTCOMES AND DISCUSSION

Kambin and coworkers performed a prospective, randomized study of 60 patients with a single-level posterolateral herniation of a lumbar disk. Patients were randomized to Group 1, which underwent open laminotomy and diskectomy, and Group 2, which underwent PTELD.

Group 1 had 93% satisfactory outcome and Group 2 had 97% satisfactory outcome. An excellent or good result is considered a satisfactory outcome. The outcome was excellent if the radicular symptoms had ceased, the tension signs had become negative, the patient had returned to their previous occupation or to normal activity, and the patient expressed satisfaction with the result of the operative procedure. The outcome was good if the criteria just mentioned were met but the patient had residual back pain and had to change their occupation.

The time to return to work was 49 days for Group 1 and 27 days for Group 2. In addition, Group 1 used narcotics in greater quantities and for a longer duration postoperatively than Group 2 which used narcotics for 7 days.

Yeung and Tsou reported a retrospective review of their series of 307 consecutive cases of posterolateral endoscopic excision for lumbar disk herniation. At an average follow-up of 19 months, 81.4% of the whole group was found to have an excellent or good result.[2] With increasing experience, this author was able to achieve results close to 95%.

Complications included deep infection (0.65%), thrombophlebitis (0.65%), dysesthesia (1.9%), and dural tear (0.3%). The patients with deep infection and dural tear required reoperation. In total, 4% of patients underwent reoperations. Other reasons for reoperation included congenital short pedicles, foraminal/lateral recess stenosis, recurrent herniation, and missed fragments.

Ahn et al. reported the results of posterolateral endoscopic diskectomy for recurrent lumbar disk herniations. 43 consecutive patients with recurrent disk herniation at the same level after a previous conventional open diskectomy with an intervening pain free interval of >6 months underwent PTELD. Surgical outcomes were assessed using the MacNab criteria and visual analog scale. Based on the MacNab criteria, excellent or good outcomes were noted in 81.4% of patients. It should be noted that the rate of excellent/good outcomes for recurrent disk herniations was equivalent to that obtained by Yeung and Tsou for primary disk herniations. Risk factors for poor outcome included age of >40 years old, symptoms >3 months, and the presence of lateral recess stenosis.

Other applications of the posterolateral endoscopic technique have also been described. Knight et al. described posterolateral endoscopic foraminal decompression in the management of symptomatic isthmic spondylolisthesis. Patients with at least a 1-year history of disabling low back and buttock pain with or without referred pain, unresponsive to conservative treatment of at least 6 months, were included in the study. It should be noted that all except one patient in the study had some degree of radicular leg pain. Endoscopic foraminal decompression with laser-assisted bone and soft tissue ablation was performed with grades I–III isthmic spondylolisthesis. Excellent/good outcomes were noted in 79% of patients. No slip progression was detected postoperatively.[4]

A prospective evaluation of endoscopic diskectomy in 30 consecutive patients with posterolateral or far lateral lumbar disk herniations was performed. All patients were treated by a single surgeon. Using the MacNab criteria, we observed 73.2% good/excellent results for the group overall. When the group was divided into two subgroups, we observed 60% good/excellent results in the first 15 patients and 87.7% good/excellent results in the second 15 patients who underwent the procedure. This difference in outcome between the two groups likely represents the learning curve associated with endoscopic diskectomy.[4]

CONCLUSION

The advantages of PTELD include the absence of epidural fibrosis and tethering of nerve roots, the preservation of intact epidural venous systems, which prevents postoperative venous stasis and chronic nerve root edema, and, finally, the minimal operative trauma to normal structures. Results of PTELD are comparable to traditional open diskectomy for soft, nonextruded posterolateral disk herniations. Results are superior with extraforaminal disk herniations in experienced hands. Experienced endoscopic surgeons are able to remove sequestered herniations with less surgical morbidity. The minimal bony resection required by this technique also potentially reduces the likelihood of surgically induced spinal instability. Endoscopic decompression in symptomatic unilateral radicular spondylolisthesis can be successful without postoperative slip progression. PTELD, though technically challenging, is safe and effective. Access to the pathology is limited to a narrow channel, and a herniated fragment is accessible only when the operating instrument is placed in the optimal trajectory. As a result, there remains a long and shallow rather than steep-learning curve that requires repetition and the recognition of the foraminal anatomy. The advent of special tools, such as bipolar radiofrequency ablation, endoscopic burrs, and articulating graspers small enough to pass through the endoscopic working channel, improves access to a wider variety of disk fragments. For simple posterolateral or far lateral disk herniations, endoscopic diskectomy produces results at least equivalent to open diskectomy while potentially allowing a faster post-operative recovery. Further improvements in instrumentation and refinements in technique will improve surgical access and decrease the learning curve of this promising technique.

REFERENCES

1. Hermantin FU, Peters T, Quartararo L, Kambin P. A prospective, randomized study comparing the results of open diskectomy with those of video-assisted arthroscopic microdiskectomy. J Bone Joint Surg Am. 1999;81(7):958-65.
2. Yeung AT, Tsou PM. Posterolateral endoscopic excision for lumbar disc herniation: surgical technique, outcome, and complications in 307 consecutive cases. Spine (Phila Pa 1976). 2002;27(7):722-31.
3. Chang MA, Talac R, Kim CW. The endoscopic diskectomy learning curve. Submitted for publication.
4. Ahn Y, Lee SH, Park WM, Lee HY, Shin SW, Kang HY. Percutaneous endoscopic lumbar diskectomy for recurrent disc herniation: surgical technique, outcome, and prognostic factors of 43 consecutive cases. Spine. 2004;29:E326-32.

54 CHAPTER

Intrathecal Implantable Devices

Samyadev Datta

ABSTRACT

Spinal opioids for pain management have been used for more than 40 years. The technology of delivery has improved in the last few decades. Implantable pumps have been shown to be very reliable and dependable, with a very high degree of accuracy in delivery of medication. Understanding of physiology of spinal opioids and introduction of newer medications have made this a more practical and commonly used modality for control of pain.

This chapter will introduce readers to this modality and will highlight the science of spinal medications, selection criteria of patients, technique of trialing patients, with some guidelines, implantation techniques, complications, and their management.

As the procedure is not used very commonly, caution is recommended. It is to be noted that with proper selection of patients, pain can be well controlled, and patients can have improved functionality and quality of life.

INTRODUCTION

Spinal opioids were found in the 1970s. Since then, there has been a need to deliver medications into the intrathecal and epidural space. Intrathecal pumps have been in use for more than 40 years and have a proven record for safety, reliability, and efficiency.[1] It is hoped that this chapter will stimulate its better acceptance and use by trained practitioners.

SCIENTIFIC RATIONALE

The primary mechanism of action of opioids is activation of opioid receptors present in various parts of the nervous system. The concentration of medications reached is much higher at this level, and the result is adequate analgesia with significantly reduced side effects. Medications may be administered orally, but higher doses may result in significant side effects and inadequate pain relief.

- Opioids work on receptors that are present in high concentrations in dorsal root ganglion (DRG). They work via the C-reactive protein that finally results in reduction in production of substance P. Opioids affect both pre- and postsynaptically by reducing neurotransmitter release, hyperpolarizing the membranes, and inhibiting pain.
- Local anesthetics act by inhibiting the sodium channel and prevent transmission along the nodes of Ranvier. Bupivacaine appears to work on calcium channels at very low concentrations.
- Clonidine is an α-2 agonist that depresses release of C-fiber neurotransmitters, substance P, and calcitonin gene-related peptide. It has not been approved for intrathecal use, but there is extensive literature supporting its safe and effective use. It has been approved for epidural use.
- Ziconotide is a calcium N-channel inhibitor specific to the dorsal horn of the spinal cord. It has been approved for intrathecal use.
- Baclofen, a γ-aminobutyric acid agonist, is used in spasticity to restore balance between active and passive muscles. It has been approved for intrathecal use and has been used quite extensively.
- Literature does mention that many other drugs have been tried. Among the class of opioids, hydromorphone, fentanyl, sufentanil, meperidine, and methadone have

been used. Hydromorphone has been used extensively and appears to be well tolerated.
- Other drugs used include ketamine, an *N*-methyl-*D*-aspartate (NMDA) receptor antagonist; droperidol, to help with nausea; gabapentin, effective on the calcium channel; ketorolac, a cyclooxygenase-1 and -2 inhibitor; midazolam; and neostigmine. None of these medications have been approved by the Food and Drug Administration (FDA) and the literature about their use is limited.

PATIENT SELECTION

The single-most key factor that decides the success of intrathecal drug delivery systems (IDDS) **(Figs. 1 and 2)** is proper patient selection. It cannot be emphasized enough that patient selection is critical for good results, and results are very rewarding and gratifying.[2,3] The opposite is also true. IDDS therapy requires long-term care. There are a limited number of trained practitioners, so choose carefully. Patients on stable regimens are easy to deal with.

Category of Patient

Spasticity Due to Multiple Sclerosis, Cerebral Palsy, and Dystonia

These patients are usually referred by neurologists and will have been on muscle relaxants of various sorts. These include baclofen, tizanidine, and diazepam. They are for placement of a pump with baclofen as medications have caused many intolerable side effects or inadequate muscle relaxation. It is usually possible to control spasticity in these patients using small doses of intrathecal baclofen. Occasionally, patients need exceedingly high doses of baclofen. Adding other medications such as bupivacaine and an opioid may potentiate the effect of baclofen.

Cancer-related Pain

Patients with cancer-related pain may have a short life expectancy of 6 months or less or may have chronic pain secondary to cancer and its treatment.

Patients with Short Life Expectancy

These patients are looking for pain relief with reduction in side effects due to medications. They wish to have an excellent quality of life during the terminal phases of their lives. The approach here is extremely aggressive as time is of the essence. Practitioners need to make changes rapidly to get quick results. A discussion with patient and family needs to clearly outline expectations. The use of tetracaine to achieve intense analgesia with associated motor weakness may be an acceptable choice for some patients. It will allow for significant reduction of pain medications with hopeful reduction in side effects, allowing for a dignified and peaceful death.[4]

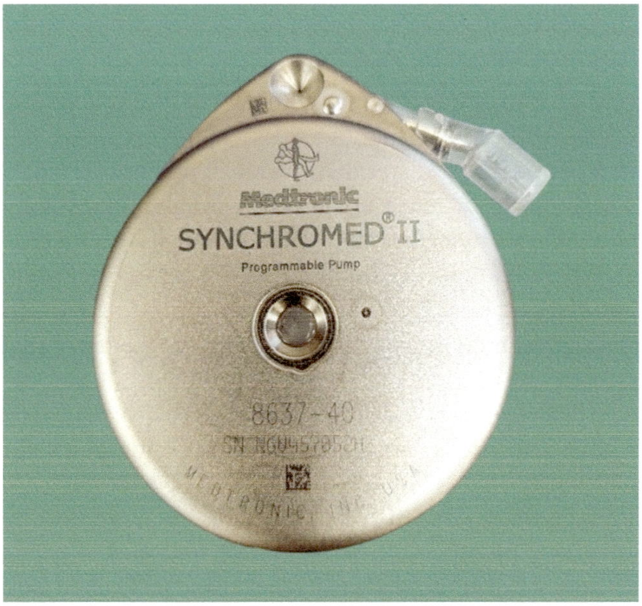

Fig. 1: Medtronic SynchroMed II pump.

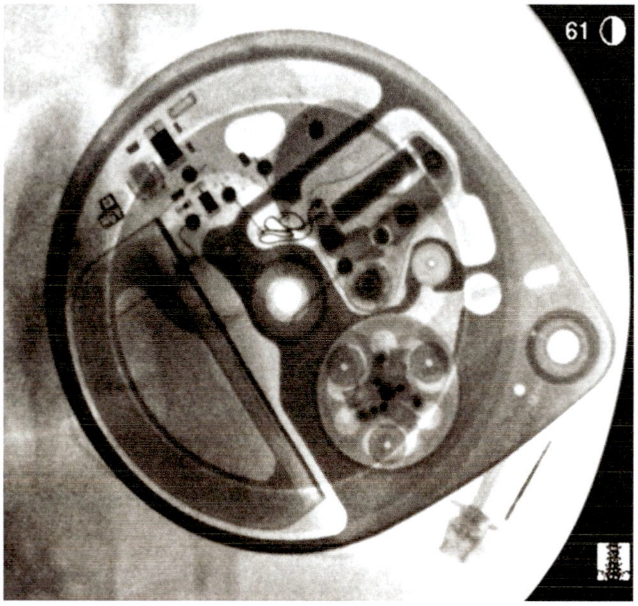

Fig. 2: X-ray view of Medtronic intrathecal pump.

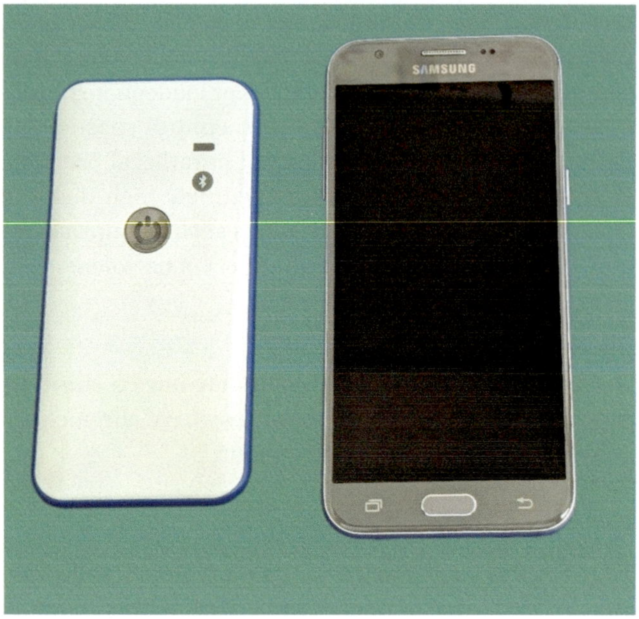

Fig. 3: Personal therapy manager.

In an excellent section on the management of this category of patients, Lynch discusses management of complex cancer pain and use of IDDS.[5] She makes every effort to try and categorize types of patients seen. She also tries to show what would be an approximate medication regimen with IDDS in the category of patients found. Many practitioners will find this as an extremely useful guide.

Use of personal therapy manager (PTM) allows patient control **(Fig. 3)**. This allows patients to rapidly titrate their medications. This allows patients' significant control. Terminal cancer patients fear loss of control, and this is a small, but highly effective modality to allow them control of their medications. It has allowed for rapid titration of medications to get good control of pain. Rapid titration may occasionally cause opioid-induced hyperalgesia. Oral methadone may help reduce medication dosage.

Patients with Chronic Pain Secondary to Cancer

This category of patients are cancer survivors, and the numbers have expanded very significantly in the last decade. Life expectancy of cancer survivors in the United States has increased dramatically. This group of patients has made every effort to live as normal a life as possible. It is very important to identify these patients and treat them with the same strict guidelines as mentioned for chronic nonmalignant pain patients. A large number of these patients have residual pain from cancer and its treatment and are expected to live normal lives. A point of note among this category of patients is that the issues related to addiction and abuse are similar with patients with chronic nonmalignant pain.[4,6,7]

Chronic Nonmalignant Complex Pain

These are mostly patients who have IDDS devices implanted. They will hopefully live a normal life and so, very careful attention must be paid to ensure that end results are favorable. Most chronic pain processes are mixed with both neuropathic and nociceptive pain, and patients need a combination of medications to help control pain. It is the ease with which admixtures can be administered via the intrathecal pump that makes this delivery system so attractive and effective. Admixtures allow for synergy of drug actions, thus providing effective analgesia with reduced dose of medications and hopefully reduced side effects. The usual type of patients includes postlaminectomy pain syndrome, complex regional pain syndrome, chronic abdominal pain secondary to multiple operative procedures, chronic pain-related pancreatitis, and so on. These patients will usually need a combination of medications for adequate control of symptoms. It is also extremely encouraging to note that adequate control of pain may help with patient's symptoms of mood and depression. In addition, patients with diabetic polyneuropathy will find that diabetic status is better controlled. A proportion of these patients may be able to keep a job. In addition, these patients are more active and tend to lose weight, an added benefit.[2,3,8]

Psychological Evaluation

All pain practitioners will have to deal with psychological issues of patients. Most often, they can be managed. It is very important to remember that as implanting an IDDS device results in establishing a long-term relationship, it is mandatory that all patients have a preoperative psychological evaluation. As pain practitioners, we may consider ourselves adequately trained to make a good psychological assessment, but it is best left to experts to make that assessment.[2,3]

The presence of significant psychiatric or psychological comorbidity may be a relative contraindication for placement of IDDS device. In addition, working with a psychologist trained in pain management will be extremely beneficial. It is recommended that an open discussion takes place with all parties, and they agree with the decision to move ahead with spinal opioid trial.[2,3]

Psychologists usually use various tests for evaluation and assessment and make a final recommendation about the feasibility of placing an intrathecal delivery device. Psychologists may occasionally recommend that there is a high risk associated with placement of IDDS. They also recommend patient follow-up for psychological treatment after placement of intrathecal pump. Occasionally, they will recommend against placement of an IDDS. It is important for practitioners to ensure that recommendations made by psychologists are understood and followed by physicians and patients.

TYPES OF PUMPS

There are two types of pumps. These are: programmable and fixed volume delivery pumps. They have their pros and cons.

Constant flow pumps are used to deliver steady dose medications in stable patients and do not have much flexibility. Increasing the dose requires higher concentrations of medications. These pumps tend to have a much longer lifespan. Occasionally, these pumps are used in multiple sclerosis patients. In addition, chemotherapy delivered into the hepatic artery can also be administered via this device.

Programmable pumps have a lot more flexibility. The main advantage of these pumps is that the dose can be changed conveniently. In addition, new models of Medtronic SynchroMed II pump can pair with a personal therapy manager. Programing is done with SynchroMed Clinical Program application **(Fig. 4)**. This allows for more flexibility about dosing and giving the patient control. It is safe and allows patients to wean from oral medications. These pumps are very reliable.

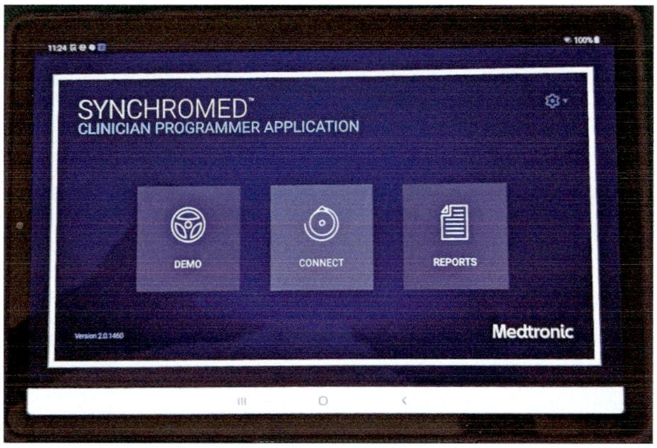

Fig. 4: SynchroMed Clinical Programmer Application.

CHOICE OF MEDICATIONS

In an excellent article in 2024, the Polyanalgesic Consensus Conference statement on the use of medications in the intrathecal pump, the authors have reviewed and described various medications that can and have been used. It is of note that there are only three medications that have been approved by the Food and Drug Administration (FDA) for intrathecal use, morphine, baclofen, and ziconotide. Other medications mentioned have been used but have not been approved. It does appear that there is significant experience in use for most of the common medications, including hydromorphone, fentanyl, clonidine, and bupivacaine.[9-12]

Some of the medications mentioned in the article have been used very infrequently and have very little literature to support their use.

TRIALING PROCEDURES

After proper selection of patient, performing an adequate trial is the most important aspect that ensures adequate success with IDDS.[1,3] All patients must have a trial. There are various trial options. Trialing can be done with a single-dose intrathecal injection, epidural, or intrathecal catheter approaches. Various articles also show that trialing procedures may be done on opioid-naive patients. It is difficult to evaluate this statement as one of indications for trialing for an intrathecal pump for pain management and administration of opioids is that oral or transdermal opioids have provided pain relief but have not been adequate and/or are causing intolerable side effects. So, the author does not perform spinal opioid trial on opioid-naive patients. Trialing with baclofen may be done in patients who are not on baclofen or other muscle relaxants.

Patient with severe spasticity is likely to have baclofen as the primary drug in IDDS. Trialing process is done in collaboration with a neurologist using single dose of baclofen. Medication is administered intrathecally. The starting dose is usually 25–50 μg and if that is inadequate, a second dose of 100 μg is given. This is usually done about 1 week apart. If the second dose is not adequate, it is unlikely that patient would benefit from intrathecal baclofen. Spasticity score is then measured in the postinjection period using Ashworth Spasticity Scale. It may take a few hours for the maximum effect of baclofen to be noted. If there has been a significant decrease in spasticity, the daily starting dose of intrathecal baclofen is the test dose that was effective.

Single dose of ziconotide has also been used for trialing process. Initially, ziconotide was administered as an epidural infusion. This caused significant side effects. As a result, this technique has been abandoned. Updated trialing process recommends intrathecal administration of single dose of 1–2 μg of ziconotide. If this is not adequate, a second bolus dose of 4 μg can be repeated. If patient shows no benefit from the second dose, it is unlikely that ziconotide will be beneficial. If successful, ziconotide can be used as a primary drug or in conjunction with other medications. One of the goals of therapy of IDDS in chronic pain patients is reduction in pain and improvement in functional status. It is difficult to appreciate any improvement in functional status with a single bolus dose of the ziconotide. So, there are no clearly defined end points for testing ziconotide.[10]

Spinal opioids can be tried as a single bolus dose. The recommendation is to try and give the approximate daily dose of medication of either morphine or hydromorphone as a single dose intrathecally. The patient is then evaluated for adequacy of pain relief. If the patient reports more than a 50% decrease in pain processes, the recommendation is to place an intrathecal catheter and pump. It is not possible to make an adequate assessment about functional improvement after intrathecal administration of single dose of medication.[1,3] In addition, in interventional pain management, placebo response up to 30–35%. We must try to truly establish adequacy of pain control and improvement in functional status, therefore this technique is not recommended. In addition, often patients will have continued with their oral medications before the trial and so will have potentially received a large dose of medication resulting in pain relief. This can result in false positive results.[1,3,9]

The other choice is placement of either a temporary epidural or intrathecal catheter. These catheters are always attached to two end-to-end 22 μm antimicrobial filters. This reduces the likelihood of infection significantly. The catheter is attached to a programmable external epidural PCA pump. The pump is programed to deliver only a continuous rate with no breakthrough doses. The dose of medications given usually reflects the entire daily dose of oral opioids. During spinal opioid trial, it is extremely important to use the same conversion guide for various routes of administration and various medications. Practitioners need to be comfortable with a conversion guide. Patients are instructed to take only short-acting pain medications for breakthrough pain. They are instructed to keep detailed notes. Patient is evaluated in the office every few days to ensure that there is adequate pain relief, no infection at the epidural insertion site, and to replenish epidural bag. An epidural catheter is usually kept for about 7–10 days. During this trial period, the patient must assess the adequacy of pain relief, improvement in functional status, decrease in side effects, and significant reduction in use of oral medications. If a patient is having side effects from medications, it may be necessary to adjust or change medications. There are only very few medication choices, so do not be in a rush to change medications.

The patients are requested to find three parameters that will be used during the trial. As every patient is different and their expectations are different, it is important to try and find specific goals for each patient. It is extremely important for the practitioner to clarify to the patient that the ultimate decision to place a permanent intrathecal catheter and pump is based completely on the patient's assessment. It is very helpful to involve the spouse and other family members in this decision-making. Chronic pain does affect more than just the patient. Seeing the patient improve during the trial is a significant positive reinforcement for the spouse and the family. The practitioner should not force their view on patients. This can result in a dissatisfied patient.

The final choice is to place an intrathecal catheter. The catheter is then infused with expected medication as would be in IDDS. Patient is admitted to the hospital and checked during their stay for about 3–5 days. It is important to understand that there is a very high risk of infection because of direct access to the intrathecal space and an exteriorized catheter. Two 22-μm antimicrobial filters are attached to the catheter. In addition, it is important to understand that this may be as close as possible to an intrathecal pump, but the minimum volume delivered in standard PCA pump is 0.1 mL/hour or 2.4 mL/day, which is far more than the amount delivered by intrathecal pump. In addition, this technique does not allow for adequacy of assessment about improvement in their functional status. Most hospitals do not allow patients to freely move around with either an intrathecal or epidural catheter in place. As a result, it is difficult to make an adequate assessment. In addition, sometimes it is difficult as the duration of trial is extremely short. The customary practice is for physical therapy to assess the patient during hospital stay. In addition, as it is an expensive option, insurance companies are reluctant to pay for hospital stays.

After proper selection of the patient, adequate trialing process will give practitioners the best idea and assessment about the possibility of success with IDDS. If an IDDS is placed for wrong reasons, then the goal of placing an intrathecal pump will not be fulfilled and it will leave patient dissatisfied and very frustrated. In a small number of patients, IDDS may need to be removed due to patient dissatisfaction or intolerable side effects.

IMPLANTATION TECHNIQUE

Implantation technique is a surgical skill. Practitioners must have surgical skills to undertake this procedure. If not, it is proper to seek help from a surgeon. Placement of intrathecal catheter can be performed by practitioner and every effort must be made to position catheter tip appropriately. In patients with neck and shoulder pain secondary to neck surgery, catheter tip should be placed at about C7-T1 level. In patients with postlaminectomy lumbar pain, catheter tip can be positioned at about T9-T10 level. It is important to try and remember these points, as it will allow us to find and position catheter tip accordingly. It is also extremely important to remember that if patients have multiple pain processes, find the most painful process, so that intrathecal therapies can be directed toward that process. The lesser pain processes may still require oral medications. That is not considered to be a failure of intrathecal therapies.

The intrathecal pump needs to be tethered to fascia adequately. If the pump is not tethered properly, there is a potential for it to flip within the cavity resulting in catheter being twisted. If that happens, refill of pump becomes extremely difficult. Twisting of catheter may result in occlusion. The other important point to remember is orientation of pump placement. The author prefers to draw a diagram with the pump template for each patient. This knowledge of exact orientation improves ease during refill.

As part of surgical protocol, it is important to administer perioperative dose of antibiotics. It is not necessary to routinely administer postoperative antibiotics. In addition, if adequate technique for placing intrathecal catheter and securing the same has been followed, postdural puncture headache is unlikely to be a problem. Placement of intrathecal catheter may result in postdural puncture headache. Most often, this can be treated conservatively, but occasionally it may be necessary to perform an epidural blood patch under fluoroscopy. The Ascenda catheter is barely visible under fluoroscopy.

In the postoperative period, the application of an abdominal binder is recommended. Occasionally, there may be a small fluid collection around the pump. Keeping the abdominal binder on for about 7–10 days allows fluid to be absorbed. It also allows the pump to settle onto the new pocket a lot better. Thin patients may occasionally complain that the pump is protruding.

An incision is usually made on the right anterior abdomen as most patients are right handed. An occasional patient may need it placed on the left abdominal wall. In addition, thin patients can have the pump placed on their back. Refill for these patients is done with them sitting. The author usually tends to place a smaller capacity 20 mL pump in thin patients. But routinely, a 40 mL pump is placed. This allows a longer interval between refills.

COMPLICATIONS

Placement of an intrathecal catheter and pump are surgical procedures. Complications are likely to happen. It is important for practitioners to be aware of potential complications and how to manage them. Having a complication is not the problem. Failure to identify and manage complications is the problem. Be prepared to seek help if the situation is beyond your ability.

Early complications are usually surgical. These include the possibility of hematoma and infection. In addition, patients who are overweight, the incidence of bleeding is slightly higher. Use of an abdominal binder is extremely beneficial in this situation. Very rarely the wound requires exploration for hematoma to be drained and bleeding stopped.

- *Infection:* Infection of wound can happen occasionally. Superficial infection can be treated with antibiotics. If you have any concerns about the choice and duration of antibiotics, it is recommended that you discuss this matter with infectious disease.

  If on the other hand, the infection is within the pump cavity, the matter is extremely serious. The pump may require to be removed. Recommendation of infectious disease is that if there is a foreign object with an infection, foreign object needs to be removed for infection to be adequately treated. During the management of infected intrathecal pump in a terminally ill patient, getting excellent pain relief may be necessary to try and salvage the pump.
- *Postdural puncture headache:* This complication can happen in a small number of patients. Most often, this is resolved with the use of conservative measures. If not, epidural blood patch may be extremely beneficial

and likelihood of resolution is very high. This must be done under fluoroscopy.

- *Drug overdosage:* In the immediate postoperative period, the most serious complication is drug overdosage. This happens because of wrong calculations. It is necessary to start with correct information about preoperative medication and dosage, make a proper dosage conversion, then start daily dose about 50% of expected dosage. It is safe to increase the dose as needed at 10–15% increments every 2–3 weeks. For control of pain, oral medications can be supplemented during this period. The transition away from oral medications may take a few months. Cancer patients with short life expectancy will require a more aggressive approach and rapid titration to effect.

Delayed Complications

These complications are usually related to the catheter and pump. During placement of intrathecal catheter, it is very important to try and follow the guidelines on tethering catheter. This reduces the likelihood of catheter migration.

- *Catheter migration:* Catheter migration can happen in a very small number of patients. Occasionally, a catheter may migrate and be partially in intrathecal space. This may give the patient partial pain relief.

  The most common symptomatology of a migrated catheter is an increase in the requirement of pain medication with inadequate pain relief. In patients who have been very stable, this should be an immediate consideration. The recommendation is to perform a dye and rotor study. This will allow evaluation of pump, reviewing positioning of intrathecal catheter, and noting adequacy of flow of dye through the catheter. If the catheter has migrated, it is recommended that it should be repositioned as soon as possible **(Figs. 5 to 7)**.

During repositioning of intrathecal catheter, it is quite important to remember that duration of catheter migration is unknown. As a result, patients may need a significantly lower amount of medication when the catheter is repositioned and pump attached. This is for safety reasons. The PTM can be programed to make up for difference in dosage. In addition, it might be necessary to see the patient overnight in hospital to prevent any overdose due to medications.

- *Catheter occlusion:* Intrathecal catheter occlusion is rare but documented. There appears to be increasing concerns about the use of very high concentrations of medications. Medications are used at high concentrations to try to increase the duration between refills. In one case, the patient did report significant difficulty with control of pain that happened over a period of 6 months. Fluoroscopic guidance showed that the catheter was in a good spot. A dye and rotor study showed that there was no free aspiration of cerebrospinal fluid (CSF) from the side port. No dye could be injected through the catheter showing an occlusion. Magnetic resonance imaging (MRI) of the thoracic spine excluded granuloma formation. Patient

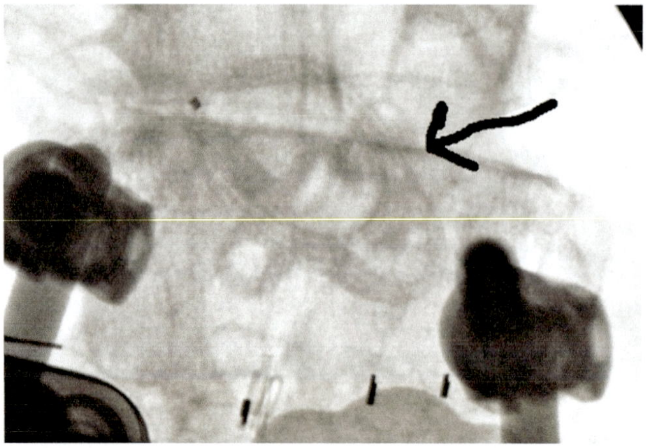

Fig. 5: Catheter migrated and curled up.

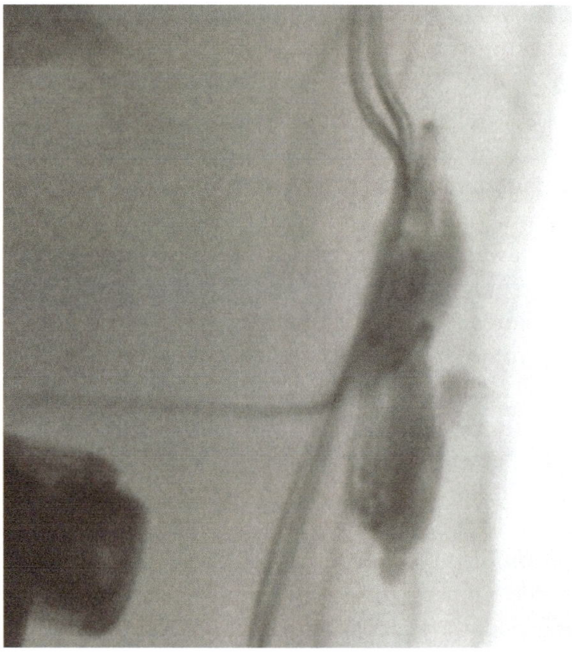

Fig. 6: Catheter in subcutaneous space with extravasation of dye.

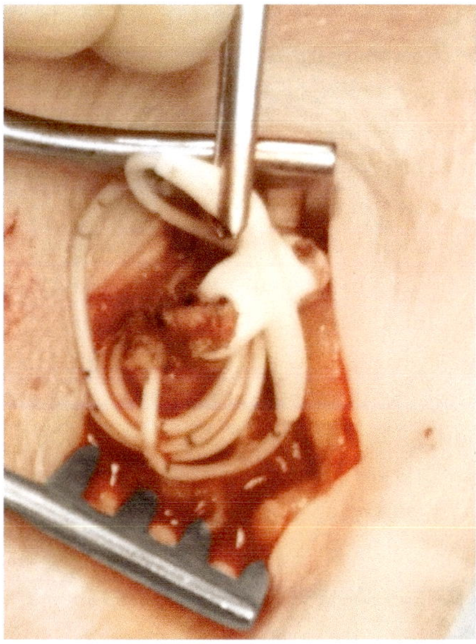

Fig. 7: Catheter migration.

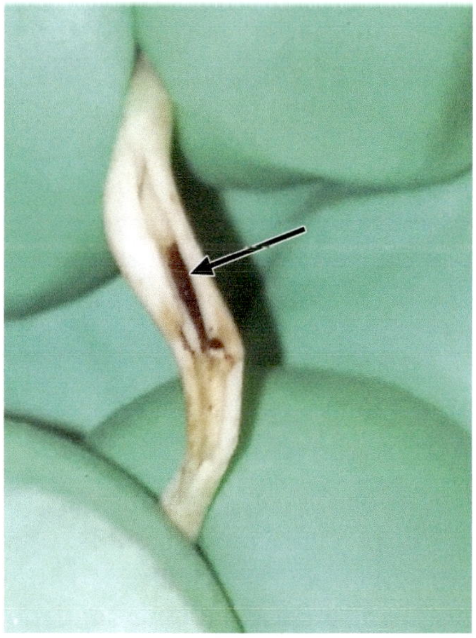

Fig. 8: Catheter dissected to show debris causing occlusion.

did have her catheter replaced. The old catheter was evaluated, and it was quite clearly noted that there appeared to be a significant amount of debris within catheter that caused an occlusion **(Fig. 8)**. This is more than likely related to high concentrations of medications used in solutions. The recommendations about the maximum concentration of medications should always be carefully considered.[9] Also try and keep a minimum daily flow of volume through catheter. About 0.3 mL/day is suggested.

- *Granuloma formation:* This is a rare complication mentioned in literature. It is usually related to the use of very high concentration of medications at very low flow rates. The presentation is that of increased pain and a negative aspiration from the side port of pump. It may be possible to inject via side port of pump. High-resolution MRI of spine will usually find the problem. If granuloma is not causing any neurological deficit, a choice to consider is to dilute medication in IDDS and increase flow. If there are neurological deficits, surgery is recommended for removal of catheter and granuloma. Use of clonidine in medication mixture may reduce likelihood of granuloma formation.[5]

Complications Related to the Intrathecal Pump

Medtronic SynchroMed II intrathecal pump is an extremely reliable medical device.[11,13,14] Occasionally, a pump that has not been tethered to the fascia properly may flip. In addition, motor stall can occur occasionally. If this does happen, the patient is likely to have opioid or baclofen withdrawal and pump will require to be replaced urgently. Sudden pump failure in patients with high-dose baclofen needs to be addressed urgently as death has been reported. It is also important to remember that when you replace the pump, the daily dose of opioids needs to be reduced to prevent overdose of medications.

New intrathecal pumps from Medtronic are all MRI compatible. If there is a motor stall at once after an MRI, it is strongly recommended that the patient be evaluated by practitioner and telemetry performed to ensure that the pump is running properly.

The literature provided by Medtronic does show that these intrathecal pumps are extremely reliable. Occasionally, there will be a significant amount of residual volume left during the refill process If this is a recurrent issue, it may be necessary to consider replacing the pump as it may not be working properly.

Medication-Related Complications

In the article from 2024,[9] there is mention about the medications used in IDDS. As mentioned earlier, there are only three medications that have been approved by the FDA. Multiple other medications have been used and literature suggests that there is good clinical experience with some of them.

Based on practitioners' experience and comfort levels, combination medications have been used very successfully. Opioids in combination with clonidine is commonly. There appears to be evidence to indicate that the addition of clonidine is less likely to result in granuloma formation.[5] In addition, patients who have baclofen as primary medication for relief of spasm, occasionally, addition of an opioid or local anesthetic may help to reduce amount of pain as spasm is associated with significant increased pain.

After the initial process of placing intrathecal catheter and pump, the problems are medication related. It is important to understand that all medications used in intrathecal pumps can cause complications. Opioids can cause nausea, vomiting, constipation, and so on. In addition, opioids can cause significant suppression of hypothalamic-pituitary-gonadal axis and results in reduced testosterone production. It is important to keep all these in mind, as even though Smith et al.'s paper from 2002 shows that there has been a significant reduction in side effects, side effects do happen.[4]

Managing side effects can become bothersome. It is also important to remember that there is limited choice of medications. It is important to try and work with your patients and explain to them that not every side effect requires change in medications. We need to try and manage the side effects.

MANAGEMENT OF INTRATHECAL PUMPS

After the intrathecal catheter and pump has been placed, managing intrathecal pump can be done either by practitioner or physician extenders. Issues can arise anytime during the maintenance of the pump.

It is important to try and follow standard procedures for maintenance of these intrathecal pumps. This starts with writing a prescription correctly, including drug, concentration, and total volume. The compounding pharmacist needs to be trained in compounding medications for intrathecal pumps. The compounding facility needs to meet all standards. They need to be able to test for sterility and stability of compounded medications.

It is also recommended that pharmacists occasionally send sample of medication for high-pressure liquid chromatography to confirm accuracy of concentration of medications.

Once the medication has been received in the practitioner's office, it is mandatory to check that medication in syringe is as prescribed. Medication needs to be stored in a secure place. This is to prevent tampering. It may need to be refrigerated.

At the time of pump refill, the area needs to be prepped and draped adequately. The pump is accessed under aseptic precautions using a 22G Huber tipped needle, emptied, and refilled with medication as prescribed. It is important to verify medication being used for refill. Use a 22 g micron filter during refill. Also, the rate of refill needs to be slow to prevent any issues. At the end, telemetry and reprograming is done. Patients are given the date for next refill. Changes can be made, if necessary. Practitioners need to be aware of risk of infection during refill of intrathecal pump.

Use of Compounded Medications

As mentioned above, there are only a few medications that have been approved for use in IDDS. It is important to understand that any combination of medication requires compounding. It is strongly recommended that compounding pharmacist be trained and facility be up to code and certified for compounding intrathecal medications.[11,12]

The single most important benefit of compounding medications is that combination can be suited for patient's requirement and response. Compounding allows for synergistic effects. This improves pain control with reduced side effects.

COST EFFECTIVENESS OF INTRATHECAL THERAPY

Intrathecal drug delivery systems are extremely expensive.[15,16] The entire process of initial evaluation, psychological evaluation, spinal opioid trial and surgical placement of intrathecal catheter and pump, and continued maintenance and refill of the intrathecal pump is expensive.

There have been multiple studies that have investigated the issue as regards cost effectiveness. The approximate time when the entire process becomes cost effective is between 6 and 12 months.[15,16] This is quite acceptable in chronic nonmalignant pain patients.

As regards cancer patients, cost effectiveness may be extremely difficult to calculate. It is reported that about 80% of entire healthcare expense of each individual patient is spent in the last 1 year of life. Based on this assessment and fact that patient have an intrathecal pump, it can potentially provide significant relief of pain and improve quality of life for these patients, and cost effectiveness may not be the most important consideration in these cases.

Ziconotide as a medication has not been studied as regards cost effectiveness. This medication is extremely expensive and average cost of medications based on an average daily dose of about 4 μg of ziconotide costs about 10–15 times the average cost of an intrathecal compounded solution. As a result, this becomes a difficult situation to justify whether this medication really has significant potential for use. Studies do show that it is an effective medication, but extremely difficult to handle and must be used with extreme caution because of side effects.[10]

CONCLUSION

Intrathecal drug delivery systems are an established modality of treatment for pain in selected patients. It is extremely important to understand that utilization of this resource must be limited to trained professionals, selection of patients must be extremely careful, trialing process must be adequate to ensure that patients selected are most likely to benefit, the surgical technique should be highest quality, and maintenance of pumps should be done by practitioners well versed in managing intrathecal pumps. A large number of patients with intrathecal pumps can expect to lead normal lifestyle. They are not likely to require any extra oral pain medications. In addition, they are likely to have very few side effects.

REFERENCES

1. Hayek SM, Deer TR, Pope JE, Panchal SJ, Patel VB. Intrathecal therapy for cancer and non-cancer pain. Pain Physician. 2011;14(3):219-48.
2. Bolash R, Mekhail N. Intrathecal pain pumps: indications, patient selection, techniques, and outcomes. Neurosurg Clin N Am. 2014;25(4):735-42.
3. Prager J, Deer T, Levy R, Bruel B, Buchser E, Caraway D, et al. Best practices for intrathecal drug delivery for pain. Neuromodulation. 2014;17(4):354-72.
4. Smith TJ, Staats PS, Deer T, Stearns LJ, Rauck RL, Boortz-Marx RL, et al. Randomized clinical trial of an implantable drug delivery system compared with comprehensive medical management for refractory cancer pain: impact on pain drug-related toxicity, and survival. J Clin Oncol. 2002;20(19):4040-9.
5. Lynch L. Intrathecal drug delivery for cancer pain. In: Sharma ML, Gupta S, Bennett MI, Simpson K (Eds). Practical Management of Complex Cancer pain. New York: Oxford University Press; 2014.
6. Deer TR, Smith HS, Burton AW, Pope JE, Doleys DM, Levy RM, et al. Comprehensive consensus-based guidelines on intrathecal drug delivery systems in the treatment of pain caused by cancer pain. Pain Physician. 2011;14(3):E283-312.
7. Upadhyay SP, Mallick PN. Intrathecal drug delivery system (IDDS) for cancer pain management: a review and updates. Am J Hosp Palliat Care. 2012;29(5):388-98.
8. Patel VB, Manchikanti L, Singh V, Schultz DM, Hayek SM, Smith HS. Systematic review of intrathecal infusion systems for long term management of chronic non-cancer pain. Pain Physician. 2009;12(2):345-60.
9. Deer TR, Prager J, Levy R, Rathmell J, Buchser E, Burton A, et al. Polyanalgesic Consensus Conference 2012: recommendations for the management of pain by intrathecal (intraspinal) drug delivery: report of an interdisciplinary expert panel. Neuromodulation. 2012;15(5):436-64.
10. Kress HG, Simpson KH, Marchettini P, Ver Donck A, Varrassi G. Intrathecal therapy: what has changed with the introduction of ziconotide? Pain Pract. 2009;9(5):338-47.
11. Deer TR, Caraway DL, Kim CK, Dempsey CD, Stewart CD, McNeil KF. Clinical experience with intrathecal bupivacaine in combination with opioid for the treatment of chronic pain related to failed back surgery syndrome and metastatic cancer pain of the spine. Spine J. 2002;2(4):274-8.
12. Rudich Z, Peng P, Dunn E, McCartney C. Stability of clonidine in clonidine-hydromorphone mixture from implanted intrathecal infusion pumps in chronic pain patients. J Pain Symptom Manage. 2004;28(6):599-602.
13. Wesemann K, Coffey RJ, Wallace MS, Tan Y, Broste S, Buvanendran A. Clinical accuracy and safety using the SynchroMed II intrathecal drug infusion pump. Reg Anesth Pain Med. 2014;39(4):341-6.
14. Wilkes D. Programmable intrathecal pumps for the management of chronic pain: recommendations for improved efficiency. J Pain Res. 2014;7:571-7.
15. Kumar K, Rizvi S, Bishop S. Cost effectiveness of intrathecal drug therapy in management of chronic nonmalignant pain. Clin J Pain. 2013;29(2):138-45.
16. Guillemette S, Witzke S, Leier J, Hinnenthal J, Prager JP. Medical cost impact of intrathecal drug delivery for noncancer pain. Pain Med. 2013;14(4):504-15.

55 CHAPTER

Percutaneous Cervical Cordotomy for Cancer Pain

Ramkumar Kalaiyarasan, Manohar L Sharma

ABSTRACT

Cordotomy means disrupting spinothalamic pathway in the spinal cord to stop sensation of pain. It has been described by open surgical means from the early 1910s, but the surgical morbidity has been high. However, effective pain relief from open surgical cordotomy has been reported to last for many years in case studies. In the 60s and 70s, there was further refinement in imaging techniques and radiofrequency lesion generators including heat lesioning technique to facilitate this procedure by a needle-based technique in cervical spinal cord, termed percutaneous cervical cordotomy (PCC). This has reduced the morbidity associated with this technique with better patient-reported outcomes and over period of time refinement in indications for this procedure. In the 1980s, the World Health Organization (WHO) analgesic ladder was published and it was misinterpreted as if neuroablative procedures will not be needed to manage refractory cancer pain. Benefits and limitations of the WHO analgesic ladder have now been realized and there has been resurgence of interest in this technique. Careful patient selection, meticulous technique, and aftercare of these patients in an appropriate environment within a setup of close collaboration with palliative medicine are essential for optimum outcome for the patients and the treating teams. These patients even if free of pain after this procedure still need ongoing input from palliative medicine for nonpain-related symptoms and further management. In carefully selected patients with unilateral medically refractory cancer-related pain, PCC is now an established advanced pain-relieving technique in the United Kingdom and Europe. Further support for this is provided by a national cordotomy registry which collects prospective multicenter data in the United Kingdom to assess the safety and efficacy of cervical cordotomy. Early results from this registry are encouraging and will be published in near future.

INTRODUCTION

Pain in 70–80% of the patients with cancer can be controlled with the World Health Organization (WHO) analgesic ladder.[1] However, 8–10% of patients still require advanced pain management techniques.[2,3] There is a growing interest in percutaneous cervical cordotomy (PCC) as an effective pain relief technique in the United Kingdom because of an expected increase in mesothelioma cases. Various publications and manuals have recommended access to a cordotomy service for difficult-to-control cancer pain syndromes.[4] Cordotomy is very effective for unilateral cancer-related pain below 4th cervical dermatome.[5-11] Incident pain (no pain at rest and worst imaginable pain on slight movement) responds poorly to opioids and adjuvant analgesics but may respond very well to cordotomy. Although nociceptive pain is a well-established indication, neuropathic pain does also respond very well in the author's opinion even if there is complete deafferentation (e.g., brachial plexopathy resulting from breast cancer metastasis to axillary lymph nodes or pancoast tumor infiltrating brachial plexus) in the painful area.[9] These pains are usually poorly responsive to usual painkillers including the ones usually used for neuropathic pain. The American Society of Pain and Neuroscience (ASPN) - Best Practices and Guidelines for the Interventional Management of Cancer-Associated Pain provides grade 2b recommendation for cordotomy in refractory unilateral nociceptive cancer pain.[12]

HISTORICAL PERSPECTIVE

Anterolateral open cordotomy was first performed by Spiller and Martin in 1912.[13] It was initially deemed acceptable as it offered long-term pain relief albeit with some disadvantages and complications. However, it never became popular due to associated high morbidity/mortality secondary to the open neurosurgical procedure. Of late, there seems to be resurgence in interest in this technique as well and this is offered in the author's unit by his neurosurgical colleagues for carefully selected patients. The percutaneous technique was described by Mullan, Rosomoff, and Lin in the mid-1960s. Mullan described the method of delineating the dentate ligament (a fine ligament which holds the spinal cord in place laterally and is halfway between the anterior and posterior half of the spinal cord) by myelography. Rosomoff developed the concept of radiofrequency (RF) current thermocoagulation to generate a quick and reliable heat lesion at the time. Lesion generation by direct current usually took very long and was not reliable, and hence the RF lesion technique was an advance. Sam Lipton popularized the percutaneous cordotomy technique in Liverpool in the United Kingdom and Europe in the 1960s.[5] However, initially patients with chronic pain with or without cancer were offered this procedure; this is usually not the case now. The percutaneous approach is difficult to tolerate, but patients recover quicker in comparison with open surgical cordotomy. This is a palliative, pain relief procedure now used to help cancer patients with medically refractory pain with limited life expectancy. It is most useful in nociceptive and mixed cancer pain syndrome, which is unilateral, and localized to a region of the body below the shoulder.

CONCEPT

Percutaneous cervical cordotomy involves interruption of the lateral spinothalamic tract at the spinal C1/C2 level by a RF heat lesion in the anterolateral quadrant of the spinal cord. Traditionally, it has been believed that the success of the procedure depends on focal thermal coagulation of the lateral spinothalamic tract. Work done by Gebarski et al. using diffusion tensor imaging (DTI) in patients with successful percutaneous cordotomy showed reduced rostrocaudal directional DTI signal in the spinothalamic tract. This suggests that the analgesic potential is not only due to the thermal focal coagulation but also due to microscopic anterograde degeneration in the cervical spinal cord through pons and mesencephalon.[14]

Percutaneous cervical cordotomy can be invaluable in patients where adequate pain control cannot be achieved by conventional analgesics including opioid therapy, and where techniques such as intrathecal or epidural drug delivery are ineffective or inappropriate or not available. The success of PCC in the treatment of costopleural pain syndrome in malignant mesothelioma has been described and established. The procedure is very effective for the management of particular types of breakthrough pain (incident pain) in cancer, e.g., from bone metastases, plexus invasion which is usually poorly responsive to opioids.

Patients must have adequate respiratory reserve due to the rare risk of respiratory failure after the procedure and can be a cause of mortality. Patients are counseled about the risk of technical failure to perform cordotomy and hence absence of pain relief. Concerns about the potential serious side effects of the procedure have led to underuse, but the procedure is very safe with good patient selection and meticulous technique in expert hands.

INDICATIONS AND PATIENT SELECTION

This procedure has been used in the past for various indications including pain due to malignant disease (rectum, lung, and breast) or benign disease (postherpetic neuralgia, nerve root pain, and phantom limb pain). The current recommendation is restricted to patients with terminal cancer **(Figs. 1 and 2)**.

The following patient selection criteria are used:

- Biopsy-proven progressive malignant disease with life expectancy <1 year

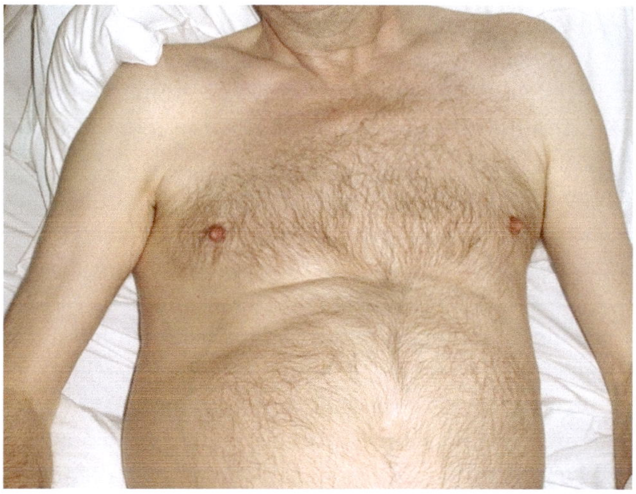

Fig. 1: Typical patient with mesothelioma on the right side, a recognized indication of cordotomy.

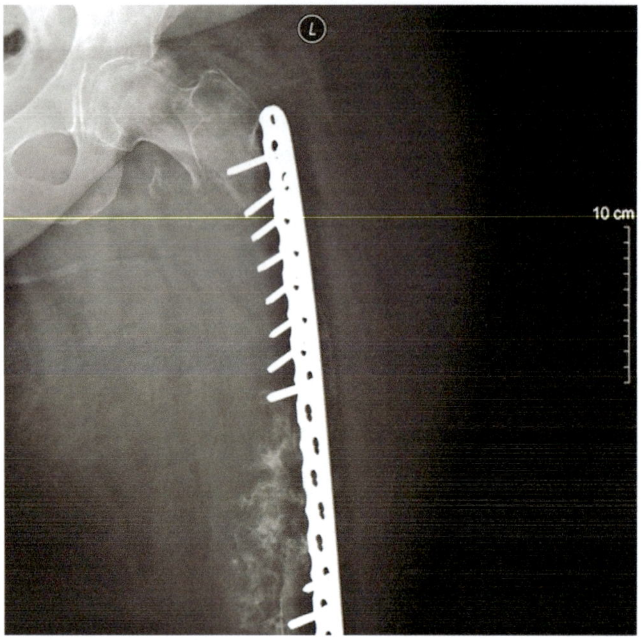

Fig. 2: Pathological fracture with internal fixation, but this patient has severe incident pain on any movement because of poor fixation of metal work.

- Increasing requirement of opioids or adjuvant analgesics with poor pain control
- Unilateral pain below 4th cervical dermatome (below shoulder)
- Patient can lie supine for at least 30–45 minutes.

Patients are excluded or the procedure is deferred if:
- Life expectancy is >1 year
- Nonprogressive nature of the disease
- Fitness issues for the procedure (poor respiratory reserve, severe anxiety, inability to lie supine).

It is important to be aware that many of these patients with severe pain are very complex and pain is just one of the symptoms apart from lethargy, poor appetite, depression, helplessness, etc. Hence, close collaboration between specialties would help manage these patients more appropriately and effectively. In our institution, palliative and pain medicine collaborates to deliver a holistic management (including physical and psychological support to the patient and their family) of these complex cases. The author conducts weekly joint pain and palliative care clinic and ward round at hospice to assess and follow up the patients who may benefit from interventional pain techniques. If suitable, patients are explained the procedure and expected benefits and risks and are given a patient information leaflet. They are also explained that this procedure only helps the pain and not the other issues which they may have because of cancer, e.g., frailty, fatigue, poor appetite, psychological sequelae because of terminal disease diagnosis, etc.

Technique

Percutaneous cervical cordotomy has been well described in many sources.[15-18] PCC can be performed by fluoroscopic or computed tomography (CT) guidance. Fluoroscopic technique is most commonly used and will be described in this chapter. It is a technically challenging procedure requiring considerable skill, dexterity, patient cooperation, and attention to detail. The procedure is performed in the operating theater. The patient is awake and has intravenous access to facilitate a small dose of sedation and prophylactic antibiotic administration. It is a usual practice to perform this procedure through C1-C2 foramen as it is the largest foramen and allows for adjustment in needle trajectory changes much easily than other foramens. The anterior transdiscal approach has been described but is not currently used.

Patient Preparation

- Consent includes discussion of likely success rate, need for cooperation during the procedure, risk of failure to perform, likely recovery period, expected discharge time, analgesic medications reduction, and potential complications. Patients are also given a patient information leaflet for cervical cordotomy as given in **Appendix 2**.
- All patients must be warned about the rare risks of failure to achieve pain relief, motor weakness, sensory loss, especially inability to discriminate temperature sensation in the area affected by cordotomy, bowel or bladder impairment, mirror pain, headache, neck pain, and feeling unwell for 24–48 hours after cordotomy
- Prepare the patient for general anesthesia, though the procedure is performed under local anesthesia. Sedation is very often required. Intravenous access, oxygen administration by nasal speculum, and routine monitoring by another doctor or anesthetist are essential.
- Strict asepsis is essential. It is usual to administer one dose of prophylactic antibiotic according to local hospital guidance.
- Another experienced team member must be dedicated to monitoring patient comfort and allay their anxiety related to the procedure.

EQUIPMENT

- X-ray machine
- Radiolucent Rosomoff headrest **(Fig. 3)** or any other suitable adapted headrest (Pounders headrest; **Fig. 4**) and needle-holding device **(Figs. 5 and 6)**
- RF lesion generator with cordotomy option in lesion settings
- 20G, 100 mm spinal needle **(Fig. 7)**
- Cordotomy RF probe with a 2 mm active tip **(Fig. 7)**
- Oil-based (lipoidal) or water-soluble radio-opaque contrast (Omnipaque 300)
- Local anesthetic
- Simple equipment for sensory examination after the heat lesion, e.g., ice cubes and Neurotips.

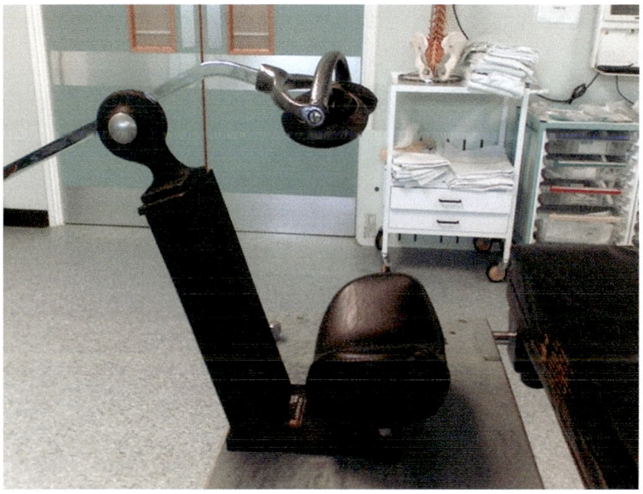

Fig. 3: Rosomoff head clamp to support head during cordotomy.

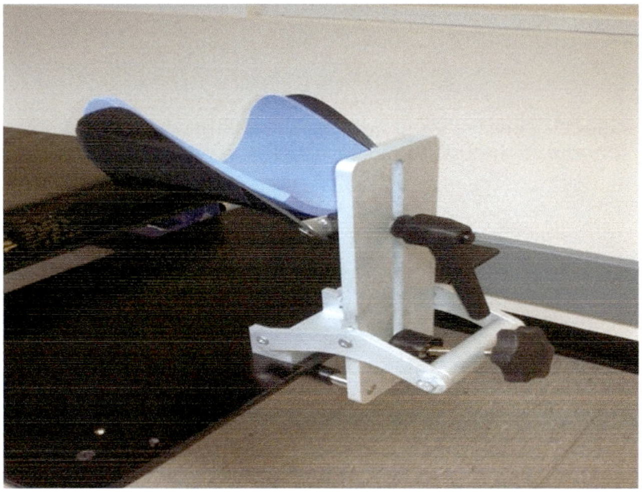

Fig. 4: New cordotomy headrest (Manufacturer: Wolverson X-Ray Limited, UK).

PATIENT POSITION

Position the patient supine on a radiolucent table with the head held in special headrest, the height of which if can be adjusted is helpful **(Fig. 8)**.

- Head is held in position by straps or part of the headrest so as to prevent extremes of neck movements
- Some patients need extra support or protection for the painful area and this should be considered and allows the patient's comfort and improve their ability to cooperate with the procedure.

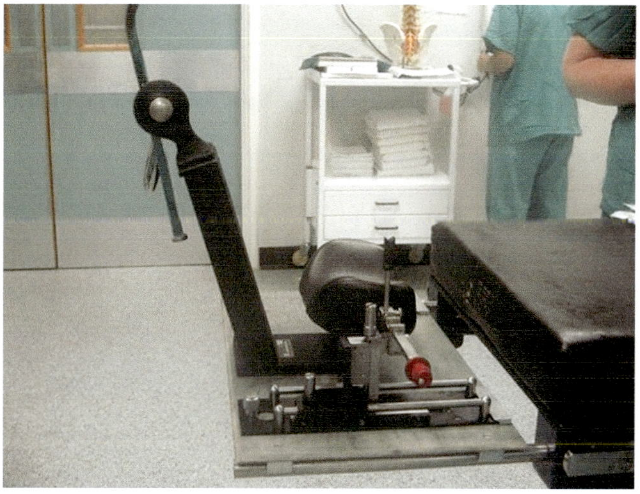

Fig. 5: Part of Rosomoff head clamp along with needle-holding device.

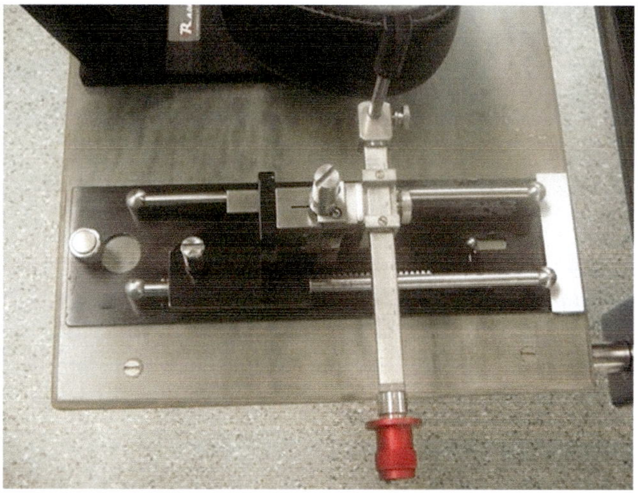

Fig. 6: Another view of the needle-holding device (can be maneuvered sideways and up and down and showing the groove in a black needle holder).

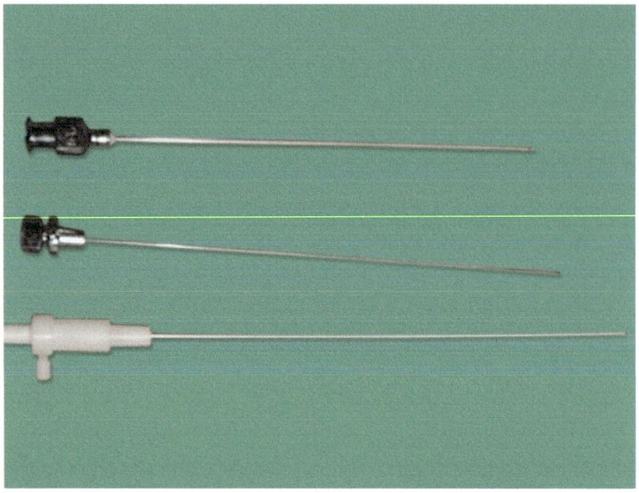

Fig. 7: 20G spinal needle and cordotomy probe.
Note: Cordotomy probe (white) has a 2 mm active tip.

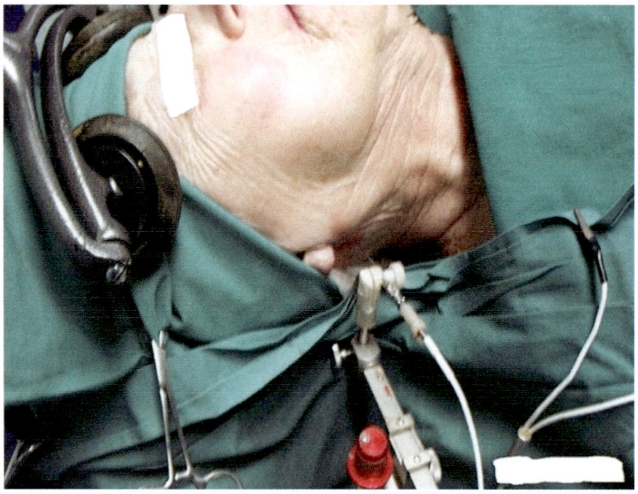

Fig. 8: Spinal needle in situ at C1-C2 spinal level with the cordotomy probe in the anterolateral quadrant of the spinal cord.

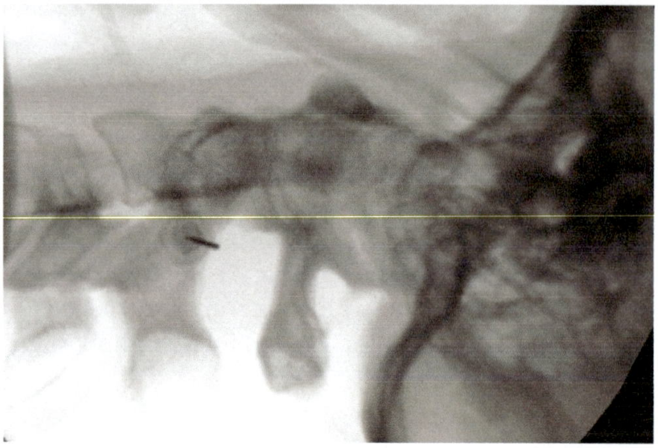

Fig. 9: Spinal needle being introduced between C1 and C2 intervertebral foramen, lateral approach (note the shape of the foramen, the needle being introduced at the point where the roof meets the wall).

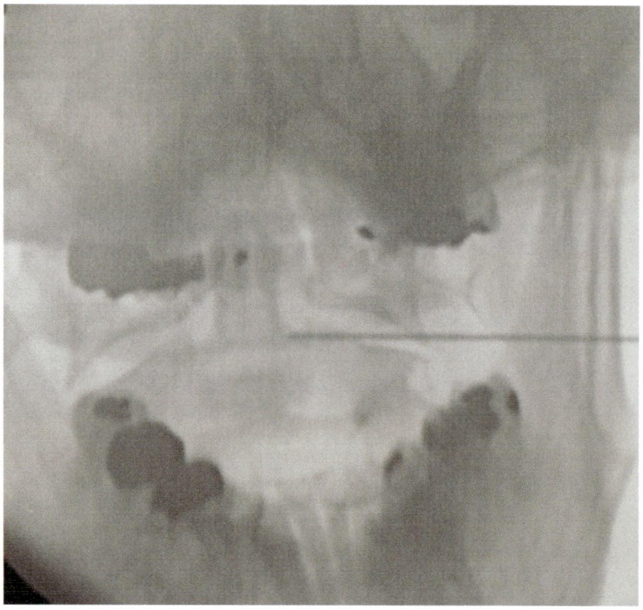

Fig. 10: Spinal needle in subarachnoid space. Cordotomy probe introduced through the spinal needle should not cross midline.

IMAGING

- The C arm should be positioned to obtain a lateral view of the cervical spine
- Minor adjustments may be needed to clearly define the margins of the 1st and 2nd cervical foramen **(Fig. 9)**
- Care should be taken to adjust the C arm angle in a way to square or remove double shadow from the upper margin of C2 vertebrae while taking a lateral X-ray of the cervical spine **(Fig. 9)**
- The anterior-posterior (AP) view should be checked during the procedure to minimize chances of the spinal needle crossing the midline, i.e., going too far across in the substance of spinal cord to the other side **(Fig. 10)**.
- During the procedure, any slight rotation of head and tilt of head to either side will distort the X-ray image and may misdirect the needle trajectory and hence, care should be taken to minimize any neck movement.

Needle Insertion

- To find the target point, the operator should imagine the boundaries of the 1st and 2nd cervical foramen as the roof and walls of a hut.

- Needle entry point is just superior to lamina of the 2nd cervical vertebrae where the roof seems to join the walls of imaginary picture **(Fig. 9)**.
- Under local anesthesia, a 20G spinal needle is inserted between the 1st and the 2nd cervical vertebrae, aiming for a needle approach to the dural sac at 90°.
- There will be need to administer local anesthesia with advancing needle to avoid pain, but be careful and aspirate before injecting a small volume of local anesthetics so as to avoid any intravascular or intrathecal injection.

Myelogram

- After free flow of cerebrospinal fluid (CSF), a myelogram is obtained using a lipid-based radiopaque or water-soluble contrast **(Fig. 11)**. The author uses lipoidal and CSF mixture 1–2 mL at a time (3 mL mixture of lipoidal mixed with 5 mL of CSF).
- Satisfactory myelogram shows the needle to be correctly positioned by visualizing dentate ligament **(Figs. 11 and 12)**.
- If the needle is posterior to the dentate ligament, then the myelogram will not show the dentate ligament.
- In this situation, the spinal needle has to be redirected anteriorly so that its tip lies just anterior to the dentate ligament.
- It is helpful at times to use needle supportive devices **(Figs. 5 and 6)**, which can also be used to redirect the needle to adjust its trajectory so as to enter the anterolateral quadrant of the spinal cord.

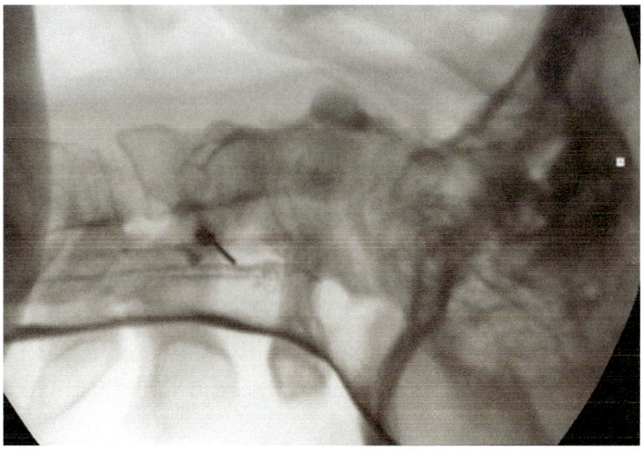

Fig. 11: Myelogram obtained with lipoidal mixed with cerebrospinal fluid (CSF), showing anterior border of the spinal cord and dentate ligament.
(Note: The tip of the spinal needle just anterior to dentate ligament.)

- If the first spinal needle on the myelogram is seen to be too anterior and it is anticipated that cordotomy probe entry in the spinal cord may be difficult, then the second spinal needle may be introduced just anterior to the dentate ligament to enter the subarachnoid space. This has been described by some authors as a double-needle technique.
- Quality of myelogram is very important in helping to direct cordotomy probe entry into the anterolateral quadrant of the spinal cord. So, all attempts should be made to obtain a good-quality myelogram. In author's view, mixing lipoidal 3 mL with 5 mL of CSF gives high-quality myelogram
- If lipoidal is mixed with saline, then one may still get a good-quality myelogram but it shows globules of contrast in a nonhomogeneous pattern **(Fig. 12)**.
- If Omnipaque (water-soluble contrast) is used for this purpose, then the quality of myelogram is good, but as Omnipaque disperses in CSF quickly, the operator does not have the advantage of continued visualization of dentate ligament so as to target cordotomy probe just anterior to it into the anterolateral quadrant of the spinal cord.

Inserting Cordotomy Probe into Spinal Cord

- Once the correct image is obtained with the spinal needle just anterior to dentate ligament **(Fig. 11)**, the cordotomy probe with a 2 mm active tip is passed just

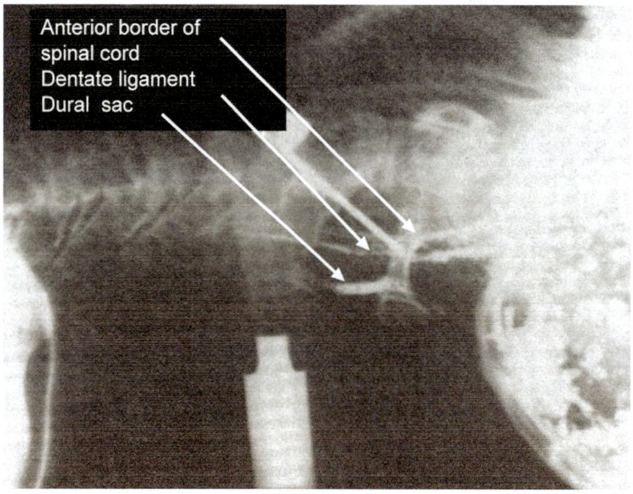

Fig. 12: Myelogram produced with lipid-based dye mixed with normal saline (showing globule in the posterior fossa and cervical spine image) showing various landmarks (dentate ligament is the most important marker and cordotomy probe has to be introduced just anterior to it into the spinal cord).

anterior to the dentate ligament through the spinal needle into the anterolateral quadrant of the spinal cord **(Fig. 8)**.

- The correct position of the electrode in the spinal cord is confirmed by a change in the audible pitch of impedance tone and impedance change from 400 to 1,200Ω as well as by sensory and motor stimulation findings.
- Patients usually report severe burning or icy cold sensation in the contralateral side of body; this is usually below the shoulder area and at stimulation settings around 0.05 V or so.
- On motor stimulation, there should be no motor twitch on the ipsilateral side of the body, except in neck muscles at about 0.5 V.
- If the probe tip is close to corticospinal tracts (meaning cordotomy probe trajectory is posterior, i.e., toward dorsal column), then motor stimulation is ipsilateral and on sensory stimulation patients will perceive vibrations.
- In some cases, localizing the spinothalamic tract can be very difficult and painful or distressing to the patient. This is helped by sedation at this stage.

Radiofrequency Lesioning Technique

- There is no established and recommended algorithm of RF heat lesioning, i.e., starting temperature and duration.
- There is no recommended endpoint as to when to stop doing a further RF lesion.
- Described technique is used by the author as learned from his mentor, Dr Tim Nash.
- Once satisfactory cordotomy probe position is confirmed as above, a gradual RF lesion is created in incremental steps, starting at 75°C and titrating up to 85°C. Each lesion is for 30 seconds.
- At each lesioning step, the patient is asked to raise the arm and bend knee and raise foot on the ipsilateral side of cordotomy **(Fig. 13)**.
- The reason for the above step is to identify any suggestion of motor weakness so as to avoid further lesioning at the wrong place. In practice, this is highly unusual if careful sensory and motor testing has been carried out before starting a RF lesion.
- After each RF lesion, sensory and motor power testing is repeated so that there is no motor weakness. Sensory testing is carried out to demonstrate loss of perception of sharpness of pin prick and temperature discrimination; that is, patients cannot accurately perceive hot or cold sensation in the cordotomy-affected area. The author prefers testing with an ice cube and it is usual for the patient to report ice cube as warm if there is effective loss of spinothalamic tract function in the painful area.

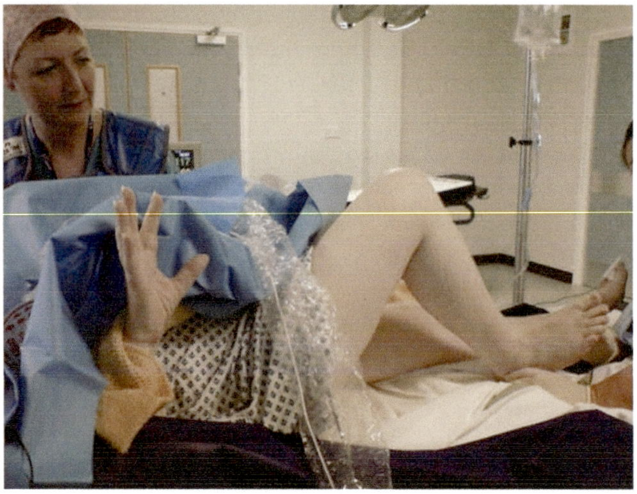

Fig. 13: Patient raising arm and feet at the time of radiofrequency lesion in the spinothalamic tract.

- Small doses of opioid can be used to make RF lesion less distressing.
- Patients usually report immediate and complete relief of pain on the operating table.
- For beginners, it may be beneficial to have experienced colleagues in the theater, including an experienced radiographer.

Points to Ensure Safety and Efficacy

- Try to direct the spinal needle to the dural sac using an end on or gun barrel approach. This maximizes chances of localizing the spinothalamic pathway by entering the spinal cord at the right angle.
- Once the spinal needle is intrathecal, make sure there is free flow of CSF when introducing a cordotomy probe. If not, there is possibility of the spinal needle being in the substance of spinal cord or touching the surface of spinal cord.
- It may be worthwhile checking AP images **(Fig. 10)** through an open mouth view to see the depth of needle or probe. There is no need to cross the midline (midline of odontoid peg).
- It is beneficial to reduce opioid dose by half on the day of the procedure, particularly if the patient is taking very high doses; this helps to minimize opioid toxicity in the postprocedure period.

- One needs a very cooperative patient and pertinence and experienced team for this procedure.
- It is a technically challenging procedure requiring considerable skill, dexterity, patient cooperation, and attention to detail. This procedure should not be embarked upon just reading this chapter, but one should seek training from the department with experience doing significant numbers.
- There have been various methods suggested to improve the safety of the percutaneous cordotomy procedure. One such method is optimizing the radiofrequency needle using electromyography in deeply sedated patients. This has been tried with good outcomes in a limited number of patients under control settings.[19]

PRE- AND POSTPROCEDURE CARE

Patients are admitted a day before the procedure to further counsel regarding the procedure and allay any concerns or anxiety and to supplement initial assessment to confirm their suitability for the cordotomy. It is also important to detect any deterioration which may have happened between initial assessment and admission. Patients are usually admitted for 3–4 days for supportive care either in hospice or in the hospital. After cordotomy, patients are usually advised bed rest for a day (see **Appendix 3**: Cordotomy care pathway). Any initial movement out of bed is carefully monitored in case there is any proprioception or motor weakness or frailty-related issues. They may need intravenous fluids, antibiotics, and oxygen for a day or two depending on their preprocedure condition. Usually, opioids are reduced by half immediately postcordotomy and this reduction is very well tolerated by the patient. Generally, it is difficult to completely wean off opioids as these may be needed for other pains. Too quick a reduction in various painkillers may precipitate withdrawal reaction which generally presents as overall feeling unwell. The author in his practice leaves the rest of the analgesic titration to the referring team after initial opioid reduction. Discharge planning, hospital transfer, and appropriate location of destination are carefully decided in conjunction with the palliative care team so as to ensure smooth transfer of care and responsibilities.

SIDE EFFECTS AND COMPLICATIONS

Patients are warned of the risks which are: 1 in 20 chance of leg weakness, taking up to 1 month to resolve, 1 in 5 chance of temporary leg weakness lasting 24–48 hours and rapidly resolving. Interference with bladder function has been extremely rare in the author's experience (once in last 100 patients and resolved in 2 days). Difficulty with perception of contralateral warm or cold sensory modality is to be expected and there is a risk of burns and patients are warned regarding this. Rarely patients find this troublesome. There is a 1 in 10 chance of failure to achieve adequate spinothalamic cordotomy. Serious complications can include death (6% incidence in earlier studies but 0.5% with meticulous patient selection) or serious hemiplegia. Rarely, severe mirror pain has occurred in a very few patients, but mild mirror pain occurs in about 15–25% of patients. Respiratory inadequacy after cordotomy because of preexisting poor respiratory reserve could be a problem, but this has not been the case in the author's experience because of meticulous patient selection. A study carried out in the Portsmouth Unit, UK, concluded that cordotomy was well tolerated with regard to lung function. Other minor side effects of the procedure include postdural puncture headache and neck pain (usually of short duration and easily controlled). Patients do feel a bit rough for a couple of days afterward, possibly as a result of systemic response to the procedure and reduction of opioids.

OUTCOME FROM PROSPECTIVE AUDIT FROM THE AUTHOR'S UNIT

A prospective review of 45 consecutive cases undergoing PCC was conducted over a 3-year period from 2009 to 2012 ($n = 45$).[18] All patients were suffering from severe, refractory unilateral pain secondary to malignancy with poor pain relief or intolerable side effects of conventional analgesics including opioids and adjuvants. Variables recorded preprocedure at 2 days and at 28 days postprocedure were: Numerical rating scale for maximum and average pain, oral morphine equivalent dose, and global impression of change. Adverse events were noted, and survival data were collected in April 2012 from the patient's general practitioner.

Survival postprocedure ranged from 7 days to 33 months. There was a statistically significant reduction in pain scores from baseline at 2 days and at 28 days postprocedure. About 70–80% of patients in this series experienced immediate pain relief on day 2 **(Fig. 14)**. Improvement in pain scores was sustained at 28 days **(Fig. 15)**. Oral morphine equivalent dosages and adjuvant analgesics were reduced by more than 50% in patients undergoing successful cordotomy. There was significant improvement in global impression of change noted by majority of patients. Majority felt that it was worthwhile

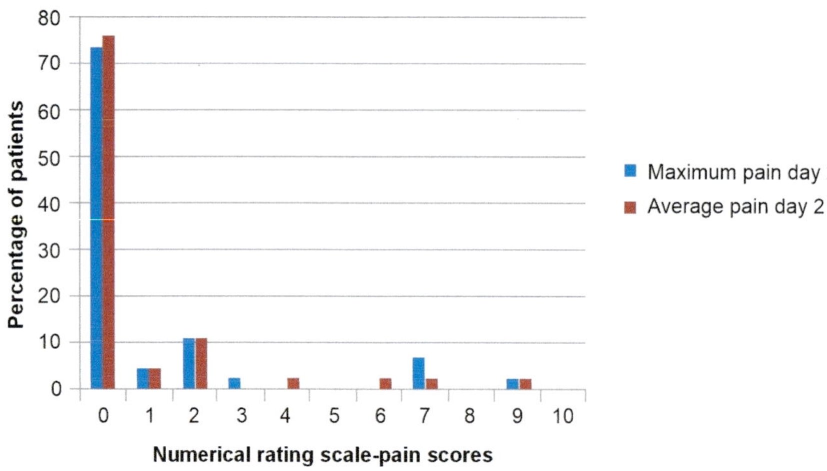

Fig. 14: Pain score 2 days postprocedure.

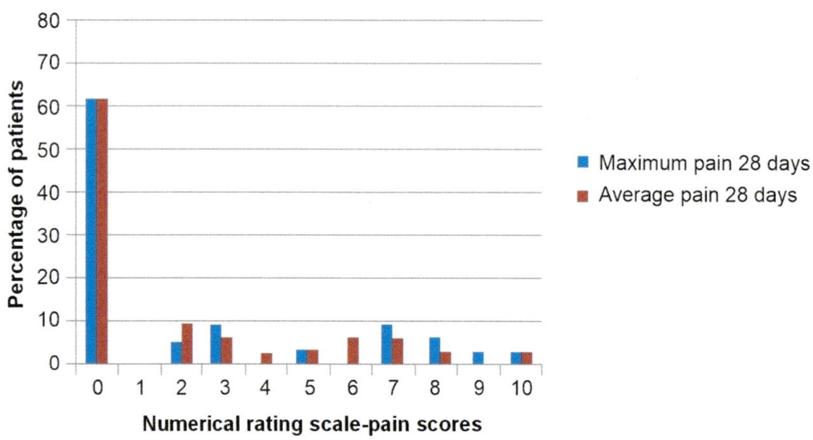

Fig. 15: Pain scores 28 days postprocedure.

undergoing cordotomy. In 45 cases, there were no serious adverse events such as respiratory failure. These results generally match with other units performing very good numbers per annum.[11] A recent systematic review supported the role of cordotomy for mesothelioma-related refractory cancer pain but concluded that evidence base was anecdotal and of limited quality.[20]

BILATERAL CORDOTOMY

Percutaneous cervical cordotomy has been described in the literature, and some practitioners still offer this in Europe as a staged procedure. Author prefers not to offer bilateral PCC because of perceived risk of Ondine's curse. If the patient develops severe pain on the side opposite to initial pain and if the pain is below T6 dermatome, then they are offered open surgical cordotomy at the T1-T3 level. This is well tolerated as it is carried out under general anesthesia, but there is a very high risk of bowel and bladder impairment. This may be acceptable in a patient who is terminally ill and has very severe uncontrollable pain. Open bilateral surgical cordotomy has been described recently with good outcome for pain relief. Rarely open surgical cordotomy can be offered to a patient who may not be able to tolerate PCC and if the pain is below T6 dermatome.

FUTURE DIRECTIONS

Training and maintenance of skills in the technique of PCC are crucial. The learning curve in this procedure is not as steep as that for other pain relief interventional techniques. As the number of centers offering this procedure is very small, the training opportunities are very limited with the risk of this technique becoming extinct. This important issue needs to be addressed by national organizations responsible for training in pain medicine in various countries. Magnetic resonance imaging (MRI) and CT-guided technique for PCC have been described and may have some advantages, especially in cases with difficult anatomy. This, however, does not seem to be popular. The endoscopic technique of cordotomy under direct vision has also been recently described. This may have some advantages, especially in carrying out lesion under direct vision. Noninvasive lesioning technique may be a possibility in future using emerging technologies so as to avoid the risks of invasive procedures. One of these techniques involves causing a lesion using stereotactic radiation with gamma knife or *Linear Accelerator* (LINAC)-based systems using high-energy protons aimed at the target site. Another is use of percutaneous ultrasound methods. MRI-guided thermal lesions can be generated and there is ability to create initial test lesion to assess efficacy before progressing to definitive lesion of the spinothalamic tract. The author expects good progress in this field in near future.

CONCLUSION

Percutaneous cervical cordotomy is a safe and highly effective procedure to treat intractable unilateral cancer pain. It offers significant advantages over other pain control methods, especially for incident pain and pain in focal areas on one side and poorly controlled otherwise with the conventional WHO analgesic ladder. Patient selection and attention to detail and delivering this service in close collaboration with palliative medicine are paramount for a successful outcome. It is underused at the moment. Various guidelines and manuals support application of this technique in medically refractory cancer pain which is predominantly below shoulder. It is mandatory to have good collaboration with palliative care to have better outcome and to deal with other nonpain related issues. Good evidence base is now developing and the author expects an increase in application of this technique to suitably selected patients as at the moment the uptake of this technique is patchy.

APPENDIX 2

Patient Information Leaflet for Cervical Cordotomy

What is percutaneous cervical cordotomy?—This means selectively heating pain carrying nerve fibers in your spinal cord. This procedure needs your cooperation in helping to localize the pain sensation carrying nerve fibers. There can be some discomfort or pain, although we will help you by administering sedation. This procedure is performed in the upper part of your neck, on the side opposite to your pain. This is normally done in cases where it is not possible to control the pain by less invasive methods including various drugs, other treatments for cancer and complementary therapies.

How is it done?—Percutaneous cervical cordotomy is performed after you have been admitted to hospital as an inpatient. For this procedure you will be needed to lie on your back. A plastic cannula (needle) will be placed in a vein on the back of your hand and sedation will be given to relax you. You will be attached to a monitor to keep a close eye on your breathing and circulation. Your head will be placed in a special headrest, which will prevent sudden movement of your head, so as to minimize chances of any complications during the procedure.

This procedure is performed by your doctor under X-ray control, which helps identify the precise location of the injection site. Local anesthetic is injected into the skin to numb the area. Nerve fibers carrying the pain sensation are located by passing a mild electrical current through a special needle.

Once you feel a sensation of warmth or cold in your painful area, the needle tip is electrically heated to burn these particular nerve fibers.

During the actual process of the needle tip being heated, you will be asked to lift your arm and toes to the ceiling, so as to detect any evidence of arm or leg weakness. This process will be repeated until there is objective change in your perception of sharp and blunt pin prick sensation.

What are the side effects?—You may feel unwell for a day or two because of neck stiffness and headache. There is a rare risk of permanent arm or leg weakness, although generally it is temporary.

There can be weakness of bowel and bladder control, but generally it is more common if the procedure is done on both sides. Very rarely, death has been reported as a result of this procedure.

What is the success rate?—In 10% of patients, the pain pathway cannot be identified and the procedure has to be abandoned. In another 10% of patients, they will not gain pain relief, despite apparent initial success. This means that 80% of patients can expect a significant reduction in pain and need for taking pain killers.

Contact Numbers:

Palliative Care, XXXXX,

Department of Pain Medicine, XXXXXXXX

APPENDIX 3

Cordotomy care pathway (guidance for the referrers, ward staff including nurse and doctors caring for patients in units doing this procedure as used in author's hospital and hospice)

Please complete goals as achieved "a" or variance "v". If any goal on this pathway is completed as variance please complete on variance sheet accordingly.

Rationale

Cervical cordotomy involves radiofrequency lesioning (by heat) of the spinothalamic tract between 1st and 2nd cervical vertebrae. It is very effective for refractory pain caused by mesothelioma. It can also be a helpful procedure for other refractory unilateral cancer pain e.g. incident pain due to bone metastases; however, the evidence for the effectiveness of cordotomy in non-mesothelioma related pain is less established, but, good in author's opinion. The patient should have good respiratory reserve so as to avoid any respiratory morbidity in post-procedure period.

Indications for Percutaneous Cervical Cordotomy

1. Unilateral pain below 4th cervical dermatome
2. Reasonable respiratory reserve (sufficient if ability to lie flat for about 45 minutes as this is the length of the procedure)
3. Expected survival more than 3 months and less than 1 year.
4. Medically refractory unilateral pain syndrome
5. Pain caused by cancer or metastatic spread (should have a confirmed tissue diagnosis).

Referral and Assessment

Patients should be referred by letter. Patients are assessed jointly by Dr XXX and Dr XXX from the chronic pain team at the Walton Centre and Dr XXX from the specialist palliative care team at University Hospital Aintree and Woodlands Hospice at Woodlands Hospice OPD. If patients are deemed suitable for percutaneous cordotomy, they should receive a copy of the information leaflet attached to this pathway.

Goal 1: Referral letter filed in case notes ☐

Goal 2: Copy of information leaflet given to patient ☐

Admission for Procedure

Patients will be admitted to Woodlands Hospice Inpatient Unit if a bed is available a few days prior to the procedure. If no bed is available at Woodlands Hospice, patients have to be admitted to the Walton Centre. To arrange this please liaise with Dr XXX's secretary XXX ext. 8294. Occasionally, patients on general wards at Aintree reviewed by the Palliative Care Hospital Support Team may undergo a cordotomy as well.

Goal 3: Patient listed for bed at Woodlands Hospice Inpatient Unit or at Walton Centre (Dr XXX's secretary 8294) ☐

Care pre-procedure

Goal 4: FBC, U&E, clotting checked (INR needs to be below 1.5) ☐

Goal 5: Patient not on warfarin ☐

Goal 6: If patient on low molecular weight heparin, this needs to be stopped 24 hours prior to procedure and restarted 8 hours after procedure ☐

Goal 7: Patient not on clopidogrel/warfarin. If on those medications they need to have been stopped ideally for seven days prior to procedure ☐

Goal 8: Baseline observations recorded

Goal 9: Review by senior doctor and opioid dose adjusted prior to procedure ☐

Goal 10: Appropriate transport booked to Walton Centre Jefferson ward (hospital taxi to go if patient fit enough if not stretcher ambulance, stretcher ambulance for return; if Tuesday list patient needs to arrive before 9 am, if Wednesday list patient needs to arrive before 1:30 pm) ☐

Care after-procedure

Goal 11: Hourly observations for the first four hours on return. Then 4 hourly for first 24 hours ☐

Goal 12: Patients should be nursed flat in bed for six hours post-procedure ☐

Goal 13: Patients should be free of headache and neck pain. However, this is frequent after cordotomy and if present should be managed with plenty of oral fluids as well as paracetamol PO or IV and breakthrough analgesia ☐

Goal 14: Opioid toxicity not present. If opioid toxicity suspected discuss with senior palliative care medical staff ☐

Goal 15: Maintain IV access for 24 hours post-procedure ☐

Goal 16: Patient should remain afebrile. If patients develop a temperature take blood cultures and discuss with senior medical staff or palliative or pain medicine consultant ☐

Goal 17: Respiration: if there are difficulties with respiration give 24% Oxygen via mask and inform the on-call palliative care doctor ☐

Goal 18: Patient able to pass urine. If not able to pass urine catheterise ☐

Goal 19: Patients will have a small wound on the side of the neck with a simple dressing. This should be changed daily for the first two days ☐

Discharge

Goal 20: Patients discharged back to the referring team

Goal 21: To take home medications (TTO) complete

Goal 22: Discharge letter completed within 48 hours

Goal 23: Copy of discharge letter sent to Dr XXX at Walton Centre, the referrer, palliative medicine consultant, general practitioner and the patient

Variance Sheet for Cordotomy Care Pathway

Date	Time	Variance and reason	Action taken

REFERENCES

1. World Health Organization. Cancer Pain Relief. Geneva: WHO; 1986.
2. The British Pain Society. Guidelines on cancer pain management. [online] Available from http://www.britishpainsociety.org/book_cancer_pain.pdf. [Last accessed August, 2024].
3. Scottish Intercollegiate Guidelines Network. Control of pain in patients with cancer. SIGN Publication No. 44; 2000.
4. Mesothelioma Framework. [online] Available from http: webarchive.nationalarchives.gov.uk/20130107105354/http:/www.dh.gov.uk/prod_consum_dh/groups/dh_digitalassets/documents/digitalasset/dh_072347.pdf. [Last accessed August, 2024].
5. Lipton S. Percutaneous electrical cordotomy in relief of intractable pain. Br Med J. 1968;2:210-2.
6. Horrax G, Price WT Jr. High cervical chordotomy for relief of intractable pain in the arm shoulder and upper chest. Ann Surg. 1954;139(5):567-85.
7. Loeser JD, Butler SH, Chapman R, Turk DC (Eds). Bonica's Management of Pain, 3rd edition. Philadelphia: Lippincott Williams & Wilkins; 2001.
8. Hugel H, Sharma ML. Symptom control at end of life in cancer patients. Indian J Pain. 2010;24:28-31.
9. Gupta S, Hugel H, Sharma ML. Percutaneous cervical cordotomy: a viable option for unilateral medically refractory neuropathic cancer pain. Indian J Pain. 2009;23:256-9.
10. Hugel H, Sharma ML. Cancer pain management: overview and personal perspective. Indian J Pain. 2009;23:272-7.
11. Jackson MB, Pounder D, Price C, Matthews AW, Neville E. Percutaneous cervical cordotomy for the control of pain in patients with pleural mesothelioma. Thorax. 1999;54:238-41.
12. Aman MM, Mahmoud A, Deer T, Sayed D, Hagedorn JM, Brogan SE, et al. The American Society of Pain and Neuroscience (ASPN) best practices and guidelines for the interventional management of cancer-associated pain. J Pain Res. 2021;14:2139-64.
13. Spiller WG, Martin E. The treatment of persistent pain of organic origin in lower part of body by division of anterolateral column of spinal cord. JAMA. 1912;58:1489-90.
14. Gebarski SS, Chiravuri S, Foerster BR, Patil PG. Microstructural mechanisms of analgesia in percutaneous cervical cordotomy revealed by diffusion tensor imaging. J Clin Neurosci. 2017;45:311-4.
15. Hester J, Sykes N, Peat S (Eds). Interventional Pain Control in Cancer Pain Management. Oxford: Oxford University Press; 2012.
16. Sharma M, Simpson KH, Bennett MI, Gupta S (Eds). Practical Management of Complex Cancer Pain. Oxford: Oxford University Press; 2014.

17. Joshi M (Ed). Textbook of Pain Management. Hyderabad: Paras Medical Publishers; 2014.
18. Bains E, Hugel H, Sharma M. Percutaneous cervical cordotomy for the management of pain from cancer: a prospective review of 45 cases. J Palliat Med. 2013;16(8);901-7.
19. Gabay S, Sapir Y, Korn A, Hochberg U, Tellem R, Zegerman A, et al. Optimization of radiofrequency needle placement in percutaneous cordotomy using electromyography in the deeply sedated patient. Oper Neurosurg. 2024;26(1):22-7.
20. France BD, Lewis RA, Sharma ML, Poolman M. Cordotomy in mesothelioma-related pain: a systematic review. BMJ Support Palliat Care. 2014;4:19-29.

56 CHAPTER

Subarachnoid or Intrathecal Neurolysis

Kritika M Doshi

ABSTRACT

Nerve destruction using chemicals to promote analgesia was extensively used in the early part of the 20th century for management of pain—both cancer and noncancer. However, with the advent of newer analgesics and the development of more advanced interventional [spinal cord stimulation (SCS) and intrathecal pump (ITP)] techniques for pain management, this procedure has been neglected and has not gained recognition.

This procedure can be extremely beneficial in developing countries to help with cancer pain as it can reduce the quantum of pain and side effects of oral analgesic drugs. Intrathecal neurolytic drugs (absolute alcohol, phenol) for chemoneurolysis of selected nerve roots can give excellent analgesia in the respective body area.

INTRODUCTION

Intrathecal neurolysis is an invasive intervention that involves destruction of sensory nerve root axons or other elements of the subarachnoid space using chemical means. With the advent of newer analgesics and the development of safer more advanced interventional [spinal cord stimulation (SCS) and intrathecal pump (ITP)] techniques for pain management, this procedure has not gained recognition and its use has markedly diminished. As a result, there is paucity of literature on indications, reports of long-term outcome, or details of the procedure.

At present, these procedures are again viewed as a useful choice in the armamentarium of the pain physician as SCS and ITP are expensive and not readily available everywhere. Also, their use is usually based on the ability of the pain specialist. Pain physicians should become familiar with chemical neurolysis as this is an inexpensive choice, especially for the severe unrelieved pain of a selected group of patients, especially cancer patients who come from remote places in developing countries.

It is an accepted fact that cancer pain is prevalent at all stages of the disease. This pain can progress over time and can have a neuropathic, nociceptive, or mixed etiology. The World Health Organization (WHO) ladder for cancer pain treatment is a practical, easy to implement tool for managing cancer pain.[1] Despite correct adherence to the WHO ladder, 10 20% patients may still suffer unacceptable pain.[2,3] These patients may benefit from interventional methods to reduce the quantum of pain as well as side effects of drugs.[4] Intrathecal neurolytic drugs (absolute alcohol, phenol) for chemoneurolysis of selected nerve roots can give excellent analgesia in the respective body area.

Neurolysis can be performed at the cervical, thoracic, or lumbosacral levels. Neurolytic subarachnoid blocks are safest in mid-thoracic region as they are distant from fibers that subserve limb, bowel, and bladder function,[5] so any motor loss would be of little consequence.

Refractory cancer pain localized to an extremity is most suited to this procedure.

The reason is that the sensory and motor roots of the somatic nerve are physically separated in the spinal canal **(Fig. 1)**. Hence, intrathecal rhizotomy or rhizolysis is the only neurolytic procedure where sensory block can be achieved without concomitant motor block.

Though this appears to be a simple routine procedure for anesthetists carrying out subarachnoid blocks for anesthesia, correct execution of the technique with neurolytic drugs determines its safety and success.

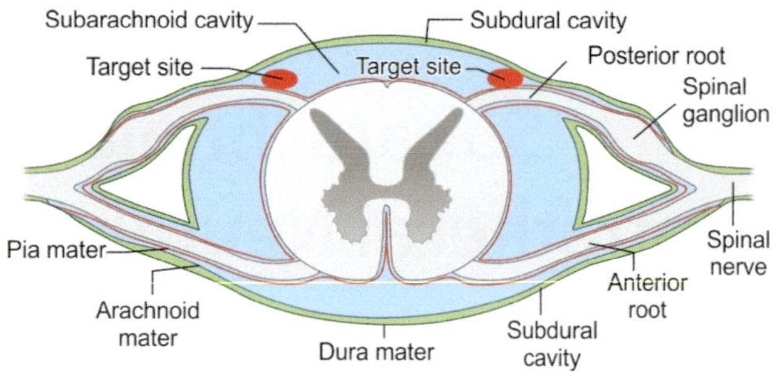

Fig. 1: Diagrammatic depiction of physically separate motor and sensory roots in subarachnoid space. Red spot shows site for depositing neurolytic drug.

Subarachnoid neurolysis is conducted at the level where the dorsal root block exits the spinal cord. The prolonged duration of action of the neurolytic drug requires a detailed and careful review of the dermatome and sclerotome to figure out which nerves are subserving the patient's pain.

PATIENT SELECTION

This procedure carries the potential risk of motor nerve dysfunction, bladder/bowel dysfunction, and dysesthesia in the denervated dermatomes.

The patient and relatives should be educated and counseled on the difference between "relief from pain" versus "numbness and loss of sensation". A prognostic block with a local anesthetic (LA) can help patients choose if they desire the procedure.

Ideal candidate for subarachnoid neurolysis should have:

- Well-established diagnosis[6]
- Short life expectancy
- Pain unresponsive to antineoplastic treatment (chemotherapy, radiotherapy)
- Pain score high despite adequate analgesics, intolerable/excessive adverse effects of drugs
- Predominant somatic pain localized to two to three dermatomes
- Unilateral pain.

AGENTS USED AS NEUROLYTIC DRUGS

Neurolytic agents have been used for interrupting pain pathways for >100 years. Luton[7] is credited with the first reported use of neurolytic solution used subcutaneously for pain relief. Doppler used phenol for neurolysis in 1925.[8] Maher reported use of phenol for subarachnoid neurolysis in 1955.[9] Today, the commonly used agents are ethyl alcohol and phenol. Both agents have different properties in the intrathecal compartment—alcohol is hypobaric and "floats" upward while phenol is hyperbaric and "sinks".

Phenol

It is not available commercially. It must be prepared in the pharmacy. Phenol is a chemical composite having carbolic acid, phenic acid, phenylic acid, phenyl hydroxide, hydroxybenzene, and oxybenzene. It is soluble in organic solvents such as alcohol and glycerol. The solution can be diluted with saline. It can be mixed with radiocontrast dye to allow fluoroscopic guidance during injection to check spread of the solution—this is very useful in peripheral neurolytic blocks, e.g., celiac plexus block.

When mixed with glycerol, it is viscous and hyperbaric with respect to cerebrospinal fluid (CSF) and diffuses slowly from the mixture. This has an advantage during intrathecal procedures as this ensures a limited spread with high local tissue fixation.

Various concentrations of phenol give varying actions. At a concentration of 2–3% in saline, phenol has a motor sparing function. The efficacy of 3% phenol in saline is comparable to that of 40% alcohol. It has an immediate LA effect due to its immediate selective effect on smaller nerve fibers; 5% is needed for sensory blockade and stronger concentrations produce motor block. Phenol concentrations of >5% produce Wallerian degeneration. Higher concentrations can cause spinal cord infarcts and arachnoiditis.

Phenol can be injected intrathecally and epidurally. The neurolytic effect may be clinically clear only after 3–7 days.

It has a shelf life of 1 year when the solution is refrigerated and not exposed to light. Phenol turns red on exposure to sunlight and air because of oxidation.

It is metabolized in the liver and excretion of metabolites occurs via the kidneys. Phenol has systemic side effects including central nervous system stimulation, cardiovascular depression, nausea, and vomiting. Systemic doses of >5 g can cause convulsive seizures and central nervous system depression. Doses <100 mg are less likely to cause serious side effects.

Ethyl Alcohol

It is a clear, hypobaric solution with respect to CSF. It is used as an absolute solution, i.e., >95% concentration.

Injection of alcohol causes severe burning, followed by a warm, numb sensation. It acts by extracting lipids (cholesterol, phospholipids, and cerebrosides) from the nerve tissues, resulting in sclerosis of nerve fibers and myelin sheath with demyelination and Wallerian degeneration. The patient positioning is crucial to ensure alcohol is deposited near the sensory target as injection of larger volumes can result in degeneration of the spinal cord.[10]

EQUIPMENT

- 20G, 22G spinal needle
- 25G local infiltration needle
- 1 mL tuberculin syringe.

DRUGS

- 2% lidocaine for local infiltration
- Absolute alcohol
- 6% phenol in glycerol refrigerated.

PATIENT PREPARATION

Position

The patient is positioned as below depending on the choice of drug.

The patient is gently strapped, so that the position is stable and patient comfortable. After clear CSF flow, "test dose" of LA should not be given.

Position for Alcohol Neurolysis

Due to hypobaric nature of alcohol, patients are made to lie with painful side uppermost, so that the dorsal root is superior as depicted in **Figure 2A**.

Then, the patient is rolled 45° anteriorly (away from operator), such that the dorsal root is superior **(Figs. 2B and C)**.

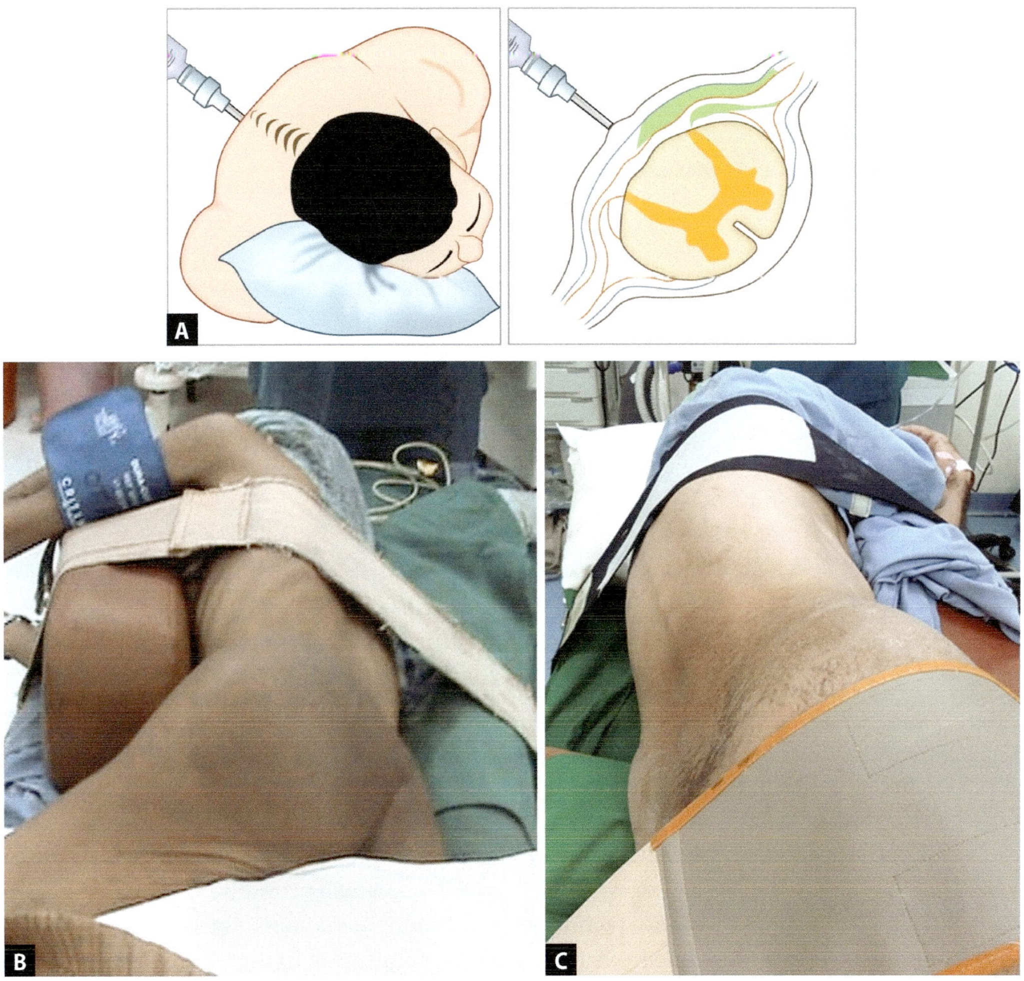

Figs. 2A to C: (A) Position for neurolysis with hypobaric drug; (B) Position for left-sided, hypobaric drug neurolysis; (C) Position for right-sided, hypobaric drug neurolysis.

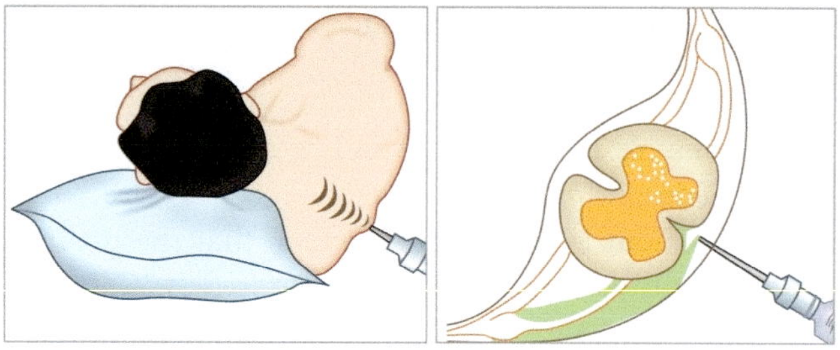

Fig. 3: Diagrammatic position for hyperbaric neurolytic drug.

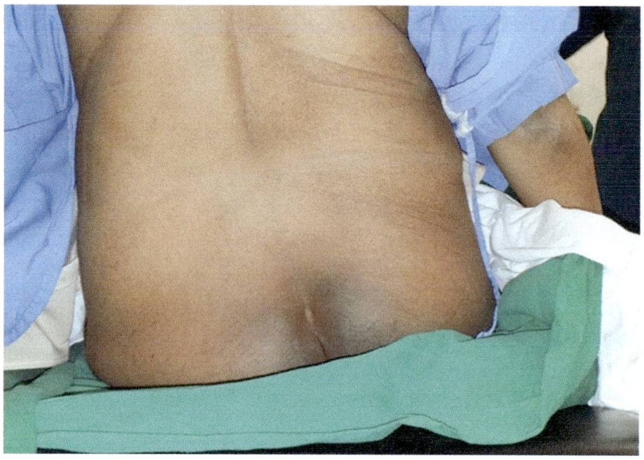

Fig. 4: Position for hyperbaric drug saddle block.

Position For Phenol Neurolysis

Due to hyperbaric nature of phenol, patient must lie with the painful side dependent and rolled posteriorly by 45° (toward the operator), so that the dorsal root is dependent **(Fig. 3)** as shown in adjoining picture.

In this position, the patient usually is extremely uncomfortable and unable to lie with painful side dependent. Hence, this drug is not commonly used for subarachnoid neurolysis of cervical, dorsal, or lumbar roots. It is mostly used for saddle block neurolysis **(Fig. 4)** as shown further.

PROCEDURE

Patients and relatives need to be educated on the necessity and risk-benefits of the procedure. Alongside, documentation of the severity of pain, other analgesics and blocks used, and pain drawing of the distribution of pain need to be done. A diagnostic procedure with LA should confirm that the pain is responsive to subarachnoid neurolysis. It also gives the patient a chance to experience pain relief versus loss of sensation they may have after the procedure.

Neurolysis with Alcohol

With complete aseptic precautions, a 22G spinal needle with bevel facing superiorly is used to enter the subarachnoid space at the level of the dorsal root to be blocked. After clear flow of CSF, alcohol is injected in 0.1 mL aliquots and the patient is told to report any burning sensation. This is a confirmation of the drug acting on the correct dorsal root. If burning occurs above or below the level of pain, another needle is inserted, and the procedure is repeated with 0.1 mL aliquots of alcohol. Total volume of alcohol needed is 0.4–0.7 mL per nerve root. No more than three or four nerves should be blocked at each session. After the injection, 0.2–0.3 mL air or saline is injected to clear the hub and shaft of alcohol and prevent fistula formation at skin, stillete reintroduced, and needle withdrawn. Though alcohol "fixes" quickly and does not float to adjacent levels, it would be prudent to maintain patient position for 15–20 minutes.

Neurolysis with Phenol

With complete aseptic precautions, a 20G spinal needle (phenol-glycerol is highly viscous) with bevel facing inferiorly is used to enter the subarachnoid space at the level of the dorsal root to be blocked. After clear flow of CSF, phenol is injected in 0.1 mL aliquots. As phenol has LA properties, the patient does not experience any burning sensation. They may feel warmth or dysesthesia along the nerve. The volume of injection is decided by the volume used during the diagnostic block. After injecting phenol, 0.1–0.3 mL air or saline is injected, stillete reintroduced, and needle withdrawn, keeping patient position for 15–20 minutes.

SUCCESS OF BLOCK

It is most rewarding to see the patient pain free and requiring no supplemental analgesics. This, however, may not be possible in all patients. Even if the patient has moderate pain relief, this will help reduce analgesic consumption and its related adverse effects.

CONTRAINDICATIONS

Subarachnoid or intrathecal neurolysis should not be done in following conditions:

- Patient has spinal tumor at the selected level
- Skin infection locally
- Patients are unable to lie in the proper position
- Some definitive treatment is available for pain.

COMPLICATIONS

The potential complications seen with subarachnoid or intrathecal neurolysis include:

- Temporary bladder and bowel dysfunction after lumbosacral neurolysis with urinary incontinence is seen. Many of these resolve within 10–15 days.
- *Deafferentation pain:* This is a poorly understood manifestation, whereby the patient complains of distressing numbness caused by an imbalance in afferent input.
- Headache
- Rarely infection, spinal cord damage, and posterior spinal artery thrombosis with paraplegia
- *Sloughing of skin, necrosis of nontarget tissues:* This can be avoided by careful attention to clearing needle tract of chemical neurolytic agent by injecting saline before withdrawing the needle.
- *Neuritis:* The reported incidence of neuritis is up to 10%. It is caused by partial destruction of somatic nerves and later regeneration. Neuritis would occur only if the nerve cell body were not destroyed. It is less likely to occur with a subarachnoid or ganglion neurolytic block. Clinically, it manifests as hyperesthesia and dysesthesia that may be worse than the original pain problem. It is one of the limiting factors in the use of chemical neurolysis. But in advanced malignancy, this is less of a problem due to the limited life expectancy.

CONCLUSION

Subarachnoid neurolysis is an extremely satisfying procedure, both for the physician and the patient. However, these techniques require specialized training, in-depth knowledge of neural anatomy, and understanding of chronic pain physiology. This procedure should be used only in painful conditions, where conventional conservative management has failed to give adequate pain relief.

REFERENCES

1. World Health Organisation. Cancer Pain Relief. Geneva, Switzerland: WHO; 1986. p. 51.
2. Cleeland CS, Gonin R, Hatfield AK, Edmonson JH, Blum RH, Stewart JA, et al. Pain and its treatment in outpatients with metastatic cancer. N Eng J Med. 1994;330(9):592-6.
3. Meuser T, Pietruck C, Radbruch L, Stute P, Lehmann KA, Grond S, et al. Symptoms during cancer pain treatment following WHO guidelines: a longitudinal follow-up study of symptom prevalence, severity and etiology. Pain. 2001;93(3):247-57.
4. Eisenberg E, Carr DB, Chalmers TC. Neurolytic coeliac plexus block for treatment of cancer pain: A meta-analysis. Anesth Analg. 1995;80(2):290-5.
5. Patt RB, Cousins MJ. Techniques for neurolytic neural blockade. In: Cousins MJ, Bidenbaugh PO (Eds). Neural Blockade. Philadelphia: J. B. Lippincott; 1998. p. 1007.
6. Katz J. Current role of neurolytic agents. Adv Neurol. 1974;4:471.
7. Luton A. Etudes sur la medication substitutive. Premiere partie, de la substitution parenchymapeuse. Arch Gen Med. 1863;2:57.
8. Jain S. The role of neurolytic procedures. In: Parris WCV (Ed). Cancer Pain Management: Principles and Practice. Boston: Butterworth-Heinemann; 1997. pp. 231-44.
9. Arter OE, Racz GB. Pain management of the oncologic patient. Semin Surg Oncol. 1990;6:162.
10. Jain S, Gupta R. Neurolytic agents in clinical practice. In: Waldman SD (Ed). Interventional Pain Management, 2nd edition. Philadelphia: WB Saunders; 2001. pp. 220-5.

57 CHAPTER

Radiofrequency Ablation of Spinal Metastasis

Samyadev Datta

ABSTRACT

Bony metastasis is well documented and more common in certain types of primary tumors. These tumors may or may not be painful. Many treatment options are available for the treatment of these tumors. The availability of targeted radiofrequency ablation of these tumors has been very successful. This technique can be used in patients who have previously undergone radiation therapy (RT).

INTRODUCTION

The current oncologic literature describes in detail that advanced diseases are associated with metastasis and poorly controlled pain. The incidence of pain was 39.3% after curative treatment; 55.0% during anticancer treatment; and 66.4% in advanced, metastatic, or terminal disease. Moderate-to-severe pain was reported by 38.0% of all patients.[1] This is despite multiple initiatives and guidelines of various organizations. Metastasis to bone is one of the most common areas after lungs and liver.[2]

It is very commonly seen in primary cancers of the lung, breast, prostate, and some radiation-resistant tumors such as sarcomas. The incidence of bony metastasis is about 0.05%. Often, bony metastasis may be present at multiple levels. Thus, it is recommended that every effort be made to treat pain and associated comorbidity that accompanies poorly or uncontrolled pain.

The standard of care for pain related to bony metastasis varies based on complexity. It includes some combination of medication, nerve blocks, radiation therapy, chemotherapy, and surgical procedures. This chapter will describe the use of targeted radiofrequency ablation (t-RFA) of painful vertebral metastasis not amenable to present standard of care.

SCIENTIFIC RATIONALE AND INDICATIONS

It is important to note that t-RFA does not cure cancer. Rather, it is indicated for palliative treatment of painful metastatic malignant lesions in the bone. Bony metastasis can be painful for many reasons, including tumor-causing microcompression fractures in susceptible weight bearing bones like those in the vertebra, biological pain from stretching/irritation of the periosteum, direct tumor growth into surrounding nerve structures, and endosteal nerve stimulation caused by osteoclastic-mediated bone resorption and its associated cytokine release.[3,4]

According to the National Comprehensive Cancer Network's 2019 guidelines regarding adult cancer pain, survival is linked to symptom control and prevention of expected analgesic side effects.[5] t-RFA has been shown to provide clinically significant pain relief in multiple studies. In addition, over 50% of those treated with t-RFA have had decreased usage of pain medications. Therefore, t-RFA should be considered in any complex pain patient suffering from bony metastasis.

Types of Devices

Anchala et al. presented retrospective data on treatment of metastatic posterior vertebral spinal lesions using a navigational bipolar radiofrequency ablation device (Dfine Star) via a transpedicular approach with excellent results. There were occasional radicular symptoms that resolved with transforaminal epidural steroids **(Fig. 1)**.[6]

The OPuS One study (Medtronic OsteoCool) showed a statistically significant decrease in patient's worst pain within 3 days postprocedure, self-reported quality of life,

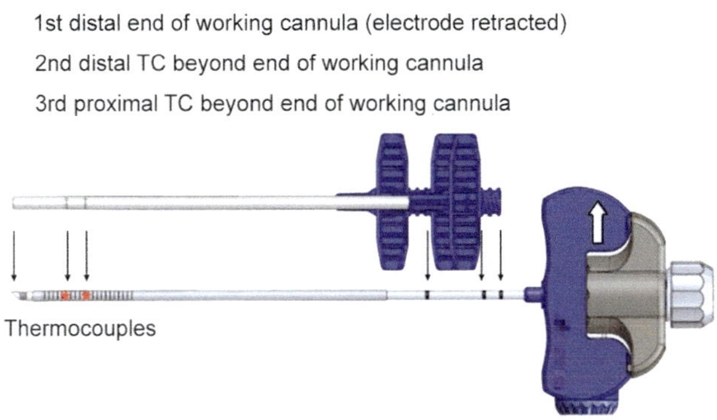

Fig. 1: Dfine Star.

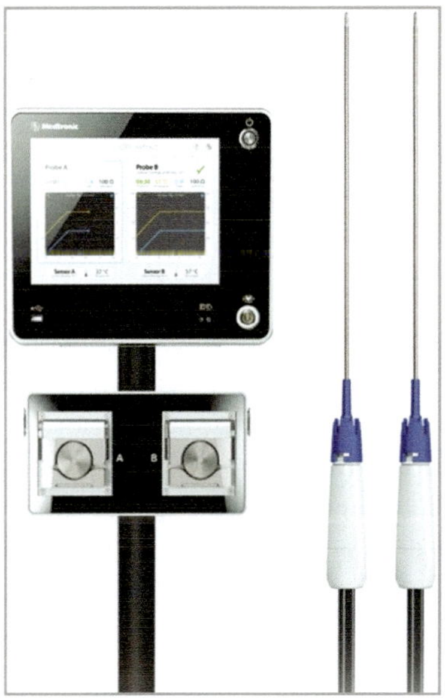

Fig. 2: Medtronic OsteoCool.

and long-term pain relief through 6 months **(Fig. 2)**.[7] Specifically, it has shown to decrease morbidity and have positive outcomes in specific patient categories.

Although t-RFA has been shown to have good outcomes, it is usually reserved for patients who have failed other more traditional treatment.[8] It is important therefore to have a thorough discussion with patient and family members before any intervention is planned.

Focal Palliative Treatment of Bone Metastases

The 2019 National Comprehensive Cancer Network (NCCN) guidelines clearly outline the available options for treatment of bony metastasis. In the management of bony metastasis and associated pain, they recommend that in general, cancer pain is treated with opioids; and other pain medications or interventions are meant only to complement management.

In patients with bony pain without oncologic emergency, recommendations include use of nonsteroidal anti-inflammatory drugs (NSAIDs) and other analgesic medications titrated to effect. Adjuvants including bone-modifying agents such as bisphosphonates and denosumab may be considered. In treating diffuse bone pain, consider hormonal therapy or chemotherapy, corticosteroids, and/or systemic administration of radioisotopes.

Local Bone Pain

Pain related to vertebral metastasis is a common cause for local bony pain. The NCCN guidelines recommend local radiation therapy. External beam radiation therapy (EBRT) is presently the standard of care. The results of therapy may take a few weeks to months before the pain relief is appreciated by patients. In addition, EBRT needs to be administered over many sessions. Patients with severe pain may not be able to tolerate this intervention. In addition, chemotherapy needs to be withheld during therapy.

Stereotactic body radiation therapy (SBRT), a newer technique of radiation therapy, allows for a faster and more efficient pain relief. This technique requires planning. Patient needs to be immobilized for the same, a very painful and unpleasant process. Also, there is a higher risk of fracture as patient needs to be positioned for radiation. Interruption to chemotherapy is limited. In a Cochrane review of literature on radiation therapy for metastatic cancer, authors find that there is no difference between single fraction compared to multiple fraction therapy.[9] There was however a significantly higher retreatment rate with single fraction therapy. The results do indicate that there is significant room for improvement.

Surgery is a more aggressive and invasive option. These patients are usually very sick and major surgical intervention is not an option to be considered lightly. A few patients may have very severe extension of diseases causing neurologic deficit. Patients will require corpectomy with decompression and stabilization.[10] This is a high-risk procedure, especially in these very sick patients. Various nerve blocks with neurolytic agents such as alcohol, (e.g., rib pain) may also be considered. Cryoablation of vertebral tumors has also been mentioned as another approach to treatment in this patient population.[11]

Finally, vertebral augmentation or kyphoplasty with or without t-RFA is an option well worth considering.[12,13]

There are many benefits to this procedure including added mechanical stability, acute pain relief, short procedure time in the hands of trained practitioners, safety, and good safety track record. Another very important benefit of this procedure is that it does not require interruption of chemotherapy and can be complementary to any ongoing radiation therapy. Targeted radiation therapy using the Star system followed by vertebral augmentation appears to be more effective with reduced likelihood of tumor recurrence.[14]

Any concerns of spinal instability or cord compression will require surgical consultation. If pain continues to be a problem, consultation with an interventional pain management physician can be very useful. Reduction in pain by any method is likely to help the patient, and this has been proven by various society guidelines, including the NCCN.

In a retrospective review of cases performed in multiple institutions, Anchala et al. have shown that this procedure is very safe and well tolerated. The majority of patients had immediate and sustained pain relief. There were no major complications. It does appear that using the t-RFA system allows us to provide patients with previously difficult to treat bony metastasis another option. In a critical review on interventional oncology, authors indicate that the process is well tolerated and can be used in both benign and metastatic tumor with good results. In another retrospective study, the results show that t-RFA can be safely used for posterior-placed vertebral spinal tumors, and complications were minor and easy to treat. In a recent systematic review with a large sample size, authors indicated clinically relevant improvement in pain, Oswestry disability index (ODI), and Karnofsky Performance score (KPS). Cement leakage was common and rarely symptomatic.[15] Dawood et al. report that there was improvement in pain scale, but not quality of life. Sample size was small.[16] As mentioned earlier, posterior spine tumors can be tough to treat by conventional methods, and t-RFA provides these patients another option.

CONTRAINDICATIONS

Targeted RFA is, in general, a well-tolerated and safe procedure. Even patients with fractures can be candidates. However, as with any intervention, there are certain patients who are ineligible. Pacemakers and other implanted electronic device implants are contraindications to t-RFA therapy as there is risk of radiofrequency therapy interfering with these devices. t-RFA should be done with caution in the cervical vertebrae (C1-C7).

Anticoagulation guidelines as set by the American Society of Regional Anesthesia (ASRA) need to be followed. This procedure is very high risk and may need to be delayed complying with recommended guidelines.[17]

DEVICE SELECTION

There are two device options for t-RFA: Dfine and Medtronic **(Figs. 1 and 2)**. The DFINE STAR system is a steerable device and has controlled and monitored temperature delivery that automatically shuts off at 50°C. Temperature is monitored at two levels. It comes in two sizes that allow for tailoring to the specific patient. The Medtronic OsteoCool features an active steering tip, which allows increased access to the tumor. In addition, energy delivery is controlled and temperature is monitored at two levels continuously to help with safe tumor debulking.

SELECTION OF PATIENTS

Like with any procedure, good results are based on careful patient selection. Many of these patients have a limited life expectancy and so the primary reason to perform this procedure is to reduce pain and improve quality of life. It must be clearly stated that t-RFA of vertebral metastasis does not result in cure of diseases. This discussion must take place with patient and family members before any intervention.

The following categories of patients are most suitable for this procedure:

- Patients with radio-resistant tumors, including sarcomas
- Patients with persistent and/or recurrent pain after radiation therapy
- Patients with metastatic tumors in the posterior aspect of vertebral body. However, anterior-positioned tumors may also be treated using this method. Posteriorly positioned tumors are much more dangerous to radiate due to the high risk of complications involving the spinal cord and therefore are good candidates for t-RFA.
- Patients with painful vertebral metastasis who have reached their maximum radiation dose limit and need further palliative treatment. Coordination with radiation oncologist is necessary.
- Patients with focal pain and symptoms that are preventing palliative radiation.

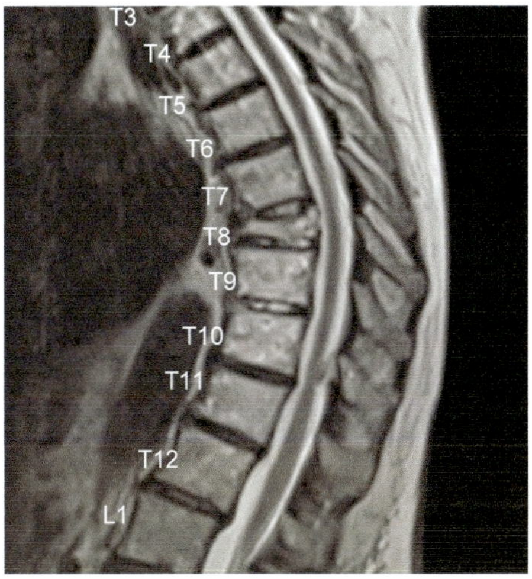

Fig. 3: Multiple myeloma with thoracic metastasis.

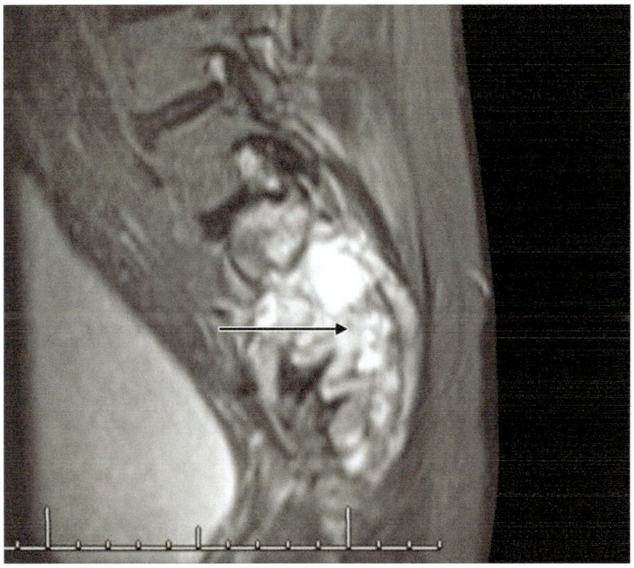

Fig. 4: Colon cancer with sacral metastasis.

- Patients who cannot undergo other palliative treatments due to concurrent systemic treatments
- Patients in whom myelosuppression is a serious concern **(Figs. 3 and 4)**.

Technical Details of Procedure

Targeted radiofrequency ablation of spinal metastasis is performed by practitioners trained in interventional procedures. If practitioners have skills in performing other procedures such as vertebral augmentation or kyphoplasty, this procedure can be performed. It is necessary to complete a history and physical examination, review magnetic resonance imaging (MRI) of spine with and without contrast, and identify the target level for t-RFA. In addition, it is necessary to identify if metastases are in the anterior or posterior aspect of vertebral body. Also review involvement of pedicles. Presence of diseases in pedicle will necessitate use of opposite pedicle. There may be two levels where the patient is complaining of pain. Also, after patient has been positioned prone on fluoroscopy table, and before receiving any analgesia and sedation, confirm level of procedure using fluoroscopy. It is a good practice to palpate and recreate pain before the patient is sedated. Metastasis may be present at more than one level, but efforts need to be directed toward the painful levels only. ASRA guidelines on anticoagulation need to be followed as this is a high-risk procedure.

The entire device consists of various introducer needles with trocar, a 10G cannula, a flexible reaming stylet, a biopsy needle, flexible RFA tip, temperature monitoring device, and finally polymethyl methacrylate (PMMA) bone cement with delivery system. Temperature is monitored in real time and is done both at proximal and distal tip of RFA probe.

If there are two or more lesions, a bipedicular approach may be better. In case of diffuse lesions, it is recommended to ablate as much of lesion as possible. Based on the size and location of lesion, probe size may be different. Smaller probes allow more control and reduce the possibility of causing trauma to the spinal cord. In case of a posterior lesion, introduce cannula up to the posterior margin of vertebra as seen on lateral view of fluoroscopy. This will improve access to tumor **(Figs. 5 and 6)**.

Vertebral augmentation is also recommended to improve pain control for these patients **(Figs. 7 and 8)**.

It is preferred that this procedure be done under sedation with local anesthesia. These patients are all on pain medications and may be very tolerant to pain. Use of general anesthesia has the risk that if there are any problems, it may be difficult to notice during the procedure.

Complications

No procedure is without complications, and t-RFA is often considered on patients who are already very sick and have significant comorbid conditions. Bleeding during the procedure can be a problem. ASRA guidelines need to be followed to reduce the risk. If the introducer cannula is compromised at all, a dose of antibiotics is warranted. If the trocar is directed too medially, trauma to the spinal

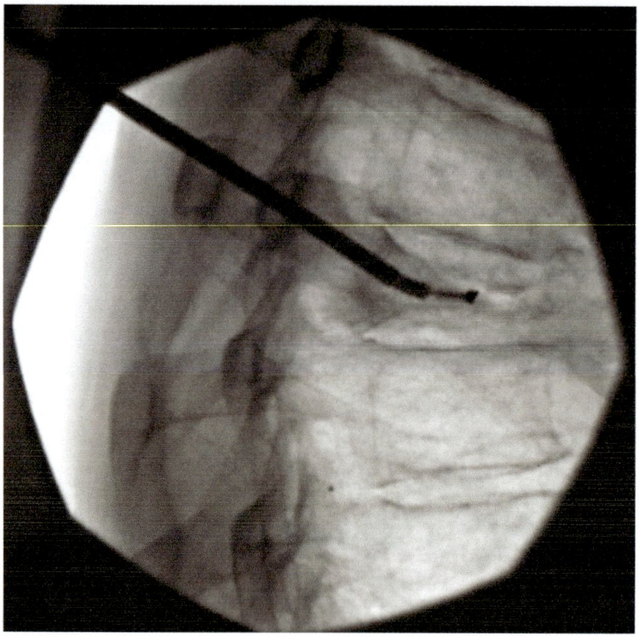

Fig. 5: Placement of radiofrequency ablation (RFA) device in thoracic vertebra.

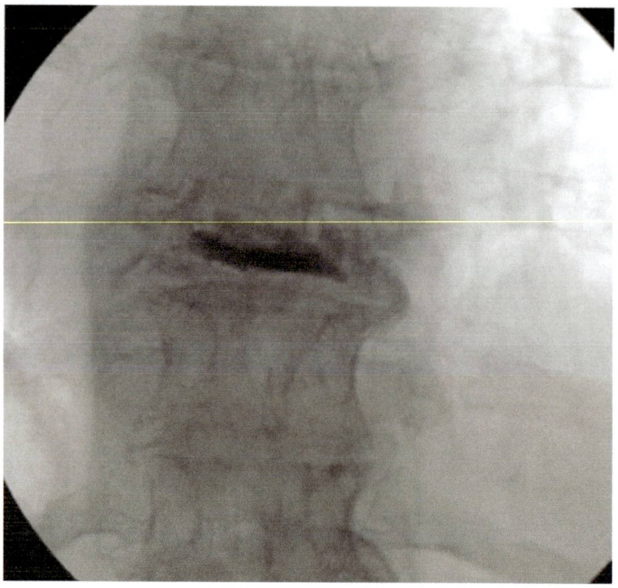

Fig. 7: Anteroposterior (AP) view of thoracic vertebra after vertebral augmentation.

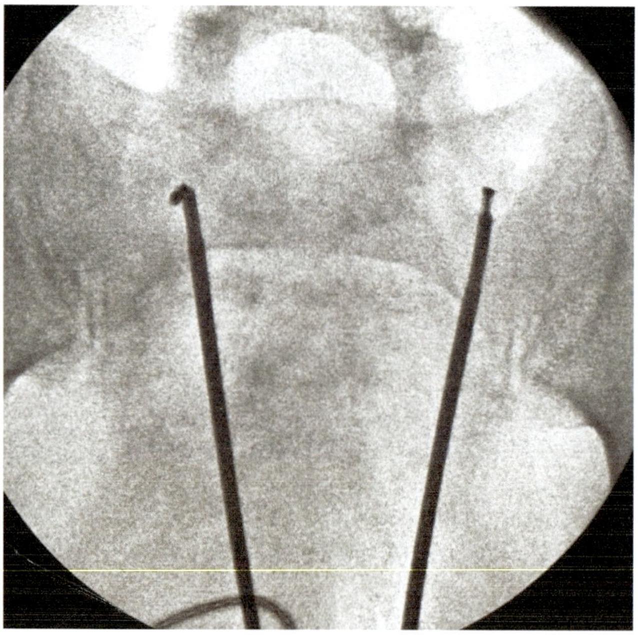

Fig. 6: Placement of two probes in sacrum.

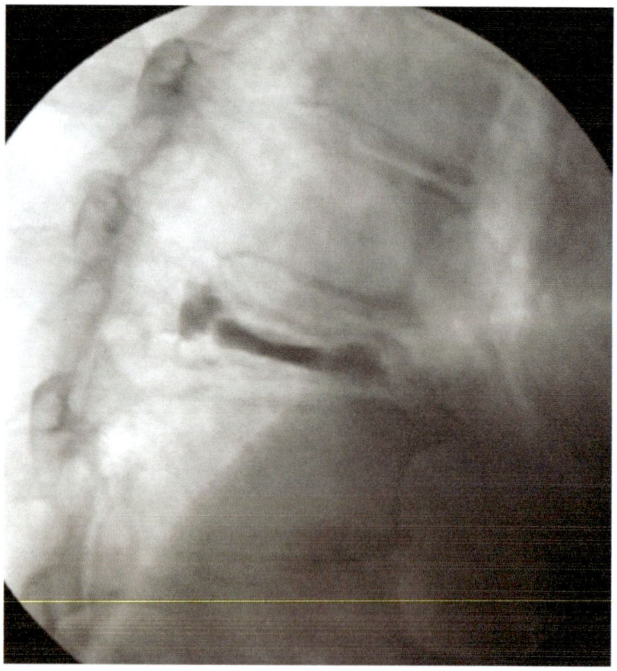

Fig. 8: Lateral view of thoracic vertebra after vertebral augmentation.

cord is possible. Patients may also have cerebrospinal fluid (CSF) leakage and resultant postdural puncture headache requires a blood patch. These complications can be decreased by using good technique.

Vertebral metastasis may extend into the pedicle and be a risk factor for pedicle fracture. Reviewing the preprocedural MRI will help determine the side from which to approach. Spinal surgical consultation may be needed to evaluate for spinal instability.

Extension of cement into the epidural space is also possible. Even though the procedure is done under direct vision and continuous monitoring, extension of cement

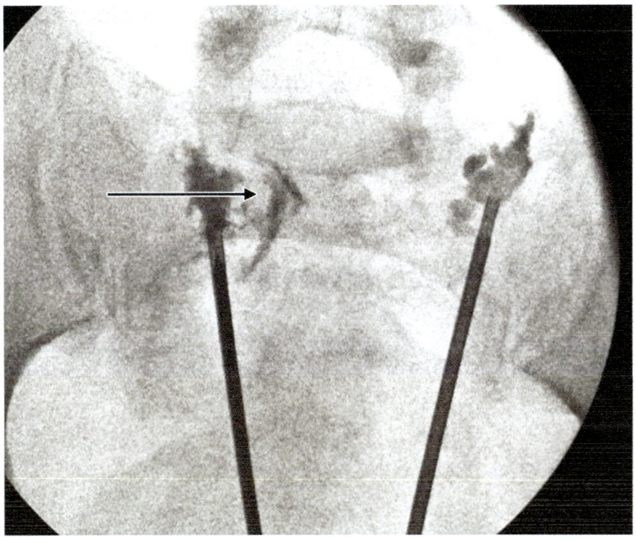

Fig. 9: Epidural extension of cement.

into posterior spinal canal may occur and can be a very serious problem (**Fig. 9**). If suspected, stop the procedure immediately and review under X-ray for any further extension. If there has been a massive leak of cement because of an unstable, undetected, posterior vertebral wall, resulting in major neurological deficit, surgical intervention may be needed to decompress the spinal cord. This option needs to be considered but not taken lightly. Meta-analysis of risk factors for cement leakage suggests that patients with intravertebral cleft, cortical disruption, low cement viscosity, and high volume of injected cement may be at high risk for cement leakage after vertebroplasty or kyphoplasty. Rigorous patient selection may reduce the occurrence of cement leakage.[18]

Another complication detected postprocedurally is neurological deficits as a result of heat generated by the probe. However, the probe temperature is measured at two levels during the procedure, this complication is rare. Occasionally, patient develops radicular pain symptoms. These can be treated with transforaminal epidural steroid injections. If major neurological deficits are noted, it is best to document the changes and treat aggressively with a combination of high-dose steroids and possible surgery. Patients may have an exacerbation of pain that needs to be addressed aggressively.

A rare but important complication to recognize is azygos and/or pulmonary vein embolism of cement. Presentation is with shortness of breath, pleuritic chest pain, and decreased oxygen saturation. Pulmonary embolism of PMMA cement is a common complication after orthopedic hip procedures. Azygos vein embolization is a much rarer complication but is very important to recognize (**Fig. 10**).

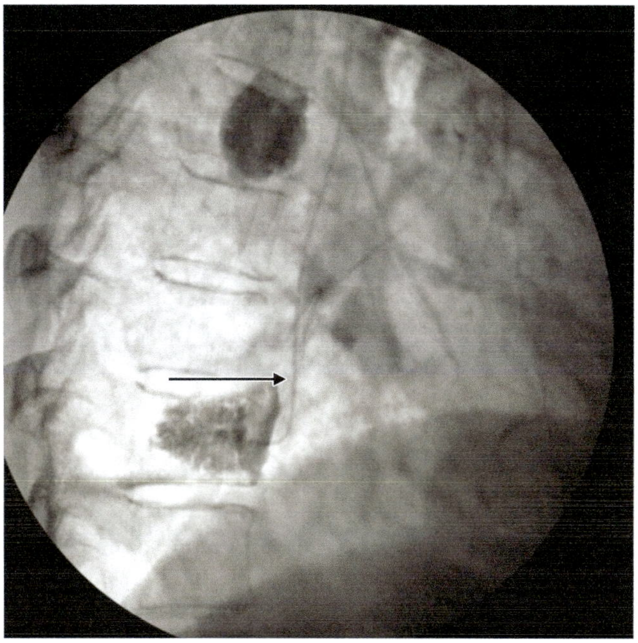

Fig. 10: Azygos vein embolization.

Patient with a recent history of t-RFA presenting with shortness of breath and lightheadedness should have a computed tomography (CT) of chest to evaluate for cement embolization. Consideration should also be given to anticoagulation according to severity of patient symptoms and location of the embolus. Other diagnoses on the differential should include postoperative pneumonia and pneumothorax.

OUTCOMES

Targeted radiofrequency ablation has been performed worldwide, with overall good results as documented in multiple publications. Very few patients needed retreatment at the same level, and a significant percentage of patients had pain relief, improvement of Oswestry disability Index, and Karnofsky performance scale. A majority of these patients had continued pain relief at 6 months. t-RFA has been used successfully in combination with conventional radiation therapy and vertebral augmentation. t-RFA permitted access to vertebral lesions and real-time accurate monitoring of the ablation zone temperature. Postprocedure MRI and positron emission tomography (PET) examinations correlated with a favorable tumor response and helped to monitor tumor growth and the timing of adjuvant therapy.[19] t-RFA combined with cement deposition in the posterior vertebral body demonstrates significantly more stable vertebrae under axial loading.[20]

Ragheb et al. in a recent publication of retrospective data of patients with metastatic breast cancer speculate that the addition of radiofrequency ablation to kyphoplasty may reduce the incidence of local recurrence of tumor. It is suggested that this may benefit metastases from other primary tumors.[21]

In 2021, The American Society of Pain and Neuroscience (ASPN) Best Practices and Guidelines for the Interventional Management of Cancer-Associated Pain Evidence Evaluation and Best Practice Statement published recommendations for spinal bony metastasis. The recommendations are that vertebral augmentation should be strongly considered for patients with symptomatic compression fractures from spinal metastases. In addition, percutaneous radiofrequency ablation is indicated with or without cement augmentation for back pain from spinal metastasis.[22]

CONCLUSION

Bony metastasis is a common and painful consequence of many types of cancer. Vertebra is the most common site. These lesions can be very painful and will contribute greatly to poor quality of life. Many options have been mentioned in the most recent NCCN guidelines for treating bony pain that is localized or generalized. These include opioids, bisphosphonates, RANKL inhibitors, and NSAIDs. For individuals with inadequate analgesia, or with intolerable effects, pain management referral for t-RFA with or without vertebral augmentation should be considered. t-RFA along with vertebral augmentation has been shown to provide increased likelihood of return to ambulatory status when compared to traditional radiation therapy alone. The scope of t-RFA has been limited mainly toward treating metastasis in the anterior vertebral body but can be considered for posterior metastasis as well with the advent of new devices.

Analysis of safety data indicates that there are few complications when done by trained interventional physicians. This can be further reduced by choosing the correct patient and correct approach. It is important to monitor patients in the postoperative period for complications such as neuropathy, cement embolism, and pneumonia.

By providing significant relief of pain almost immediately after the procedure, targeted RFA has indeed changed the outlook and functional status for patients suffering from vertebral metastasis. The technology is actively expanding and the future is promising.

REFERENCES

1. van den Beuken-van Everdingen MH, Hochstenbach LM, Joosten EA, Tjan-Heijnen VC, Janssen DJ. Update on prevalence of pain in patients with cancer: systematic review and meta-analysis. J Pain Symptom Manage. 2016;51(6):1070-90.e9.
2. Harel R, Angelov L. Spine metastases: current treatments and future directions. Eur J Cancer. 2010;46:2696-707.
3. Smith HS. Painful boney metastases. Ann Palliat Med. 2012;1(1):14-31.
4. Rybak LD. Fire and ice: thermal ablation of musculoskeletal tumors. Radiol Clin North Am. 2009;47(3):455-69.
5. Swarm RA, Paice JA, Anghelescu DL, Are M, Bruce JY, Buga S, et al. Adult Cancer Pain, Version 3.2019, NCCN Clinical Practice Guidelines in Oncology. J Natl Compr Canc Netw. 2019;17(8):977-1007.
6. Anchala PR, Irving WD, Hillen TJ, Friedman MV, Georgy BA, Coldwell DM, et al. Treatment of metastatic spinal lesions with navigational bipolar radiofrequency ablation device: a multicenter retrospective study. Pain Physician. 2014;17(4):317-27.
7. OsteoCool Tumor Ablation Post-Market Study. [online] Available from clinicaltrials.gov/ct2/show/results/NCT03249584. [Last accessed August, 2024].
8. Levy J, Hopkins T, Morris J, Tran ND, David E, Massari F, et al. Abstract No. 346. Radiofrequency ablation for the palliative treatment of bone metastases: outcomes from a multicenter study in 100 patients. J Vasc Intervent Radiol. 2020;31:S158.
9. Chow E, Harris K, Fan G, Tsao M, Sze WM. Palliative radiotherapy trials for bone metastases: a systematic review. J Clin Oncol. 2007;25(11):1423-36.
10. Lau D, Chou D. Posterior thoracic corpectomy with cage reconstruction for metastatic spinal tumors: comparing the mini-open approach to the open approach. J Neurosurg Spine. 2015;23(2):217-27.
11. Callstrom MR, Dupuy DE, Solomon SB, Beres RA, Littrup PJ, Davis KW, et al. Percutaneous image-guided cryoablation of painful metastases involving bone: multicenter trial. Cancer. 2013;119(5):1033-41.
12. Kam NM, Maingard J, Kok HK, Ranatunga D, Brooks D, Torreggian WC, et al. Combined vertebral augmentation and radiofrequency ablation in the management of spinal metastases: an update. Curr Treat Options Oncol. 2017;18(12):74.
13. Lane MD, Le HBQ, Lee S, Young C, Heran MKS, Badii M, et al. Combination radiofrequency ablation and

cementoplasty for palliative treatment of painful neoplastic bone metastasis: experience with 53 treated lesions in 36 patients. Skeletal Radiol. 2011;40(1):25-32.

14. Bollen L, Dijkstra SPD, Bartels RHMA, Graeff A, Poelma DLH, Brouwer T, et al. Clinical management of spinal metastases—The Dutch National Guideline. Eur J Cancer. 2018;104:81-90.
15. Sørensen ST, Kirkegaard AO, Carreon L, Rousing R, Andersen MØ. Vertebroplasty or kyphoplasty as palliative treatment for cancer-related vertebral compression fractures: a systematic review. Spine J. 2019;19(6):1067-75.
16. Sayed D, Jacobs D, Sowder T, Haines D, Orr W. Spinal radiofrequency ablation combined with cement augmentation for painful spinal vertebral metastasis: a single-center prospective study. Pain Physician. 2019;22(5):E441-9.
17. Narouze S, Benzon HT, Provenzano D, Buvanendran A, De Andres J, Deer T, et al. Interventional spine and pain procedures in patients on antiplatelet and anticoagulant medications (second edition): guidelines from the American Society of Regional Anesthesia and Pain Medicine, the European Society of Regional Anaesthesia and Pain Therapy, the American Academy of Pain Medicine, the International Neuromodulation Society, the North American Neuromodulation Society, and the World Institute of Pain. Reg Anesth Pain Med. 2018;43(3):225-62.
18. Zhan Y, Jiang J, Liao H, Tan H, Yang K. Risk factors for cement leakage after vertebroplasty or kyphoplasty: a meta-analysis of published evidence. World Neurosurg. 2017;101:633-42.
19. Reyes M, Georgy M, Brook L, Ortiz O, Brook A, Agarwal V, et al. Multicenter clinical and imaging evaluation of targeted radiofrequency ablation (t-RFA) and cement augmentation of neoplastic vertebral lesions. J Neurointerv Surg. 2018;10(2):176-82.
20. Pezeshki PS, Davidson S, Murphy K, McCann C, Slodkowska E, Sherar M, et al. Comparison of the effect of two different bone-targeted radiofrequency ablation (RFA) systems alone and in combination with percutaneous vertebroplasty (PVP) on the biomechanical stability of the metastatic spine. Eur Spine J. 2016;25(12):3990-6.
21. Ragheb A, Vanood A, Fahim D. The addition of radiofrequency tumor ablation to kyphoplasty may reduce the rate of local recurrence in spinal metastases secondary to breast cancer. World Neurosurg. 2022;161:e500-7.
22. Aman M, Mahmoud A, Deer T, Sayed D, Hagedorn JM, Brogan SE, et al. The American Society of Pain and Neuroscience (ASPN) best practices and guidelines for interventional management of cancer-associated pain. J Pain Res. 2021;14:2139-64.

CHAPTER 58

Cryoablation in Pain Management

Amod Manocha, Shefali Panjwani, Puneet Sharma

ABSTRACT

This chapter explores the use of cryoneuroablation, a minimally invasive technique for managing a variety of pain conditions including acute, chronic, neuropathic, cancer-related, and musculoskeletal pain. Cryoneuroablation employs extreme cold to temporarily disable nerve function, offering immediate and prolonged pain relief with minimal complications and no risk of neuroma formation. The development of portable cryoablation devices and high-definition ultrasound machines has enabled its application in various clinical settings, including office-based practices. This technique is particularly valuable for perioperative pain management and for patients with persistent postsurgical pain, offering significant reductions in opioid use and improved functional outcomes. This chapter discusses the mechanisms, clinical applications, and advantages of cryoneuroablation, highlighting its potential to enhance pain management strategies and improve patient's quality of life.

INTRODUCTION

Cryoneurolysis, also referred to as cryoneuroablation or cryoanalgesia, is a cutting-edge pain management technique that involves applying extreme cold to target nerves. This process aims to interrupt the transmission of pain signals from the peripheral nervous system to the central nervous system.[1,2]

The origins of modern cryoanalgesia trace back to the work of Cooper et al.,[2,3] who developed a hollow tube filled with liquid nitrogen capable of reaching temperatures as low as –190°C. The term "cryoanalgesia" was later coined by Lloyd et al.,[2,4] who recognized this technique's distinct advantages over other nerve destruction methods such as alcohol and phenol neurolysis or surgical lesions. These traditional methods often result in postprocedure neuritis or neuralgia, whereas cryoanalgesia does not.[2] Despite the disruption to the nerve structure, the myelin sheath and endoneurium remain intact, preventing permanent damage or neuroma formation.[2] Initially, the treated nerve undergoes Wallerian degeneration, followed by regeneration at a consistent rate. While the nerve structure may recover sooner, the functionality of the sensory nerve might remain impaired, leading to prolonged pain relief. Complete recovery typically takes between 6 and 12 months. The effects of cryoablation are akin to a conduction block observed with local anesthetics, but with a significantly longer duration of pain relief.

Recent advancements in the understanding of sonoanatomy and ultrasound technology, alongside the development of sophisticated cryoablation devices, have broadened the applications of this technique. Modern high-resolution ultrasound systems allow for precise, real-time localization of nerves, facilitating targeted treatment delivery and expanding treatment options. Currently, cryoablation is employed to manage various pain conditions, including neuropathic, neoplastic, musculoskeletal, and postsurgical pain. The minimally invasive nature of percutaneous techniques, enhanced by image guidance, makes them safe[5] and suitable for outpatient or daycare procedures. In certain scenarios, cryoneurolysis offers a viable alternative to open surgical methods and pharmaceutical pain management, thereby reducing the risks associated with opioid use.

This chapter provides a broad overview of cryoablation including the indications, mechanism of action, equipment and procedure, and advantages and limitations.

MECHANISM OF ACTION (FIGS. 1A TO C)

Cryoneuroablation for treating chronic pain involves direct application of extreme cold to targeted nerves, causing reversible neuronal injury[1] that disrupts the ability of the nerve to transmit pain signals. In percutaneous cryoneuroablation, a cryoprobe is placed near the target neural structure under image guidance. The cryoprobes have a smaller inner tube with pressurized gas (usually carbon dioxide or nitrous oxide at 600–800 psi) that travels through a fine aperture into the larger outer tube at a lower pressure of 10–15 psi. This rapid expansion causes a significant temperature drop (Joule-Thomson effect), forming an iceball at the probe's tip. The gas is then cycled back to the machine, ensuring no gas enters the patient's tissues.[1,5]

Cold temperatures between –20 and –100°C cause reversible disruption of the axonal continuity and the myelin sheath, resulting in conduction block and Wallerian degeneration distal to the ablation site. The endoneurium remains intact, reducing the risk of neuroma formation and the Schwann cell basal lamina is spared, facilitating regeneration.[2,6] This second degree of neuronal injury or axonotmesis is the goal in cryoneuroablation.[2] Subsequent axonal regeneration occurs at a rate of approximately 1–2 mm/day,[1] with the time to full regeneration depending on the rate of axonal regrowth and the distance of the cryo-produced lesion from the end organ.[6] Eventually, axonal regrowth restores sensation, resolving the conduction block.[1]

Beyond direct cold-induced injury, indirect mechanisms via changes in the cellular microenvironment and impaired tissue viability also cause cellular damage, death, and necrosis of tissues.[7] These mechanisms include the following processes:

Freezing Phase (Fig. 1A)

As the cryoprobe absorbs heat from the tissue and the tissues cool, the following events take place.

- *Ice crystals formation:* These are initially formed in the extracellular space.
- *Extracellular osmolarity increase:* Due to ice crystal formation[7]
- *Intracellular dehydration:* Increased extracellular osmolality draws water out of cells, causing dehydration and cell shrinkage. The increased intracellular solute concentration damages cytoplasmic enzymes and destabilizes cell membranes.[7]
- *Intracellular ice crystals:* Rapid cooling traps water inside cells, leading to intracellular ice crystal formation and immediate cell death[7]
- *Intracellular damage:* Ice crystals can form pores in the plasma membrane, disrupting electrochemical gradients and allowing cellular components to diffuse if the pores are large.[7]

Thawing Phase (Fig. 1B)

- *Reduced extracellular osmolality:* Melting extracellular ice reduces tonicity, causing a shift of fluid into cells leading to cell swelling and/or bursting.
- *Increased intracellular ice crystals:* Influx of water into the cell can increase the size of intracellular crystals, and this can continue to happen even while the extracellular space ice is melting as high extracellular osmolarity lowers the freezing point of extracellular water. During the thawing phase, maximum intracellular ice crystal growth occurs at –20 to –25°C.[7]

Delayed Effects (Fig. 1C)

- *Apoptosis:* Cells in the peripheral zone with less temperature exposure may undergo programmed cell death due to mechanisms such as proteases (caspases) activation secondary to mitochondrial damage and unfavorable microenvironment for cellular survival.[7]
- *Intravascular damage:* Intracellular ice crystal formation in blood vessels damages vascular endothelial cells, leading to thrombus formation and ischemia upon reperfusion in the post-thaw period.[7]
- *Inflammatory response:* Cryoablation triggers an inflammatory response, releasing cytokines that increase vascular permeability and tissue edema. Macrophages and other immune cells clear cellular debris and promote tissue repair, leading to coagulation necrosis in the ablation zone.

Factors Influencing Cellular Injury

Cellular injury, both indirect and direct, can be influenced by the following factors[7]:

- *Target temperature:* The temperature varies across the iceball, being lowest adjacent to the cryoprobe and highest at the periphery.[7] This is measured by a thermistor at the probe tip, with the gas type determining the lowest possible temperature as it cannot be lower than the boiling point of the gases

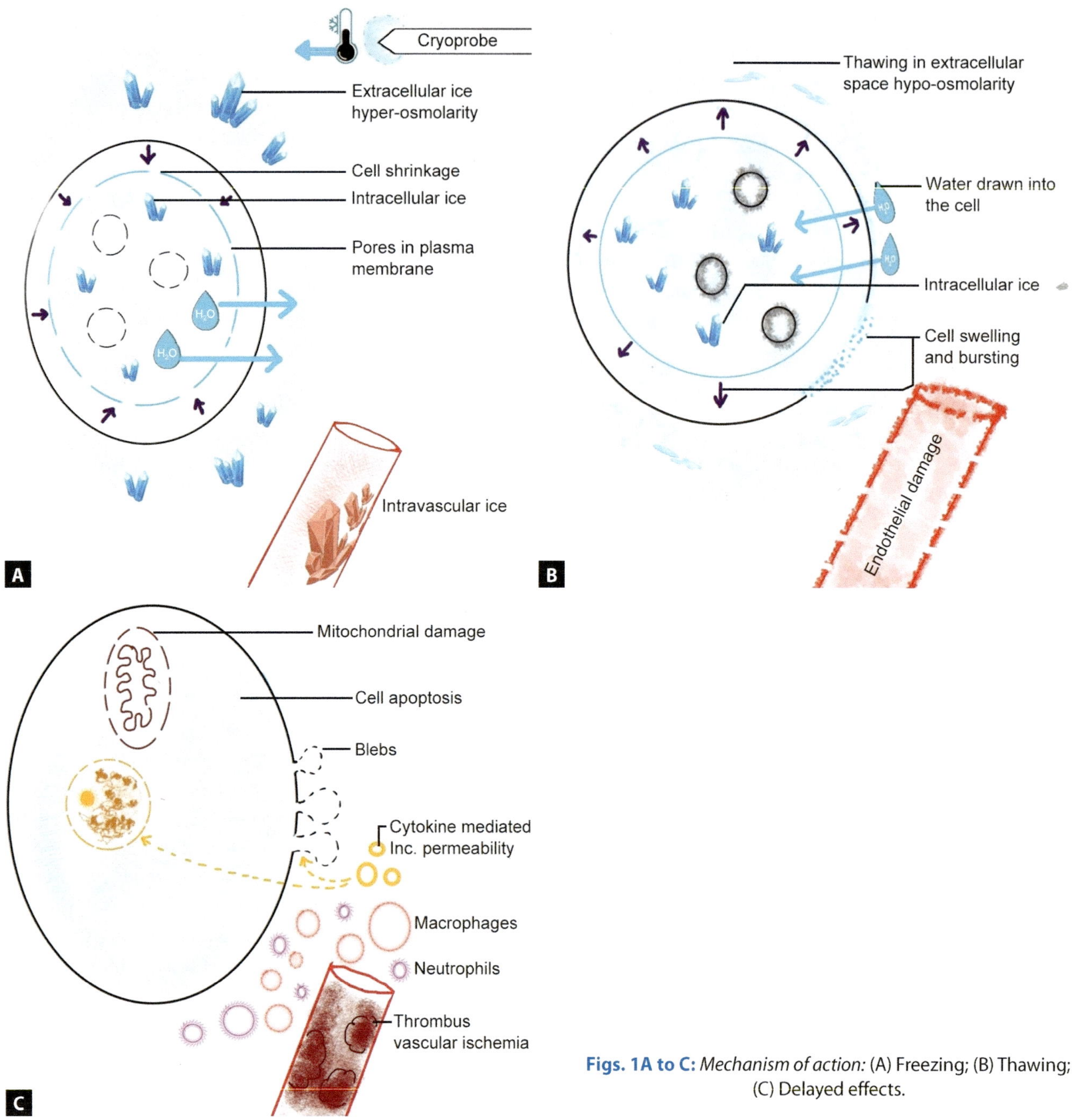

Figs. 1A to C: *Mechanism of action:* (A) Freezing; (B) Thawing; (C) Delayed effects.

used (nitrous oxide: –88°C; carbon dioxide: –79°C). This provides a safety margin as irreversible nerve damage is less likely at temperatures above –100°C.[1]

- *Time at target temperature:* Longer exposure increases intracellular ice formation, enhancing damage even in the peripheral portion of the iceball. Typical cryoneurolysis cycles involve 2- to 3-minute freezes with 30 seconds defrosting between cycles.[1]
- *Cooling rate:* Faster cooling leads to a higher intracellular water content before freezing, increasing intracellular ice crystal formation and causing more damage. Cooling is most rapid near the cryoprobe and slower at the periphery of the iceball.[7] Cells from different organs have different thresholds for cold-induced cell death, but most will exhibit subsequent cell death when cooled rapidly below –40°C.[7]

- *Thawing rate:* Rapid thawing limits intracellular ice crystal size, increasing cell survival. Passive thawing and repeated freeze–thaw cycles result in more cell death and liquefactive necrosis.[7] Adequate thawing for 20–40 seconds between freezes increases the freeze zone size.[1]
- Besides the factors mentioned above, the extent of nerve damage is also influenced by the proximity of the probe to the nerve, the size of the cryoprobe as this impacts the size of the iceball formed, and the temperature of the tissues in proximity to the probe.[2]

CLINICAL APPLICATIONS

Cryoneuroablation offers a unique, versatile solution for managing a wide range of pain conditions, from acute and chronic to neuropathic, cancer-related, and musculoskeletal pain. Its minimally invasive nature, combined with the potential for nerve regeneration, makes it particularly valuable when other treatments are ineffective or unsuitable. The development of handheld cryoablation devices and high-definition portable ultrasound machines has enabled its use in office-based clinical settings. The common indications include the following:

- *Peripheral neuropathies/neuropathic pain syndromes:*
    - *Peripheral nerves* are common target for cryoneuroablation **(Table 1)** and used to control pain in their respective territories, regardless of whether the nerves are themselves the pain generators or not. It is easier to target the nerve if it can be identified with advanced imaging or nerve stimulator. A successful block with local anesthetic can increase confidence in recommending cryoneuroablation. If the involved nerve carries motor fibers, then an analysis of the risk-benefit ratio needs to be performed before considering cryoneuroablation.
    - *Neuromas* including Morton's and stump neuromas
- *Musculoskeletal pain:* Large joints chronic degenerative conditions such as arthritis have a significant prevalence in the community with a wide range of individuals not keen for surgery or unfit for surgery or with persisting pain despite surgery. Cryoneuroablation is a reasonable option to consider in such situations and targeting the articular branches specifically can help achieve analgesia without causing motor dysfunction. Common musculoskeletal indications include:
    - *Shoulder pain:* Arthritis, rotator cuff repair, adhesive capsulitis, bursitis
    - *Knee pain:* Osteoarthritis, persistent postsurgical pain
    - *Hip pain:* Osteoarthritis, avascular necrosis, trochanteric bursitis
    - *Chest pain:* Post-rib fracture and persisting costochondritis pain
- *Acute and perioperative pain:* Cryoneuroablation for acute pain offers significant advantages over other traditional alternatives, including:
    - *Immediate effect:* Essential in acute pain situations where rapid relief is required, unlike options that take longer to work.
    - *Prolonged analgesia:* Emerging evidence suggests that cryoanalgesia provides longer-lasting pain relief and a better side effect profile compared to regional anesthesia.[1] This leads to improved functional performance and quality of life. Besides prolonged pain reduction, improved functional performance and quality of life are other possible benefits.
    - *Low complication rates:* There is no risk of neuroma formation.
    - *Benefits from nonusage of alternatives:* These include reduction in opioid requirements and associated side effects, reduced risk of local anesthetic toxicity, and infections.[1]
    - *Reduced patient, family, and healthcare burden:* This is due to decreased need for monitoring,

TABLE 1: Nerve targets for cryoneuroablation as per pain distribution.

Region affected	***Target nerves***
Craniofacial	Occipital nerves,[5] trigeminal nerve and its branches[2] (supraorbital, infraorbital, mandibular, maxillary, mental, auriculotemporal), posterior auricular,[2] and glossopharyngeal nerve[2]
Shoulder and upper extremity	Suprascapular nerve, superficial radial nerve, and digital nerves
Chest wall	Intercostal nerves
Abdominopelvic	Ilioinguinal, iliohypogastric, genitofemoral,[2] and pudendal nerves[2,5]
Buttock and lower extremity	Lateral femoral cutaneous nerve,[5] cluneal nerve, sural nerve and neuromas, saphenous nerve and its infrapatellar branch, obturator nerve, genicular nerves,[5] and digital nerves

catheter or pump care, and shorter hospital stays, as seen in procedures such as total knee arthroplasty (TKA).[1]

Perioperative cryoneurolysis is used in situations with a high risk of persistent postsurgical pain and procedures expecting significant moderate-to-severe postoperative pain. Initially applied to intercostal nerves in thoracotomy surgery, data now supports its use in mastectomy, shoulder surgery, and TKA, demonstrating safety, efficacy, and long-lasting pain control.[1]

- *Thoracotomy and rib fractures:* Thoracotomy surgery often results in severe pain which correlates with increased postoperative morbidity and a high incidence of persistent postsurgical pain. Thoracic epidural analgesia traditionally used for post-thoracotomy pain has its own limitations and may not be suitable for all. Recent studies suggest that intercostal nerve cryoneurolysis provides significant, long-lasting postoperative pain relief, comparable to epidural analgesia, with reduced monitoring and catheter care requirements.[1] A randomized trial on patients undergoing the Nuss procedure for pectus excavatum correction showed decreased hospital stays (by 2 days) and lower opioid requirements with intercostal nerve cryoablation compared to thoracic epidural analgesia while offering equivalent pain control.[8]

  Rib fractures also benefit from cryoablation of the involved intercostal nerves, providing prolonged pain relief and potentially improving respiratory parameters and ventilator weaning.
- *Mastectomy:* Cryoneuroablation of ipsilateral intercostal nerves (T2-T5) can be performed for pain relief. Currently, there are no direct studies directly comparing paravertebral or erector spinae plane blocks with percutaneous intercostal nerve cryoneurolysis.

Total knee arthroplasty: Cryoneurolysis of the genicular nerves, infrapatellar branch of the saphenous nerve, and anterior femoral cutaneous nerve has been used to provide prolonged postoperative pain relief.[1] It has been shown to be reduce postoperative pain scores, opioid consumption, and hospital length of stay, while improving functional performance, reducing stiffness, and enhancing the quality of life.

- *Shoulder arthroplasty:* Cryoneurolysis of the suprascapular nerve has been used for postoperative analgesia. Although motor blockade of unpredictable duration could be a limiting factor, it has not been shown to affect rehabilitation. Also, with better anatomical understanding of the articular branches, this concern is further mitigated.

▪ *Spine-related pain:*
  - *Facet joint pain (cervical, thoracic and lumbar):* Medial branches are suitable targets for cryoablation.
  - *Sacroiliac joint pain:* Special sacroiliac cryoprobes create continuous lesion to increase success rates and procedure time.

▪ *Chronic postsurgical pain:* Cryoablation is frequently used for treating persisting pain postthoracotomy, herniorrhaphy, or amputation. Postsurgical pain secondary to nerve injuries and entrapments in scar tissue or mesh may be amenable to cryoablation. Direct cryoneuroablation of nerves under vision at the time of surgery has been reported especially with surgeries such as thoracotomies and herniorrhaphy.

▪ *Chronic pain syndromes:* These include a variety of conditions such as:
  - *Chest wall pain:* Including post-thoracotomy, postherpetic pain, and intercostal neuralgia
  - *Chronic groin and pelvic pain:* Including conditions such as chronic orchialgia
  - *Headache disorders:* Those with positive response to nerve blocks such as the occipital, supraorbital, or supratrochlear nerves can be considered for cryoablation for prolonged effect.
  - *Facial pain* include temporomandibular disorders (TMD) and trigeminal neuralgia: Trigeminal nerve or its branches can be targets for cryoneuroablation. This auriculotemporal nerve derived from the third division of the trigeminal nerve can be targeted for painful TMD as it supplies the lateral capsule of the joint.[1]
  - *Phantom limb pain:* This may involve treatment of peripheral nerves or neuromas or both. Local anesthetic blocks can help in identifying the targets.

▪ *Cancer pain:* Percutaneous cryoanalgesia has been used for relief from intractable pain related to abdominal, pelvic, and thoracic neoplasms.[5] It can be used for pain associated with tumor infiltration of nerves, for localized pain in the distribution of a nerve, or for painful bone metastases.

Cryoprobes used for tumor ablation are different from those used for nerve analgesia as explained in the subsequent text. Those using liquid nitrogen for tumor ablation can have temperatures reach up to –196°C at the center of the iceball.

CRYOABLATION EQUIPMENT

There are two different types of products available for percutaneous cryoanalgesia: Those for tumor ablation and those for nerve lesions. Tumor ablation cryoprobes are generally larger, lack an inbuilt neurostimulator, and may or may not use the Joule-Thomson effect like argon-based systems use, whereas the liquid nitrogen systems do not. In contrast, cryoprobes for nerve lesions are smaller, utilize the Joule-Thomson effect, and have an inbuilt nerve stimulator for precise nerve localization.[1] Additionally, the Food and Drug Administration (FDA) approved handheld devices are available for convenience. This section focuses on nonhand-held devices used for cryoneuroablation.

Cryoprobes

Cryoprobes operate on the Joule-Thompson effect, where a pressurized gas (such as N_2O or CO_2) rapidly expands through a very fine aperture, cooling down as it expands and forming an iceball by drawing energy from the surrounding tissues.[2]

The cryoprobe consists of a smaller inner tube carrying high-pressure gas and a larger outer tube which transfers the gas to the machine, creating a "closed system" that prevents gas from escaping into the patient's tissues **(Fig. 2)**.

Cryoprobes come in various sizes from 14 to 21G with different lengths and tips (sharp or blunt).

The size of cryoprobe affects the iceball size produced on targeted nerves.[1] Specialized probe with high echogenicity for improved ultrasound visibility and specific treatments such as for sacroiliac joint cryoablation are available. The sacroiliac probes can create *continuous lesion with no gaps* in less time. These probes can be single use or reusable and easy to sterilize **(Fig. 3)**.

Most probes have a built-in nerve stimulator for nerve localization, covered by Teflon, to ensure that stimulation occurs only at the tip and include a thermistor to measure the tip's temperature **(Fig. 4)**.[2]

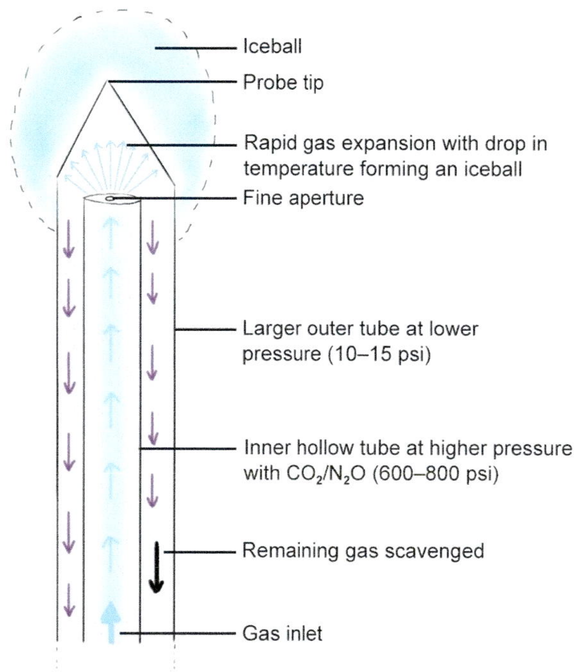

Fig. 2: Cryoprobe demonstrating Joule–Thompson effect.

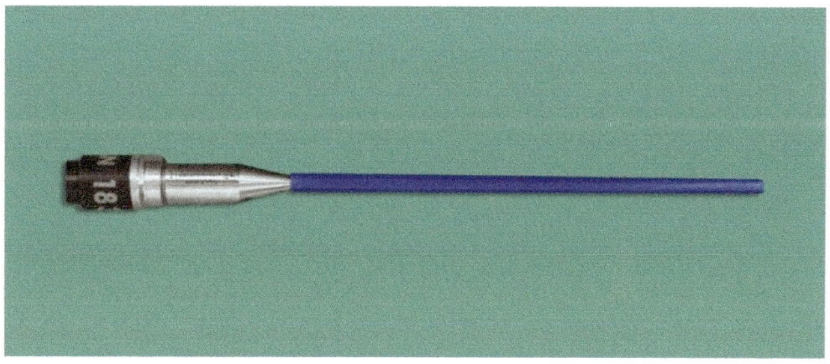

Fig. 3: Cryoprobe with RFID attached. (RFID: radiofrequency identification)

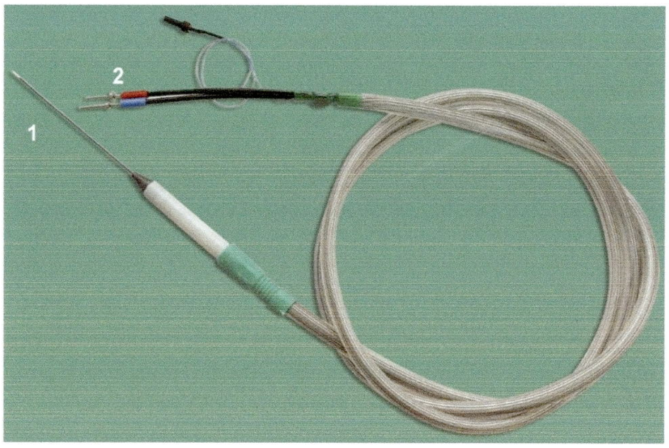

Fig. 4: Single-use cryoprobe. (1) 0.8 mm tip, (2) Connections for attaching to machine.

Cryoablation Machine (Fig. 5)

Modern cryoablation machines typically feature:

- A liquid crystal display (LCD) touchscreen displaying and monitoring all parameters including cylinder pressure, gas flow, cryoprobe temperature, and procedure time
- Various operational modes, such as probe cleaning, nerve stimulation, and freezing, selectable via the touchscreen and footswitch
- An inbuilt nerve stimulator requires a grounding pad connected to the patient, allowing selection of sensory (50, 100, 150, and 200 Hz) and motor stimulation (1 and 2 Hz) frequencies and impulse width (0.1, 0.2, 0.5, 1, 2–5 ms).
- Operator-defined treatment cycles, including freezing and thawing times, with a microprocessor-controlled cooling source. Other parameters and cryoprobe characteristics, such as the gas flow and pressure, are auto-configured for optimal operation.

Gas Source

Pain management procedures typically use CO_2 (–78°C) or N_2O (–89°C) as the working medium, with a 10 L cylinder sufficient for approximately 60 procedures.

Image Guidance

Ultrasound, X-ray, and computed tomography (CT) scan as appropriate for guiding the cryoprobe to the correct location are required. For cryoneuroablation, real-time, high-resolution ultrasound guidance has significantly enhanced the precision of targeting specific nerves and deeper structures.[1]

PROCEDURE TECHNIQUE

Indications and contraindications for cryoablation are covered in the chapter elsewhere. If a cryoneuroablation is planned, a prior local anesthetic block, done on a separate occasion, can help obtain critical diagnostic information and define therapeutic goals. It is essential that a small volume of local anesthetic be used for the diagnostic block to avoid a false-positive result, secondary to blocking of any other nearby structures. A diagnostic block can help in giving the patient a real-time experience of what to expect post procedure. This section describes a stepwise approach to performing cryoablation.

Preparation (Fig. 6)

- *Informed consent:* Obtain informed consent after discussing the procedure's benefits, risks, and possible complications.[1]
- *Diagnostic block review:* If a prior diagnostic block was performed, review the old images/notes. If not, perform a preliminary ultrasound scan to localize the target nerve and plan the cryoprobe trajectory.
- *Sterility measures:* Ensure extended room and local procedure site sterility as per local protocols.[1]
- *Intravenous (IV) access and monitoring:* Establish IV access and use monitoring according to recommended standards. Cryoanalgesia is typically performed with local anesthesia or conscious sedation; however,

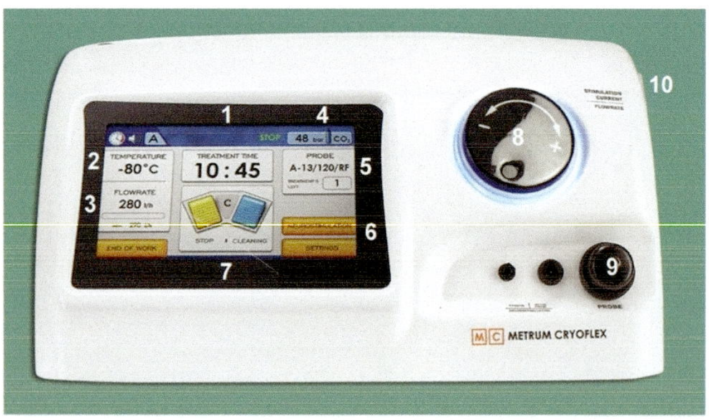

Fig. 5: Cryo-S painless machine (Metrum Cryoflex Warsaw, Poland). (1) LCD screen, (2) Temperature, (3) Gas flow rate, (4) Cylinder pressure and the gas used, (5) Probe specifications, (6) Machine mode and settings, (7) Machine controls, (8) Stimulation regulator, (9) Probe connection, (10) RFID sensor. (LCD: liquid crystal display; RFID: radiofrequency identification)

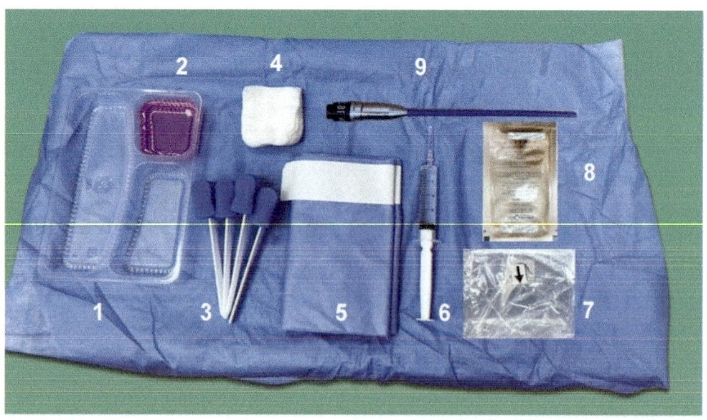

Fig. 6: Sterile procedure tray. (1) Sterile plastic tray with: (2) chlorhexidine solution for skin preparation, (3) Sterile sponges for skin cleaning, (4) Sterile gauze pieces, (5) Sterile drape, (6) Syringe with local anesthetic for skin infiltration, (7) Camera Cover, (8) Sterile ultrasound gel, (9) Cryoprobe.

general anesthesia or deep sedation may be required for some sessions, especially in cancer patients.[1]

- *Antibiotics:* The authors do not use prophylactic antibiotics, though practices may vary globally.
- *Imaging guidance:* Place cryoablation probes under imaging guidance (ultrasound, fluoroscopy, CT).[1] Ensure the functionality of the imaging equipment before starting the procedure.

Cryoablation Machine Preparation

- *Gas source:* Ensure that an adequately filled CO_2 or N_2O cylinder is available for use. The authors use a Cryo-S Painless Machine (Metrum Cryoflex, Warsaw, Poland), and this description pertains to that setup.
- The machine is connected to the gas source and switched on. Once the cylinder has been opened, the cylinder pressure reflects on the machine screen.
- *Footpad and foot switch:* Connect the footpad to the patient and machine to complete the neurostimulation circuit. Attach the foot switch for operating the inbuilt nerve stimulator to the machine.
- *Machine and gas connection:* Connect the machine to the gas source and switch it on. Check that the cylinder pressure is displayed on the machine screen and is in the required range.
- *Cryoprobe* ***(Fig. 7)****:* Have an appropriately sized cryoprobe available, with a backup ready. For reusable probes, ensure sterility. The reusable probes have a detachable back end which serves as a radiofrequency identification (RFID) for the machine to identify the probe and ensure that it is not used more than the recommended times. This back end with RFID is detached and presented to the sensor on the side of machine for probe recognition.
- *Cryoprobe connections* ***(Fig. 8)****:* Connect the cryoprobe to the probe hose/tubing and then to the cryomachine. Maintain sterility using a sterile camera cover for the cryoprobe tubing or sterilize the full assembly as needed.
- *Probe testing:* Modern machines will automatically test the probe to ensure that it is clear of any moisture and in a functional state with adequate gas flow. Set the treatment cycles as per operator preference (e.g., two 2-minute freeze cycles with a 30-second defrost cycle and a final 10-second defrost).
- *Freeze mode activation:* Once testing is completed, the freeze option on the machine becomes active, allowing for sensory and motor testing and lesion creation.

Performing Cryoablation (Fig. 9)

- *Local anesthetic and sedation:* Administer a small amount of local anesthetic at the needle/probe insertion site and use sedation as required.

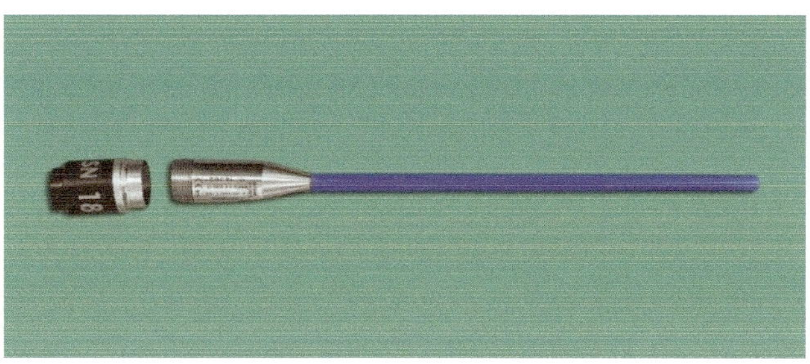

Fig. 7: Cryoprobe with RFID detached.
(RFID: radiofrequency identification)

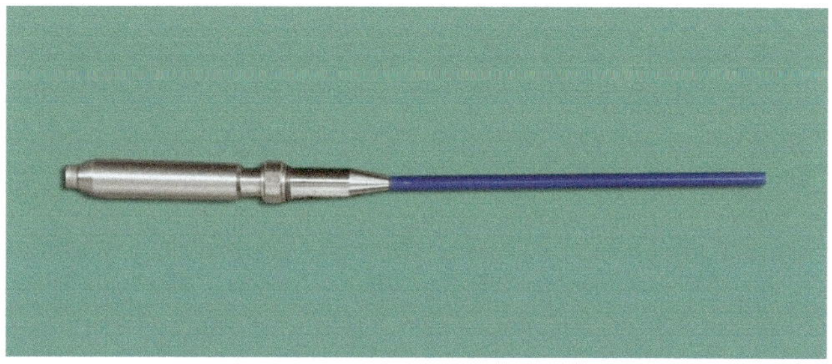

Fig. 8: Cryoprobe attached to the hose.

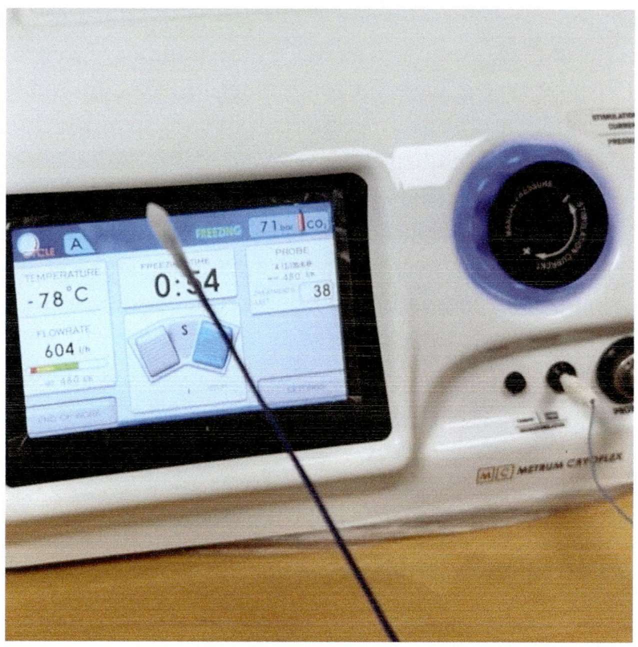

Fig. 9: Iceball formation on cryoprobe tip with machine in cryoablation background.

- *Using an introducer:* Use an appropriately sized cannula/angiocath as an introducer for the size of cryoprobe being used. For example, for a standard-sized cryoprobe (12 cm, 18G, 0.7 mm tip), a 14G IV cannula (orange color) can be used as an introducer. The introducer pierces tissues easily, helps to infiltrate local anesthetic, isolates electrical current, and protects the skin from the iceball, especially when targeting superficial structures.[2]
- *Image-guided introducer placement:* Place the introducer/cannula close to the target neural tissue under image guidance (e.g., ultrasound). Remove the stylet and introduce the cryoprobe through the cannula, advancing it using a coaxial technique close to the target tissue (nerve or neuroma). Slightly withdraw the cannula sheath to expose the cryoprobe tip completely.
- *Nerve stimulation confirmation:* Use the inbuilt nerve stimulator to confirm correct positioning of cryoprobe and proximity to the targeted neural tissue, with sensory (100 Hz) or motor (2 Hz) testing as appropriate for the target tissue.
- *Freeze–thaw cycles:* Activate the cryoprobe freezing mode for carrying out the lesion. Monitor the temperature drop to –75 to –80°C and iceball formation can be observed via an ultrasound if used.[6] The number of iceballs or lesions required varies depending on the indication and target size and the optimal freeze and thaw durations, as well as the number of freeze–thaw cycles, have yet to be determined. Commonly performed percutaneous cryoneuroablation techniques utilize a freeze cycle of 30–120 seconds' duration followed by a thaw of 30–60 seconds and this is frequently repeated one or two times.[9] Some experts recommend creating at least three contiguous iceballs along the nerve under fluoroscopy guidance if no lesion is visualized.[7]
- *Final defrost and probe removal:* Perform a final short defrost cycle to thaw the iceball before withdrawing the cryoprobe to avoid tissue damage or nerve avulsion.[2] Regardless of the number of cycles administered, it is imperative that after each freeze the probe remains fixed until iceball resolution to avoid tearing of involved tissues.[10]
- *Postprocedure assessment:* Monitor for frostbite/skin ischemia, especially when treating superficial structures. Evaluate pain relief and motor function postprocedure. Discharge them once they recover from sedation/anesthesia with written, standardized postprocedure instructions.
- *Follow-up:* Arrange follow-up reviews according to local protocols, typically 2–4 weeks post procedure or sooner if complications are anticipated.

ADVANTAGES

Cryoneuroablation simply can be viewed as a long-lasting nerve block. It offers several advantages over traditional pain management techniques:

- *Immediate effectiveness:* Cryoablation works almost instantaneously, allowing for immediate assessment of treatment adequacy. This quick onset mitigates suffering almost instantly, unlike other treatments that may take longer to achieve full effect.[7]
- *Real-time monitoring:* During cryoablation, the formation of the iceball around the nerve can be visualized in real time using ultrasound, CT, or magnetic resonance (MR) imaging.[7] Real-time sonographic visualization of the probe, nerve, and its proximity to the iceball ensures precise targeting and effective treatment of the nerve,[6] which is a significant advantage over thermal ablation techniques such as radiofrequency ablation. In ultrasound, the iceball appears as a hyperechoic rim; in CT, it shows as a hypoattenuating zone; and in MR T1- or T2-weighted sequences, it appears as a dark signal void.[7]
- *Safety*: Cryoablation is a safe procedure with low complication rates. Freeze-induced cellular injury is less destructive to tissue compared to radiofrequency thermal ablation.[7] It minimizes the risk of vascular obliteration, neuroma formation, or scar tissue and secondary pain. The built-in neurostimulator enhances safety by differentiating between motor and sensory nerves. Repeat treatments can be carried out as necessary without increased risks.[5]
- *Efficacy and duration*: The analgesic effects of cryoablation can last from 6 months to 2 years, providing long-term pain relief without causing motor blockade. This extended duration of relief is highly beneficial for chronic pain management. Results from numerous prospective studies show favorable results with 50–60% of patients experiencing significant pain reduction for 6–12 months, and one randomized controlled trial evaluating the efficacy and safety of cryoanalgesia showed symptomatic relief for up to 150 days.[5]

- *Minimally invasive*: The procedure is minimally invasive, especially when performed percutaneously under image guidance. It can often be done as an outpatient or a daycare procedure, facilitating a quicker return to normal activities without the need for hospitalization.[7]
- *Reduced procedural pain*: Compared to heat-based thermal ablation techniques like radiofrequency ablation, cryoablation is less painful. The cooling effect on tissues and nerves acts as an anesthetic, allowing the procedure to be comfortably performed under local anesthesia or sedation.[7]
- *Nonopioid and nonsteroid pain relief*: By providing effective pain relief without the use of opioids, cryoablation reduces the need for opioid analgesics and their associated side effects. Steroid side effects such as cutaneous and subcutaneous atrophy, altered pigmentation, and systemic disturbances such as hypertension and glycemic disorders can also be avoided. Compared to alternatives like nerve block catheters, cryoablation carries a reduced risk of local anesthetic toxicity, catheter dislodgement, leakage, and infection.
- *Compatibility with equipment*: Cryoablation does not interfere with CT or MR imaging machines or monitoring equipment, as it operates primarily through mechanical mechanisms rather than electronic ones.
- *Other uses*: Besides pain relief, cryoablation is also used in other treatments such as tumor ablation.

COMPLICATIONS AND CONSIDERATIONS

Cryoablation, although regarded as a safe procedure, can be associated with complications. Careful consideration and planning can help in minimizing these potential complications. These can be broadly categorized into general and cryoablation-specific issues.

General Complications

- *Bruising and/or bleeding:*[1,2,5] Bruising and bleeding can occur at the procedure site. Since cryoablation does not use heat, it lacks cautery effects, which can exacerbate bleeding. Frozen tissues are more brittle, increasing the risk of organ injury and bleeding with excessive displacement of cryoprobes while in tissues.[7] It is important to maintain vigilance in cases like intercostal cryoneurolysis (bleeding into the thorax) or obturator nerve cryoneurolysis (bleeding into the pelvis), where bleeding might go unnoticed.
- *Infection:*[1,2] Infection is a rare complication, although there is one case report of myonecrosis and abscess formation following cryoneurolysis for chronic right knee pain requiring IV antibiotics.[5,10] Placing the probe through infected tissue could seed the infection into deeper tissues.[2]
- *Damage to adjacent structures:* Such as the risk of pneumothorax with intercostal cryoablation. Skin and hair changes such as hyperpigmentation, depigmentation, and alopecia may be observed, especially when treating superficial structures.

Cryoablation-Specific Complications

- *Skin complications:* Skin and hair in the proximity of treatment site may be affected, especially when targeting superficial structures[1] like digital and supraorbital nerves. Apart from the changes mentioned previously, skin ischemia, which manifests as skin blanching during the treatment, may be seen. Some clinicians consider terminating the freeze cycle if blanching is observed during treatment as this can later lead to skin necrosis.[7] Altering the needle path and monitoring the ice formation can help in avoiding damage to the surrounding nontarget structures to some extent. Frostbite to the skin with full-thickness damage resulting in depigmentation may also be observed. Vascular thrombotic events may be seen during the treatment of superficial structures.
- *Numbness*: Numbness in the distribution of targeted nerve is commonly observed after cryoneuroablation and can be distressing for some. The patients should be made aware of the same, and a diagnostic local anesthetic nerve block can give them a preview of what to expect after the treatment.[1,2]
- *Neurological complications*: Currently, there are no published reports of neuroma formation or permanent nerve injury.[1] Any motor damage if observed is usually reversible. There is no risk of deafferentation with cryoneuroablation. There is only one reported case of neuritis following cryoneuroablation.[11] Partial ablation may result in symptoms such as allodynia and/or acute worsening of pain,[5] and hence care must be taken to perform a uniform thermal lesion for adequate time. One of the limitations of the currently available technology is the lack of real-time knowledge of

BOX 1: Contraindications to cryoablation.

- Patient refusal
- Local/systemic infection
- Anticoagulation or bleeding disorders
- Anatomy-related issues precluding safe access to region of interest[5]
- Cryoglobulinemia, cold urticaria, and Raynaud's syndrome[1,5]

in vivo temperatures as a function of time and individual patient characteristics to specifically impart the desired lesion and avoid over- or underablation.[5]

- *Cryoshock:* This refers to a systemic inflammatory response syndrome mediated by cytokine production and is typically seen with large-volume liver cryoablation. Symptoms include hypotension, respiratory compromise, multiorgan failure, and disseminated intravascular coagulation.[7]

While considering cryoablation treatment, costs need to be considered and any contraindications **(Box 1)** need to be ruled out.

CONCLUSION

Cryoneuroablation emerges as an effective and versatile technique for managing a broad-spectrum of pain conditions, ranging from acute and chronic to neuropathic, cancer-related, and musculoskeletal pain. Its safety profile and minimally invasive nature, combined with the potential for nerve regeneration and the advent of portable and user-friendly equipment, have significantly expanded its clinical applications. The technique offers immediate and prolonged analgesia with low complication rates and reduced reliance on opioids, making it particularly valuable in perioperative settings and for patients with persistent postsurgical pain. By targeting specific nerves without causing motor dysfunction, cryoneuroablation provides targeted pain relief, improves functional outcomes, and enhances the quality of life for patients who are unsuitable for, or have not responded to, other treatments. As the understanding of cryoneuroablation mechanisms and applications continues to grow, its role in pain management is likely to become increasingly prominent, offering new hope for patients suffering from debilitating pain conditions.

REFERENCES

1. Biel E, Aroke EN, Maye J, Zhang SJ. The applications of cryoneurolysis for acute and chronic pain management. Pain Pract. 2023;23(2):204-15.
2. Trescot AM. Cryoanalgesia in interventional pain management. Pain Physician. 2003;6(3):345-60.
3. Cooper IS, Lee AS. Cryostatic congelation: a system for producing a limited, controlled region of cooling or freezing of biologic tissues. J Nerv Ment Dis. 1961;133:259-63.
4. Lloyd JW, Barnard JD, Glynn CJ. Cryoanalgesia. a new approach to pain relief. Lancet. 1976;2(7992):932-4.
5. Filippiadis D, Efthymiou E, Tsochatzis A, Kelekis A, Prologo JD. Percutaneous cryoanalgesia for pain palliation: current status and future trends. Diagn Interv Imaging. 2021;102(5):273-8.
6. Friedman T, Richman D, Adler R. Sonographically guided cryoneurolysis: preliminary experience and clinical outcomes. J Ultrasound Med. 2012;31(12):2025-34.
7. Erinjeri JP, Clark TW. Cryoablation: mechanism of action and devices. J Vasc Interv Radiol. 2010;21(8 Suppl.):S187-91.
8. Graves CE, Moyer J, Zobel MJ, Mora R, Smith D, O'Day M, et al. Intraoperative intercostal nerve cryoablation during the Nuss procedure reduces length of stay and opioid requirement: a randomized clinical trial. J Pediatr Surg. 2019;54(11):2250-6.
9. Ilfeld BM, Finneran JJ. Cryoneurolysis and percutaneous peripheral nerve stimulation to treat acute pain. Anesthesiology. 2020;133(5):1127-49.
10. Cahani D, Chacko J, Hahn B. Myonecrosis: a rare complication of cryoneurolysis. J Emerg Med. 2019;57(3):e73-6.
11. Johannesen N, Madsen G, Ahlburg P. Neurological sequelae after cryoanalgesia for thoracotomy pain relief. Ann Chir Gynaecol. 1990;79(2):108-9.

8 SECTION

Ultrasound-guided Procedures

59 CHAPTER

Which One is Better: Ultrasonography or Fluoroscopy?

Omobonike O Olowosuko, Steve M Aydin

ABSTRACT

Interventional techniques for pain management have advanced over the years. The advent of fluoroscopic guidance for injection into areas of pain generation has been paramount in safely and effectively treating patients. Although fluoroscopy is extremely useful in patients, it has limitations in evaluating soft tissues. Ultrasound has become a mainstay in the interventional pain management world. It has allowed the ability to visualize a field of soft tissue, such as ligaments and bones, and allow interventions to be done. Both are extremely useful and the proper setting for each should be considered.

INTRODUCTION

Over the past two or three decades, the field of interventional pain management has evolved. As we advance, new techniques and imaging tools have developed to help us provide optimal and precise care without treatments. Fluoroscopy has been a mainstay for much of the injections done in interventional pain management, and with the advent of ultrasound use in many of the injections, more options have been provided to patients in regard to injection techniques and options.

ULTRASOUND

The earliest use of ultrasound in the musculoskeletal system was first described by McDonald and Leopold, where it was used to differentiate Baker's cyst from thrombophlebitis.[1] Since then, the applications of ultrasound to musculoskeletal conditions have continued to broaden and may soon become the standard of practice for most musculoskeletal conditions.

Ultrasound guidance is of great use in joint evaluation and arthrocentesis, where it serves a dual function as a diagnostic and therapeutic tool. It can be used to diagnose and evaluate suspected septic joints, identify crystal arthropathies, among other musculoskeletal conditions.[2] As a therapeutic tool, ultrasound use can provide pain relief via aspiration of synovial fluid or blood, and intra-articular injection of drugs (e.g., corticosteroids and anesthetics).

Ultrasound use may show some benefit in these regions: The glenohumeral joint (**Figs. 1A to C**), subacromial bursa, elbow joint, wrist, DeQuervain's tendinopathy, knee joint (**Figs. 2A and B**), hip (**Figs. 3A and B**), and tibiotalar joint.

Advantages

Ultrasound offers the following advantages in interventional pain management:

- Its ease of use, portability, and real-time dynamic examination makes it possible to provide diagnostic services within the community
- No exposure to ionizing radiation
- Can explore multiple joints during the same appointment
- Noninvasive
- Permits contralateral examination and has no limitations owing to metal artifacts, which may be issues when using other imaging modalities.

Disadvantages/Limitations

Limitations of the use of ultrasound include the following:

- To be proficient in ultrasound use, demands time depending on the trainee's hand-eye coordination
- It is operator-dependent, with poor repeatability
- Deeper structures are difficult to visualize, because higher frequency transducers have lower tissue penetration

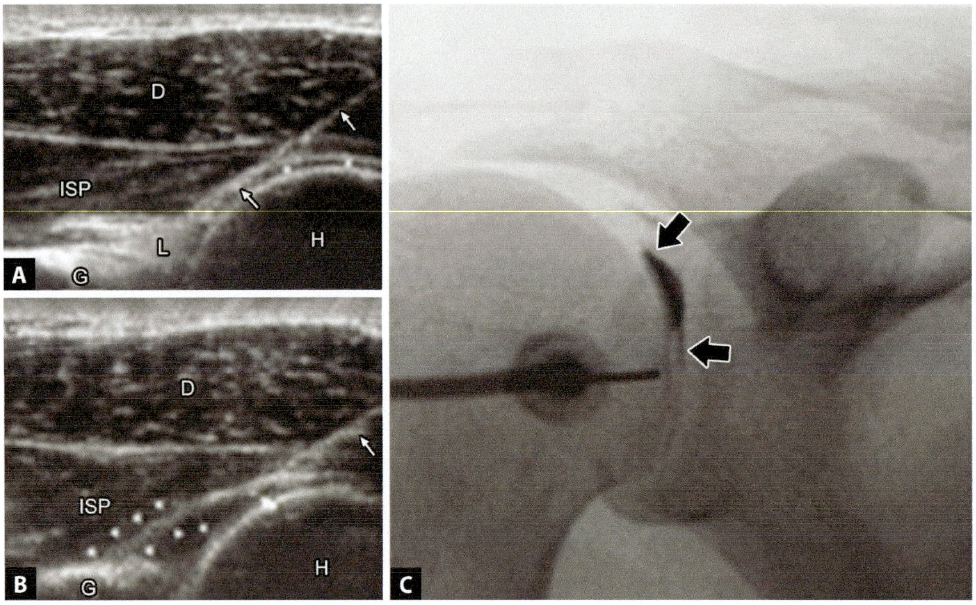

Figs. 1A to C: Ultrasound imaging of the glenohumeral (GH) joint injection next to a fluoroscopic-guided GH injection. (D: deltoid; G: glenoid; H: humerus; ISP: infraspinatus tendon; L: posterior labruming)

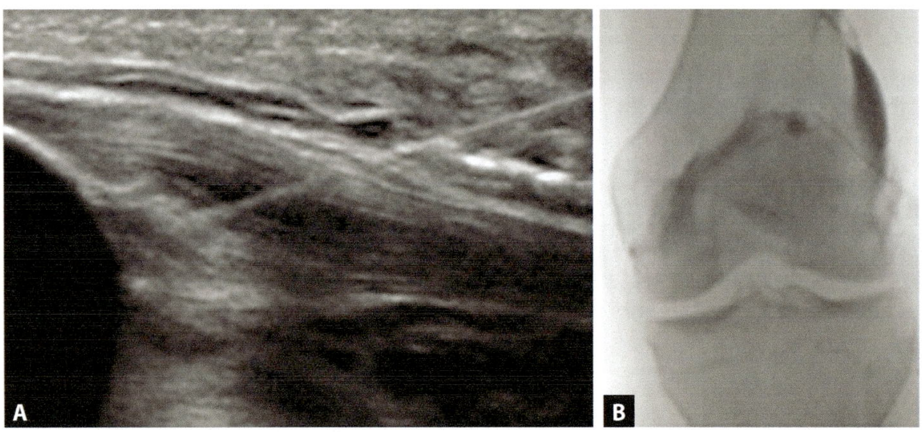

Figs. 2A and B: Ultrasound imaging of the knee joint injection next to a fluoroscopic-guided knee joint injection.

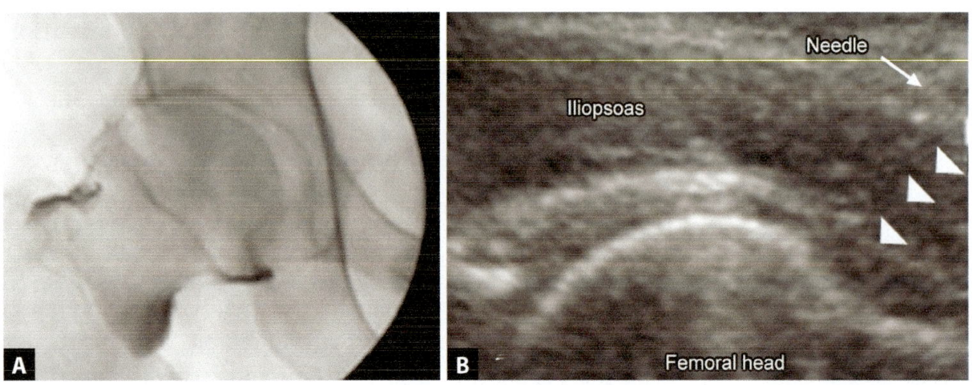

Figs. 3A and B: Ultrasound imaging of the hip joint injection next to a fluoroscopic-guided hip joint injection.

- Although complications from ultrasound use are quite minimal, potential complications include allergic reactions to local anesthetics. In addition, damage to cartilage, tendon, and blood vessels may occur with improper needle placement.

Required Equipment for Ultrasound

- Ultrasound machine with 7–15 MHz linear array broadband probe, and a 5 MHz convex array probe **(Fig. 4)**
- Sterile or nonsterile gel
- Needles of different sizes
- Sterile gloves and drapes
- Syringes (5 mL and 25 or 27G needle for lidocaine injection), 30 mL and 18G needle for synovial fluid aspiration.

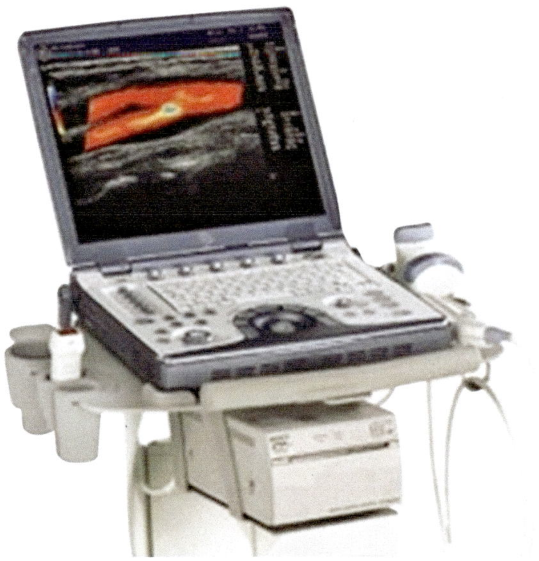

Fig. 4: A typical ultrasound machine.

Ultrasound transducers operate via emitting sound waves within a specific frequency range. The higher the frequencies yielding, the better the image resolution. However, this results in poorer penetration of deeper tissue structures. On the contrary, a transducer with lower frequency will penetrate deeper tissue structures, but will produce lower image resolution **(Fig. 5)**.[2,3]

The two most used transducers are the linear and curvilinear probes, the former being a high-frequency probe, whereas the latter is a low-frequency probe.

The ultrasound machine processes the intensity of returning echoes to create an image on the screen according to a grayscale spectrum of black, white, and many shades of gray. A structure will appear black, white, or gray on the screen based on the tissue's echogenicity. Echogenicity is defined as the ability of tissue to reflect or transmit ultrasound waves in the context of surrounding tissue, which in turn depends on the tissue's density, water content, and elasticity.[3]

FLUOROSCOPY

This is an imaging technique that uses X-rays, a form of ionizing radiation to generate real-time still images of a patient's body. It is a commonly used technique that aids in diagnostic and interventional procedures **(Fig. 6)**.

Indications

Fluoroscopy is indicated for the following:

- Interventional pain management (e.g., epidural steroid injection to the spine and sacroiliac joints)
- Orthopedic procedures (e.g., manipulation of broken bones in fracture reduction)
- Cardiovascular and interventional radiology procedures.

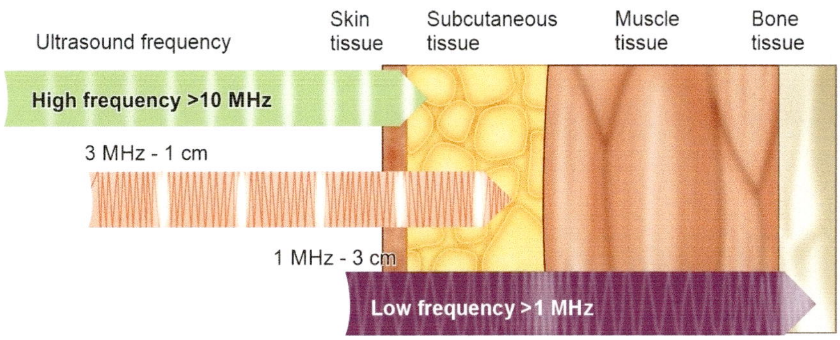

Fig. 5: Demonstration of ultrasound frequencies and their tissue penetration. Higher frequency reaches more superficial tissues, but greater detail in imaging. Lower frequencies can get to deeper structures but have less image detail.

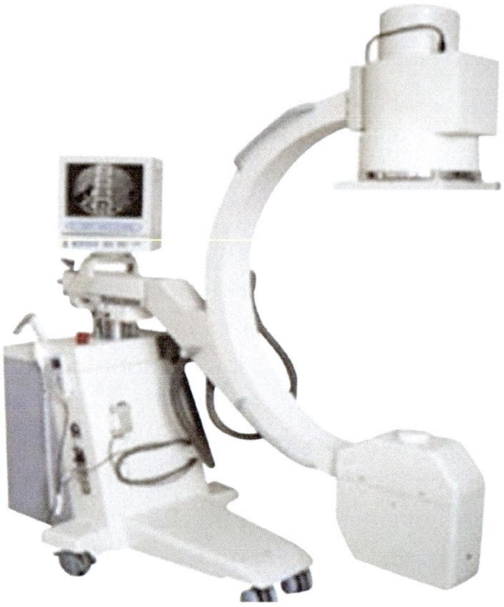

Fig. 6: A typical C-arm fluoroscopic machine.

Contraindications

A relative contraindication is pregnancy, as it contains ionizing radiation, which may be harmful to the fetus.

Equipment

The fluoroscope contains an X-ray source at one end and a fluorescent screen at the other end. The part of the body to be imaged is placed between these ends. The X-rays pass through the body, create an image on the detector, which is then transmitted to a monitor for viewing by the physician. To visualize a body part, it must be radiopaque, or made radiopaque with a dye or contrast agent.[4]

Advantages

Fluoroscopy offers the following advantages:

- It is preferred over ultrasonography because of its ability to penetrate deeper tissue structures.
- Live-contrast spread can be used to show vascular or epidural injection spread in a larger field.

Disadvantages

Disadvantages of using fluoroscopy in interventional pain management include:

- *Exposure to ionizing radiation:* Although low-dose radiation is used, fluoroscopy carries the same risk as other X-ray procedures. One should note that the radiation dose a patient receives depends also on the body part being examined and the duration of the procedure[4]
- Expensive
- Limited soft tissue evaluation.

CONCLUSION

When looking at both the options, and which is a better choice, an answer may not be available. Many would argue that fluoroscopy is still required and needed for many spinal procedures given the ability of having a better appreciation for bony structures, and live fluoroscopy with contrast injections. Although, in the more peripheral joints and soft tissue injection, ultrasound may be a better option due to the ability of ultrasound to provide visualization of multiple types of tissue. In many cases, the choice of which guidance to use will be left to the comfort level of the treating doctor.

REFERENCES

1. Mcdonald DG, Leopold GR. Ultrasound B-scanning in the differentiation of Baker's cyst and thrombophlebitis. Br J Radiol. 1972;45(538):729-32.
2. Dasgupta B, Patil P. Role of diagnostic ultrasound in the assessment of musculoskeletal diseases. Ther Adv Musuloskeletal Dis. 2012;4(5):341-55.
3. Lewis M, Gunabushanam G. Joint assessment using bedside ultrasonography. Medscape; 2013.
4. Daley EL, Bajaj S, Bisson LJ, Cole BJ. Improving injection accuracy of the elbow, knee, and shoulder. Am J Sports Med. 2011;39(3):656-62.

60 CHAPTER

Introduction to Ultrasound in Interventional Pain Medicine

Ritesh Roy, Gaurav Agarwal

ABSTRACT

Interventional techniques for pain management have advanced over the years. The advent of fluoroscopic guidance for injection into areas of pain generation has been paramount in safely and effectively treating patients. Although fluoroscopy is extremely useful in patients, it has limitations in evaluating soft tissues. Ultrasound has become a mainstay in the interventional pain management world. It has allowed the ability to visualize a field of soft tissue, such as ligaments and bones, and allow interventions to be done. Both are extremely useful and the proper setting for each should be considered.

INTRODUCTION

Interventional pain medicine has evolved from landmark-guided procedures, computed tomography (CT)-guided procedures, to X-ray/fluoroscopy-guided and now to ultrasound/ultrasonography (USG)-guided interventions. There has been development in imaging adjuncts such as three-dimensional rotational angiography (3D-RA), flat detector CT (FDCT), or cone beam CT (CBCT), and digital subtraction angiography, with need for additional setup for imaging-oriented specification for optimum intervention results. The national focus on safety and precision in clinical practice has created a need for advanced imaging tools for interventional pain physicians. Physicians have always weighed the cost–benefit risks for imaging modalities in intervention pain medicine, which has been an emerging branch in patient care with increasing awareness among patients and fellow clinicians, for the best outcomes.[1]

Ultrasonography has been studied extensively as an imaging modality, and the advantages of USG have been proven over others in several pain procedures in acute perioperative suites, such as peripheral nerve blocks (e.g., the brachial or lumbar plexus), especially when required for distal branches of the plexus proximal to neural trauma, entrapment, or neuroma formation. Small sensory or mixed nerves blockades such as ilioinguinal (posthernia surgery nerve entrapment), lateral femoral cutaneous (meralgia paresthetica), suprascapular (shoulder pain, frozen shoulder), pudendal (pudendal neuralgia), intercostal (thoracic herpetic neuralgia), trigeminal nerve branches (trigeminal neuralgia), median nerve (carpal tunnel syndrome), and various others have been performed. USG has proven as beneficial aid for intra-articular injections, trigger point injections, myofascial pain syndrome interventions, and many neuraxial procedures including caudal epidurals, selective spinal nerve blocks, facet joint, medial branch blocks, and third occipital nerve blocks, as well as sympathetic blocks (stellate ganglion, hypogastric plexus, and celiac ganglion). USG has also been used as an imaging modality for peripheral neuromodulation electrode placement.[1-3]

The advantages of USG over existing modalities have also been proven to be:

- *Affordable:* As it can be used in office-based or clinic-based practice, the same machine can be shared by different departments of the unit/institution.
- *Portable:* As it can be easily moved around for different procedures, provides convenience and accessibility. USG proves to be comfortable for the operator as well as the patient.
- *Safer alternative:* As it is associated with no radiation exposure, allows for real time visualisation of structures, and dynamic needle placement. It can be

used for scanning and identification of neurovascular structures in the needle path and aid in reducing complications of inadvertent injuries.

- *Advantages in diagnostics:* USG is also used in diagnostics in pain management such as shoulder, knee, and ankle pathologies and aids in definitive management.
- *Accuracy:* As it can show real-time visualization of the needle tip and the anatomical landmark, it improves the accuracy of procedures such as peripheral nerve blocks, radiofrequency ablation, and cryoablations of nerves.[4,5]

Ultrasonography, like all other imaging modalities, needs a learning skill and the basics; hence, we describe the basics of USG in this chapter.

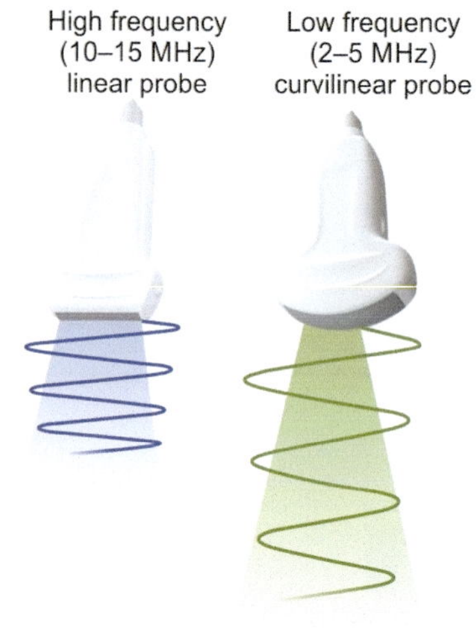

Fig. 1: Probes showing waves for different types of probes.

PHYSICS OF ULTRASONOGRAPHY AND TECHNICAL ASPECTS OF ULTRASONOGRAPHY MACHINE

Ultrasound waves are generated in pulsed manner (pulse echo) by piezoelectric crystals placed symmetrically in USG transducer or probe, on application of electrical current (*reverse piezoelectric effect*), which traverses various tissues of the body to get absorbed, refracted, scattered, or reflected (based on their individual tissue density or acoustic impedance) back to the probe which receives them to generate electrical impulses (*piezoelectric effect*) in turn to create echoes (images) on the screen. USG machine has basic settings, which need attention prior to use for optimum image production and intervention.

The medical ultrasound machine generates sound waves in the frequency of 1–20 MHz (human audible sound waves lie between 2 and 20 kHz). The higher the frequency, the shorter the wavelength. This property is important in the selection of *the probe* used for USG-guided interventions. The high frequency (10–15 MHz) linear probes will generate higher resolution (spatial or two-point differentiation) and are used for superficial target scanning. The low frequency (2–5 MHz) curvilinear probes in turn are used for deeper target scanning and produce lower resolution but better penetration of ultrasound waves, with wider footprint (more tissue coverage under the probe) **(Fig. 1)**.

Ultrasonography produces various echoes called hyperechoic structures (such as nerves, muscles, and procedure needles), hyperechoic with shadow (such as bones and lungs), hypoechoic structures (such as fat and subcutaneous tissue), and anechoic structures (all fluid-filled structures such as artery and vein). The knowledge of the echogenicity of each structure makes correlation of the anatomy easier.

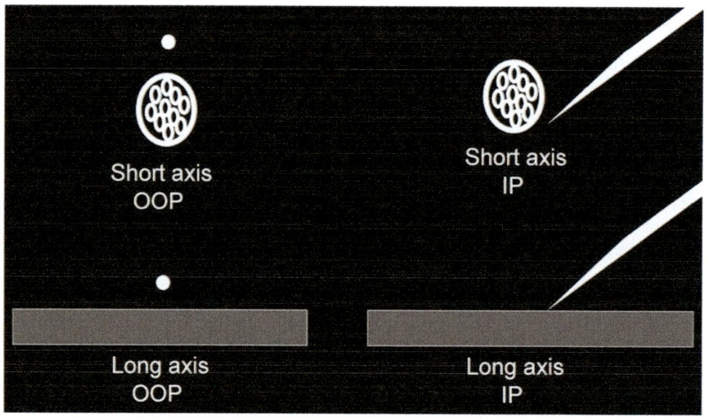

Fig. 2: Orientation of target and needle.
(IP: in-plane; OOP: out-of-plane)

The *probe marker* is the raised part of the probe, which corresponds to the center of the probe used and is used for orientation of the side of patient and screen. The probe marker is the point below which USG produces a *credit card thin* beam of ultrasound, and the structures lying under this thin beam will be visible on the image created on the screen.

The *orientation of procedure needle* with respect to the probe helps in visualization of the target **(Fig. 2)** and needle tip for optimal outcome. The needle when placed parallel to the probe the needling is called in-plane (IP) needling where the movement of the needle can be seen in real time in whole length of needle. The advantages of IP needling are the real-time visualization, accuracy of tip placement, and less complications, whereas the disadvantages being longer needle path causing greater discomfort to the patient. While the out-of-plane (OOP) needling is associated with shorter needle path and less discomfort when needle is placed perpendicular to the probe but has longer learning curve and associated with inadvertent injuries.

The *orientation of probe* when placed transverse to target structures, the view is called *short axis view* of the target and is especially used for single shot nerve blocks and identification of anatomical structures. Whereas the longitudinal view of the target structure under the probe is known as *long axis view* of target and is used for continuous catheter placements, various chronic pain interventions, and vascular access.

The *depth* setting is of paramount importance to enhance the resolution. The focal depth is the location of the screen where the spatial and axial resolution (two-point discrimination) of USG beam is the best. The target should be placed at the focal length for the best resolution and outcome **(Fig. 3)**.

Ultrasonography has a *gain* (or literally brightness) setting for the image produced under the probe, where the optimal gain or setting of time gain compensation produces desired target resolution, with least of noise or artifacts (aberrant echogenicity produced due to limitations of the ultrasound beams).

Modern machines provide various *presets* with these settings optimized for best visualization of images. USG needs stability of the operator's hands and probe,

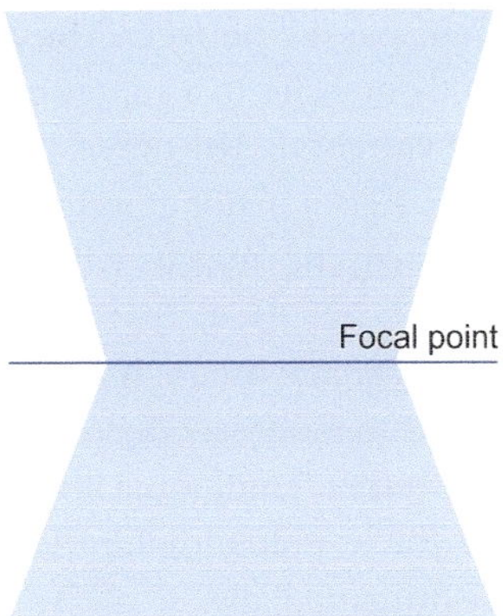

Fig. 3: Image showing concept of focal length with respect to : ultrasonography (USG) image.

and good hand-eye coordination for an optimum procedure outcome; hence, *ergonomics* is eminent. The placement of patient between the machine and operator (on the ipsilateral side) is the best ergonomic position for interventions for a direct gaze to screen, probe, needle, and patient.[6-8]

CONCLUSION

The advent of technology mandates up skilling in clinicians. The technology should be used as an adjunct to the knowledge of anatomy, and learning of technical skills to co-relate the same. USG has been a great and safe tool for imaging modality for intervention which needs upskilling and should be used with adequate training and practice.

REFERENCES

1. Huntoon, MA. Imaging in Interventional Pain Management. In: Narouze S (Eds). Atlas of Ultrasound-Guided Procedures in Interventional Pain Management. Springer, New York; (2018) NY.
2. Simpson G, Nicholls B. Use of ultrasound in chronic pain medicine. Part 1: neuraxial and sympathetic blocks. Contin Educ Anaesth Crit Care Pain. 2013;13(5):145-51.
3. Simpson G, Nicholls B. Use of ultrasound in chronic pain medicine—Part 2: musculoskeletal and peripheral nerve applications. Contin Educ Anaesth Crit Care Pain. 2014;14(4):176-84.
4. Korbe S, Udoji EN, Ness TJ, Udoji MA. Ultrasound-guided interventional procedures for chronic pain management. Pain Manag. 2015;5(6):465-82.
5. Narouze SN, Provenzano D, Peng P, et al. The American Society of Regional Anesthesia and Pain Medicine, the European Society of Regional Anaesthesia and Pain Therapy, and the Asian Australasian Federation of Pain Societies Joint Committee Recommendations for Education and Training in Ultrasound-Guided Interventional Pain Procedures: Reg Anesth Pain Med. 2012;37(6):657-64.
6. Basics of Musculoskeletal and Doppler Ultrasound Imaging for Regional Anesthesia and Pain Medicine. In: Karmakar MK, Soh E, Chee V, Sheah K. eds. Atlas of Sonoanatomy for Regional Anesthesia and Pain Medicine. McGraw-Hill Education; 2018.
7. Lin E, Gaur A, Jones M, Ahmed A. Introduction. In: Sonoanatomy for Anaesthetists. Cambridge University Press; 2012:1-11.
8. Chan, V., Perlas, A. (2018). Basics of Ultrasound: Pitfalls and Limitations. In: Narouze, S. (Eds) Atlas of Ultrasound-guided procedures in interventional pain management. Springer, New York, NY.

CHAPTER 61

Ultrasound-guided Greater Occipital and Third Occipital Nerve Block

Surbhi Bhagat, Kritika M Doshi

ABSTRACT

An ultrasound-guided greater occipital nerve (GON) and third occipital nerve (TON) block is a minimally invasive procedure used to diagnose and treat headaches and chronic neck pain, particularly in conditions like occipital neuralgia and cervicogenic headaches. The procedure involves using real-time ultrasound imaging to accurately locate and inject local anesthetic, with or without corticosteroids, near the GON and TON. Ultrasound guidance enhances precision, reduces the risk of complications, and avoids radiation exposure.

INTRODUCTION

The occipital nerves are a group of nerves that arise from the C2 and C3 spinal nerves. There are three major occipital nerves in the human body: The greater occipital nerve (GON), the lesser occipital nerve (LON), and the third occipital nerve (TON).[1]

The medial branch of the dorsal ramus of C2 known as the greater occipital nerve is a purely sensory nerve. The TON is the medial branch of the dorsal ramus of C3. The TON innervates the facet joint between the C2 and C3 spinal nerves and a portion of the semispinalis capitis.[2]

These nerve blocks are indicated in occipital neuralgia, chronic refractory migraine, and headaches with pain around the occipital and cervical region.

Traditionally, GON block was done using landmarks and as a blind procedure. The TON block was done under fluoroscopy guidance. Ultrasonography (USG)-guided blocks are gaining popularity as they have the advantage of direct visualization of injection, vascular structures, and it avoids complications of fluoroscopy. A high-frequency ultrasound transducer is used to perform these blocks. Identification of anatomical structures under ultrasound is important for a successful block.

INDICATIONS

- Occipital neuralgias
- Other headaches, such as migraines, cluster headaches, and cervicogenic headaches[3]
- Patients with whiplash injuries may also suffer from TON headache (54% incidence of head/neck pain after whiplash injury).

GREATER OCCIPITAL NERVE BLOCK

Anatomy

The occipital region is innervated by three nerves: GON, LON, and TON. The medial branch of the dorsal ramus of C2 nerve is the GON **(Fig. 1)**. After emerging from the suboccipital triangle, it passes beneath and posterior to the obliquus capitis inferior muscle (OCIM) **(Fig. 2)**.[4] It, then, passes between the OCIM and the semispinalis capitis muscles in a superomedial fashion at the level of C1-C2 vertebrae. The nerve, then, crosses over the rectus capitis posterior major muscle and arises medial to the semispinalis capitis muscle, which it occasionally pierces.[5]

Along with the occipital artery, it pierces the trapezius muscle and ascends to innervate the occipitoparietal part of the scalp to the vertex. Traditional landmark technique for GON block involves palpating for the occipital artery and injecting the drug medially.

Sono Anatomy and Technique

Using USG to accurately locate the GON improves short-term efficacy.[6]

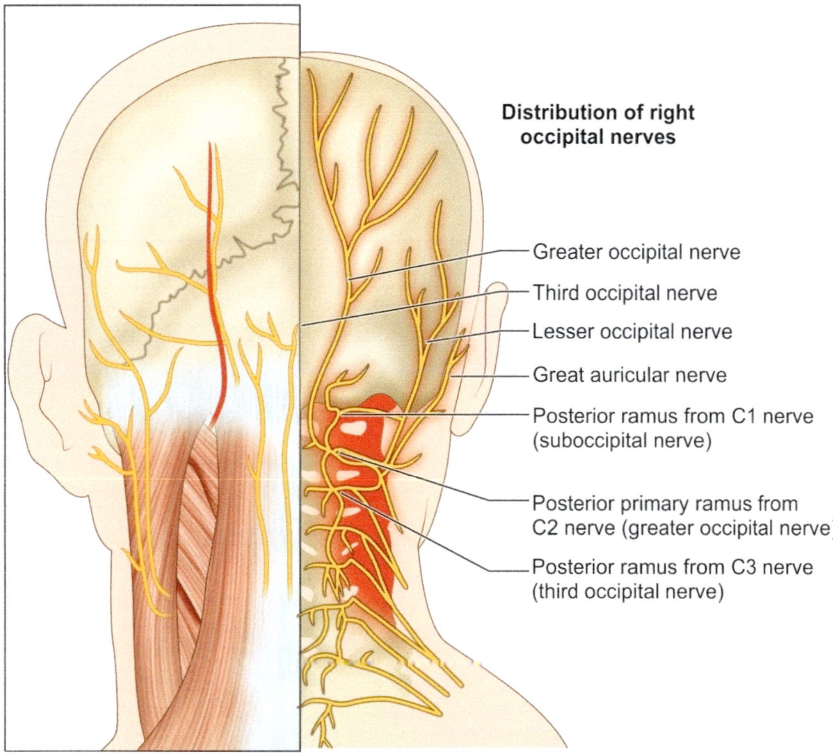

Fig. 1: Distribution of occipital nerves.

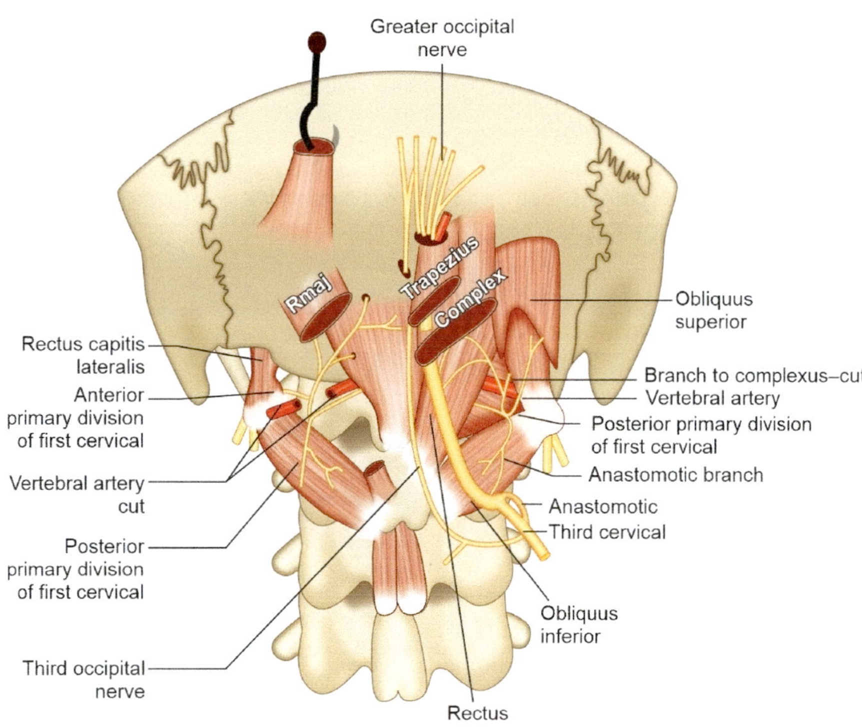

Fig. 2: Greater occipital nerve course: After emerging from below the suboccipital triangle beneath the obliquus capitis inferior muscle, it passes through the trapezius muscle.[4]

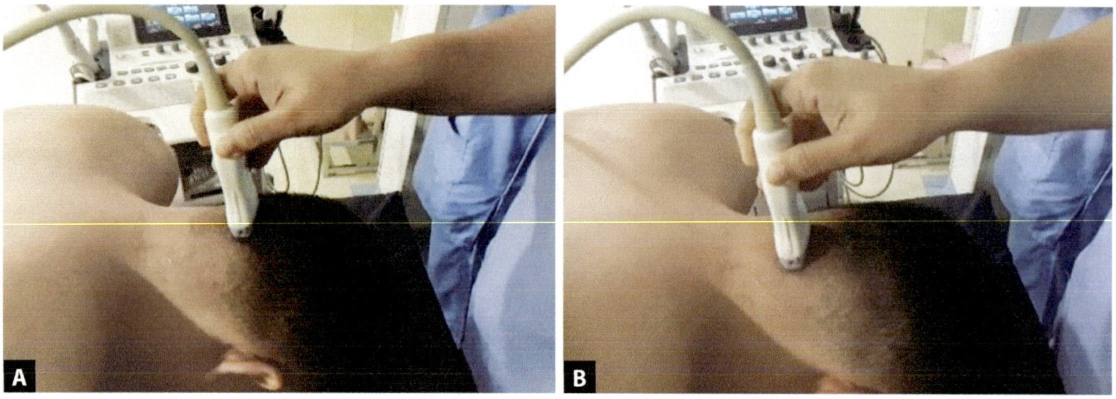

Figs. 3A and B: (A) Probe placement and (B) probe moved caudad.

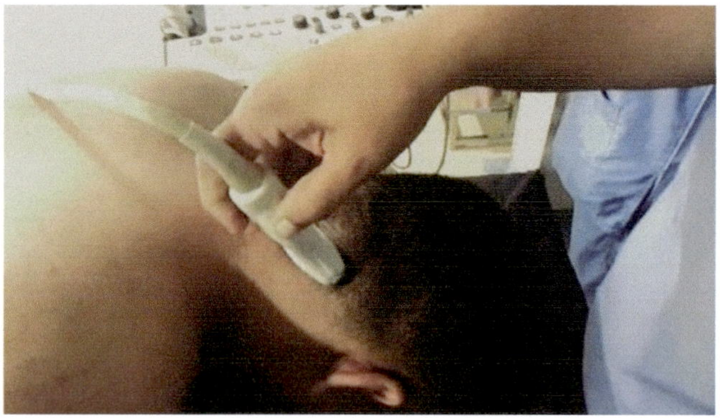

Fig. 4: Lateral end of probe rotated cranially.

Greater occipital nerve block procedure is performed with the patient lying in lateral or prone position and using a high-frequency linear transducer. The area of interest is at the level of C1-C2 vertebrae, where the nerve runs between the OCIM and the semispinalis capitis muscles.

Begin scanning by placing the transducer in a transverse orientation over the occiput **(Figs. 3A and B)** and gently move caudad.

The first acoustic shadow encountered is the bifid spinous process of the C2 vertebra (the two tubercles of the massive spinous process of the axis) as the C1 vertebra does not have a true spinous process. This is the most important osseous Sono anatomic landmark to locate the OCIM.

As the transducer is moved laterally, to a position between C2 spine and the mastoid process, the suboccipital muscle layer seen immediately overlying the lamina is the OCIM. Immediately superficial to this muscle is the semispinalis capitis muscle. GON is located in between these two muscles—the oval-shaped GON is clearly seen "on top of" the OCIM **(Fig. 4)**. To improve visualization, rotate the lateral end of the probe cranially to lie between the spinous process of C2 and the mastoid process **(Figs. 4 to 6)**.

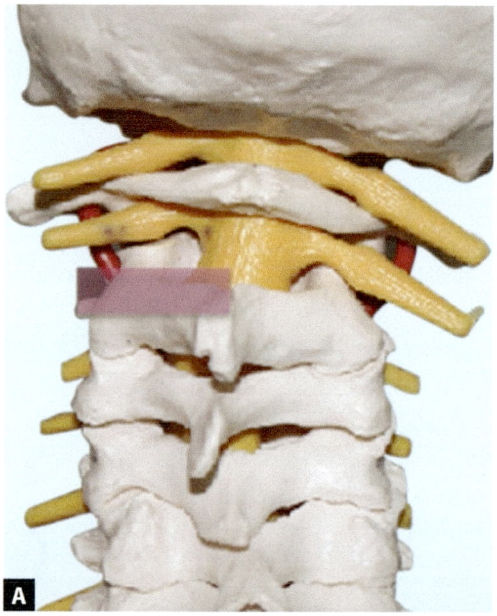

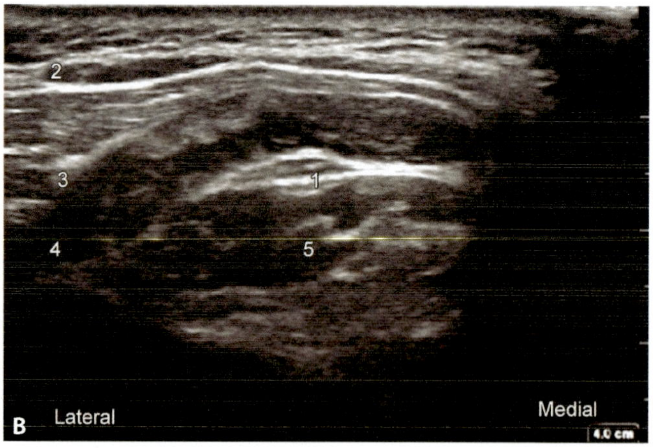

Figs. 5A and B: (A) Transducer position—transverse at C2 and (B) ultrasonographic image of the left greater occipital nerve. 1—Greater occipital nerve, 2—trapezius muscle, 3—splenius capitis muscle, 4—semispinalis capitis muscle, and 5—obliquus capitis inferior muscle.

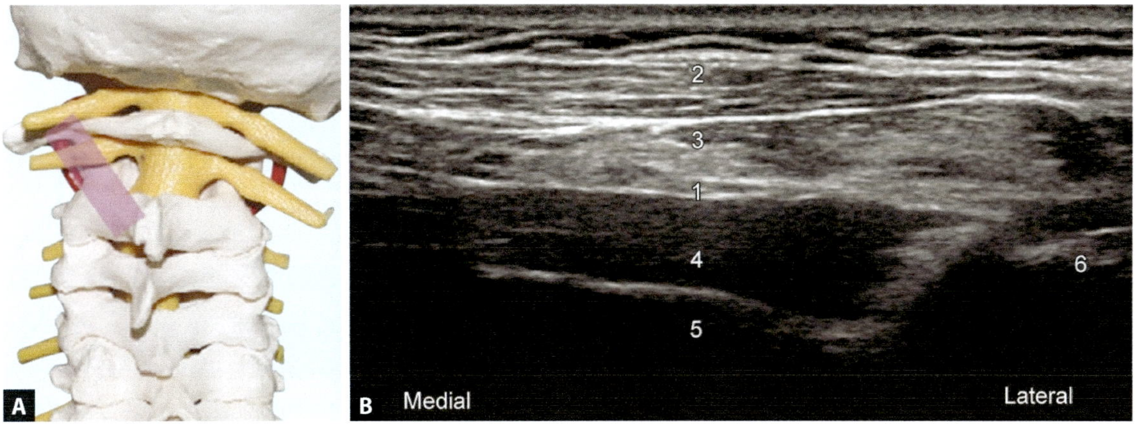

Figs. 6A and B: (A) Transducer position—oblique between mastoid and C2 spinous process and (B) ultrasonographic image of the left greater occipital nerve. 1—Greater occipital nerve, 2—trapezius muscle, 3—semispinalis capitis muscle, 4—obliquus capitis inferior muscle.

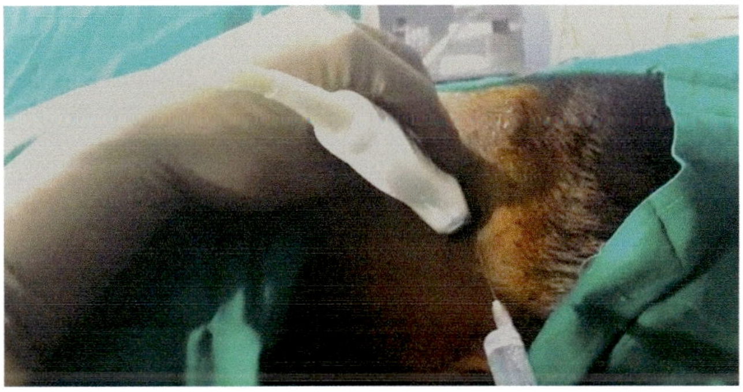

Fig. 7: In-plane injection.

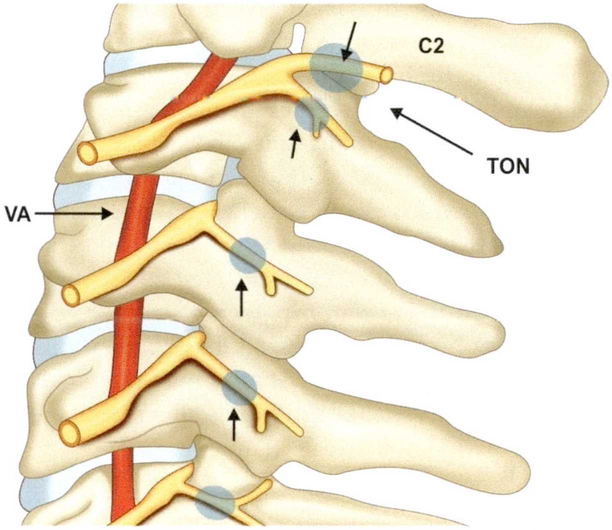

Fig. 8: Third occipital nerve (TON): Note the larger superficial and medial branch of C2 is the TON. (VA: vertebral artery)

The block needle is always introduced in-plane **(Fig. 7)** and the medication is deposited between these two muscle layers (long-acting local anesthetic 0.5 mL for a diagnostic block).

Caution is advised against deeper advancement of the needle as the vertebral artery travels cranially over the acoustic window between the C2 and C1.

THIRD OCCIPITAL NERVE BLOCK

Anatomy

The medial branches of the C3 dorsal rami have a unique course compared to the other cervical medial branches. After emerging from the C2-C3 intervertebral foramen, the dorsal ramus divides into two branches **(Fig. 8)**. The deep medial branch passes around the waist of the C3 articular pillar like other cervical medial branches and supplies the C3-C4 zygapophyseal joint. The larger superficial medial branch of C3 is also known as TON. This nerve runs close to the C2-C3 zygapophyseal joint giving articular branches to the joints. Continuing further, the TON provides the cutaneous innervation to the suboccipital region **(Figs. 1 and 2)**. This branch of C3 nerve has also been implicated in cervicogenic headache.

Sono Anatomy

A coronal (long-axis) scan is used for level confirmation in both the upper and lower cervical spines. In the long axis, the articular pillars appear as a series of peaks (zygapophyseal joints lines) and valleys (convex shapes of the articular pillars). Above the C2-C3 joint, the slope of the inferior articular process of C2 creates a characteristic

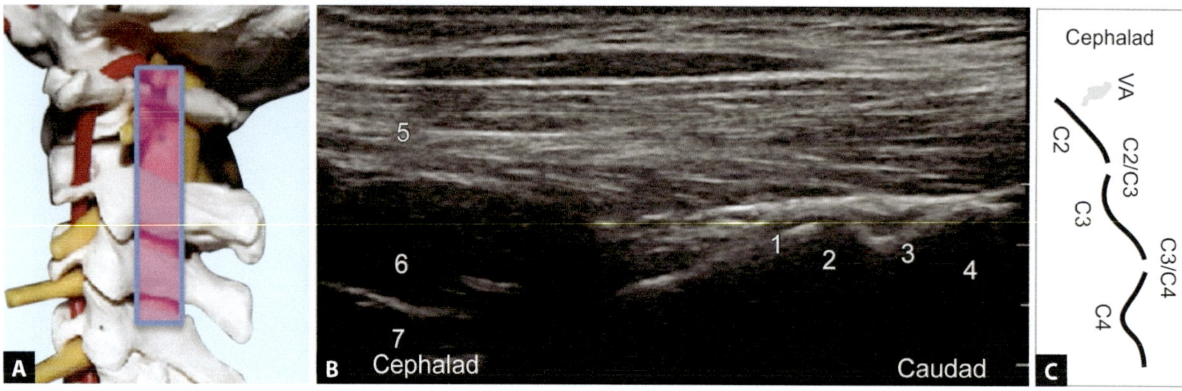

Figs. 9A to C: (A) Transducer position—vertical orientation over the C2/3 zygapophyseal joint; (B) ultrasonic image of the third occipital nerve; and (C) Line drawing of Peaks and troughs of Cervical ZA joints. (VA: vertebral artery)

drop off with the vertebral artery visible immediately cephalad to it.

The TON can be visualized and blocked under ultrasound guidance. Position and scanning technique for the TON follow the basic principles as for the other cervical medial branch blocks. Position the patient in the lateral position with the blocking side up. A high-frequency linear transducer is placed in longitudinal orientation until "saw pattern" is identified below the level of mastoid process. Close to the first peak, which corresponds to the C2-C3 articulation, the TON is located as a 2 mm oval hypoechoic structure with hyperechoic spots inside like a typical peripheral nerve **(Figs. 9A to C)**. Cephalad to the C2-C3 articulation, the arch of atlas may be visualized. Occasionally, the vertebral artery pulsation can be seen in the acoustic window between C1 and C2.

Procedure

Adequate aseptic precautions are to be followed. Patients are in a lateral position with head support and in neutral position.

A 5–11 MHz linear probe, a 2.5-inch 24G or 25G Block needle is used. After identifying the level, the needle is introduced in-plane manner from anterior to posterior direction till periosteum is reached (because all the vulnerable structures, such as vertebral artery and neural foramen are situated more anteriorly to the facet joint line). Real-time imaging is used to inject 0.3–0.5 mL of long-acting local anesthetic like ropivacaine for diagnostic blocks.

CONCLUSION

Universal aseptic precautions are mandatory while performing interventional pain procedures. Ultrasound-guided GON and TON blocks are to be performed after careful identification of anatomical structures. Care is needed to avoid intra-arterial and intraneural injections.

REFERENCES

1. Yu M, Wang SM. Anatomy, head and neck, occipital nerves. In: StatPearls [Internet]. Treasure Island (FL): StatPearls Publishing; 2024.
2. Kemp WJ 3rd, Tubbs RS, Cohen-Gadol AA. The innervation of the scalp: a comprehensive review including anatomy, pathology, and neurosurgical correlates. Surg Neurol Int. 2011;2:178.
3. Kim DD, Sibai N. Prolongation of greater occipital neural blockade with 10% lidocaine neurolysis: a case series of a new technique. J Pain Res. 2016;9:721-5.
4. Gray H. Anatomy of the Human Body. Philadelphia: Lea and Febiger; 1918.
5. Tubbs RS, Watanabe K, Loukas M, Cohen-Gadol AA. The intramuscular course of the greater occipital nerve: novel findings with potential implications for operative interventions and occipital neuralgia. Surg Neurol Int. 2014;5:155.
6. Palamar D, Uluduz D, Saip S, Erden G, Unalan H, Akarirmak U. Ultrasound-guided greater occipital nerve block: an efficient technique in chronic refractory migraine without aura? Pain Physician. 2015;18(2):153-62.

62 CHAPTER

Ultrasound-guided Cervical Medial Branch Block

Surbhi Bhagat, Kritika M Doshi

ABSTRACT

Cervical medial branch (MB) block is performed to diagnose whether the cervical facet joints are contributing to neck pain. Although fluoroscopy constitutes the imaging standard for these procedures, recently Ultrasound-guided cervical medial branch block (CMBB) are used to manage chronic neck pain associated with facet joint arthritis or dysfunction. Using real-time ultrasound imaging, the procedure involves the precise injection of a local anesthetic, often combined with steroids, near the cervical medial branches of the dorsal rami nerves that innervate the facet joints. Ultrasound guidance enhances precision, reduces the risk of complications, and avoids radiation exposure.

INTRODUCTION

Cervical medial branch (MB) block is performed to diagnose whether the cervical facet joints are contributing to neck pain. It is imperative to remember that MB blocks are not indicated for acute neck pain and that universal aseptic precautions must be taken while performing the procedure. Although fluoroscopy constitutes the imaging standard for these procedures, recent evidence suggests that ultrasound guidance (USG) can provide similar accuracy coupled with shorter performance times. USG is helpful to avoid both intraneural and intra-arterial injections.

ANATOMY

The cervical facet (zygapophysial) joint is a diarthrodial synovial joint oriented at a 45° angle in the coronal plane at C3 in posteromedial direction.[1] The superior and inferior articular facets are joined by articular pillars of the cervical vertebra.[2] These articular pillars correspond to the pars interarticularis of the lumbar spine **(Figs. 1A and B)**.

Each cervical spinal facet joint receives innervation from the MB nerves both above and below the joint. The dorsal ramus of the spinal nerve root divides into medial and lateral branches. The MB gives out an ascending branch which innervates the facet joint above while a descending branch innervates the joint below, providing dual innervation for each facet joint. For example, the C5-C6 facet joint receives innervation from both C5 and C6 medial nerve branches. **Table 1** lists the target nerves for each facet joint. For performing a MB block, the "waist" of the articular pillar acts as an important target.

Indications: The facet joint as a pain generator is suspected when there is a history of dull, achy, and paravertebral neck pain that is provoked on ipsilateral facet loading, with reduced range of motion and associated with morning stiffness.[3] This pain can also be referred to the shoulder or the arm or both. There is a nondermatomal distribution of pain pattern **(Fig. 2)**. Occasionally, headaches are noticed when upper cervical level facets are involved. Blocking of the cervical MBs is the reference while diagnosing facet-related pain in the neck.[4]

PROCEDURE UNDER ULTRASOUND GUIDANCE

Several anatomic features unique to the neck offer an ideal canvas for USG. For instance, cervical targets are relatively shallow (usually ≤3 cm under the skin surface:[5] This falls within the range of high-resolution linear array probes. A major advantage of using ultrasound in the neck is its ability to identify and avoid vascular and neural structures while maintaining accuracy (*see* **Fig. 6**). A high-frequency

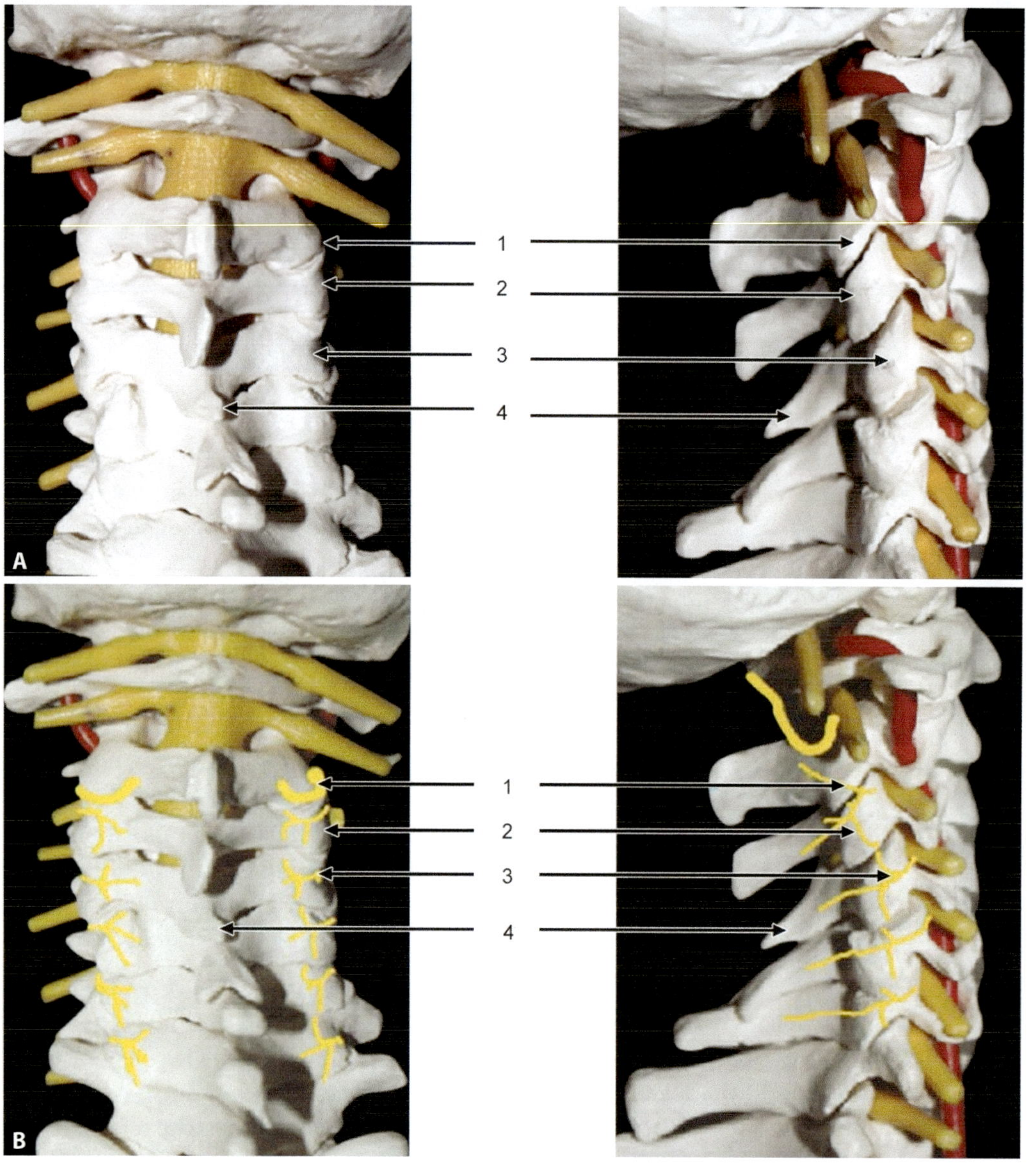

Figs. 1A and B: Cervical spine: posterior and lateral views, 1—Zygapophysial joints, 2—Articular pillars, 3—Medial branches, 4—Spinous process.

TABLE 1: Target for medial branch block (MBB).

Facet joint	*Anatomy*	*Target nerve for block*
C1-C2	Inferior articular process of C-1 with Superior articular process of C-2	Greater Occipital Nerve
C2-C3	Inferior articular process of C-2 with Superior articular process of C-3	Third Occipital Nerve
C3-C4	Inferior articular process of C-3 with Superior articular process of C-4	Medial Brach of C3 and C4
C4-C5	Inferior articular process of C-4 with Superior articular process of C-5	Medial Brach of C4 and C5
C5-C6	Inferior articular process of C-5 with superior articular process of C-6	Medial Brach of C5 and C6
C6-C7	Inferior articular process of C-6 with superior articular process of C-7	Medial Brach of C6 and C7
C7-T1	Inferior articular process of C-7 with superior articular process of T-1	Medial Brach of C7 and T1

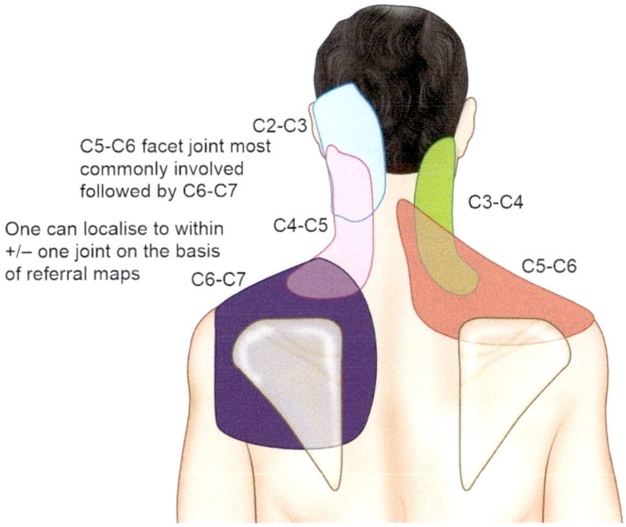

Fig. 2: Cervical facetogenic referral pain pattern; C5-C6 is most commonly involved followed by C6-C7.

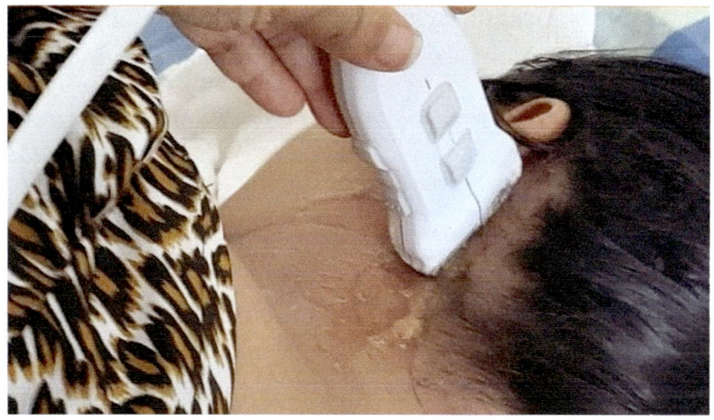

Fig. 3: Patient position with painful side up.

linear transducer is commonly used for most ultrasound-guided interventions in the neck.

The MBs at C4-C7 levels are often difficult to visualize in clinical practice, therefore, the validated landmark-based technique relies on identifying target points on the bony contours of the cervical spine. For C3 to C6 MBs, the centroid of the AP is targeted and a small injectate deposited between the periosteum and the tendinous insertions of the semispinalis capitis (SSC) muscle.[6] This plane contains the MB and small local anesthetic volumes can efficiently spread to cover the entire surface of the AP.

The patient can be positioned prone or lateral with the operating side in nondependent position **(Fig. 3)**.

The prone position is helpful to perform bilateral injections without altering patient position. Curvilinear or linear transducer can be used depending on the patient habitus. Linear transducers are helpful for superficial scanning in lean subjects. Ultrasound scanning is started in the posterior midline with the transducer in sagittal orientation **(Figs. 4A and B)**. The most superficial acoustic shadow is that of the spinous processes. The superior most bifid spinous process is that of the C2 vertebra as the atlas (C1) vertebra has no true spine.

Although the bifid spinous process of the C2 is often used as a sonographic landmark, considerable variation in the morphology makes precise identification of the level difficult.[7] From the C2 spinous process, vertebrae are counted downward while scanning to the required level. Scanning laterally identifies the laminae with the

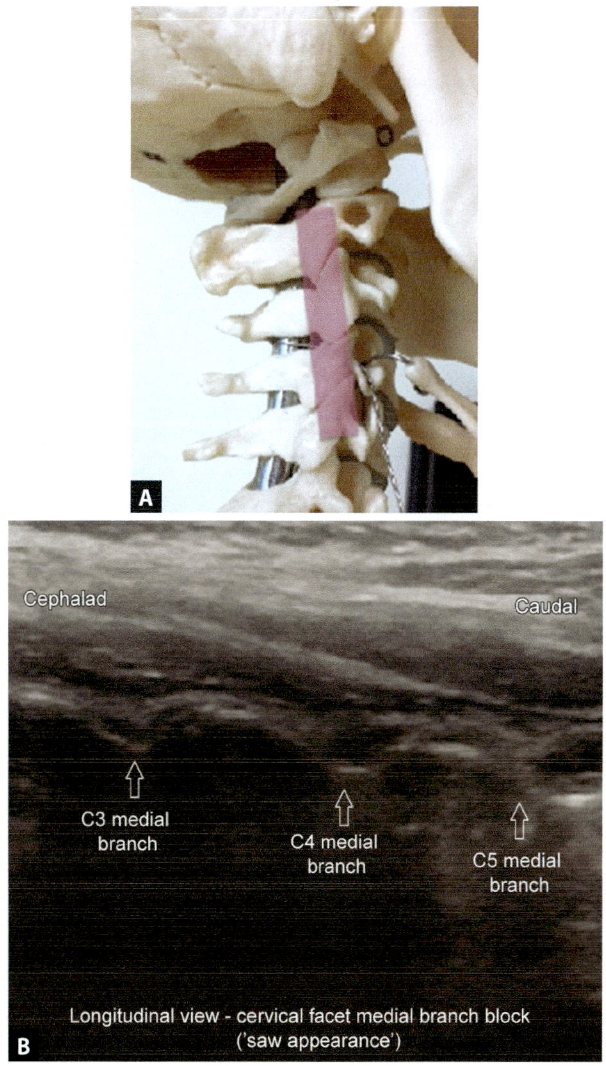

Figs. 4A and B: Cervical facet medial branch. (A) Linear transducer position—vertical orientation over the cervical zygapophysial joints; (B) Ultrasonic image of the cervical facets with saw appearance and medial branches in the troughs.

facet joints located above and below the articular pillars giving an anechoic "saw sign" **(Figs. 5 to 7)**. The first peak represents C2/3 facet articulation **(Figs. 4 and 5)**. The trough or the waist of the articular pillar is the target for the MB block **(Fig. 5)**.

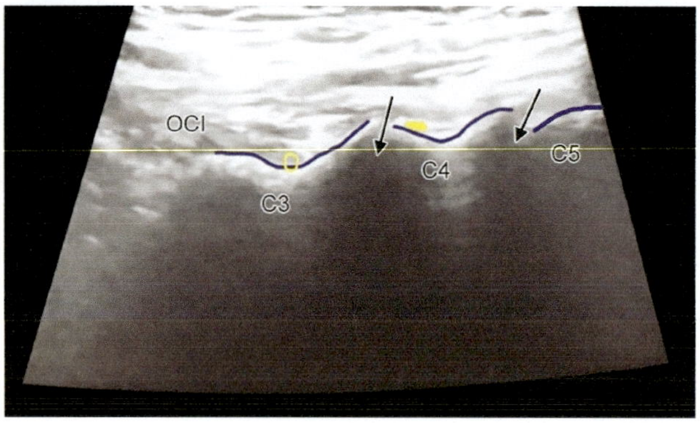

Fig. 5: Saw-toothed appearance with yellow dot indicating the target point for the medial branch.

INJECTION PROCEDURE

A posterolateral in-plane approach is used. The needle is advanced until contact with the periosteum. The probe is then rotated to obtain a coronal scan, and the needle tip confirmed to be in the middle of the targeted AP. Although in-plane approach is possible, some find it challenging as the shoulder obstructs maneuvering of the needle. Depending on one's sonoanatomic comfort, an out-of-plane approach can be more practical. The needle is advanced preferably in anterior to posterior (AP) direction until the needle tip hits the articular waist or the troughs

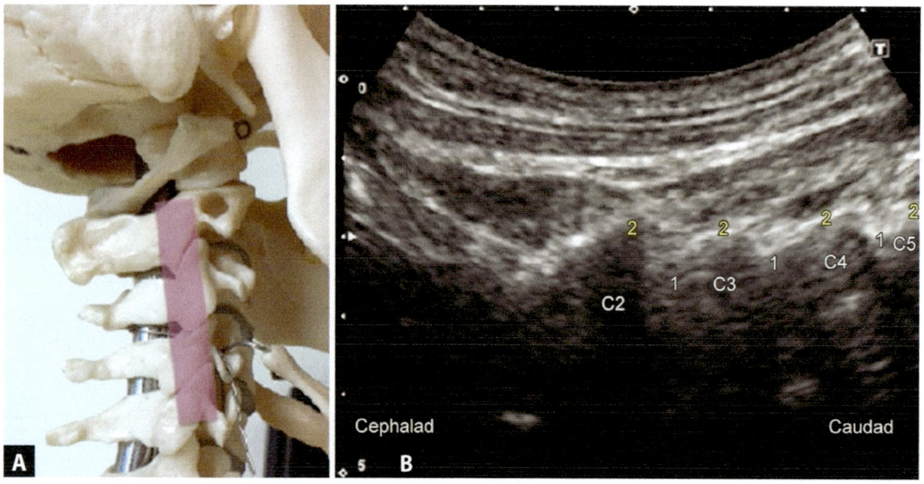

Figs. 6A and B: Cervical facet medial branch. (A) Curvilinear transducer position—vertical orientation over the cervical zygapophysial joints; (B) Ultrasonic image of the cervical facets with saw-toothed appearance and medial branches in the troughs. 1—Medial branch and 2—Facet joints.

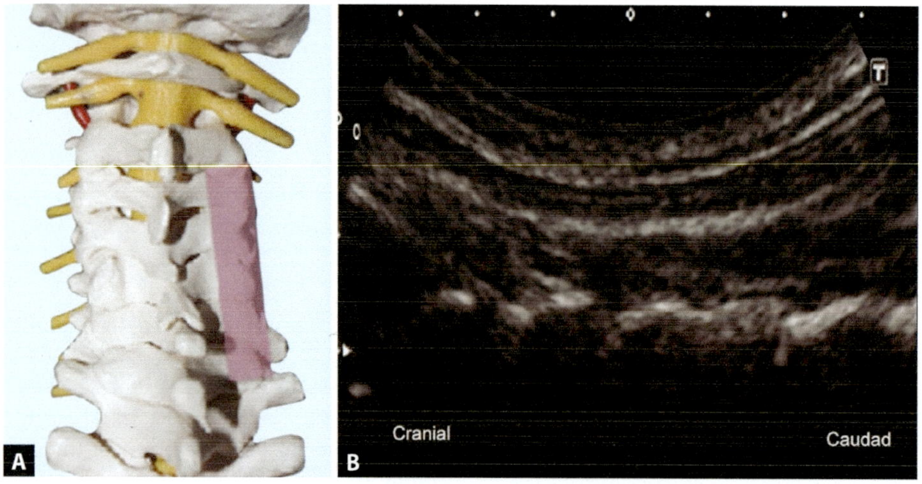

Figs. 7A and B: Cervical facet medial branch. (A) Linear transducer position—sagittal orientation over the cervical zygapophysial joints; (B) Ultrasonic image of the cervical facets with saw-toothed appearance.

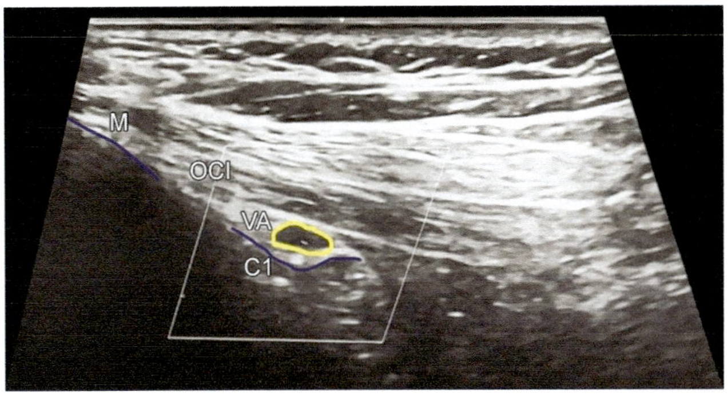

Fig. 8: Visualizing the position of vertebral artery.

of the saw. The rationale for this AP navigation is to avoid inadvertent trauma to the vertebral artery or the cervical nerve roots. Prior scanning with a color Doppler can help to identify and avoid blood vessels in the needle trajectory **(Fig. 8)**. After touching the periosteum, slightly withdraw the needle to inject the drug mixture.

COMPLICATIONS

The complications associated with cervical MB block include:

- Postprocedure flare-up of pain
- Bruising
- Hematoma
- Infection
- Intravascular injection
- Nerve damage
- Allergic reactions to medication used.

CONCLUSION

Identification of the correct vertebral level is important in injecting the appropriate articular pillar before injection.

Color Doppler can be used to avoid intra-articular injection and prevent nerve damage.

REFERENCES

1. Pal GP, Routal RV, Saggu SK. The orientation of the articular facets of the zygapophyseal joints at the cervical and upper thoracic region. J Anat. 2001;198(4):431-41.
2. Lewis WH. Anatomy of the Human Body, 20th edition. New York: Bartleby.Com; 2000.
3. Fukui S, Ohseto K, Shiotani M, Ohno K, Karasawa H, Naganuma Y, et al. Referred pain distribution of the cervical zygapophyseal joints and cervical dorsal rami. Pain. 1996;68(1):79-83.
4. Barnsley L, Bogduk N. Medial branch blocks are specific for the diagnosis of cervical zygapophyseal joint pain. Reg Anesth. 1993;18(6):343-50.
5. Finlayson RJ, Etheridge JP, Chalermkitpanit P, Tiyaprasertkul W, Nelems B, Tran DQ, et al. Real-time detection of periforaminal vessels in the cervical spine: an ultrasound survey. Reg Anesth Pain Med. 2016;41(2):130-4.
6. Finlayson RJ, Gupta G, Alhujairi M, Dugani S, Tran DQ. Cervical medial branch block: a novel technique using ultrasound guidance. Reg Anesth Pain Med. 2012; 37(2):219-23.
7. Ji-Hong F, Li-Ping W, Yi-Kai L, Bo-Jin L, Das M, Xiao-Yong F. Variable morphology of the axis vertebrae in 100 specimens: implications for clinical palpation and diagnostic imaging. J Manipulative Physiol Ther. 2010;33(2):125-31.

63 CHAPTER

Ultrasound-guided Shoulder Injections

Thomas P Lione, Steve M Aydin

ABSTRACT

Shoulder injuries and inflammatory conditions are common, and injections can serve both diagnostic and therapeutic purposes. Typically, joint injections should only be considered after other, more conservative therapeutic modalities have been tried such as nonsteroidal anti-inflammatory drugs (NSAIDs), activity modification, and physical therapy. Traditionally, injections are performed using anatomical landmarks with or without ultrasound guidance to guide needle placement into the subacromial space, acromioclavicular (AC) joint, scapulothoracic joint, long head of the bicep tendon, or glenohumeral joint. Indications for each vary, but may include osteoarthritis, adhesive capsulitis, rheumatoid arthritis, and rotator cuff pathology. Injections are most often performed using a combination of local anesthetic and corticosteroid. More recently, the use of ultrasound guidance has become more commonplace maximizing accuracy and optimizing response and outcomes.

INTRODUCTION

The shoulder is a common site of pain due to injury and/or inflammatory conditions. Chronic shoulder pain is a prevalent condition that can be due to multiple factors or causes. In addition to causing pain and affecting quality of life, shoulder disorders can be associated with high societal cost and patient burden. As people age, shoulder pain becomes more common. It is estimated that 6.9–34% of the general population will experience shoulder pain from various causes, and up to 21% in those over 70 years of age will experience shoulder derangements.[1] Interventional treatments such as joint injections may be considered after other therapeutic interventions such as nonsteroidal anti-inflammatory drugs, physical therapy, and activity modification have been trialed. Proper techniques, choice and doses of injectates, and appropriate follow-up are essential for effective outcomes.[2] Traditionally, injections have been performed using anatomical landmarks to guide needle placement into the subacromial space and/or glenohumeral (GH) joint.[3] However, with the increased use of ultrasound, more people are referred for injections using image guidance **(Fig. 1)**.

GLENOHUMERAL JOINT

The GH joint represents the articulation of the humerus with the glenoid fossa.[4] It is the most mobile joint in the body and is not considered a true ball-and-socket joint. The joint articulation is stabilized by soft tissues including multiple ligaments and muscles. These include the four muscles of the rotator cuff (supraspinatus, infraspinatus, teres minor, and subscapularis) which serve as stabilizers of the joint. Static stabilizers include the joint capsule, the glenoid labrum, and the GH ligaments.

ACROMIOCLAVICULAR JOINT

The acromioclavicular (AC) joint is a diarthrodial joint that connects the acromion to the distal clavicle.[5] The AC ligament is relatively weak and provides little joint stability. The coracoclavicular ligament (trapezoid and conoid ligaments) provides the major structural support of the joint and is the primary and most commonly injured ligament in an AC joint sprain/strain.

SCAPULOTHORACIC JOINT

The scapulothoracic joint is not a true joint but rather represents the position of the scapula on the posterior

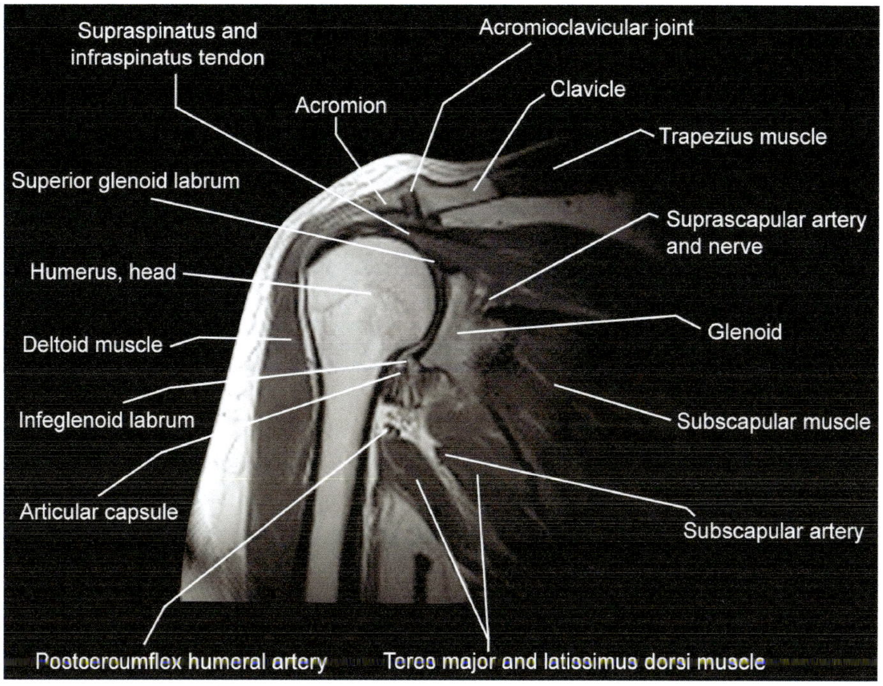

Fig. 1: Shoulder joint anatomy on magnetic resonance imaging.

thoracic cage on which it freely moves. Located lateral to the inferior medial border of the scapula is a bursa that can become inflamed.[5]

LONG HEAD OF THE BICEPS TENDON

The long head of the bicep tendon travels through the bicipital groove to insert on the head of the humerus.[5] Inflammation may be caused with any repetitive motion involving flexion of the shoulder. Pain and tenderness of the long head of the biceps tendon commonly occur concomitantly with rotator cuff tendinosis.

INDICATIONS

Glenohumeral Joint

- Osteoarthritis
- Adhesive capsulitis (frozen shoulder)
- Rheumatoid arthritis.

Acromioclavicular Joint

- Osteolysis of the distal clavicle
  - Degenerative process that results in chronic pain, may be made worse with adduction movements of the shoulder
  - Typically seen secondary to traumatic injury or in persons who perform repetitive exercises involving the shoulder
- Osteoarthritis.

Subacromial Space

- Subdeltoid bursitis
- Rotator cuff impingement
- Rotator cuff tendinosis
- Adhesive capsulitis.

CONTRAINDICATIONS

Shoulder injections are contraindicated in the following:

- Coagulopathies
- Local or systemic infection.

PRECAUTIONS

Precautions should be taken while administering shoulder injections in the following:

- Diabetes
- Treatment with anticoagulant or antiaggregation drugs
- Glaucoma: Ophthalmological opinion should be obtained prior to injection
- Previous corticosteroid injection(s).

EQUIPMENT AND DRUGS

Glenohumeral joint

- 5–10 mL syringe
- 25G needle
- 4–7 mL of 1% lidocaine or 0.25% or 0.5% bupivacaine
- 1–2 mL betamethasone sodium phosphate and acetate, 0.5–1 mL triamcinolone (20–40 mg), or 1–2 mL methylprednisolone.

Acromioclavicular joint

- 3–5 mL syringe
- 25G needle
- 0.5 mL of 1% lidocaine
- 0.25–0.5 mL betamethasone sodium phosphate or acetate, 0.5–1 mL of triamcinolone (20–40 mg), or 0.25–0.5 mL methylprednisolone.

Subacromial space

- 5–10 mL syringe
- 25G needle
- 4–7 mL of 1% lidocaine or 0.25% or 0.5% bupivacaine
- 1–2 mL betamethasone sodium phosphate and acetate, 0.5–1 mL of triamcinolone (20–40 mg), or 1–2 mL methylprednisolone.

PROCEDURE AND TECHNIQUE

Glenohumeral Joint

The GH joint is typically injected from an anterior or a posterior approach using anatomical landmarks as guidance or with ultrasound imaging. The patient may be placed in the prone position with a pillow placed under the ipsilateral shoulder or more commonly in the sitting position with the forearm across the body.[4]

The ultrasound-guided posterior approach uses a linear array transducer positioned over the long axis of the myotendinous junction of the infraspinatus muscle, located inferior to the spine of the scapula. The infraspinatus may be differentiated from the teres minor by its superior location, its larger size, and longer tendon length. The needle is advanced between the head of the humerus and the labrum into the GH joint.[6] After aspiration, injection should proceed without resistance. If resistance is encountered, repositioning of the needle is necessary[7] **(Figs. 2A and B)**.

Acromioclavicular Joint

The patient is placed in a supine or seated position with the affected arm resting at their side. First, the AC joint is identified by palpating the clavicle distally until its terminal end point where a slight depression will be appreciated.[8] The needle is then inserted from a superior and an anterior approach into the joint and directed inferiorly **(Figs. 3A to C)**.

Subacromial Bursa

The distal, lateral, and posterior aspects of the acromion are identified and palpated. Insert the needle just inferior to the posterolateral edge of the acromion. The needle is then directed toward the coracoid.[6]

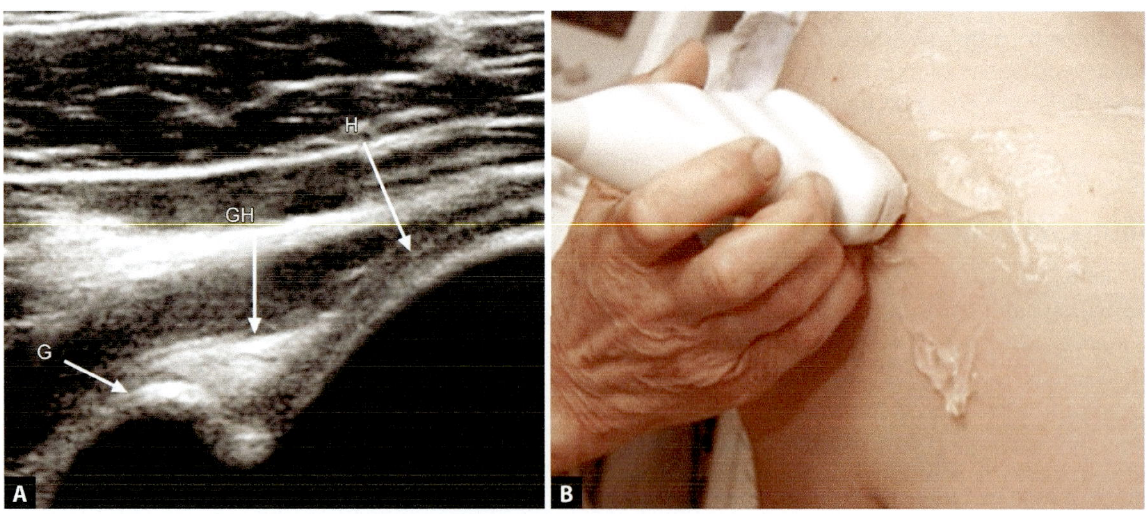

Figs. 2A and B: Ultrasound evaluation of the glenohumeral (GH) joint. Arrow labeled GH is the joint region that the needle would be directed under ultrasound. Arrow labeled H is the humorous and arrow labeled G is the glenoid.

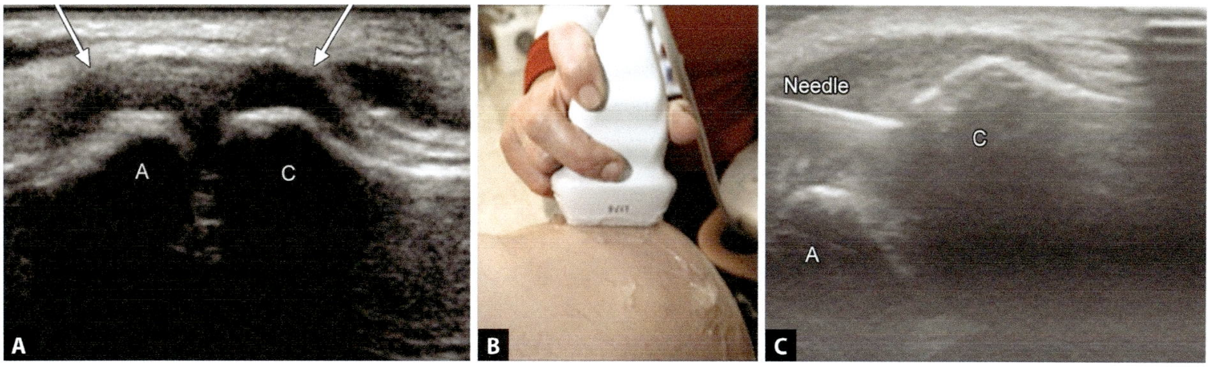

Figs. 3A to C: Ultrasound evaluation of the acromioclavicular joint, with "A" noting the acromial region and "C" the clavicular region. Needle placement is shown as well.

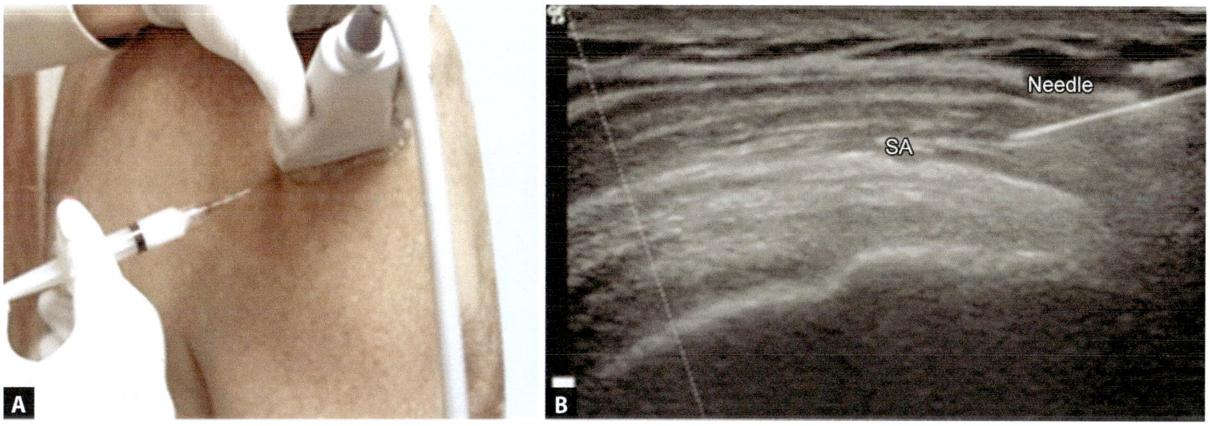

Figs. 4A and B: The posterior approach to injection of the subacromial bursa (SA) bursa with ultrasound. The labeled area SA is the bursa and the needle is demonstrated as well entering.

If using ultrasound guidance, the patient's arm should be flexed at the elbow, arm supinated, and palm of hand placed over ipsilateral hip. For the posterolateral approach, the linear array transducer is aligned along the longitudinal axis of the supraspinatus tendon. This approach allows visualization of the acromion, deltoid muscle, and supraspinatus tendon.[9,10] Using a sterile technique, the needle is advanced under ultrasound guidance into the subacromial space and bursa **(Figs. 4A and B)**.

CONCLUSION

Shoulder pain is a very common cause of pain and dysfunction in patients, which can limit function and quality of life. Often, proper evaluation and diagnosis can be done with physical examination. Interventions and injections can be performed in multiple regions of the shoulder joint; however, proper diagnosis and needle placement are essential for optimal response. Ultrasound guidance maximizes the ability for proper needle placement resulting in a higher probability for pain and functional improvement, as well as lower risk and complication.[10]

REFERENCES

1. Blair B, Rokito AS, Cuomo F, Jarolem K, Zuckerman JD. Efficacy of injections of corticosteroids for sub- acromial impingement syndrome. J Bone Joint Surg Am. 1996; 78:1685-9.
2. Chard MD, Hazleman R, Hazleman BL, King RH, Reiss BB. Shoulder disorders in the elderly: a community survey. Arthritis Rheumatol. 1991;34:766-9.
3. Cheng PH, Modir JG, Kim HJ, Narouze S. Ultrasound-guided shoulder joint injections. Tech Reg Anesth Pain Manage. 2009;13:184-90.
4. Gross C, Dhawan A, Harwood D, Gochanour E, Romeo A. Glenohumeral Joint Injections: A Review. Sports Health. 2013;5(2):153-9.

5. Gruson KL, Ruchelsman DE, Zuckerman JD. Subacromial corticosteroid injections. J Shoulder Elbow Surg. 2008;17:118S-130S.
6. Meislin RJ, Sperling JW, Stitik TP. Persistent shoulder pain: epidemiology, pathophysiology, and diagnosis. Am J Orthop (Belle Mead NJ). 2005;34(12 Suppl):5-9.
7. Molini L, Mariacher S, Bianchi S. US guided corticosteroid injection into the subacromial-subdeltoid bursa: Technique and approach. J Ultrasound. 2012;15:61-8.
8. Kerlan RK, Glousman RE. Injections and techniques in athletic medicine. Clin Sports Med. 1989;8:541-60.
9. Tallia AF, Cardone DA. Diagnosis and therapeutic injection of shoulder region. Am Fam Physician. 2003;67(6): 1271-8.
10. Travis RD, Doane R, Burkhead WZ Jr. Tendon ruptures about the shoulder. Orthop Clin North Am. 2000;31: 313-30.

CHAPTER 64

Ultrasound-guided Lumbar Medial Branch Block

Kritika M Doshi, Surbhi Bhagat

ABSTRACT

The Facet/Zygoapophyseal joints have been recognized as a source for low back pain; these joints are supplied by the medial branches of the dorsal rami of somatic nerves L1 to L5. A lumbar medial branch block (LMBB) is a minimally invasive procedure used to diagnose and treat chronic lower back pain. The procedure to block the medial branch involves injection of a local anesthetic sometimes combined with a steroid and is performed under imaging- fluroscopy and USG are used. In the lumbar region, each facet joint is supplied by the medial branch above and at the same level. Example: the L3-L4 Facet joint is supplied by the medial branches of the dorsal rami of L2 and L3. Ultrasound guidance enhances precision, reduces the risk of complications, and avoids radiation exposure.

INTRODUCTION

Lumbar medial branch block is a common interventional pain procedure for pain originating from the lumbar zygapophyseal joints. Fluoroscopic guidance is routinely used, although ultrasound is slowly gaining popularity. Ultrasound-guided approaches for lumbar medial branch block are described in this chapter along with relevant anatomy and associated complications. The correct nomenclature of the median nerve supplying the facet joint needs to be appreciated and recorded.

ANATOMY

Lumbar facet joints are synovial joints formed by the inferior articular process of the vertebra above and superior articular process (SAP) of the vertebra below.[1] It has been demonstrated that both the capsule[2,3] and synovial folds[2,3] of facet joints possess nociceptive nerve endings. The lumbar facet joints in axial view have a "C"-shaped configuration with concavity facing inwards.[2] The posteriormost portion of the joint is the most accessible portion of the vertebral facet for an intra-articular injection.

Lumbar zygapophyseal (facet) joints are innervated by articular branches arising from the medial branches of the lumbar dorsal rami.[2] Each zygapophyseal joint receives an articular branch from the medial branches above and at the joint, resulting in a dual innervation. For example, the L4-L5 facet joint receives innervation from both the L4 and L5 medial branches **(Fig. 1)**. **Table 1** lists the nomenclature of each lumbar facet joint and its innervation.

There is no specific clinical test for making a diagnosis. Clinically, lumbar back pain of zygapophyseal (facet) origin is suspected when there is dull, achy, paravertebral low back pain, with reduced range of motion and morning stiffness. Pain could be provoked on extension, twisting motion, or on ipsilateral facet loading. Sometimes, pain is also referred to the buttocks, hips, thighs, and rarely into the calves with a nondermatomal and nonradicular distribution[2] **(Fig. 2)**.

The gold standard test to confirm diagnosis of facet joint as the pain generator is a controlled local anesthetic block of the medial branch.[2] Traditionally, facet medial branch block injections are performed under fluoroscopic guidance. Currently, the use of ultrasound is gaining popularity.

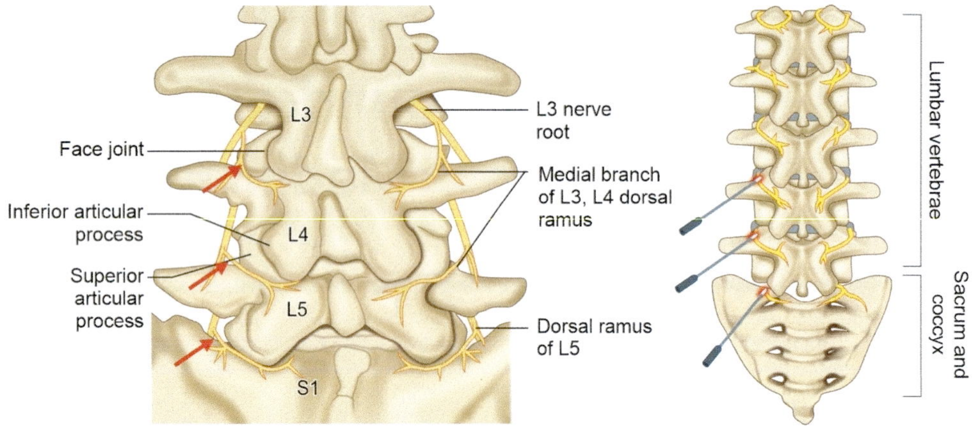

Fig. 1: Lumbar medial branch course.

TABLE 1: Nomenclature of each lumbar facet joint and its innervation.

Facet joint	*Anatomy*	*Target nerve for block*
L1-L2	Inferior articular process of L1 with superior articular process of L2	Medial branch of T12 and L1
L2-L3	Inferior articular process of L2 with superior articular process of L3	Medial branch of L1 and L2
L3-L4	Inferior articular process of L3 with superior articular process of L4	Medial branch of L2 and L3
L4-L5	Inferior articular process of L4 with superior articular process of L5	Medial branch of L3 and L4
L5-S1	Inferior articular process of L5 with sacral ala	Medial branch of L4 and dorsal ramus of L5

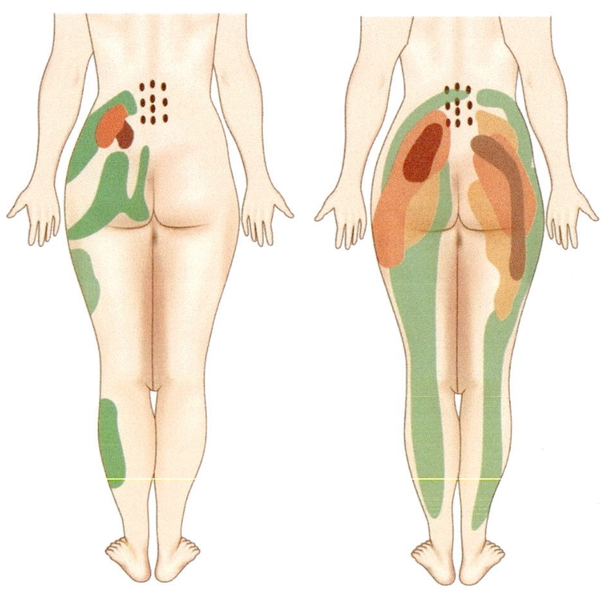

Fig. 2: Lumbar facetogenic referred pain pattern.

ULTRASOUND-GUIDED LUMBAR MEDIAL BRANCH BLOCK

Position: The patient is placed prone **(Fig. 3)** with pillows under the abdomen to improve visualization by reducing the lumbar lordosis.

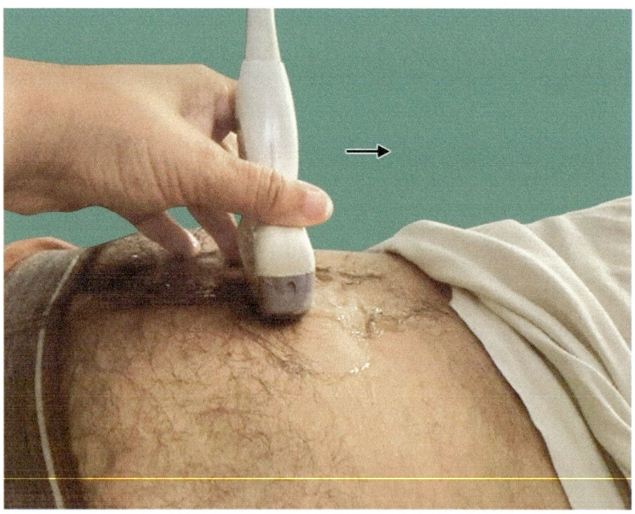

Fig. 3: Prone position, low-frequency (LF) curvilinear probe.

Ultrasound transducer: A low-frequency, higher penetration, curvilinear transducer is more appropriate for most lumbar ultrasound-guided procedures.

Sonoanatomy

The ultrasound transducer is placed in sagittal orientation in the midline. First, identify the dorsal surface of the

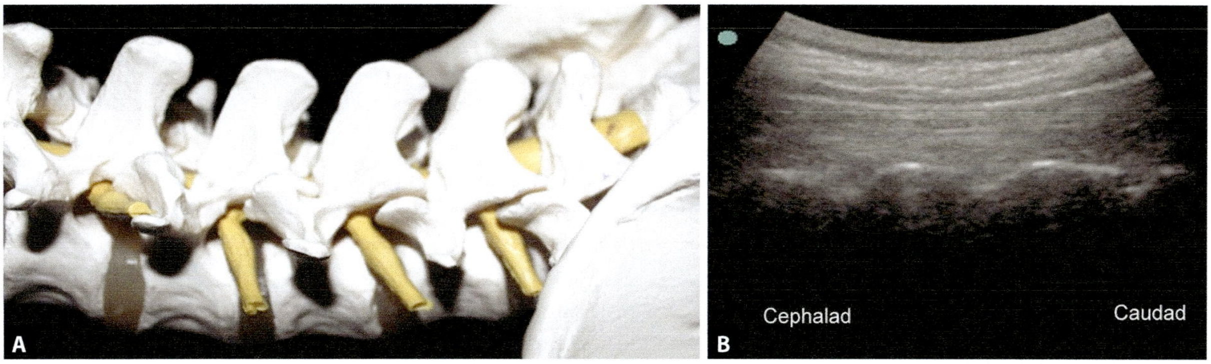

Figs. 4A and B: Lumbar spinous processes. (A) Transducer midline sagittal orientation over lumbar spine; (B) Ultrasonographic view of lumbar spine in midline.

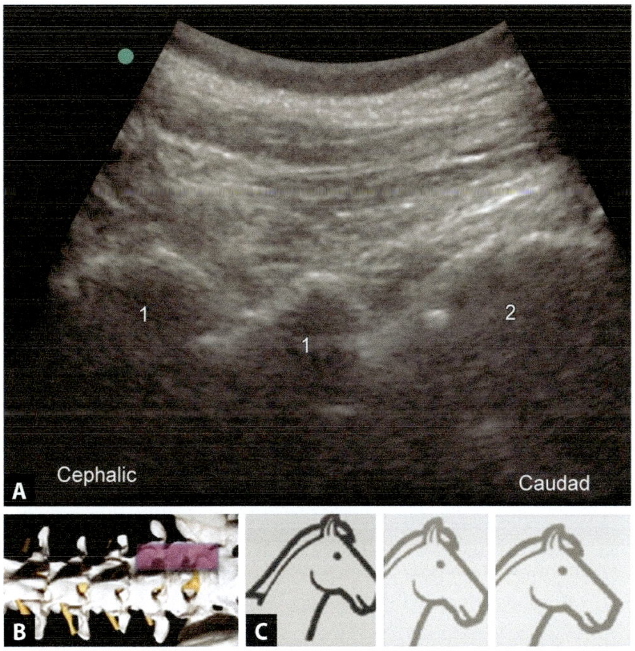

Figs. 5A to C: Lumbar laminar view. (A) Ultrasonographic view of lumbar spines; (B) Transducer in parasagittal position with slight medial oblique tilt; (C) "Horse-head" appearance. Lamina (1) and sacral ala (2).

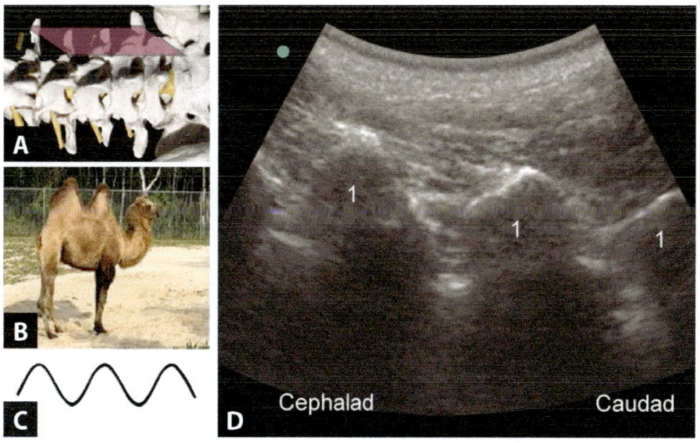

Figs. 6A to D: Lumbar facet view. (A) Transducer in vertical orientation parasagittal position; (B) "Camel-hump" appearance; (C) "Saw-tooth" appearance; (D) Ultrasonographic view of lumbar spine over the facet joints (1).

sacrum as a hyperechoic reflection and then, scan cephalad while counting the spinous processes to the required vertebral level. Over the spines, no satisfactory acoustic window is noticed **(Figs. 4A and B)**.

After ascertaining the level to be blocked, gently move the transducer laterally with a slight medial oblique tilt to show the laminae with a discontinuous "acoustic window". This produces "horse-head" appearance between the contiguous laminae by the hyperechoic reflections of ligamentum flavum and posterior longitudinal ligaments[2] **(Figs. 5A to C)**. Realigning the transducer into a sagittal orientation in a paramedian position over the laminae gives a "saw tooth" appearance. Just lateral to this, the facet joints formed by the superior and inferior articular processes appear as a "camel hump" **(Figs. 6A to D)**. Scanning further laterally reveals transverse processes (TP) as "trident" like discontinuous acoustic shadows with the psoas muscle in the acoustic window **(Figs. 7 and 8)**.

After identifying the desired level to block, turn the transducer into transverse orientation. Locate the spinous process, move into the interspinous space to visualize a "flying bat" appearance, formed by the articular processes and the TP. The target for the medial branch block is the angle formed by the SAP and the TP **(Figs. 9A and B)**.

After centralizing the SAP and TP, the needle is inserted in-plane and adjacent to the transducer directed into the angulation of the SAP and TP. After touching bone and confirming negative aspiration for blood or cerebrospinal

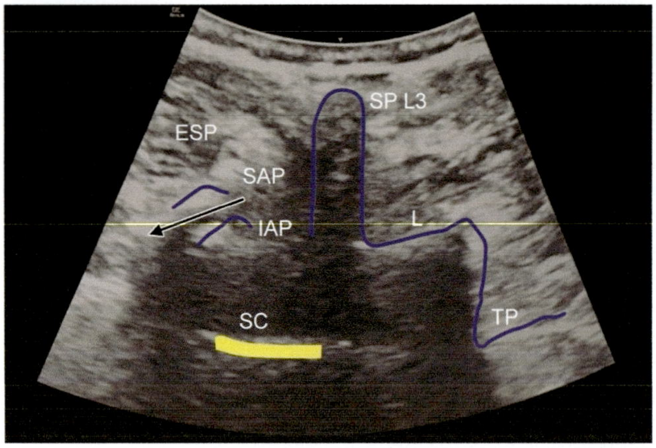

Fig. 7: Lumbar spinous process (SP), transverse process (TP).

fluid, 0.5 mL of chosen drug is injected while assessing its spread in real time.

L5 dorsal ramus anatomy and block: The dorsal ramus of L5 has a longer course. Instead of crossing the TP, its medial branch crosses the groove formed by the SAP and ala of the sacrum, before coursing medially around the base of the facet joint **(Fig. 10)**. The L5 dorsal ramus continues caudally over the posterior surface of sacrum to supply the sacroiliac joint. Performing an L5 dorsal ramus block under ultrasound guidance is technically more difficult due to its anatomical position and its depth from the skin **(Figs. 11A and B)**. An in-plane approach is followed, using a technique similar to the lumbar facet injection. Identification of the

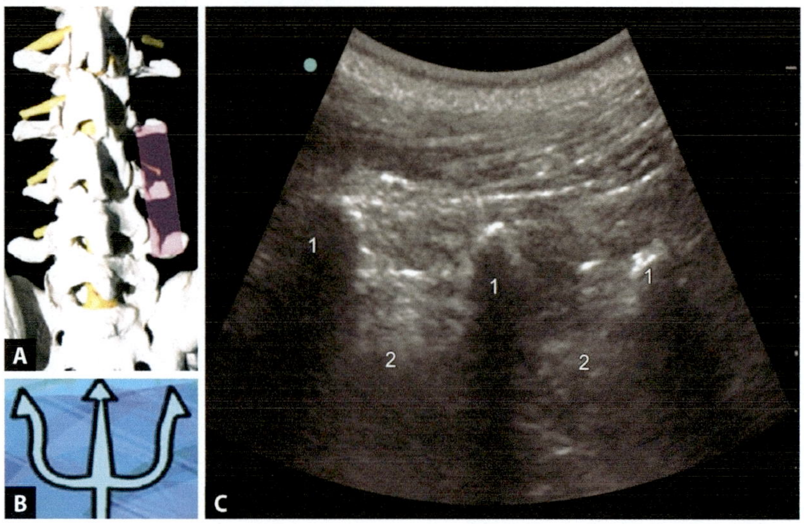

Figs. 8A to C: Lumbar transverse process (TP) view. (A) Transducer in vertical orientation parasagittal position; (B) "Trident" appearance; (C) Ultrasonographic view of lumbar spine over the TP (1) with psoas muscle (2) in the acoustic window.

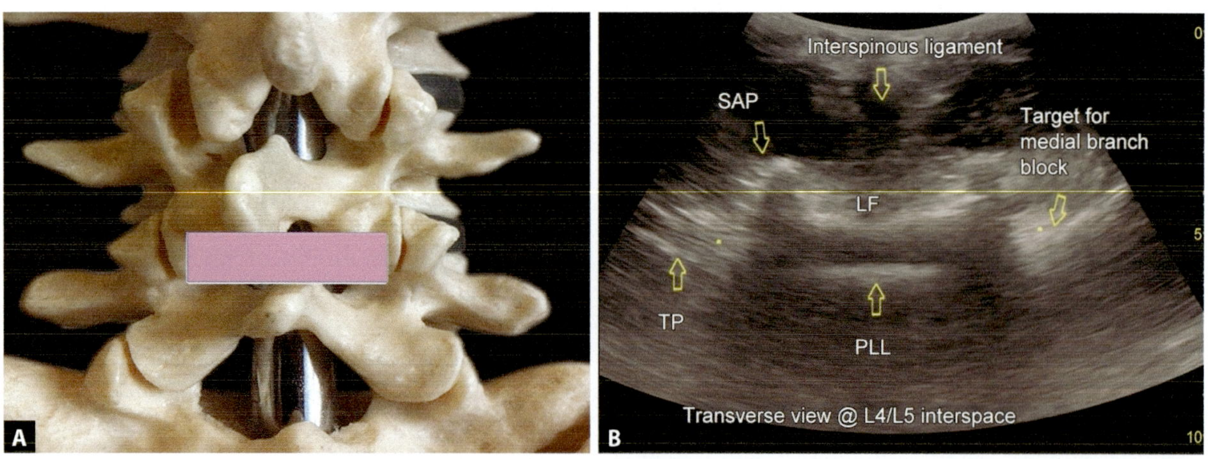

Figs. 9A and B: Lumbar facet medial branch L4/L5 level. (A) Transducer in horizontal orientation parasagittal position; (B) Ultrasonographic view of lumbar spine showing the location of the medial branch at the angle of the superior articular process (SAP) and transverse process (TP).

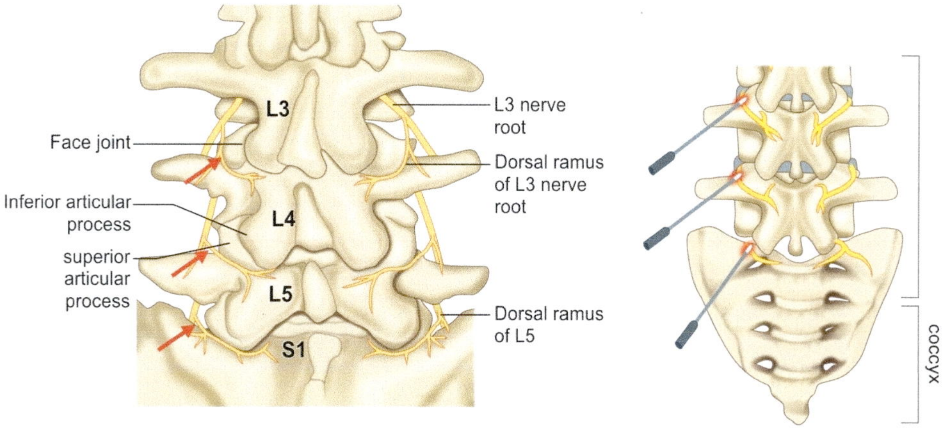

Fig. 10: Course of the L5 dorsal ramus branching into the medial branch to L5/S1 facet joint and also continuing to supply the sacroiliac joint laterally.

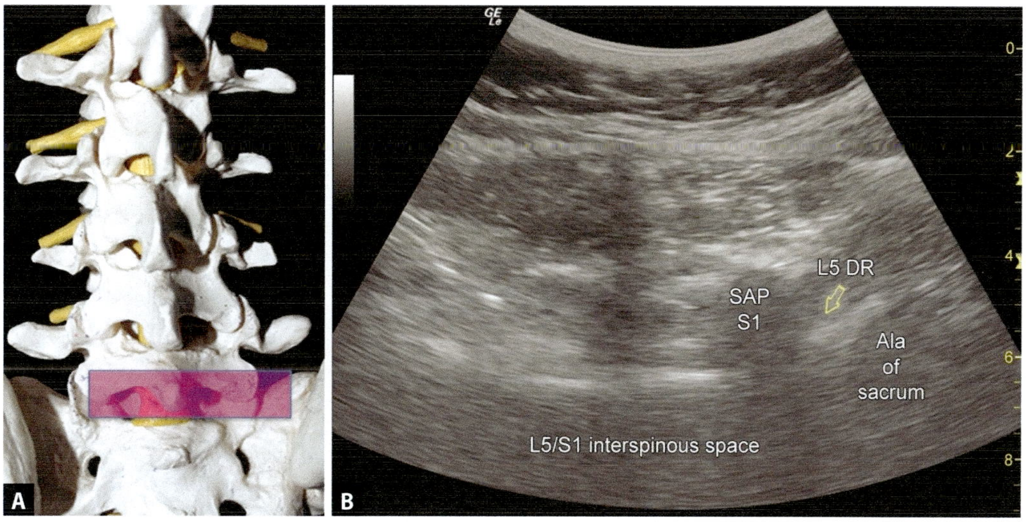

Figs. 11A and B: L5/S1 dorsal ramus branch. (A) Transducer in horizontal orientation parasagittal position; (B) Ultrasonographic view of lumbar sacral spine showing the location of the dorsal ramus branch at the angle of the SAP of S1 and ala of sacrum.

needle tip can be difficult sometimes. If the access to the SAP of the sacrum and sacral alar angle is obscured by the iliac crest, then an out-of-plane approach from a caudal direction can help reaching the target.

Limitations of USG:
- Utility of an ultrasound is limited in obese patients, degenerative spines, kyphoscoliosis, and with some anatomical variations.
- Ultrasound guidance cannot detect intravascular spread or inadvertent root blocks.

COMPLICATIONS

Some of the recognized complications include:
- Allergic reactions to the injected drugs
- Postprocedural pain
- Bruising
- Hematoma
- Intravascular injection
- Transient increase in blood sugar levels due to steroids
- Nerve damage and intrathecal injection.

CONCLUSION

Lumbar medial branch block under ultrasound guidance requires identification of anatomical structures. This may be difficult in obese individuals. L5 dorsal ramus block can be particularly difficult as the nerve lies farther from the skin. Ultrasound-guided lumbar medial branch block is preferably performed in an in-plane approach after identifying the level to be blocked in the sagittal plane.

REFERENCES

1. Laplante BL, DePalma MJ. Spine osteoarthritis. PM&R. 2012;4(Suppl 5):S28-36.
2. Karmakar MK, Ho AM, Li X, Kwok WH, Tsang K, Ngan Kee WD. Ultrasound-guided lumbar plexus block through the acoustic window of the lumbar ultrasound trident. Br J Anaesth. 2008;100(4):533-7.
3. Chin KJ, Karmakar MK, Peng P. Ultrasonography of the adult thoracic and lumbar spine for central neuraxial blockade. Anesthesiology. 2011;114(6):1459-85.

65 CHAPTER

Ultrasound-guided Sacroiliac Joint Injection

Kritika M Doshi, Surbhi Bhagat

ABSTRACT

The sacroiliac joint is a common cause of low back pain. A sacroiliac joint (SIJ) injection is a procedure to prove the clinical diagnosis of SIJ as the pain generator. Ultrasound-guided sacroiliac (SI) joint injection is a minimally invasive procedure performed to diagnose and treat pain originating from the sacroiliac joint using real-time ultrasound imaging to guide the accurate placement of a needle into the SI joint, ensuring precise delivery of corticosteroids and local anesthetic. Ultrasound guidance enhances precision, reduces the risk of complications, and avoids radiation exposure.

ANATOMY

Sacroiliac joint (SIJ) is a diarthrodial joint between the sacrum and the iliac bone. It supports the spine at the base of the vertebral column and forms an integral part of the pelvic girdle. The joint space is enclosed by a fibrous capsule and protected by strong ligaments **(Fig. 1)**, namely the anterior sacroiliac ligament arising from the anterior capsule and the posterior sacroiliac, sacrotuberous, and sacrospinous ligaments posteriorly. The muscular and fascial support of the SIJ is derived from the gluteus maximus and medius, the erector spinae, the latissimus dorsi and thoracolumbar fascia, the biceps femoris, the piriformis and oblique muscles, and the transversus abdominis. The gluteus maximus, biceps, and piriformis attach to the sacrotuberous ligament, while the thoracodorsal fascia connects to the remaining muscle groups.[1] This joint has synovium, especially at the superior and inferior aspects. Advancing age, intra-articular fibrosis, and large interdigitating osteophytes reduce the joint space.[2,3]

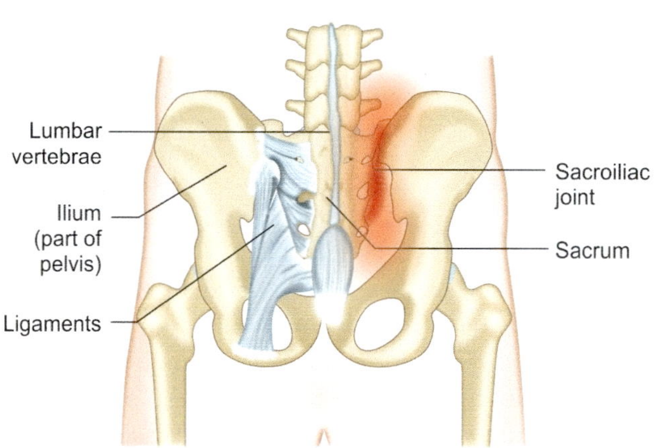

Fig. 1: Sacroiliac joint (SIJ) and its ligaments.

The innervation of the SIJ is complex. The posterior SIJ is predominantly innervated by lateral branches of the L4-S2 nerve roots with contributions from S3 and the superior gluteal nerve. The anterior SIJ innervation is from the L2-S2 segments.[4,5] The synovial capsule and ligaments contain free nerve endings as well as mechanoreceptors that transmit proprioceptive and pain sensation from the joint. Referral patterns from the SIJ pain are very variable due to the multiple nerves supplying the joint **(Figs. 2A and B)**.

Low back pain can arise from the SIJ since there is a wide variation in the nerve supply to the joint. Clinical and radiological tests help in the diagnosis of SIJ involvement, whereas a SIJ injection can confirm pain arising from the joint. Ultrasound guidance can be used to perform these injections.

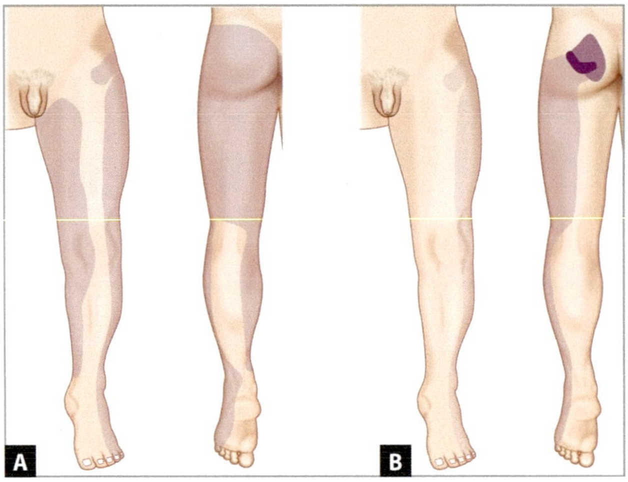

Figs. 2A and B: Pain referral from the sacroiliac joint. (A) Overall pain map and (B) Intensity map.
Source: Modified from vander wurff et al. (2006).

INDICATIONS

Sacroiliac joint is implicated in 17–30% cases of pain of lumbar origin.[6,7] Pain around the posterior superior iliac spines without pain near the ischial tuberosity may indicate SIJ pain.

Numerous clinical tests are described to aid early clinical decision-making and to reduce the number of unnecessary minimally invasive diagnostic SIJ procedures:

- The most commonly performed test for SIJ pain is Patrick's test. It is done by provoking pain in the SIJ by Flexion, Abduction, and External Rotation maneuver of the hip, hence also referred to as FABER test.
- *Thigh thrust test:* Patient is supine. The examiner places the hip in 90° flexion and adduction. The examiner then applies posteriorly directed force through the femur at varying angles of abduction/adduction. (Reproduction of buttock pain)
- *Gaenslen test:* Patient is supine with both legs extended. The test leg is passively brought into full knee flexion, while the opposite hip remains in extension. Overpressure is then applied to the flexed extremity. (Reproduction of pain)
- *Distraction test:* Patient is supine. The examiner applies posterolateral directed pressure to bilateral ASIS. (Reproduction of pain)
- *Compression test:* Patient lies on his painless side. The examiner compresses pelvis with pressure applied over the iliac crest directed at the opposite iliac crest. (Reproduction of symptoms)

Even though each individual tests lack specificity, SIJ pain is suggested when three or more of the five tests are positive with one of three positive results being thigh thrust or compression tests, in the absence of centralization of pain.[8-10] The pooled tests provide an overall sensitivity of 85% and specificity of 76%. When none of the tests are positive, SIJ pain is ruled out. As described above, since the clinical tests or radiological investigations do not confirm the SIJ as the pain generator, diagnostic injection in the SIJ has become the gold standard.

POSITION

Patient is positioned prone with a pillow under the hips.

SONOANATOMY

The linear or curvilinear transducer is placed on the middle of the sacrum at the level of the sacral hiatus in transverse orientation.

The two bony prominences of the sacral cornua are seen as acoustic shadows ("frog eye" appearance) **(Fig. 3)**. From here, the transducer is moved cranially paying attention to the lateral margin of the sacrum—the lateral edge of the sacrum is identified. Then the transducer is moved laterally and cephalad till the bony contour of the ileum is clearly identified **(Figs. 4 and 5)**. At the level of the SIJ, an acoustic window of the joint is identified between the acoustic shadows of the sacral bone medially and iliac bone laterally **(Figs. 6 to 8)**.

TECHNIQUE

Accurate intra-articular needle placement and drug injection can be facilitated by ultrasound guidance. A block needle is inserted in plane into the joint space (acoustic window) from the medial end of the transducer. The volume of the SIJ is 0.5–1 mL. A small volume of local anesthetic is injected under all aseptic precautions for a diagnostic block.

LIMITATIONS

The potential for periarticular rather than intra-articular injection may be increased compared to fluoroscopic or CT-guided SIJ injections because an arthrogram with contrast agent injection can be reliably obtained in most cases with the latter technique. Also, ultrasound is not very reliable in detecting intravascular injection while performing SIJ injections. Due to the irregular shape of the

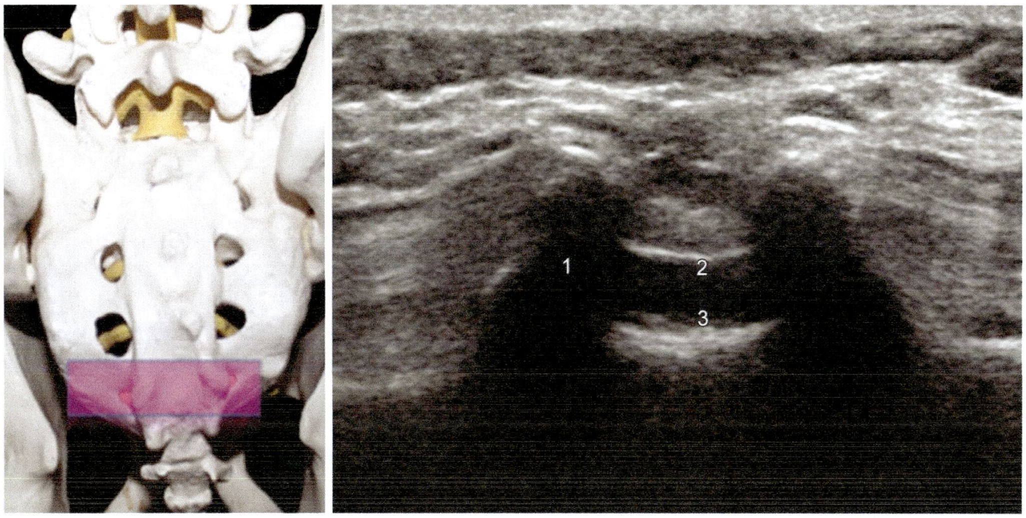

Fig. 3: Sacral cornu seen as "frog eye" on USG.

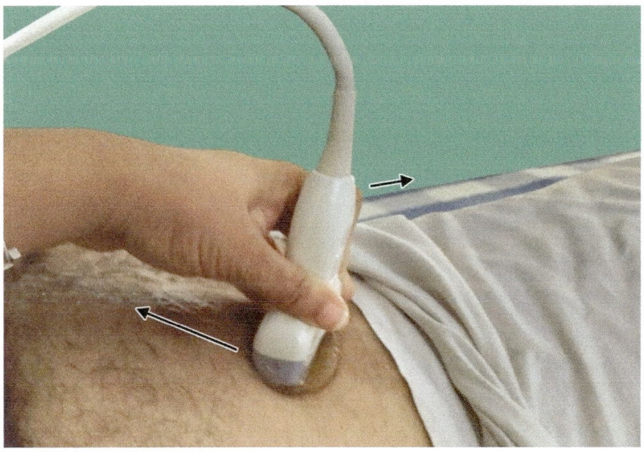

Fig. 4: Transducer moved cranially.

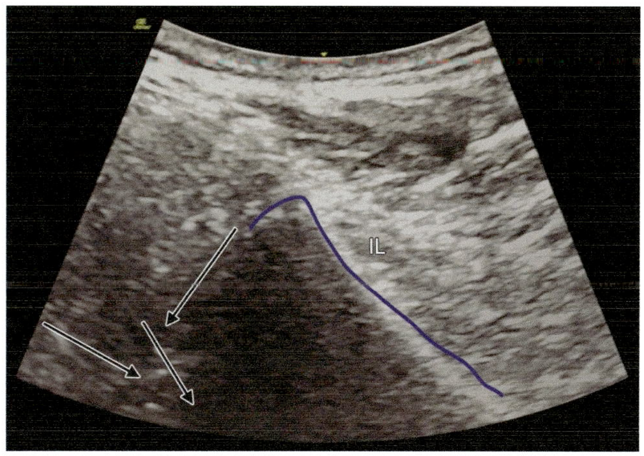

Fig. 5: Contour of ileum (IL) identified.

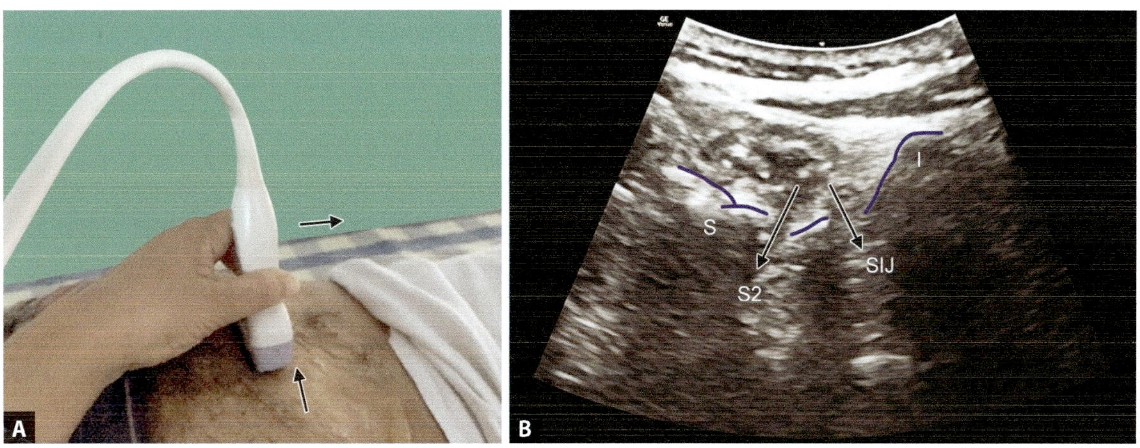

Figs. 6A and B: Acoustic window of the joint is identified between the acoustic shadows of the sacral bone medially and iliac bone laterally.

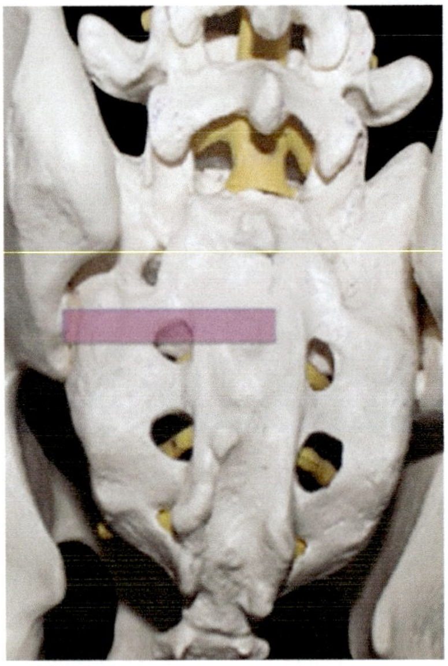

Fig. 7: Probe placement at S2.

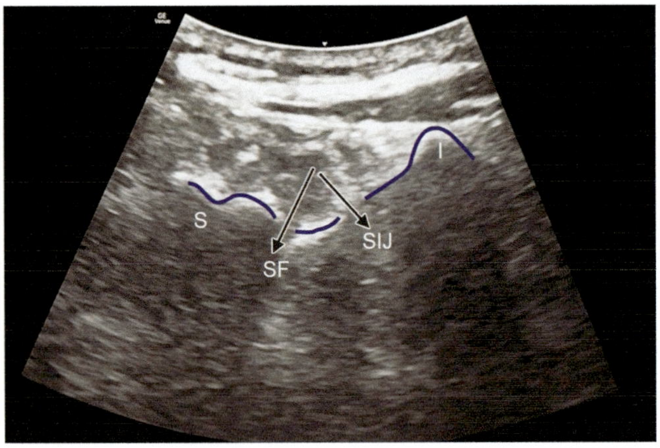

Fig. 8: USG image at S2. (I: iliac bone; SF: sacral foramen; S: sacrum; SIJ: sacroiliac joint)

SIJ, real-time visualization of the spread of the medication is not possible during ultrasound-guided SIJ injection.

COMPLICATIONS

Some of the common complications include:

- Allergic reactions to the injected drugs
- Postprocedural pain
- Bruising
- Hematoma
- Intravascular injection
- Transient increase in blood sugar levels due to steroids
- Nerve damage

CONCLUSION

Ultrasound-guided SIJ injections should be performed under strict aseptic precautions. They are diagnostic of pain arising from the SIJ. Identification of the anatomical structures is important in performing a successful injection.

REFERENCES

1. Vydyanathan A, Narouze SN. Ultrasound-guided sacroiliac joint injection. In: Narouze S (Ed). Atlas of Ultrasound-Guided Procedures in Interventional Pain Management. New York: Springer; 2018.
2. Bowen V, Cassidy JD. Macroscopic and microscopic anatomy of the sacroiliac joint from embryonic life until the eighth decade. Spine. 1981;6(6):620-8.
3. Dreyfuss P, Dreyer SJ, Cole A, Mayo K. Sacroiliac joint pain. J Am Acad Orthop Surg. 2004;12(4):255-65.
4. Ikeda R. Innervation of the sacroiliacjoint. Macroscopical and histologicalstudies. Nihon Ika Daigaku Zasshi. 1991;58:587-96.
5. Horwitz M. The anatomy of (A) the lumbosacral nerve plexus—its relation to variations of vertebral segmentation, and (B), the posterior sacral nerve plexus. Anat Rec. 1939;74:91-107.
6. Slipman C, Whyte W, Chow D, Chou L, Lenrow D, Ellen M. Sacroiliac join syndrome. Pain Physician. 2001;4(2):143-52.
7. Bernard TN Jr, Kirkaldy-Willis WH. Recognizing specific characteristics of nonspecific low back pain. Clin Orthop Relat Res. 1987;217:266-80.
8. Szadek KM, van der Wurff P, van Tulder MW, Zuurmond WW, Perez RS. Diagnostic validity of criteria for sacroiliac joint pain: a systematic review. J Pain. 2009;10(4):354-68.
9. Laslett M, Aprill CN, McDonald B, Young SB. Diagnosis of sacroiliac joint pain: validity of individual provocation tests and composites of tests. Man Ther. 2005;10(3):207-18.
10. Laslett M. Evidence-based diagnosis and treatment of the painful sacroiliac joint. J Man Manip Ther. 2008;16(3):142-52.

66 CHAPTER

Ultrasound-guided Hip Injections

Madouna G Hanna, Edward Papa, Steve M Aydin

ABSTRACT

The hip joint is often the driver of pain in the groin area. Its symptoms can develop from inflammation or degeneration of the joint or other structures that support it. It is an extremely stable joint. When the joint is painful for a patient, it can limit ambulation and functions. Many times, evaluation can be done with X-ray and treatment, if indicated with an injection, can be done with fluoroscopic guidance. With the use of ultrasound, evaluation of the joint and soft tissues around can be visualized. This helps to limit the need for a fluoroscope, reduces radiation exposure to patients, as well as may help avoid neurovascular structures, which can be marked and avoided by ultrasound evaluation.

INTRODUCTION

Intra-articular hip injections are challenging due to the difficulty of palpating the hip joint secondary to its deep anatomic location in the body. In addition, the femoral nerve, artery, and veins lie in close proximity to the anterior hip joint. As a result, image guidance is typically recommended. Over the last decade, ultrasound has proven to be a useful tool in the assessment of tendons, ligaments, muscles, nerves, and joint capsules.[1] The goals of ultrasound imaging are to detect and localize pathological processes, to differentiate between intra-articular and extra-articular pathology, to perform diagnostic and therapeutic interventional procedures, and to monitor the efficacy of therapy. High-resolution ultrasound of the hip is commonly used for the assessment of hip pathology as well as direct visualization of the joint for guided procedures in the joint and periarticular soft tissues.[2]

ANATOMY

Each hip bone consists of three separate bones—the ileum, ischium, and pubis that are fused in the adult, and it is difficult to see any signs of their junction. All three elements help form the deep receptacle for the head of the femur, the acetabulum. The bone of the thigh, the femur, has a rounded upper end, or head, that is attached to the shaft by a neck that does not continue in the direction of the shaft but rather projects medially at an angle of inclination. A large protuberance, the greater trochanter, projects upward where the neck joins the shaft.[3] On the posteromedial side at the junction of the neck and shaft is a smaller protuberance, the lesser trochanter. The acetabulum receives the rounded head of the femur to form the hip joint, which is the best example in the body of a ball-and-socket joint. The smooth articular surface of the head of the femur occupies considerably more than a hemisphere and ends at the neck, but it is interrupted at one point by a pit, or fovea, into which the ligament of the head of the femur attaches. The acetabulum is made deeper by a fibrocartilaginous mass, the acetabular labrum, attached to its edge.[4]

The joint capsule of the hip joint is very strong. It attaches lower on the anterior femur than it does posteriorly. The capsule is composed mainly of longitudinally oriented fibers. The most prominent features of the capsule are three thickenings, the iliofemoral, pubofemoral, and ischiofemoral ligaments, that run a somewhat spiral course from the hip bone to the femur.[5] The iliofemoral ligament is attached to the ileum below the anterior inferior iliac spine and covers most of the front of the joint. It is shaped like an inverted Y, also known as the "ligament of Bigelow".

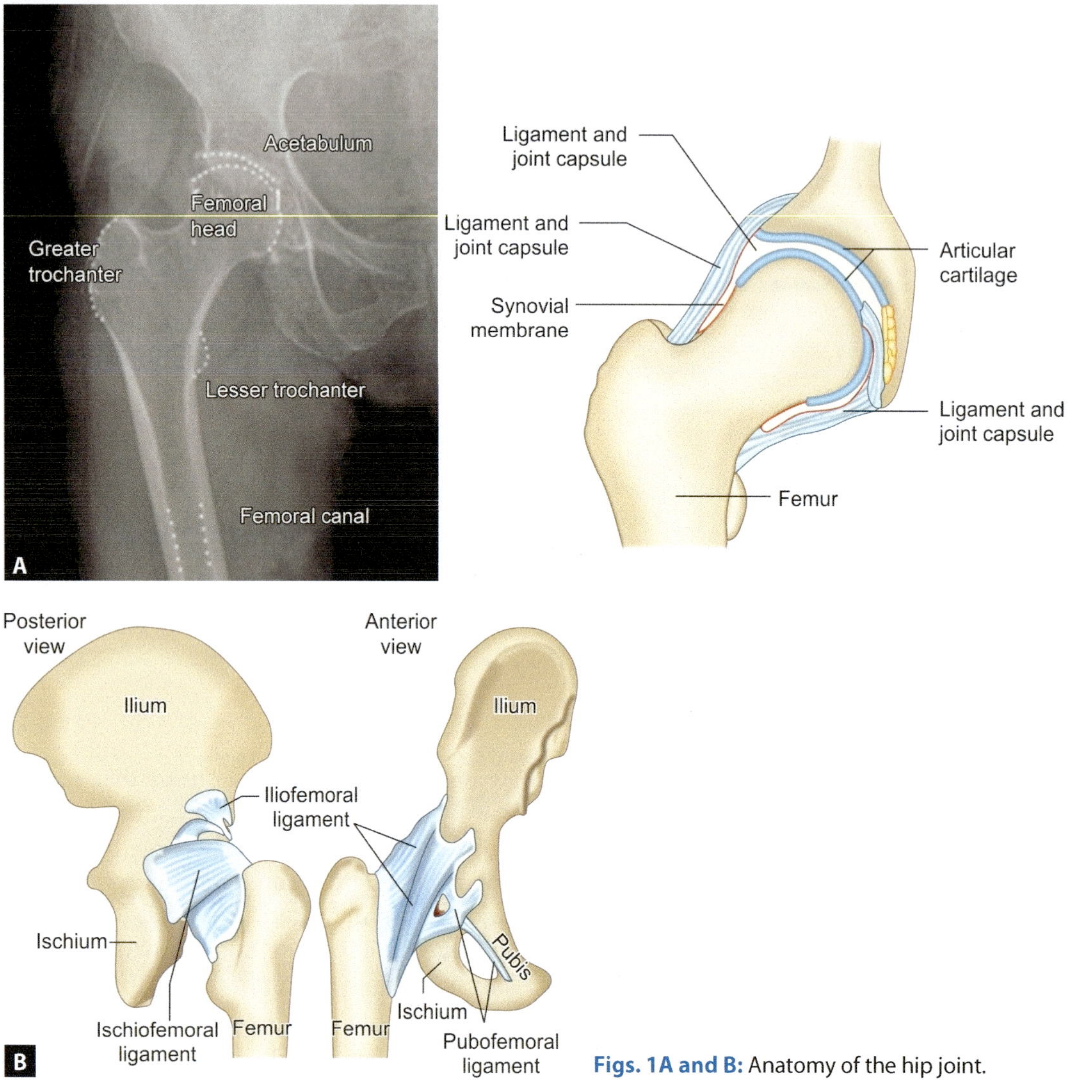

Figs. 1A and B: Anatomy of the hip joint.

The special function of this ligament is the maintenance of the erect posture without constant muscular action **(Figs. 1A and B)**.

INDICATIONS

Since hip pain is a common symptom with a number of possible causes, ultrasound of the hip joint is a commonly performed investigation used to guide intervention around the hip joint for both diagnostic and therapeutic purposes, after a focused history and physical examinations are performed. Injections of the hip joint are undertaken for a variety of reasons. Ultrasound is the imaging modality of choice for detection of fluid collections inside the hip joint, with osteoarthritis being the most common cause of effusions. In patients with osteoarthritis, ultrasound can demonstrate thickening of the joint capsule due to fibrotic change, with anterior osteophytes visualized as hyperechoic projections arising from the junction between the head and the neck of the femur.[1,6]

Although for many decades, fluoroscopic guidance has been the standard for intra-articular hip injections, due to its disadvantages, ultrasound has been more recently accepted as the routine method for injections. Compared with fluoroscopy, ultrasound produces no radiation and does not require contrast. Also, ultrasound offers good visualization of the joint cavity, possibility of multiple joint scanning, speed of performance, rapid side-to-side anatomic comparison, relative low cost as well as dynamic real-time study of multiple planes.[7]

CONTRAINDICATIONS

There are no risks or contraindications to the use of ultrasound guidance in hip injections, but a careful attention should be paid to an antiseptic approach. Bleeding into the joint is minimized by ensuring the international normalized ratio is below 1.5. Patients on anticoagulation therapy should be advised to stop the therapy before the procedure is performed. Also, allergy status should be reviewed, since an allergic reaction to the local anesthetic may present with systemic symptoms of headaches, dizziness, tachycardia, and local symptoms related to nerve damage.[5,8]

EQUIPMENT

Either a portable ultrasound unit with 4–15 MHz linear array transducer or a compact ultrasound machine with a 6–12 MHz, 40 mm long linear array transducer, and standard B-mode imaging can be used. Hip injections are typically performed with the transducer frequency set at 9 or 12 MHz. The 12 MHz setting provides better spatial resolution than the 9 MHz setting but with less penetration. The image is optimized with the use of appropriate depth and focal zones.[4]

Intra-articular hip injections are performed under aseptic conditions. A 27G needle is usually used to anesthetize the skin and superficial tissues with 2 mL of 1% lidocaine. A 22G spinal needle is then advanced into the joint capsule at the femoral head-neck junction. For hip joint aspiration, a larger bore needle, such as 16 or 18 g may be needed.

The instilled material for intra-articular hip injections usually consists of a standard volume of 7 mL: 4 mL of 0.25% bupivacaine and 3 mL of 1% lidocaine or 4 mL of 0.25% bupivacaine, 2 mL of 1% lidocaine, and 1 mL of 40 mg/1 mL methylprednisolone acetate or 40 mg/1 mL of triamcinolone.

PROCEDURE

Intra-articular Hip Injection/Aspiration

Informed consent must be obtained. Patients should be informed of the risk of infection and bleeding as potential complications. They should be made aware that signs of infection may present as ongoing or worsening symptoms accompanied by redness and swelling around the joint.

The patient is placed in the supine position with the hip in neutral or slight internal rotation. The anterior superior iliac spine (ASIS) is palpated, and the long linear array transducer is oriented in a sagittal plane with the superior end just medial to the ASIS. While the sagittal orientation is maintained, the transducer is moved medially until the hyperechoic (i.e., bright) rounded surface of the femoral head is visualized. The penetration depth and transducer orientation are next adjusted to an optimal view of the anterior hip joint, including the anterior labrum. The transducer is then rotated into the transverse plane and moved medially to clearly identify the femoral nerve and vessels using the color Doppler. After confirming the position of the neurovascular structures, the transducer is moved back to the anterior hip joint in the sagittal plane, and the inferior end of the transducer is then rotated laterally while maintaining the superior portion on the femoral head. After the inferior transducer is rotated approximately 30° laterally, the femoral neck should come into view. In this long-axis femoral head-neck view, the ultrasound settings (gain setting, time gain compensation) and transducer orientation are optimized to provide a clear picture of the target the femoral head-neck junction, and overlying hyperechoic iliofemoral ligament and hip capsule. Maintaining this orientation, the examiner sweeps the transducer slightly superolaterally, while keeping both the head and neck in view, to place the transducer as far laterally on the head-neck junction as possible. At this point, the skin at the inferior end of the transducer is marked with an indelible ink marker.[7]

Before the area is prepared, any excess ultrasound gel needs to be removed from the side of the transducer closest to the planned needle insertion site with the use of gauze and then alcohol swabs. Also, it should be ensured that the skin entry site is at least 4 cm from the transducer and that no contact with the transducer or gel occurs.[6]

Next, sterile gloves are donned by the physician and sterile technique is used. The "needle hand" must remain sterile throughout the procedure. The skin entry site is then triple prepped with chlorhexidine alcohol swab covering an 8–10 cm diameter region.

When first performing this technique, a sterile probe cover and a thin layer of sterile gel should be used. With the transducer repositioned to once again visualize the head-neck junction, a 27G needle is used to anesthetize the skin and superficial tissues with 2 mL of 1% lidocaine.

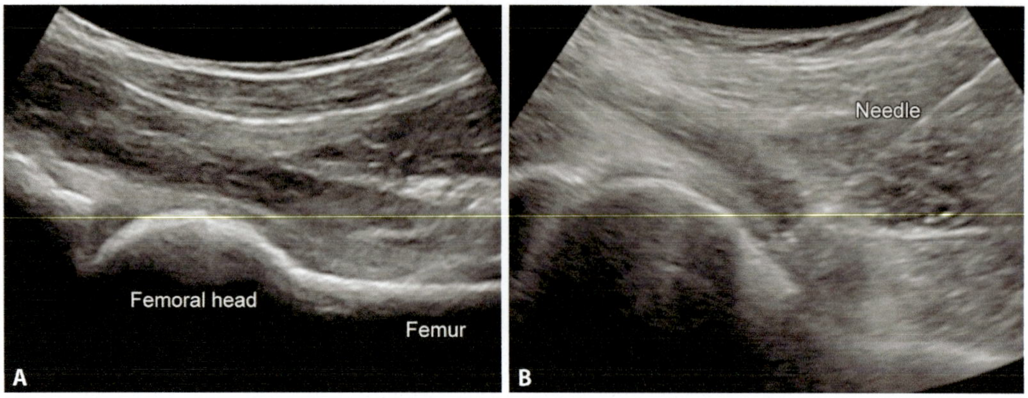

Figs. 2A and B: Ultrasound evaluation and needle placement of the hip joint.

Next, a 22G spinal needle with stylet (3.5 or 6 inches) should be slowly advanced down to the target site at the femoral head-neck junction under the inguinal ligament toward the anterior or inferior capsule below the femoral head via the use of the long-axis (in-plane) approach. A slight increase in resistance is appreciated as the needle reaches the iliofemoral ligament. With further advance, the needle can be felt to pop through the ligament and enter the hip joint. If the patient has a joint effusion, this can be visualized and aspirated if necessary, in order to offer relief of symptoms and send fluid for culture and sensitivity to screen for possible infectious/inflammatory etiology.[7]

Direct visualization of the needle tip and a test injection of 1–2 mL of local anesthetic or normal saline confirms intra-articular placement. On this scan, when the needle is perpendicular to the ultrasound beam, it appears as a sharply defined echoic band with strong posterior reverberations. Any further injectate (local anesthetic or local anesthetic and corticosteroid) is then delivered while visualizing the capsular distention with ultrasound. Fluid appears anechoic (i.e., dark) on ultrasound, and therefore, as the hip is injected, the relatively hyperechoic iliofemoral ligament and anterior hip capsule can be visualized peeling away from the femoral neck and head.[8]

After delivery of the injectate, the needle is removed, the area is cleaned, a small bandage applied, and postinjection care follows the standard protocols **(Figs. 2A and B)**.

Greater Trochanteric Bursa Injection

The trochanteric bursa is best approached with the patient lying in the lateral decubitus position with the symptomatic hip up, and hips and knees gently flexed in a position of comfort. The bursa is relatively superficial structure and therefore, readily accessible. With the transducer in the transverse plane perpendicular to the long axis of the femur, the patient's site of maximal pain over the gluteus medius insertion on the greater trochanter is localized and marked along the posterior aspect of the transducer. Both axial and sagittal imaging will show fluid within the bursa secondary to inflammation. Once again, the overlying skin should be prepared and draped in a sterile manner as mentioned previously. Anesthetize the superficial and deep soft tissues with buffered 1% lidocaine. Under ultrasound guidance, a 22G, 3.5 inches needle is directed in plane with the transducer from posterior to anterior and placed within the peritendinous soft tissues of the greater trochanter. The transducer is positioned in the longitudinal plane in relation to the greater trochanter. A combination of local anesthetic and steroids (typically 40 mg triamcinolone) should be prepared and injected into the fluid collection. After delivery of the injectate, the needle is removed and the area is cleaned **(Figs. 3A to C)**.[5,7]

POSTPROCEDURAL CARE AND EVALUATION

The procedures can be completed in 10–15 minutes, depending on the extent of the preinjection diagnostic scan and the technical challenges of an individual patient. Immobilization after injection is not necessary, but the examiner should recommend the patient to keep the joint relatively immobile for maximizing the therapeutic effect of the injected drugs and reduce their possible diffusion into the adjacent tissues. The patient should be warned that there might be an aching sensation in the hip in the 24 hours after injection, and when cortisone has been

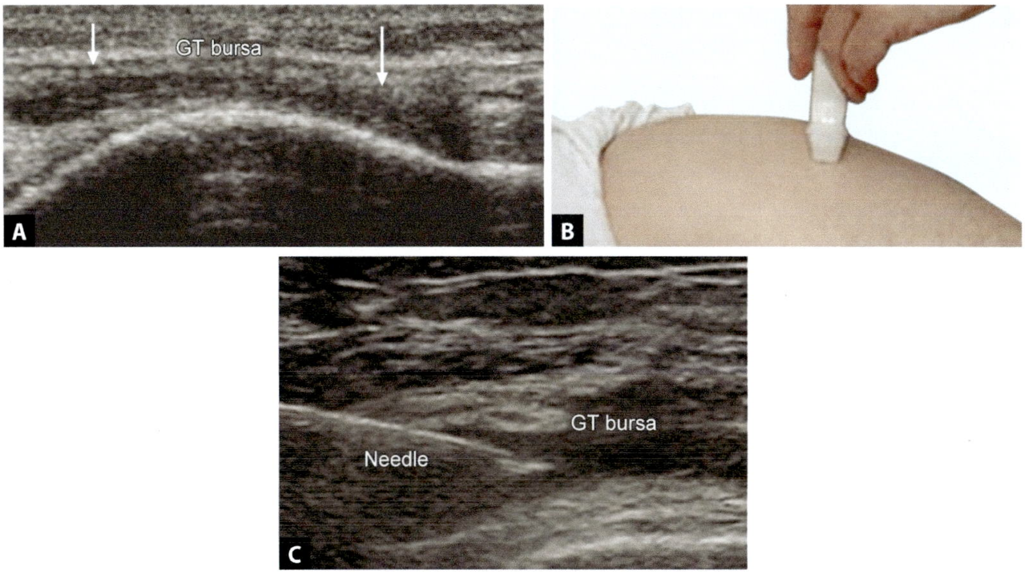

Figs. 3A to C: GT bursa ultrasound view and needle placement. (GT bursa: greater trochanteric bursa)

injected, the maximal therapeutic benefit may not be experienced for several days after the procedure.[7,8]

CONCLUSION

High-frequency ultrasound is a bedside diagnostic/therapeutic tool that can be used for patients with hip pain and limited range of motion. As was shown throughout this chapter, ultrasound is an ideal method for guiding interventional intra-articular hip injections in an office setting with a compact, portable, and affordable equipment. The procedure is safe, with no serious complications or risk of exposure to ionizing radiation, which makes it applicable across a broad patient population, including adolescent and pregnant patients. Most importantly, it allows the physician to identify and avoid important neurovascular structures and ensure accurate placement of the needle intra-articularly. Nevertheless, performing an ultrasound-guided hip injection requires an intermediate level of skill at a minimum.

REFERENCES

1. David JB. Functional Anatomy of the Limbs and Back, 9th edition. Canada: Saunders/Elsevier; 2009. pp. 245-57.
2. Nestorova R, Vlad V, Petranova T, Porta F, Radunovic G, Micu MC, et al. Ultrasonography of the hip. Med Ultrasono. 2012;14(3):217-24.
3. Sofka CM, Saboeiro G, Adler RS. Ultrasound-guided adult hip injections. J Vasc Interv Radiol. 2005;16:1121-3.
4. Rowbotham EL, Grainger AJ. Ultrasound-guided intervention around the hip joint. Am J Roentgenol. 2011;197:W122-7.
5. Smith J, Hurdle MF. Office-based ultrasound-guided intra-articular hip injection: technique for physiatric practice. Arch Phys Med Rehabil. 2006;87(2):296-8.
6. Byrd JW, Potts EA, Allison RK, Jones KS. Ultrasound-guided hip injections: a comparative study with fluoroscopy-guided injections. Arthroscopy. 2014;30(1):42-6.
7. Levi DS. Intra-articular hip injections using ultrasound guidance: accuracy using a linear array transducer. PM R. 2013;5(2):129-34.
8. Carson BW, Wong A. Ultrasonographic guidance for injections of local steroids in the native hip. J Ultrasound Med. 1999;18(2):159-60.

67 CHAPTER

Ultrasound-guided Knee Injections

Edward Papa, Steve M Aydin

ABSTRACT

Knee pain is one of the most common joint pains that patients will present with. In the older population, it is the number one degenerative joint complaint patients will seek medical care for. Intra-articular knee injections can be used primarily for the treatment of osteoarthritis of the knee and help palliate the pain and allow patients to return to previous level of function. There are currently two different approaches to treat osteoarthritis of the knee with injections. There is a variety of approaches and compositions to inject into the knee. We will discuss primarily the technique and approach of providing an effective knee injection.

INTRODUCTION

Intra-articular knee injections are used primarily for the treatment of osteoarthritis (OA) of the knee. There are currently two different approaches to treat OA of the knee with injections. The first is by injecting a local anesthetic along with a corticosteroid with the primary goal of decreasing inflammation and thus reducing pain in the joint. The second treatment option is injecting hyaluronic acid into the joint in order to increase joint lubrication and reduce pain.[1]

ANATOMY

The knee is a synovial hinge joint; it is formed by the interaction of the femur and tibia on each other.

The knee joint is covered by a joint capsule that does not form a complete covering around the joint. The capsule covering is replaced anteriorly by the insertion of the quadriceps muscle on the patella, the patella itself, and the patellar ligament. On the sides of the quadriceps tendon, between the patella and the tibial and femoral condyles are the medial and lateral patellar retinacula, which are fibers from the deep fascia of the thigh and expansions from the quadriceps tendon.

The joint cavity of the knee starts inferiorly below the patella and between the femur and tibia and continues proximally anterior to the femur between the femur and quadriceps muscle and is continuous with the suprapatellar bursa. The knee joint can further be divided into medial and lateral parts that communicate with each other only anteriorly and are separated by the cruciate ligaments. Within the joint are two semilunar, wedge-shaped cartilages, the medial and lateral menisci.[2] The inner layers are continuous with the joint capsule, whereas the outer layer of menisci is attached to the synovial and fibrous layers of the joint capsule **(Fig. 1)**.

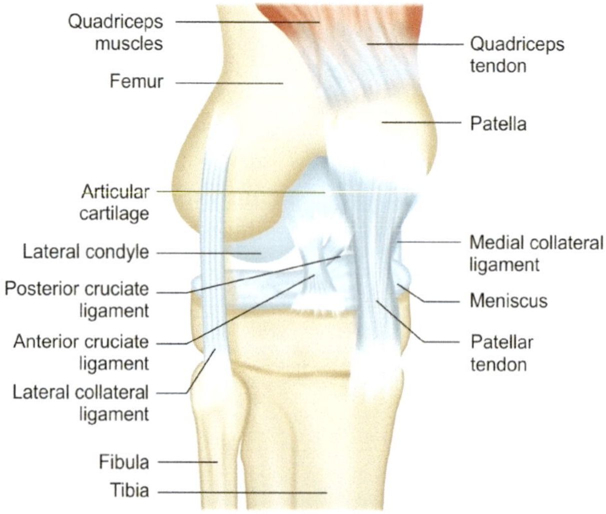

Fig. 1: Anatomy of the knee joint.

INDICATIONS

It is important to know for knee injections that the pain is arising from the knee joint and not from a joint above or below or radiating pain into the knee. OA is the biggest indicator for intra-articular knee injections. Both corticosteroids and viscosupplementation with high molecular weight hyaluronic acid are indicated for knee injections in individuals with knee OA, multi-joint OA, and OA with multiple comorbidities. It has been shown that intra-articular corticosteroid injections are more effective at short-term pain relief of knee pain with the greatest benefit at 2 weeks. Whereas, viscosupplementation with hyaluronic acid was more effective for long-term relief of knee pain with significant pain reduction at 4 weeks, peak at 8 weeks, and a residual benefit up to 24 weeks post injection.[3]

History and physical examination may give us an idea if the pain is arising from the knee joint. Pain is one of the top complaints with pain localized to the knee and worse with increased usage. Joint stiffness is also noted, more commonly in the morning and improves after movement. Swelling can also be present from an effusion within the joint or commonly in the suprapatellar bursa. Crepitis and positive patellar grind test may lead to the diagnosis of knee OA. Other indications of knee OA are bony enlargement and bony tenderness. You can further confirm diagnosis by obtaining knee radiographs and severity can be graded using the Kellgren-Lawrence grading scale, which grades severity based on joint space architecture, osteophyte severity, and amount of sclerosis.[1]

CONTRAINDICATIONS

Systemic or localized bacterial infections, total knee replacements, uncontrolled coagulopathy, hemarthrosis, and allergy to the medication.[2]

EQUIPMENT

- Ultrasound is optional but has been shown to have increased accuracy and decreased risk of complications. Use a linear transducer with 6–12 MHz.
- The procedure is performed under aseptic or sterile conditions.
- 21 or 23 G, 1.5–3.5 inches hypodermic needles, and 5 or 10 mL syringes are preferred.
- Intravenous solutions, sedation, or antibiotics are not required.
- Lidocaine (1%) is used with depo-medrol for corticosteroid injection.
- High-molecular-weight hyaluronic acid for viscosupplementation.

PROCEDURE

Information about the location and severity of the patient's knee pain should be obtained prior to the injection. Movements and activities of daily living that can exacerbate pain should also be documented in order to know how the patient responded to the injection.

Informed consent needs to be obtained. The patient should be explained the risks of infection, bleeding, and allergic reaction from the injection procedure.

There are six different approaches to aspirate and inject either lidocaine with corticosteroids or hyaluronic acid viscosupplementation into the knee. The six portals include the lateral and medial mid-patellar, superolateral, superomedial, anterolateral, and anteromedial. All injections should be performed with aseptic technique. An ultrasound machine can also be utilized, using the free-hand technique with the needle in plane with the ultrasound probe, allowing the physician to visualize the needle tip as it travels through the knee tissue into the joint space, thus reducing the risk of a traumatic injection. Injections under ultrasound have been shown to have significantly greater accuracy over blind intra-articular knee injections, as well as lower rate of traumatic injection.

For the medial and lateral mid-patellar approach, the patient is supine with the knee fully extended. Then use the ultrasound machine to locate an adequate portal by having the probe parallel to the patella and shifting the ultrasound probe up and down examining the articular surfaces of the patellofemoral joint, which is located just lateral or medial to the middle of the patella. An adequate portal can be selected with an intra-articular space with less of a fat pad. For both approaches the ultrasound probe is visualizing the portal and the needle is inserted just below the probe and visualized entering the portal and joint. In a blind medial injection, the needle enters the medial aspect of the knee joint under the middle of the patella (mid-pole), and is directed toward the lateral patellar mid-pole, while your free hand is putting pressure on the lateral patella medially to open the portal. For the lateral blind injection the needle is directed at 45° toward the middle of the medial aspect of the joint, while the free hand is on the medial aspect of the patella pushing medially to open the joint.[3] Even though the most common site of entry to the knee is mid-patellar, the superolateral and superomedial approaches can be used if those poles have an abundance of patellofemoral arthritis or if there is a large effusion in the suprapatellar bursa.[1] The technique is performed with the patient supine and the knee extended. Locate the pole of entry for needle placement superior to the patella and either lateral or medial to the quadriceps tendon. Hold the ultrasound probe in a mid-longitudinal position, locating the tendons of the quadriceps and the suprapatellar bursa. Insert the needle allowing the needle to pass underneath the articular surface of the patella while aiming for the suprapatellar pouch. Under ultrasound follow the needle tip into the suprapatellar bursa **(Figs. 2A and B)**.

Anterolateral and anteromedial portal approaches are useful in patients who cannot fully extend their knee. With the knee flexed to 90° locate the pole either medial or lateral to the patellar tendon and inferior to the patella. Use the ultrasound probe in a mid-longitudinal position to accurately locate the needle tip. Then insert the needle directing it upward toward the femoral notch.[2] The approach traverses Hoffa's fat pad, which can be localized with ultrasound. The ultrasound can monitor the needle tip in order to avoid hitting the anterior horns of the menisci and transverse patellar ligaments **(Figs. 3A and B)**.

Once the needle tip is in the joint space, using the attached connector and syringe, attempt to aspirate the fluid out of joint space. If there is an assistant present, he/she can milk the joint to remove more fluid. Once all fluid is removed, disconnect the syringe. Then, take your prepared syringe of either hyaluronic acid or corticosteroid with lidocaine and connect it to your needle setup, and inject the medication. If using an ultrasound machine, you can use a 3-way stop cock connector and aspirate with an empty syringe, then close that syringe off and open the

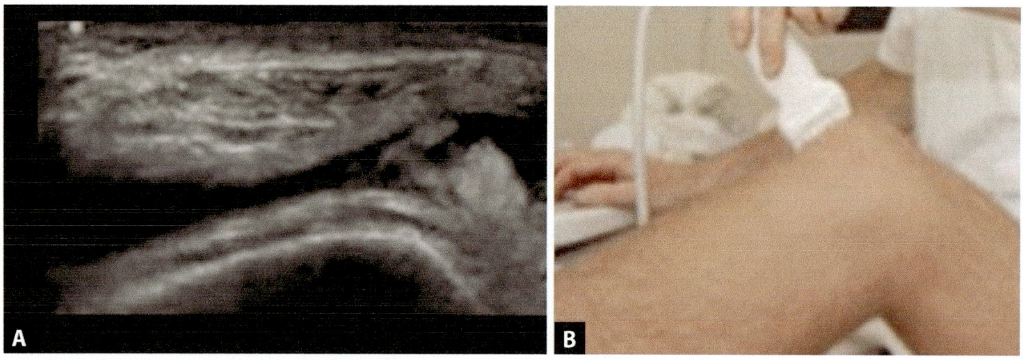

Figs. 2A and B: This is the suprapatellar approach, and evaluation with ultrasound of the knee.

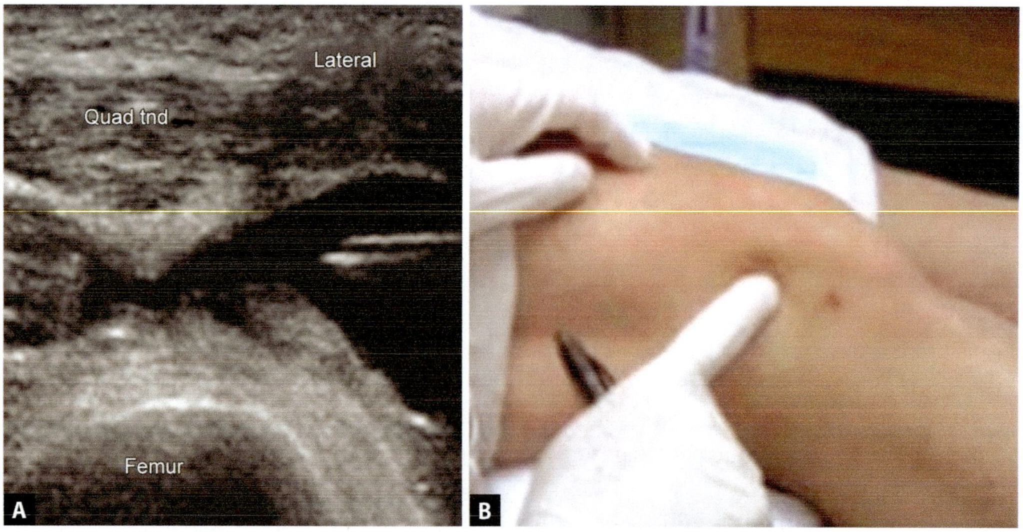

Figs. 3A and B: This is the ultrasound lateral approach of the knee injection.

syringe with your medication and inject the medication all while holding your probe with the other hand. While injecting the medication you can confirm injection accuracy with color Doppler analyzing the direction of drug injected.[2]

POSTPROCEDURAL CARE

After the knee joint is injected, apply pressure to the injection site to prevent hematoma formation. Ask the patient to move his/her leg up and down in order to move the medication throughout the knee joint. If lidocaine with steroid was injected, ask the patient if there was a significant pain reduction to assess the success of the injection.[1]

CONCLUSION

Both intra-articular knee injections of lidocaine with corticosteroid and hyaluronic acid for OA are frontline treatments to provide pain reduction and improved quality of life. Both can be performed blind or with an ultrasound machine. Accuracy results vary, but overall accuracy is improved when using ultrasound, thus reducing complications such as fat atrophy and traumatic injections.

REFERENCES

1. Douglas RJ. Aspiration and injection of the knee joint: approach portal. Knee Surg Relat Res. 2014;26(1):1-6.
2. Im SH, Lee SC, Park YB, Cho SR, Kim JC. Feasibility of sonography for intra-articular injections in the knee through a medial patellar portal. J Ultrasound Med. 2009;28(11):1465-70.
3. McAlindon TE, Bannuru RR, Sullivan MC, Arden NK, Berenbaum F, Bierma-Zeinstra SM, et al. OARSI guidelines for the non-surgical management of knee osteoarthritis. Osteoarthritis Cartilage. 2014;22(3):363-88.

9 SECTION

Alternate Therapies

68 CHAPTER

Dry Needling and Ultrasound-guided Dry Needling

Sushama R Phanse, Madhavi Joshi

ABSTRACT

Dry needling (DN) (in this chapter used specifically to denote dry needling without ultrasound guidance), and ultrasound-guided dry needling (USGDN) are safe, effective, easy, and economical methods to address myofascial pain. Fine 32 G, solid filiform needles of varying lengths are inserted into muscles. They are kept in situ for a few minutes and removed, without injection. The targets are the taut bands of muscle and the myofascial trigger points (MTrPs).

Myofascial pains are known to occur not only in acute pain conditions but are also a part of all chronic pain syndromes. They are not always completely relieved by conventional therapeutic methods, which do not address the myofascial component of pain and consequent disability. DN is one of the modalities which addresses these issues and hence plays a significant role in pain relief.

Both DN and USGDN are based on the same principles and exert the same effects for pain relief.

Ultrasound-guided dry needling is a highly evolved, sophisticated version of traditional DN. It has more accuracy, safety, and scope compared to traditional DN.

Knowledge of anatomy and muscle kinesiology is an important prerequisite for both DN and USGDN. In addition, USGDN also demands a fair skill with ultrasonography as well as a sound knowledge of sonoanatomy.

By addressing the muscles, these modalities play an important role not only in pain relief but also in restoration of activity. They are thus important, indispensable components in the armamentarium for pain relief.

INTRODUCTION

Dry needling (DN) is a specific modality which addresses the myofascial component of pain. It was formerly termed as intramuscular stimulation (IMS).

Insertion of a needle for treating trigger points in muscle was first introduced by Czech physician Karel Lewit in 1979. He called it Dry Needling.[1] In the 1980s Dr Chan Gunn of Vancouver, Canada used the term intramuscular stimulation, which moved away from targeting only trigger points and proposed the "radiculopathy" model to explain the various manifestations of chronic pain.[2]

Traditionally, DN is a modality which is extensively used by healthcare providers, particularly physiotherapists, in many countries in the management of patients with myofascial pain. The technique of DN has evolved immensely because of its ease and usefulness in the treatment of both acute and chronic pain. DN is a blind technique based on surface anatomy, whereas today it is performed under Ultrasound Guidance, hence the term ultrasound-guided dry needling (USGDN). The targets, the indications, and the effects on pain are identical, both for DN as well as USGDN. However, there are differences in their technique, efficacy, and scope. USGDN is a more sophisticated modality as compared to DN. The initial part of the chapter is dedicated to DN. The merits and technique of USGDN are discussed later in the chapter.

CHANGING PARADIGMS

It is now universally recognized that "Pain" is a complex phenomenon with multifactorial etiopathology.

Dry needling has been hitherto used only in myofascial pain syndrome (MPS). This is because MPS has been only associated with muscle strains, tendonitis, or inflammation. Muscle pain has been variously described by different terms, including fibrositis, interstitial myofibrositis, myogeloses, nonarticular rheumatism, myofascial pain, myalgia, perineuritis, myofascitis, and fibromyalgia.

Hitherto, myofascial involvement was not considered as a component of neuropathy, because neuropathy has always been described as a disorder of the somatosensory system.[3] However, in clinical practice, myofascial pain is also seen to occur in many chronic neuropathic pain conditions such as radiculopathies, joint dysfunction, disk pathology, craniomandibular dysfunction, migraines, tension-type headaches, carpal tunnel syndrome, computer-related disorders, whiplash associated disorders, spinal dysfunction, cancer, pelvic pain, and other urologic syndromes, visceral pain syndromes, postherpetic neuralgia, complex regional pain syndrome (CRPS), nocturnal cramps, phantom pain, and other relatively uncommon diagnoses such as Barre–Lieou syndrome and neurogenic pruritus. According to a current study, MPS has been known to affect up to 95% of people with chronic pain disorders,[4] including all neuropathic and central pain syndromes. According to Vas et al., MPS can be considered as a neuromuscular problem and neuropathies can be considered as neuromyopathies which manifest with MPS.[5]

This new emerging concept of *Neuromyopathy* recognizes muscles as the expressors and sustainers of pain in all neuropathic conditions.

Most pain interventions such as epidurals, nerve blocks, and radiofrequency (RF) ablations address the sensory, motor, or sympathetic nerves. DN is the modality which addresses the myofascial component of pain. DN can be used alone or as an integral part of the multi-modality regime (MMR) along with nerve blocks, epidurals, or other interventions.

TARGETS OF DRY NEEDLING

Dry needling targets the taut band in a muscle, and more specifically the myofascial trigger points (MTrPs).[6] The taut band is formed by a group of contracted muscle fibers and is readily palpable. The trigger point (MTrP) is defined as a tender region in a taut band of a skeletal muscle (Sola 1990).[7]

An MTrP is associated with an increased spontaneous electrical activity (SEA).[8]

A local twitch response (LTR) is a spinal reflex that is unique to MTrPs. It is characterized by a sudden contraction of muscle fibers within a taut band when the taut band is strummed manually or needled. MTrPs are known to sustain the pain cycle by an independent process of central sensitization.[9] Hence, addressal and resolution of MTrPs is an important goal in the reversal of pain.

Dry needling emphasizes the fact that muscles seldom act in isolation, but each action is a composite action involving other agonists, antagonists, and fixators.[10] LTRs which are pathognomonic of MTrPs are routinely visualized in coworking muscles indicating that there is a much wider distribution of MTrPs than is currently assumed. For example, MTrPs in agonist muscles (flexors) cause strain leading to reactive MTrPs in coworking muscles such as antagonists (extensors), other agonists (synergists), and fixators.

A taut band mechanically alters the function in all coworking muscles. DN targets not only the pain but also the disability resulting from the structural impairment caused by the taut band. This makes DN a specific treatment option for all chronic nociceptive and neuropathic pain conditions, cancer pains, and arthritic pains, all of which manifest with MPS.[11]

Trigger points are broadly divided into active and latent trigger points.[6,8] Active trigger points are tender and present with a taut band and feature spontaneous pain. The pain is referred away from the trigger point on direct compression and sometimes mediates an LTR. Latent trigger points do not cause spontaneous pain but eventually have a propensity to develop all the clinical characteristics of an active trigger point including a taut band. Both active and latent MTrPs contribute to general motor dysfunction comprising stiffness and restricted range of motion.

Myofascial trigger points in muscles also generate reactive MTrPs in other agonists, antagonists, synergists, and fixators. They are variously described with different nomenclatures such as associated trigger point, attachment trigger point, and satellite trigger point.[12-14] Despite a thorough clinical examination, there is neither a way to identify evolving, yet-to-become painful MTrPs, nor the presence of taut bands, which are still too fine to be felt by gross clinical examination. MTrPs in coworking muscle groups are neither acknowledged nor elicited.

Myofascial trigger points and muscle abnormalities are also normally not picked up by computed tomography (CT) or magnetic resonance imaging (MRI).

INDICATIONS OF DRY NEEDLING/ ULTRASOUND-GUIDED DRY NEEDLING

- Acute myofascial pain of direct trauma due to intense physical exercise[15] or whiplash injury[16,17] or work-related, because of low-load repetitive tasks and sustained postures[18,19]
- Chronic neuropathic pain conditions such as Herpes zoster,[20,21] trigeminal and other neuralgias,[22] radicular and nonradicular low back pain in spondylitis,[23,24] phantom pain,[25] chronic postsurgery pain,[26] and cancer[27]
- Joint dysfunction as in osteoarthritis (OA) knee, frozen shoulder, cervical or lumbar facet dysfunction[28]
- Visceral pain and dysfunction[29,30]
- Vascular pain syndrome like peripheral arterial diseases associated with ischemic neuropathy[31]
- Headaches and migraines[32-34]
- Complex regional pain syndrome[35]
- Fibromyalgia syndrome.[36]

ROLE OF MUSCLES IN CERVICAL AND LUMBAR RADICULAR PAINS

In the classical radiculopathy syndromes, pain distribution is myotomal rather than dermatomal **(Tables 1 and 2).** For example, cervical radicular pain, though originating in the neck, can be perceived in the shoulder or arm depending on the level. A neuropathy at C5/C6 can affect muscles like deltoid and supraspinatus resulting in a frozen shoulder.

In lumbar radiculopathy, compression of the motor nerve root at spinal level due to a protruded disk, osteophytes, facetal pathology, etc. can cause pain in the myotomes supplied by it. Nerve entrapment at foramen or MTrPs in erector spinae muscles can cause entrapment of primary rami of spinal nerves causing pain in the relevant myotomes.

In addition to myotomes as mentioned above, DN is also advocated in paraspinal muscles in all cases of neck and back pains, as MTrPs in erector spinae muscles are always present in these conditions. The shortening of the paraspinal muscles, particularly the deeper muscles of the spine (multifidi, rotatores and intertransversarii), leads to disk compression and narrowing of the intervertebral foramina, or exerts direct pressure on the nerve root. DN is done bilaterally as the segmental spread of referred pain may be bilateral as noted by Janet Travell.[37] In addition, a list on one side due to a radicular pain invariably leads to additional stress on the contralateral erector spinae muscles with development of MTrPs.

TABLE 1: Muscles supplied by cervical nerve roots.

Muscles	*Nerve roots*
Deltoid	C5
Biceps, brachialis	C5, C6
Triceps	C7
Flexors of wrist	C8
Extensor of wrist	C6
Flexors of fingers	C8
Extensors of fingers	C7
Intrinsic muscles of hand	T1

TABLE 2: Muscles supplied by lumbar nerve roots.

Muscles	*Nerve Roots*
Gluteus Maximus	L5, S1
Gluteus Medius/Minimus/Tensor Fascia Lata	L4, L5
Piriformis	L4, L5, S1
Quadriceps	L3, L4
Hamstrings	S1
Tibialis Anterior	L4
Gastrocnemius/Soleus	S1
Peronei	L5, S1

Bilateral paraspinal DN is especially indicated in spondylolisthesis which is caused by a shortening of the intermediate and deep layers of the erector spinae.

PAIN REFERRAL SYNDROMES

According to Simons and Travels,[37] the MTrPs in muscles can also refer pain to other distant areas in the body. Some common pain referral maps are shown in **Figures 1A to D**.

In visceral pain syndromes the trigger points develop in the thoracolumbar paraspinal muscles and abdominal wall muscles due to viscerosomatic convergence.[38] In trigeminal neuralgia, MTrPs in the trapezius and sternocleidomastoid muscles can refer pain to the facial muscles supplied by the trigeminal nerve and sustain the pain even after gasserian ganglion block and opioid medication.[39] In cervicogenic headache syndromes, MTrPs in trapezius and sternocleidomastoid muscles can refer pain to the head and face.[40]

PREREQUISITES FOR DRY NEEDLING

A sound knowledge of structural anatomy and muscle kinesiology is mandatory. A sound knowledge of surface anatomy of muscles is also needed.

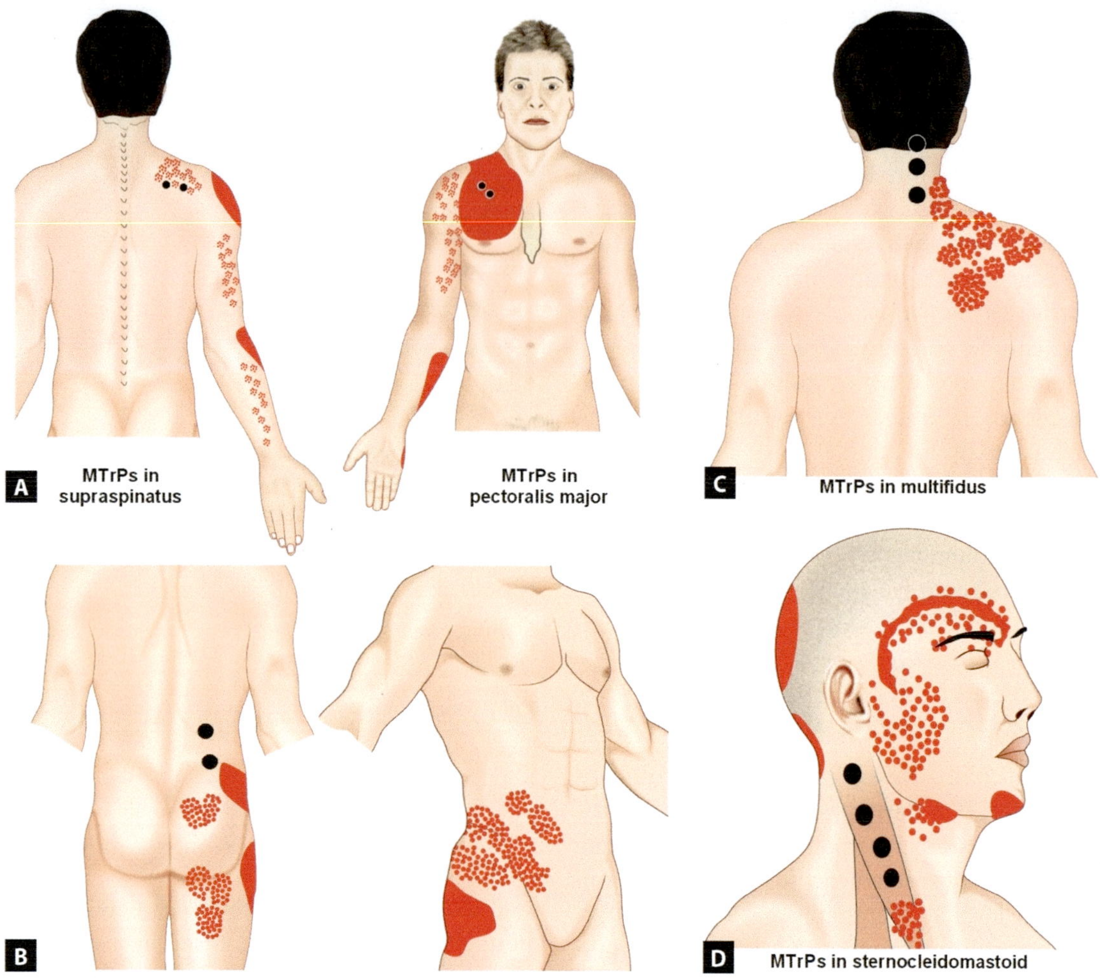

Figs. 1A to D: Some common pain referral patterns. The black dots indicate myofascial trigger points (MTrPs), solid and stippled areas indicate locations of pain and radiation patterns, respectively.

A detailed history of pain and current illness is mandatory.

This should be followed by a detailed clinical examination to establish a diagnosis—whether the myofascial pain is nociceptive or a contributor to neuropathic pain. Once the original source of neuropathy is established after a detailed clinical examination and relevant investigations, the muscles in all the relevant myotomes of the affected nerve must be addressed. It is important to address not only the relevant agonist muscles, but also the antagonists and synergist muscles. The possibility of pain referral with respect to the prevalent pain condition should be kept in mind, before performing the procedure. The pain referral maps given above can serve as a useful guide.

CLINICAL EXAMINATION

Clinical examination includes palpation, which is the primary tool for identifying trigger points. The presence of a taut band with exquisite spot tenderness is diagnostic for MTrPs **(Fig. 2)**. A painful spasmodic taut band of muscle is best characterized as a palpable, ropey structure, and is typically a group of tense muscle fibers extending from a trigger point to the muscle attachments.

There are different methods of palpation.

- *Flat palpation method:* In which a clinician applies finger or thumb pressure to muscle against underlying bone tissue **(Fig. 3)**.
- *Pincer method:* In this, the muscle belly is palpated between the thumb and fingers, which act like a pincer **(Fig. 4)**.

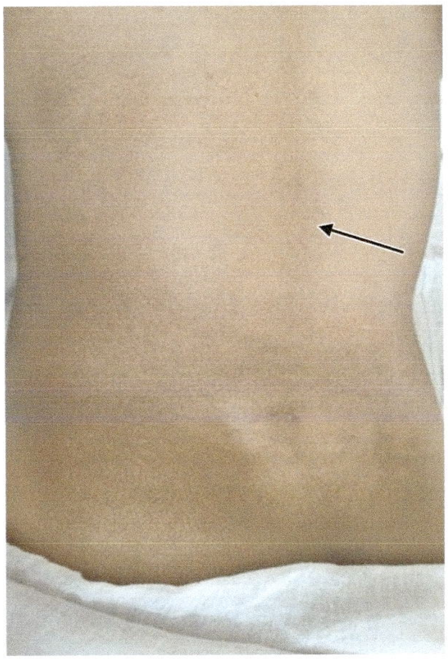

Fig. 2: The taut band in erector spinae secondary to disk prolapse.

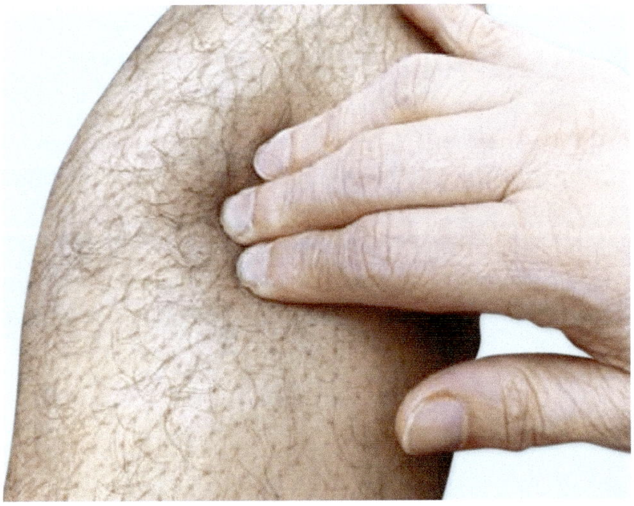

Fig. 3: Flat palpation method.

- *Elicitation of jump sign or LTR*: "Jump sign" is a jump in the muscle elicited when a taut band is strummed with the examiner's fingertips at 90° to the muscle. This is the manifestation of the LTR, which is a spinal reflex that is pathognomonic of an MTrP.

EQUIPMENT FOR DRY NEEDLING

Acupuncture needles **(Fig. 5)***:* 32G acupuncture needles of varying lengths are available. The advantages of acupuncture needles are:

- The fine gauge (G) renders them atraumatic.
- They are flexible with pointed tip.

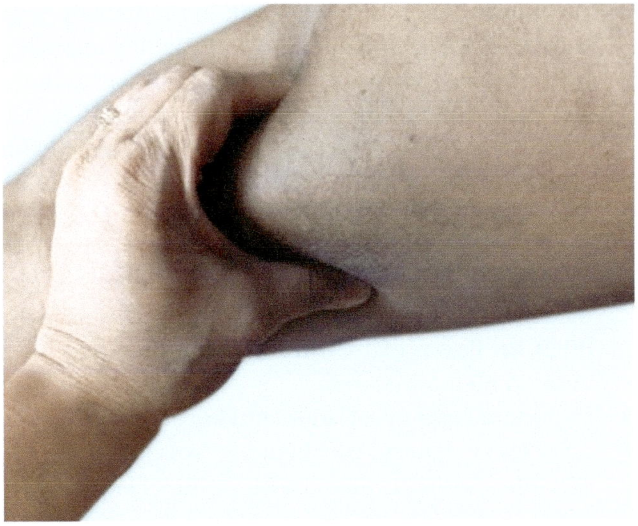

Fig. 4: Pincer palpation method.

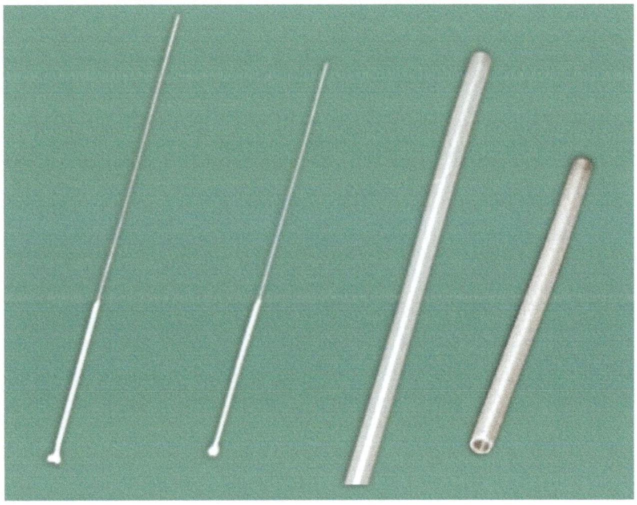

Fig. 5: Traditional filiform solid acupuncture needles.

- They have a spring-like quality.
- They are available in varying lengths.
- They are easy to sterilize.
- They transmit the nature and consistency of tissues penetrated to the experienced hand.

PREPARATION OF THE PATIENT

- The procedure is well explained to the patient to allay needle phobia or anxiety. The patient should be informed that any movement of the concerned part of the body is to be avoided during the procedure.
- An informed consent is taken.
- Monitoring of vital signs is done.
- Resuscitation facilities should be available if required.

- An appropriate position is given to the patient. Care is taken to make the patient comfortable, and props or support can be provided as required, for example, a prone position is given for paraspinal needling. For selective needling of an extremity, a lateral position is preferred with the affected side up, as in frozen shoulder. The advantage of this position is that it promotes easy access to both the anterior and posterior muscles. A supine position is good for needling the muscles on the anterior aspect, for example, the quadriceps in the thigh, the flexors of the arm and forearm, or muscles of anterior abdominal wall.
- Important anatomical landmarks are noted.
- The area is prepared with betadine/spirit.
- The interventionist should wear sterile gloves.

TECHNIQUE OF DRY NEEDLING (FIGS. 6 TO 8)

A needle of appropriate length is chosen according to the estimated depth of the target muscle from the skin. The needle in the plastic sheath is held in the left hand and a gentle tap is given at the hub so that the needle pierces the skin **(Fig. 6)**.

After piercing the skin, the needle is guided deeper by a gentle twirling motion. A sudden giveaway or a loss of resistance is felt by the hand when a needle enters a taut muscle. At this point the patient may experience pain or discomfort as the needle is gripped by the tight muscle. An LTR or jump sign may be seen when the needle enters an MTrP. This is likely to cause some discomfort to the patient. The patient should be informed as such, prior to the procedure. This is followed by a relaxation of the muscle and relief of the trigger point. Elicitation of LTR is a sure sign of having entered the MTrP and ensures improved outcome.[1,30] LTRs are elicited only in the regions of active MTrPs. They may not always be elicited in areas of latent or satellite trigger points.

The method which is usually followed in clinical practice is described by Chann Gunn. DN is done in the synergist as well as antagonist muscles because a restricted range in the agonist can lead to MTrP formation in the antagonist muscle. A satellite trigger point may develop in the zone of reference of the key trigger point, in an overloaded synergist, or in an antagonist.

In the case of sensitive patients, prilocaine gel can be applied over the concerned area half an hour prior to the procedure. The needles are kept in situ for 20–30 minutes and removed.

ULTRASOUND-GUIDED DRY NEEDLING

As stated earlier, the indications and usefulness of USGDN are the same as DN. However, USGDN is done under vision with USG guidance, unlike DN which is a blind procedure.

A detailed history, clinical examination, and informed consent are mandatory for the DN. All the initial steps for preparation of the patient are also the same as described under DN.

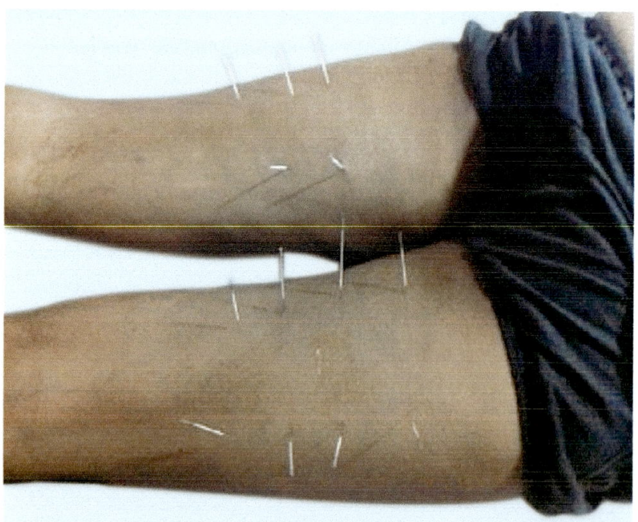

Fig. 7: Dry needling of hamstring muscles of the thigh.

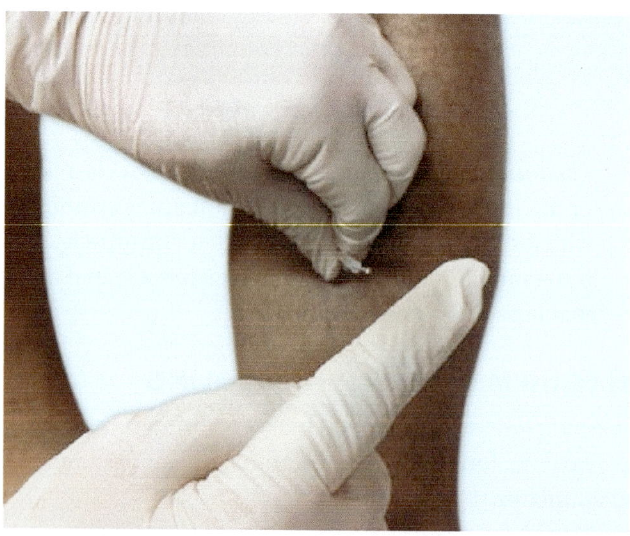

Fig. 6: Tapping for insertion of needle in dry needling.

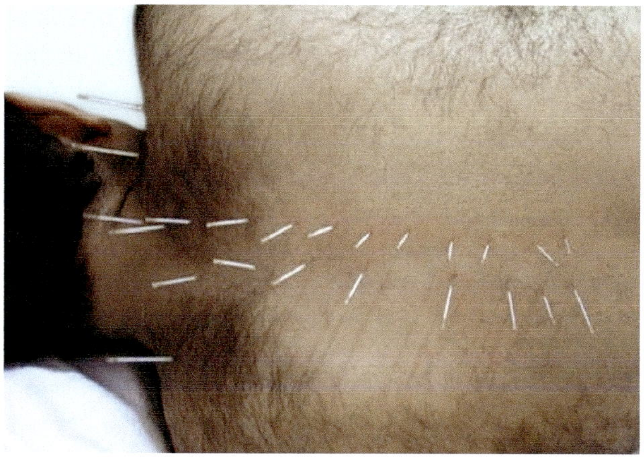

Fig. 8A: Paraspinal needling cervicothoracic region.

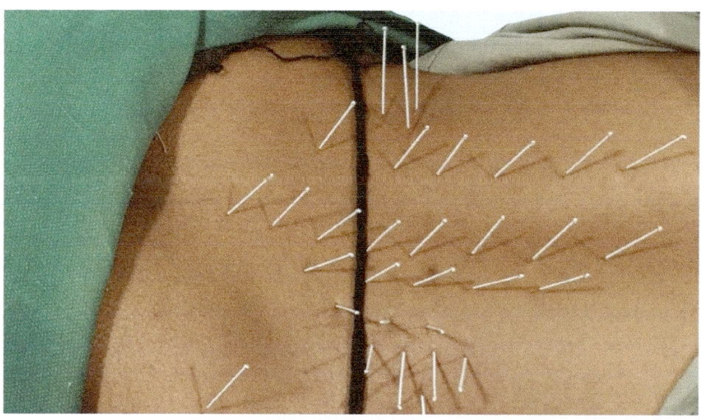

Fig. 8B: Paraspinal needling in lumbosacral area.

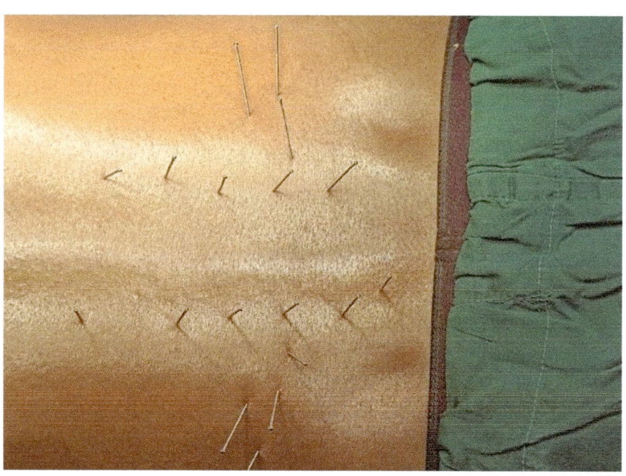

Fig. 8C: Paraspinal needling in lumbar area.

PREREQUISITES FOR ULTRASOUND-GUIDED DRY NEEDLING

In addition to a sound knowledge of structural anatomy and muscle kinesiology, a knowledge of sonoanatomy is mandatory **(Figs. 9 and 10)**.

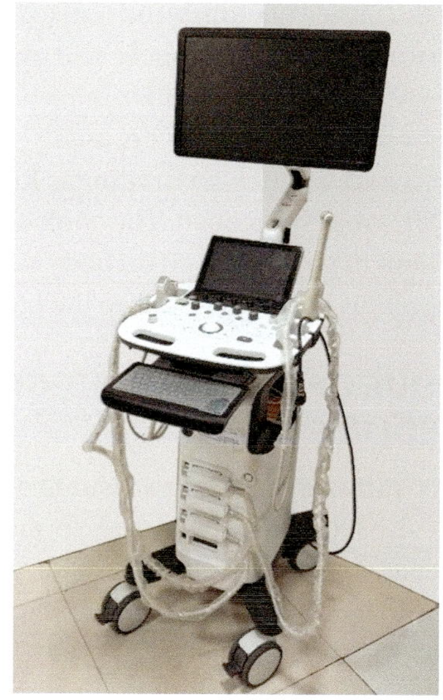

Fig. 9: Ultrasonography machine.

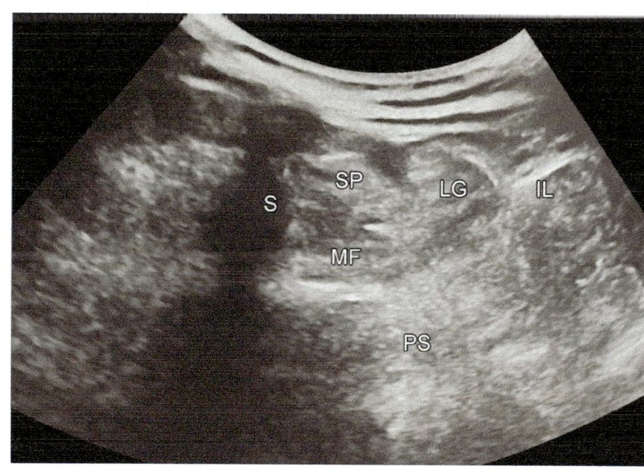

Fig. 10A: Lumbar paraspinal muscles. (IL: iliocostalis muscle; LG: longissimus muscle; MF: multifidus muscle; PS: psoas muscle; S: spinous process; SP: spinalis muscle)

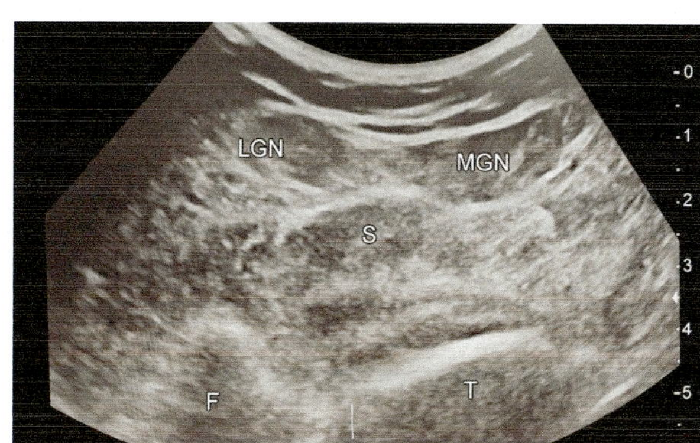

Fig. 10B: Calf muscles. (F: fibula; LGN: lateral gastrocnemius muscle; MGN: medial gastrocnemius muscle; S: soleus muscle; T: tibia)

Knowing the basics of ultrasound is also helpful.

For the upper extremity back and neck, a high-frequency linear probe of 10–18 MHz is used. For the knee multifrequency probe of 4-20 MHz is used.

For the hip and buttock a curvilinear low-frequency probe of 6-1 MHz may be needed. The choice of probe may vary from patient to patient based on body structure.

Color Doppler is useful to visualize the blood vessels.

TECHNIQUE OF ULTRASOUND-GUIDED DRY NEEDLING

A preliminary ultrasound scan to visualize and identify the relevant muscles and to visualize any structural abnormalities is performed. This may be followed by a dynamic examination to identify the deeper muscles and functional abnormalities.

The USG probe is cleaned and covered with sterile probe cover. After appropriate positioning of the patient, the area of interest is cleaned with antiseptic solutions and draped well with sterile covers. After noting the depth of the muscle, a needle of appropriate length is selected. The probe is firmly placed on the muscle and the needle is introduced in plane. Care is taken to keep the tip in view in case the entire needle is not visualized. Out-of-plane technique can also be used for deeper muscles or if there is lack of space. The LTRs denote active trigger points. Many needles are placed along the length of the muscle at regular intervals.

Few pictures of USGDN are shown in **Figures 11A to C**.

ADVANTAGES OF ULTRASOUND-GUIDED DRY NEEDLING

- The use of ultrasound ensures direct visualization of the needle as it enters the muscle.
- It is thus a safer technique, as not only does it ensure the accuracy of needle insertion, but also helps in avoiding important structures such as blood vessels, nerves, and pleura.
- Longer needles, even of 100 mm size can be inserted wherever required.
- MTrPs, which are normally not picked up by CT or MRI, can be detected with a high-resolution ultrasound machine. They can be seen on ultrasound as hypoechoic spots and are usually abundant in the deeper muscles.
- LTRs in deeper muscles, which may not be visible, can be seen only with ultrasound **(Video 15)**.
- The use of ultrasound enables the study of changes in muscle morphology, which can occur in long-standing chronic pain syndromes. A normal muscle is hypoechoic on ultrasound and the connective tissue gives a bright curvilinear echo of oblique and parallel fibers. Atrophy of muscle occurs in chronic neuropathies, there may be calcifications seen in certain arthritides, or a complete disruption of morphologic structure in CRPS.
- USGDN thus has immense scope for further research into myopathies and the contribution of muscles to chronic pain.

To summarize, USGDN has opened new vistas and provided new insights into the hitherto unexplained and little-known mechanisms of pain, particularly the huge role played by muscles in the propagation of all types of chronic pain.

EFFECTS OF NEEDLE INSERTION IN DRY NEEDLING AND ULTRASOUND-GUIDED DRY NEEDLING

Both modalities cause deactivation of MTrPs, thereby leading to relief of muscle spasm and pain. This is achieved by various mechanisms.[41]

- Karett Lewitt called the immediate analgesic effect of the needle which was distinct and independent of any injection as a "needle effect".
- The effect of LTR is a decrease in the spontaneous electrical activity by depletion of acetylcholine stores leading to a relief of spasm and pain.[41,42]
- The twirling or insertion of the needle has a mechanical effect of breaking fibrous contractures in the spasmodic muscle due to disruption of the muscle cell wall by the needle, causing alterations of calcium influx into the cytoplasm. It also activates fibroblasts and promotes collagen synthesis.
- Release of vasoactive substances, such as calcitonin gene-related peptide,[43] substance P as well as vascular endothelial growth factors which increase blood supply and muscle oxygenation, and promote healing.
- Reversal of peripheral and central sensitization by segmental inhibition/gate control,[44] accompanied with the release of endogenous opioids and neurogenic transmitters like serotonin and noradrenaline, which have a descending inhibitory effect.[45]
- Central effects due to stimulation of anterior cingulate cortex have been noted.

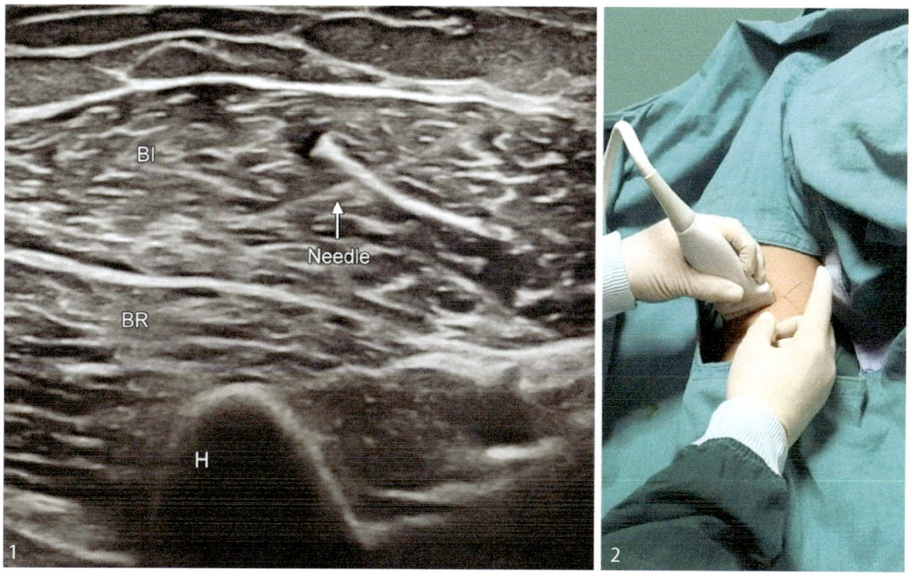

Fig. 11A: (1) Ultrasound-guided dry needling (USGDN) of biceps muscle; (2) Probe and needle placement. (BI: biceps muscle; BR: brachialis muscle; H: humerus)

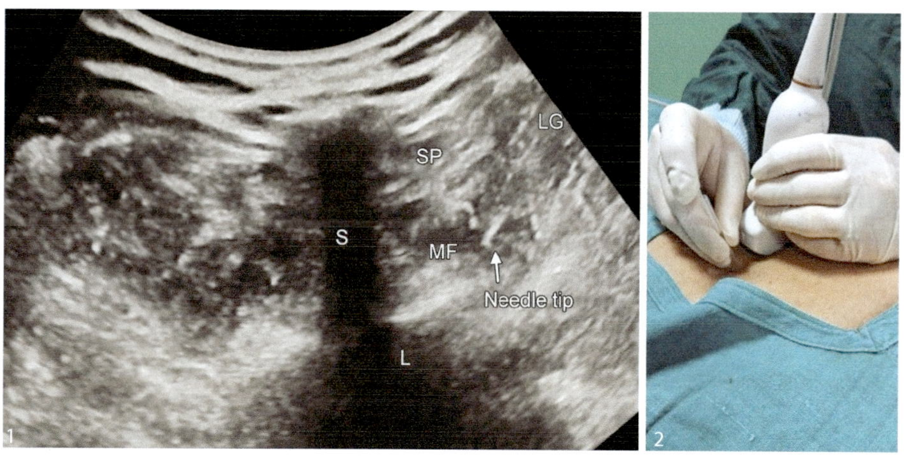

Fig. 11B: (1) Ultrasound-guided dry needling (USGDN) of multifidus muscle; (2) Probe and needle placement. (L: lamina; LG: longissimus muscle; MF: multifidus muscle; S: spinous process of vertebra; SP: spinalis muscle)

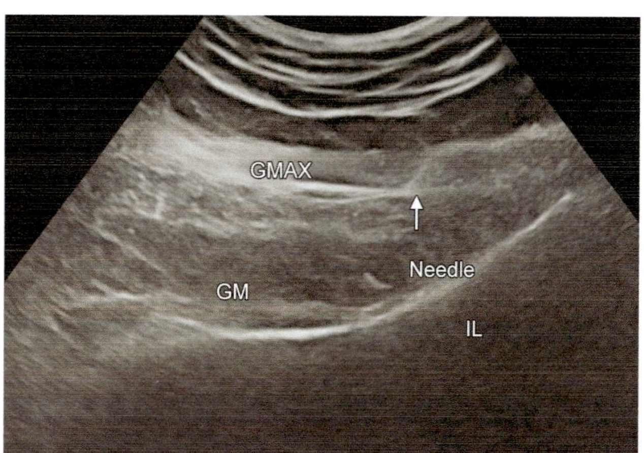

Fig. 11C: Ultrasound-guided dry needling (USGDN) of gluteus medius and gluteus maximus. (GM: gluteus medius muscle; GMAX: gluteus maximus muscle; IL: ileum)

- There is also evidence of release of oxytocin, which has an analgesic effect as well as a sense of well-being.

CONTRAINDICATIONS

Relative Contraindications

- *Fear of needles:* A detailed prior explanation of the procedure helps in allaying patient's fear.
- *Severe allodynia or hyperalgesia:* This can be overcome by prior application of lignocaine or prilocaine gel, 20–30 minutes prior to the procedure.
- *Patients on anticoagulant therapy*: The needles are 32G, so there are no reported major complications even in patients on anticoagulants.

Absolute Contraindications

These are very few.

- It is best avoided in the first trimester of pregnancy though there is no evidence of any abortifacient effects.
- Local or systemic infection
- Patients who cannot communicate directly or via communicator
- Local skin lesions.

COMPLICATIONS AND SIDE EFFECTS

They are seen very rarely.

- Pain on needle insertion occurs on penetration of a tight muscle.
- Localized bleeding or hematoma formation due to accidental piercing of a blood vessel. It is usually minimal even with DN and resolves within a day or two. It can be totally avoided with USGDN as it is done under vision.
- Postneedling soreness is common, especially after the initial sessions.
- Wheal formation occurs in individuals with hypersensitivity or is obvious in light-skinned individuals.
- Transient vasovagal reaction which can manifest as momentary giddiness with sweating and bradycardia. In such cases the procedure may have to be paused temporarily and then resumed once the vital parameters return to normal.

DRY NEEDLING/ULTRASOUND-GUIDED DRY NEEDLING VERSUS ACUPUNCTURE

These modalities are often confused with acupuncture, which also employs similar needles.

It is to be noted that the concept of trigger points and the modality of DN were developed by Dr Travell independently of already existing acupuncture concepts.

Acupuncture is based on the Chinese philosophy of meridians and knowledge of anatomy is not essential. DN and USGDN, on the other hand, require a detailed medical history and examination. A medical diagnosis is an essential prerequisite. A thorough knowledge of muscle kinesiology is mandatory.

Prompt subjective and objective effects are seen with DN and USGDN but are not evident with acupuncture.

DRY NEEDLING/ULTRASOUND-GUIDED DRY NEEDLING VERSUS TRIGGER POINT INJECTIONS

Trigger point injections (TPI) are done usually using lidocaine (1–2%) for injection into the MTrP along with a steroid-like triamcinolone or depo-medrol. Cummings and White[46] reviewed 23 papers and found that there was no difference between DN and injection. In clinical practice, it is found that the resolution of MTrPs by DN/USGDN completely eliminates the need for TPIs.

CONCLUSION

- Dry needling and USGDN are directed at inactivating MTrPs in muscles which continue to sustain the pain cycle by central sensitization long after cessation of the original painful stimulus. Thus, they exert a positive impact on central processes by removing a common and peripheral source of persistent nociceptive input found in all chronic and neuropathic pain syndromes.
- They address the interrelated functions of various structures in the body that work together as a whole, by recognizing the role of muscles in expressing and sustaining pain in all neuropathic pain syndromes.
- The goal of pain management is not just pain relief, but also a return to activity. Both *pain* and *disability* are addressed by these modalities.
- They are *safe*. They do not interfere with the physiological mechanisms in the body, as no injections are involved. Side effects and complications are very rare due to the small diameter of the acupuncture needles.
- Most importantly, they significantly *reduce the dose of opioids and narcotics*, especially in cancer pain syndromes.

- Both modalities have a high *efficacy*. They provide immediate pain relief and there is less waiting time between treatments.

In the current scenario of pain management, ultrasound is being very widely used as a tool in all pain interventions. DN should always be performed under ultrasound (US) guidance wherever possible for the obvious advantages described earlier.

However, DN (even without ultrasound) is safe and economically viable, especially in low-resource settings where ultrasound machine may not be available. If performed with proper knowledge and skills, it can yield the same results as USGDN. Thus, these modalities are an indispensable part of the armamentarium of pain management, which aims at a holistic approach. DN is being widely practiced all over the world, and there is increasing evidence about its efficacy. USGDN can provide further insight into MPS and its biomechanical and neurophysiological mechanisms of action. Large-scale, good quality, placebo-controlled, double-blinded, randomized controlled trials are needed, to support clinical evidence of USGDN, because of the limited sample size and poor quality of studies conducted so far.

ACKNOWLEDGMENT

We would like to thank Dr Lakshmi Vas for the training we have received, her constant support and encouragement.

REFERENCES

1. Lewit K. The needle effect in the relief of myofascial pain. Pain. 1979;6(1):83-90.
2. Gunn CC. The Gunn Approach to the Treatment of Chronic Pain: Intramuscular Stimulation for Myofascial Pain of Radiculopathic Origin, 2nd edition. Churchill Livingstone; 1996.
3. Dommerholt J, Bron C, Franssen J. Myofascial trigger points: an evidence-informed review. J Man Manip Ther. 2006;14(4):203-21.
4. Shah JP, Danoff JV, Desai MJ, Parikh S, Nakamura LY, Phillips TM, et al. Biochemicals associated with pain and inflammation are elevated in sites near to and remote from active myofascial trigger points. Arch Phys Med Rehabil. 2008;89(1):16-23.
5. Vas L, Phanse S, Pai R. A new perspective of neuromyopathy to explain intractable pancreatic cancer pains; dry needling as an effective adjunct to neurolytic blocks. Indian J Palliat Care. 2016;22:85-93.
6. Gerwin RD. Myofascial pain syndrome. In: Gerwin RD (Ed). Muscle Pain: Diagnosis and Treatment. Springer; 2010. pp. 15-83.
7. Sola AE, Bonica JJ. Myofascial pain syndromes. In: Bonica JJ, Loser JD, Chapman CR, Fordyce WE, (Eds). The Management of Pain, 2nd edition. Philadelphia: Lea & Febiger; 1990. pp. 352-67.
8. Simons DG, Hong CZ, Simons LS. Prevalence of spontaneous electrical activity at trigger spots and at control sites in rabbit skeletal muscle. J Musculoskelet Pain. 1995;3(1):35-48.
9. Sengupta JN. Visceral pain: the neurophysiological mechanism. Handb Exp Pharmacol. 2009;(194):31-74.
10. Vas LC. Ultrasound guided dry needling: relevance in chronic pain. J Postgrad Med. 2022;68(1):1-9.
11. Vas LC. Effectiveness of ultrasound guided dry needling in chronic pain. Pain News. 2019;17:202-12.
12. Gibson W, Arendt-Nielsen L, Graven-Nielsen T. Referred pain and hyperalgesia in human tendon and muscle belly tissue. Pain. 2006;120(1-2):113-23.
13. Hsieh YL, Kao MJ, Kuan TS, Chen SM, Chen JT, Hong CZ. Dry needling to a key myofascial trigger point may reduce the irritability of satellite MTrPs. Am J Phys Med Rehabil. 2007;86(5):397-403.
14. Simons DG, Travell J. Myofascial trigger points: a possible explanation. Pain. 1981;10(1):106-9.
15. Vecchiet L, Vecchiet J, Bellomo R, Giamberardino MA. Muscle pain from physical exercise. J Musculoskelet Pain. 1999;7(1/2):43-53.
16. Curatolo M, Arendt-Nielsen L, Petersen-Felix S. Evidence, mechanisms, and clinical implications of central hypersensitivity in chronic pain after whiplash injury. Clin J Pain. 2004;20:469-76.
17. Dommerholt J. Persistent myalgia following whiplash. Curr Pain Headache Rep. 2005;9:326-30.
18. Huguenin LK. Myofascial trigger points: the current evidence. Phys Ther Sport. 2004;5:2-12.
19. Hagg GM. The Cinderella hypothesis. In: Joahnsson H, Windhorst U, Djupsjöbacka M, Passatore M (Eds). Chronic Work-Related Myalgia: Neuromuscular Mechanisms behind Work-related Chronic Muscle Pain Syndromes. Gävle: Gävle University Press; 2003. pp. 127-32.
20. Chen SM, Chen JT, Kuan TS, Hong CZ. Myofascial trigger points in intercostal muscles secondary to herpes zoster infection of intercostal nerve. Arch Phys Med Rehabil. 1998;79:336-8.
21. Weiner DK, Schmader KE. Postherpetic pain: more than sensory neuralgia? Pain Med. 2006;7:243-50.
22. Ichida MC, da Silva LA, Teixeira MJ, de Siqueira JT, de Siqueira SR. Functional and sensory evaluation of patients with idiopathic trigeminal neuralgia: comparison with controls. Clin Neurol Neurosurg. 2015;130(3):114-21.
23. Rosomoff HL, Fishbain DA, Goldberg M, Rosomoff RS. Myofascial findings with patients with chronic intractable benign pain of the back and neck. Pain Manag. 1989;3:114-8.
24. O'Neill S, Manniche C, Graven-Nielsen T, Arendt-Nielsen L. Generalized deep-tissue hyperalgesia in patients with chronic low-back pain. Eur J Pain. 2007;11:415-20.

25. Kern U, Martin C, Scheicher S, Müller H. Does botulinum toxin A make prosthesis use easier for amputees? J Rehabil Med. 2004;36(5):238-9.
26. Vas L, Pai R. Reversal of complex regional pain syndrome type 2 and the subsequent management of complex regional pain syndrome type 1 occurring after corrective surgery for residual ulnar claw. Pain Med. 2014;15(6):1059-63.
27. Lacomba MT, del Moral OM, Zazo JL, Gerwin RD, Goñí AZ. Incidence of myofascial pain syndrome in breast cancer surgery: a prospective study. Clin J Pain. 2010;26:320-5.
28. Bajaj P, Graven-Nielsen T, Arendt-Nielsen L. Trigger points in patients with lower limb osteoarthritis. J Musculoskelet Pain. 2001;9(3):17-33.
29. Sikandar S, Dickenson AH. Visceral pain: the ins and outs, the ups and downs. Curr Opin Support Palliat Care. 2012;6(1):17-26.
30. Gerwin RD. Myofascial and visceral pain syndromes: visceral-somatic pain representations. J Musculoskelet Pain. 2002;10(1/2):165-75.
31. Bartoli V, Dorigo B, Grisillo D, Beconi D. Fibrositic myofascial pain in intermittent claudication: significance of trigger areas in the calf. Angiology. 1980;31(1):11-20.
32. Giamberardino MA, Tafuri E, Savini A, Fabrizio A, Affaitati G, Lerza R, et al. Contribution of myofascial trigger points to migraine symptoms. J Pain. 2007;8:869-78.
33. Calandre EP, Hidalgo J, García-Leiva JM, Rico-Villademoros F. Trigger point evaluation in migraine patients: an indication of peripheral sensitization linked to migraine predisposition? Eur J Neurol. 2006;13:244-9.
34. Fernández-de-las-Peñas C, Cuadrado ML, Barriga FJ, Pareja JA. Active muscle trigger points as sign of sensitization in chronic primary headaches. J Musculoskelet Pain. 2009;17:155-61.
35. Rashiq S, Galer BS. Proximal myofascial dysfunction in complex regional pain syndrome: a retrospective prevalence study. Clin J Pain. 1999;15(2):151-3.
36. Affaitati G, Costantini R, Fabrizio A, Lapenna D, Tafuri E, Giamberardino MA. Effects of treatment of peripheral pain generators in fibromyalgia patients. Eur J Pain. 2011;15(1):61-9.
37. Simons DG, Travell JG, Simons LS. Travell and Simons Myofascial Pain and Dysfunction: The Trigger Point Manual, 2nd edition. Baltimore: Lippincott Williams and Wilkins; 1999.
38. Vas L, Phanse S, Pai R. A new perspective of neuromyopathy to explain intractable pancreatic cancer pains; Dry needling as an effective adjunct to neurolytic blocks. Indian J Palliat Care. 2016;22:85-93.
39. Vas L, Phanse S, Pawar KS, Pai R, Pattnaik M. Ultrasound-guided dry needling of masticatory muscles in trigeminal neuralgia - A case series of 35 patients. J Postgrad Med. 2023;69:11-20.
40. Simons DG, Travell JG. Cervicogenic headache. In: Simons LS (Ed). Travell & Simons' Myofascial Pain and Dysfunction: The Trigger Point Manual: Volume 1: Upper Half of the Body. Baltimore, MD: Lippincott Williams and Wilkins; 1999.
41. Cagnie B, Dewitte V, Barbe T, Timmermans F, Delrue N, Meeus M. Physiologic effects of dry needling. Curr Pain Headache Rep. 2013;17:348.
42. Chen JT, Chung KC, Hou CR, Kuan TS, Chen SM, Hong CZ. Inhibitory effect of dry needling on the spontaneous electrical activity recorded from myofascial trigger spots of rabbit skeletal muscle. Am J Phys Med Rehabil. 2001;80(10):729-35.
43. Sato A, Sato Y, Shimura M, Uchida S. Calcitonin gene-related peptide produces skeletal muscle vasodilation following antidromic stimulation of unmyelinated afferents in the dorsal root in rats. Neurosci Lett. 2000;283(2):137-40.
44. Facco E, Ceccherelli F. Myofascial pain mimicking radicular symptoms. Acta Neurochir Suppl. 2005;92:147-50.
45. Butts R, Dunning J, Perreault T, Mourad F, Grubb M. Peripheral and spinal mechanisms of pain and dry needling mediated analgesia: a clinical resource guide for health care professionals. Int J Phys Med Rehabil. 2016;4:327.
46. Cummings TM, White AR. Needling Therapies in the management of myofascial trigger point pain: a systematic review. Arch Phys med Rehabil.2001; 82:986-92.

69 CHAPTER

Myofascial Pain Syndrome and Trigger Point Injections

Vince Z Si, Mona Mirchandani, Kevin K Bernard, Emilia Ravski, Dellene E Troy, Christopher V Boudakian, Nayeema Chowdhury, Jason D Freeman

ABSTRACT

This chapter will describe the clinical presentation, physiology, and pathophysiology of myofascial pain syndrome (MPS) and the role of trigger point injections in its management. MPS is characterized by abnormal taut bands of skeletal muscle referred to as myofascial trigger points (MTrPs), which are often pain generators. Trigger point injections are procedures that can be done in the office by healthcare professionals and target these abnormal taut bands to help eliminate painful MTrPs. This chapter will outline how to perform trigger point injections on the most common muscles encountered in clinical practice.

INTRODUCTION

Skeletal muscle in the human body accounts for approximately 40% or more of body weight. Therefore, it is not surprising that there is a high prevalence of myalgia in the general population. Approximately, 23 million people in the US have one or more chronic disorders of the musculoskeletal system. Myofascial pain syndrome (MPS) is among the most common muscle disorders seen by clinicians.[1] The MPS is a painful condition with sensory, motor, and autonomic symptoms caused by myofascial trigger points (MTrPs). The MTrPs are located in tender skeletal muscle associated with a hypersensitive palpable nodule in a taut band. The MTrP is characteristically painful when compressed and is often associated with a pattern of referred pain, referred tenderness, motor dysfunction, and autonomic phenomena.[2,3] MPS occurs alone but can also be present with other pain generators (i.e., osteoarthritis, rheumatologic conditions, radiculopathy, and tendinopathies). MPS affects the quality of life and places an economic burden upon societies. Therefore, it is important to identify, diagnose, and treat MPS to improve patients' quality of life and reduce the cost of lost productive time. Patients afflicted with chronic pain syndromes, such as low back pain, have a high prevalence of MTrPs in the quadratus lumborum, iliocostalis lumborum, and gluteus medius muscles and exhibit a greater disability and worse sleep quality when compared with healthy controls.[4] Musculoskeletal complaints are the second most common cause of short-term sickness absences in developed countries and are also a common reason for disability pension claims, early retirement, or long-term sick leave. In most developed countries, musculoskeletal complaints are the second most common presenting complaint to a doctor and make up 10–20% of primary care consultations. It is estimated that the healthcare costs for musculoskeletal complaints account for 1.2% of the gross national product in the US.[5] Furthermore, 13% of the total workforce had a loss in productive time secondary to a common pain condition, with headache, back pain, arthritis pain, and other musculoskeletal pain being the most common conditions accounting for the reduced performance. This loss in productive time is estimated to cost $61.2 billion per year.[6]

Myofascial trigger points have been a well-established medical condition and can contribute significantly to acute and chronic musculoskeletal pain conditions. It places a burden on an individual's quality of life, healthcare costs, and economic costs. Therefore, it is the purpose of this chapter to describe briefly the pathophysiology of MTrPs and the role of trigger point injections as an effective treatment of MPS. This chapter will focus on the mechanism of action of trigger point injections, how to identify trigger points, and outline how to perform them in the most commonly affected muscles.

NORMAL ANATOMY/PHYSIOLOGY

Muscle Structure and Function

Skeletal muscles are composed of fascicles, which contain hundreds of muscle fibers. Muscle fibers are made up of 1,000–2,000 myofibrils, each of which consists of sarcomeres connected end to end in a chain-like pattern. Sarcomeres are the basic contractile units of skeletal muscles, consisting of actin and myosin molecules. Skeletal muscle contraction occurs when actin and myosin filaments slide over one another according to the sliding filament theory.[7] Adenosine triphosphatase is an enzyme in the myosin head of the myosin filament that interacts with actin to produce a contractile force and shortening of the sarcomere. In the absence of adenosine triphosphate (ATP), the myosin heads remain attached to the actin filaments, causing muscles to become stiff as in rigor mortis. Calcium is normally sequestered in the sarcoplasmic reticulum and is released when an action potential reaches the T-tubules in the muscle fiber. Calcium binds to tropomyosin and causes an allosteric change in the protein that removes it from the actin filament and unblocks the myosin head-binding site. In the absence of calcium, the contractile activity of sarcomeres is terminated.[2,7]

The central nervous system (CNS) controls voluntary muscle activity through a motor unit. The motor unit consists of an alpha motor neuron cell body in the anterior horn of the spinal cord, its axon, the motor endplates, and the muscle fibers supplied by the alpha motoneuron.[2] The action potential is transmitted down the axon of the alpha motor neuron toward the neuromuscular junction. When the action potential reaches the neuromuscular junction, there is an influx of calcium that causes vesicles containing acetylcholine (Ach) to fuse with the plasma membrane, releasing it into the extracellular space. Ach diffuses across the neuromuscular junction to the postsynaptic muscle fiber. The random release of Ach from a nerve terminal causes individual miniature endplate potentials. A mass release of Ach from multiple vesicles in response to an action potential is required to achieve the threshold for excitation, depolarize the postjunctional membrane, and initiate an action potential throughout the muscle fiber.[2]

PATHOPHYSIOLOGY OF MYOFASCIAL TRIGGER POINTS

Biopsies of trigger points showed contraction knots that were large, rounded, darkly staining muscle fibers with a larger diameter than surrounding muscle fibers. Currently, there are no pathologic or laboratory tests to identify trigger points. There are several theories of trigger point formation, and much of the research on pathophysiology has been directed toward verifying common theories. The integrated hypothesis is the most widely accepted theory of trigger point formation that combines two lines of trigger point investigation, electrodiagnostic and histopathological.[2] According to the integrated hypothesis, there is an abnormal increase in the production and release of Ach from the motor nerve terminal that causes a sustained depolarization of the muscle fibers in response to trauma or abnormal stress.[2] This causes a continuous release and uptake of calcium ions from the sarcoplasmic reticulum, with insufficient ATP to return calcium to the sarcoplasmic reticulum, resulting in sustained shortening of sarcomeres. This leads to an "energy crisis" where there is an increased metabolic demand and impaired metabolic supply. The sustained sarcomere shortening compresses local blood vessels, diminishing blood flow, and causes localized ischemia and tissue hypoxia. Eventually, this leads to a vicious cycle causing the formation of a taut band.[2,8]

Electromyographic studies of trigger points have shown that trigger points have spontaneous electrical activity and healthy muscle tissue does not.[2,9,10] Trigger points develop secondary to an abnormal increase in the production and release of Ach from the motor nerve terminal under resting conditions. These increased miniature end-plate potentials produce "endplate noise" and sustained depolarization of the postjunctional membrane of the muscle fiber characteristic of trigger points.[2,8]

Clinical Characteristics

Musculoskeletal History

When evaluating a patient, it is important to get a complete history to guide the physical examination. Location will help to focus the physical examination on a particular region of the body, while onset or duration will help characterize the pain as acute, subacute, or chronic. It is important to determine if the pain was a result of a fall or trauma prompting additional evaluation and work-up. Characteristics of the pain, such as its quality, radiation, alleviating and exacerbating factors, and associated symptoms, will further aid in developing a differential diagnosis.

Review of systems is important to rule out more serious causes of musculoskeletal pain when formulating a differential diagnosis. For example, fevers, night sweats, and weight loss may point to underlying malignancy. Pain, weakness, muscle weakness, or wasting may infer a neuropathic or radicular pattern.

Physical Examination Findings

Classically, trigger points are divided into two broad categories that may cause muscle dysfunction—latent and active MTrP. Latent MTrPs do not cause pain at rest but may present with weakness or restrictions in movement. Active MTrPs cause pain at rest and present with clinical symptoms and characteristic referral patterns. Physical examination should begin by inspecting the area in question. Care should be taken to compare the contralateral side for evidence of asymmetry. Range of motion (ROM) should also be performed to evaluate for muscle dysfunction or restriction. If muscle dysfunction or asymmetry is noted, the area should be gently palpated. Increase in muscle tone or muscle tenderness may indicate that an MTrP is present. Applying pressure to this area will reproduce the patient's pain and possibly the referral pattern. Perpendicularly, palpating the finger gently across the fiber can aid in identifying the rope-like taut band that runs the length of the muscle.[2]

General Approach to Management

When managing a patient with myofascial pain, it is important to address the underlying muscle dysfunction. A course of physical therapy may be appropriate for therapeutic exercise and functional evaluation. Modalities such as ultrasound, acupressure, myofascial release, osteopathic manipulative treatment, acupuncture, and cold spray and stretch techniques may be useful to relieve pain and reduce tension. Studies have also shown that dry needling is also an effective method for the treatment of MTrPs.[11] The use of Botox for myofascial pain remains controversial with a need for more high-quality studies to be performed before definitive conclusions can be drawn.[12,13]

Trigger Point Injections

Mechanism of Action

The exact mechanism of action of trigger point inactivation with injections is unknown. Travell and Simons have suggested several mechanisms, including mechanical disruption of the self-sustaining MTrP mechanism; depolarization block of the nerve fibers by the released intracellular potassium; a wash-out process of the nerve-sensitizing substances by the injected fluid or local hemorrhage; and focal necrosis of the area of the MTrP by the injected drug. Since an injection usually produces immediate pain relief, it is likely that local mechanical disruption of the MTrP may play a key role in the interruption of the pain reflex.

One MTrP has many different loci that can generate pain and a local twitch response (LTR) when palpated. These loci are thought to be sensory receptors or sensory nerve fibers that need to be inactivated to achieve pain relief.[14,15] In addition, a proper diagnosis of an MTrP in combination with a proper technique is necessary to achieve pain relief. The diagnosis of an MTrP on physical examination is based on four factors—(1) palpable nodule/taut band; (2) referred pain; (3) LTR; and (4) satellite trigger points. With snapping palpation of the MTrP, the area elicits a twitch response referred to as the LTR that is associated with a sharp pain or discomfort at the site, as well as a referred pain pattern. This same response and referral pain pattern can be seen when a needle is inserted into an MTrP. When an LTR is seen on insertion, it is associated with better pain relief than when an LTR is not seen on needle insertion.[16]

Goal of Trigger Point Injections

Injections are indicated in cases when MTrPs remain unresponsive to noninvasive approaches; treatment time is limited, and when a muscle cannot be stretched for mechanical reasons. The purpose of an injection is to increase ROM, restore muscle length and function, and eliminate pain. When a trigger point is precisely identified and injected with accuracy, one injection can be sufficient to inactivate the trigger point. Contraindications to injections include anticoagulation therapy and local skin infection.[2]

Injection content: The trigger point injection can be performed using the dry-needling technique or "wet-needling" with an injection of a solution such as local anesthetics, isotonic saline, steroids, nonsteroidal anti-inflammatory drugs (NSAIDs), or Botox.

Several studies have investigated the benefits of dry needling versus wet needling and have not shown one to be superior to the other. There was also no significant difference between the solutions used in the wet-needling approach, though Botox remains controversial.[17] Some benefit has been reported with a local anesthetic compared to dry needling. In a study by Hong et al., when an upper trapezius trigger point was injected and an LTR was present, those injected with lidocaine reported less soreness at 2–8 hours postinjection and lower pain scores at 2 weeks compared to the dry-needling group. However, both groups had similar improvements in immediate pain.[11]

Injection Approach

Preparation: Before beginning the procedure, appropriate informed consent should be obtained, and the patient should be aware that injecting the MTrP can cause pain at the MTrP site and in its referral pattern. The clinician must ask if the patient is taking any oral anticoagulants or vitamin C, which can increase the risk of bleeding. If possible, the patient should be positioned in a recumbent position in order to avoid syncope and minimize patient anxiety. Appropriate needle size must be chosen so that the needle length is sufficient enough to reach the depth of the MTrP. The size of the needle diameter is typically dependent on the clinician's preference. Larger diameter needles are less likely to bend within the tissue and be redirected by the taught bands. On the other hand, smaller diameter needles cause less tissue damage and are well-suited for a "fast-in, fast-out" technique which will be described in the following sections.

Skin preparation/cleansing: The skin should be prepared with an antiseptic. If using alcohol, the alcohol should be allowed to dry prior to injecting the needle as it can sting as the needle penetrates the skin. A vapocoolant spray can be used to provide cold anesthesia and decrease the pain of needle insertion by decreasing the temperature to below 10°C. After cleansing the skin, the vapocoolant spray is applied from a distance of about 45 cm for 5–6 seconds just before frosting. After stopping the vapocoolant and allowing a moment for the vapocoolant to evaporate from the skin, the needle is then quickly introduced into the skin.

Localization and injection: Localizing an MTrP is essential for accurate injection and pain relief. The trigger point is identified by first palpating a taut band, followed by a firmer nodule within the taut band, and finding the spot of highest tenderness. The area of most tenderness is the location that is most likely to elicit LTR by snapping palpation or by needle insertion. There are several palpation techniques that can be used to localize the MTrP—flat palpation, pincer palpation, and deep palpation. With flat palpation, an MTrP nodule is pushed back and forth between the fingers and then fixed between fingertips for injection. Using the pincer palpation technique, the nodule is located by rolling the taut band between the fingers. For injection, the MTrP is held between the thumb and fingertips. Lastly, deep palpation can also be used to locate points of maximal tenderness.

Injection technique: In preparation for injection, the skin is pulled taut to hold the MTrP in position and prevent it from rolling. The needle is then inserted into the skin and the trigger point. Trigger points can also be located at the muscle attachment and are injected in similar fashion. During the procedure, bleeding should be prevented which can be achieved by spreading the skin during the injection and applying pressure postinjection for hemostasis. Each taut band can have multiple MTrPs that should be inactivated to achieve maximal pain relief. In this situation, the needle can be redirected (without being removed from the skin) to inject all the painful foci.[18] If an LTR and referred pain were present prior to the injection, then they are also expected to be present during the injection. Injections that elicit LTR are much more likely to achieve pain relief than those that do not. The hand holding the syringe must be supported by the body to allow adequate control of the needle while injecting. The "fast in, fast out" injection technique has been shown to be effective for injecting MTrP. With this technique, the needle is quickly inserted to fully penetrate the taut band and then is pulled back to the subcutaneous tissue layer while still remaining in the skin. With this technique, LTRs are more likely to be elicited and the needle is more likely to follow a straight path rather than be deflected by the contracted knots.

Postprocedure: Following an injection, the symptoms of MTrP, such as the LTR, tense band spot tenderness, and referred pain, should disappear. The number of MTrPs that should be injected at one time depends on practitioner preference. Acute MTrPs with no additional tissue damage or perpetuating factors are expected to resolve with one or two injections. Chronic MTrPs may require many injections over months of treatment. In such instances, the period of relief should become longer with each injection. When multiple active MTrPs are present in functionally related muscles, it is advantageous to inactivate all the MTrP in that muscle group. Postinjection treatment is important for successful pain relief. A full active stretch of the muscle should be performed immediately postinjection. Elimination of underlying factors modified and a stretching or strengthening protocol should be implemented in order to prevent recurring MTrPs.[2]

The following sections will focus on specific muscle groups commonly seen in MPS with typical referral patterns, injection approaches, and precautions, if applicable.

Head and Neck

Upper Trapezius

Typical pain pattern: Pain refers to the posterolateral neck, posterior ear, and the temple.

Injection approach ***(Figs. 1A to D)****:*

- Trigger point 1 can be located with the patient supine and the examiner pinching the upper trapezius, lifting it superiorly off of the underlying tissue, and palpating the trigger point nodule, which will reproduce the patient's pain. When injecting, start anteriorly and direct the needle tip posterosuperiorly toward the trigger point.
- Trigger point 2 can be located with the patient side-lying on the opposite side or prone. It is located at the level of the spinous processes of C5-C6, midway between the acromion and cervical spine. When injecting start posteriorly and direct the needle tip anterosuperiorly into the trigger point.

Precautions: It is important to direct the needle tip superiorly while advancing to avoid lung puncture with both upper trapezius trigger point injections. Advancing too deeply when injecting trigger point 2 can also result in the injection of the supraspinatus muscle instead of the trapezius.

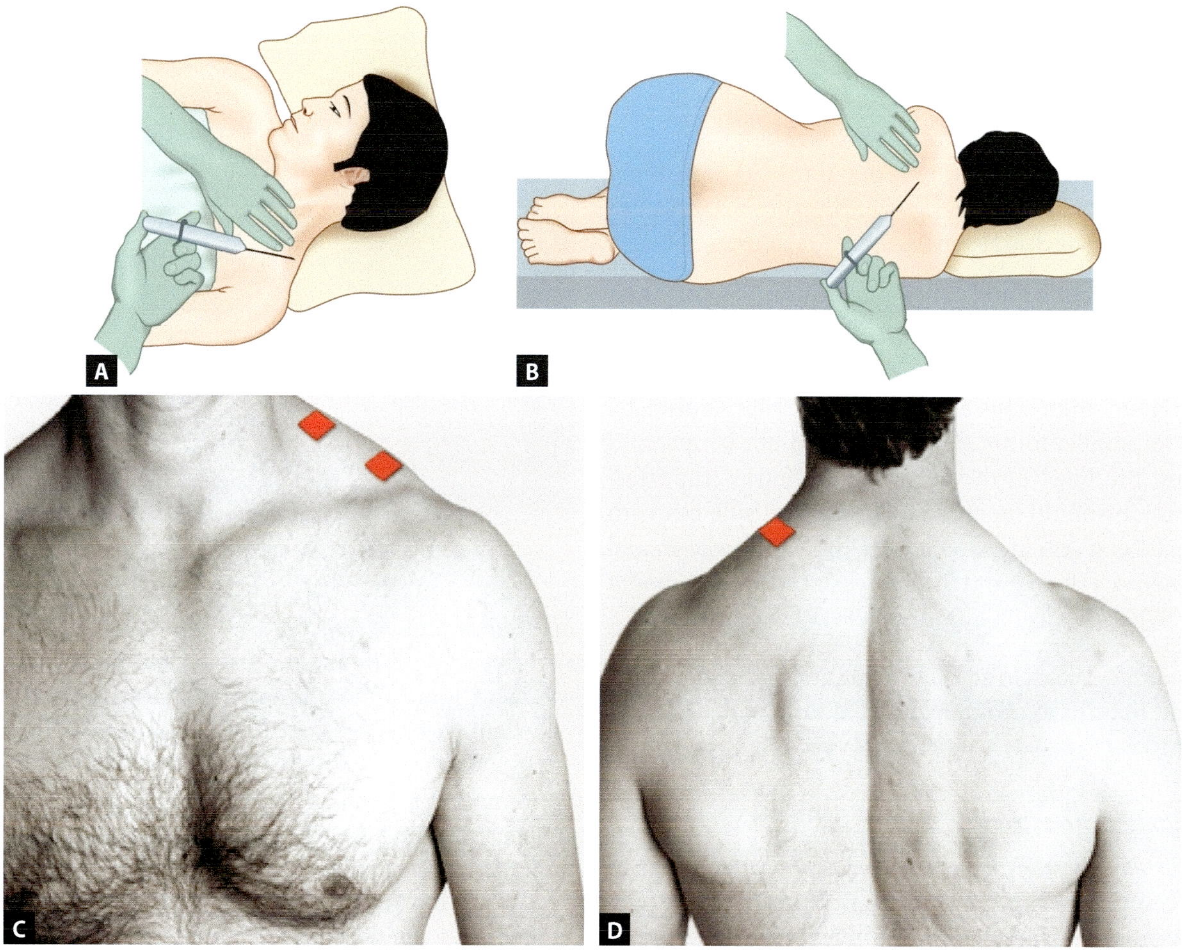

Figs. 1A to D: Upper trapezius.

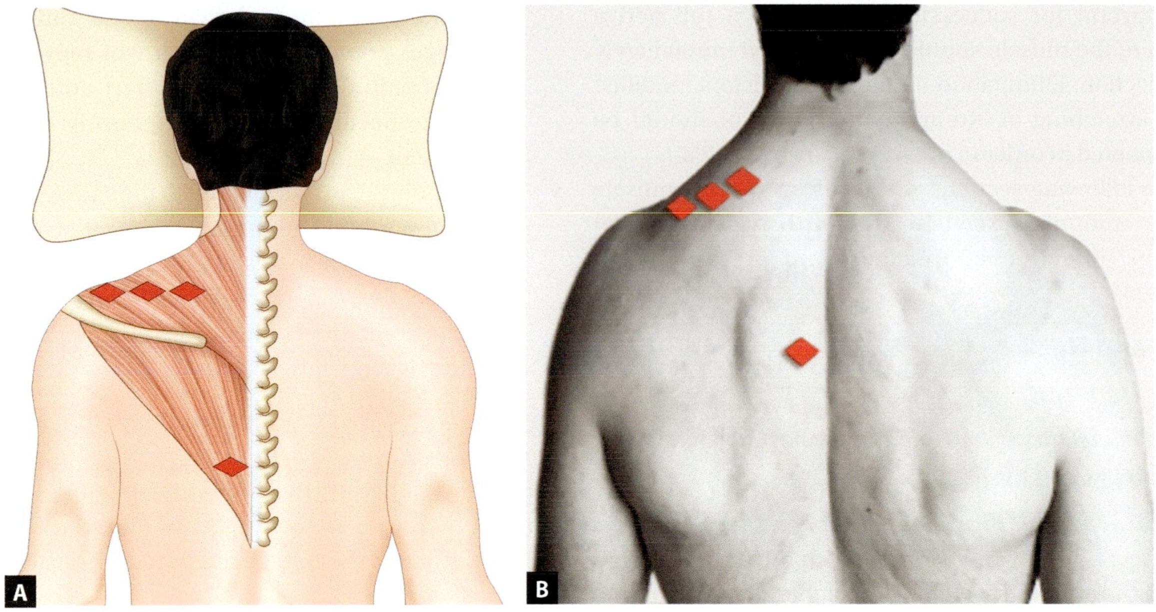

Figs. 2A and B: Middle and lower trapezius.

Middle and Lower Trapezius

Typical pain pattern: Pain from the middle trapezius trigger points refers to the upper thoracic paraspinal region ipsilaterally. Lower trapezius trigger points refer to posterolateral neck and suprascapular region.

Injection approach ***(Figs. 2A and B)****:* For the middle trapezius, the patient should lie on the contralateral side with hands between the knees. While aiming toward the trigger point, the angle of the needle should be close to parallel to the skin and should not be inserted beyond the level of the ribs. For the lower trapezius, the patient should lie on the contralateral side but with the ipsilateral arm in front of the body. The needle should be aimed at a rib to avoid the intercostal space and should also not be advanced beyond the level of the ribs.

Precautions: Maintain an acute angle and do not penetrate beyond the ribs to avoid inadvertent lung puncture. Aim toward a rib to avoid the intercostal space.

Sternocleidomastoid

Typical pain pattern: The sternal division often refers to the occiput, over the maxilla, periorbitally, and to the sternum. The clavicular component can cause frontal headaches and pain posterior to and in the ear.

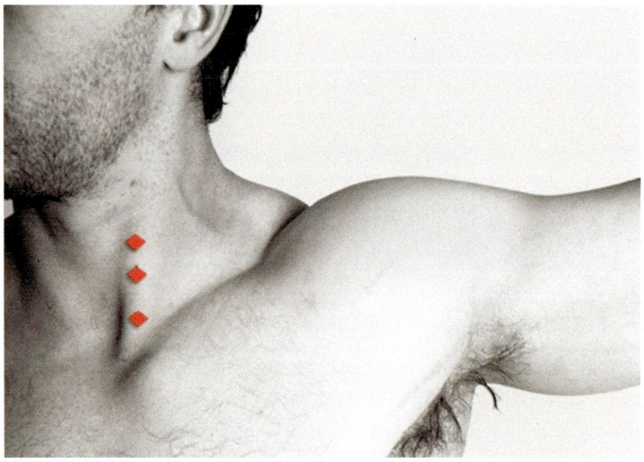

Fig. 3: Sternocleidomastoid.

Injection approach ***(Fig. 3)****:*

- Trigger points along the sternocleidomastoid can be found by encircling the entire muscle belly between the examiner's fingers, starting from the sternoclavicular attachment and continuing up to the mastoid, while identifying areas of tenderness, tightness, and/or referred pain. The examiner must be sure to evaluate both heads of the sternocleidomastoid muscle (SCM).
- For the injection, the patient should lie supine with the head slightly rotated toward the side that will be injected. The entire muscle belly should be grasped

within the examiner's fingers and lifted off of any underlying neuromuscular structures. The external jugular vein can be located by compressing it just above the clavicle. Avoid injection of the external jugular vein while inserting needle and inject once the area of most tenderness is reached. The examiner can at that point reassess for any more trigger points of the SCM and inject them with redirection or if necessary can pull the needle out and repeat on another trigger point of the SCM.

Precautions:

- It is frequent to have worsening local pain and headache after the injection of sternocleidomastoid trigger points. Heat packs and gentle ROM initially after and for the following 1–3 days are advised.
- Occasionally, the injected solution may infiltrate and block the posterior branch of the greater auricular nerve during SCM trigger point injection. It is advised to warn the patient that they may experience a sensation of numbness or prickling pain at the jaw, cheek, and ear initially after the injection, which will subside usually in about 15–20 minutes depending on the injectate used.
- Avoid bilateral sternocleidomastoid injections on the same visit. If patient has bilateral sternocleidomastoid trigger points, it is recommended to assess improvement of the first injection prior to proceeding with the second.
- Avoid excessive straining after the injection. Educate patient on techniques to avoid strain on the SCM (for example, while rising from lying to a sitting position, have the patient turn his/her head slightly in the ipsilateral direction).

Splenius Capitis/Splenius Cervicis

Typical pain pattern: Pain is experienced diffusely throughout the cranium, most intensely at the vertex and posterior to the orbit.

Injection approach ***(Figs. 4A and B)****:*

- The patient should lie down on the contralateral side in neutral cervical position. The trigger point is usually located in the middle of the muscle belly. To locate the splenius capitis, the examiner should first locate the sternocleidomastoid at its mastoid origination and then palpate just posteriorly while asking the patient to rotate ipsilaterally and slightly extend the neck. The patient must then relax the neck while the examiner palpates along the direction of the splenius capitis fibers and locates any tight bands with associated pain.
- To avoid injecting the vertebral artery, it is safest to inject the mid-muscle trigger points and the needle must be angled caudally, aiming below the level of the C1-C2 junction. The needle should also be angled close to the plane and the direction of the muscle fibers since it is a relatively thin muscle.

Precautions: Be aware of the anatomical location of the vertebral artery. Slightly cephalad to the C1 spinous process, the vertebral artery is poorly protected. Therefore, aim caudad from the level of the C1-C2 vertebral junction.

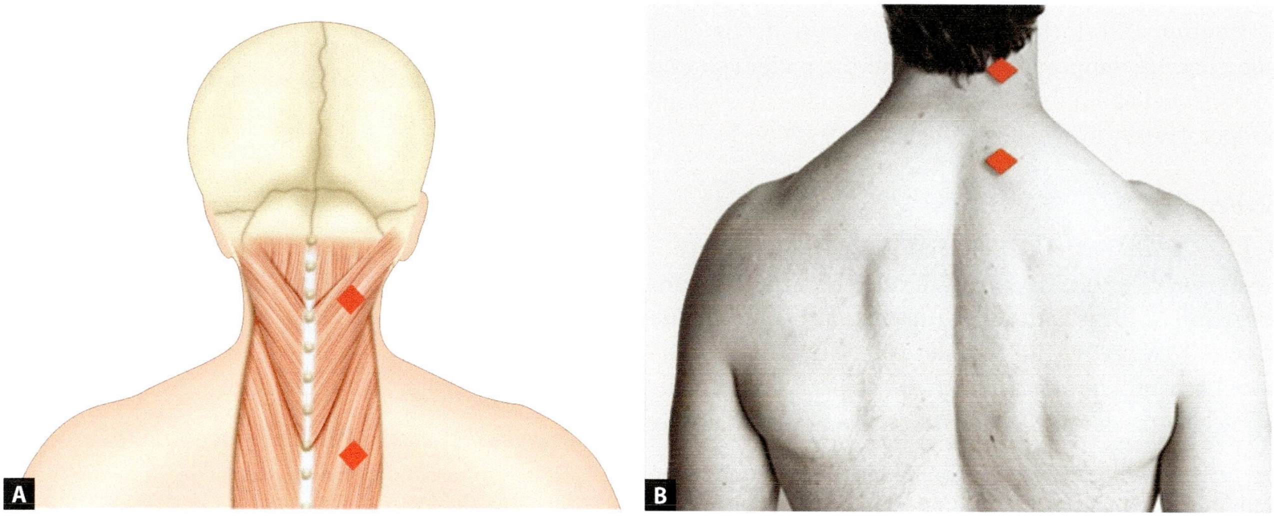

Figs. 4A and B: Splenius capitis/cervicis.

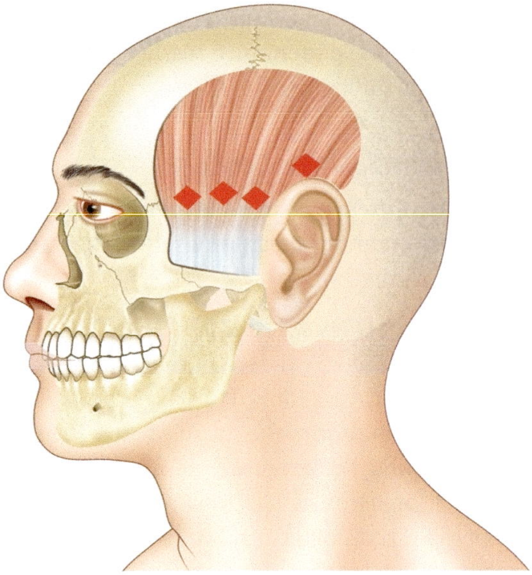

Fig. 5: Temporalis muscles.

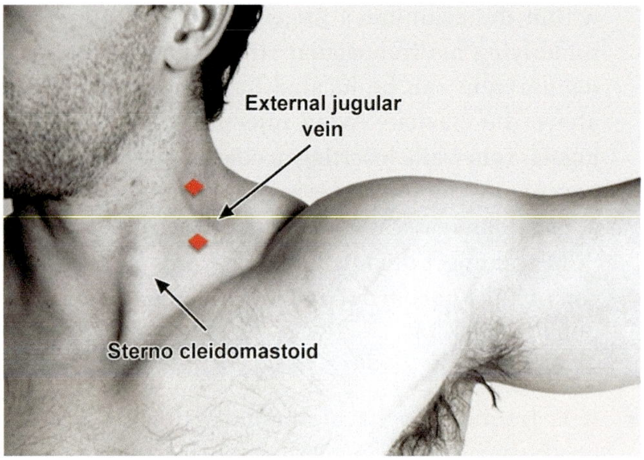

Fig. 6: Trigger points of the scalene muscles.

Temporalis

Typical pain pattern: Patients can present with complaints of temporal headaches, temporomandibular joint pain, and maxillary toothaches.

*Injection approach **(Fig. 5)**:* The jaw should be partially open and flat palpation can be used to localize the trigger points. They can be located along the musculotendinous junction or near the mid fibers. Place one finger over the temporal artery and one over the trigger point to localize the injection site and advance the needle cephalad during the injection to hit the intended trigger point.

Precautions: Periorbital ecchymosis may occur after injecting the temporalis muscle and the patient should be educated about this. Place one finger directly over the temporal artery to avoid injecting it.

Scalenes

Typical pain pattern: Referred pain can be present posteriorly, anteriorly, or laterally. In the posterior direction, pain is felt along the medial border of the scapula. Laterally, the pain is experienced along the upper arm and forearm, though the elbow is not typically involved. Anteriorly, the pain projects to the pectoral area.

*Injection approach **(Fig. 6)**:* The patient should be supine with the head rotated slightly in the contralateral direction with the use of a pillow to allow for slight cervical flexion. The most common trigger points for the anterior and middle scalenes are located around the jugular vein and can be located by occluding the vein with a finger slightly above the clavicle. The needle should be inserted at least 4 cm above the clavicle to avoid lung puncture and should be directed superiorly. The brachial plexus is located in the vertical groove (between the anterior and middle scalene muscles). During injection, one digit should be placed in the groove, and the other on the other side of the trigger point being injected so that the trigger point lies in between the fingers. To inject the anterior scalene, the needle should be angled anteriorly from the groove. To inject the middle scalene, the needle should be angled posteriorly from the groove.

Precautions: All injections to the scalene muscles should be inserted at least 4 cm above the clavicle and directed superiorly (and not inferiorly) to avoid lung puncture. Avoid deep injection or too far anterior since this may cause a block of the stellate ganglion or sympathetic trunk and cause a transient Horner syndrome. Avoid injecting into the groove to avoid direct injection of the brachial plexus. Proper injection of the scalenes may still cause transient numbness in the upper extremity due to infiltration by the anesthetic. Referral pain down the upper extremity is common during trigger point injection of the scalenes.

Levator Scapulae

Typical pain pattern: Pain is concentrated along the length of the muscle in the posterior neck to the medial scapula and can project to the posterior shoulder joint and interscapular area.

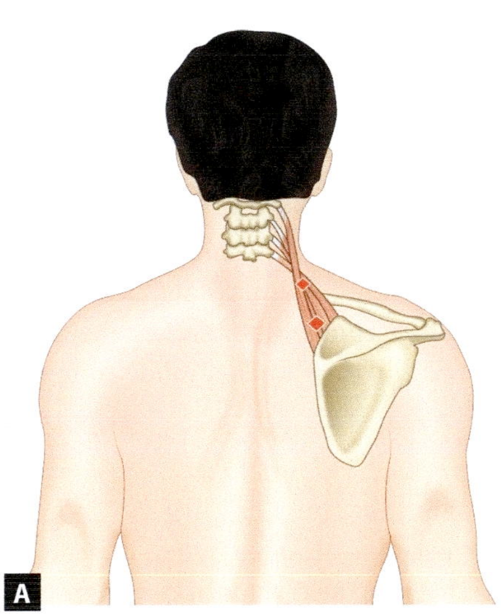

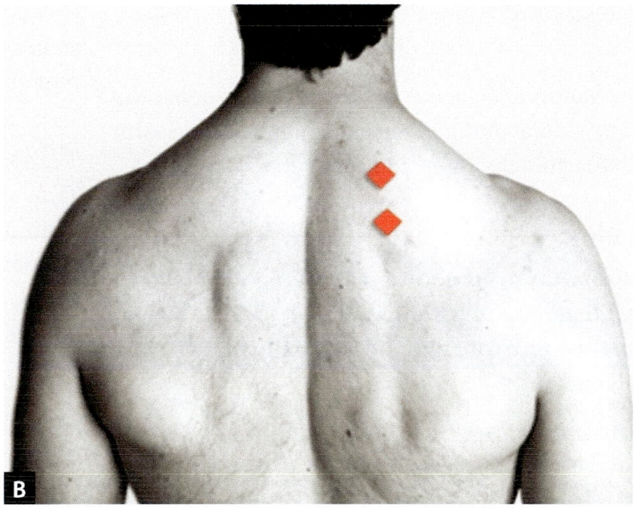

Figs. 7A and B: Trigger points of the levator scapulae muscles.

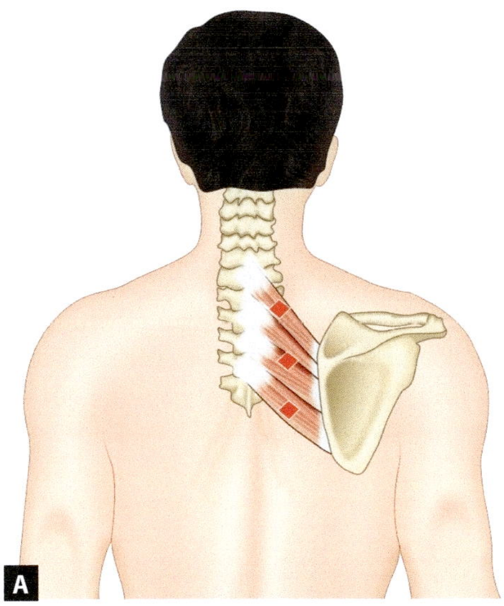

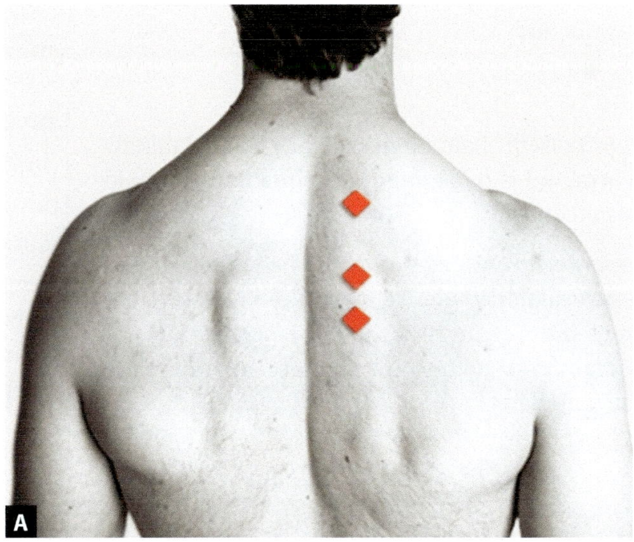

Figs. 8A and B: Trigger points of the rhomboid major and minor muscles.

Injection approach ***(Figs. 7A and B)****:* The patient should lie on the contralateral side with a pillow supporting the head and the ipsilateral arm lying on the body. The levator scapula can be located by pushing the upper trapezius inferiorly out of the way and palpating the tight levator scapula directly anterior to the trapezius. The needle should be directed from posterior to anterior toward the trigger point.

Precautions*:* Avoid injecting inferiorly into the rib cage to avoid lung puncture and avoid injecting too deeply to avoid brachial plexus injection.

Upper Back and Torso

Rhomboid Major/Minor

Typical pain pattern: The pain pattern of the rhomboids typically stays localized along the course of the muscles, most concentrated at the insertion along the medial scapula.

Injection approach ***(Figs. 8A and B)****:* After palpating the trigger point, it should be held between the operator's digits and injected as tangentially as possible to avoid injecting into the intercostal space and lungs. The approach is similar to that described for the middle trapezius trigger point.

Precautions: Maintain an acute angle and do not penetrate beyond the ribs to avoid inadvertent lung puncture. Aim toward a rib to avoid the intercostal space.

Pectoralis Major

Typical pain pattern: In addition to being localized in the pectoral region, pain can be referred to the anterior shoulder, medial forearm, and, occasionally, the 4th and 5th digits of the hand.

Injection approach ***(Figs. 9A and B)****:* After palpating the trigger point, it should be held between the operator's digits and injected as tangentially as possible to avoid injecting into the intercostal space and lungs.

Precautions: Avoid perpendicular or deep injections to avoid lung puncture.

Supraspinatus

Typical pain pattern: Pain often typically refers laterally down the arm and is most intense at the middle deltoid and lateral epicondyle.

Injection approach ***(Figs. 10A and B)****:* The patient should lie on the contralateral side. To inject the medial trigger point, direct the needle into the suprascapular fossa, inferior and posterior to the trapezius, just superior to the spine of the scapula.

Precautions: Avoid injecting too medially or superiorly as this may cause injection of the upper trapezius or lung puncture.

Infraspinatus

Typical pain pattern: The referral pattern for this muscle is similar to that of the supraspinatus muscles, except that the pain is more concentrated along the anterior deltoid and deeper within the shoulder joint rather than along the middle deltoid.

Injection approach ***(Figs. 10A and B)****:* The patient should lie on the contralateral side with the shoulder in 45° of flexion and propped elevated by a pillow. The trigger point should be located and remain between the operator's fingers during the injection.

Precautions: As long as the needle is inserted directed toward the infraspinous fossa, there are no precautions to a trigger point injection to the infraspinatus muscle.

Lower Torso and Lower Limb

Lumbar Paraspinal Muscles: Iliocostalis, Longissimus, Multifidi

Typical pain pattern: Pain from the iliocostalis refers to the mid-buttock area, while the longissimus refers to the low-buttock and sacroiliac region. Pain from the multifidi remains localized along the spinous processes and paraspinal region.

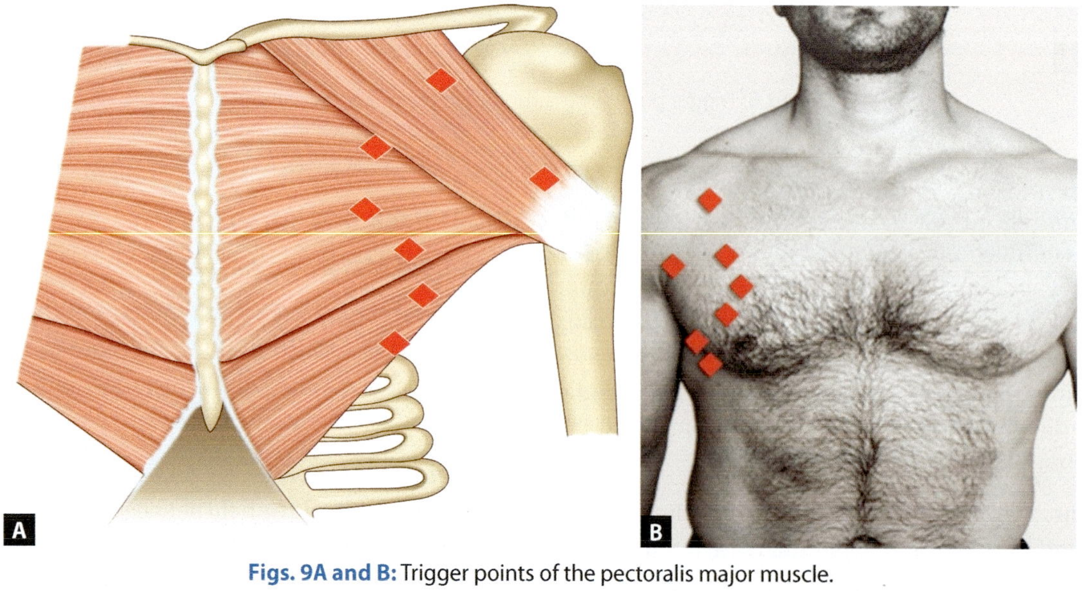

Figs. 9A and B: Trigger points of the pectoralis major muscle.

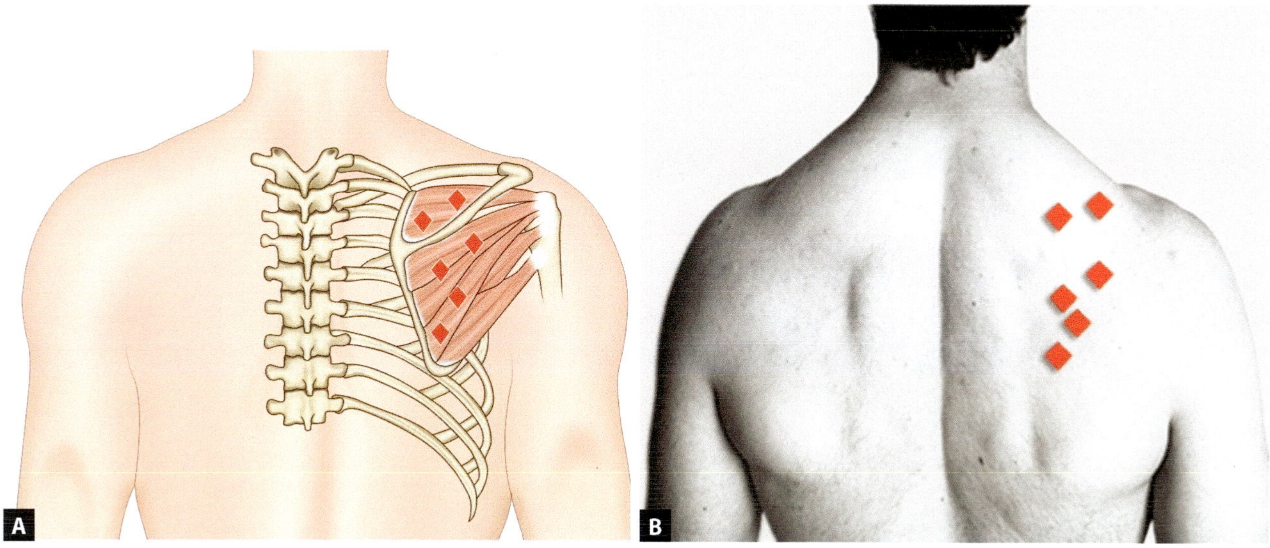

Figs. 10A and B: Trigger points of the supraspinatus (superior 2 points) and infraspinatus (inferior 4 points).

Injection approach ***(Fig. 11)****:* To locate the trigger points, the patient should lie prone with a pillow supporting the abdomen or should be seated and leaning forward to allow for slight flexion of the spine. Tenderness along the spinous processes will reveal associated trigger points in the associated paraspinal musculature upon deeper finger pressure. The deep and superficial muscles are injected and treated as a group. The needle should be tangential to the frontal plane of the patient.

Precautions: Avoid deep penetration in the upper lumbar region and entrance into the intervertebral space by directing the needle in a caudal direction, similar to the injection approach outlined in the thoracic region to avoid entering the intercostal space.

Quadratus Lumborum

Typical pain pattern: Pain refers posteriorly to the sacroiliac region and lower buttock. It can also radiate anteriorly along the iliac crest and greater trochanter.

Injection approach ***(Figs. 12A and B)****:*

- When palpating, the patient should be positioned side lying on the unaffected side. The ipsilateral upper limb should be positioned cephalad with the lower limb dropped to the table or hanging off to accentuate a contralateral side bending of the torso as tolerated by the patient. A pillow may be placed between the costal cage and iliac crest. Three key regions are palpated: (1) Deep into intersection of the paraspinal mass and iliac crest (iliocostal and iliolumbar fibers); (2) Medial iliac crest (iliocostal fibers); and (3) At the angle of the paraspinal mass and 12th rib (iliocostal and lumbocostal fibers).
- Injection of the superficial iliocostal fiber trigger point can be performed by palpatory control. Deeper trigger points should be performed on the side lying, with the plane of the back perpendicular to the table. Insert the needle at the lateral edge of the paraspinal mass directed toward the lumbar transverse process.

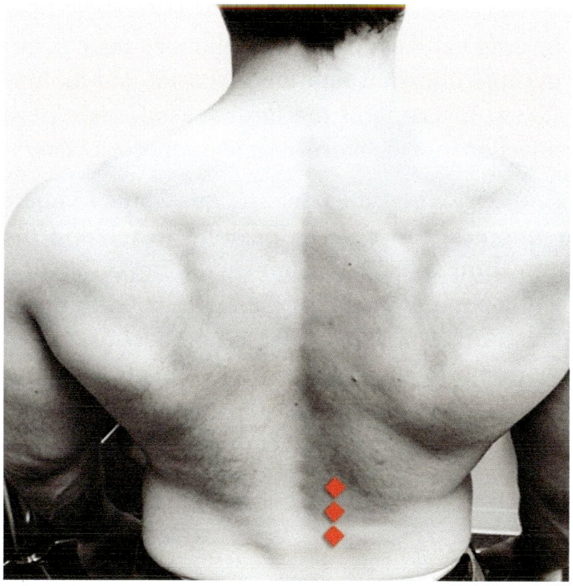

Fig. 11: Trigger points of the lumbar paraspinal muscles.

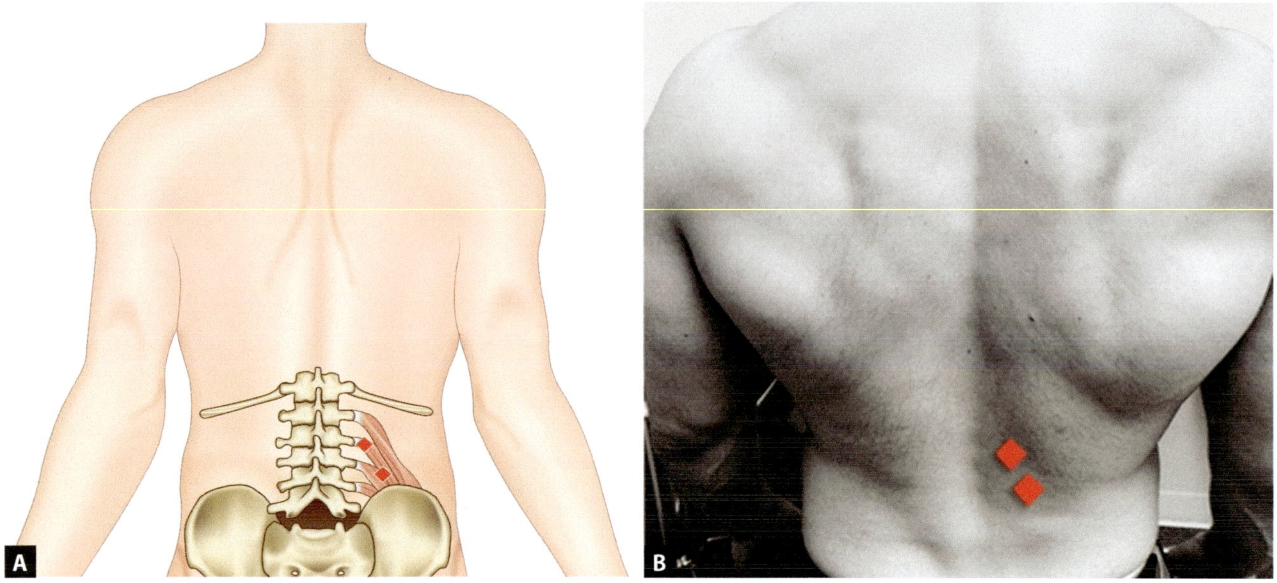

Figs. 12A and B: Trigger points of the quadratus lumborum muscle.

Insertion at the level of the iliolumbar angle (L4 level) permits injection into the iliocostal and iliolumbar fibers. Inserting at the lumbocostal angle permits injection into the iliocostal and lumbocostal fibers.

Precautions: When injecting the quadratus lumborum, it is important to note its position in relation to the retroperitoneal space. Superficial injection needle selection should be appropriate in relation to the body habitus of the patient to reach the fibers of quadratus lumborum through the paraspinal musculature. Caution should also be exercised when attempting to inject iliocostal and lumbocostal fibers, keeping the needle between the levels of L2 and L3 to prevent pneumothorax.

Gluteus Maximus

Typical pain pattern: Pain typically remains in the buttock region.

Injection approach **(*Fig. 13*)***:* This superficial muscle is best examined with the patient's side-lying hip partially flexed to stretch the muscle. Superior fibers may be palpated by moving the pad of the thumb parallel to the imaginary line from the sacroiliac joint to the greater trochanter. Inferior fibers may be assessed by pinching the muscle mass along the same imaginary track. The superficial location of gluteus maximus allows isolation of the trigger point between the 2nd and 3rd digits with direct injection into the taut band. *Note:* A vigorous twitch response may occur.

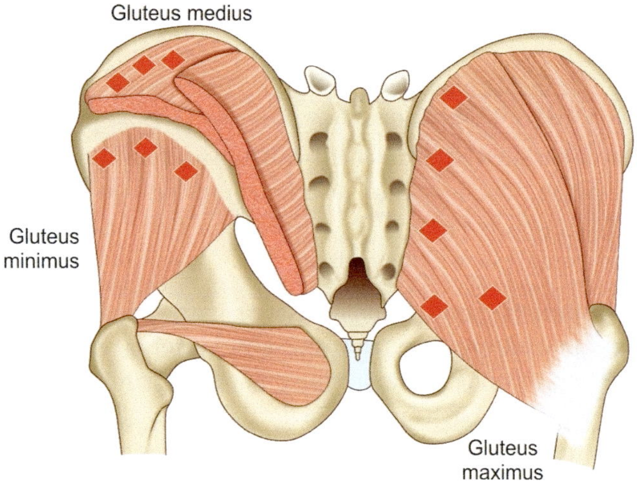

Fig. 13: Trigger points of the gluteus maximus, medius, and minimus.

Precautions: Avoid injecting too deeply as the sciatic nerve lies directly deep in this muscle.

Gluteus Medius, Minimus

Typical pain pattern: Gluteus medius pain may refer to the lumbar region, extending into the posterior iliac crest, sacrum, and posterolateral aspect of the buttocks. Gluteus minimus may refer to pain down the lateral aspect of the thigh, knee, and leg to the ankle.

Injection approach **(*Fig. 13*)***:* Examination of the gluteus medius and minimus is best performed with the patient in a side-lying position, course the thumb in a fan-like distribution from the iliac crest toward the greater trochanter, paralleling its fibers. The 2nd and 3rd digits can be utilized to isolate the trigger point. Given their anatomy and underlying ilium, injection is directed toward the trigger point keeping in mind that the medius overlies the minimus muscle.

Precautions: Depth should be adjusted based on the targeted muscle; the needle may be advanced to oculus sinister (OS) and retracted to the desired depth.

Tensor Fascia Latae

Typical pain pattern: Pain is primarily referred to down the lateral thigh and can mimic trochanteric bursitis.

Injection approach ***(Fig. 14)****:* The muscle is best examined in the supine position by palpating the fibers starting at the anterior iliac crest, traversing over the hip joint, and ending into the iliotibial band. The muscle can be identified by asking the patient to internally rotate the thigh against resistance. It may be helpful to induce slight flexion at the hip by using a pillow under the knee. The trigger point is isolated between the fingertips to prevent movement while injecting.

Precautions: Although there are not any major blood vessels or nerves immediately superficial or deep to the tensor fascia latae, care must be taken to avoid the femoral neurovascular bundle lying medial to the muscle.

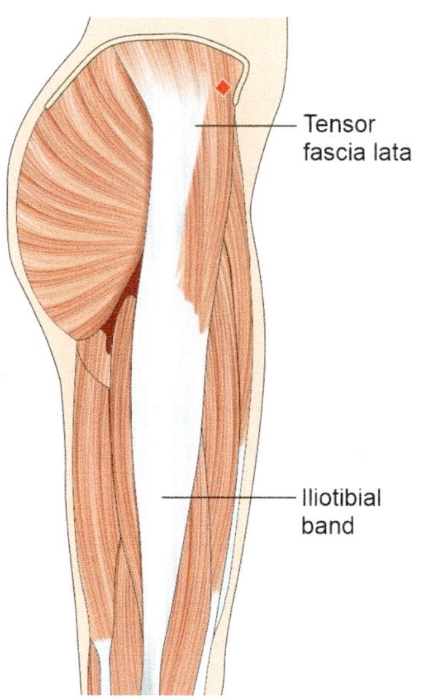

Fig. 14: Trigger points of the tensor fascia latae muscle.

Adductor Longus, Brevis, Magnus

Typical pain pattern: Trigger points in this muscle group can cause referred pain in the groin.

Injection approach ***(Fig. 15)****:* The adductors are best examined with the patient in the supine position. Trigger points can be palpated along the length of the medial thigh overlying the femur. Injection of the adductor longus and brevis is best done by grasping the muscle belly in a pincer grip with the patient supine. The thigh should be in partial abduction to allow slack in the muscle.

Precautions: Care should be taken to avoid the neurovascular bundle, especially the femoral artery which lies in close proximity to the adductor longus and brevis. The above technique will help prevent trauma to the femoral neurovascular bundle. Also, it should be noted that the sciatic nerve passes posterior to and runs the length of the adductor magnus, traversing anteriorly through the adductor hiatus distally.

Quadriceps (Rectus Femoris, Vastus Lateralis, Intermedius, Medialis)

Typical pain pattern: Trigger points cause referred pain to the lateral, anterior, and medial thighs. Pain can be referred to the distal thigh and into the knee.

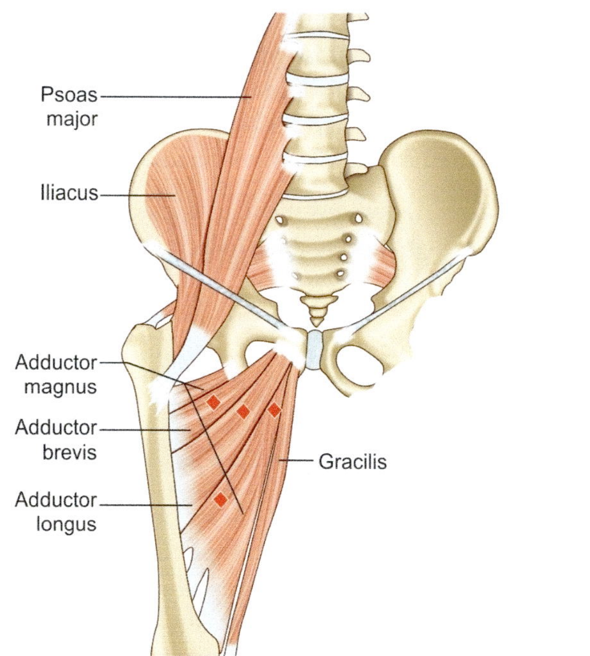

Fig. 15: Trigger points of the adductor longus, adductor brevis, and adductor magnus muscles.

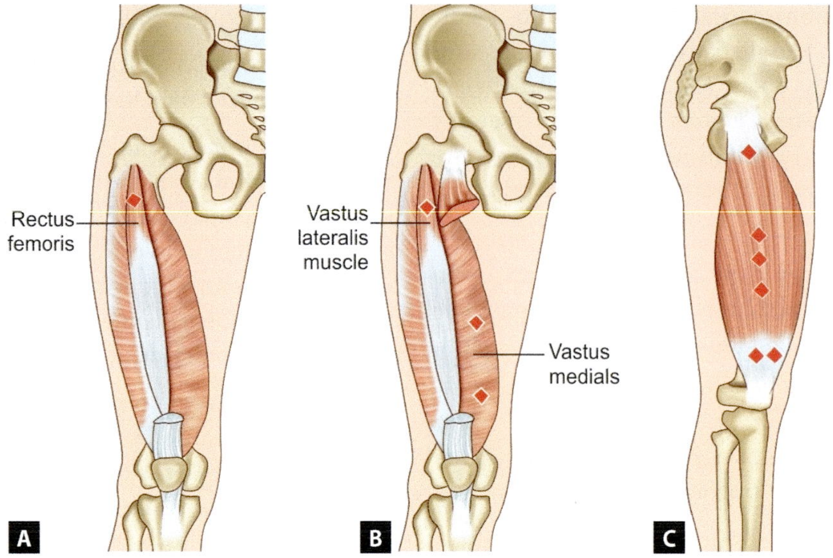

Figs. 16A to C: (A) Trigger points of the rectus femoris; (B) Vastus intermedius and vastus medialis; (C) Vastus lateralis.

Injection approach ***(Figs. 16A to C)****:* To examine the quadriceps, the patient may be supine with the leg draped off the examination table inducing hip extension and the practitioner flexing the knee joint. This maneuver will tighten the fibers of the quadriceps to accentuate tender points. Injection is performed with the patient in the supine position with the hip in slight extension and knee in flexion to reduce slack in the muscle fibers. The trigger point is palpated and isolated between two digits of the noninjecting hand. If trigger points in the rectus femoris are inactivated and pain persists, one may infer the trigger point lies in the deep vastus intermedius.

Precautions: The vastus medialis is palpable in the distal half of the thigh; the proximal half consists of the adductor muscles.

Hamstrings (Biceps Femoris, Semitendinosus, Semimembranosus)

Typical pain pattern: Trigger points cause referred pain to the buttocks, posterior thigh, and into the knee.

Injection approach ***(Fig. 17)****:* Injection of semitendinosus and semimembranosus can be performed in the supine position with the hip partially flexed and abducted and the knee flexed. Distal trigger points are best injected with a pincer grasp using the noninjecting hand. It is important to keep the needle between the digits grasping the muscle belly. When injecting biceps femoris, the patient should be in a side-lying position on the unaffected side. The needle should be inserted midline in the posterior thigh and directed laterally.

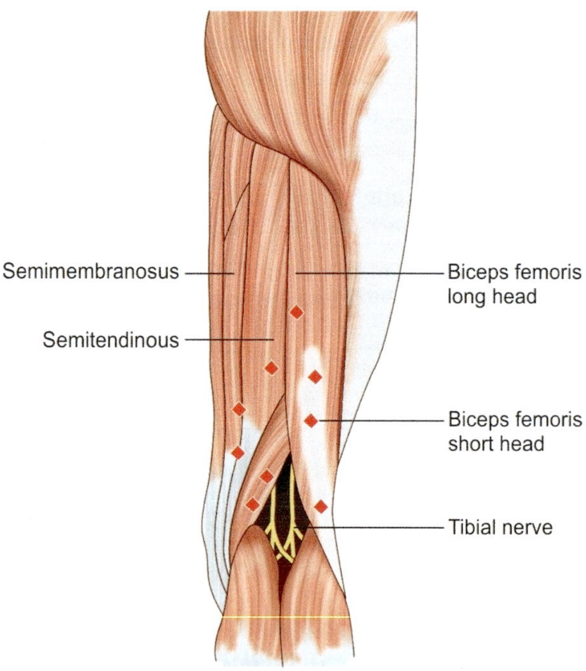

Fig. 17: Trigger points of the biceps femoris, semitendinosus, and semimembranosus.

Precautions: It is important to review the anatomy of the sciatic nerve to avoid trauma. Care should be taken to avoid the neurovascular bundle at the distal thigh. When treating the hamstrings, it is recommended to treat one side per visit as the patient may experience significant postinjection discomfort.

CONCLUSION

Myofascial pain syndrome and its associated trigger points have been well-documented in the medical literature and comprise a significant proportion of presenting complaints to physicians' offices. A multitude of options exist, both invasive and noninvasive, for managing MPS, including physical therapy, stretching, massage, spray and stretch, and trigger point injections. The ultimate goal when treating MPS is to correct the underlying abnormality that perpetuates the trigger points, such as poor posture, gait biomechanics, bony abnormalities (osteoarthritis, facet arthropathy), soft tissue abnormalities (diskogenic disease), and neuropathies (radiculopathy).

Trigger point injections are commonly utilized by clinicians, and an MTrP is localized via physical examination. However, physical examination skills can be varied and often unreliable. Moreover, objective clinical measurements are currently lacking in evaluating the efficacy of the afore-mentioned therapeutic options. Current research is examining the utility of ultrasound in providing objective real-time data in identifying MTrPs, especially in the deep back and cervical neck muscles.[19-22] Studies have shown that MTrPs appear as focal, hypoechoic elliptical regions.[19] In addition to guiding and confirming proper needle placement into the muscle and MTrP of interest, ultrasound may also demonstrate postprocedural changes in the surrounding tissue. A recent randomized controlled pilot study demonstrated improvement in tissue conditions seen on 2D ultrasound after dry needling with acupuncture.[23] This recent implementation of ultrasound in objectively evaluating MPS and MTrP injections is a promising area of ongoing research and may aid in optimizing MTrP injections in the future.

REFERENCES

1. Alvarez DJ, Rockwell PG. Trigger points: diagnosis and management. Am Fam Physician. 2002;65(4):653-60.
2. Simons D, Travell J, Simons L. Myofascial Pain and Dysfunction: The Trigger Point Manual, 2nd edition. Baltimore: Williams and Wilkins; 1999.
3. Simons DG, Hong CZ, Simons LS. Endplate potentials are common to midfiber myofascial trigger points. Am J Phys Med Rehabil. 2002;81(3):212-22.
4. Iglesias-González JJ, Muñoz-García MT, Rodrigues-de-Souza DP, Alburquerque-Sendín F, Fernández-de-Las-Peñas C. Myofascial trigger points, pain, disability, and sleep quality in patients with chronic nonspecific low back pain. Pain Med. 2013;14(12):1964-70.
5. Woolf AD, Pfleger B. Burden of major musculoskeletal conditions. Bull World Health Organ. 2003;81(9):646-56.
6. Stewart WF, Ricci JA, Chee E, Morganstein D, Lipton R. Lost productive time and cost due to common pain conditions in the US workforce. JAMA. 2003;290(18):2443-54.
7. Huxley AF, Niedergerke R. Structural changes in muscle during contraction: interference microscopy of living muscle fibers. Nature. 1954;173(4412):971-3.
8. Shah JP, Gilliams EA. Uncovering the biochemical milieu of myofascial trigger points using in vivo microdialysis: an application of muscle pain concepts to myofascial pain syndrome. J Bodyw Mov Ther. 2008;12(4):371-84.
9. McPartland JM. Travell trigger points: molecular and osteopathic perspectives. J Am Osteopath Assoc. 2004; 104(6):244-9.
10. Hubbard DR, Berkoff GM. Myofascial trigger points show spontaneous needle EMG activity. Spine (Phila Pa 1976). 1993;18(13):1803-7.
11. Tekin L, Akarsu S, Durmuş O, Cakar E, Dinçer U, Kıralp MZ. The effect of dry needling in the treatment of myofascial pain syndrome: a randomized double-blinded placebo-controlled trial. Clin Rheumatol. 2013;32(3):309-15.
12. Soares A, Andriolo RB, Atallah ÁN, da Silva EM. Botulinum toxin for myofascial pain syndromes in adults. Cochrane Database Syst Rev. 2014;2014(7):CD007533.
13. Zhou JY, Wang D. An update on botulinum toxin A injections of trigger points for myofascial pain. Curr Pain Headache Rep. 2014;18(1):386.
14. Hesse J, Møgelvang B, Simonsen H. Acupuncture versus metoprolol in migraine prophylaxis: a randomized trial of trigger point inactivation. J Intern Med. 1994;235(5): 451-6.
15. Hong CZ. Lidocaine injection versus dry needling to myofascial trigger point. The importance of the local twitch response. Am J Phys Med Rehabil. 1994;73(4):256-63.
16. Hong CZ, Simons DG. Response to standard treatment for pectoralis minor myofascial pain syndrome after whiplash. J Musculoskel Pain. 1993;1(1):89-131.
17. Cummings TM, White AR. Needling therapies in the management of myofascial trigger point pain: a systematic review. Arch Phys Med Rehabil. 2001;82(7):986-92.
18. Hong CZ, Simons DG. Pathophysiologic and electrophysiologic mechanisms of myofascial trigger points. Arch Phys Med Rehabil. 1998;79(7):863-72.
19. Sikdar S, Shah JP, Gebreab T, Yen RH, Gilliams E, Danoff J, et al. Novel applications of ultrasound technology to

visualize and characterize myofascial trigger points and surrounding soft tissue. Arch Phys Med Rehabil. 2009;90(11): 1829-38.

20. Rha DW, Shin JC, Kim YK, Jung JH, Kim YU, Lee SC. Detecting local twitch responses of myofascial trigger points in the lower-back muscles using ultrasonography. Arch Phys Med Rehabil. 2011;92(10):1576-80.e1.
21. Thomas K, Shankar H. Targeting myofascial taut bands by ultrasound. Curr Pain Headache Rep. 2013; 17(7):349.
22. Turo D, Otto P, Shah JP, Heimur J, Gebreab T, Zaazhoa M, et al. Ultrasonic characterization of the upper trapezius muscle in patients with chronic neck pain. Ultrason Imaging. 2013;35(2):173-87.
23. Müller CE, Aranha MF, Gavião MB. Two-dimensional ultrasound and ultrasound elastography imaging of trigger points in women with myofascial pain syndrome treated by acupuncture and electroacupuncture: a double-blinded randomized controlled pilot study. Ultrason Imaging. 2015;37(2):152-67.

10

SECTION

Miscellaneous

70 CHAPTER

Understanding Implications and Handling of Medicolegal Aspects for Pain Physicians

Manjiri N Ranade

ABSTRACT

Pain medicine is a rapidly expanding specialty that focuses on relieving and controlling pain in patients with various conditions. Medicolegal awareness is essential for pain physicians to navigate the complexities of their profession, ensure ethical practice, prevent malpractice claims, maintain licensure, and improve patient safety. Informed consent is a critical aspect of medical practice, particularly in pain medicine, allowing patients to make decisions about their bodies and establishing a legal basis in case of disputes. Professional liability risks are inherent in pain medicine, and pain physicians must take steps to mitigate and manage these risks, such as maintaining honesty and professionalism with patients. Accurate and comprehensive documentation is crucial in pain medicine for effective communication, continuity of care, and medicolegal purposes. Pain physicians should adhere to their scope of practice, maintain accurate documentation, and prioritize patient safety and treatment outcomes. Overall, this paper highlights the importance of medicolegal awareness, informed consent, professional liability management, and documentation in pain medicine.

INTRODUCTION

Pain management is a complex field that intersects medicine, law, and ethics. Understanding the medicolegal aspects is crucial for pain physicians to navigate potential legal challenges, ensure compliance with regulations, and provide high-quality care.

The medicolegal landscape for pain physicians is multifaceted, requiring a balance of clinical expertise, ethical considerations, and legal awareness. By staying informed and proactive, pain specialists can enhance their practice while minimizing legal risks and improving patient outcomes. Continued education in these areas is essential for delivering safe and effective pain management.

MEDICOLEGAL CONSIDERATIONS IN PAIN MEDICINE

Definition and Scope of Pain Medicine

Pain medicine is a rapidly expanding multidisciplinary specialty that focuses on relieving and controlling pain in patients with various painful conditions. It requires personalized and evidence-based treatment approaches, considering each patient's needs.[1] Pain medicine has struggled with fragmentation and lack of interdisciplinary agreement, leading to confusion regarding who speaks for pain medicine.[2] However, efforts are being made to increase awareness and education in pain management, including dedicated awareness programs, continuing medical education programs, and conferences.[3] In the future, new pain medicines are expected to reach the market, expanding the options available for clinicians in managing persistent ongoing pain.[4]

Importance of Medicolegal Awareness for Pain Physicians

Medicolegal awareness is essential for pain physicians to navigate the complexities of their profession, prevent potential legal issues, and maintain a high standard of care for their patients. Some of the reasons why medicolegal awareness is important for pain physicians are discussed here.

- *Ensuring ethical practice:* Medicolegal awareness helps pain physicians understand the ethical guidelines

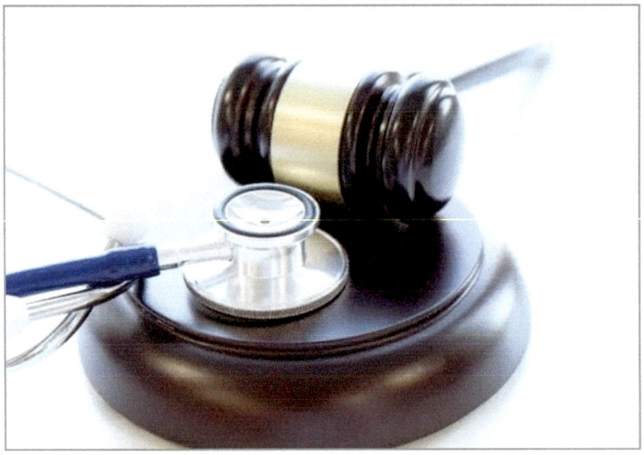

Fig. 1: Medicolegal awareness for pain physicians.

set forth by their profession and the broader medical community. This knowledge ensures that they make informed decisions and maintain high standards of care for their patients.

- *Preventing malpractice claims:* By being aware of the legal implications of their actions, pain physicians can minimize the risk of malpractice claims. This is crucial for maintaining a successful practice and protecting their professional reputation.
- *Enhancing patient trust:* A pain physician who demonstrates a strong understanding of medicolegal issues is more likely to gain the trust of their patients. This trust is vital for establishing a strong patient–physician relationship and promoting better outcomes.
- *Maintaining licensure:* Pain physicians must adhere to the laws and regulations set forth by their licensing boards. Medicolegal awareness ensures they comply with these requirements and avoid potential disciplinary actions.
- *Improving patient safety:* Pain physicians can identify potential risks and implement strategies to mitigate them by being mindful of medicolegal issues. This ultimately leads to a safer patient environment and a more effective healthcare system **(Fig. 1)**.

Overview of the Topics Covered in the Chapter

The chapter discusses the importance of medicolegal awareness for pain physicians, including ensuring ethical practice, preventing malpractice claims, maintaining licensure, and improving patient safety. It emphasizes the significance of informed consent in pain medicine, highlighting its role in respecting patient autonomy, establishing a clear understanding of medical procedures, and providing a legal basis in case of disputes. The chapter also addresses the management of professional liability risks in pain medicine, including the role of federal regulations and state laws in shaping the practice and the importance of teamwork, collaboration, and sharing knowledge among healthcare professionals. Accurate and comprehensive documentation in pain medicine is discussed, covering the essential components such as patient history, physical examination, diagnostic tests, treatment plan, and follow-up for effective communication, continuity of care, and medicolegal purposes. The chapter also highlights the need for documenting informed consent discussions in pain medicine, exploring various methods such as video recordings and opioid treatment agreements (OTAs), to minimize legal and ethical liability. Overall, the chapter covers medicolegal awareness, informed consent, professional liability management, and documentation in pain medicine.

INFORMED CONSENT AND SHARED DECISION-MAKING

Definition and Importance of Informed Consent

Informed consent is critical to medical practice, particularly in pain medicine. It is obtaining the patient's consent before any medical action is taken, ensuring that the patient is fully informed about their illness, treatment options, risks, and costs.[5] Informed consent is based on respect for individual autonomy, allowing patients to decide about their bodies.[6] It serves as a safeguard for doctors and patients, clearly understanding the potential outcomes of medical procedures and establishing a legal basis in case of any disputes.[7] In pain medicine, informed consent is particularly important due to the potential risks and complications associated with opioid therapy.[8] It allows for open communication between doctors and patients, ensuring that treatment goals are mutually agreed upon and patients actively manage their pain.

Elements of Informed Consent in Pain Medicine

When obtaining informed consent for pain management procedures, several key elements must be addressed.

These include:

- *Disclosure of diagnosis:* Patients must be provided with an accurate and clear diagnosis, including the nature and severity of their pain and any contributing factors.

- *Explanation of proposed treatment:* Providers must explain the proposed treatment or procedure, including its purpose, anticipated benefits, and potential risks.
- *Alternatives and consequences:* Patients should be informed about alternative treatments, their potential benefits and risks, and the consequences of not undergoing any treatment.
- *Patient understanding and decision-making:* Providers should engage in a dialog with the patient to ensure that they have understood the information presented and have had an opportunity to ask questions and express their preferences.

Shared Decision-making Process and Its Role in Reducing Legal Risks: Practical Medicolegal Implications

Shared decision-making (SDM) is a collaborative process that involves patients and healthcare professionals working together to make decisions about the patient's healthcare. In pain medicine, SDM plays a crucial role in reducing legal risks by ensuring that patients are actively involved in the decision-making process regarding their treatment options. In this, we will explore the significance of the SDM process and its impact on mitigating legal risks in pain medicine.

- *Importance of shared decision-making in pain medicine:* In pain medicine, SDM is essential as it acknowledges the patient as an integral part of the decision-making process. Patients suffering from chronic pain often face complex treatment choices, including medication management, interventional procedures, physical therapy, and psychological interventions. Involving patients in these decisions empowers them and ensures that their preferences, values, and goals are considered when determining the most appropriate treatment plan.[9]

  Moreover, SDM fosters a sense of trust and transparency between the healthcare provider and the patient. By engaging in open discussions about treatment options, potential risks, benefits, and uncertainties, healthcare professionals can build a stronger rapport with their patients. This transparent approach can help mitigate legal risks by reducing the likelihood of misunderstandings or allegations of medical negligence.[10]
- *Reducing legal risks through informed consent:* In pain medicine, informed consent is critical to SDM. When patients actively participate in treatment decisions, they are more likely to understand their condition and the proposed interventions comprehensively. This understanding is fundamental to obtaining valid informed consent, a legal and ethical requirement for medical interventions.[11]

  By engaging in SDM and obtaining informed consent, healthcare providers can reduce legal risks associated with allegations of medical malpractice or lack of patient autonomy. Patients well-informed about their treatment options are less likely to pursue legal action based on claims of inadequate disclosure or lack of involvement in decision-making processes.
- *Enhancing patient satisfaction and compliance:* SDM has been linked to higher levels of patient satisfaction and adherence to treatment plans. Satisfied and compliant patients are less likely to resort to litigation or complaints against healthcare providers in pain medicine. By involving patients in the decision-making process, healthcare professionals can promote a sense of ownership over their treatment journey, leading to improved outcomes and reduced legal risks.[12]

  Furthermore, when patients actively participate in treatment decisions, they are more likely to adhere to prescribed regimens and follow-up appointments. This increased compliance can contribute to better pain management outcomes while minimizing the potential for legal disputes related to alleged negligence or inadequate care.

Documenting Informed Consent Discussions

In pain medicine, there is a need to document informed consent discussions. Obtaining informed consent involves explaining the benefits and risks associated with a specific research project or therapeutic design.[13,14] Various methods have been proposed for documenting informed consent, including obtaining video recordings of patient encounters and storing them in a computer-readable data storage medium. In the context of opioid therapy for pain, OTAs have been used to promote safe use and may include documentation of informed consent.[8] However, studies have shown that surgeons often do not meet basic informed consent standards, highlighting the need to improve documenting discussions.[15] It is important to ensure that the information discussed between patients and providers is accurately documented to minimize legal and ethical liability.

MEDICAL RECORDS AND DOCUMENTATION

Significance of Accurate and Detailed Documentation

Accurate and detailed documentation in pain medicine ensures optimal patient care and outcomes. In this, we will explore the significance of accurate and detailed documentation in pain medicine, including its impact on patient safety, clinical decision-making, and research advancements.

- *Ensuring patient safety:* Accurate and detailed documentation is essential for patient safety in pain medicine. By maintaining a comprehensive record of a patient's medical history, including previous treatments, allergies, and potential contraindications, healthcare providers can minimize the risk of medication errors and adverse reactions. This information is particularly important when prescribing opioids or other potentially harmful medications, as it helps providers make informed decisions about appropriate dosing and monitoring.[16]
- *Informed clinical decision-making:* Detailed documentation is vital for tracking a patient's progress and identifying trends or patterns that may inform clinical decision-making. By maintaining thorough records of pain assessments, interventions, and outcomes, healthcare providers can better understand the efficacy of various treatment options and make more informed decisions about which treatments to recommend. This information can also help providers identify patients who may benefit from additional resources, such as referrals to pain specialists or pain management programs.[17]
- *Advancing pain medicine research:* Accurate and detailed documentation is crucial for advancing pain medicine research. By compiling comprehensive data on patient outcomes, healthcare providers can contribute to the growing body of knowledge on pain management and contribute to developing new treatments and interventions. Furthermore, well-documented cases can serve as valuable teaching tools for medical students, residents, and practitioners, helping to disseminate best practices and improve patient care.[18]

Essential Components of Pain Medicine Documentation

Pain medicine documentation is crucial to patient care, as it provides a comprehensive record of the patient's condition, treatment, and progress. Accurate and detailed documentation is essential for effective communication among healthcare providers, continuity of care, and medicolegal purposes. The essential components of pain medicine documentation encompass various aspects of the patient's history, physical examination, diagnostic tests, treatment plan, and follow-up. In this, we will outline the key components of pain medicine documentation to ensure comprehensive and accurate record-keeping for patients with pain-related conditions.

- *Patient history:* The patient's history is fundamental to pain medicine documentation. It should include a detailed account of the patient's pain symptoms, including the onset, duration, location, intensity, quality, aggravating and alleviating factors, and associated symptoms. Additionally, the history should encompass the patient's medical history, surgical history, medication history (including current medications and previous treatments for pain), allergies, social history (such as occupation and lifestyle factors), and family history of pain-related conditions.[19]
- *Physical examination:* A thorough physical examination is essential in pain medicine documentation to assess the patient's overall health status and identify any specific findings related to the pain condition. The physical examination should encompass vital signs, neurological assessment, musculoskeletal evaluation, sensory testing, motor function assessment, and any relevant physical findings associated with the pain complaint.[20]
- *Diagnostic tests:* Documentation of diagnostic tests is critical in pain medicine to provide objective data supporting the diagnosis and management of pain conditions. This may include imaging studies such as X-rays, magnetic resonance imaging (MRI) scans, computed tomography (CT) scans, or other specialized tests like electromyography (EMG) or nerve conduction studies. The results of these tests should be accurately recorded in the patient's medical record, along with interpretations and implications for the treatment plan.[21]
- *Pain assessment tools:* In addition to subjective descriptions of pain provided by the patient, standardized pain assessment tools can be valuable in documenting the severity and impact of pain on the patient's daily activities. Commonly used tools include visual analog scales (VAS), numerical rating scales (NRS), McGill Pain Questionnaire, Brief Pain Inventory

(BPI), and Pain Disability Index (PDI). These tools can provide quantifiable measures of pain that are useful for tracking changes over time and evaluating treatment effectiveness.[22]

- *Treatment plan:* Documenting a comprehensive treatment plan is essential in managing patients with pain conditions. This should include details on pharmacological interventions (medications prescribed), nonpharmacological interventions (physical therapy, acupuncture, cognitive-behavioral therapy), interventional procedures (injections or nerve blocks), surgical interventions if applicable, and referrals to other specialists or multidisciplinary pain management programs. The rationale for each treatment modality and informed consent discussions should also be documented.[23]
- *Follow-up and progress notes:* Regular follow-up visits require detailed progress notes documenting the patient's response to treatment interventions, any changes in symptoms or functional status, medication adjustments, or adverse effects experienced by the patient. These progress notes are essential for tracking the trajectory of the patient's condition over time and modifying the treatment plan accordingly.[24]
- *Medicolegal considerations:* Accurate and comprehensive documentation in pain medicine is crucial from a medicolegal standpoint. It serves as a legal record that can be used to justify clinical decisions made by healthcare providers and defend against potential malpractice claims. Therefore, the responsible healthcare provider must ensure that all documentation is clear, legible, dated, timed, and authenticated.[25]

Best Practices for Medical Record Keeping

Pain medicine is a specialized field that requires meticulous record-keeping to ensure accurate diagnosis, effective treatment, and optimal patient care. Proper medical record-keeping in pain medicine involves adhering to best practices prioritizing patient privacy, data security, and regulatory compliance. Some of the key best practices for medical record-keeping **(Fig. 2)** in pain medicine are mentioned here.

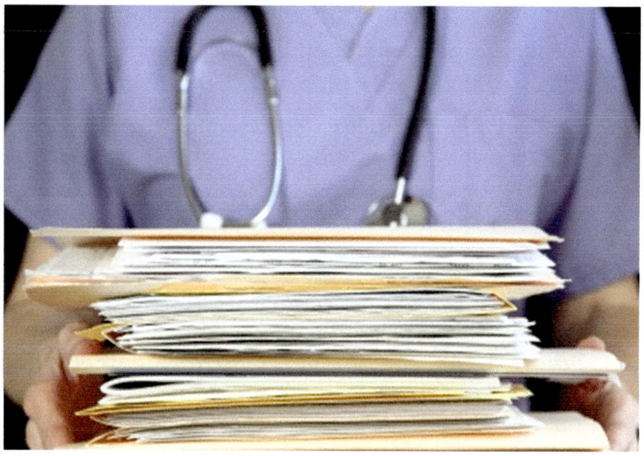

Fig. 2: Medical health records.

- *Standardized documentation:* Standardized documentation helps ensure consistency and accuracy in medical records. This can be achieved using established templates and guidelines for recording patient demographics, medical history, pain assessment, treatment plans, and follow-up care. Standardized documentation also allows for easier comparison and analysis of patient data, which can aid in research and quality improvement efforts.
- *Confidentiality and privacy:* Maintaining patient confidentiality and privacy is essential in pain medicine, as healthcare providers and patients often share sensitive information. Adhering to HIPAA (Health Insurance Portability and Accountability Act) regulations and other relevant privacy laws ensures that patient information is protected and only accessed by authorized individuals.
- *Electronic health records (EHRs):* EHRs are an efficient and secure method for storing and managing medical records. EHRs allow for easy access to patient information, streamlined communication between healthcare providers, and real-time updates to medical records. Utilizing EHRs can help reduce the risk of errors and improve overall patient care.

Importance of Timely and Comprehensive Documentation

Timely and comprehensive documentation plays a crucial role in pain medicine, as it helps healthcare providers to assess, diagnose, and treat patients effectively and accurately. This will discuss the importance of timely and comprehensive documentation in pain medicine, including its benefits and challenges.

Benefits of Timely and Comprehensive Documentation in Pain Medicine

- *Accurate assessment and diagnosis:* Proper documentation allows healthcare providers to understand the patient's medical history, symptoms, and previous treatments. This information is essential in making an accurate assessment and diagnosis of the patient's pain condition, which ultimately helps in developing a tailored treatment plan.

- *Effective communication:* Timely and comprehensive documentation ensures that all healthcare providers involved in a patient's care have access to the necessary information. This promotes effective communication among the team, leading to better coordination of care and improved patient outcomes.
- *Quality improvement and research:* Documentation is a valuable data source for quality improvement initiatives and research in pain medicine. By analyzing and comparing patient outcomes, healthcare providers can identify best practices and develop evidence-based guidelines to improve patient care.
- *Legal and regulatory compliance:* Proper documentation is essential for maintaining legal and regulatory compliance in pain medicine. Accurate records help protect healthcare providers from lawsuits and ensure they comply with relevant regulations governing opioid prescribing and monitoring.

Challenges in Timely and Comprehensive Documentation in Pain Medicine

- *Time constraints:* Healthcare providers often face time constraints, making it difficult to document all the necessary information promptly. This may lead to incomplete or inaccurate documentation, negatively impacting patient care.
- *Documentation burden:* EHRs have increased the documentation required by healthcare providers. This documentation burden can be overwhelming, leading to potential errors and inefficiencies in the documentation process.
- *Variation in documentation practices:* There is often a lack of standardization in documentation practices among healthcare providers, which can lead to inconsistencies in the information available for patient care.

REGULATORY COMPLIANCE AND LEGAL FRAMEWORK

Federal, State, and Local Laws Affecting Pain Physicians

- *Federal laws affecting pain physicians:* The federal government has enacted several laws to regulate the prescription and distribution of medications, particularly those with potential for abuse, such as opioids. The Controlled Substances Act (CSA),[26] enacted in 1970, classifies drugs based on their potential for abuse, medical use, and physical and psychological dependence. Pain physicians must adhere to the strict regulations set forth by the CSA when prescribing controlled substances.

  Another federal law impacting pain physicians is the Drug Enforcement Administration (DEA),[27] which enforces the CSA. The DEA regulates the manufacturing, distribution, and dispensing of controlled substances, ensuring that practitioners follow proper protocols to prevent diversion and abuse. Furthermore, the Narcotic Drug and Psychotropic Substances Act, 1986 regulates the manufacture, possession, sale, purchase, transport, warehousing, use, consumption, import inter-state, export inter-state, import into India, export from India or transshipment of narcotic drug and psychotropic substances.

  Medical Council of India (MCI) Regulations, which have been replaced by the National Medical Commission (NMC) in recent years, set the standards for medical education and practice in India. Pain management and the use of certain drugs may be covered by these regulations. According to State Medical Councils, each state in India has its own State Medical Council, which may have additional regulations or guidelines that affect the practice of medicine, including pain management. The Drug and Cosmetics Act, 1940, governs the import, manufacture, distribution, and sale of drugs and cosmetics in India. Pain medications and anesthetics fall under the purview of this act. Some states in India have adopted the Clinical Establishments (Registration and Regulation) Act, 2010 to regulate clinical establishments, including pain clinics and hospitals. According to State-Specific Laws, some states may have specific laws or regulations related to healthcare, medical practice, or the use of certain drugs. It is important for pain physicians to be aware of any state-specific regulations that may apply to their practice.
- *State laws affecting pain physicians:* In addition to federal regulations, state laws also play a significant role in shaping the practice of pain medicine. States have enacted various laws to address the opioid epidemic, such as prescription drug monitoring programs (PDMPs).[28] These programs require

practitioners to consult a centralized database before prescribing controlled substances, helping to prevent overprescribing and patient shopping for medications.

- *Local laws affecting pain physicians:* Local governments may also enact ordinances and regulations that impact pain physicians' practices. These laws may address clinic zoning restrictions, licensing requirements, and other operational aspects of pain management facilities. For example, a city may require a specific setback distance between a pain clinic and schools or residential areas or mandate that clinics obtain a conditional use permit before opening.

Compliance with Controlled Substance Regulations and Prescription Drug Monitoring Programs

Compliance with controlled substance regulations and PDMPs has been shown to have various impacts. PDMP usage has been associated with reducing or eliminating controlled substance prescriptions and changing them to nonopioid pharmacologic therapy or nonpharmacologic therapy.[29] Implementation of PDMPs with mandated provider review has been associated with a reduction in benzodiazepine prescription dispensing among adolescents and young adults.[30] "Must access" PDMP mandates have led to fewer retail opioid prescriptions in counties compared to "voluntary access" PDMP states.[31] Establishing centralized controlled substances compliance and drug diversion programs in healthcare facilities has been found to have organizational benefits, including standardization of processes and effective risk mitigation.[32]

Impact of Health Insurance Portability and Accountability Act Regulations on Patient Confidentiality

- *Enhanced privacy protection:* HIPAA regulations require that covered entities, such as healthcare providers, maintain the privacy of patients' protected health information (PHI). This includes restricting access to patient records and ensuring that only authorized personnel can view or disclose sensitive information.
- *Improved security measures:* The Security Rule mandates that covered entities implement reasonable and appropriate security measures to protect electronic PHI from unauthorized access, use, or disclosure. This includes using encryption, access controls, and regular security audits.
- *Increased accountability:* HIPAA regulations hold covered entities accountable for compliance with privacy and security rules. Noncompliance can result in fines, corrective action plans, and criminal penalties. This has led to a greater emphasis on training and education for healthcare professionals to ensure they understand their responsibilities under HIPAA.
- *Streamlined communication:* HIPAA regulations have facilitated the sharing of patient information between healthcare providers, as long as the sharing is necessary for treatment, payment, or healthcare operations. This can lead to improved coordination of care and more efficient communication among providers.
- *Patient empowerment:* HIPAA regulations give patients more control over their PHI by granting them the right to access, amend, and obtain a copy of their medical records. This can help to foster trust between patients and healthcare providers and promote a more collaborative approach to pain management.

The Preconception and Prenatal by Act of 2003

Diagnostic Techniques (Prohibition of Sex Selection) Act 1994.

Received the Assent of the President in May 2003.

- *Definition of Pre-Conception and Pre-Natal Diagnostic Techniques (PCPNDT):* An act to provide for the prohibition of sex selection, before or after conception, and for regulation of prenatal diagnostic techniques for the purposes of detecting abnormalities or metabolic disorders or chromosomal abnormalities or certain congenital malformations or sex-linked disorders and for the prevention of their misuse for sex determination leading to female feticide
- *Pre-Conception and Pre-Natal Diagnostic Techniques and Pain Management:* All facilities and clinics including hospitals/intensive care units or wherever a USG machine is used need to register with the appropriate authorities at least 3 months in advance, irrespective of whether the machine is being used for prenatal diagnostic tests or not. All doctors using the ultrasonography (USG) machine also need to be registered and should be appropriately qualified to perform sonography. This law basically centers around radiologists/sonologists and obstetricians who are regularly involved with prenatal or preconception testing.

Qualification to perform sonography and the training required. The act defines a "sonologist or imaging specialist" as a doctor having a postgraduate degree or diploma, or 6 months of training or 1 year of experience in USG or image scanning. In this context, the place and role of anesthesiologists, surgeons, cardiologists, intensive care and trauma physicians along with other specialist physicians within this law are ambiguous and a matter of continuous debate and changing laws. According to a Delhi High Court ruling in 2016, doctors and institutes owning and using a USG machine may register and could be exempt from complying with the provisions of the PCPNDT Act and other paperwork if they provide a declaration or undertaking stating that the machine is not intended for conducting prenatal diagnostic procedures and to not use or allow the use of the same for prenatal diagnostic procedures. This should also be displayed clearly outside the premises where USG is being used.

RISK MANAGEMENT STRATEGIES

Importance of Risk Assessment in Pain Medicine

Risk assessment plays a crucial role in pain medicine. It helps identify patients at a higher risk of adverse outcomes and allows for targeted interventions. Risk assessment tools such as the NSQIP (National Surgical Quality Improvement Program) and Modified-DASI (Duke Activity Status Index) have been developed to aid this process. However, accurately estimating the probability of adverse events can be challenging, and uncertainty is often involved. Understanding the social dimension of risk is essential in clinical practice and public health to implement effective risk management strategies. In the field of chronic pain, a biopsychosocial model has been developed to predict the number of coexisting pain sites and various pain-related medical conditions. This model can aid in tailoring research protocols, optimizing patient randomization in clinical trials, and improving pain management. Overall, risk assessment in pain medicine helps in informed decision-making, resource allocation, and improving patient outcomes.

Strategies for Identifying and Managing Risks Associated with Treatments and Procedures

Medical treatments and procedures are essential for diagnosing and managing various health conditions.

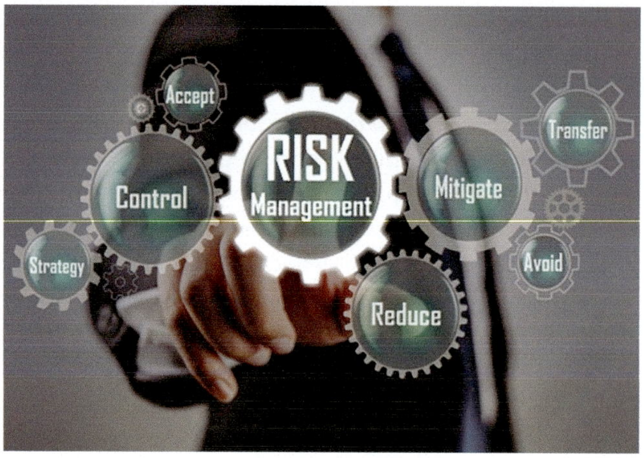

Fig. 3: Risk management.

However, they also have inherent risks that can impact patient safety and well-being. Therefore, healthcare professionals must employ effective strategies for identifying and managing these risks to ensure patient outcomes. Managing risks effectively is paramount in safeguarding patient safety and optimizing treatment outcomes. The following strategies can aid in the proactive management of risks **(Fig. 3)** associated with medical treatments and procedures:

- *Implementation of standardized protocols:* Establishing standardized protocols for high-risk procedures promotes consistency in care delivery and reduces the likelihood of errors or adverse events.
- *Continuous monitoring and surveillance:* Utilizing advanced monitoring technologies and surveillance systems enables real-time tracking of patient status during treatments or procedures, allowing for prompt intervention in case of any deviations from expected outcomes.
- *Quality improvement initiatives:* Continuous quality improvement efforts foster a safety culture within healthcare organizations, leading to enhanced risk management practices and better patient outcomes.
- *Risk mitigation strategies:* Developing specific strategies to mitigate identified risks, such as infection control measures, medication reconciliation processes, or fall prevention protocols, contributes to overall risk reduction.
- *Adherence to evidence-based practices:* Embracing evidence-based guidelines and best practices ensures that treatments and procedures align with established standards, minimizing unnecessary risks.

- *Open communication and reporting systems:* Encouraging open communication channels for reporting near-misses or potential risks cultivates a culture of transparency and accountability within healthcare settings.
- *Posttreatment follow-up:* Implementing structured posttreatment follow-up protocols allows for early detection of any complications or adverse effects, enabling timely intervention and management.

Prompt Recognition and Management of Complications

Prompt recognition and management of complications in pain medicine is crucial for patient safety and optimal outcomes. Interventional pain management procedures can have potential iatrogenic complications, including cardiovascular and neurologic complications.[33,34] In addition, there is a risk of serious, life-threatening infectious complications associated with interventional pain procedures and surgeries.[35] It is important for physicians to thoroughly understand potential complications, their pathophysiology, and appropriate management strategies. Complications can range from minor infections to more severe outcomes such as hematomas, paralysis, and even death.[36] Preoperative screening and using tools like fluoroscopy are essential in preventing complications.[37] In pain medicine, prompt recognition and management of complications is crucial to ensure patient safety and improve outcomes.

Implementing Protocols for Patient Safety

Implementing protocols for patient safety in pain medicine is crucial to prevent medical errors and improve patient outcomes. Multidisciplinary checklists and physician-led time-outs, such as the World Health Organization (WHO) Surgical Safety Checklist, have significantly improved patient safety in interventional pain procedures.[38] Standardized pain management protocols, including multimodal, sliding scale protocols, are more effective than traditional analgesic prescribing in achieving meaningful analgesia, reducing opioid use, and improving safety measures.[39] Training programs incorporating simulated patients and bedside teaching have been shown to increase student competence in pain medicine dramatically.[40] Implementing protocols and algorithms for the rational use of opioid analgesics, along with knowledge and expertise among healthcare professionals, can improve patient safety in pain management.[41] While some recommended protocols are available, developing standardized protocols specific to the Indian population is needed in pain medicine.[42]

ETHICAL CONSIDERATIONS IN PAIN MEDICINE

Ethical Principles Guiding Pain Physicians

Pain medicine requires a strong foundation in ethical principles to ensure the best possible care for patients. Pain physicians must adhere to these principles to maintain the trust of their patients and the medical community. There are several ethical principles **(Fig. 4)** that pain physicians must follow, including the following:

- *Autonomy:* Pain physicians must respect their patients' autonomy by allowing them to make informed decisions about their care. This involves providing accurate information about treatment options, risks, and benefits and discussing the potential outcomes of each choice.
- *Nonmaleficence:* Pain physicians must not harm their patients. This principle requires them to weigh the potential risks and benefits of treatments and interventions and only proceed with those likely to benefit the patient.
- *Beneficence:* Pain physicians must act in their patients' best interests, providing care likely to maximize their well-being. This includes offering appropriate treatments, managing side effects, and addressing any emotional or psychological issues that may arise during treatment.

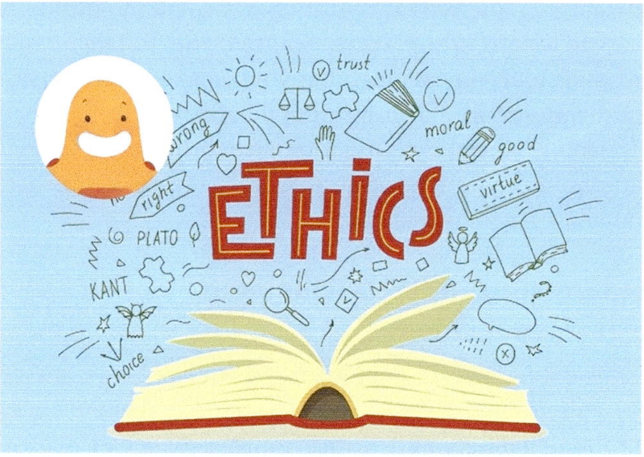

Fig. 4: Professional ethics.

- *Justice:* Pain physicians must ensure their care is distributed fairly and equitably among all patients. This involves equal access to care, regardless of socioeconomic status, race, or gender.
- *Confidentiality:* Pain physicians must protect the privacy of their patients by maintaining confidentiality and only sharing information with other healthcare providers when necessary or with the patient's consent.
- *Truth-telling:* Pain physicians must be honest and transparent with their patients, providing accurate information about their condition and treatment options. This includes discussing various treatments' potential risks, benefits, and limitations.
- *Professionalism:* Pain physicians must maintain high standards of professionalism, including adhering to professional codes of conduct and demonstrating empathy and compassion toward their patients.

Balancing Patient Autonomy and Physician Responsibility

Balancing patient autonomy and physician responsibility in pain medicine requires a shift toward a relational approach to patient autonomy. This approach allows physicians to understand patients in a broader social and cultural context, supporting patient autonomy in diverse healthcare settings.[43] It is important to integrate the expertise and ideas of physicians while respecting patient autonomy. Patients should be seen as experts on their values, goals, and preferences, while physicians are experts on the medical means to honor the patient's perspective.[44] By incorporating the lessons of moral virtue in medical practice, physicians can make informed decisions and offer considered therapeutic options to patients.[45] The excessive deference to patient autonomy can inadvertently place unwanted and unreasonable responsibility on patients, depriving them of expert advice and potentially harming their healthcare decisions.[46] Therefore, a balance must be struck between patient autonomy and physician responsibility to ensure the best outcomes in pain medicine.

Addressing Ethical Dilemmas in Pain Management

Ethical dilemmas in pain management can be addressed by redefining the principles of autonomy, beneficence/nonmaleficence, and justice to agency, social justice, and solidarity. The principles of respect for autonomy, nonmaleficence, beneficence, and justice are essential in biomedical ethics and should be applied in pain medicine. Pain specialists face day-to-day challenges in managing chronic pain, and ethical considerations must be considered based on guidelines, clinical practice, and evidence. Nurses working with patients with substance dependence and pain encounter ethical issues such as trust, paternalism, coercion, failure to respect autonomy, advocacy, and withholding. Ethical applications in pain research involve sound design, informed consent, population selection, and availability of alternative pain treatments. Collaborative approaches, awareness of power differentials, and ethical guidance can help address ethical dilemmas in pain management.

Ethical Decision-making Frameworks

Ethical decision-making in pain medicine involves complex considerations due to the subjective nature of pain, potential for misuse of medications, and the need to balance patient autonomy with societal interests. Several ethical frameworks guide healthcare professionals in navigating these complexities to ensure the delivery of high-quality care while upholding ethical principles.

- *Principles of bioethics:* As outlined by Beauchamp and Childress, the principles of bioethics provide a foundational framework for ethical decision-making in healthcare. These principles include respect for autonomy, beneficence, nonmaleficence, and justice.[47] In pain medicine, these principles guide physicians in respecting patients' autonomy in treatment decisions, promoting their well-being (beneficence), avoiding harm (nonmaleficence), and ensuring fair distribution of pain management resources (justice).
- *Shared decision-making:* SDM is essential to ethical practice in pain medicine. It involves collaborative discussions between healthcare providers and patients to make informed decisions about treatment options based on the best available evidence and the patient's values and preferences.[9] In pain management, SDM empowers patients to actively participate in their care while considering the ethical principles of respect for autonomy and beneficence.
- *Palliative care:* Principles in cases where pain management intersects with end-of-life care, palliative care principles play a crucial role in ethical decision-making. The World Health Organization's definition of palliative care emphasizes the relief of pain and other

distressing symptoms while affirming life and regarding dying as a normal process.[48] Ethical frameworks in pain medicine often integrate these palliative care principles to ensure compassionate and holistic care for patients with advanced or terminal illnesses.

- *Risk-benefit:* Analysis of ethical decision-making in pain medicine involves a thorough risk-benefit analysis of treatment options. This approach requires healthcare providers to assess the potential benefits of pain interventions against the risks, including adverse effects and the potential for misuse or addiction. By carefully weighing these factors, clinicians can make ethically sound decisions prioritizing patient safety and well-being.
- *Cultural competence:* Cultural competence is an integral aspect of ethical decision-making in pain medicine, particularly in addressing disparities in pain management among diverse patient populations. Healthcare providers must be attuned to cultural beliefs about pain and treatment approaches while ensuring equitable access to effective pain care. Ethical frameworks emphasize the importance of cultural competence to uphold the principle of justice and mitigate disparities in pain management.

EFFECTIVE COMMUNICATION AND DOCUMENTATION

Importance of Clear and Effective Communication with Patients and Colleagues

Pain medicine is a specialized field that requires a high level of precision, empathy, and understanding. As healthcare professionals in this field, it is crucial to establish clear and effective communication with patients and colleagues to ensure the best possible outcomes for those in our care. This heading will discuss the importance of clear and effective communication in pain medicine and how it can positively impact patient care and professional relationships.

- *Effective communication with patients:*
  - Enhancing patient understanding and compliance: When patients fully understand their diagnosis, treatment options, and expected outcomes, they are more likely to adhere to their treatment plan. This can lead to better pain management and overall well-being.
  - Building trust and rapport: Trust is a fundamental aspect of the patient-provider relationship. Providers can establish trust and rapport by communicating effectively, leading to better patient satisfaction and improved outcomes.
  - Reducing anxiety and stress: Patients with chronic pain often experience high levels of anxiety and stress. By clearly communicating with patients, providers can help alleviate these feelings and create a more comfortable environment for discussing their concerns.
- *Effective communication with colleagues:*
  - Enhancing teamwork and collaboration: In pain medicine, collaboration between various healthcare professionals is essential for providing comprehensive and effective care. Clear communication among team members can improve coordination and patient care.
  - Sharing knowledge and best practices: Effective communication among colleagues allows for sharing knowledge and expertise, which can lead to the implementation of best practices and improved patient outcomes.
  - Identifying and addressing gaps in care: Through open communication, healthcare professionals can identify gaps and work together to develop strategies to address these issues, ultimately leading to improved patient care.

Strategies for Improving Communication Skills

Pain medicine is a critical aspect of healthcare that requires effective communication between patients and healthcare providers to ensure proper diagnosis, treatment, and pain management. Improving communication skills in pain medicine can lead to better patient outcomes and increased patient and provider satisfaction. In this, we will discuss various strategies for enhancing communication skills in pain medicine.

- *Active listening:* Active listening is a crucial skill in pain medicine as it helps providers understand the patient's perspective and concerns. By fully engaging in the conversation and asking open-ended questions, healthcare providers can better assess the patient's pain and develop an appropriate treatment plan.[49]
- *Empathy and compassion:* Empathy and compassion are essential in pain medicine, as patients often experience significant distress and suffering. By expressing genuine concern and understanding of the

patient's situation, providers can help alleviate their emotional pain and build trust.[50]

- *Cultural competence:* Cultural competence is vital in pain medicine as it ensures that providers can effectively communicate with patients from diverse backgrounds. By understanding and respecting cultural differences, providers can better assess and manage pain while minimizing the risk of cultural misunderstandings.[51]
- *Patient education and shared decision-making:* In pain medicine, patient education and SDM empower patients to take an active role in their care. By providing clear information about their condition, treatment options, and potential side effects, providers can help patients make informed decisions about their care.[52]
- *Continuous quality improvement and training:* To improve communication skills in pain medicine, healthcare providers must continually assess their skills and seek opportunities for training and professional development. Continuous quality improvement and training can help providers stay up-to-date with the latest evidence-based practices and enhance their communication skills.[53]

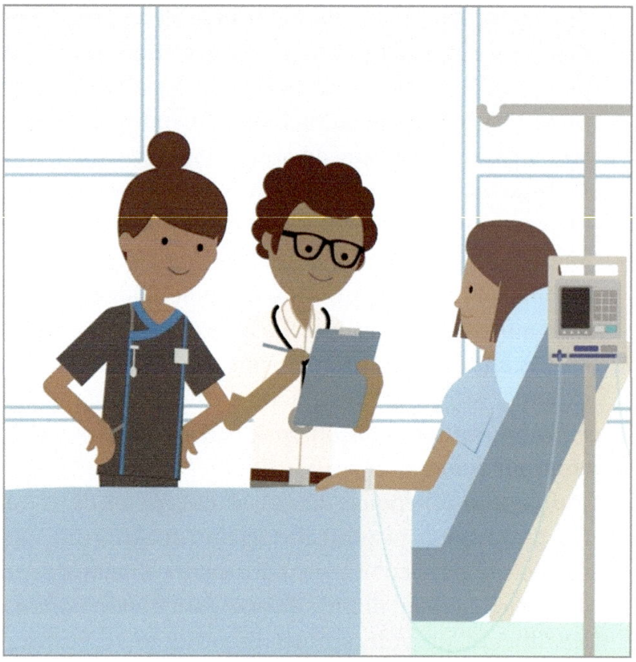

Fig. 5: Patient interaction.

Documentations of Communications and Interactions

Documentation of communication and interactions in pain medicine is an important aspect of patient care. Limited English proficiency (LEP) and language barriers can contribute to poorer patient assessment and inadequate pain control. Studies have shown that pain documentation and management vary based on patient language and race/ethnicity. In a pain management program (PMP) context, patient-to-patient interactions about chronic pain were found to be strongly prosocial and inclusive, potentially enhancing clinical outcomes. Effective documentation of pain scores and care plans is crucial for improving pain management in cancer patients. Overall, understanding and documenting communication and interactions in pain medicine **(Fig. 5)** can help improve patient outcomes and enhance the quality of care.

Addressing Language and Cultural Barriers in Communication

Addressing language and cultural barriers in communication in pain medicine is crucial for providing quality care to culturally and linguistically diverse (CALD) populations.[54] Communication barriers between healthcare providers and patients, including differences in language, cultural beliefs, and historical factors, can lead to poor access to pain management services and disparities in care.[55,56] To overcome these barriers, healthcare providers need to become culturally adept in practice and acknowledge the impact of cultural and historical factors on patients' trust and care.[56] Developing cultural competence and practicing a patient-centered approach are promising ways to address these challenges.[57] Additionally, the use of culturally appropriate pain terminologies and addressing differences in pain perceptions and beliefs among ethnic groups can improve the acceptability and equity of digital pain self-report tools. Addressing language and cultural barriers is essential for effective communication and equitable pain medicine for diverse populations.

PROFESSIONAL LIABILITY AND INSURANCE

Understanding Professional Liability Risks for Pain Physicians

Pain physicians play a crucial role in managing and treating patients with chronic pain. However, like any medical professional, they face professional liability risks that can arise from various aspects of their practice.

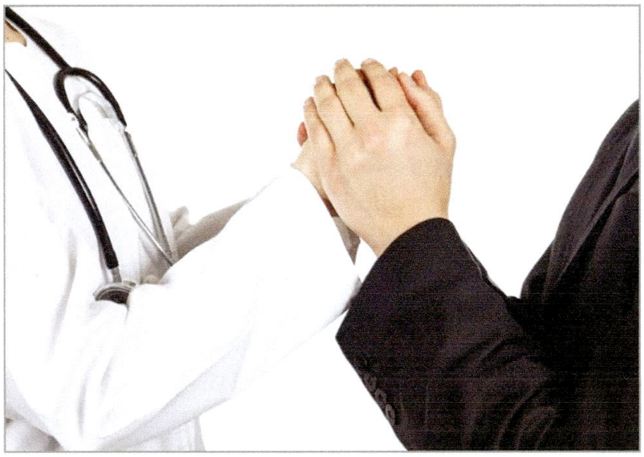

Fig. 6: Understanding of professional liability and insurance.

Understanding these risks is essential for pain physicians to mitigate potential liabilities and ensure the delivery of high-quality care to their patients **(Fig. 6)**.

- *Scope of practice and standard of care:* Pain physicians are expected to adhere to a certain standard of care when diagnosing and treating patients. Deviating from this standard can lead to allegations of medical malpractice. Pain physicians must stay updated with the latest guidelines and best practices in pain management. Additionally, clear documentation of patient assessments, treatment plans, and informed consent is crucial in demonstrating adherence to the standard of care.[58]
- *Informed consent and communication:* Obtaining informed consent is fundamental to medical practice. Pain physicians must ensure patients are fully informed about the risks, benefits, and alternatives to proposed treatments or procedures. Failure to obtain valid informed consent can lead to legal challenges. Moreover, effective communication with patients regarding their condition, treatment options, and potential outcomes is essential in minimizing misunderstandings and dissatisfaction that could result in liability claims.[59]
- *Prescription practices and controlled substances:* Pain management often involves the use of controlled substances such as opioids. Physicians must exercise caution in prescribing these medications to avoid allegations of overprescribing, inappropriate prescribing, or diversion. Compliance with state regulations, prescription monitoring programs, and guidelines from organizations such as the Centers for Disease Control and Prevention (CDC) is critical in mitigating the risks associated with opioid prescriptions.[60]
- *Documentation and record-keeping:* Comprehensive and accurate documentation is vital for pain physicians. Detailed records of patient encounters, assessments, treatment plans, discussions of risks and benefits, and follow-up care can be crucial evidence in defending against malpractice claims. Incomplete or inadequate documentation may undermine the physician's ability to demonstrate the rationale behind their clinical decisions.
- *Collaboration and referrals:* Pain management often requires collaboration with other healthcare providers. Referring patients to specialists or ancillary services should be done judiciously and with clear communication to ensure continuity of care. Failure to make appropriate referrals or coordinate care effectively can lead to allegations of negligence.[61]

Importance of Professional Liability Insurance

Professional liability insurance is crucial to practicing medicine, especially in pain medicine. This insurance covers claims arising from alleged errors or negligence in healthcare services. Professional liability insurance significantly protects healthcare providers from potential legal and financial repercussions in pain medicine, where patient care often involves complex treatments and procedures.

- *Risk management and patient safety:* Professional liability insurance serves as a risk management tool, allowing physicians to focus on providing high-quality care while mitigating the financial risks associated with potential malpractice claims. By maintaining adequate coverage, healthcare providers demonstrate their commitment to patient safety and accountability in their practice.[62]
- *Legal protection and financial security:* Professional liability insurance provides a layer of defense against such scenarios, ensuring physicians can continue their practice with confidence and peace of mind.[63]
- *Preservation of professional reputation:* In the event of adverse outcomes, professional liability insurance can facilitate open communication with patients and their families, demonstrating a proactive approach to addressing concerns and resolving issues while upholding professional standards.[64]

Tips for Mitigating and Managing Professional Liability Risks

Professional liability risks are inherent in any medical profession, including pain medicine. Pain management's complex and sensitive nature can expose practitioners to lawsuits and legal claims. This will discuss various tips for mitigating and managing professional liability risks in pain medicine.

- *Understand the scope of practice and adhere to it:* This includes knowing the limitations of the training and expertise and understanding the legal and ethical implications of providing care outside the scope.[65]
- *Maintain accurate and comprehensive documentation:* Practitioners should document patient histories, assessment findings, treatment plans, and progress notes in a timely and detailed manner.
- *Obtain informed consent:* Informed consent is the foundation of ethical medical practice. Pain management professionals must ensure that patients understand the benefits, risks, and alternatives to proposed treatments and provide their consent voluntarily.[66] This process should be documented in the patient's chart.
- *Communicate effectively with patients and colleagues:* Clear and open communication is vital in pain medicine. Practitioners should discuss treatment options, prognosis, and potential risks with patients and consult other healthcare professionals when necessary. Good communication can help prevent misunderstandings and miscommunications leading to legal disputes.
- *Stay updated on clinical guidelines and best practices:* Pain management professionals should regularly review clinical guidelines and best practices to ensure they provide the most current and evidence-based care. This can help reduce the risk of malpractice claims and improve patient outcomes.[67]
- *Implement risk management strategies:* Risk management is an ongoing process that involves identifying, assessing, and mitigating potential risks in pain medicine. This can include regular self-assessments, peer review, and quality improvement initiatives.
- *Educate patients on proper use of medications and other treatments:* Patient education is crucial in pain management. Practitioners should ensure patients understand the proper use of medications, alternative treatments, and self-management strategies. This can help reduce the risk of medication errors and adverse events.[68]

Seeking Legal Counsel and Support

Seeking legal counsel and support in pain medicine is important due to the legal and social infrastructure involved in the field. Pain physicians must clearly understand the law of consent and may be called upon to provide expert evidence in personal injury and medical negligence claims.[69,70] Understanding the situations where complications leading to lawsuits may arise is crucial, as not all complications will result in legal action.[71] Pain physicians may also face legal issues in administrative and other hearings, making it important to be knowledgeable about medicolegal issues.[72] Seeking legal counsel and support can help pain physicians navigate these complex legal and regulatory issues to effectively and safely manage their patients.

CONCLUSION

Medicolegal awareness is crucial for pain physicians to navigate the complexities of their profession, ensure ethical practice, prevent malpractice claims, maintain licensure, and improve patient safety. Informed consent is a critical aspect of medical practice, particularly in pain medicine, as it allows patients to make decisions about their bodies and serves as a safeguard for both doctors and patients. Professional liability insurance plays a significant role in protecting pain physicians from potential legal and financial repercussions arising from alleged errors or negligence in the delivery of healthcare services. Empathy, compassion, cultural understanding, patient education, and SDM are essential in pain medicine to alleviate emotional pain, build trust, minimize cultural misunderstandings, and empower patients to take an active role in their care. Enhanced privacy protection and improved security measures, such as HIPAA regulations and the Security Rule, are necessary to safeguard patient information in pain medicine. Pain physicians must be well-informed about medicolegal considerations, ensure proper documentation, engage in SDM, and adhere to ethical principles to navigate the complex medicolegal landscape in pain medicine.

REFERENCES

1. Chansoria M, Das G. Scope of pain clinics in India. J Recent Adv Pain. 2017;3(2):59-60.

2. Dubois MY, Follett KA. Pain medicine: the case for an independent medical specialty and training programs. Acad Med. 2014;89(6):863-8.
3. Cheng J. Overview of pain states. In: Jianguo Cheng, Richard W. Rosenquist (Eds). Fundamentals of Pain Medicine. Springer Cham; 2018. pp. 3-6.
4. Smith MT, South SM. Pain pharmacology and analgesia. In: Majewski H (Ed). Encyclopedia of Life Support Systems. Oxford, UK: EOLSS Publishers; 2008. pp. 1-80.
5. Rizka A, Khairunnisa CZ, Annabila ZI, Windiani S. Pelaksanaan informed consent Dalam Pelayanan Medik. Manuju. 2023;5(4):1284-94.
6. Shaha KK, Patra AP, Das S. The importance of informed consent in medicine. Sch J App Med Sci. 2013;1(5):455-63.
7. Mammucari M, Lazzari M, Maggiori E, Gafforio P, Tufaro G, Baffini S, et al. Role of the informed consent, from mesotherapy to opioid therapy. Eur Rev Med Pharmacol Sci. 2014;18(4):566-74.
8. Cheatle MD, Savage SR. Informed consent in opioid therapy: a potential obligation and opportunity. J Pain Symptom Manage. 2012;44(1):105-16.
9. Elwyn G, Frosch D, Thomson R, Joseph Williams N, Lloyd A, Kinnersley P, et al. Shared decision making: a model for clinical practice. J Gen Intern Med. 2012;27(10):1361-7.
10. Charles C, Gafni A, Whelan T. Shared decision-making in the medical encounter: what does it mean? (or it takes at least two to tango). Soc Sci Med. 1997;44(5):681-92.
11. Faden RR, Beauchamp TL. A History and Theory of Informed Consent. Oxford University Press; 1986.
12. Stiggelbout AM, Van der Weijden T, Wit MPT, Frosch D, Légaré, F, Montori VM, et al. Shared decision making: really putting patients at the centre of healthcare. BMJ. 2012;344:e256.
13. Compagnone C, Michael ES, Rauck RL, Zundert JV, Kraus M, Primorac D, et al. Past, present, and future of informed consent in pain and genomics research: challenges facing global medical community. Pain Pract. 2017;17(1):8-15.
14. Celis MA, Halabe J, Arrieta O, Burgos R, Campillo C, De la Llata M, et al. El consentimiento informado: recomendaciones para su documentación. Gaceta Medica De Mexico. 2018;154(6):716-8.
15. Hall DE, Hanusa BH, Fine MJ, Arnold RM. Do surgeons and patients discuss what they document on consent forms. J Surg Res. 2015;197(1):67-77.
16. Institute for Safe Medication Practices. (2018). Improving medication safety: a practical guide to implementing the principles of the national coordinating council for medication error reporting and prevention's medication error prevention and reduction program. [online] Available from https://www.ismp.org/ [Last accessed August, 2024].
17. American Academy of Pain Medicine. (2019). Pain management in the 21st century: a vision for the future. [online] Available from https://www.aspan.org/ [Last accessed August, 2024].
18. International Association for the Study of Pain. (2020). The IASP taxonomy: a classification of pain-related terms and concepts. [online] Available from https://www.iasp-pain.org/ [Last accessed August, 2024].
19. Smith A. Patient history documentation in pain medicine. J Pain Manag. 2018;25(2):87-94.
20. Brown C. Physical examination findings in chronic pain patients. Pain Medicine Reports. 2019;36(4):301-10.
21. Johnson E. Role of diagnostic tests in pain medicine documentation. J Med Imaging. 2020;18(3):145-52.
22. Williams B. Use of pain assessment tools in clinical practice. J Pain Res. 2017;12:89-96.
23. Garcia D. Comprehensive treatment planning in pain medicine. J Anesth Analg. 2019;28(1):45-52.
24. Patel S. Follow-up documentation practices in chronic pain management. J Clin Outcomes Manag. 2018;22(4):201-8.
25. Doe J. Legal Aspects in Healthcare Documentation: A Practical Guide for Healthcare. Medical Legal Press; 2021.
26. DEA. (2018). The Controlled Substances Act. [online] Available from https://www.dea.gov/drug-information/csa [Last accessed August, 2024].
27. DEA. (2021). About. [online] Available from https://www.dea.gov/who-we-are/about [Last accessed August, 2024].
28. Centers for Disease Control and Prevention. Prescription Drug Monitoring Programs. 2021.
29. Ravanpak R. The ethics of prescription drug monitoring programs. Voices in Bioethics. 2023;9.
30. Mehta S, Brown W, Ferguson E, Najera J, Pantell MS. The association between prescription drug monitoring programs and controlled substance prescribing: a cross-sectional study using data from 2019 National Electronic Health Records Survey. J Am Med Inform Assoc. 2023; 30(6):1042-6.
31. Toce MS, Michelson KA, Hudgins JD, Olson KL, Monuteaux MC, Bourgeois FT. Association of prescription drug monitoring programs with benzodiazepine prescription dispensation and overdose in adolescents and young adults. Clin Toxicol (Phila). 2023;61(4):234-40.
32. Shakya S, Ruseski JE. The effect of Prescription Drug Monitoring Programs on county- level opioid prescribing practices and spillovers. Contemp Econ Policy. 2023; 41(3):435-54.
33. Bautista A, Chang Chien GC, Abd-Elsayed A. Identification and management of iatrogenic complications in interventional pain management. In: Abd-Elsayed A (Ed). Pain. Cham: Springer; 2019.
34. Grille M, Chien GCC, Wu J. Management of Iatrogenic emergencies in interventional pain management. In: Pope J, Deer T (Eds). Treatment of Chronic Pain Conditions. New York: Springer; 2017. pp. 163-71.
35. Provenzano D, Hanes M, Deer TR. Interventional pain procedures and the risk of infection. In: Hurley RW (Ed). Essentials of Pain Medicine, 4th edition. Elsevier; 2018.
36. Erdine S. The importance of studying complications in pain medicine. In: Erdine S, Staats PS (Eds). Complications of

Pain-Relieving Procedures: An Illustrated Guide. Wiley; 2022. pp. 1-7.
37. Bolander S, Post G. Prompt Recognition: 5 pediatric elbow fractures not to miss. J Orthop Phys Assist. 2023;11(2):e23.00001.
38. Senthilkumar A, AlFarra T, Chopra H, Chhatre A. ASK! Preoperative safety checklist protocol in interventional spine procedures: a quality improvement study thirty month follow-up. J Rehab Pain Med. 2023;1(2):74-9.
39. Pawasauskas J, Kelley M, Gill C, Facente M. Comparison of multimodal, sliding scale acute pain protocols with traditional prescribing in non-surgical patients. Postgrad Med. 2020;132(1):37-43.
40. Kurz S, Lohse J, Buggenhagen H, Schmidtmann I, Laufenberg-Feldmann R, Engelhard K. Improving competence and safety in pain medicine: a practical clinical teaching strategy for students combining simulation and bedside teaching. BMC Med Educ. 2021;21(1):1-7.
41. Caycedo MAB, José, Silva JND, Brecher GS, Garzón LB. Protocolo uso seguro de opioides en Clínica Universitaria Colombia. Revista Médica Sanitas. 2017;20(2):93-102.
42. Gurumurthi R, Das G. Need of Indian protocol in pain management. Indian J Pain. 2015;29(2):59-60.
43. Guevremont N, Barnes M, Haupt E. Physician autonomy and the opioid crisis. J Law Med Ethics. 2018;46(2):203-19.
44. Learch R, Cumberledge J. Physicians' responsibility to understand patients' pain. Virtual Mentor. 2013;15(5):430-3.
45. Mavroudis C, Cook JT, Mavroudis CD. Autonomy and the principles of medical practice. In: Mavroudis C, Cook JT, Mavroudis CD (Eds). Bioethical Controversies in Pediatric Cardiology and Cardiac Surgery. Cham: Springer; 2020: pp. 29-37.
46. Feldman MD. From the editors' desk: patient autonomy and medical decisions: getting it just right. J Gen Intern Med. 2010;25(7):639.
47. Beauchamp TL, Childress JF. Principles of Biomedical Ethics. Oxford University Press; 2009.
48. World Health Organization. National Cancer Control Programs: Policies and Managerial Guidelines, 2nd edition. World Health Organization; 2002.
49. Clarfield MA. Active listening: a key skill in pain management. Pain Manag Nurs. 2012;13(3):149-58.
50. Katz AM. Empathic communication and its impact on patient satisfaction in pain management. J Pain Symptom Manage. 2004;28:250-5.
51. Wade LE, Gil KA. Cultural competence in pain management: a review of the literature. J Pain Symptom Manage. 2016;47(1):1-15.
52. Ferrell LR. Patient education and shared decision-making in pain management: a systematic review. J Pain Symptom Manage. 2016;51.
53. Gil KA, Wade LE. Continuous quality improvement and training in pain management: a review of the literature. J Pain. 2018;19:1234-56.
54. LaGue L. Cultural Perspectives in Pain and Palliative Care. San Jose State University; 2023.
55. Bernardes CM, Houkamau K, Lin I, Taylor M, Birch S, Claus A, et al. *Communication and access to healthcare*: Experiences of Aboriginal and Torres Strait Islander people managing pain in Queensland, Australia. Front Pain Res (Lausanne). 2022;3:1041968.
56. Ali SM, Lee RR, McBeth J, James B, McAlister S, Chiarotto A, et al. Exploring the Cross-Cultural Acceptability of Digital Tools for Pain Self-reporting: Qualitative Study. JMIR Hum Factors. 2022;10:e42177.
57. Zhura VV, Utesheva AP, Yremeba A. Crosscultural communication in medical settings. Bioethics. 2020; 13(2):14-7.
58. Jones B. Legal Considerations in Pain Medicine. Academic Press; 2019.
59. Johnson D. Effective Communication in Healthcare. Oxford University Press; 2017.
60. Miller F. Controlled Substances Regulations. Legal Publications; 2021.
61. Adams H. Interprofessional Collaboration in Healthcare. Jones and Bartlett Learning. 2020.
62. Smith A. Risk management in pain medicine practice. J Pain Med. 2018;15(2):87-94.
63. Jones B, Brown C. Professional liability insurance: safeguarding your practice. Medical Risk Management Quarterly. 2019;25(4):301-15.
64. Garcia D. Ethical considerations in pain medicine: preserving patient trust. J Med Ethics. 2020;32(3): 189-204.
65. Canadian Centre for Occupational Health and Safety. (2021). Scope of Practice: A Guide for Health Professionals. [online] Available from https://www.ccohs.ca/oshanswers/health_care/scope_practice.html [Last accessed August, 2024].
66. Canadian Centre for Occupational Health and Safety. Informed Consent: A Guide for Health Professionals. [online] Available from https://www.ccohs.ca/oshanswers/health_care/informed_consent.html
67. Canadian Centre for Occupational Health and Safety. Clinical Practice Guidelines: A Guide for Health Professionals. [online] Available from https://www.ccohs.ca/oshanswers/health_care/clin_pract_guide.html
68. Canadian Centre for Occupational Health and Safety. Patient Education: A Guide for Health Professionals. Available from https://www.ccohs.ca/oshanswers/health_care/patient_education.html
69. de Gray LE. Legal and social aspects of pain medicine. Anaesth Intensive Care Med. 2022;23(7):409-12.
70. de Gray L. Medicolegal and social implications of practicing in pain medicine. Anaesth Intensive Care Med. 2019;20(8):446-9.
71. Racz GB, Noe C, Munglani R. Medico-legal aspects of pain medicine. In: Racz GB, Noe C (Eds). Pain and Treatment. InTech; 2014.
72. Erdine S. Medical legal issues in pain management. In: Erdine S, Staats PS (Eds). Complications of Pain Relieving Procedures: An Illustrated Guide. Wiley-Blackwell; 2022.

Index

Page numbers followed by *b* refer to box, *f* refer to figure, *fc* refer to flowchart, and *t* refer to table

D

E

T